Introduction to DIAGNOSTIC MICROBIOLOGY for the Laboratory Sciences

Maria Dannessa Delost, PhD, MT(ASC-P)

Professor and Director of Medical Laboratory Programs

Department of Health Professions

The Bitonte College of Health & Human Services

Youngstown State University

Youngstown, OH

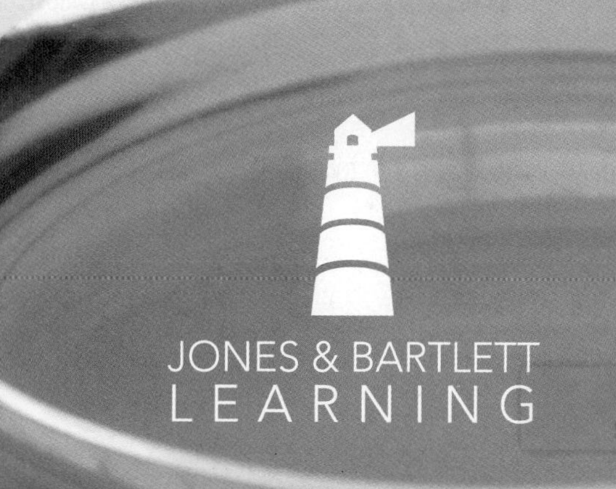

World Headquarters
Jones & Bartlett Learning
5 Wall Street
Burlington, MA 01803
978-443-5000
info@jblearning.com
www.jblearning.com

Jones & Bartlett Learning books and products are available through most bookstores and online booksellers. To contact Jones & Bartlett Learning directly, call 800-832-0034, fax 978-443-8000, or visit our website, www.jblearning.com.

Substantial discounts on bulk quantities of Jones & Bartlett Learning publications are available to corporations, professional associations, and other qualified organizations. For details and specific discount information, contact the special sales department at Jones & Bartlett Learning via the above contact information or send an email to specialsales@jblearning.com.

Production Credits
Executive Publisher: William Brottmiller
Publisher: Cathy L. Esperti
Acquisitions Editor: Ryan Angel
Associate Editor: Kayla Dos Santos
Editorial Assistant: Sean Fabery
Production Manager: Tracey McCrea
Marketing Manager: Grace Richards
Art Development Editor: Joanna Lundeen
Production Assistant: Eileen Worthley
VP, Manufacturing and Inventory Control: Therese Connell
Composition: Cenveo® Publisher Services
Cover Design: Scott Moden
Photo Research and Permissions Coordinator: Amy Rathburn
Cover and Title Page Image: © Alex011973/Shutterstock, Inc.
Printing and Binding: Courier Companies
Cover Printing: Courier Companies

Library of Congress Cataloging-in-Publication Data
Delost, Maria Dannessa, author.
Introduction to diagnostic microbiology for the laboratory sciences / Maria Dannessa Delost.
p. ; cm.
Includes bibliographical references and index.
ISBN 978-1-284-03231-4 (pbk.)
I. Title.
[DNLM: 1. Clinical Laboratory Techniques—Problems and Exercises. 2. Microbiological Techniques—Problems and Exercises. QY 18.2]
RB38.25
616.07'5076—dc23

2013034746

6048

Dedication

To the memory of my Dads, Amil M. Dannessa and George Delost, Jr., who served their country in World War II as members of our Greatest Generation and who taught me the values of hard work, loyalty, and honesty

Contents

Preface

Introduction to Diagnostic Microbiology for the Laboratory Sciences provides a concise study of clinically significant microorganisms for the medical laboratory science student and the laboratory professional. This text is on the recommended reading list to prepare for the ASCP MLT (American Society for Clinical Pathology, Medical Laboratory Technician) exam. Although comprehensive textbooks for diagnostic microbiology abound, this text is unique in its focus on what is most essential for the beginning student. The concept of this text was originally suggested by my medical laboratory technology students who were frustrated by the length and depth of other microbiology textbooks. Students became discouraged with the vast amount of information included in these texts, which serve as excellent learning resources but were inappropriate for the beginning student.

This text provides an overview of diagnostic microbiology that is relevant and essential to medical laboratory students and entry level medical laboratory technicians. Chapters 1 through 6 begin by providing an overview of the infectious process, including disease transmission and host immunity. The importance of specimen collection is emphasized with both general and specific requirements, instilling in the student the importance of pre-analytical factors in specimen management and quality laboratory testing. The goal is to provide a thorough yet succinct discussion of isolation media, as well as the basics of preliminary testing in the microbiology laboratory.

Essential manual methods are addressed both in theory and method so the student can understand, practice, and apply each laboratory procedure. The chapters mesh didactic theory with laboratory testing and interpretation, creating an orderly and complete presentation. Additional testing methods, such as serology, immunoassay, antibiotic susceptibility testing, and molecular diagnostics are also presented with pertinent applications. Current modes of antibiotic resistance and the required testing are included which introduce the student to the increased attention required in antibiotic testing, as well as the identification of resistance patterns. The expanded information on molecular diagnostics provides the student with the essential framework and examples of the expanding use of molecular technologies in the microbiology laboratory. The text also introduces the student to current automation in the microbiology laboratory, including contemporary instrumentation used in microbial identification, antibiotic susceptibility testing, and blood culture technologies.

Chapters 7 through 18 address medically important bacteria, including their isolation, identification, and treatment. Each chapter focuses on major divisions of bacteria, including gram-positive cocci, gram-negative cocci, gram-negative bacilli, gram-positive bacilli, mycobacterium, anaerobes, spirochetes, chlamydia, and rickettsia. Each chapter includes concise information on the isolation, identification, and clinical relevance of those microorganisms that a microbiologist may encounter in the clinical setting. These chapters also include news pieces that describe a timely concern related to a specific microorganism and its associated public health concern. Examples include antibiotic resistance in *Staphylococcus aureus*, meningococcoal disease, listeriosis, Lyme Disease, and legionellosis. These items attempt to instill in the student the relevance of clinical microbiology in their everyday life by relating contemporary events to the lessons presented in the chapter.

Chapters 19 through 21 provide an orderly presentation of clinical virology, mycology, and parasitology that can be realistically covered in an introductory course. These topics are often overwhelming in both quantity and depth of information in most microbiology texts, leading to frustration in many students. These important topics are summarized in a format that encourages the student to review and apply central concepts in each discipline. Chapter 19,

Introduction to Virology summarizes viral replication, classification of DNA and RNA viruses, and the isolation and identification of medically important viruses. This chapter also summarizes and describes significant viral infections and the role of the laboratory in the diagnosis of viral infections. Chapter 20, Introduction to Medical Mycology discusses the classification of mycoses, specimen collection, and fungal culture media. Clear identification schemes utilizing both macroscopic colonial appearance and microscopic characteristics as well as biochemical methods for medically important fungi are included. Superficial, subcutaneous, systemic, and opportunistic mycoses are addressed. This chapter includes images that are vital in the correct identification of the fungi. Chapter 21, Introduction to Medical Parasitology provides an organized classification outline of medically relevant parasites and infections. Specimen collection requirements unique to parasitology are described as well as concentration methods and stains. The chapter is divided into units which discuss protozoans such as the amebae, sporozoans and hemoflagellates, nematodes, cestodes, and trematodes. Extensive, clearly drawn life cycles with images of the infectious stage and diagnostic stage are included for clinically relevant parasites.

The final chapter, Chapter 22, Clinical Specimens, ties the components of the text together by summarizing the medically important pathogens typically found in clinical specimens with identification schemes. Complete work-ups of microorganisms from major clinical sites are included with flowcharts and suggested laboratory protocols. Students are able to apply the didactic and laboratory concepts presented throughout the text to evaluate clinical specimens and develop appropriate testing schemes to correctly identify pathogens and differentiate these from normal flora.

The goal of the text is to provide the medical laboratory student with the information and skills necessary for entry into the medical laboratory profession. The information is organized into a format that facilitates learning through the use of integrated text, charts, figures, and laboratory exercises. This format also provides a quick reference to the most frequently utilized manual procedures and most commonly referred topics in clinical microbiology.

Key Features

Introduction to Diagnostic Microbiology for the Laboratory Sciences includes learning objectives, laboratory exercises, news features, and review questions. Both didactic and psychomotor skills are presented and reinforced in each chapter.

- *Learning Objectives*–Clearly outlines for the reader the desired outcomes of the chapter, focuses reading, and provides a basis to gauge learning.
- *Laboratory Exercises*–Engages the reader by having them apply what they learned in a lab activity, record their results, and push their analysis further with critical thinking questions.
- *News Feature*–Highlights current issues that face the contemporary medical laboratory technician, grounding the information in a real-word context.
- *Review Questions*–Provides a way to apply what has been learned in the chapter and also provides practice for preparation for the Medical Lab Technician (MLT) certification examination.

Many reference texts in clinical microbiology are available with complex descriptions and highly detailed methods which can intimidate the beginning student. The purpose of *Introduction to Diagnostic Microbiology for the Laboratory Sciences* is to provide a condensed and practical approach for students and novice microbiologists. A mastery of the material and procedures in this text will provide students with a strong background for pursuing higher levels in clinical microbiology. Additionally, the text is an excellent resource to prepare for the ASCP certification examination. It further serves as a valuable review for laboratory professionals who are returning to the microbiology field after an absence. The concise format provides a quick and thorough review mechanism for students and laboratory professionals who may need a refresher course in diagnostic microbiology.

Acknowledgments

Special thanks to my husband, Raymond, and my sons, Gregory and Michael, and my entire family for their encouragement and support during this project. Also, thank you to all of my medical laboratory students at Youngstown State University from whom I have learned so much during my thirty years of teaching.

Reviewers

Angela R. Bell, MS, MLS(ASCP)SM, DLM
Tidewater Community College
Virginia Beach, VA

Janet E. Cooper, MSNS, BSMT(ASCP)H
Instructor in Medical Laboratory Technology
Mississippi Delta Community College
Moorhead, MS

Katrina P. Ghazanfar, PhD, MT(ASCP)
University of Hawaii-Kapiolani Community College
Honolulu, HI

Michelle M. Hill, MS, MT(ASCP)
Instructor, MLT Program
Southwest Tennessee Community College
Memphis, TN

Benjamin F. Newsome Jr., MA/MS, MT(AMT), CM
Director
San Jacinto College
Pasadena, TX

Dale Telgenhoff, PhD, HTL(ASCP)
Associate Professor
Tarleton State University
Fort Worth, TX

CHAPTER 1

Introduction to Clinical Microbiology

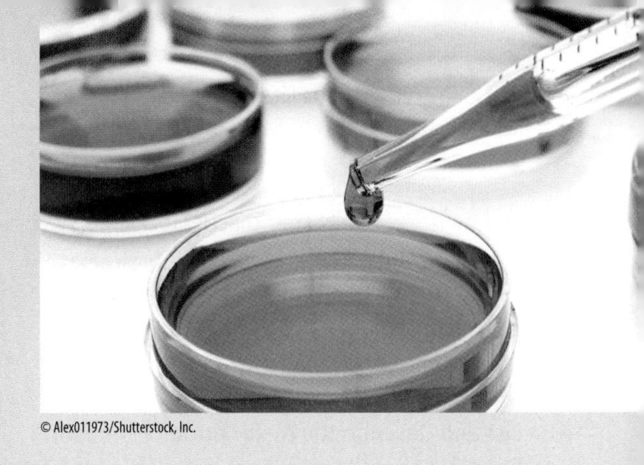

CHAPTER OUTLINE

Classification and Taxonomy
Characteristics of Eukaryotes and Prokaryotes
The Role of Clinical Microbiology
The Infectious Process

KEY TERMS

Acquired immunity
Antibody
Antigen
Asymptomatic carrier
Cell-mediated immunity (CMI)
Colonization
Endotoxin
Exotoxin
Humoral immunity
Immunoglobulin
Immunosuppressive
Infection
Infectious disease
Inflammatory response
Innate immunity
Normal flora
Nosocomial
Pathogen
Phagocytosis
Pili
Superinfection

LEARNING OBJECTIVES

1. Discuss the purpose of clinical microbiology.
2. Describe the binomial system of taxonomy and discuss how phenotypic and molecular characteristics are used to classify bacteria.
3. Identify and give the function of the bacterial cell components.
4. Differentiate the gram-positive cell wall from the gram-negative cell wall.
5. State the function of pili, fimbriae, flagella, and the capsule.
6. Describe the important metabolic activities of the bacterial cell.
7. Define the following terms:
   a. Infection
   b. Infectious disease
   c. True pathogen
   d. Opportunistic pathogen
   e. Nosocomial infection
   f. Endogenous infection
   g. Exogenous infection
   h. Asymptomatic carriage (carriers)
   i. Colonization
8. Define and contrast:
   a. endemic and epidemic
   b. disease prevalence and incidence

9. Define normal flora and discuss its role in each of the following sites:
   a. Mouth and oral cavity
   b. Nasopharynx
   c. Stomach and small intestine
   d. Colon
10. List and describe the major routes of infection.
11. Describe the following host defense mechanisms:
    a. Innate (natural) immunity
    b. Inflammatory response
    c. Acquired immunity
    d. Humoral immunity
    e. Cell-mediated immunity
12. Describe the function of B and T cells in the immune response:
    a. List and summarize the characteristics of the human immunoglobulin classes.
    b. List and state the function of four populations of T cells.
13. Define and describe endotoxins and exotoxins.
14. List the signs of microbial infection.
15. List the laboratory procedures that might be requested to identify infectious disease.

The purpose of clinical microbiology is to isolate and identify pathogenic microorganisms. Clinical microbiologists work with clinicians and other personnel to assist in the diagnosis, management, and treatment of infectious disease. The microbiology laboratory can provide the physician with information from direct smears and stains, cultures, molecular analysis, serological testing, and antibiotic susceptibility testing. The physician also relies on the patient's medical history; physical examination; and results of X-rays, laboratory tests, and epidemiological information (such as previous infections, travel, and illness in the family) to aid in the diagnosis of infectious disease.

This chapter provides an introduction to clinical microbiology, including a review on taxonomy, bacterial structure, and metabolism. Also discussed are the concepts of pathogens and normal flora and the infectious process, including symptoms and routes of infection. A summary of the inflammatory process and immunity is discussed and important definitions provided.

Classification and Taxonomy

The classification of organisms into categories based on genotypic and phenotypic characteristics is known as taxonomy. Historically, classification has been based mostly on observable properties such as morphology, biochemical characteristics, and antigenic relationships. Examples of phenotypical characteristics used to classify microorganisms are shown in BOX 1-1.

This phenotypical classification is being replaced with systems based on genetic homology. Although these systems are more precise, at times, they do not conform to classification based on phenotypic characteristics. Genetic homology includes classification based on DNA base composition and ratio. The cytosine and guanine content (CG) to total base content is used as an indicator of relatedness. Nucleic acid sequence analysis uses the order of bases along the DNA or RNA sequence and determines similar sequences between two organisms.

BOX 1-1 Phenotypical Classification Characteristics

Macroscopic morphology: Size, texture, color, elevation

Microscopic morphology: Size, shape (cocci, bacilli), arrangement (pairs, chains, clusters)

Staining characteristics: Gram-stain reaction (positive/negative), acid fastness

Environmental requirements: Temperature optimum, oxygen needs, pH needs, carbon dioxide needs, need/able to withstand NaCl

Nutritional requirements: Use carbon or nitrogen substrates

Resistance profiles: Inherent resistance to antibiotics, chemicals

Antigenic properties: Serological or immunological methods (Lancefield groups of *Streptococcus*, properties of capsules)

When identifying microorganisms, the key features are outlined based on genotypic characteristics, including genes and nucleic acids and phenotypic characteristics, which are observable. The hierarchy for classification is summarized below, beginning with the largest division, or kingdom, and ending with the smallest division, or species.

Kingdom
Division
Class
Order
Family
Genus
Species

The species is the most basic taxonomic group and encompasses bacterial strains with common genetic, physiologic, and phenotypic characteristics. There may be subgroups within the species, which are known as subspecies. Below the subspecies level, there may be microorganisms that share specific minor characteristics; these are known as biotypes, subtypes, or strains or genotypes. Strains or subtypes are genetic variants of the microorganism. Different species with many important features in common are known as a genus (genera). Genera are based on genetic and phenotypic characteristics among several species. It is usually not practical in microbiology to classify similar genera into higher taxonomic levels. However, at times, grouping into families may be helpful.

In the binomial system of nomenclature, two names, the genus and species, are used. These are generally derived from the Latin or Greek language. Both the genus and species names should be italicized or underlined; the genus name is always capitalized and the species name is never capitalized. Accepted abbreviations include the uppercase form of the first letter of the genus with a period. Informal names are written in lower case without italics or underlining.

Proposed changes in nomenclature are examined by the *International Journal for Systematic Bacteriology*. New information on the organism is investigated, and the organism may or may not be reclassified or renamed. When a new name is accepted, the written format is "new name (old name)" until sufficient time has elapsed to recognize the change. For example, *Enterococcus faecalis* was formerly classified in the genus *Streptococcus*; when it was reclassified, *Enterococcus (Streptococcus) faecalis* was written for clarification. BOX 1-2 gives an example of nomenclature.

BOX 1-2 Example of Classification

Family:	Micrococcoceae
Genus:	*Staphylococcus*
Species:	*aureus*
Accepted abbreviation:	*S. aureus*
Informal:	staphylococci

Characteristics of Eukaryotes and Prokaryotes

Eukaryotic cells contain membrane-enclosed structures, which have specific functions. Fungi and parasites are categorized as eukaryotes. Eukaryotic cells have a cytoskeleton that supports the cell and also various organelles, such as the nucleus, mitochondria, endoplasmic reticulum, Golgi bodies, and lysosomes. Bacterial cells are prokaryotic, which means that they do not contain organelles enclosed in membranes. Prokaryotes are unicellular organisms without a nuclear membrane, mitochondria, endoplasmic reticulum, or Golgi bodies. Bacteria multiply asexually, and all cellular functions occur in either the cytoplasm or cytoplasmic membrane of the bacterial cell.

TABLE 1-1 summarizes the characteristics of eukaryotic and prokaryotic organisms.

TABLE 1-1 Comparing the Characteristics of Eukaryotic and Prokaryotic Cells

	Eukaryotes	Prokaryotes
Microorganisms included	Algae, fungi, protozoa	Bacteria
Nucleus	Enclosed in nuclear membrane	No nuclear membrane
Mitochondria	Present	Absent
Golgi bodies	Present	Absent
Endoplasmic reticulum	Present	Absent
Ribosomes	80S (60S + 40S)	70S (50S + 30S)

Bacterial cells range from 1 μm to 3 μm in length and thus are not visible to the human eye without the aid of a microscope. Bacteria that are round are known as cocci; cocci may arrange in pairs, chains, or clusters. Bacteria that have a rod shape are known as bacilli, and those with a spiral form are known as spirochetes.

Typical morphologies of bacteria are shown in **FIGURE 1-1**.

BACTERIAL COMPONENTS

Bacterial cells contain a number of components that are located within the interior of the cell, known as the **cytoplasm** or **cytosol**. These cytoplasmic structures include ribosomes, the DNA chromosome, mRNA, proteins and metabolites, nucleoid, and plasmids. The cytosol contains many enzymes and is the site of most metabolic processes for the bacterial cell. The bacterial chromosome is one double-stranded circle contained in a discrete area of the cytoplasm, known as the nucleoid. The DNA is not contained within a nucleus, and there are no histones. Plasmids, which are small, circular extrachromosomal DNA may also be found in the cytoplasm. Plasmids play a role in the development of antibiotic resistance.

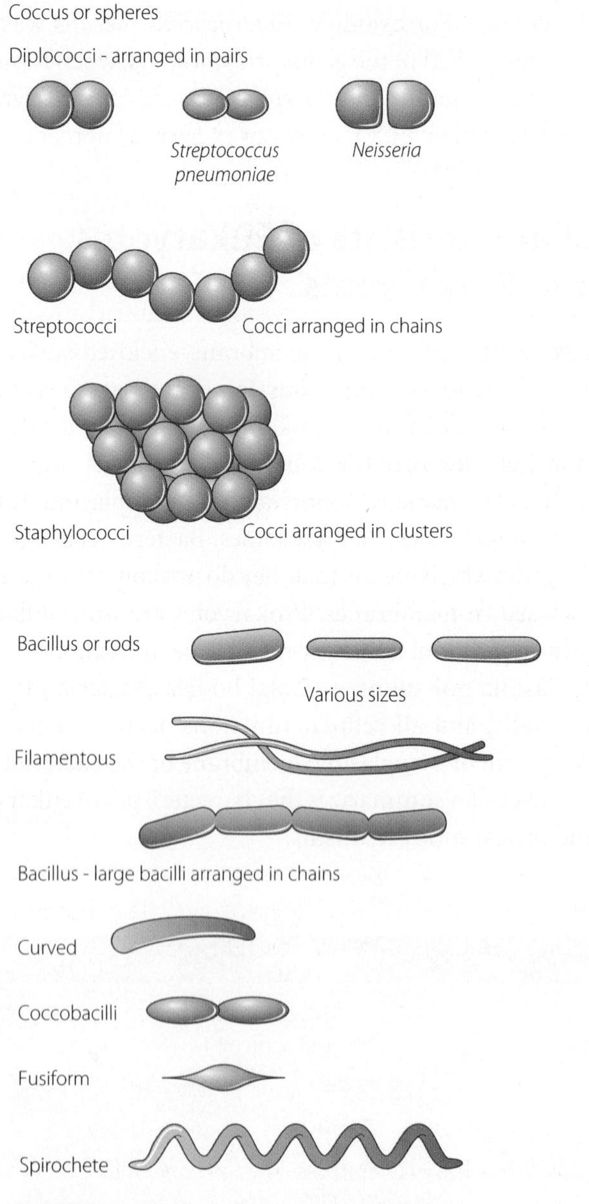

FIGURE 1-1 Bacterial shapes and morphology.

The cytosol has a granular appearance as a result of the presence of polysomes and inclusions. The polysomes contain messenger RNA bound to ribosomes, serving as the site of protein formation. Transcription and translation occur as a coupled reaction in the cytoplasm; ribosomes bind to mRNA, and protein is made at the same time that the mRNA is being synthesized and is still bound to the DNA. The Svedberg unit (S) expresses the sedimentation coefficient for macromolecules and serves as a measure of particle size. It is used to describe the complex subunits of ribosomes. The bacterial ribosome consists of 30S and 50S subunits that form a 70S ribosome. By contrast, the eukaryotic ribosome contains 40S and 60S subunits that form an 80S ribosome.

The inclusions contain glycogen and inorganic phosphates. Other inclusions may be present depending on the specific bacterial species.

The bacterial cell may convert to an endospore form under poor environmental conditions. The spore state is inactive but is able to resist the adverse conditions. When the situation becomes favorable, the spore can germinate into the bacterial cell.

The cytosol is enclosed by the **cellular envelope**, which includes the **cytoplasmic membrane** and **cell wall**. There is also periplasmic space and an outer membrane in gram-negative bacteria. The cytoplasmic, or inner membrane, is found in both gram-positive and gram-negative bacteria. It consists of a lipid bilayer intermixed with protein molecules including enzymes. The functions of the cytoplasmic membrane include generation of ATP, transport of solutes in and out of the cell, cell motility, chromosomal segregation, and sensors for detecting environmental changes. Enzymes involved in cell-wall and outer-wall formation and the synthesis and secretion of various compounds are also located here.

Cellular structures or appendages also are located in the cellular envelope. These include pili or **fimbriae**, which are hair-like extensions that extend into the environment.

There are common pili, which permit the organism to attach to the host cells, and sex pili, which are involved in conjugation. Flagella are connected to the cellular envelope and found in those bacteria that are motile. Monotrichous flagella are located at one end of the cell, while lophotrichous flagella are located on both ends of the cell. Peritrichous flagella cover the entire bacterial surface. The presence or absence and location of flagella are important identification characteristics.

Other bacteria have **capsules**, which are composed of polysaccharide or protein layers. When these materials are more loosely arranged, it is known as a **slime layer**. Capsules are poor antigens and are antiphagocytic and important virulence factors for bacteria. Capsules also may serve as barriers to hydrophobic compounds such as detergents and can enable the bacteria to adhere to other bacteria or to host surfaces.

The periplasmic space contains the murein layer and a gel-like structure that assists the bacteria in obtaining nutrients. There are also enzymes that can break down large molecules in this area. It is located between the inner part of the outer membrane and the outer external membrane and is found only in gram-negative bacteria.

The cell wall, or murein layer, is more commonly known as peptidoglycan; it serves as the external wall of most bacteria. This layer provides stability and strength to the bacterial cell and blocks the passage of some macromolecules. It is composed of the disaccharides N-acetylglucosamine and N-acetylmuramic acid, which are cross-linked to form peptidoglycan sheets when they are bound by peptide molecules. These peptidoglycan sheets further cross-link to form a multilayered structure. The peptidoglycan is much thicker in the gram-positive cell wall when compared to that of gram-negative bacteria. In addition, there are also techoic acids linked to the cellular membrane in the gram-positive cell wall. Techoic acids are water-soluble polymers of polyol phosphates bound to peptidoglycan and essential for the viability of the cell. Lipoteichoic acids contain a fatty acid and are important as surface antigens to differentiate bacterial serotypes. Lipoteichoic acids also aid the attachment of the organism to host receptors. Techoic acids also play a role in virulence. The mycobacteria contain a waxy substance, mycolic acid, in their cell walls, which enables them to resist the actions of acid. Other compounds that contribute to the acid-resistance and waxy character of the mycobacterial cell wall are cord factor, wax D, and sulfolipids.

Gram-negative bacteria also have an outer membrane, which acts as a barrier for the cell against the external environment and contains important enzymes and proteins. This outer membrane is external to the cytoplasmic membrane and is made up of **lipopolysaccharide** (LPS). LPS, also known as **endotoxin**, has several biological functions important in the disease process. When LPS is released upon cell lysis into the environment of the host, B cells are activated, which stimulates macrophage and other cells to release interleukin-1, interleukin-2, tumor necrosis factor, and other cytokines. LPS can also induce fever and cause shock; disseminated intravascular coagulation (DIC) is one severe consequence of large amounts of LPS released into the blood. DIC is characterized by systemic activation of blood coagulation with the formation of fibrin clots, which may result in thrombi, or clots, within the blood and organs of the body. This may ultimately result in multiple organ failure and bleeding from consumption of the coagulation proteins and platelets. There are several causes of DIC that include severe infection and sepsis, trauma, malignancy, hepatic failure, and transfusion reactions.

LPS consists of three sections: lipid A, core polysaccharide, and O antigen. Lipid A is associated with endotoxin activity; its structure is similar for closely related bacteria. Core polysaccharide is important structurally and for the viability of the bacterial cell. The O antigen is important in differentiating serotypes or strains of a bacterial species. For example, there are over 150 types of O antigen for *E. coli*; one particularly important type is O157. Porins present in the outer membrane contain water and help regulate the passage of nutrients, antibiotics, and other hydrophilic compounds into the cell.

The cell walls of gram-positive and gram-negative bacteria are compared in **FIGURE 1-2**.

CELLULAR METABOLISM

Cellular metabolism of bacteria is important when determining how bacteria cause disease and also for the biochemical identification of bacteria. Bacteria must obtain nutrients from the environment through the cell envelope; water, oxygen, and carbon dioxide diffuse across the cell membrane. Active transport is needed to move other molecules such as organic acids, amino acids, and inorganic ions into the bacterial cell. These processes are facilitated through carrier molecules. Other compounds such as sugars, fatty acids, and nucleotide bases are chemically modified through group

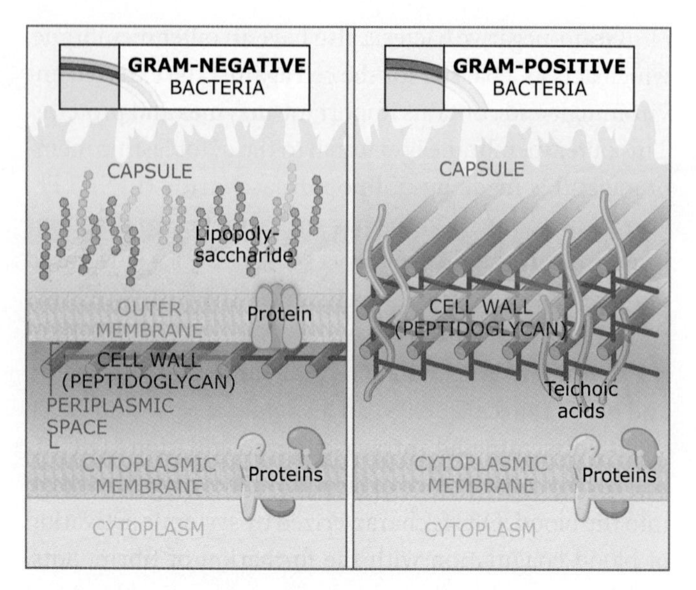

FIGURE 1-2 Cell wall comparisons.

translocation to enter the cell. Nutrients also include nitrate, phosphate, hydrogen sulfide, sulfate, potassium, magnesium, calcium, sodium, iron, and ammonia.

Precursor molecules are formed from the nutrients once they are within the bacterial cell. These compounds are produced through the pentose phosphate shunt, Embden-Meyerhof-Parnas (EMP) pathway, and the tricarboxylic acid (TCA) cycle. These metabolites include acetyl CoA, glucose-6-phosphate, pyruvate, oxaloacetate, and other compounds. Through biosynthesis, these molecules form fatty acids, sugars, amino acids, and nucleotides, which then polymerize to form larger macromolecules. Macromolecules include lipid, lipopolysaccharide, glycogen, murein, protein, DNA, and RNA. The final step is assembly whereby inclusions; cytosol; polyribosomes; pili; flagella; and the cellular envelope, nucleoid, and capsule are formed from the macromolecules.

Energy is required for all bacterial metabolism and occurs through the breakdown of chemical substrates. The substrate is oxidized and donates electrons to an electron-acceptor molecule, which is reduced. Carrier molecules such as nicotinamide-adenine-dinucleotide (NAD+) and nicotinamide-adenine-dinucleotide-phosphate (NADP+) mediate this process. The energy released is transferred to phosphate-containing compounds such as ATP, where high-energy phosphate bonds are found. This provides the needed energy for the biochemical reactions for the cell.

Fermentative processes within the cell do not require oxygen; typical end products produced from fermentation include alcohols, acids, hydrogen, and carbon dioxide. Fermentative processes vary with each bacterial species and can be used to identify bacteria. For example, all members of the Enterobacteriaceae family possess the necessary enzymes to ferment the carbohydrate glucose. Identifying the production of acid end products from a specific substrate is useful in the identification of bacteria.

Bacteria can also use oxidative phosphorylation to generate energy. In this process, carrier molecules transport electrons from a reduced carrier molecule to a terminal electron acceptor. In the process, ATP is generated from ADP. In aerobic respiration, oxygen is used as the terminal electron acceptor. In anaerobic respiration, an electron acceptor other than oxygen is used.

Bacteria that totally rely on aerobic respiration and cannot grow in the absence of oxygen are known as obligate (strict) aerobes; those that cannot tolerate any amount of oxygen are known as obligate (strict) anaerobes. Facultative anaerobic bacteria can use aerobic respiration or fermentative processes.

EXOTOXINS AND ENDOTOXINS

Bacteria produce systemic effects of infection through the production of **toxins**. **Exotoxins** are associated with gram-positive organisms and are secreted by the living bacterial cell. Exotoxins are usually found in high concentration in fluid media and are not associated with the production of fever. Examples include leukocidin, produced by *S. aureus*, which inhibits white blood cells (WBCs); the toxic shock syndrome toxin of *S. aureus*; diphtheria toxin of *Corynebacterium diphtheriae*; and theta toxin, a necrotizing toxin produced by *Clostridium perfringens*. Other exotoxins are extracellular enzymes such as DNAse, which inhibits the host deoxyribonucleic acid (DNA); coagulase, which converts fibrinogen into fibrin; hemolysins, which lyse red blood cells (RBCs); proteases, which break down protein; and fibrinolysins, which lyse fibrin clots. Endotoxins are usually associated with gram-negative bacteria and consist of lipopolysaccharide (LPS), the component of the cell wall. Endotoxins are released at cell lysis or death and are capable of inducing fever in the host.

The Role of Clinical Microbiology

Clinical microbiology begins when the patient presents signs of infection to the physician. An initial diagnosis is made, and the physician then orders diagnostic medical and laboratory procedures. A direct stain, a culture, and an antibiotic susceptibility test are typical tests that may involve the microbiology laboratory. The appropriate laboratory specimens are collected, labeled, and sent to the laboratory with a requisition or laboratory order form. The laboratory performs direct stains, plates the specimen on appropriate culture media, and incubates the plates at the suitable temperature and atmosphere. The plates are examined and interpreted for the presence of pathogens, most often at 24 and 48 hours. Subcultures are performed as needed, and any biochemical, serological, molecular, antibiotic susceptibility, and automated procedures are performed. These tests are interpreted and the organisms are identified. The final report of the identification and antibiotic susceptibility tests is sent to the physician. The physician interprets the report and treats the patient appropriately.

Early diagnosis is associated with early treatment and a better prognosis for the patient. Testing must be performed in a timely, yet accurate, manner. Often, a presumptive identification can be sent to the physician so that antibiotic therapy can be initiated. A final, definitive identification is then sent to update the report.

The Infectious Process

An **infection** is the entrance and multiplication of a microorganism in or on a host. The microorganism may enter the host through many routes including the respiratory tract, gastrointestinal tract, or breaks in the skin. The microorganism next establishes itself and multiplies. Infections can spread directly through tissues or the lymphatic system into the blood. **Infectious disease** refers to an infection with functional and structural harm to the host that usually is accompanied by signs and symptoms.

In this process, the pathogen first must come in contact with and colonize the host. Colonization refers to the state when the microbe has established itself in a particular niche or body site. This generally corresponds with the incubation period, and the host has no signs of infection. Next, the pathogen breaks the host's protective barrier and multiplies. This coincides with the first signs of clinical infection, known as the prodromal stage, during which time the host is particularly infective. The clinical symptoms peak during the clinical sage of infection. At this time the pathogen continues to multiply, attacking deeper tissues and eventually disseminating through the blood to other organs. The pathogen is met by the host's inflammatory and immune system, which have been stimulated by the microbe and its products. Depending on the immune status of the host and severity of the infection, there may be various outcomes. The host may destroy the pathogen, or the pathogen may destroy the host; in some cases, the pathogen may remain latent within the host. If the host recovers, the signs of infection decline, and the host eventually enters the convalescent phase of infection. Consequences of infection may remain as a result of toxins or other compounds produced by the microbe. If the host continues to deteriorate, the symptoms may worsen, eventually resulting in permanent damage or even death.

All **pathogens** in a specimen must be identified and reported to the physician. A pathogen is a microorganism, including bacteria, viruses, fungi, and parasites, that is capable of causing infectious disease. The identification of pathogens may be difficult because many microorganisms are present in the normal microbial flora. **Normal flora** refers to those microorganisms normally residing in a particular body site or niche that do not generally cause infection. Normal flora may also be known as indigenous or resident flora or microbiota; these bacteria may perform important functions and compete with pathogenic microorganisms.

NORMAL FLORA

A limited number of organisms can be categorized as normal flora. The slightly acidic pH of the **skin** (5.5 to 6.0) results from the presence of acids produced by a number of bacteria. For example, *Propionibacterium acnes* produces large amounts of propionic acid. Other normal skin flora include *Staphylococcus epidermidis*, viridans streptococcus, and enterococcus. In addition, a number of contaminating organisms may be found transiently on the skin, such as intestinal tract and soil contaminants.

In the **mouth and oral cavity**, the major normal flora is the viridans streptococcus, a collection of streptococcal species exhibiting alpha hemolysis or greening of sheep blood agar. In addition, *S. epidermidis*, nonpathogenic *Neisseria* species, *Moraxella catarrhalis*, lactobacilli, and diphtheroids may be present. Members of the anaerobic normal flora in this area include *Actinomyces, Veillonella*, and *Bacteroides* species.

The **nasopharynx** may serve as a site for asymptomatic carriage of several microorganisms. **Asymptomatic**

carriers maintain a reservoir for the microorganism but do not have an infectious disease. The carrier state may be transient or permanent, and these individuals may serve as an infectious source to transmit the pathogen to others. Bacteria that may be carried asymptomatically in the nasopharynx include *Staphylococcus aureus* and *Neisseria meningitidis*.

The **stomach** and **upper small intestine** are usually sterile, containing less than 1,000 organisms per milliliter. Organisms entering the stomach are usually killed by the hydrochloric acid and resulting low pH of the stomach, as well as by gastric enzymes. Other organisms are passed to the small intestine, where they may be destroyed by bile and pancreatic enzymes. When the gastric pH increases over 5.0, colonization from bacteria of oral, nasopharyngeal, or colon origin may occur.

The **colon** is heavily colonized and serves as a reservoir for infection for numerous body sites, including the urinary tract and peritoneal cavity. Major components of the normal bowel flora include *Bacteroides, Lactobacillus, Clostridium, Eubacterium*, coliforms such as *Escherichia coli*, aerobic and anaerobic streptococci, and yeast.

The normal flora of the distal **urethra** in both males and females may contain diphtheroids, alpha and nonhemolytic streptococci, *Peptococcus, S. epidermidis*, and *Bacteroides*.

Those sites considered to be sterile in the body, containing no normal flora, include the **blood**, **cerebrospinal fluid**, and **urinary bladder**. Normal flora can become pathogenic if they are moved to another site. Thus normal flora *E. coli* of the colon is an important cause of urinary tract infection (UTI) once it enters the bladder or kidneys. Likewise, although viridans streptococcus is considered to be normal flora of the oral cavity, the organism is a significant cause of subacute bacterial endocarditis when established in the heart.

MODES OF TRANSMISSION—ROUTES OF INFECTION

Infectious disease can be transmitted by several routes, which can be categorized as direct or indirect modes of transmission. The etiologic agent is the microorganism that has caused the infection. The reservoir of infection refers to the origin of the etiologic agent or its location such as contaminated food, another human, or an infected animal. Types of **direct transmission** include congenital contact, sexual contact, hand-to-hand contact, and droplet infection.

Congenital contact may occur across the placenta or as the baby passes through the vaginal canal during delivery. Rubella virus and syphilis may be acquired during pregnancy, whereas *Streptococcus agalactiae* and *Neisseria gonorrhoeae* are examples of bacteria that may be transmitted to the infant during delivery.

Sexual contact may be the route of infection for several sexually transmittable diseases, including gonorrhea (*N. gonorrhoeae*); syphilis (*Treponema pallidum*); chlamydia (*Chlamydia trachomatis*); acquired immunodeficiency syndrome, or AIDS (human immunodeficiency virus, or HIV); and herpes (herpes simplex virus).

Hand-to-hand transmission is the mode of direct contact seen with the spread of the common cold from rhinovirus. This route is also involved in the transmission of various GI infections when the hands are not properly washed and are fecally contaminated.

Infectious respiratory secretion or droplet infection serves as a route for several respiratory viruses as well as for bacterial pathogens including *Streptococcus pyogenes* (the agent in streptococcal pharyngitis throat) and *N. meningitidis*. Infectious secretions include coughing, sneezing, kissing, and nasal drainage. Respiratory secretions can become dried on clothing, bedding, or floors and converted to dust, which may serve as a route of indirect transmission.

Indirect routes of infection include fomites, ingestion of contaminated food and water, airborne routes, and animal or arthropod vectors.

Fomites are inanimate objects such as eating utensils, drinking devices (water bottles and cups), hospital instruments, clothing, money, doorknobs, and tampons. Sometimes, these inanimate objects may serve as a route of **nosocomial** (hospital-acquired) infection. Fomites may also be referred to as vehicles of infection, which refers to nonliving objects that have been contaminted with the infectious agent.

Water may be contaminated as a result of improper sanitary measures or after it has been treated. Microorganisms that may be associated with contaminated water include *Shigella, Salmonella*, enteropathogenic *E. coli*, and hepatitis A virus (HAV). Improperly prepared, processed, preserved, or stored **food** may become contaminated with various microorganisms, including *Salmonella, Listeria, E. coli* O157:H7, and *S. aureus*. Milk and milk products may be contaminated through improper or lack of pasteurization, while undercooked meats may serve as sources of contamination. Ingestion of the microorganisms or of preformed toxins plays a role in infections acquired through contaminated foods.

Infections may be incidentally transmitted to humans through infected **animals** or **insect** or **arthropod vectors**. Rabies, pasteurellosis (*Pasteurella multocida*), and tularemia (*Francisella tularensis*) are examples of infections that can be acquired through the bite or scratch of an infected animal. Arthropod vectors such as flies, mites, lice, ticks, and mosquitoes may transmit microorganisms from an infected animal to a human host. Malaria (*Plasmodium*) is transmitted by mosquitoes, whereas Lyme disease (*Borrelia burgdorferi*) is transmitted by the bite of an infected tick.

Airborne routes of infection include the **inhalation** of infectious particles that may be suspended in the air. **Infectious aerosols** can be formed in the laboratory that can serve as a route for laboratory-acquired infection. *Mycobacterium tuberculosis*, the agent in tuberculosis, can remain suspended in droplets that serve as infectious aerosols. Dimorphic fungi, which cause systemic infections such as *Coccidioides immitis*, can cause airborne infections through the inhalation of infectious spores.

FIGURE 1-3 summarizes routes of infection for microorganisms.

Once established in a particular area, the microorganism may multiply and spread from its original site of entry to contiguous tissue or disseminate through the blood to other, distant sites. Microorganisms spread and multiply when host defense mechanisms are overcome.

The **incidence** of a disease refers to the number of those individuals infected in a population, whereas the disease **prevalence** describes the percentage of infected individuals in a given population at a given time. An **endemic** is when a disease consistently occurs at a constant rate in a given location. An **epidemic** occurs when there are larger numbers of cases of a disease in a given location. **Pandemics** are epidemics that occur around the world. **Outbreaks** generally refer to instances where there is a disproportionately larger number of infected individuals in a fairly short amount of time.

TRUE VERSUS OPPORTUNISTIC PATHOGENS

A true pathogen has the ability to cause an infection under all conditions in all types of individuals. By contrast, an opportunistic pathogen refers to an organism that is pathogenic only under particular, favorable conditions. Under other conditions, opportunisms are nonpathogenic and generally harmless and are often members of the human normal flora. **Opportunistic infections** are infections that occur when there are preexisting conditions that increase the susceptibility of the host to infection. Generally, opportunistic pathogens do not cause disease in individuals with a normal immune system. These infections are increasing as a result of a number of factors including the widespread use of broad-spectrum antibiotics that can alter the normal flora, the increased use of immunosuppressive drugs to prevent organ transplant rejection, the use of chemotherapeutic agents to treat cancer, and the increased and prolonged use of urethral catheters. Thus an **opportunistic pathogen** is one that attacks an already debilitated host but usually presents no danger to an individual with an intact immune system.

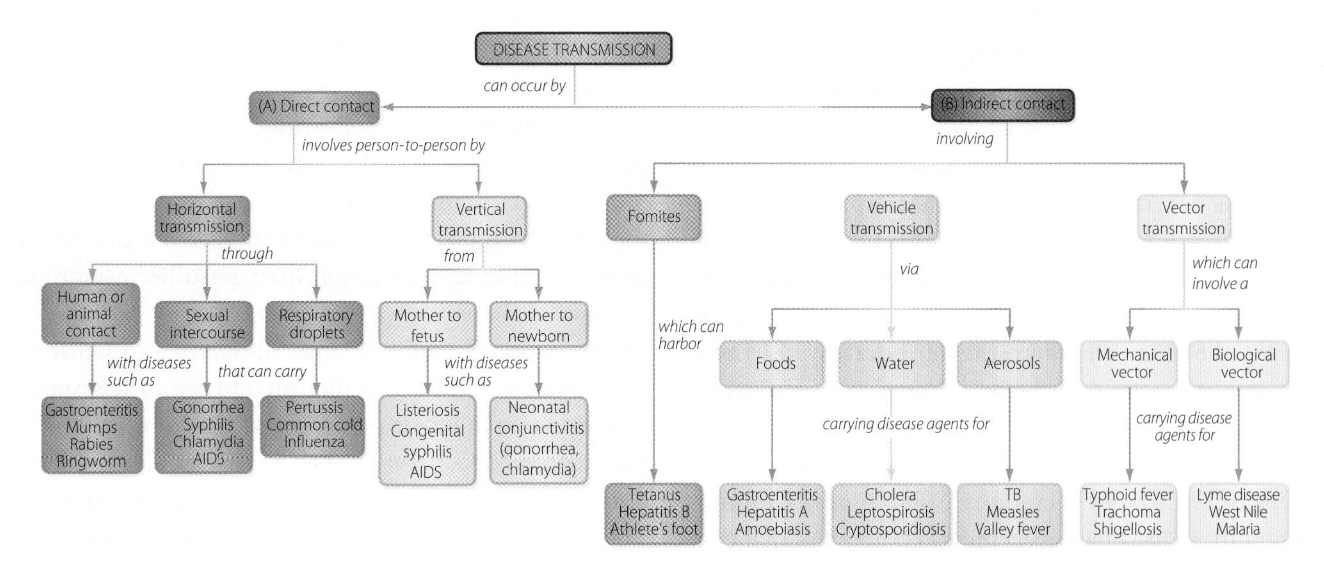

FIGURE 1-3 Routes of infection.

In immunosuppressive conditions the host immune system is unable to effectively battle those microorganisms considered to be normal flora for the general population. Other individuals at risk for opportunistic pathogens include dialysis patients, those with HIV-AIDS, burn victims, diabetics, and any individual who has chronic medical problems or is undergoing invasive medical techniques. Those individuals with foreign body implants including heart valves, prosthetic devices, and indwelling intravenous catheters; alcoholics; and intravenous drug users are also at increased risk of opportunistic pathogens.

By contrast, a **true pathogen** has the ability to infect those individuals with a healthy immune system as well as those with an immunosuppressed state.

HOST DEFENSE MECHANISMS

Host defense mechanisms include innate, or natural, immunity; acquired immunity; and phagocytosis. **Immunity** refers to host properties that confer resistance of the host to foreign substances. It is the sum of all mechanisms used by the body as protection against environmental agents that are not normally present in the body.

Innate or Natural Immunity

Innate, or **natural**, **immunity** is inborn, mainly genetically determined, and nonspecific. It is not acquired through previous contact with an infectious agent. The skin acts as a protective barrier, and a limited number of microorganisms can penetrate the intact skin barrier. Many microorganisms, however, can enter the body through breaks in the skin resulting from bites, wounds, cuts, or needles. In addition, microorganisms can enter through the sweat and fat glands. The normal flora bacteria of the skin produce free fatty acids from oil, which will produce low pH on the skin and thus prevent the establishment of infection.

Mucus covers the surfaces of the **respiratory tract**. The mucus can trap bacteria and, with the assistance of **cilia**, which are also present in the nasal cavity, can trap many microorganisms. The bacteria are either swallowed, entering the stomach where they are destroyed by the acidic environment, or removed through external openings such as the nose and mouth by sneezing or coughing. **Lysozyme**, an enzyme that lyses bacterial cell walls, is also present in respiratory secretions. Some types of immunoglobulin A (IgA) have a secretory component that can prevent attachment of the microorganisms to the mucous membranes of the respiratory tract. Those bacteria that are phagocytized are transported through the lymphatic system and eventually removed from the body.

The respiratory tract is a common portal of entry for several microorganisms, including *Streptococcus pneumoniae, M. tuberculosis, Mycoplasma pneumoniae*, and several respiratory viruses. Those microorganisms possessing pili, appendages for attachment, are able to attach to the mucous membranes.

Saliva in the oral cavity possesses various hydrolytic enzymes that can break down bacteria. The low pH of the stomach and the presence of gastric enzymes result in a limited amount of microorganisms that can sustain life in the stomach. The rapid peristalsis in the **small intestine**, together with the presence of enzymes and bile, keeps the microbial population in this site at very low levels. The **large intestine** has a large amount of normal flora that competes with pathogens, thus decreasing the chance for establishment of infection. The anaerobic normal flora of the large intestine produces fatty acids, while facultative anaerobes produce bacteriocins, which also hinder the multiplication of pathogens.

The constant flushing action and low pH of **urine** prevent pathogens from establishing in the urinary system. Females, who have shorter urethras, are more prone to UTIs than are males, who have longer urethras. Bacteria have easier access to the female bladder from the GI and vaginal tracts.

Lactobacilli, a major normal flora in the female vaginal tract, produce large amounts of lactic acid, which results in a low pH. This acidic environment decreases the amount of other microorganisms that can cause infection in this area.

The **eyes** are protected through the constant flushing provided by tears as well as the presence of lysozyme in tears.

Other elements of innate immunity include fever, interferon, phagocytosis, and various serum proteins. These components are described with the inflammatory response.

Natural immunity can be affected by a number of factors. For example, very young and very old persons are more susceptible to infection than are other age groups. Hormonal changes such as those occurring during pregnancy, diabetes mellitus, and Addison's and Cushing's diseases can alter the metabolism and immune response, which results in increased susceptibility to infection. The use of broad-spectrum antibiotics, which alter the host's normal flora, can also promote the growth of pathogens. The normal flora is no longer present in large amounts to compete with the pathogenic organisms. Such infections

BOX 1-3 Hallmark Signs of Inflammation

Sign	Latin Derivation	Description
Redness	Rubor	Dilation of small blood vessels in area of injury
Heat	Calor	Increased blood flow through the inflamed area in peripheral parts of body; fever as a result of chemical mediators of inflammation
Swelling	Edema	Fluid accumulates outside of blood vessels
Pain	Dolar	As a result of edema because tissues are inflamed; effects of serotonin, bradykinin, and prostaglandins

are termed **secondary infections** or superinfections because the infection results from the use of an antibiotic.

Inflammatory Response

The inflammatory response can be activated by trauma or tissue injury. **Inflammation** is the total of the changes occurring in tissue factors upon injury. There are four hallmark signs of inflammation: redness, heat, swelling, and pain. These are described in BOX 1-3. Hemodynamic changes, such as increased vascular permeability, dilation of arterioles and capillaries, and increased blood flow to the injured area, occur. Plasma proteins, such as complement, interferon, and antibodies, are also released. Edema may occur as a result of vasodilation, while there is also an influx of red blood cells to the area.

Phagocytic white blood cells, which include neutrophils (PMNs) and macrophages, have four functions: **migration, chemotaxis, ingestion**, and **killing**. These cells may **adhere** to the vascular endothelium or migrate from the blood to the affected tissues in a process known as **diapedesis**. Chemotaxis refers to the attraction of the phagocytes to the affected area by the microorganisms or its products from the blood to the injured site. Neutrophils and monocytes are attracted by bacterial products such as endotoxins and enzymes. **Attachment** initiates the phagocytic process. The microorganism must be coated with opsonins such as IgG or complement units for effective phagocytosis. Those microbes that have a capsule are resistant to the effects of phagocytosis. The next step is ingestion, which involves the formation of a **phagosome** that undergoes a respiratory burst. The respiratory burst results in the release of superoxide anion and peroxide, both of which are toxic to microorganisms. Lysosomes within the cell combine with phagosomes to form phagolysosomes, which eventually release hydrolytic enzymes.

Neutrophils are formed in the bone marrow and enter the blood and tissue. Monocytes, also formed in the bone marrow, are known as macrophages once the cells have entered the tissue. Macrophages are present in tissues but are also fixed to the blood vessels of the liver, spleen, and lymph nodes. Macrophages can become activated by microorganisms, endotoxins, and antigen–antibody complexes. Once activated, macrophages produce an increased number of lysosomes that produce interleukin-1. Interleukin-1 is associated with the stimulation of fever and activation of phagocytosis.

Inflammation caused by microorganisms may be initiated through activation of the complement system or the blood coagulation cascade. These systems initiate the release of several chemical mediators of inflammation, which are summarized in TABLE 1-2.

Acquired Immunity

Acquired immunity can be either passive or active. **Passively acquired immunity** refers to the temporary resistance to infectious agents by administration of antibodies preformed in another host. Examples include gamma globulin and antitoxin to *Clostridium botulinum* toxin. Passive acquisition is also seen in the fetus, who acquires antibodies from the mother's blood during pregnancy. These antibodies remain active in the newborn until 4 to 6 months of age. Newborns may also acquire immunity passively from their mothers through antibodies carried in breast milk.

Actively acquired immunity is a state of resistance built in an individual following contact with foreign antigens such as microorganisms. The immunity may result from clinical or subclinical infection, through injection of live or inactivated microorganisms, their antigens, or nucleic acids, or through the absorption of bacterial products such as toxins or toxoids. In active immunity the host actively produces antibody in reaction to a foreign antigen.

TABLE 1-2 Chemical Mediators of Inflammation

Compound	Effect
Histamine	Dilates blood vessels, increases permeability of blood vessels
Kinins	Increase vascular permeability and initiate or enhance release of other mediators from white blood cells; derived in the clotting cascade from activation of the precursor **kininogen** by **kallikrein**
Leukotrienes	Affect white blood cell mobility and metabolism
Prostaglandins	Formed in the hypothalamus in the thermoregulation center; induce fever
C-reactive protein, serum amyloid A, antitrypsin	Liver proteins playing a role in the acute response
Interleukin-1	Stimulates cells of immune response, increases fever by interaction with prostaglandins, increases adhesion of neutrophils to endothelium, promotes T cell proliferation
Interleukin-2	Causes proliferation of activated T and B cells
Cytokines	Stimulate white blood cells, promoting their growth and differentiation
Gamma interferon	Promotes growth of T and B cells

Acquired immunity involves contact with a foreign agent or **antigen**. This process is known as **immunization**, and it initiates a series of reactions that lead to the activation of **lymphocytes** and the synthesis of specialized serum proteins known as **antibodies**. Thus antigens are substances foreign to the body that initiate the production of antibodies.

Three major cell types are involved in the immune response: T lymphocytes, B lymphocytes, and macrophages. **T** and **B lymphocytes** arise from a common lymphoid precursor cell but mature in different areas of the body. T cells mature in the thymus, while B cells, named for the bursa of Fabricius (the area in the chicken where the cells were first isolated), mature in the bone marrow. Although B and T cells have different functions, both play a role in the recognition of antigen and reaction to it. The third type of cells, **macrophages**, are phagocytic cells that ingest, process, and present antigens to T cells.

Humoral immunity is mediated by serum antibodies secreted by B cells. These antibodies are known as **immunoglobulins**. There are five major classes of immunoglobulins: IgG, IgM, IgA, IgD, and IgE. Each immunoglobulin class has unique biological abilities.

IgG is able to cross the placenta and is most active at 37°C. It is the major immunoglobulin in normal serum. IgG is primarily involved in the secondary, or anamnestic, immune response.

IgM is involved mainly in the primary immune response and appears in the serum following initial exposure to an antigen. IgM has its greatest activity at 20°C to 25°C.

IgA is unique in that it is the only immunoglobulin found in secretions such as tears, saliva, and of the respiratory tract. Important characteristics of the immunoglobulins are summarized in **TABLE 1-3**, and a summary of their primary functions is found in **BOX 1-4**.

The **complement system** is another important aspect of humoral immunity. The complement system involves more than 20 serum proteins and enzymes that can be activated by immune (antigen–antibody) complexes or nonimmune routes such as lipopolysaccharide. If the complement

TABLE 1-3 Summary of Human Immunoglobulins

	IgG	IgM	IgA	IgD	IgE
Percentage in normal serum	75%–85%	5%–10%	5%–15%	0.001%	0.0003%
Molecular weight (approximate)	150,000	900,000	160,000 (serum), 400,000 (secretory)	180,000	190,000
Heavy chain class	gamma (γ)	mu (μ)	alpha (α)	delta (δ)	epsilon (ε)
Heavy chain subclasses	$\gamma_1\gamma_2\gamma_3\gamma_4$	$\mu_1\mu_2$	$\alpha_1\alpha_2$	None	None
Cross placenta	Yes	No	No	No	No
Activate complement	Yes for IgG-1, -2, -3	Yes	No	No	No

BOX 1-4 **Primary Functions of Human Immunoglobulins**

IgG: Passive immunity for newborns, neutralization of viruses and exotoxins; responds best to protein antigens, mainly involved in secondary (anamnestic) immune response

IgM: Endotoxin neutralization, bacterial agglutination, complement-mediated bacteriolysis, strong opsonization ability; responds best to polysaccharide antigens, mainly involved in primary immune response

IgA: Prevention of bacterial and viral invasion of mucous membranes through interference with adherence of microorganism to site; found in tears, milk, saliva, and respiratory and GI secretions

IgD: Little is known; may serve as a B cell receptor or play a role in autoallergic diseases

IgE: Major role in allergic response; found on surface of mast cells

cascade is activated, the target cell may be lysed, or phagocytic cells may be stimulated.

Cell-Mediated Immunity

Cell-mediated immunity (CMI) involves the T lymphocytes, which circulate to the antigen to perform their function. There are several populations of T cells including:

- **T helper (inducer) cells**
  - Enhance proliferation and differentiation of B cells and precursors to cytotoxic T cells
  - Increase ability of macrophages to ingest and destroy pathogens
  - Enhance the production of antibody by B cells
  - Release lymphokines, including interleukin-1 (IL-1) and interleukin-2 (IL-2) and B cell–stimulating factor, which helps to activate B cells
- **Cytotoxic T cells**—destroy targets on direct contact through the recognition and destruction of antigen-bearing cells
- **T suppressor cells**—suppress or regulate the response of T and B cells
- **Null cells (natural killer [NK] and killer [K] cells)**—kill tumor or viral-infected cells, although not with the specificity of cytotoxic T cells

Although presented as separate functions, the humoral and cell-mediated immune systems interact in the immune response.

SIGNS OF INFECTION

The need for clinical microbiology begins with a patient who is exhibiting one or more signs of infection. Some common general or systemic signs of acute infection include a high-grade, spiking fever; chills; vasodilation with flushing; and an increased pulse rate. Chronic or subacute infections may be accompanied by the following systemic signs: intermittent, low-grade fever; weight loss; and fatigue. Local signs of infection include pain, heat, redness, and swelling. The hallmark signs of inflammation are found in Box 1-3.

In the laboratory, specific procedures are used to diagnose infection. These include the **leukocyte count**, which is elevated for most infectious processes, and the **differential white blood cell count**, which enables the clinician to determine the type of infection. In general, but not always, bacterial infections are associated with an elevated white blood cell count and an increased percentage of **neutrophils**. By contrast, lymphocytes are the predominant WBC in most viral infections. The **erythrocyte sedimentation rate** (ESR) is a nonspecific indicator of inflammation and is frequently increased in infectious disease and numerous other inflammatory states. **C-reactive protein** is another plasma protein that is present during infectious disease. Finally, the presence of **type-specific antibodies** in a patient's serum can be used to identify the presence of a particular pathogen. On exposure to a bacterial or viral pathogen, the patient produces antibodies against the antigens of the organism. The antibodies then can be detected through use of antigenic markers.

Radiographic signs of infectious disease that a clinician would note include pulmonary infiltrates, gas and swelling in the tissues, and the accumulation of fluid in a body cavity.

Gastrointestinal signs such as nausea, vomiting, and diarrhea, as well as various neuromuscular and cardiopulmonary signs, are also noted by the clinician.

NOSOCOMIAL AND HEALTH CARE–ASSOCIATED INFECTIONS

A **nosocomial**, or **health care–associated**, **infection** is acquired in a hospital or other health care setting. The organism is not present and not incubating in the patient on entry or admission into the health care facility. A **community-acquired infection** is present or incubating at the time of admission into the health care facility. Community-acquired infections also are those that are acquired within an individual's community such as her or his school, workplace, or athletic or social setting. As with other infections, nosocomial and community-acquired infections can be categorized as endogenous or exogenous. **Endogenous infections** result from organisms that are a part of the patient's normal flora, whereas **exogenous infections** result from organisms from external sources. These sources may include contaminated medical instruments or equipment or inanimate objects in the health care setting or from contact with health care personnel. Individuals, including health care providers, may be colonized with an organism. **Colonization** is defined as the presence and multiplication of a microorganism in a host, with no clinical signs of infection. Such individuals may serve as a reservoir of infection and transmit the organism to susceptible individuals.

The most common types of nosocomial infections are urinary tract infections (35% to 40%), surgical wound infections (20%), lower respiratory tract infections (15%), and bacteremia (5%–10%). These percentages may vary with each health care setting. Those bacteria most often associated with nosocomial infections include *S. aureus, E. coli, Enterococcus*, and *Pseudomonas aeruginosa*. Many nosocomial pathogens are resistant to multiple antimicrobial agents.

Nosocomial urinary tract infections may be the result of catheterization or the presence of indwelling catheters or other urological techniques such as cystoscopy. The organism is frequently of endogenous origin, as with *E. coli*, which is a member of the normal flora of the large intestine. Exogenous sources include the contaminated hands of health care providers or contaminated equipment or solutions.

Nosocomial surgical wound infections usually involve *S. aureus, Enterococcus*, or gram-negative bacilli. These infections may be endogenous or exogenous.

Nosocomial pneumonia may result from aspiration of the organisms from the stomach or upper respiratory tract. The airways or stomach may become colonized with bacteria including *S. aureus, P. aeruginosa*, and *Klebsiella pneumoniae*. Respiratory care procedures, such as endotracheal suctioning and inhalation therapy, also present a greater risk for nosocomial pneumonia. A high mortality rate is associated with nosocomial infections of the lower respiratory tract.

Bacteremia may result from the patient's own flora as well as that of the health care provider. In addition, intravenous devices or solutions may be contaminated.

Host factors that lead to increased susceptibility to nosocomial infections include a compromised immune system, underlying medical disease or diseases, age, trauma, burns, poor nutritional status, anatomical abnormalities, use of medical instrumentation, and diagnostic procedures.

Some, but not all, nosocomial infections can be prevented. The universal use of gloves and practice of aseptic techniques, including thorough hand washing, can decrease the incidence of nosocomial infections. The routine disinfection of inanimate surfaces and prevention of aerosols are also important factors.

Review Questions

Matching

Match the following terms with the correct definition:

_______ 1. Infection
_______ 2. Infectious disease
_______ 3. Opportunistic infection
_______ 4. Nosocomial infection
_______ 5. Colonization

a. Condition associated with functional and structural harm to the host, accompanied by signs and symptoms
b. Infection in an immunocompromised host that does not cause infection in an immunocompetent individual
c. Infection acquired in a health care setting
d. Presence and multiplication of a microorganism in a host with no clinical signs of infection
e. Entrance and multiplication of a microorganism in a host

Multiple Choice

6. All the following sites contain normal flora *except*:
   a. Oral cavity
   b. Skin
   c. Colon
   d. Cerebrospinal fluid
7. Which of the following is *not* classified as a direct route of infection?
   a. Ingestion of contaminated food or water
   b. Sexual contact
   c. Hand-to-hand contact
   d. Congenital contact
8. Droplet infection through contact with infectious respiratory secretions may be described as:
   a. Inhalation of infectious aerosols during laboratory procedures
   b. Transmission of rhinovirus through failing to wash hands
   c. Spread of respiratory viruses and *Streptococcus pyogenes* through coughing or sneezing
   d. Inhalation of bacteria or viruses that have dried on bedding or clothing
9. Which of the following organisms are typically spread through the ingestion of contaminated food or water?
   a. *Neisseria meningitidis* and *S. pyogenes*
   b. *Salmonella* and *Shigella*
   c. Herpes simplex virus and *Treponema pallidum*
   d. *Plasmodium* and *Borrelia*
10. Which of the following organisms are spread through arthropod vectors?
    a. *N. meningitidis* and *S. pyogenes*
    b. *Salmonella* and *Shigella*
    c. Herpes simplex virus and *T. pallidum*
    d. *Plasmodium* and *Borrelia*
11. Innate, or natural, immunity involves which of the following mechanisms?
    a. Mucus and cilia in the respiratory tract that help to trap and clear microorganisms
    b. Humoral immunity
    c. Cell-mediated immunity
    d. Immunity resulting from vaccination
12. The movement of neutrophils and monocytes from the blood to injured tissue is known as:
    a. Diapedesis
    b. Chemotaxis
    c. Ingestion
    d. Hematopoiesis
13. Antibody-producing white blood cells are:
    a. Macrophages
    b. Neutrophils
    c. T lymphocytes
    d. B lymphocytes
14. Which of the following cells play a major role in cell-mediated immunity?
    a. Macrophages
    b. Neutrophils
    c. T lymphocytes
    d. B lymphocytes
15. The immunoglobulin found in the highest concentration in normal serum is:
    a. IgA
    b. IgD
    c. IgE
    d. IgG
    e. IgM
16. Which of the following immunoglobulins is involved mainly in the primary immune response?
    a. IgA
    b. IgD
    c. IgE
    d. IgG
    e. IgM
17. Gram-negative bacteria contain ________________, which are not found in gram-positive bacteria.
    a. Capsules
    b. Periplasmic space and outer membrane
    c. Teichoic acids
    d. Cross-linked peptidoglycan
18. Which of the following is true for bacterial cells?
    a. The DNA is contained within a nuclear membrane.
    b. Their mitochondria, Golgi bodies, and endoplasmic reticulum are present in the cytoplasm.
    c. The DNA is found in the nucleoid.
    d. The ribosomes are 80S.
19. The ________________ are important for motlity of the bacterial cell.
    a. pili
    b. capsules
    c. flagella
    d. LPS
20. Phenotypic properties used to classify bacteria include all of the following *except*:
    a. DNA relatedness
    b. Colonial morphology
    c. Biochemical properties
    d. Antibiotic resistance patterns

Bibliography

Bower, S., & Rosenthal, K. S. (2006). Bacterial cell walls: The armor, artillery and Achilles heel. *Infectious Diseases in Clinical Practice, 15*, 309–316.

Casadevall, A., & Pirofski, L. (2001). Host-pathogen interactions: The attributes of virulence. *The Journal of Infectious Diseases, 184*, 337–344.

Diekema, D. J., & Pfaller, M. A. (2007). Infection control epidemiology and clinical microbiology. In P. R. Murray, E. J. Baron, J. H. Jorgensen, M. L. Landry, & M. A. Pfaller (Eds.), *Manual of clinical microbiology*, 9th ed. (pp. 118–128). Washington, DC: American Society for Microbiology.

Finlay, B. B., & Falkow, S. (1989). Common themes in microbial pathogenicity. *Microbiology and Molecular Biology Reviews, 53*, 210.

Forbes, B. A., Sahm, D. F., & Weissfeld, A. S. (2007). Bacterial genetics, metabolism and structure. In *Bailey and Scott's diagnostic microbiology*, 12th ed. St. Louis, MO: Mosby.

Klevins, R. M., Edwards, J. R., Richards Jr., C. L., Horan T. C., Gaynes, R. P., Pollock, D. A., & Cardo, D. M. (2007). Estimating health care-associated infections and deaths in U.S. hospitals, 2002. *Public Health Reports, 122*, 160–166.

Murray, P. R., Rosenthal, K. S., & Pfaller, M. A. (2009). Mechanisms of bacterial pathogenesis. In *Medical microbiology*, 6th ed. (pp. 179–187). Philadelphia, PA: Mosby.

Parham, P. (2009). Antibody structure and the generation of B-cell diversity. In *The immune system*, 3rd ed (pp. 1–31). New York, NY: Garland Science Taylor & Francis Group.

Parham, P. (2009). Elements of the immune system and their roles in defense. In *The immune system*, 3rd ed (pp. 1–31). New York, NY: Garland Science Taylor & Francis Group.

Schaechter, M. (2012). Biology of infectious diseases. In N. C. Engleberg, T. Dermody, & V. DiRita (Eds.), *Schaechter's mechanisms of microbial disease*, 5th ed. (pp. 18–37). Philadelphia, PA: Lippincott Williams & Wilkins.

Soule, B. M., & LaRocco, M. T. (1993). Nosocomial infections: An overview. In B. J. Howard, J. F. Keiser, A. S. Weissfeld, & F. Thomas (Eds.), *Clinical and pathogenic microbiology*, 2nd ed. (pp. 83–99). St. Louis, MO: Mosby.

Turgeon ML (2003). Antigens and antibodies. In *Immunology and serology in laboratory medicine*, 3rd ed. (pp. 15–35). St. Louis, MO: Mosby.

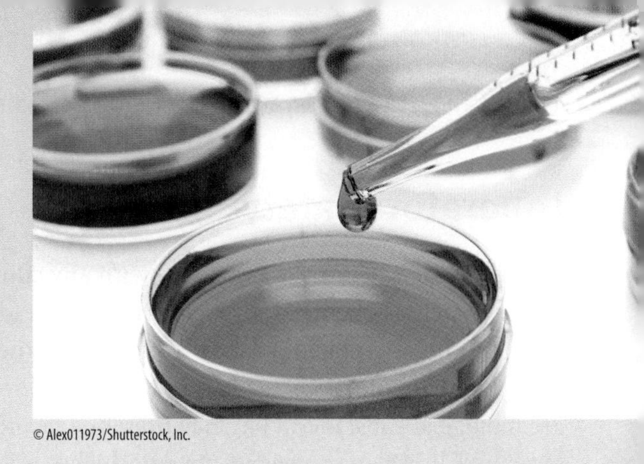
© Alex011973/Shutterstock, Inc.

CHAPTER 2

Safety in the Clinical Microbiology Laboratory

CHAPTER OUTLINE

Laboratory Safety
Exposure Control
Fire Safety
Chemical Safety

KEY TERMS

Biohazard
Biosafety Level
Disinfection
Standard precautions
Sterilization
Universal precautions

LEARNING OBJECTIVES

1. Describe the elements of a laboratory safety program as applicable to the student microbiology laboratory.
2. List and describe the possible routes of laboratory-acquired infections.
3. Name the agencies that recommend policy for laboratory safety.
4. Discuss the concepts of standard precautions and universal precautions.
5. Describe and practice the general guidelines for safety in the clinical laboratory:
   a. Discuss personal protective equipment and its purpose in the clinical laboratory.
   b. Describe safety precautions with specific applications to the microbiology laboratory.
6. Summarize the criteria for and differentiate Biosafety Levels 1, 2, 3, and 4.
7. Describe and differentiate the various types of biological safety cabinets.
8. Define and give examples of sterilizers, disinfectants, and antiseptics.
9. State the principle of the autoclave.
10. List and define the five types of hazardous chemicals.

Laboratory Safety

In addition to safety risks associated with any clinical laboratory, such as chemical, fire, electrical, and radioactive hazards, the microbiology laboratory presents the hazard of exposure to infectious agents, or biohazards. Biohazards are biological substances that may present a health risk to humans. Clinical specimens are potential biohazards to laboratory personnel because the specimens may contain human immunodeficiency virus (HIV); hepatitis B virus (HBV); and numerous other bacterial, viral, and fungal agents.

Possible routes of infection that may occur in the microbiology laboratory include airborne, ingestion, direct inoculation, mucous membrane contact, and arthropod vectors. Each of these routes is summarized in BOX 2-1.

Guidelines to ensure safety in the clinical laboratory have been compiled by several agencies, including the Occupational Safety and Health Administration (OSHA), the Centers for Disease Control and Prevention (CDC), the College of American Pathology (CAP), and the Joint Commission (JC). Of particular significance is the publication of standards for bloodborne pathogens by OSHA, which were published in the *Federal Registry* in 1991. Standards for bloodborne pathogens are updated periodically by OSHA. The recommendations of these agencies can be used to develop safety regulations for the student microbiology laboratory.

Exposure Control

Each facility is required by law to have a laboratory safety officer and an exposure control plan. The safety officer oversees the development and implementation of a safety program, orientation of laboratory employees, preparation of a laboratory safety manual, and the development and implementation of the exposure plan. In the education setting, this officer may be a faculty member or an individual designated by the institution to oversee the general safety and well-being of employees and students. The **exposure control plan** describes the risk of exposure to infectious agents for all job classifications and explains exposure-reduction methods. The exposure plan must include procedures and documentation related to the following:

- Safety education
- Universal precautions and standard precautions
- Engineering controls
- Personal protective equipment
- Disposal of hazardous waste
- Postexposure procedures

SAFETY EDUCATION

Safety education includes orientation of new employees and continuing education for current employees regarding laboratory safety policies. In addition, current employees must receive continuing education regarding safety. All safety must be documented. Information may be compiled within a **safety manual**, which must contain policy and procedures concerning fire prevention and control, electrical safety, radiation safety, biohazard control, chemical hazards, hazardous waste disposal, and internal and external disaster preparedness. Safety policies should be posted or readily available to all individuals in the laboratory setting. The policy should be periodically reviewed and revised as needed. Employees who handle infectious

BOX 2-1 **Possible Routes of Infection in the Microbiology Laboratory**

Airborne: Aerosols may form during centrifugation of unstoppered tubes or from heating cultures or specimens too rapidly (sterilization of inoculating loops in the Bunsen burner flame), removing stoppers from tubes, or leakage from a container that holds contaminated specimens.

Ingestion: Infection may occur as a result of failure to wash hands or eating, drinking, smoking, applying cosmetics, or pipetting with the mouth.

Direct inoculation: Infection may result from needlesticks, broken glass, animal bites, or small scratches on the fingers.

Mucous membrane contact: Infection may occur if the organism can directly enter through the mucous membranes, such as through the conjunctiva of the eye.

Arthropod vectors: Infectious sources include ticks, fleas, and mosquitoes, which may harbor various microorganisms.

materials on a daily basis and those who have limited exposure, such as cleaning personnel, should be educated in the current safety recommendations of the facility.

UNIVERSAL PRECAUTIONS AND STANDARD PRECAUTIONS

Universal precautions are recommendations that describe the handling of clinical specimens by health care personnel, first introduced by the Centers for Disease Control (CDC) in 1987. According to the Clinical Laboratory and Standards Institute (CLSI), universal precautions are a set of preventive measures designed to reduce the risk of transferring HIV, hepatitis B virus, and other bloodborne pathogens in the health care setting. Universal precautions apply to all human blood and all other body fluids that contain visible blood (semen, vaginal secretions, and tissue and cerebrospinal, synovial, pleural, peritoneal, pericardial, and amniotic fluids). However, universal precautions do not apply to feces, nasal secretions, saliva except in the dental setting, sputum, sweat, tears, urine, and vomitus unless they contain visible blood. **Standard precautions** are a set of preventive measures, applied to all patients, that are designed to reduce the risk of infection in the health care setting. All blood, tissue, body fluids, secretions, and excretions (except sweat) are considered potentially infectious. A basic premise of standard precautions is that because the infectivity of any patient's blood and body fluids cannot be known, all patient blood and body fluid specimens must be treated as if they are potentially infectious.

All laboratory accidents, illnesses, and injuries must be reported immediately and recorded on the appropriate forms. Faculty, laboratory assistants, and students must complete the required incident reports in a timely fashion and follow the recommendations of the laboratory safety officer, including serological and clinical follow-up.

General guidelines to be followed in any clinical laboratory are summarized in BOX 2-2.

BOX 2-2 Safety Guidelines for the Clinical Laboratory

- **No food or drink** is permitted in the laboratory; no eating or drinking is permitted in the laboratory. Specimens may contain microorganisms that can induce infectious disease. No food or drink should be stored in clinical refrigerators. Separate refrigerators are required for food storage. These refrigerators should not be located in the clinical setting and should be labeled as to their contents.
- **No smoking** is permitted in the clinical laboratory. Smoking can ignite flammables and also may serve as a vehicle for exposure to microorganisms. Smoking is generally prohibited in most health care facilities.
- **Cosmetics**, including lip balm, are not to be applied in the laboratory because contamination is possible.
- **Protective eyewear** with side guards must be worn in all laboratories using hazardous chemicals or etiologic agents, in laboratories where animals are dissected, or if the threat of eye injury from flying debris may be a risk. The eyewear should be equipped with side shields. Regular prescription lenses are not suitable unless goggles are worn over the top of the prescription glasses. Contact lenses in those laboratories where volatile fumes are present are not recommended because the lenses may absorb the volatile fumes. Protective eyewear does not prevent this problem, and thus contact lens wearers should be advised to wear prescription glasses with protective eyewear over their glasses.
- **Face shields** with goggles and masks are recommended when working with agents that can infect through the skin or mucous membranes and when splashing may occur.
- **Clothing** should be clean and neat, and the use of **gowns**, **aprons**, or **laboratory coats** is required if splashing of blood or other body fluids onto the skin or clothing is likely to occur. Long-sleeved gowns with a closed front or long-sleeved laboratory coats that are buttoned are required. Disposable gowns, which can be autoclaved at the facility, are recommended. All protective clothing should be worn only in the laboratory or patient areas and is *not* to be worn in nonlaboratory areas. For example, laboratory gowns or coats must not be worn into the cafeteria or to the individual's home. Nondisposable gowns and coats must be properly **disinfected** and cleaned when contaminated, whereas disposable gowns and coats should be properly decontaminated and disposed of.
- **Shoes** should cover the entire foot; no open shoes, such as sandals, are permitted.

(*continues*)

BOX 2-2 **Safety Guidelines for the Clinical Laboratory (Continued)**

- **Hair** should be worn in a manner that prevents contact with contaminated materials as well as with moving instruments or equipment, such as centrifuges, in which it can become tangled. Those with **beards** must observe the same guidelines. **Jewelry** should not dangle, to prevent contamination or tangling into equipment.
- **Frequent and thorough hand washing** is required. The hands should be washed after removing gloves, before leaving the laboratory area, before and after patient contact, and before eating or smoking. The hands should be washed immediately after contact with blood or other contaminated specimens or materials. Care must be taken to scrub thoroughly, including areas beneath the fingernails.
- **Eyewash stations** must be located within 100 feet or 10 seconds of travel from any area in which hazardous chemicals (irritants, corrosives, acids, or toxic compounds) are used. The emergency eyewash must be plumbed into the fixtures; plastic wash bottles are not acceptable. The eyewash stations must be tested weekly to ensure proper working order and to flush out stagnant water.
- **Emergency showers** are required whenever corrosive or caustic chemicals are used. The shower should be tested periodically to ensure proper functioning.
- **Respirators** must be made available to those working in areas where the air may be contaminated with gases, fumes, vapors, or other harmful compounds.
- **Mouth pipetting** is strictly prohibited because of the possible ingestion of microorganisms and caustic chemicals. Pipette bulbs and automated devices are available for all pipetting needs.
- **Glassware** should be discarded in puncture-resistant containers when broken or chipped. **Sharp objects** should be handled with care. Needles should never be recapped, bent, or broken. All sharp objects must be placed immediately in puncture-resistant containers that are labeled as to the contents. Typical puncture-resistant containers for sharps disposal are illustrated in **FIGURE 2-1**. More information on sharp objects is found in the next section.
- **Centrifuges** must minimize the production of aerosols. Uncovered tubes or flammables should not be centrifuged; sealed tubes must be centrifuged at low speeds only. Sealed centrifuge tubes in covered cups or rotors are recommended for centrifugation of specimens containing microorganisms likely to become infectious through the production of aerosols.

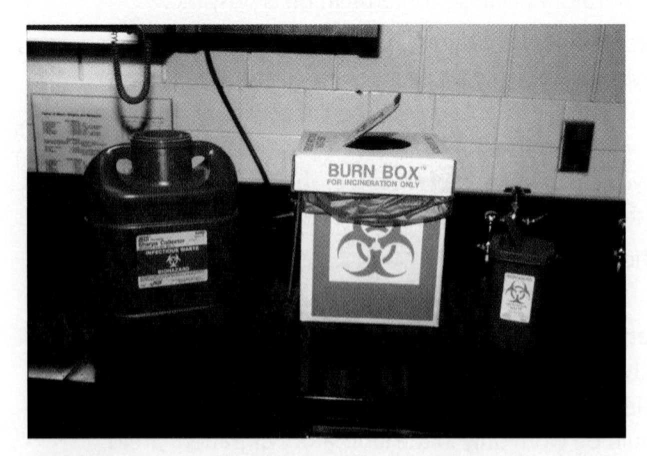

FIGURE 2-1 Puncture-resistant sharps containers.

PERSONAL PROTECTIVE EQUIPMENT

Personal protective equipment (PPE) is a significant part of standard precautions; OSHA requires that employees must be protected from hazards encountered during work. In the laboratory, PPE includes protective laboratory clothing, disposable gloves, eye protection, and face masks. **Barrier protection** should be used to prevent skin and mucous membrane contamination with those specimens that adhere to universal precautions. **Gloves** should be worn when there is potential for skin contact with potentially infectious materials. Thus gloves should be worn when performing routine laboratory work and when handling materials contaminated with blood or other body fluids, such as instruments and specimen containers. Gloves also are recommended when performing phlebotomy and capillary puncture. Gloves should be changed between patients, and hands should be washed immediately after removing gloves. Gloves must fit properly, be replaced immediately if torn or contaminated, and not be washed and reused. Facial protection and a protective body covering should be worn when splashes with blood or other fluids may occur.

High-efficiency particulate air (HEPA) respirators should be fit tested for each person; those who encounter mycobacteria through contact with either the patient or specimen should have access to a HEPA respirator. Laboratory employees who have contact with body fluids must be offered the hepatitis B vaccinations free of charge.

ENGINEERING CONTROLS

Engineering controls are needed to protect employees from the hazards that may occur during the performance of laboratory procedures. All laboratories must adhere to a minimum of **Biosafety Level 2 guidelines**. The CDC has classified microorganisms into various biosafety categories. These categories are based on several factors including number of occupational infections, infectious dose, and route of infection and are summarized in BOX 2-3.

Hazardous areas should be identified and labeled accordingly. The **biohazard** label (**FIGURE 2-2**) should be used to identify those areas of the laboratory where infectious specimens or cultures are stored or present. Needles, lancets, and other sharp objects should be placed immediately into puncture-resistant biohazard containers. Needles should not be recapped, bent, cut, broken, or removed from disposable syringes, to prevent an accidental needlestick.

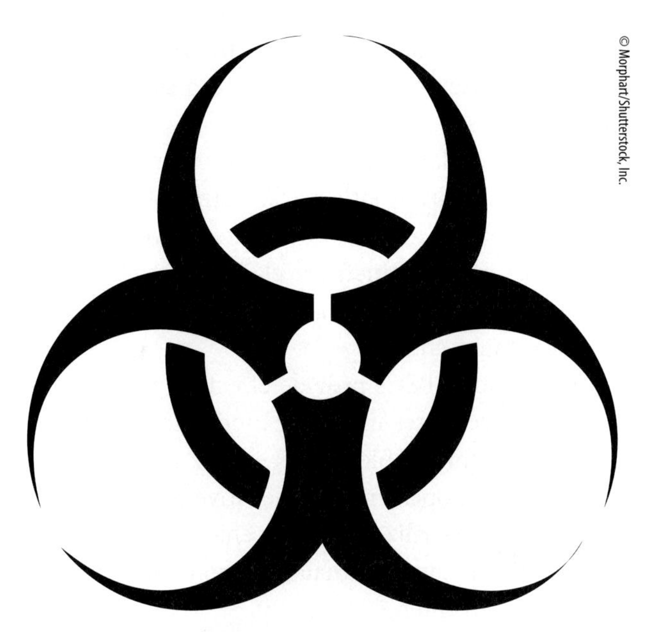

FIGURE 2-2 Biohazard label.

Air in the microbiology laboratory should move from areas of low risk to high risk and should not be recirculated after it passes through the microbiology laboratory. Procedures known to create aerosols must be performed in a biological safety cabinet (BSC). Infectious particles from microorganisms may become suspended in the air; these infectious aerosols may be inhaled by the laboratory worker. These procedures include the preparation

BOX 2-3 Summary of Biosafety Levels (BSLs) for Infectious Agents

Biosafety Level 1 (BSL 1): No known pathogenic potential for immunocompetent individuals. Typical examples include *Bacillus subtilis*. Most undergraduate laboratory courses operate under BSL 1 precautions. Precautions include adherence to standard laboratory techniques.

Biosafety Level 2 (BSL 2): Level 1 practices plus laboratory coats, protective gloves, limited access, decontamination of all infectious waste, and biohazard warning signs. Apparatus includes partial containment equipment (such as classes I and II biological safety cabinets) when procedures may lead to the production of infectious aerosols. This category includes the most common microorganisms associated with laboratory-acquired infections, including HBV, HIV, *Staphylococcus*, and enteric pathogens such as *Salmonella* and *Shigella*.

Biosafety Level 3 (BSL 3): Level 2 procedures plus special laboratory clothing and controlled access are recommended for handling clinical material suspected of containing *Mycobacterium tuberculosis, Brucella, Coccidioides immitis, Rickettsia*, and specific viruses such as arbovirus. The air movement must be carefully controlled to contain the infectious materials.

Biosafety Level 4 (BSL 4): Level 3 practices plus entrance through a separate room in which street clothing is changed and replaced with laboratory clothing. Maximum containment includes the use of a class II biological safety cabinet and the decontamination of all personnel and materials before leaving the area. This level is primarily used in research facilities and includes a limited number of exotic viruses including filovirus and arenavirus.

of smears, flaming inoculating loops and needles in the burner flame, vortexing, grinding tissue, and subculturing blood cultures.

BSCs protect laboratory workers from aerosols through **sterilization** by either heat, ultraviolet light, or passage of air through a HEPA filter that removes particles larger than 0.3 mm. Cabinets are classified as class I, II, or III based on performance characteristics with regard to biological containment.

Classes I and II BSCs provide effective partial containment for procedures involving moderate- and high-risk microorganisms or Biosafety Levels 2 and 3 agents. Class I cabinets are open-fronted, negative-pressure, ventilated cabinets. Unsterilized room air enters and circulates within the cabinet, and the exhaust air from the cabinet is filtered by a HEPA filter.

Class II BSCs sterilize both the air entering and circulating within the cabinet and the exhaust air. Type II vertical laminar-flow biological cabinets are open-fronted, ventilated cabinets. Type II cabinets have HEPA-filtered, recirculated airflow within the workspace. The exhaust air from the cabinet also is filtered by a HEPA filter. HEPA filters trap particulates and infectious agents but do not trap volatile chemicals or gases. There are two major types of type II BSCs, based on the inlet flow velocity and percentage of air filtered. Type II-A BSCs are self-contained with 70% of the air recirculated; type II-A BSCs are not required to be vented and are acceptable for low- to moderate-risk agents. A class II BSC is illustrated in **FIGURE 2-3**. Class II type B cabinets must be vented with 30% of the air exhausted from the cabinet and 70% recirculated back into the room.

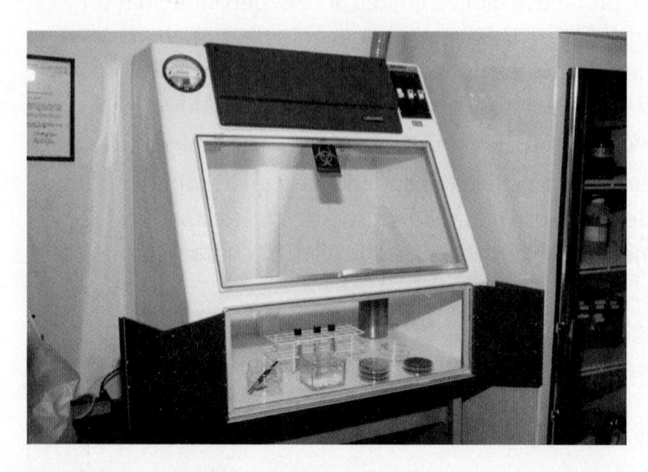

FIGURE 2-3 Class II biological safety cabinet.

Class III BSCs provide the highest level of safety, and all air entering and leaving the cabinet is sterilized with a HEPA filter. Supply air is drawn through a HEPA filter while exhaust air is filtered through two HEPA filters. The system is entirely enclosed, and all infectious materials are handled with rubber gloves that are sealed to the cabinet.

Most hospital microbiology laboratories routinely use class II-A BSCs.

Biosafety Level guidelines as applicable to the microbiology laboratory are found in BOX 2-4.

POSTEXPOSURE PLAN

All laboratory accidents or safety incidents must be reported to the laboratory safety officer or supervisor. Appropriate medical treatment must be given immediately. Percutaneous, mucous membrane, or abraded skin exposure to hepatitis B or HIV should be followed clinically and serologically. This includes the administration of immunizations, hepatitis B immune globulin (HBIG), and hepatitis B vaccinations. Collection of blood specimens for serological testing may also be indicated. This includes collection of serum samples at 6 weeks, 3 months, and 6 months for antibodies to HIV or abraded skin exposure to HBV or HIV. Appropriate serological and clinical follow-up of the employee must be provided.

There must be documentation of the accident with a report verifying the incident and follow-up. The accident also should be reviewed to determine how it could have been prevented. Finally, corrective actions must be given so that the accident can be prevented in the future.

Disposal of Hazardous Waste

Microbiological waste must be **decontaminated** before disposal. These waste materials include patient specimens, patient cultures, sharp instruments (needles, lancets) that have been placed in puncture-resistant containers, inoculated media, and other contaminated laboratory supplies. All contaminated materials should be placed into two leak-proof plastic bags; double bagging protects against infectious materials from leaking or falling from a single bag. Contaminated pipettes, swabs, and glass should be placed into puncture-resistant burn boxes. Contaminated needles, scalpels, and other implements that have a puncture risk should be placed into sharps containers. The **autoclave** (**FIGURE 2-4**) is often used to decontaminate these materials. The autoclave, which uses saturated steam, is operated

BOX 2-4 **Biosafety Level 2 Criteria for Standard Microbiology Practices**

1. Limit access to the laboratory when working with infectious agents.
2. Decontaminate work surfaces at least once daily and after any spill of potentially infectious material.
3. Use mechanical pipetting devices.
4. Do not eat, drink, smoke, or use cosmetics in the work area. Store food only in refrigerators so designated that are not in the work area.
5. Thoroughly wash hands after handling infectious materials when leaving the laboratory.
6. Minimize the creation of aerosols in all work procedures.
7. Wear laboratory coats, gowns, or smocks in the laboratory and remove before leaving the laboratory for nonlaboratory areas.
8. Avoid skin contamination by covering cuts in skin with occlusive bandages and using gloves when working with potentially infectious substances.
9. Do not use needles that are bent, cut, or recapped. Used needles should be placed immediately into a puncture-resistant container. Minimize the use of needles for laboratory procedures, such as aspiration of body fluids. A negative pressure may exist between the contents of the bottle and the atmosphere, which may lead to spraying of the contents. A needlestick injury is also a potential consequence in this situation.
10. Handle *M. tuberculosis* at Biosafety Level 3 in a class II biological safety cabinet while wearing a solid-front gown and personal respirator (or face-molding mask). Use sealed safety cups for centrifugation.
11. Handle all mold-like fungi in a biological safety cabinet. All plated media for mycology should be sealed with a cellulose band or cellophane or labeling tape to prevent the dispersion of spores.

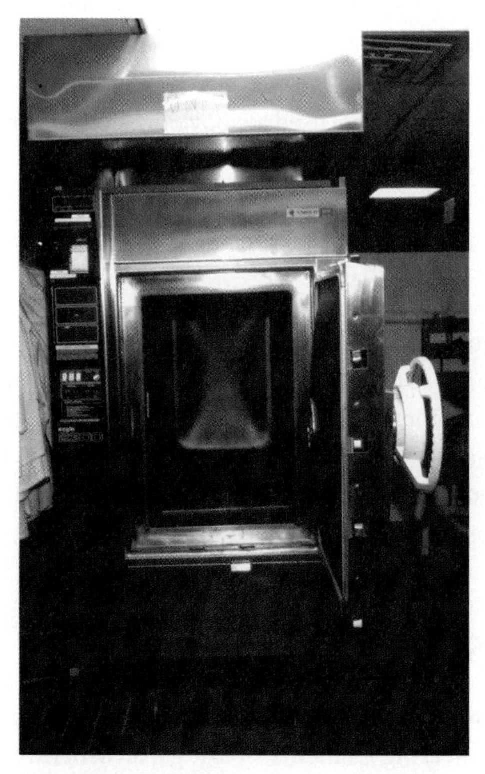

FIGURE 2-4 Autoclave.

at 121°C and 15 psi (pounds per square inch) of pressure for 1 hour to sterilize most contaminated microbiological materials. All known pathogens, including spores, vegetative cells, fungi, and viruses, are killed under these conditions. Infectious medical waste is usually autoclaved at 132°C for 1/2 hour to 1 hour.

The autoclave must be monitored periodically to measure its effectiveness. *Bacillus stearothermophilus* spore indicator strips, which are quite resistant to the effects of the autoclave, can be used for this purpose. The strips are wrapped in a fashion similar to those articles that are autoclaved. Weekly monitoring is recommended.

Sterilization is a physical or chemical process that kills all microorganisms, including the spores. **Disinfection** destroys most microbes but does not kill the spores.

Biocides are chemical agents that inactivate microorganisms; these agents may be either static and inhibit growth of the microbe or cidal and kill the target organism.

Liquid decontaminants, such as 70% ethanol or a 10% solution of household bleach (sodium hypochlorite), can be used to decontaminate laboratory workbenches. Bleach is

BOX 2-5 **Chemical Germicide Categories**

1. **Sterilizer:** purpose is to destroy all microorganisms (bacteria, viruses, fungi, prions, viroids) and their spores on inanimate surfaces
   - Moist heat or steam under pressure (autoclave): 121°C for 1 hour at 15 psi of pressure
   - Dry heat: 171°C for 1 hour, 160°C for 2 hours, 121°C for 16 hours
   - Liquid: glutaraldehyde (variable strength), hydrogen peroxide (6% to 30%), formaldehyde (6% to 8%), chlorine dioxide (variable strength)
2. **Disinfectant:** purpose is to destroy or irreversibly inactivate bacteria, viruses, and fungi (but not necessarily the spores) on inanimate objects
   - Moist heat: 75°C to 100°C
   - Liquid: glutaraldehyde (variable strength, bacteriocidal, health care risks including asthma), hydrogen peroxide (3% to 6%), formaldehyde (1% to 8%), chlorine compounds, 70% isopropyl alcohol
   - Liquid household bleach (sodium hypochlorite) can be used as an intermediate-level disinfectant and has bactericidal, fungicidal, virucidal, and tuberculocidal activity. Concentrations of 500 mg to 1,000 mg of chlorine per liter have rapid activity. Concentrations are made based on the nature of the contaminated surface. Porous surfaces should be cleaned with a 1:10 dilution and smooth, hard surfaces with a 1:100 dilution. Time of exposure to the diluted bleach solution may be short. For example, a 1:100 dilution inactivates HBV in 10 minutes and HIV within 2 minutes. Large spills or concentrated infectious agents should be flooded and cleaned with a concentrated (1:5 dilution) solution of bleach. All dilutions should be made up weekly with tap water to prevent the loss of germicidal activity on storage.
   - Quaternary ammonium compounds such as benzalkonium chloride are effective as low-level disinfectants when in concentrated forms. Newer formulations are very effective disinfects with quick activity against bacteria, viruses, fungi, and mycobacteria.
3. **Antiseptic:** chemical germicide for use on the skin or tissues and not to be substituted for a disinfectant
   - **Alcohols:** 70% ethyl or isopropyl alcohol; exhibit rapid broad-spectrum actvity against microorganisms but not against the spores
   - **Iodophors:** iodine combined with an organic carrier molecule; most widely used are povidone-iodine and poloxamer-iodine in both antiseptics and disinfectants
   - **Hexachlorophene:** bactericidal and broad spectrum but may be toxic

an effective antiviral agent and should be in contact with the surface for a minimum of 10 minutes to increase its ability to decontaminate. Contaminated spills first should be diluted with a detergent and then decontaminated. BOX 2-5 summarizes laboratory sterilization and disinfectant measures.

Specimens or infectious materials shipped to reference laboratories must be packaged according to the requirements of the Interstate Shipment of Etiologic Agents code. Specimens must be packaged to protect them in transit and to protect the personnel handling them. Specimens should never be mailed in petri plates and instead should be shipped in thick glass or plastic culture bottles. Culture caps must be sealed with waterproof tape and packed in material that can absorb the entire culture if necessary. This container is then inserted into a second container, usually a metal tube. The second container is inserted into a cardboard mailing tube, which is labeled with an official Etiologic Agents label.

Fire Safety

Ignition sources in the laboratory may include open flames; heating elements; spark gaps, which may result from light switches or static electricity; and electrical instrumentation. Ignitable liquids include flammable and combustible liquids. When possible, a separate storage room should be used to store these liquids. Flammables and combustibles must be stored in approved containers and should not be stored or positioned by open flames or heat sources. Areas where flammable liquids are used must be properly ventilated for fire protection as well as to protect the laboratory worker. Flammable or combustible liquids may be stored in safety cabinets or safety cans. The supply of these liquids should not be excessive, and up to 60 gallons can be stored in a properly designed safety cabinet (**FIGURE 2-5**) per 5,000 square feet of laboratory space. Up to 25 gallons may be stored in safety cans (**FIGURE 2-6**), while up to 10 gallons may be stored on open shelving per 5,000 square feet of laboratory space.

Flammables should not be stored in refrigerators or within corridors. Transfer of combustible liquids from stock solutions to working solutions must be performed in a storage room when available or within a fume hood. The transport of hazardous liquids should be performed using rubber or plastic safety carriers.

Various types of fire extinguishers (BOX 2-6) are available, including dry chemical, carbon dioxide (CO_2), and halon. Solid wood or paper combustibles can be extinguished with water or CO_2, whereas dry chemical extinguishers are needed for flammable liquids. Halon is most suitable for electrical fires, although CO_2 and halon also can be used. Fire blankets and heat-retardant gloves also should be readily accessible within the laboratory. All electrical receptacles must be inspected at least annually. Laboratory instruments and appliances should be checked for electrical hazards at least once every 12 months.

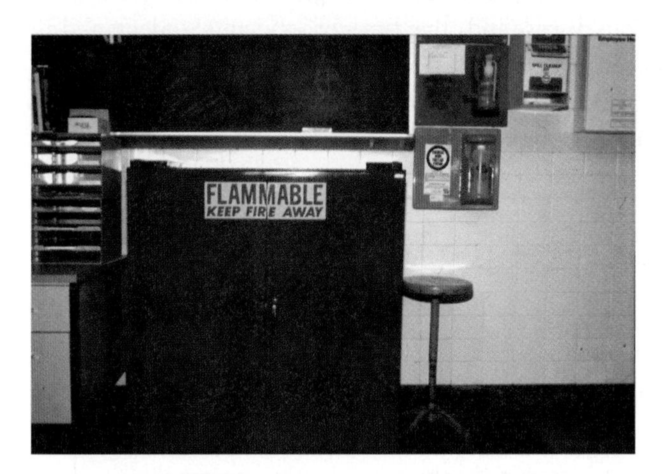

FIGURE 2-5 Chemical storage cabinet.

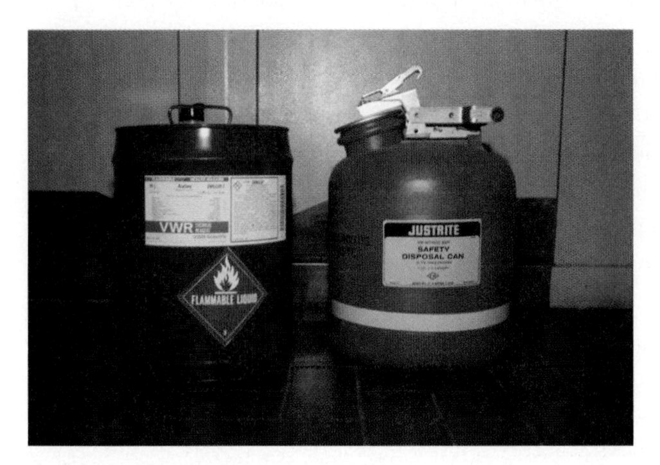

FIGURE 2-6 Safety cans.

BOX 2-6 Types of Fires and Fire Extinguishers

Type A, Water Fire Extinguisher

Used on combustible materials for fires in paper, wood, rubber, cloth, and certain plastics. Extinguish fire with cooling effect.

Type B, Carbon Dioxide (CO_2) Fire Extinguisher

Used on extremely flammable liquids or electrical fires including fires of oil, kerosene, or gasoline and some paints, fats, grease, solvents, or other types of flammable liquids.

Extinguish fire by eliminating oxygen.

Type C, Dry Chemical Extinguishers

Used on electrical fires in wiring and other electrical sources or equipment. Extinguish electrical fires because chemicals don't conduct electricity.

Type D, Combustible Metals

Used for fires involving combustible metals, such as sodium, potassium, magnesium, and sodium-potassium alloys. There are a variety of types including sodium-chloride salt which forms a metal layer over the fire which occludes the oxygen. Other types include graphite, sodium carbonate based, and copper based.

Class K, Dry and Wet Chemical Extinguishers

Used for kitchen fires involving combustible materials such as oil or fat.

Extinguish fire by using various wet or dry chemical agents.

Chemical Safety

All hazardous chemicals must be clearly labeled. **Material Safety Data Sheets** (MSDS) outline the characteristics of hazardous compound chemicals. These must be available to all laboratory workers, who are then responsible for following the safety measures given. OSHA dictates the required information for MSDS; this is summarized in BOX 2-7. **Precautionary labels** must be applied to the containers of all hazardous chemicals, including flammables, combustibles, corrosives, carcinogens, and potential carcinogens. The permissible exposure limit, or PEL, is the legal limit for exposure of an employee to a chemical substance or physical agent. It is usually expressed in parts per million (ppm) or in milligrams per cubic millimeter. PEL limits are established by OSHA and are the result of the 1970 Occupational Health Act, which first established OSHA. Short-term exposure limits, or STEL, refer to the maximum limits that a worker can be continuously exposed to a chemical for up to 15 minutes without danger to health.

Hazardous chemicals can be grouped into five categories as follows:

1. **Corrosive**: causes visible destruction or irreversible damage to human skin on contact
2. **Toxic**: serious biological effects after inhalation, ingestion, or skin contact with relatively small amounts
3. **Carcinogenic**: ability of chemical to induce a malignant tumor
4. **Ignitable**: any chemical that can burn and includes both **combustible** and **flammable liquids**
5. **Explosive**: reactive and unstable substances that readily undergo violent chemical change

Individuals who handle chemicals must be knowledgeable about the risks of chemical hazards and must follow established safety protocols. Appropriate preventive measures must be in place and an action plan for exposure must be documented.

Laboratory safety measures prevent transmission of infectious disease and other types of accidents. Students and all laboratory personnel should be knowledgeable of and follow the safety guidelines of their institutions. When an accident occurs, it is important to report and document appropriately.

BOX 2-7 MSDS Required Information

Section	Required information
I	Manufacturer's name and address, emergency telephone number, telephone number for information, date prepared
II	Hazardous ingredient's identity information, components, specific chemical identity common name(s), PEL
III	Physical/chemical characteristics: boiling point, specific gravity, vapor pressure, vapor density, melting point, evaporation rate, solubility in water, appearance and odor
IV	Fire and explosion hazard data: flash point, flammable limits extinguishing media, special firefighting procedures, unusual fire and explosion hazards
V	Reactivity data: stability incompatibility, hazardous decomposition by-products, hazardous polymerization
VI	Health hazard data: route(s) of entry—inhalation, skin, ingestion, health hazards (acute and chronic), carcinogenicity, signs and symptoms of exposure, medical conditions, generally aggravated by exposure, emergency and first-aid procedures
VII	Precautions for safe handling and use: waste-disposal method, precautions to be taken in handling and storing, action if material is released or spilled
VIII	Control measures: respiratory protection, ventilation, eye protection, gloves, work/hygienic practices

Review Questions

Multiple Choice

1. An infection that may occur as a result of accidental needlesticks or through broken glass is classified as which of the following routes?
   a. Airborne
   b. Ingestion
   c. Direct inoculation
   d. Mucous membrane contact
2. Standard precautions state:
   a. Handle only known HBV-positive or HIV-positive specimens as infectious.
   b. Personal protective equipment is required for only direct patient contact.
   c. Blood and body fluid precautions must be observed for all patients' blood and body fluid specimens.
   d. Infectious specimens must be labeled with the biohazard symbol.
3. The Biosafety Level that includes most common laboratory microorganisms and involves organisms such as HBV, HIV, and enteric pathogens is:
   a. BSL 1
   b. BSL 2
   c. BSL 3
   d. BSL 4
4. Which of the following biological safety cabinets sterilize both the air entering and leaving the cabinet and utilize a HEPA filter?
   a. Class I
   b. Class II
   c. Class III
   d. Class IV
5. Autoclave standards for decontamination of most microbiological materials are:
   a. 100°C at 15 psi for 45 minutes
   b. 121°C at 15 psi for 45 minutes
   c. 121°C at 15 psi for 60 minutes
   d. 100°C at 10 psi for 60 minutes
6. Which germicide is intended to destroy all microorganisms and their spores on inanimate surfaces?
   a. Sterilizer
   b. Disinfectant
   c. Antiseptic
   d. Antibiotic
7. Which of the following types of hazardous chemicals causes serious biological effects following inhalation, ingestion, or skin contact with even small amounts?
   a. Corrosive
   b. Toxic
   c. Carcinogenic
   d. Ignitable
   e. Explosive

Discussion

1. List the items of an exposure plan, giving an example of each.
2. Prepare a list of guidelines for laboratory safety to be observed in your microbiology laboratory.
3. Identify the following in your microbiology laboratory:
   a. Sharps containers
   b. Biohazard symbol
   c. First-aid station (or kit)
   d. Eyewash station
   e. Fire extinguisher and fire blanket

Bibliography

Centers for Disease Control and Prevention. (2009). *Biosafety in microbiological and biomedical laboratories (BMBL)*, 5th ed. Available at http://www.cdc.gov/biosafety/publications/bmbl5/index.htm

Centers for Disease Control and Prevention. (2011). Occupational HIV transmission and prevention among health care workers. Available at http://www.cdc.gov/hiv/resources/factsheets/PDF/hcw.pdf

Centers for Disease Control and Prevention. (2011). Workplace safety and health. Available at http://www.cdc.gov/Workplace/

Centers for Disease Control and Prevention, National Center for Infectious Disease, & the World Health Organization. (2003). Appendix 1: Standard safety practices in the clinical microbiology laboratory. In *Manual for the laboratory identification and antimicrobial susceptibility testing of bacterial pathogens of public health importance in the developing world.* Washington, DC: WHO. Available at http://www.who.int/csr/resources/publications/drugresist/WHO_CDS_CSR_RMD_2003_6/en/

Clinical and Laboratory Standards Institute. (2005). *Protection of laboratory workers from occupationally acquired infections; Approved guideline*, 3rd ed. (M29-A3). Available at http://utahflowcytometry.files.wordpress.com/2012/11/blood-borne-2.pdf

Clinical and Laboratory Standards Institute. (2012). *Clinical laboratory safety; Approved guideline*, 3rd ed. (GP17-A3).

Department of Health and Human Services, Centers for Disease Control and Prevention. (2008). Exposure to blood: What healthcare personnel need to know. Available at http://www.cdc.gov/HAI/pdfs/bbp/Exp_to_Blood.pdf

Duetsch, B. S., & Malley, C. B. (1992). Safety standards and laboratory procedures for exposure to chemicals. *Laboratory Medicine*, *23*, 482.

Emmert, E. A. B., & the ASM Task Committee on Laboratory Biosafety (2013). Biosafety guidelines for handling microorganisms in the teaching laboratory: Development and rationale. *Journal of Microbiology and Biology Education*, *14*, 78–83.

Miller, S. M. (1992). Chemical safety: Dangers and risk control. *Clinical Laboratory Science*, *5*, 338.

Occupational Safety and Health Administration. (2011). OSHA's bloodborne pathogens standard. Available at www.osha.gov https://www.osha.gov/pls/oshaweb/owadisp.show_document?p_table=STANDARDS&p_id=10051

Siegel, J. D., Rhinehart, E., Jackson, M., Chiarello, L., & the Healthcare Infection Control Practices Advisory Committee. (2007). Guideline for isolation precautions: Preventing transmission of infectious agents in healthcare settings. Available at http://www.cdc.gov/ncidod/dhqp/pdf/isolation2007.pdf

National Center for Infectious Diseases, Centers for Disease Control and Prevention, Division of HIV/AIDS. (1993). Surveillance for occupationally acquired HIV infection: United States 1981–1992. *Laboratory Medicine*, *24*, 107. Adapted from U.S. Department of Health and Human Services, Public Health Service, Centers for Disease Control. (1992). *Morbidity and Mortality Weekly Report*, A*1*, 823.

U.S. Department of Labor, Occupational Safety & Health Administration. Hazardous and toxic substances. Available at https://www.osha.gov/SLTC/hazardoustoxicsubstances/index.html

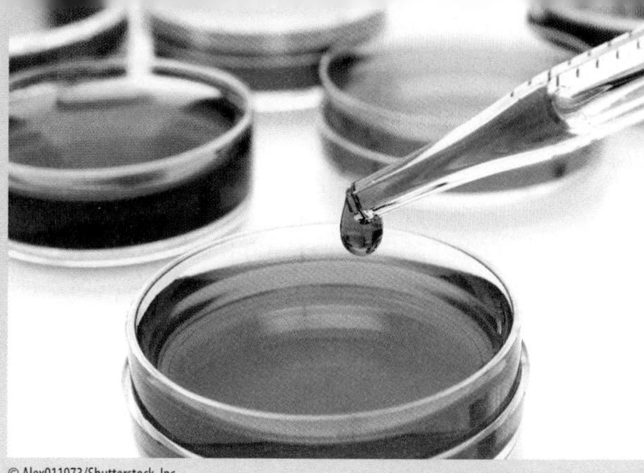

CHAPTER 3

Specimen Collection, Transport, and Processing: Preliminary Identification Methods

CHAPTER OUTLINE

- General Specimen Guidelines
- Collection Requirements for Specific Sites and Specimens
- Specimen Transport and Processing
- Initial Specimen Plating and Identification Methods
- Preliminary Biochemical Tests
- Laboratory Procedures
- Quality Control

KEY TERMS

Antibiotic media
Asymptomatic carrier
Bacteremia
Bartlett's classification
Capnophilic
Colony count
Differential media
Enrichment broth
Facultative anaerobe
Fastidious
General isolation media
Meningitis
Mesophilic
Nonselective isolation media
Normal flora
Obligate aerobe
Obligate anaerobe
Selective media
Septicemia

LEARNING OBJECTIVES

1. List and discuss the basic concepts for proper specimen collection in diagnostic microbiology. Recognize samples that are not suitable and suggest appropriate corrective action.
2. For each of the following sites, or specimens, describe specific collection requirements:
   a. Throat
   b. Nasopharyngeal
   c. Sputum
   d. Urine (clean catch, catheterized, suprapubic)
   e. Wound
   f. Stool
   g. Cerebrospinal fluid
   h. Genital (male urethral, female vaginal and cervical)
   i. Blood
3. Discuss proper specimen transport and processing methods.
4. Describe the gross examination of specimens for microbiology.
5. Using Bartlett's classification, determine whether a sputum sample is acceptable or contaminated.
6. List and discuss important quality-control measures used in the microbiology laboratory.

7. For each of the following media, state the purpose and describe the important components:
   a. Sheep blood agar
   b. Colistin-nalidixic acid
   c. Chocolate agar
   d. Modified Thayer-Martin, Martin-Lewis,
   e. MacConkey
   f. Eosin-methylene blue
   g. Gram-negative broth, selenite broth, tetrathionate broth
   h. Thioglycollate
   i. Hektoen enteric, *Salmonella–Shigella*, xylose-lysine-deoxycholate
8. Identify and describe the types of hemolysis observed on sheep blood agar.
9. Streak an agar plate correctly to obtain isolated colonies.
10. Define and differentiate the following:
    a. Aerobe and anaerobe
    b. Facultative anaerobe and obligate anaerobe
    c. Mesophile and thermophile
11. Discuss how the following tests can be used in the preliminary identification of bacteria:
    a. catalase
    b. cytochrome oxidase
    c. coagulase
    d. PYR hydrolysis
    e. carbohydrate utilization

In the clinical laboratory, proper specimen collection is essential to providing accurate and appropriate results. This is especially true in clinical microbiology; specimens collected improperly provide the physician with misleading and erroneous results that may lead to incorrect treatment or failure to appropriately treat a suspected infection. Specimen collection is included in the preanalytical phase of laboratory testing, which involves patient identification and preparation and specimen collection, labeling, transport, and storage. The analytical phase involves the testing of the specimen (reagents, procedure, quality control, interpretation), and the postanalytical phase involves the reporting of results. Thus, errors in specimen collection ultimately affect the laboratory results and outcomes for the patient. This process is summarized in **FIGURE 3-1**.

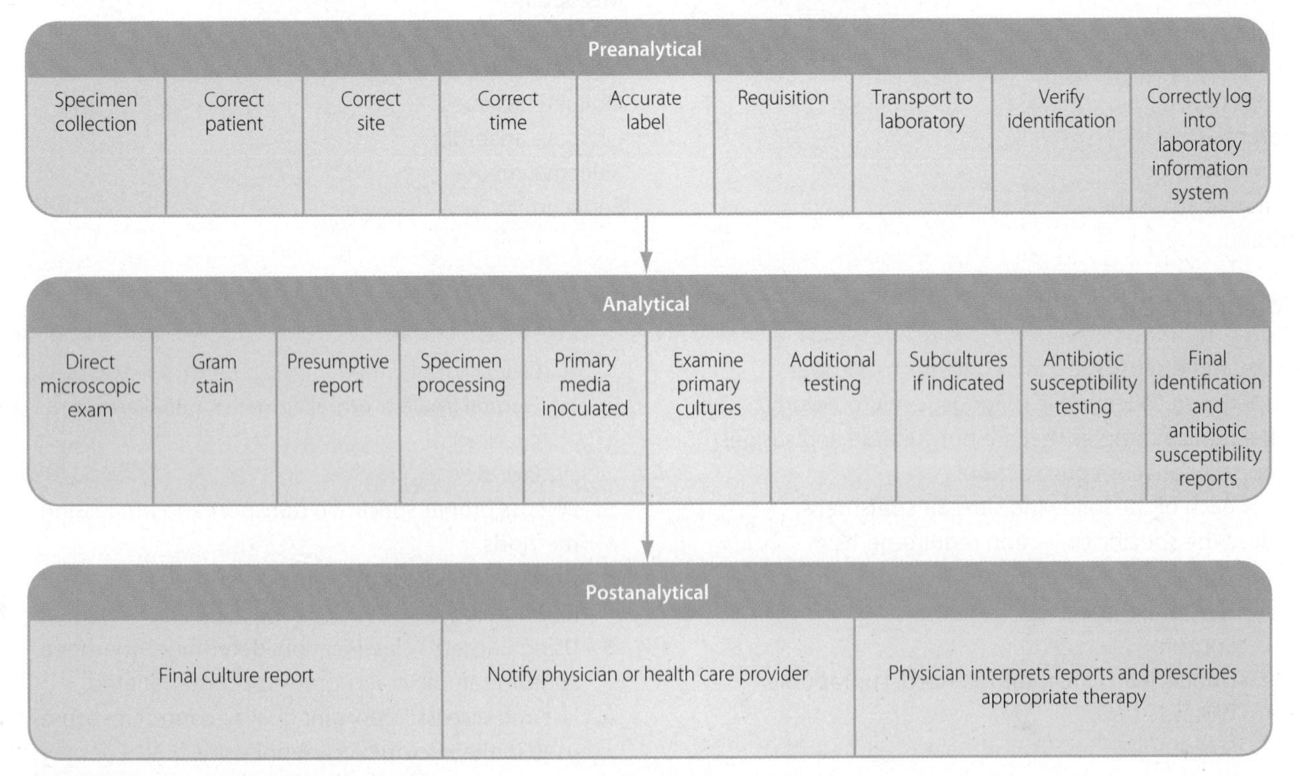

FIGURE 3-1 Laboratory testing process.

Guidelines for proper specimen collection must be established and communicated by the microbiology laboratory to other members of the health care team to provide valid, consistent results. Failure to properly collect specimens for culture may result in the failure to isolate the organism that is actually causing the infection. Also, the recovery of contaminants or indigenous flora may lead to inappropriate or unnecessary antibiotic therapy. Each microbiology laboratory establishes criteria for specimen collection and for rejecting specimens that do not meet the requirements.

This chapter discusses general guidelines for specimen collection and then specific guidelines for some common collection sites. Specimen processing and transport, as well as primary culture media and preliminary testing of bacteria, also are described.

General Specimen Guidelines

A specimen is a representative sample of a tissue, body fluid, or other site that is analyzed in the clinical laboratory. Microbiological specimens must represent the actual infected site and thus must be collected from the specific site of the infection. Contamination from adjacent tissue and any bacteria that normally colonize the site should be avoided during specimen collection. **Normal flora** may overgrow the pathogen and lead to inaccurate findings.

For example, the area adjacent to a wound infection should not be cultured. A swab of the adjacent area may lead to the isolation of *Staphylococcus epidermidis*, a normal flora of the skin Instead, a needle aspiration of the wound is recommended. If the skin or mucous membrane area is cultured, the skin surface first should be disinfected. Similarly, in the collection of a specimen for the diagnosis of bronchitis or pneumonia, the specimen collected should be representative of the lower respiratory tract. A sputum sample is representative of this area; however, saliva from the oral cavity would yield normal oropharyngeal flora.

When possible, one should culture for a specific pathogen and culture the site where a particular pathogen is most likely found. For example, if a patient has symptoms of a urinary tract infection, the urine should be collected. Sometimes this is not feasible or practical; for example, endocarditis may be diagnosed through positive blood cultures and other clinical procedures and not necessarily from a specimen collected from the heart.

Specimens for bacterial culture should be collected as soon as possible after the onset of the symptoms of infection. When possible, specimens should be collected before the initiation of antibiotic therapy. Antibiotics may inhibit the growth of pathogens, which may result in a negative culture even if the patient has a bacterial infection. When this is not possible, it is important for the health care provider to note any antibiotics prescribed for the patient on the laboratory requisition.

It is usually sufficient to collect one culture to diagnose infection from a particular site. The exception is for blood cultures, which require more than one specimen.

The history and physiology of the disease must also be considered to determine when to collect a specimen. The causative organism may be recovered from various sites at different times during the course of the illness. Also, a higher yield of the organism may be obtained during different stages of the illness. For example, the enteric pathogens associated with gastroenteritis are most efficiently cultured when the patient is in the acute diarrheal stage. When one considers viral meningitis, the optimal collection time for highest viral yield is shortly after the onset of the illness.

A good example that can be used to illustrate the importance of specimen collection related to the physiology of the disease is *Salmonella typhi*, the agent of typhoid fever. The organism first attacks the blood and therefore can be isolated from the blood during the first week of illness. During weeks 2 and 3, the highest yield is found in the urine or feces. Finally, antibody titers become positive in the fifth week. Culturing the appropriate site will initiate the process for proper isolation and identification of the infectious agent.

The specimen also should be in a sufficient quantity to perform all procedures requested. Inadequate specimens should be marked *QNS* (quantity not sufficient) and held until the health care provider determines which tests, if any, should be performed. Specimens are held and not discarded until this information is obtained. If a specimen must be re-collected, the health care provider must be notified. Although some samples are re-collected easily, others such as cerebrospinal fluid, biopsies, and catheterized urine are more difficult to obtain. There may be no guarantee that a repeat specimen can be collected. Communication with the health care provider is important for appropriate specimen collection and follow-up when the specimen is not suitable or sufficient for all requested testing.

Specimens must be collected using sterile collection methods. Contaminated containers may lead to inaccurate results. Also, when possible, swabs are not recommended for collection because organisms have a tendency to dry out. Swabs are never appropriate for anaerobic culture because the atmospheric oxygen is toxic to anaerobes. Culture tubes with semisolid Stuart's or Amies transport medium provide excellent systems for collection and transport of specimens. **FIGURE 3-2** illustrates examples of various specimen collection devices. Because cotton swabs may produce toxic fatty acids, Dacron, rayon, and calcium alginate swabs are preferred for collection.

The actual time between specimen collection and plating to media should be kept to a minimum. Any delay may lead to the decline of the pathogen and multiplication of the normal flora. Certain bacteria such as the pathogenic *Neisseria* and *Haemophilus* are very susceptible to changes in temperature and drying out. Thus, it is important immediately to culture samples suspected of harboring any fastidious organism. **Fastidious** bacteria are those organisms that require special cultivation measures, such as enriched media or special atmospheric conditions such as increased carbon dioxide (CO_2). In general, a 2-hour limit between collection and receipt of the specimen in the laboratory is established for those specimens that have not been preserved in a transport medium.

Cerebrospinal fluids should be transported immediately to the laboratory and examined. It is crucial to avoid any delay in the workup of cerebrospinal fluid when one considers the morbidity and mortality of the infection and the fastidious nature of those bacteria associated with meningitis.

Finally, a complete and accurate label is required. The label should include the patient's full name, identification number, date and time of collection, room number, and source of collection. The physician's name should be available so that the laboratory will know whom to contact if additional information is needed or a problem arises. All information on the specimen must agree with that provided on the laboratory requisition. Any discrepancies must be addressed to ensure that the specimen was collected from the correct patient.

Specimen quality assurance means that the collection of suitable specimens for the microbiology laboratory depends on proper communication among the director of the microbiology laboratory, medical staff, laboratory personnel, and nursing staff. Procedure manuals and thorough instructions for specimen collection are helpful, as is direct verbal communication between the laboratory and medical and nursing personnel. When a specimen is not suitable for culture, the health care provider must be informed of the reasons so that the error does not continue

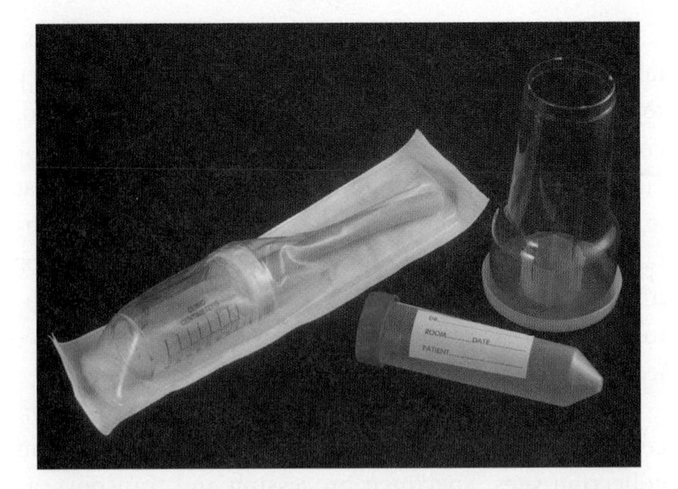

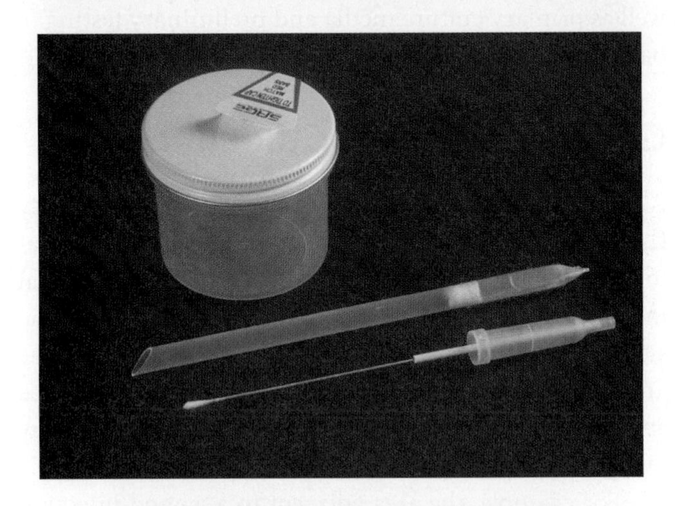

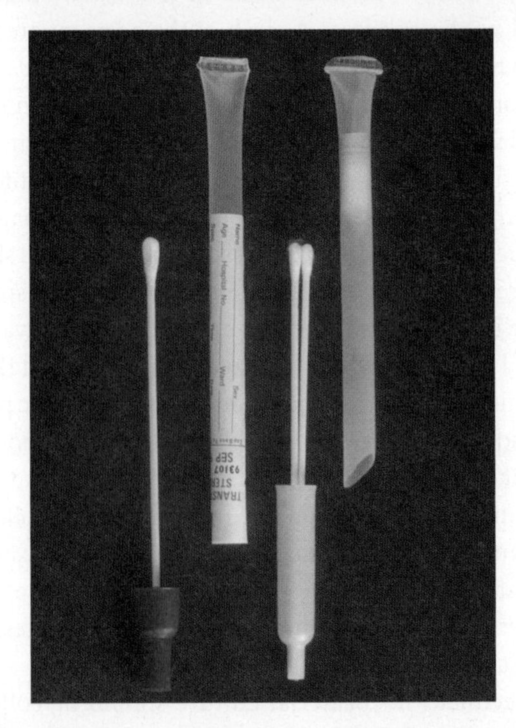

FIGURE 3-2 Specimen collection and transport devices.

to occur. In addition to improving the quality of patient care, proper specimen collection is an important factor in delivering cost-effective care.

Specimen Collection Requirements for Specific Sites

RESPIRATORY TRACT

Specimens collected from the upper respiratory tract include throat cultures, nasopharyngeal cultures, and specimens from the oral cavity. The normal flora of the upper respiratory tract includes α-hemolytic streptococci (viridans streptococci), *Staphylococcus epidermidis*, diphtheroids, nonpathogenic *Neisseria* species, some anaerobes, *Haemophilus* species, and a few *Candida albicans*. Other organisms that may be carried asymptomatically in the upper respiratory tract include *Staphylococcus aureus*, *Streptococcus pneumoniae*, *Moraxella catarrhalis*, and some anaerobes such as *Fusobacterium*. The indigenous flora of the respiratory tract may transiently change in hospitalized patients from gram-positive cocci to gram-negative bacilli, including members of the Enterobacteriaceae and Pseudomonadaceae families.

Most throat infections are caused by viruses; however, the most frequent cause of bacterial pharyngitis is group A streptococcus or *Streptococcus pyogenes*. Thus, culturing the throat is usually requested to diagnose streptococcal pharyngitis. The most important consideration in the collection of a throat culture is to avoid the normal oropharyngeal flora. The posterior pharynx between the tonsillar pillars should be firmly swabbed while the roof and sides of the mouth and the tongue should be avoided. The swab is placed in sterile transport media or immediately inoculated onto a blood agar plate. Rapid testing for group A streptococcus also is performed. Throat specimens should be transported within 24 hours and held at room temperature and plated onto blood agar in the laboratory. A chocolate agar plate is also inoculated in specific cases, for example, when *Neisseria* or *Haemophilus* are suspected.

Throat cultures also may be requested to diagnose epiglottitis from infection with *Haemophilus influenzae* type B. This infection is found less frequently because of effective immunization of infants and children.

Agents of viral pharyngitis include adenovirus, rhinovirus, and Epstein-Barr virus.

Oral candidiasis, or thrush, in infants and immunosuppressed patients from *Candida albicans* also may be identified with a throat culture. Throat cultures also may be used to identify gonococcal pharyngitis or oral gonorrhea infections caused by *Neisseria gonorrhoeae*.

The nasopharynx is cultured with a flexible thin wire swab that has been premoistened with sterile saline. The swab is gently guided into the nares and backward through the nasal septum until the posterior pharynx is reached. The swab is left in contact with the pharynx for 15 to 30 seconds if possible and then gently removed. A nasopharyngeal specimen is preferred for the diagnosis of pertussis, which is caused by *Bordetella pertussis*. Nasopharyngeal specimens may be used to identify the carrier state of *Staphylococcus aureus* or *Neisseria meningitidis*. If an individual is an **asymptomatic carrier**, the bacterium is present but does not cause infection. However, the carrier can serve as a source of infection to susceptible individuals. Nasopharyngeal swabs are occasionally collected to diagnose middle ear infections

Infections of the oral cavity include gingivitis and dental caries. Dental infections can extend into adjacent tissues, causing abscesses. Necrotizing ulcerative gingivostomatitis, also known as Vincent's angina or trench mouth, is caused by infection with multiple anaerobic bacteria but is rare today.

Middle ear, or otitis media, infections and sinusitis generally have predictable pathogens and thus, are not usually cultured. Sinus secretions collected by direct sinus aspirations or washes or biopsies collected by endoscopy may be submitted for culture. Common pathogens in ears and sinuses include *Streptococcus pneumoniae, Haemophilus influenzae,* and *Moraxella catarrhalis.*

Cultures of the lower respiratory tract are requested to diagnose bronchitis or pneumonia. Although most lower respiratory tract infections are viral, they can also be caused by several important bacterial pathogens. Specific bacterial species associated with pneumonia include *Streptococcus pneumoniae*, *Klebsiella pneumoniae*, *Serratia* species, *Pseudomonas aeruginosa*, *Escherichia coli*, *S. aureus*, anaerobes, and fungi. *Mycoplasma pneumoniae* is associated with bronchitis and also is the agent of primary atypical pneumonia.

Specimens that are used to diagnose lower respiratory tract infections include expectorated sputum, endotracheal specimens, translaryngeal aspirates, and bronchoalveolar lavage. Expectorated sputum is frequently collected to diagnose infections and is considered to be the preferred specimen to diagnose pneumonia. However, acceptable sputum samples may be difficult to collect without contamination from oropharyngeal flora which may result as the sputum passes through the mouth. It is important to obtain deep cough secretions that will yield productive results. A saline gargle or use of nebulized saline without disinfectants may enhance the collection. Brushing the teeth with water (without a mouthwash with disinfectant) also decreases the normal oropharyngeal flora. Collection of the first morning specimen is recommended, as it will contain more pooled bacteria. Twenty-four-hour collections are discouraged because of contamination and because the pathogen may be diluted out in the larger volume of specimen. Sputum is collected into a sterile wide-mouth container with a screw cap.

Saliva, oropharyngeal secretions, and sinus drainages from the nasopharynx should be rejected as lower respiratory tract specimens because of contamination.

Several classification schemes are available to assess the quality of sputum samples. In **Bartlett's classification** (BOX 3-1), the number of neutrophils and epithelial cells per low-power field (LPF) is enumerated. Based on these findings, the sputum is given a score. Scores of 0 or less indicate a lack of inflammation or the presence of saliva while scores greater than 1 indicate inflammation or infection

Other methods of determining the suitability of a sputum sample include scanning the slide for the presence of squamous epithelial cells (SECs), polymorphonuclear neutrophils (PMNs), alveolar macrophages (AMs), and columnar cells (CCs). The relative number of each cell may be semiquantitated by using the following guidelines:

- Few: fewer than 10 cells/LPF
- Moderate: 10 to 25 cells/LPF
- Abundant: greater than 25 cells/LPF

In general, PMNs are associated with acute bacterial pneumonia, whereas AMs and CCs are found in the lower respiratory tract and indicate that the specimen was collected properly. Their presence may or may not indicate infection. SECs line the mucous membranes of the oral cavity and therefore usually indicate oral flora contamination. **Purulent secretions** contain more than 25 PMNs and fewer than 10 SECs/LPF, whereas a predominance of AMs or CCs (greater than 25/LPF) indicate respiratory secretions. Oral secretions are indicated by more than 25 SECs/LPF and fewer than 10 PMNs/LPF. Other combinations are considered borderline samples. It is recommended that all specimens containing purulent secretions should be cultured, whereas those containing oral secretions should be re-collected.

BOX 3-1 **Bartlett's Classification**

Number of neutrophils per low-power field	**Grade**
Fewer than 10	0
10–25	+1
Greater than 25	+2
Mucus	+1
Number of epithelial cells per low-power field	
10–25	–1
Greater than 25	–2
TOTAL SCORE	

Scores of 0 or less indicate lack of inflammation or presence of saliva.

GASTROINTESTINAL TRACT

Specimens from the gastrointestinal tract may be cultured to diagnose the cause of gastroenteritis. Bacterial infections of the stomach are rare because of its acidic pH; thus most gastrointestinal infections involve the intestines. The clinical symptoms of gastroenteritis include nausea, vomiting, and diarrhea. The nausea and vomiting usually result from the ingestion of preformed toxins and not from bacterial invasion. There also may be fever.

The patient's history is significant in determining the cause of gastroenteritis. The food eaten and its method and location of preparation are important in determining the nature of the pathogen. Ingestion of contaminated water may be related to travel to areas where particular bacteria or viruses are endemic. Foreign travel, such as to developing countries with poor water treatment and sanitation methods, also may be associated with specific bacterial pathogens. Recent antibiotic use and hospitalization also are important clues to determine the cause of gastroenteritis. Finally, knowledge of similar symptoms with family members and contacts at school or work may also provide clues to the cause and type of infection.

Suitable cultures for gastroenteritis include freshly passed stools, washes, or feces collected during endoscopy.

Rectal swabs are acceptable in specific cases; however, stool specimens are usually preferred over rectal swabs. Other specimens include gastric aspirates, which are used for infants and children to identify acid-fast bacilli, and gastric biopsies for diagnosis of *Helicobacter pylori* infection.

When examining for ova and parasites, the specimen should be analyzed as soon as possible. For ova and parasites, three specimens are collected every other day for outpatients, while three specimens are collected on consecutive days for inpatients. When a delay is anticipated, the specimen is preserved in polyvinyl alcohol for the examination of ova and parasites and transported within 24 hours at room temperature.

Stool specimens are collected into a sterile wide-mouth container with a screw cap and transported within 24 hours and held at 4°C. Rectal swabs are placed in enteric transport media and also transported within 24 hours at 4°C.

A direct Gram stained examination of all stool specimens for fecal white blood cells, mucous, parasites, and yeast should be performed. The presence of leukocytes is often an indication of a bacterial infection. Observation of red blood cells may indicate an invasive infection such as shigellosis or verotoxic *E. coli*.

When analysis of bacterial pathogens is required, an enrichment medium such as selenite broth or gram-negative broth is inoculated to enhance the isolation of the pathogen by inhibiting the growth of the normal flora enteric bacteria. Initial inoculation of primary plating media may be modified based on probable pathogens suspected from the individual's history.

URINE

A urine culture may be requested to diagnose a urinary tract infection (UTI) of the upper or lower tract. Lower UTIs may involve the bladder (**cystitis**) or the urethra (**urethritis**). Such infections frequently ascend through the urethra and consist of normal flora coliforms that may be present in the periurethral flora. Other sources of infection include urinary catheters or other types of instrumentation, which also may involve the normal flora coliforms or contaminating bacteria from health care personnel.

Upper UTIs include infections of the kidney, such as **pyelonephritis** and **glomerulonephritis**. In addition, the renal pelvis (**pyelitis**) or ureters may be infected.

Acceptable specimens for diagnosis of a urinary tract infection include a clean-catch midstream specimen, straight catheterized urine, suprapubic aspirate, and urine collected from a cystoscopy or other surgical method. Specimens that generally are not accepted include urine collected from a Foley (indwelling) catheter or a bagged collection of urine. Foley catheters may be contaminated with urethral microflora; however, if used for specimen collection, the catheter first must be disinfected prior to collection.

In most cases, the specimen of choice for bacterial culture of urine is the **clean-catch midstream specimen**. A **routine or randomly voided specimen** is not acceptable because of the presence of contaminating bacteria from the periurethral and vaginal areas. In collection of the clean-catch midstream specimen, the periurethral area is cleansed with soap, sterile water, and sterile gauze using a front-to-back motion. The first few milliliters of the specimen are discarded to flush bacteria from the urethra. The midstream portion is collected into a sterile container.

A **straight catheterized urine** sample may be used for bacterial culture only if the patient cannot void or the catheter has been inserted for another medical reason. Urine is normally sterile in the bladder, and therefore a catheterized specimen should contain no bacteria. A **suprapubic aspiration** may be performed on infants and young children. Because this is an invasive technique, it is performed only when absolutely necessary. The skin is disinfected over the urinary bladder, and the area is locally anesthetized. A small incision with a surgical blade is made, and a needle is inserted through the abdominal wall into the bladder to withdraw the specimen. This procedure is reserved for patients who cannot provide a urine sample or be catheterized when a urine sample is urgently needed.

Uncultured urine should be refrigerated at 4°C and transported to the microbiology laboratory within 24 hours to minimize bacterial multiplication. Catheterized (Foley and straight) or suprapubic specimens are also held at 4°C but must be transported to the laboratory within 2 hours. Routine or randomly voided samples should be examined for contamination.

A **colony count** is performed on all urine samples submitted for bacterial culture. A 1 μl calibrated inoculating loop is used to deliver 1 μl (0.001 ml) of urine. The plate is incubated overnight and the number of colonies counted. The number is multiplied by 1,000 to convert microliters to milliliters. The value obtained indicates the number of colonies per milliliter of urine of colony forming units (CFU) per milliliter of urine. For example, if a 1 μl calibrated loop yields 145 colonies, the colony count is

145,000, or 1.45×10^5 CFU/ml urine. Values greater than 1.0×10^5 CFU/ml indicate infection. Values between 1.0×10^3 and 1.0×10^5 colonies/ml are considered to be contaminated or may represent cultures taken during the period of recovery from a urinary tract infection after antibiotics have been initiated. When culturing a catheterized urine specimen, some microbiologists prefer to use a 10 μl inoculating loop. In this case, the number of colonies counted is multiplied by 100 to determine the number of CFU/ml when using the 10 μl loop.

The most common cause of UTIs is *E. coli*, which is associated with approximately 90% of all UTIs in ambulatory persons and also a large percentage of those occurring in hospitalized patients. Other members of the Enterobacteriaceae family, including *Klebsiella*, *Proteus*, and *Enterobacter*, as well as *Enterococcus faecalis* and *P. aeruginosa*, are also associated with UTIs. *Staphylococcus saprophyticus* may cause UTIs with colony counts in a lower range of fewer than 1.0×10^5 CFU/ml.

BLOOD

Bacteremia refers to the presence of bacteria in blood, which is considered a sterile site. In **transient bacteremia**, normal flora bacteria may be introduced into the blood. For example, after brushing or cleaning the teeth, the viridans streptococci may be introduced into the blood from the oral cavity. In **intermittent bacteremia**, bacteria are sporadically discharged from extravascular abscesses or infections into the blood. In **continuous bacteremia**, there is a constant release of bacteria into the blood; this may occur with subacute bacterial endocarditis, from contaminated indwelling catheters, or from intravascular infections. Bacteremia is frequently accompanied by fever, chills, increased pulse rate, and decreased blood pressure.

The normal immune system clears bacteria from the blood within 30 to 45 minutes. This does not occur as readily in patients who are immunosuppressed or have overwhelming infections. In **septicemia** the circulating bacteria multiply faster than phagocytosis can occur, and multiple organs and body systems may be infected.

Even when bacteremia is significant, organisms in the blood are usually not of great enough numbers to be grown from a single blood culture specimen. As few as 1 to 10 bacteria per milliliter of blood can be associated with bacteremia. Also, the highest concentration of bacteria in the blood occurs before the fever spikes. Since this cannot be predicted, specimens should be collected when the patient is febrile. It is recommended to collect two to four specimens from separate venipuncture sites at least 1 hour apart. When possible, collect two sets from the right arm and two sets from the left arm. These actions help to increase the probability of isolating the organism.

It is imperative to prepare the patient's skin properly before phlebotomy to ensure that no skin contaminants are collected. Typical methods include a 70% to 95% alcohol rinse to remove dirt, lipids, and fatty acids. A circular motion moving in to out is needed. This is followed by either a chlorhexidine or iodophor scrub, which is left on for 1 minute. Preparations containing iodine should not be used for those who are allergic to iodine. Next, a second alcohol rinse is applied. A second method uses a wash with green soap followed by a sterile water rinse. Tincture of iodine is applied and allowed to dry. The final step is the application of 70% alcohol.

At least 20 ml of blood should be collected for each adult set of blood cultures and 1 to 10 ml per set for pediatric blood culture sets. An aerobic and anaerobic bottle should be collected. No more than three sets should be collected in any 24-hour period.

Clotted specimens for blood cultures are rejected. Also, specimens collected using only alcohol as the antiseptic should not be accepted because of contamination risks. Those specimens containing less than 20 ml for adults are also questionable. The collection of a single blood culture per day is not recommended

CEREBROSPINAL FLUID

Cerebrospinal fluid (CSF) is collected by lumbar puncture in the third or fourth lumbar vertebra by a physician. A local anesthetic is used, and a needle is inserted into the spinal canal. In most adults the collection consists of three tubes. Because the first two tubes may contain skin contaminants, it is usually recommended that the third tube is used for microbiology. However, the order of the tubes used for each procedure is determined by that facility.

A normal CSF is clear and colorless, and on receipt in the laboratory the volume, color, and appearance should be recorded. Cytocentrifugation will concentrate the specimen and enhance the detection of bacteria, fungi, and cells. The specimen should be screened immediately for the presence of bacteria or fungi by performing a methylene blue or Gram stain. Rapid antigen testing to detect bacterial or fungal antigens can also be performed. The presence of any microorganisms and blood cells is reported to the physician immediately.

There should be no delay in the processing or workup of CSF because some of the organisms associated with meningitis are fastidious and prone to chilling or drying. These include *N. meningitidis* and *H. influenzae*. Delays also must be avoided because of the high mortality rate and rapid proliferation associated with the infection. CSF can be held for up to 6 hours at 37°C for bacteria and fungi, but must be maintained at 4°C for virus detection.

GENITAL TRACT

Microorganisms associated with genital tract infections include *Neisseria gonorrhoeae*, *Treponema pallidum*, herpes simplex virus type 2, *Chlamydia trachomatis*, and the parasite *Trichomonas vaginalis*. Testing methods specific for sexually transmitted diseases for gonorrhea and chlamydia are available. *Trichomonas* may be identified by a standard wet mount procedure. *N. gonorrhoeae* requires chocolate to grow. It is imperative to inoculate the media and incubate the plates in increased CO_2 soon after specimen collection to enhance the chances of recovery. Transport media such as JEMBEC (BD Diagnostics) alternatively may be used to provide proper nutrient and atmospheric requirements.

For the diagnosis of male urogenital infections, the urethral discharge is usually collected. Prostatic fluid also may be submitted to identify specific pathogens. In female patients, specimens of the uterine cervix, urethra, or cervix may be collected. Because of the abundance of normal flora in the female genital tract, it is important to use a plate selective for *N. gonorrhoeae* such as Martin-Lewis or modified Thayer-Martin. Such media inhibit the normal flora and allow a better recovery of the pathogen. Anaerobic and aerobic media should be set up for female specimens from the endometrium, cul-de-sac, or Bartholin cysts.

WOUND AND ABSCESSES

Superficial wound specimens are collected from surface infections. Suitable specimens include pus aspirates, irrigation fluids, and swabs of purulent drainage from the dermis. It is recommended always to collect specimens for wound culture using a needle and syringe to aspirate the drainage. This avoids the collection of normal flora and also enhances the recovery of anaerobes, which are often associated with wound infections and abscesses. The isolation of normal flora may hinder the recovery of both aerobic and anaerobic bacteria in such infections. Swabs for superficial wounds should be collected along the edge of the wound after irrigation with sterile saline. Specimens from deep wound infections include any purulent drainage, necrotic tissue, or other tissue suspected of infection. These specimens usually are collected by needle aspiration and cultured for both anaerobes and aerobes.

Swabs of surface materials or specimens contaminated with surface material should not be accepted for culture. Any specimen collected with saline that contains preservatives should also be rejected.

Exogenous wound infections result from animal and human bites, burns, ulcers, and traumatic wounds (gunshot or stabbing). **Endogenous** wound infections may be attributed to indigenous bacterias within the patient and include cellulitis, dental infections, and septic arthritis. Many endogenous infections are nosocomial and occur as a result of contamination during an invasive procedure.

Specimen Transport and Processing

It is important to maintain the specimen as close to its original state as possible. Exposure to heat, cold, and drying should be avoided. In general, a 2-hour limit between collection and reception into the laboratory is required. If a delay is anticipated, a transport medium such as Stuart's or Amies should be used to increase the viability of the pathogen. The Stuart's system consists of swabs in a test tube with transport media that can be activated by crushing an ampule. The buffered semisolid agar, which contains sodium thioglycollate, can maintain bacteria for up to 72 hours. Cary-Blair medium is designed for the transport of stool specimens and is recommended for the transport of enteric pathogens.

Because cotton swabs may release toxic fatty acids, calcium alginate or Dacron swabs usually are preferred for collection. Specimen collection devices often are incorporated into a transport medium. The medium is released by crushing an ampule after the swab has been inserted into the collection tube. Systems for both aerobes and anaerobes are commercially available.

In the laboratory, the specimen is logged into the computer system or department log. There is an initial examination of the specimen, which should be performed in the biological safety cabinet to avoid laboratory acquired infections.

The specimen should be examined for adherence to collection guidelines on receipt in the laboratory. The specimen requisition and label must match. If any concerns are found, the health care provider should be notified and the specimen collected again when possible. However, the physician may request that the specimen be accepted and worked up even if collection criteria are not met. The laboratory should note any problems with collection on the requisition and report them to ensure proper communication of results.

A **gross examination** of the specimen is performed. This includes examination of the color, volume, and appearance of the specimen. The gross examination may provide initial clues. For example, a cloudy CSF may indicate infection, and a rust-tinged sputum may indicate *Streptococcus pneumoniae*.

The ultimate identification of bacteria and their designation as normal flora or pathogen depends on proper specimen collection. Guidelines must be established and followed for proper specimen workup to provide the clinician with accurate results. Specimen rejection criteria are established by each laboratory and based on general guidelines and accreditation standards. BOX 3-2 describes criteria for dealing with specimens that do not meet the established collection criteria and BOX 3-3 provides criteria for specimen rejection.

BOX 3-3 Criteria for Specimen Rejection

In general, reject the following specimens:

Twenty-four-hour sputum collections—prone to contamination and may dilute out the pathogen because of the normal flora

One swab for many requests, such as aerobes, anaerobes, and fungi

Leaking containers—may present a biohazard and be contaminated

Nonsterile or contaminated containers

Culture or agar plates that are overgrown and dry except for specific mycology request

Specimens contaminated with dyes, oils, or chemicals

Formalin in any specimen

For anaerobes, reject the following:

Gastric washes

Midstream urine

Feces, except for *Clostridium difficile* and *Clostridium perfringens*

Throat, nares, or oropharyngeal specimens

Most swabs, including superficial skin swabs

BOX 3-2 Specimen Collection/Rejection Guidelines

Requisition and specimen label must match.

Re-collect specimens that do not meet criteria when possible and whose procedures for collection are not difficult or invasive for the patient.

Document why the specimen was rejected and communicate to the individual who collected the specimen why it was rejected.

Try not to reject specimens that are difficult to collect, such as CSF or surgical biopsies.

Set up cultures when the situation cannot be resolved, but comment concerns on the report and how the results may be affected.

Communicate to and educate hospital personnel who collect specimens through laboratory directives, manuals, and other forms of communication.

Initial Specimen Plating and Identification Methods

Initial methods to work up a specimen include the selection and inoculation onto appropriate primary media. Also, staining procedures, such as the Gram stain and acid-fast staining, are performed, as are preliminary biochemical procedures.

MICROSCOPIC EXAMINATION OF CLINICAL SPECIMENS

A Gram stain on the specimen itself can provide valuable information. First, the presence of neutrophils indicates inflammation and also generally is evidence that the quality of the specimen is acceptable. By contrast, an abundance of squamous epithelial cells may be an indication that the specimen is not from the actual site of infection but instead from surrounding tissue or fluids that contain commensal bacteria. By scanning a Gram stain made directly from the specimen, the Gram stain reaction and morphology of bacteria can be determined, which can provide a preliminary identification. The morphology also can direct the microbiologist to perform specific tests to identify the suspected microorganism. The presence of yeast, fungal elements, and parasites also can be determined by evaluating a direct Gram stained specimen. Anaerobes that have distinctive microscopic morphologies also can be presumptively identified or considered through examination of a Gram stained smear. Stains also can be performed on colonies that have been isolated on media.

SELECTION AND INOCULATION OF PRIMARY MEDIA

Culture medium is a mixture of the nutrients needed by microorganisms. Most media contain an energy source, such as carbon, nitrogen, sulfur, phosphorus, hydrogen, oxygen, and buffers. In addition, various agents, such as dyes or antibiotics, may be added to either increase or decrease the viability of a particular organism or group of organisms.

Media in liquid form are known as **broth**. When the medium is in a gel or semisolid form, it is known as **agar**. Most agar is solidified by using either the red algae polysaccharide **agar agar**; **agarose** also can be used to solidify agar. Agarose melts at a temperature over 95°C but re-solidifies at a temperature less than 50°C. Thus, media can be heated high to sterilize them after the required ingredients have been added, poured into petri plates, and allowed to cool and solidify.

Bacterial cells are inoculated onto media and multiply exponentially so that they can be seen on the agar. A colony is a bacterial population that is derived from a single bacterial cell or clone. Bacterial colonies can be observed as discrete colonies on agar, which is essential to obtain isolated colonies or to enumerate colonies. Each clone or colony has identical genetic and phenotypical characteristics. All tests used to identify bacteria must be performed on isolated colonies to obtain accurate results.

Different types of media are used for specific purposes in clinical microbiology. Several classification methods for media follow.

General isolation media, also known as **supportive media**, support the growth of most nonfastidious bacteria. Examples include nutrient agar, trypticase soy agar, and nutrient broth. No growth advantage is given to any group of bacteria.

Nonselective isolation media, also known as **enriched media**, contain a nutrient supplement. Examples include **sheep blood agar** (SBA) and **chocolate agar**. SBA has a trypticase soy agar base to which has been added 5% defibrinated sheep red blood cells. Other agar bases that can be used include Columbia agar and brain-heart infusion agar. Sheep blood is the preferred source of blood cells because other sources, such as horse blood, may give different or erratic results for hemolysis. For example, the enterococci of group D streptococci are nonhemolytic on sheep blood agar but β-hemolytic on rabbit, horse, or human blood agar. Sheep blood agar does not support the growth of *Haemophilus influenzae* or *Haemophilus haemolyticus. H. influenzae* requires NAD (nicotinamide dinucleotide, coenzyme I), which is destroyed by NADase in the sheep blood agar. However, these Haemophilus will grow on horse blood agar. *H. haemolyticus* is considered to be normal flora of the oropharynx, and its β-hemolytic properties on other types of blood agar may be misinterpreted as *Streptococcus pyogenes*, a pathogen. BOX 3-4 summarizes patterns of hemolysis, which are illustrated in **FIGURE 3-3**.

FIGURE 3-3 Hemolytic patterns on sheep blood agar.

BOX 3-4 **Hemolytic Patterns**

Hemolytic patterns are best observed by passing a bright light through the bottom of the blood agar plate and looking through the top of the agar plate.

Alpha: incomplete; greening or browning of the medium

Beta: complete; total clearing of the medium

Nonhemolytic: no change in the color of the medium; may be referred to as gamma hemolysis

Chocolate agar is prepared in a manner similar to that used to produce blood agar except the agar is either heated or enzyme treated to hemolyze the red blood cells. By either heating or treating with enzymes, the red blood cells are destroyed, releasing NAD. Chocolate agar is also enriched with IsoVitaleX, which contains dextrose, cysteine, vitamin B_{12}, thiamine, and ferric nitrate and supports the growth of fastidious bacteria, such as *N. gonorrhoeae* and *H. influenzae*.

Differential media provide distinct colonial appearances of microorganisms to aid in their identification. One species or group of bacteria has a certain characteristic that separates it from other types of bacteria. Most differential media are used to isolate gram-negative bacteria through the addition of ingredients that are inhibitory for gram-positive bacteria. **MacConkey agar** contains lactose, bile salt, neutral red indicator, and crystal violet. The bile salt and crystal violet inhibit the growth of gram-positive bacteria. If the organism can ferment lactose, the colonies appear pink to red in color. If the organism is unable to ferment lactose, the colonies appear clear. Another example of agar is **eosin-methylene blue** (EMB) **agar**, which contains lactose and the dyes eosin and methylene blue. The dyes are toxic to gram-positive bacteria and isolate gram-negative bacteria. In addition, bacteria that can ferment lactose cause the pH of the medium to decrease, which decreases the solubility of the eosin-methylene blue complex. This results in a purple color. Gram-negative bacteria that cannot ferment lactose appear clear on the medium. *E. coli* produce colonies with a unique green metallic sheen caused by the precipitation of the dyes following fermentation of lactose, which produces a very acidic environment.

Some authors prefer to categorize MacConkey agar and EMB agar as **selective differential** because they *select* for gram-negative bacteria and *differentiate* lactose fermenters from lactose nonfermenters. These media are used interchangeably based on the laboratory's preference. Growth characteristics on these media must be interpreted at 18–24 hours incubation for accurate results.

Enrichment broths are used to inhibit the growth of one organism while enhancing that of another organism by providing nutrients. These broths are used for specimens that generally have a mixture of organisms. For example, enrichment broths are used for stool cultures to inhibit the normal flora bacteria, such as *E. coli*, so that pathogens, such as *Salmonella* and *Shigella*, can be isolated. Examples of these broths include gram negative, selenite, and tetrathionate. **Gram-negative broth** contains bile salt in the form of sodium deoxycholate, which is toxic to gram-positive bacteria and inhibitory to the normal flora coliforms. **Selenite broth** contains sodium hydrogen selenite, which allows for the isolation of *Salmonella* and *Shigella*. **Tetrathionate broth** contains bile salts and sodium thiosulfate, which enhance the isolation of *Salmonella* and *Shigella*. Each of these three broths has the same purpose.

Thioglycollate broth, another type of enrichment broth, contains thioglycollic acid as a reducing agent, a small percentage of agar to prevent oxygen from reaching all areas of the broth, and numerous nutrients, such as yeast and beef extracts, vitamins, and hemin. The medium allows for the differentiation of aerobes and anaerobes. For example, strict or obligate aerobes grow at the surface of the broth, whereas facultative bacteria grow throughout the media. Strict or obligate anaerobes usually grow in the deeper portion of the tube, where the oxygen level is lowest.

Selective media contain agents that inhibit the growth of all bacteria except those that are sought. These media allow one to select for pathogens through the inhibition of normal flora. Examples include **Hektoen enteric** (HE) **agar**, ***Salmonella–Shigella*** (SS) **agar**, and **xylose-lysine-deoxycholate** (XLD) **agar**. All these media selectively inhibit gram-positive bacteria and gram-negative coliform bacteria and permit the isolation of stool pathogens. HE medium contains lactose, sucrose, salicin, sodium thiosulfate, ferric ammonium citrate, and bromthymol blue indicator. Organisms that ferment one or more of the carbohydrates will appear as yellow-orange colonies, whereas nonfermenters appear green or blue in color. The medium also permits the differentiation of hydrogen sulfide–producing bacteria (black precipitate) from those that cannot produce hydrogen sulfide. SS medium contains lactose, bile salts, sodium thiosulfate, neutral red indicator, and ferric citrate. It allows for the differentiation of lactose fermenters from nonfermenters, as well as the detection of hydrogen sulfide producers. XLD contains xylose, lysine, lactose, sucrose, phenol red indicator, sodium deoxycholate, sodium thiosulfate, and ferric ammonium citrate. The medium is selective for gram-negative enteric pathogens and allows for the detection of xylose fermentation, lysine decarboxylation, and hydrogen sulfide production.

Antibiotic media are selective for a specific group of bacteria through the addition of specific antibiotics. Examples include **colistin-nalidixic acid** (CNA) and **modified Thayer-Martin** (MTM). CNA contains sheep blood agar base with the antibiotics colistin and nalidixic acid added. Colistin (polymyxin E) disrupts the cell membrane of gram-negative organisms, and nalidixic acid blocks DNA replication in gram-negative bacteria. Thus CNA allows for the selection of gram-positive bacteria.

MTM is a chocolate agar base with the antibiotics vancomycin, colistin, nystatin, and trimethoprim lactate added. The medium selectively isolates *N. gonorrhoeae*. Vancomycin inhibits gram-positive bacteria through interference with cell wall synthesis, colistin inhibits gram-negative bacteria by interfering with synthesis of the cell wall, and nystatin is inhibitory to yeast. Trimethoprim inhibits the swarming of *Proteus*. **Martin-Lewis medium**, also selective for *N. gonorrhoeae*, contains similar components to MTM, except anisomycin replaces nystatin as the yeast inhibitor.

TABLE 3-1 summarizes some of the frequently used media and their purposes.

Primary plating media are selected based on specimen type. The growth requirements of those bacteria most often isolated from a particular site must be met. For example, since most UTIs are caused by gram-negative bacilli, such as *E. coli*, a differential plate must be inoculated. Because most throat cultures are performed to determine the presence of *S. pyogenes*, it is essential to inoculate a blood agar plate.

It is also necessary to obtain isolated colonies for biochemical and serological testing. Streaking an agar plate for isolation can be accomplished using several methods. These are shown in the procedures section at the end of this chapter. When inoculating sheep blood agar, it is important to "stab" the medium and force some of the growth into the medium to observe for subsurface hemolysis.

Incubation

Most pathogenic bacteria are **mesophilic**, preferring a growth temperature of 30°C to 45°C. Most incubators are set at 35°C ± 2°C to meet the preferred temperature of most internal human pathogens. Those bacteria growing on the body surface, such as skin pathogens, prefer a lower temperature of 30°C. A limited number of pathogens are classified as **thermophiles** and prefer a growth temperature greater than 40°C. **Psychrophiles** prefer growing at lower temperatures, such as 4°C to 20°C.

Aerobic bacteria require molecular oxygen for cellular respiration and thus require incubation in the presence of atmospheric oxygen. **Strict aerobes** or **obligate aerobes** have an absolute oxygen requirement, needing it as the terminal electron acceptor for cellular respiration. An example of a strict aerobe is *Pseudomonas*. **Facultative anaerobes** can multiply in the presence or absence of oxygen and are able to use oxygen as the final electron acceptor in cellular respiration. However, they also can acquire energy through fermentation. Facultative bacteria include Staphylococcus and members of the Enterobacteriaceae. **Strict anaerobes** or **obligate anaerobes** are unable to multiply in the presence of oxygen and require incubation in an anaerobic environment, such as in an anaerobic jar or glove box. Examples of **obligate anaerobes** included Clostridium and Bacterioides.

Finally, certain bacteria prefer to grow in the presence of 5% to 10% CO_2 with small amounts of oxygen and are categorized as **capnophilic**. An environment of increased CO_2 can be obtained through piping in gases of the desired concentration or using commercially available plastic bags with CO_2 generators. An environment of approximately 3% CO_2 can be obtained by using the candle jar. A white beeswax candle is placed into a large glass jar with the plates to be incubated. The candle is lit and the jar closed with a tightly fitting lid. When the oxygen has been used

TABLE 3-1 Primary Isolation Media

Medium	Purpose
Anaerobic phenylethyl alcohol agar	Isolation of gram-positive and gram-negative anaerobes
Anaerobic kanamycin-vancomycin agar	Isolation of gram-negative anaerobes
Bordet-Gengou media	Isolation of *Bordetella pertussis*
Buffered charcoal yeast extract	Enrichment used to isolate *Legionella*
Campy blood agar	Isolation of *Campylobacter*; Brucella agar and sheep blood with antibiotics
Chocolate agar	Enriched, nonselective medium to isolate fastidious organisms, such as *Neisseria* and *Haemophilus*
Cefsulodin-Irgasin-novobiocin (CIN) agar	Isolation of *Yersinia* species
Colistin-nalidixic acid agar	Isolation of gram-positive bacteria
Eosin-methylene blue agar	Differential: isolation of gram-negative bacilli and differentiation of lactose fermenters from nonlactose fermenters
Gram-negative broth	Enrichment broth to enhance recovery of stool pathogens and inhibit normal flora coliforms
Hektoen enteric agar	Selective: isolation of stool pathogens through inhibition of normal flora coliforms
Löwenstein-Jensen medium	Primary isolation medium for *Mycobacterium*
MacConkey agar	Differential: isolation of gram-negative bacilli and differentiation of lactose fermenters from nonlactose fermenters
Martin-Lewis medium	Isolation of *N. gonorrhoeae*
Middlebrook medium	Primary isolation medium for *Mycobacterium*
Modified Thayer-Martin agar	Isolation of *Neisseria gonorrhoeae*
Petragnani's medium	Primary isolation medium for *Mycobacterium*
Regan-Lowe agar	Isolation of *Bordetella pertussis*
Salmonella–Shigella agar	Selective: isolation of stool pathogens through inhibition of normal flora coliforms
Sheep blood agar	Enriched, nonselective medium
Thiosulfate-citrate-bile salts-sucrose agar	Isolation and differentiation of *Vibrio*
Trypticase soy agar	All-purpose isolation media; subculture from primary plate
Xylose-lysine-deoxycholate agar	Selective: isolation of stool pathogens through inhibition of normal flora coliforms
Selenite broth	Enrichment broth to enhance recovery of stool pathogens and inhibit normal flora coliforms
Tetrathionate broth	Enrichment broth to enhance recovery of stool pathogens and inhibit normal flora coliforms
Thioglycollate broth	Enriched broth that permits growth at various oxygen levels

in the jar, the candle extinguishes, providing an environment with increased CO_2.

Plates are incubated at the appropriate temperature and atmosphere for 24 hours, at which time the plates are examined for growth. The identification process can begin for those plates with positive growth. These plates, along with those showing no growth at 24 hours, should be reincubated for an additional 24 hours for a total incubation of 48 hours Anaerobic cultures are incubated for a longer period, which ranges from 3 to 6 days. If slow-growing bacteria are suspected, incubation time can be lengthened past the recommended period

Observation of Growth Characteristics

Colonial characteristics are important observations in the identification of bacteria. It is essential to make the observations under direct light, preferably with a hand lens or a dissecting microscope. Some important descriptions are summarized in BOX 3-5 and illustrated in **FIGURE 3-4**.

The type of hemolysis and width of the zone of hemolysis on sheep blood agar are also noted. When differential or selective plates are used for primary plating, the growth characteristics can be used as preliminary identification tools. For example, the presence of pink colonies from a

BOX 3-5 **Colonial Characteristics**

Size: pinpoint, small, medium, large
Form: circular, filamentous, pinpoint, irregular
Elevation: flat, convex (dome shaped), raised, umbilicate (depressed center), umbonate (raised center)
Margin: smooth or entire, rough, irregular, curled, filamentous,
Surface: dull, glistening, moist
Form of margin: observe at the edge of the colony
swarming of *Proteus*, star-like appearance of yeast
Consistency: touch colony with sterile loop to determine
mucoid, creamy, viscous, butyrous, brittle, sticky, dry, waxy
Density: translucent, transparent, opaque
Color: white, golden, buff (tan), red, gray
Pigmentation: red (some *Serratia marcescens*), green—*Pseudomonas aeruginosa*

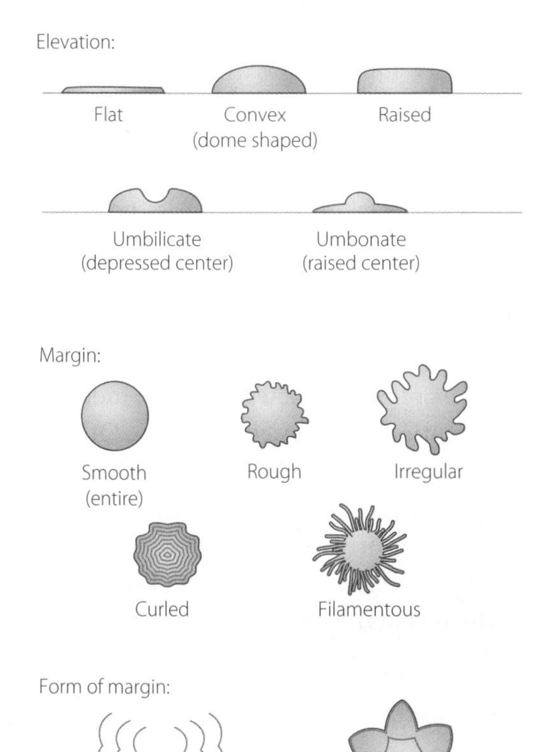

FIGURE 3-4 Colonial characteristics.

urine sample on MacConkey agar would indicate a gram-negative lactose fermenter.

Certain bacteria also have characteristic odors, such as *Pseudomonas aeruginosa*, which has been described as smelling like grapes, tortilla chips, or fruity gum. *Proteus* species have been described as smelling like burned chocolate, whereas anaerobes have very foul and putrid odors. It is not recommended that one directly smell any culture or specimen. These odors are detectable by opening the lid of the plate as it remains on the laboratory bench. Other unique characteristics of specific bacteria include the ability of Proteus species to grow in wavelike rings or swarm on sheep blood agar. Many strains of *P. aeruginosa* produce an abundant blue-green pigment.

Preliminary Biochemical Tests

Based on the colonial morphology on specific primary isolation plates and Gram stain characteristics, preliminary biochemical procedures can be performed. These results will provide a presumptive identification and guide the microbiologist in deciding which additional procedures to perform to arrive at the final identification of the isolate. A brief summary of some of these methods follows.

CARBOHYDRATE UTILIZATION

Bacteria may utilize carbohydrates if they possess the specific enzyme needed to break down that carbohydrate. When the carbohydrate is used in the absence of oxygen, the process is known as fermentation, which may be accompanied by the production of gas. If the organism can use the carbohydrate only in the presence of oxygen, the process is known as oxidation. Media may incorporate one or more carbohydrates and an acid-base indicator. If carbohydrate is utilized, the indicator changes from its neutral color to its acidic color, denoting a positive reaction. For example, to determine glucose fermentation, a media containing glucose and phenol red indicator is used. After inoculation and incubation, the change in color from pink-red to yellow would indicate a positive reaction. Bubbles or breaks in the media would indicate the production of gas. Carbohydrates commonly tested include glucose, lactose, maltose, sucrose, and fructose.

When reading reactions for carbohydrate utilization, fermentation is read from the deepest part of the tube, where oxygen content is the lowest. By contrast, oxidation is read from the uppermost part of the tube, where oxygen is most plentiful.

CATALASE

Many microorganisms produce oxygen radicals, including hydrogen peroxide, that are harmful to cells. Some bacteria are able to produce the enzyme catalase, which breaks down hydrogen peroxide by converting it to water and molecular oxygen. White blood cells also produce peroxide, which can kill those bacteria that have been phagocytized. The production of catalase by bacteria can enable them to survive within host white blood cells. Bacteria that produce catalase include *Staphylococcus* species, *Listeria monocytogenes*, *Bacillus* species, and *Bacteroides fragilis*. The test is important in the differentiation of gram-positive cocci: *Staphylococcus* are catalase positive, and *Streptococcus* are catalase negative. The catalase reaction is also important in distinguishing the gram-positive bacilli: *Bacillus*, which are aerobic and catalase positive, and *Clostridium*, which are anaerobic and catalase negative. Most bacteria are catalase positive.

The catalase test is performed by placing the bacterial colony on a microscopic slide and adding a drop of 3.0% hydrogen peroxide (H_2O_2). After mixing, a positive test is indicated by effervescent bubbling, which happens almost immediately.

CYTOCHROME OXIDASE

Those bacteria that possess the cytochrome oxidase enzyme system are able to transfer electrons to oxygen through aerobic bacterial respiration systems. Cytochromes are iron-containing heme proteins that transfer electrons to oxygen in the last reaction of aerobic respiration. In this method, oxidase reagent acts as the electron acceptor. Cytochrome oxidase in the presence of atmospheric oxygen oxidizes tetramethyl-*para*-phenylenediamine dihydrochloride (oxidase reagent) to form a colored compound—indophenol. The cytochrome system is found in the following genera: *Neisseria*, *Aeromonas*, *Pseudomonas*, *Campylobacter*, and *Pasteurella* but not in any of the Enterobacteriaceae. The test is performed by smearing the isolated organism over filter paper that has been saturated with oxidase reagent. Alternatively, the test can be performed by touching a swab to the isolated colony and then adding oxidase reagent to the swab. The development of a purple color is indicative of a positive reaction.

COAGULASE

Fibrinogen is converted to fibrin in the presence of the enzyme coagulase. *Staphylococcus aureus* produces both bound and free coagulase. Bound coagulase is detected in the coagulase slide test, which is performed by mixing the colony with a drop of rabbit plasma; a positive reaction is shown by the presence of fibrin clots. A negative control of rabbit plasma mixed with saline must be used in the slide test. The coagulase tube test detects free coagulase and is performed by mixing 0.5 ml of rabbit plasma with the organism and incubating in a water bath at 37°C for 1 to 4 hours. The presence of a clot indicates a positive reaction; negative tubes are incubated at room temperature overnight. The presence of staphylokinase may cause a false-negative reaction; thus, it is important to periodically examine the tubes for the presence of a clot.

SPOT INDOLE

The enzyme tryptophanase degrades the amino acid tryptophan into indole, ammonia, and pyruvic acid. The spot test can be performed on bacteria grown only on media that contain tryptophan, which include sheep blood agar and chocolate agar. It cannot be performed on bacterial colonies from MacConkey agar because this medium does not contain tryptophan. This test is important in the identification of *Escherichia coli*, which is the only lactose-fermenting member of Enterobacteriaceae that is indole positive. A positive indole reaction is also important in differentiation of *Proteus* species; *Proteus mirabilis* is indole negative, and *Proteus vulgaris* is indole positive. Most other members of Enterobacteriaceae are indole negative, with the exception of *Klebsiella oxytoca*. Other bacteria that are indole positive include *Aeromonas hydrophilia*, *Pasteurella multicido*, and *Vibrio* species.

The test is performed by smearing the colony across filter paper that has been saturated with Kovac's or Ehrich's reagent, which contains the chemical *para*-dimethylaminobenzaldehyde. A red to pink color indicates a positive reaction.

PYR HYDROLYSIS

Those bacteria that possess the enzyme L-pyrroglutamyl aminopeptidase can break down the substrate L-pyrrolidonyl-β-naphthylamide (PYR). This test is important in the differentiation of *Streptococcus* and

Enterococcus. Group D streptococcus includes enterococci and non-enterococci; enterococci such as *E. faecalis* are positive for PYR hydrolysis, whereas non-enterococci are negative. Group A β-hemolytic streptococcus (*Streptococcus pyogenes*) gives a positive PYR hydrolysis reaction, whereas group B streptococcus (*Streptococcus agalactiae*), which can also give β-hemolysis, is negative for PYR hydrolysis.

Quality Control

Quality control, a system used to monitor the quality of performance and results in the clinical laboratory, is an essential component in the clinical microbiology laboratory. Some basic aspects of quality control as applied to the microbiology laboratory include the following:

1. Monitoring of laboratory equipment. The temperatures of refrigerators, freezers, incubators, water baths, and heating blocks must be monitored and recorded. The concentration of gases in the various types of incubators, such as the anaerobic glove box and CO_2 incubator, also must be checked and recorded. When values are not within the accepted range, corrective action to bring the values back into acceptable limits must be taken. Anaerobic jars should be monitored for anaerobiosis by using a methylene blue indicator. The effectiveness of autoclaves should be tested using a spore strip of *Bacillus stearothermophilus*. No spores should grow in the subculture. All corrective actions must be documented.
2. Procedure manual. The department should have a thorough, organized, current procedure manual that contains all policies, regulations, procedures, and locations of reagents and supplies. In addition, the correct method to report results should be available, such as computer information or requisition forms.
3. Culture media and reagents. Each new shipment of media should be tested with control organisms with known results. Stock organisms should be chosen so that both positive and negative results can be observed. Although it is acceptable for a laboratory to accept the manufacturer's quality-control testing, it is advisable for each laboratory to perform its own testing on media. **TABLE 3-2** lists some common quality-control procedures and the organisms used for testing.
4. Personnel should be properly educated and attend continuing education courses to remain updated on the field. Orientation should be provided for new employees and updated training made available for current employees. All continuing education activities must be documented on the employee's record. Safety policies are an important component of each laboratory department.

Laboratory Procedures

Procedure
Streaking for isolation

Purpose
Isolated colonies are required for all procedures performed to identify bacteria.

Principle
Each of the methods can be used in certain situations to isolate bacteria.

Method A can be used on either liquid specimens (such as urine) or swabs.

1. Transfer a drop of the liquid specimen using a sterile pipette to a corner of the agar plate. Swabs are plated directly by rolling over an area in the corner of the plate.
2. Sterilize the wire loop and pass it through the initial inoculum several times, streaking the top quarter of the plate into the second quadrant. This is streak area 1.
3. Rotate the plate 90° and repeat the streaking from the second quadrant into the third quadrant. This is streak area 2.
4. Rotate the plate again 90° and continue the streaking from the third quadrant into the fourth quadrant. This is streak area 3. Flame between quadrants unless inoculum is light.

This method can be semiquantitated by using the following scale:

Growth rating	Quadrant		
	2	3	4
1+	Less than 10		
2+	More than 10	Less than 5	
3+	More than 10	More than 5	Less than 5
4+	More than 10	More than 5	More than 5

TABLE 3-2 Suggested Quality-Control Media and Organisms

Media or procedure	Control	Reactions
Sheep blood agar	*Streptococcus pyogenes*	β-hemolysis
	Streptococcus pneumoniae	α-hemolysis
Chocolate agar	*Haemophilus influenzae*	Growth
MacConkey agar	*Escherichia coli*	Pink growth
	Proteus vulgaris	Colorless growth
	S. pyogenes	No growth
Eosin-methylene blue agar	*E. coli*	Green metallic sheen
	Klebsiella pneumoniae	Purple growth
	P. vulgaris	Colorless growth
	S. pyogenes	No growth
Hektoen enteric agar	*Shigella sonnei*	Green growth
	Salmonella typhimurium	Green growth with black centers
	E. coli	Orange growth that is inhibited
Colistin-nalidixic acid agar	*Staphylococcus aureus*	Growth
	E. coli	No growth
Catalase	*S. aureus*	Positive
	S. pyogenes	Negative
Coagulase	*S. aureus*	Positive
	Staphylococcus epidermidis	Negative
Bile-esculin agar	*Enterococcus faecalis*	Growth/hydrolysis
	S. pyogenes	No growth
Cytochrome oxidase	*Pseudomonas aeruginosa*	Positive
	E. coli	Negative
Cystine trypticase agar	*Neisseria lactamica*	Positive for all carbohydrates: glucose, maltose, lactose
	Moraxella catarrhalis	Negative for all carbohydrates
Triple sugar iron agar	*E. coli*	A/[A] H_2S negative
	Salmonella enteriditis	K/[A] H_2S positive
	S. sonnei	K/A H_2S negative
	P. aeruginosa	K/K
Indole	*E. coli*	Positive
	Enterobacter cloacae	Negative
Voges-Proskauer reaction	*E. cloacae*	Positive
	E. coli	Negative
Urease test broth	*Proteus mirabilis*	Positive
	E. coli	Negative
X and V factors	*H. influenzae*	Growth between X and V
	Haemophilus parainfluenzae	Growth around V and between X and V

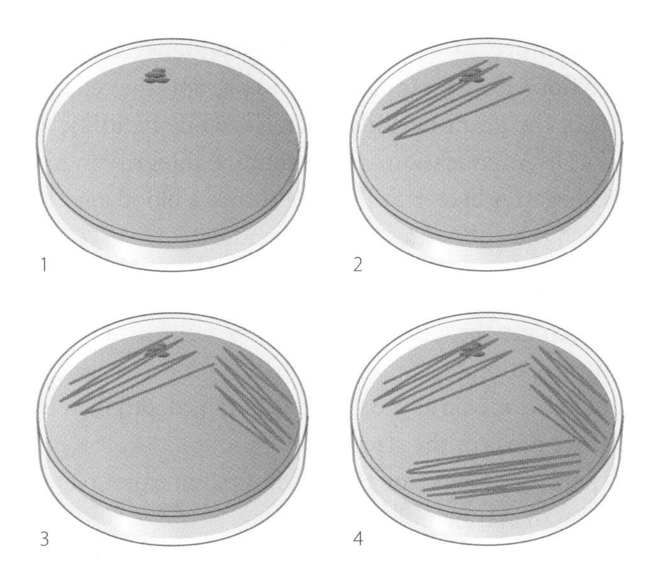

Method B can be used for cultures in heavy broth or solid media.

1. Streak specimen or inoculum in top quarter of plate.
2. With sterile loop, make a light sweep through inoculated area and streak entire top quarter of plate with parallel strokes. Sterilize loop.
3. Turn plate 90° and make a light sweep into lower portion of area streaked in step 2. Streak as in step 2, covering approximately half of remaining plate.
4. Turn plate 180° and streak remaining plate with sterilized loop. Avoid any previously streaked areas.

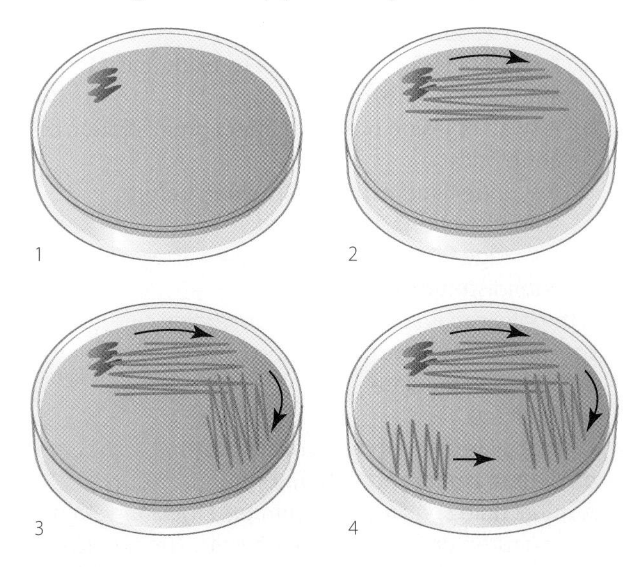

Method C is a method preferred by some microbiologists for broth cultures.

1. Apply a loopful of inoculum near periphery of plate. Cover approximately a fourth of the plate with close parallel streaks. Sterilize loop.
2. Make one light sweep through lower portion of streaked area. Turn plate 90° and streak approximately half of remaining plate.
3. Turn plate 180° and streak remainder of plate. Avoid any previously streaked areas.

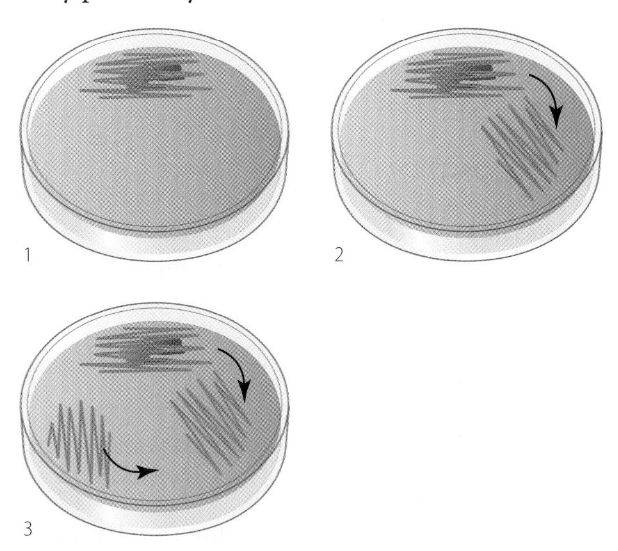

Procedure
Blood agar

Purpose
Blood agar is an example of a nonselective enriched media.

Principle
Blood agar is prepared through addition of 5% defibrinated sheep, horse, or rabbit blood to a base of either trypticase or tryptic soy agar. The soy provides peptones, which serve as a source of amino acids, carbon, nitrogen, and sulfur. Blood provides serum ingredients as well as erythrocytes, which enable detection of the hemolytic pattern. Because growth and hemolysis patterns may vary depending on the type of blood cells used, it is important to know the source of the red blood cells.

The types of hemolysis are **alpha**, incomplete or partial lysis with greening; **beta**, complete lysis with a colorless, clear zone; **gamma**, nonhemolytic; and **alpha prime**, a wide zone of β-hemolysis surrounding a small zone of α-hemolysis, which surrounds the colony. Blood agar plates should be observed for surface and subsurface hemolysis. The latter is detected by forcing a small amount of growth into approximately half of the agar's depth by stabbing the medium. Subsurface hemolysis is caused by oxygen-labile **streptolysin O**, and surface hemolysis is caused by oxygen-stable **streptolysin S**. Both hemolysins are produced by various strains of β-hemolytic streptococci, such as *Streptococcus pyogenes*.

Procedure

1. Streak the culture or specimen on blood agar to obtain isolated colonies.
2. Stab the media approximately half its depth in at least three areas of the streak.
3. Incubate at 35°C for 18 to 24 hours.
4. Interpret growth and type of hemolysis according to above descriptions.

QUALITY CONTROL

Streptococcus pyogenes: growth, β-hemolysis
Streptococcus pneumoniae: growth, α-hemolysis

Procedure

Colistin-nalidixic acid agar (CNA)

Purpose

CNA permits the selective recovery of gram-positive bacteria.

Principle

CNA is a medium that selectively inhibits the growth of gram-negative bacteria. It is useful to isolate staphylococci and streptococci from clinical specimens containing mixed flora. Colistin (polymyxin E) disrupts the cell membrane of the gram-negative bacteria, while nalidixic acid blocks DNA replication and membrane integrity in many gram-negative bacteria. The medium is a blood agar base to which the antibiotics have been added.

Procedure

1. Inoculate the CNA plate with the culture and streak for isolation.
2. Stab the media approximately half its depth in at least three areas of the streak.
3. Incubate at 35°C for 18 to 24 hours. Interpret plate for growth and hemolysis.

Quality Control

Escherichia coli: total inhibition
Proteus mirabilis: partial inhibition
Streptococcus pneumoniae: growth, α-hemolysis
Streptococcus pyogenes: growth, β-hemolysis

Review Questions

Matching

Match the medium with its classification (some responses may be used more than once):

1. Modified Thayer-Martin agar
2. Colistin-nalidixic acid agar
3. MacConkey agar
4. Hektoen enteric agar
5. Blood agar
6. Eosin-methylene blue agar
7. Chocolate agar
   a. Enriched, nonselective
   b. Differential recovery of gram-negative bacilli
   c. Selective for fecal pathogens
   d. Antibiotic, selects for gram-positive bacteria
   e. Antibiotic, selects for pathogenic *Neisseria*

Multiple Choice

8. Complete hemolysis of blood is known as:
   a. α-hemolysis
   b. β-hemolysis
   c. γ-hemolysis
   d. Synergistic hemolysis
9. The specimen of choice for bacterial culture of urine is a:
   a. Clean-catch midstream
   b. Catheterized sample
   c. Suprapubic
   d. Routine void
10. The optimal wound specimen for culture of anaerobic organisms should be:
    a. A swab of lesion obtained before administration of antibiotics
    b. A swab of lesion obtained after administration of antibiotics
    c. A syringe filled with pus obtained before administration of antibiotics
    d. A syringe filled with pus obtained after administration of antibiotics
11. A throat swab is submitted for anaerobic culture. This specimen should be:
    a. Set up immediately
    b. Rejected
    c. Inoculated into thioglycollate broth
    d. Sent to a reference laboratory
12. A spinal fluid specimen is submitted for Gram stain and culture during an afternoon shift. The physician also requests that an aliquot be saved for possible serological studies, which are performed only on day shift. The most correct action is:
    a. Inoculate culture, perform a Gram stain, and refrigerate remaining spinal fluid
    b. Inoculate culture, perform a Gram stain, and incubate remaining spinal fluid at 35°C to 37°C

c. Incubate entire specimen at 35°C to 37°C and perform culture and Gram stain the next day
d. Refrigerate entire specimen and perform culture and Gram stain the next day

13. The general guidelines for collection of blood cultures state:
a. Disinfect skin with an alcohol swab only.
b. Large amounts of bacteria are required to cause bacteremia.
c. Two to three sets per 24 hours are usually sufficient to diagnose bacteremia.
d. One specimen per 24 hours is sufficient to diagnose bacteremia.

14. Prompt delivery of specimens for microbiology is essential for accurate culture workup. Which of the following is *not a* consequence of delay in specimen delivery?
a. Normal flora may overgrow pathogen.
b. Fastidious organisms may no longer be viable.
c. Swabs may dry out, resulting in loss of pathogens.
d. Normal flora may no longer be isolated.

15. Optimal collection time to diagnose gastrointestinal infection caused by bacterial or viral pathogens is:
a. Anytime during the course of the illness
b. During the acute stage of the illness
c. During the convalescent stage of the illness
d. Through collection of serum to identify type-specific antibodies

16. Which of the following is *not* considered to be a sterile site?
a. Blood
b. Urinary bladder
c. Spinal fluid
d. Oral cavity

17. An abdominal abscess specimen received in the laboratory produced abundant growth when grown anaerobically but produced no growth when the culture plates were incubated aerobically. This culture contains:
a. An obligate aerobe
b. An obligate anaerobe
c. A facultative anaerobe
d. None of the above

18. The optimal time to collect blood cultures is:
a. Shortly before the fever spikes
b. While the fever spikes
c. Shortly after the fever spikes
d. No more than one set daily

19. Most pathogenic bacteria prefer an incubation temperature of:
a. 30°C to 32°C
b. 33°C to 35°C
c. 35°C to 37°C
d. 42°C to 45°C

20. Those bacteria that prefer growth under increased CO_2 are known as:
a. Mesophiles
b. Microaerophiles
c. Capnophilic
d. Facultative anaerobes

21. Which of the following should be monitored as part of the quality-control program in the microbiology laboratory?
a. Temperature of incubators and refrigerators
b. Plating media with known positive and negative controls
c. Oxygen content and CO_2 content of incubators
d. All the above

22. The catalase test is useful in differentiation of:
a. *E. coli* from other Enterobacteriaceae
b. β-hemolytic streptococcus
c. Differentiation of *Staphylococcus* from *Streptococcus*
d. Identification of *Staphylococcus aureus*

Bibliography

Chapin, K. C. (2007). Principles of stains and media. In P. R. Murray, E. J. Baron, J. H. Jorgensen, M. L. Landry, & M. A. Pfaller (Eds.), *Manual of clinical microbiology,* 9th ed. (pp. 182–191). Washington, DC: American Society for Microbiology.

Estevez, E. G. (1984). Bacteriologic plate media: Review of mechanisms of action. *Laboratory Medicine, 15,* 4.

Forbes, B. A, Sahn, D. F., & Weissfeld, A. S. (2007). Specimen management. In *Bailey and Scott's diagnostic microbiology,* 12th ed. (pp. 62–77). St. Louis, MO: Mosby.

Miller, J. M., Krisher, K., & Holmes, H. T. (2007). General principles of specimen collection and handling. In P. R. Murray, E. J. Baron, J. H. Jorgensen, M. L. Landry, & M. A. Pfaller (Eds.), *Manual of clinical microbiology,* 9th ed. (pp. 43–54). Washington, DC: American Society for Microbiology.

Winn, Jr., W., Allen, S., Janda, W., Konemen, E., Procop, G., Schreckenberger, P., & Woods, G. (Eds.). Guidelines for the collection, transport, processing, analysis, and reporting of cultures from specific specimen sources. In *Koneman's color atlas and textbook of diagnostic microbiology,* 6th ed. (pp. 67–110). Philadelphia, PA: Lippincott Williams & Wilkins.

Zimbro, M. J., Power, D. A., Miller, S. M., Wilson, G. E., & Johnson, J. A. (2009). *Difco and BBL manual: Manual of microbiological culture media,* 2nd ed. Sparks, MD: Becton, Dickinson and Company.

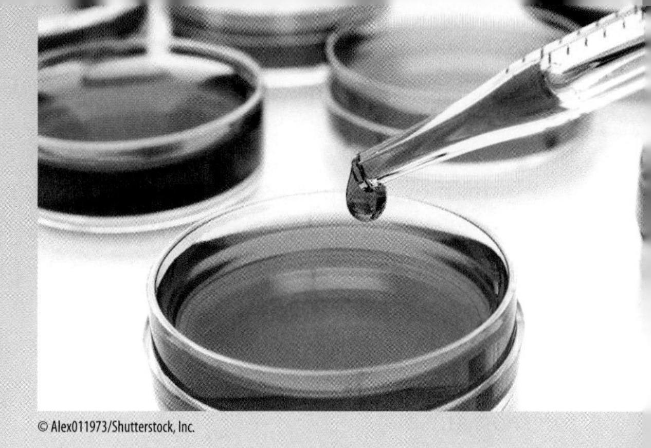
© Alex011973/Shutterstock, Inc.

CHAPTER 4

Microscopy, Staining, and Traditional Methods of Examination

CHAPTER OUTLINE

Microscopy
Direct Examination Methods
Staining Methods
Laboratory Procedures
Quality Control
Laboratory Exercises

KEY TERMS

Brightfield microscopy
Darkfield microscopy
Fluorescent microscopy
Gram stain
Phase-contrast microscopy

LEARNING OBJECTIVES

1. Recognize and state the function of the following parts of a compound microscope:
   a. Ocular
   b. Objectives
   c. Condenser
   d. Iris diaphragm
2. Describe the use of darkfield microscopy in clinical microbiology.
3. Explain the principle of fluorescent microscopy.
4. State the purpose of each of the following direct methods of examination:
   a. Saline mount
   b. Hanging drop
   c. Iodine mount
   d. Potassium hydroxide preparation
   e. Nigrosin
   f. Neufeld (Quellung) reaction
5. Prepare without error smears from stock cultures or clinical specimens.
6. State the reagents used in the Gram stain and the function of each.
   a. Perform without error Gram stains on stock cultures or clinical specimens.
   b. Interpret Gram stains to include the shape, morphology, and Gram stain reaction.
7. Name the stains used to stain *Mycobacterium* and explain why these bacteria are termed *acid-fast bacilli*.
8. Name two fluorescent stains and state the purpose of each.
9. Describe the use of antibody-conjugated stains in clinical microbiology.

The human eye cannot see bacteria and other microorganisms without the use of magnification. Microscopes are used to see bacteria whose average size is 0.5 to 2.0 μm and whose average diameter ranges from 0.3 to 1.0 μm. A variety of microscopic methods and stains are used in clinical microbiology to facilitate the identification of microorganisms.

Microscopy

BRIGHTFIELD MICROSCOPY

In **brightfield microscopy**, the specimen's image appears dark against a brighter background. The light is usually provided through a tungsten filament lamp. **Compound microscopes** have two separate lens systems: an **objective** located near the specimen that magnifies the specimen and an **ocular** or **eyepiece** that further magnifies the image presented by the objective. The total **magnification** is equal to the magnification of the objective multiplied by that of the ocular. Most brightfield microscopes have three objectives: a low-power objective of 10X, a high-power objective of 40X or 45X, and an oil-immersion objective of 100X. The ocular has a magnification of 10X. Thus the total magnification under low power is 100X; high power, 400X or 450X; and oil immersion, 1,000X. When using the oil-immersion objective, a drop of oil is placed on the microscopic slide. The oil decreases the amount of diffraction, or bending of light rays, because it has the same refractive index as glass. Immersion oil is needed to maintain resolution at 100X because resolving power is lost as magnification increases.

Resolving power refers to the ability to distinguish between two adjacent points. It depends on the **wavelength of light** and the **numerical aperture**. The human eye can see within the range of 400 nm to 700 nm. White light is composed of a mixture of colored lights of these various wavelengths. When specimens are too clear to be seen, a dye or stain can be used to form a color image that will be visible to the eye. The specimen will absorb certain wavelengths of light and transmit the other wavelengths. The numerical aperture is an expression relating the measurement of the cone of light that is delivered to the specimen by the condenser and gathered by the objective. The higher the numerical aperture of the objective, the greater is the resolving power of the microscope. The numerical aperture of the condenser must be equal to or greater than that of the aperture.

The function of the **condenser** is to gather light rays and focus these on the object to be illuminated. The **iris diaphragm** is an opaque disk with an opening that can be expanded or contracted. The result is a large range of sizes that can be adjusted to various conditions. To increase the contrast to view unstained specimens, the condenser should be closed slightly. This will increase contrast and improve the observation.

A schematic of a brightfield microscope is shown in **FIGURE 4-1**.

Advanced Microscopy

There are other types of microscopes that offer functions different from those of the standard light microscope. These include phase contrast, darkfield, and fluorescent microscopes.

Phase-Contrast Microscopy

In **phase-contrast microscopy**, light beams are deflected by different thicknesses of the object. The light beams are reflected a second time when they strike the objective. The light waves *increase* in length when in phase;

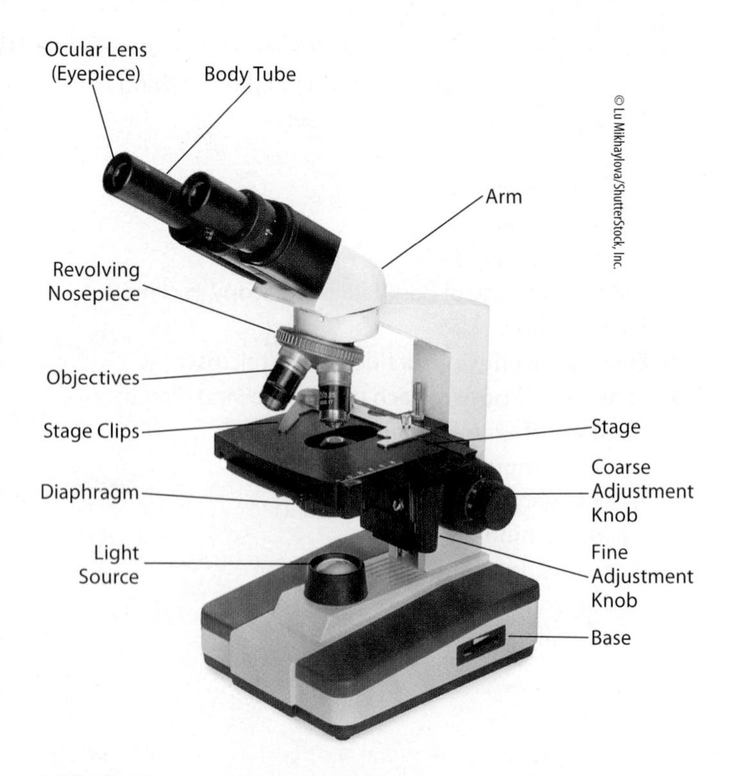

FIGURE 4-1 Light microscope schematic.

this is when the specimen is of uniform thickness. By contrast, the light waves *decrease* in length when not in phase; this is when the specimen has different thicknesses and thus different refractive indices. **Refractive index** refers to the ratio of the speed of light in air compared with the speed of light in another medium. This ratio determines the amount of bending of light rays. Phase contrast is particularly useful for direct observation of specimens that are not stained.

Darkfield Microscopy

In **darkfield microscopy**, the specimen appears luminous against a background of little or no light. The technique is used for those specimens that are so thin that they cannot be resolved using brightfield or phase-contrast microscopy. Light from below the specimen is blocked so that light from only the outer edges reaches the object at a sharp angle. The object reflects and scatters light near its edges. The scattered light is then viewed through the objective. Darkfield is used primarily to view spirochetes, which do not stain very well and are too narrow to be observed by other methods. Typical organisms viewed using this method include *Treponema*, *Leptospira*, and *Borrelia*.

Fluorescent Microscopy

Fluorescent microscopy uses dyes known as **fluorochromes**, which absorb light in the ultraviolet range, fluoresce, and then emit visible light of a greater wavelength. The fluorescing object appears bright against a dark background. Illumination is provided by high-intensity mercury arc or xenon lamps. The light passes through **excitation filters**, which select and limit the wavelength of the transmitted light. Only those wavelengths that can excite the fluorochrome being used are selected. The **dichromatic splitter** then transmits excited wavelengths to the objective. If the fluorochrome dye is bound to the specimen, fluorescence results. The longer wavelengths that are emitted pass through the **beam splitter**, and the image fluoresces. When the fluorochrome dye is not bound, no fluorescence occurs and the object remains dark. Some frequently used fluorescent stains, such as acridine orange, are discussed later in this chapter.

Direct Examination Methods

Several methods for **direct examination** of specimens exist. One example is the **saline mount**, in which the specimen (or organism) is mixed with saline and observed with the condenser lowered. This method permits one to detect the presence of bacteria in a specimen and also to observe for motility. One also can observe for trophozoite forms of pathogenic stool parasites, such as *Giardia lamblia* and *Trichomonas vaginalis* in urine sediment. The use of phase-contrast microscopy greatly enhances the results of the saline mount method.

The **hanging drop** technique, seldom used today, utilizes a slide with a depressed area that houses the specimen. A coverslip is fixed over the depression. This technique is used primarily to observe for motility of the organism, allowing for less distortion when compared with the saline mount method.

In the **iodine mount**, Lugol's iodine is mixed with the stool specimen. This technique is used to stain stools for parasitic ova whose nuclei appear orange to brown.

In the **potassium hydroxide** (KOH) **preparation**, fungal elements can be detected by mixing the tissue with 10% KOH. The KOH dissolves tissue, such as skin, hair, or nails, making the fungal elements more visible.

India ink, or **nigrosin**, once the preferred method to detect capsules, produces a black, semi-opaque background, which makes the clear capsule more visible. The **Neufeld (Quellung) reaction**, or **capsular swelling reaction**, was also used in the past to detect capsular antigen. When mixed with the corresponding antisera, the capsular antigen would bind to the antisera, causing the capsule to become more prominent. These techniques, which have proved to be cumbersome, have been widely replaced by newer methods that allow for the direct detection of capsular antigen, using serological markers, such as latex or fluorescence.

Staining Methods

Because bacteria have a refractive index similar to that of water, biological stains are often needed so that the organisms can be visualized. Stains are organic or aqueous preparations of dyes that impart a variety of colors to tissue or microorganisms.

Stains are classified as either simple or differential. **Simple stains** impart the same color to all structures, whereas **differential stains** contain more than one dye and impart different colors to various structures. An example of a simple stain is the methylene blue stain, whereas the Gram stain is a frequently used differential stain.

The first step in staining is the preparation of a **smear**. A smear is a small sample of the specimen or culture to be studied. Smears are prepared by rolling a swab on a microscopic slide and placing a drop of liquid broth or specimen on a microscopic slide or by emulsifying a colony in saline and then placing it on a microscopic slide. Smears are allowed to air dry or are dried using a slide warmer. Next, the material is fixed through the application of methanol or a pass through the opening of a sterile incinerator.

METHYLENE BLUE

In the **methylene blue** stain, the specimen can be observed for the presence of microorganisms as well as for their size, shape, and morphology. After preparing a fixed smear, the slide is flooded with stain for 1 minute and then rinsed and examined under the oil-immersion objective. This method is quick and helpful in the observation of metachromatic granules in bacteria, such as *Corynebacterium diphtheriae*.

GRAM STAIN

The **Gram stain** will differentiate **gram-positive** bacteria from **gram-negative** bacteria. The method, first introduced by Hans Christian Gram in the late 1800s, has been modified and adjusted numerous times. **TABLE 4-1** lists the basic reagents and their functions.

Bacterial morphology can be observed using the methylene blue stain or Gram stain. Bacteria can be categorized according to shape and arrangement. **Cocci** are round in shape and may appear as **diplococci** (pairs), chains, or clusters. The arrangement depends on the planes of cell division. *Streptococcus pneumoniae* is an example of lancet-shaped diplococci, whereas *Neisseria* species typically form tiny diplococci that resemble kidney beans. Staphylococci typically form grape-like clusters. whereas streptococci usually appear in pairs or short chains. **Bacilli** are rod-shaped bacteria. Some bacilli are long and square ended, such as *Bacillus*, whereas others, such as the Enterobacteriaceae family, are long with rounded ends. Very short bacilli are termed **coccobacilli**, and **fusiform** bacilli taper at both ends. Other bacilli take on a **filamentous** form and appear as long threads that do not appear to separate. Curved bacilli may be small and comma shaped, as with *Campylobacter*, or slightly coiled with one spiral, as with *Vibrio*. True **spirochetes** are coiled bacteria, such as *Treponema*, which may possess four to 20 coils. Spirochetes do not Gram stain well.

Gram stain also can be used to directly examine clinical specimens. Uncentrifuged urine samples, centrifuged cerebrospinal fluid, stool specimens, and sputum can be stained and examined for the presence of bacteria and white blood cells. Gram stain can provide valuable information about the presence of inflammation or infection, which is indicated by the presence of white blood cells.

In cultures 48 hours old or longer, gram-positive bacteria may stain as gram-negative bacteria. For this reason, it is important to use 24-hour cultures for the Gram stain.

When Gram staining for certain organisms, such as *Legionella* and *Campylobacter* and certain anaerobes, it is recommended to use carbolfuchsin instead of safranin O as the counterstain.

Typical Gram stains are shown in **FIGURES 4-2** to **4-6**. **FIGURE 4-7** summarizes the Gram stain reaction.

ACID-FAST STAINS

Acid-fast stains are used to stain mycobacteria that possess thick, waxy cell walls. Once stained, these bacteria resist decolorizing by acid alcohol, and thus the designation *acid fast*. In the **Ziehl-Neelsen technique**, **carbolfuchsin** is heated to drive the stain into the cell wall of the mycobacterium. In the **Kinyoun carbolfuchsin method**, a detergent is used with the carbolfuchsin to enable the stain to penetrate the cell wall.

TABLE 4-1 Gram Stain Reagents

Reagent	Function
Crystal violet	Primary stain: stains all bacteria blue to purple
Gram's iodine	Mordant: enhances reaction between cell wall and primary stain
Ethyl alcohol or acetone	Gram-positive bacteria retain the primary stain because of the peptidoglycan and teichoic acid cross-links. Gram-negative bacteria lose the primary stain because of the large amount of lipopolysaccharide in the cell wall.
Safranin O or carbolfuchsin	Counterstain: no effect on gram-positive bacteria; stains gram-negative bacteria pink to red

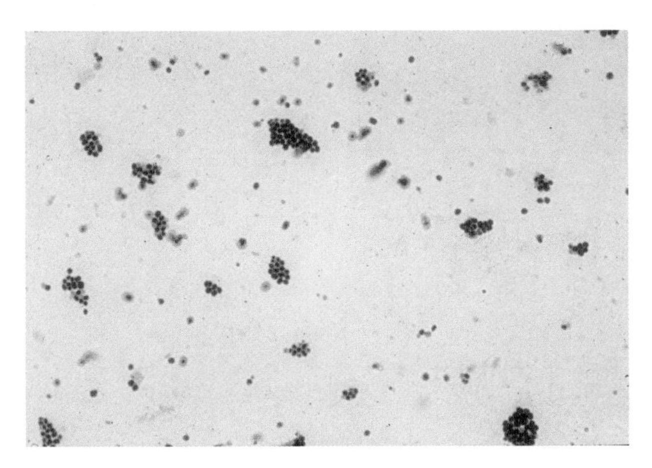

FIGURE 4-2 *Staphylococcus epidermidis* in Gram-stained smear showing typical morphology of gram-positive cocci in clusters.

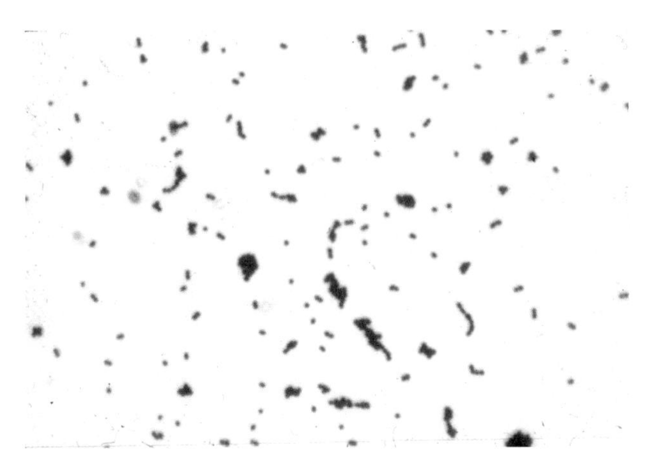

FIGURE 4-3 *Streptococcus pyogenes* in Gram-stained smear showing typical morphology of gram-positive cocci in chains.

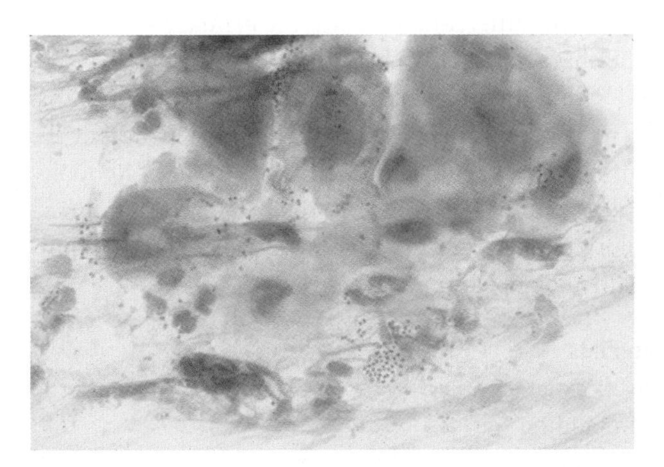

FIGURE 4-4 Vaginal smear of gram-negative diplococci and segmented neutrophils, which illustrates the typical morphology of *Neisseria gonorrhoeae* to resemble miniature kidney beans or coffee beans. Identification of the organism is confirmed through biochemical testing.

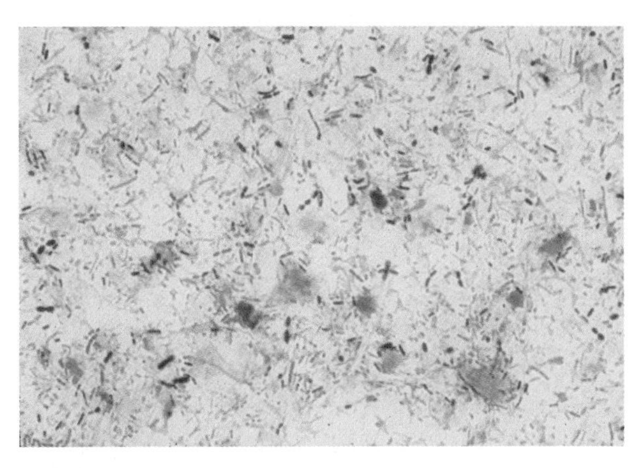

FIGURE 4-5 Normal stool specimen showing normal flora coliforms, including the gram-negative bacillus *Escherichia coli*, gram-positive diphtheroid bacilli, and gram-positive cocci.

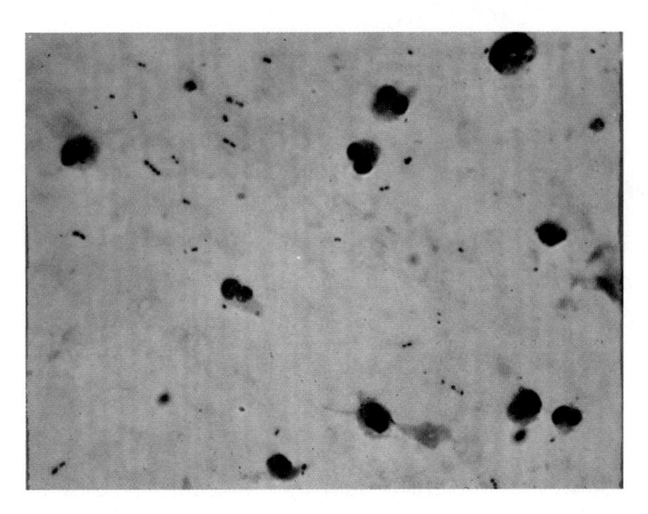

FIGURE 4-6 Sputum showing *Streptococcus pneumoniae*, a gram-positive diplococcus, and segmented neutrophils in a Gram stain.

FLUORESCENT STAINS

Rhodamine-auramine is a fluorescent stain used to stain mycobacteria. The stains bind to the mycolic acid in the organism's cell wall, staining the bacteria yellow to orange. **Acridine orange** selectively binds to any nucleic acid and is useful in demonstrating small amounts of bacteria in blood cultures, cerebrospinal fluid, urethral smears, and other exudates. It is very helpful in observing bacteria in those specimens contaminated with tissue and other debris. **Calcofluor white** is another fluorescent stain used to stain specimens directly for the presence of fungi. The fungal elements appear blue-white when observed with a fluorescent microscope.

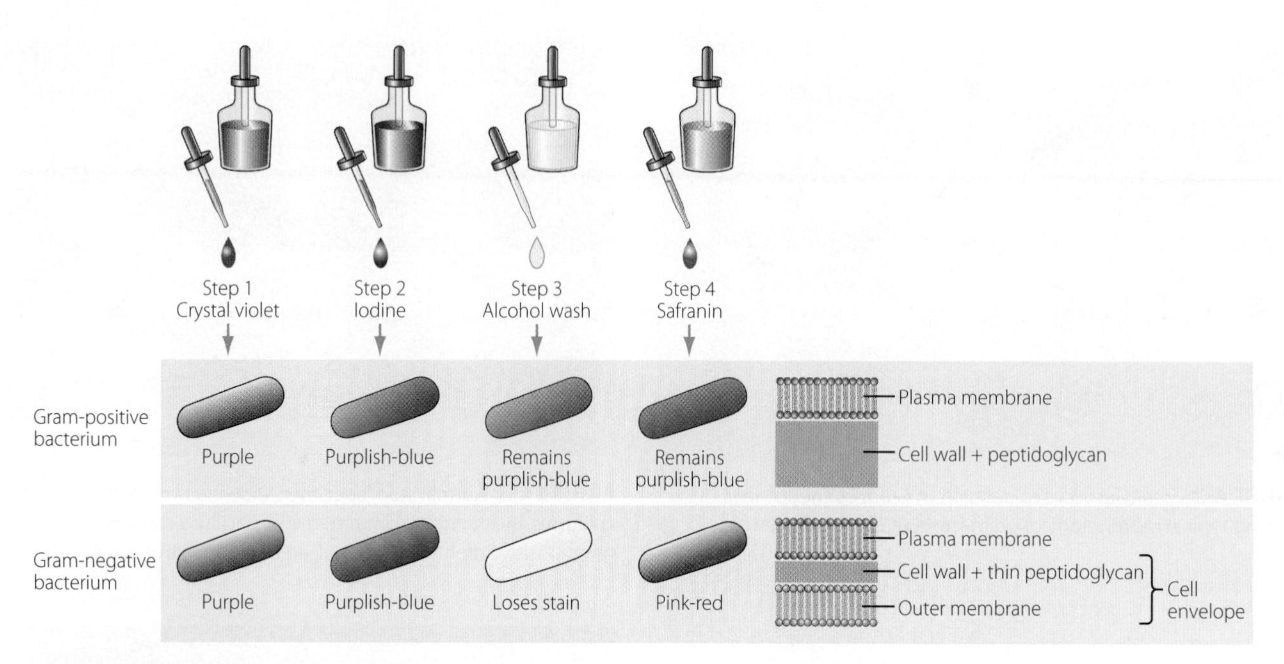

FIGURE 4-7 Gram stain method.

FUNGAL STAINS

Lactophenol cotton blue, **methenamine silver**, and **periodic acid-Schiff** (PAS) also can be used to stain fungal mycelium. The PAS stain is generally preferred for staining direct clinical material.

ANTIBODY-CONJUGATED STAINS

Antibodies are specific proteins produced in response to exposure to **antigens** of a particular organism. By binding specific antibodies to stain, one can detect the corresponding organism. Specific applications include:

- **Fluorescein-conjugated stains.** Antibodies are bound to **fluorescein isothiocyanate**, which binds to the specific antigen if it is present. Examples include the **direct fluorescent antibody** (DFA) technique used to directly detect *Legionella pneumophila* and *Bordetella pertussis* in clinical specimens.
- **Enzyme-conjugated stains.** Enzymes such as horseradish peroxidase are bound to a specific antibody. The conjugated stain will bind to the specific antigen if it is present. This enzyme produces a colored end product, which can be measured photometrically. This technique has been used primarily to detect viruses.

Immunologic procedures are discussed in more detail in Chapter 5.

Laboratory Procedures

Procedure
Gram stain

Purpose
To categorize bacteria as gram positive or gram negative and to observe the cellular morphology. Gram stain is also a valuable tool in the direct observation of clinical material.

Principle
Bacteria will differentially retain the primary stain based on the characteristics of the cell wall. Gram-positive bacteria, with a high content of peptidoglycan and teichoic acid, retain the primary stain and appear blue to purple. Gram-negative bacteria, with a high content of lipopolysaccharide in the cell wall, lose the primary stain during decolorization. Gram-negative bacteria take up the counterstain and appear pink to red.

Materials
Crystal violet
Gram's iodine
Acetone or ethyl alcohol
Safranin O
95% methanol

Procedure

1. Prepare a thin smear of the culture or specimen to be observed. Allow the smear to air dry and heat fix. Alternatively, fix the smear by flooding with 95% methanol and allowing to air dry.
2. Overlay smear with crystal violet for 30 seconds to 1 minute.
3. Rinse with distilled water, tapping off excess.
4. Flood smear with Gram's iodine for 1 minute.
5. Rinse with distilled water, tapping off excess.
6. Add acetone or ethyl alcohol to decolorize drop by drop until no violet color appears in rinse. This requires less than 10 seconds.
7. Rinse immediately with distilled water.
8. Flood smear with safranin O for 30 seconds.
9. Rinse with distilled water and allow slide to drain.
10. Blot dry with paper towel (bulbous paper) or air dry for delicate smears.
11. Examine each slide under oil-immersion objective for characteristic Gram stain reaction, morphology, white blood cells, and other important structures.

Interpretation

Gram-positive organisms stain blue-purple.
Gram-negative organisms stain pink-red.

Quality Control

Prepare a mixed suspension of *Staphylococcus* and *Escherichia coli* in saline. Place a drop on the surface of the slide and allow to air dry. Fix and stain smear as in above method.

Results

Staphylococcus appear as purple cocci in clusters. *E. coli* appear as pink bacilli.

Laboratory Exercises

1. Prepare one smear of each of the following specimens. Perform a Gram stain on each. Observe your stains under the oil-immersion lens. Record your results.
   a. *Staphylococcus epidermidis*
   b. *Streptococcus pneumoniae*
   c. *Enterococcus faecalis*
   d. *Escherichia coli*
   e. *Moraxella catarrhalis*
   f. *Bacillus subtilis*
2. Observe prepared acid-fast smears. Record your results.
3. Observe the following prepared smears and describe your findings. Note the presence of microorganisms, PMNs, red cells, mucus, and epithelial cells.
   a. Sputum
   b. Stool
   c. Wound
   d. Blood

Review Questions

Matching

Match the direct method of examination with its purpose:

1. Iodine mount
2. Nigrosin
3. Potassium hydroxide preparation
4. Hanging drop
   a. Motility
   b. Fungal elements
   c. Parasitic nuclei
   d. Capsules

Multiple Choice

5. The oil-immersion objective provides a *total* specimen magnification of:
   a. 10X
   b. 100X
   c. 450X
   d. 1,000X
6. The higher the numerical aperture, the lower the resolving power of the microscope.
   a. True
   b. False

7. The function of the ________ is to gather and focus light rays on the specimen.
   a. Objective
   b. Iris diaphram
   c. Condenser
   d. Ocular
8. Darkfield microscopy is most often used to study:
   a. Fungi
   b. Mycobacteria
   c. Parasitic nuclei
   d. Spirochetes
9. The typical morphology of *Staphylococcus* is:
   a. Cocci in chains
   b. Cocci in clusters
   c. Filamentous bacilli
   d. Coccibacilli
10. In the Gram stain technique, Gram's iodine functions as the:
    a. Primary stain
    b. Mordant
    c. Decolorizer
    d. Counterstain
11. Gram-positive bacteria stain blue to purple.
    a. True
    b. False
12. The dye used to stain *Mycobacterium* is:
    a. Methylene blue
    b. Crystal violet
    c. Carbolfuchsin
    d. Iodine
13. Which of the following is not used to stain fungal mycelium?
    a. Calcofluor white
    b. Lactophenol cotton blue
    c. Carbolfuchsin
    d. Periodic acid-Schiff

Bibliography

American Optical. (1982). American Optical series 150 reference manual. Buffalo, NY: Scientific Instrument Division, American Optical.

Chapin, K. C. (2007). Principles of stains and media. In P. R. Murray, E. J. Baron, J. H. Jorgensen, M. L. Landry, & M. A. Pfaller (Eds.), *Manual of clinical microbiology*, 9th ed. (pp. 182–191). Washington, DC: American Society for Microbiology.

Introduction to Phase Contrast Microscopy, Nikon—Micros copy U—The Source for Microscopy education. http://www.microscopyu.com/articles/phasecontrast/phasemicroscopy.html 2000–2013.

Leica. (2007). Glossary of optical terms; Leica microsystems. http://www.leica-microsystems.com/fileadmin/downloads/Leica%20DM750/Brochures/Leica_Glossary_of_optical_terms_RvD-Booklet_2012_EN.pdf

Microscope Optical Systems, Nikon—Microscopy U—The source for microscopy education. http://www.microscopyu.com/articles/optics/index.html 2000–2013.

Wiedbrauk, D. L. (2007). Microscopy. In P. R. Murray, E. J. Baron, J. H. Jorgensen, M. L. Landry, & M. A. Pfaller (Eds.), *Manual of clinical microbiology*, 9th ed. (pp. 182–191). Washington, DC: American Society for Microbiology.

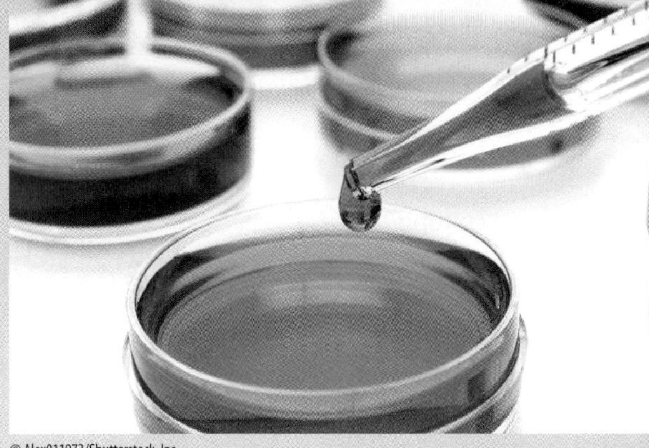
© Alex011973/Shutterstock, Inc.

CHAPTER 5

Automation, Immunodiagnostics, and Molecular Methods

CHAPTER OUTLINE

Multitest Systems
Automated Identification Systems
Immunochemical Methods
Agglutination
Enzyme-Linked Immunosorbent Assay (ELISA)
Immunofluorescence
Immunoserological Techniques
Molecular Techniques

KEY TERMS

Acute phase specimen
Affinity
Agglutination
Antibody titer
Avidity
Colorimetry
Convalescent phase specimen
Counterimmunoelectrophoresis
Direct agglutination
Direct immunofluorescence
Enzyme-linked immunosorbent assay (ELISA)
Fluorometry
Genetic probe
Immunoserological techniques
Indirect agglutination
Indirect immunofluorescence
Monoclonal antibody
Multitest systems
Nephelometry
Neutralization tests
Nucleic acid probe
Polyclonal antibody
Polymerase chain reaction (PCR)
Sensitivity
Specificity

LEARNING OBJECTIVES

1. Discuss the use of miniaturized, multitest systems in the microbiology laboratory.
2. State the principle of colorimetry, and explain how it is used in semiautomated and automated identification systems.
3. State the principle of nephelometry, and explain how it is used in semiautomated and automated identification systems.
4. For each of the following semiautomated and automated identification systems, state the principle of operation and capabilities:
   a. BD Phoenix™
   b. VITEK®
   c. MicroScan WalkAway®
5. Define the following terms as applied to immunochemical methods used in microbiology:
   a. Affinity
   b. Avidity

c. Epitope
d. Specificity
e. Cross-reactivity
6. Explain how sensitivity and specificity are determined for an immunochemical reaction.
7. For each of the following immunochemical methods, state the principle and discuss the application of the test to clinical microbiology:
a. Precipitin tests
b. Particle agglutination
c. Immunofluorescence
d. Enzyme immunosorbent assay
8. Differentiate direct immunofluorescence from indirect immunofluorescence.
9. Discuss immunoserological methods in clinical microbiology:
a. Discuss the significance of an acute phase and a convalescent phase specimen for serological testing.
b. Define titer and explain its significance in confirming an infection.
10. Define the following molecular diagnostic terms:
a. Nucleic acid probe
b. Target
c. Reporter molecule
11. List and describe the methods used to detect hybridization.
12. Explain the process of polymerase chain reaction.
13. Compare and contrast molecular methods with traditional phenotypic methods in microbiology.
14. List and discuss applications of molecular diagnostics to clinical microbiology to include identification, antibiotic resistance, and strain typing of microorganisms.
15. Briefly discuss reverse transcriptase PRCR, nested PCR, multiplex PCR, and real-time PCR.
16. Describe the theory and use of restriction fragment length polymorphisms in clinical microbiology.

Conventional methods to identify microorganisms have been the mainstay in clinical microbiology for many years. These methods rely on the use of several organic substrates, their reaction with microbial enzymes, and the determination of metabolic end products. These systems may incorporate a pH indicator, whose color changes in a positive reaction. Numerous biochemical tests are available, but because these tests are cumbersome to inoculate and often require incubation periods of 24 to 48 hours, alternative testing methods have evolved.

Several conventional methods have been adapted into a rapid format. These methods may use paper disks or strips that are impregnated with reagent or substrate and require inoculation with a large concentration of substrate or a heavy inoculum. Examples include the spot oxidase test, which can detect the enzyme cytochrome oxidase, and the spot indole test, which uses filter paper that contains *para*-dimethylaminobenzaldehyde (Kovac's reagent). These formats can provide a quick reaction result that can be used in the preliminary identification of bacteria and also can guide the laboratorian to further appropriate test methods.

Multitest Systems

Several miniaturized **multitest systems** have been developed that have converted multistep procedures into single-step procedures, which include multiple reactions. These include bioMérieux's API® systems, which utilize microtubes with dehydrated substrates that are reconstituted by adding a bacterial suspension. After interpretation of reactions, a profile number is determined, which can be matched with that in a profile index from a database. Most of the microorganisms can be identified to the species level using bioMérieux's API® identification products. A large database is accessible through the Internet-based APIweb™ service. Manual bioMérieux's API® products for gram-negative bacteria include the API® 20E for 18- to 24-hour identification of Enterobacteriaceae and other nonfastidious gram-negative bacilli, the API® Rapid 20E for 4-hour identification of Enterobacteriaceae, the API® 20NE for 24- to 48-hour identification of gram-negative non-Enterobacteriaceae, and the API® NH for 2-hour identification of *Neisseria, Haemophilus*, and *Branhamella catarrhalis*. Products to identify gram-positive bacteria from API include the API® Staph, which provides overnight identification of clinical staphylococci and micrococci; the RAPIDEC® Staph for 2-hour identification of commonly occurring staphylococci; the API® 20 Strep for 4- or 24-hour identification of streptococci and enterococci; and the API® Coryne for 24-hour identification of corynebacteria and similar organisms. The API® 20A is used for 24-hour identification of anaerobes and the Rapid ID® 32A, for 4-hour identification of anaerobes. The API® 20C AUX provides for 48- to 72-hour identification of yeasts. An API is shown in **FIGURE 5-1**.

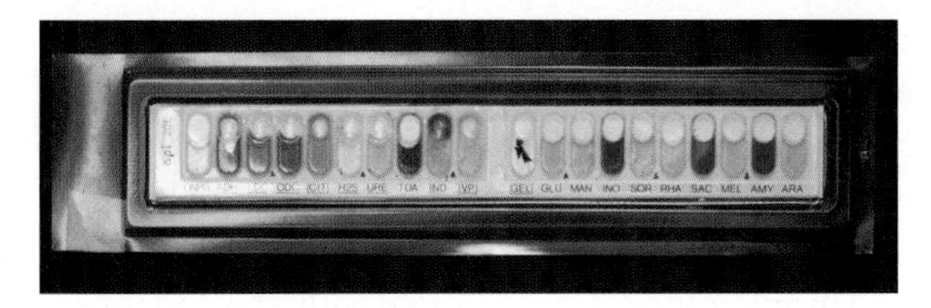

FIGURE 5-1 API identification strip.

Another multitest system is the BD BBL™ Enterotube™ II, which incorporates 15 standard biochemical tests contained in a compartmented tube designed to permit the simultaneous inoculation of 12 test media. This product system provides rapid, accurate identification of Enterobacteriaceae. This product contains several small pieces of agar substrates in a long plastic tube. The entire tube is inoculated with a long wire, which is enclosed in the system. After incubation and interpretation of results, a profile number is determined, which can be matched to a database. BD BBL Oxi/Ferm Tube™ II provides for the rapid identification of gram-negative oxidative and fermentative bacilli.

Another multitest system is the BBL Crystal System (BD BBL™ Diagnostics). The product, shown in **FIGURE 5-2**, is inoculated with one step, which then provides a closed system that is safe and easy to handle. Reagent addition and oil overlay are not needed in this panel design. This miniaturized identification system can identify almost 500 organisms. The Crystal panels may be read manually or with the BBL Crystal Auto Reader, which uses a software program to read and print reports. There are panels for the identification of gram-negative bacilli, enterics, and nonfermenters and for gram-positive aerobic organisms.

Remel's RapID™ System provides a variety of identification products that use enzyme technology; most require 4-hour incubation. Reagents are impregnated in wells in a clear plastic tray. The RapID™ One uses 19 substrates to identify over 70 oxidase-negative, gram-negative bacilli (Enterobacteriaceae), and the RapID™ NF Plus is used to identify oxidase-positive enteric organisms as well as nonfermenting gram-negative bacilli. There are also identification systems available for identification of *Corynebacterium* and other gram-positive coryneform bacilli (RapID™ CB Plus) and for *Neisseria*, *Moraxella*, *Haemophilus*, and similar organisms (RapID™ NH). The RapID™ Staph Plus provides for the identification of 40 staphylococci and related genera, and the RapID™ STR System identifies β-hemolytic streptococci and viridans streptococcus. RapID™ Yeast Plus provides for a 4-hour identification of yeasts. Databases are available for each test system.

Several of these systems have been adapted as a part of semiautomated procedures that may aid in inoculation, incubation, interpretation, and reporting of results. These systems provide for shorter incubation and reaction times and more reliable, reproducible results, with the identification of a greater number of organisms. One such system is the BIOMIC® V3 Microbiology System, which utilizes color digital imaging to automate the reading and interpretation of antibiotic susceptibility and organism identification tests for bacteria and yeast. The BIOMIC® V3, shown in **FIGURE 5-3**, is an open-system automating clinical microbiology test, including antibiotic disk diffusion, Etest® (bioMérieux), API® (bioMérieux), RapID™ (Remel), Crystal™ (BD), 96-well microtiter plates, antibiotic susceptibility testing, and colony count plates. BIOMIC® V3 provides an instant digital record of all test results and high-resolution images. It can be interfaced with the laboratory information system interface and is useful for smaller volume microbiology laboratories as well as for a backup or supplement to larger instruments.

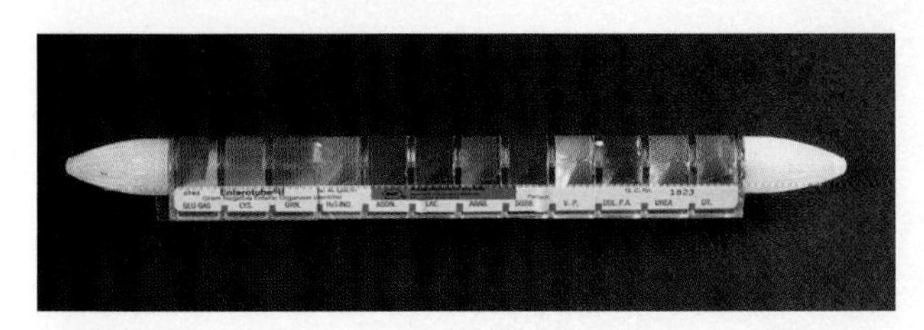

FIGURE 5-2 BD BBL™ Crystal™ Enteric/Nonfermenter ID System.

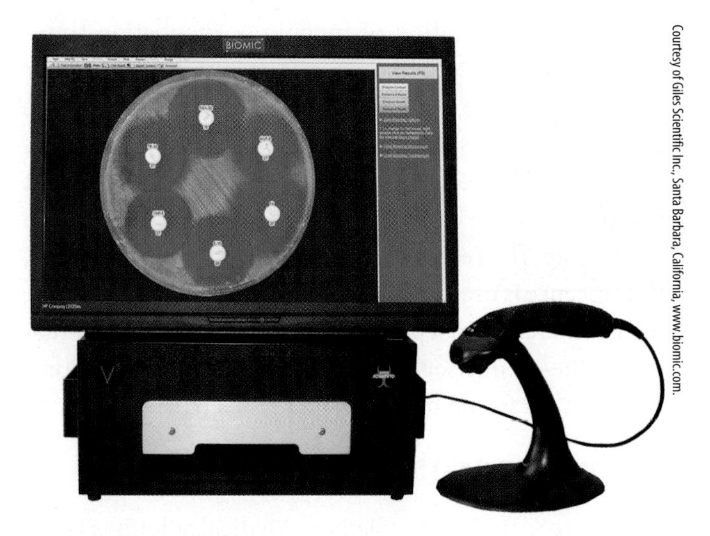

Courtesy of Giles Scientific Inc., Santa Barbara, California, www.biomic.com.

FIGURE 5-3 BIOMIC® V3.

Automated Identification Systems

Automated systems in microbiology combine the principles used in manual testing with instrumentation. These systems permit the analysis of multiple isolates and utilize several biochemical reactions; thus, clinical isolates can be more efficiently identified.

PRINCIPLES

Semiautomated systems usually involve a plastic tray with substrates contained in multiple wells. These systems are available for both the identification of microorganisms and antibiotic susceptibility testing, including qualitative results and determination of the minimal inhibitory concentration (MIC). Most of these systems have a computer module with software available from the manufacturer to aid in the reporting of results. The panels can be inoculated either manually or automatically using a multipronged inoculator.

Semiautomated and automated systems usually rely on the principles of **colorimetry**, **nephelometry**, or **fluorometry**. Colorimetry uses a spectrophotometer to measure a color change in the pH indicator or other indicator as an organism metabolizes a particular substrate. Nephelometry is based on the principle of light scattering and has been used for antibiotic susceptibility testing. As an organism grows, the well becomes turbid. Photometers are placed at angles to the turbid suspension, and the scattering of light is measured. Alternatively, the absorbance of the solution can be measured. The percentage of light transmitted through the solution is compared with that transmitted through a clear control well. Substrates are either dehydrated or freeze-dried and inoculated with a standard concentration of inoculum. Incubation times may vary from 4 to 24 hours, and results are read either manually or automatically. The identification is made through comparison with a database. Fluorometric procedures use biochemical substrates that have a fluorescent component. If the organism has the enzyme to metabolize a substrate, fluorescence is exhibited. In some reactions, fluorescence is used to detect a change in pH. For example, the pH increases in a positive decarboxylase reaction that causes the production of fluorescence. In other reactions, an acidic pH would be noted by the lack of fluorescence.

AUTOMATED SYSTEMS FOR IDENTIFICATION

The MicroScan® System (Siemens Medical Solutions Diagnostics, formerly from Dade Behring) uses plastic 96-well microtiter trays in which up to 32 substrates can be used to identify Enterobacteriaceae. Gram-positive panels, urinary tract panels, and panels for other gram-negative bacteria, as well as for antibiotic susceptibility testing, are also available. The trays are shipped in either a dehydrated or frozen form. The microtubes are inoculated with a heavy suspension of the organism and incubated for 15 to 18 hours at 35°C. The panels may be interpreted manually, and each biochemical result is converted into a seven- or eight-digit code number, which is found in a codebook. Alternatively, an automated tray reader can be used, which will detect bacterial growth or color changes as noted by changes in light transmission. A computer with software analyzes the electronic pulses and compares the reaction patterns with an internal program to identify the organism.

The Sensititre System (TREK Diagnostic Systems) can be used as a manual enteric identification system or as an auto-identification system. Each manual plate contains media to perform 23 standard biochemical tests and a control, which are dehydrated in a 96-well microtiter plate. The Sensititre is read and interpreted manually.

The BD Phoenix™ Automated Microbiology System (**FIGURE 5-4**) uses the principle of nephelometry. It is a fully automated identification instrument that also can provide antimicrobial susceptibility testing. The system consists of disposable panels that combine identification and antimicrobial susceptibility testing. The instrument automatically takes readings every 20 minutes during incubation. The system measures colorimetric changes and changes in fluorescence intensity levels depending on the type of

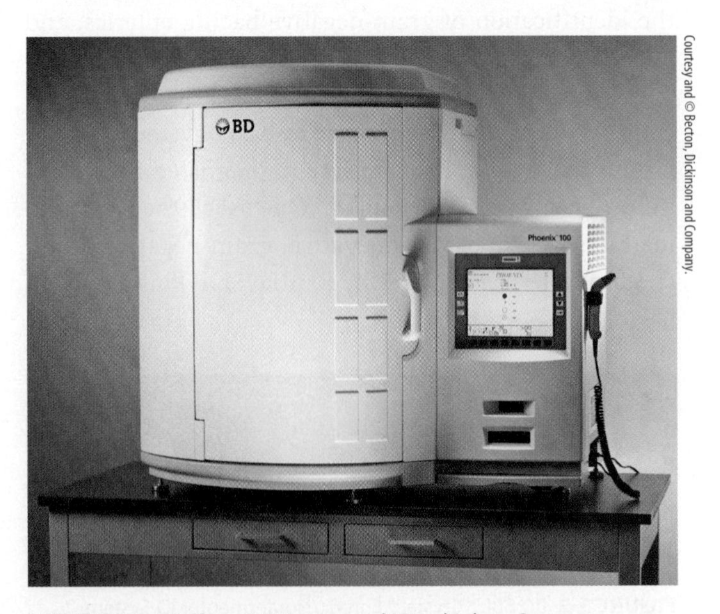

FIGURE 5-4 BD Phoenix™ Automated Microbiology System.

substrate. There are 45 biochemical reactions, which include fluorogenic, fermentative, chromogenic, and carbon source substrates, to identify gram-negative bacilli. Most organisms are identified within 2 to 12 hours; many results are available within 4 hours.

The VITEK® System (bioMérieux VITEK) (**FIGURE 5-5**) identifies most clinically significant bacteria and yeast and also performs qualitative and quantitative antibiotic susceptibility tests. The VITEK® 2 is an automated microbiology system utilizing growth-based technology and is currently available in three formats: The VITEK® 2 compact is recommended for low- to middle-volume clinical and industrial laboratories, and the VITEK® 2-60 and VITEK® 2 XL are adapted for clinical microbiology laboratories. The system uses reagent cards, which have 64 wells, each containing an individual test substrate. Substrates measure various metabolic activities such as acidification, alkalinization, enzyme hydrolysis, and growth in the presence of inhibitory substances. Four reagent cards for the identification of different organism classes are currently available—the GN card for gram-negative fermenting and nonfermenting bacilli, the GP card for gram-positive cocci and nonspore-forming bacilli, the YST card for yeasts and yeast-like organisms, and the BCL card for gram-positive spore-forming bacilli.

The VITEK® has several modules, including a reader/incubator module, which has a capacity of 30, 60, 120, or 240 cards depending on the specific VITEK® model. The card-filling unit inoculates test cards in a vacuumized repressurization procedure. The sealer module seals the test cards after the inoculation procedure. The card-filling and card-sealing modules can hold one to eight trays, each capable of holding 30 test cards. The reader/incubator processes and incubates the cards at 35°C and monitors each card optically for data collection. The computer module stores, analyzes, and interprets test data and also controls reader/incubator functions. The data terminal and printer module allow the visual examination of results and provide an automatic printed copy of results.

The inoculum is prepared from a growing isolate, and the cards are inoculated automatically. The card is placed in the reader/incubator module, where it is scanned by a series of emitted diodes. The light source directs light through the wells to the reader. The data are sent to a computer, which records and interprets the readings. Changes in absorbance, resulting from changes in turbidity as the organism grows or from color changes that occur as the pH changes, are measured. A transmittance optical system allows interpretation of test reactions using different wavelengths in the visible spectrum. During incubation, each test reaction is read every 15 minutes to measure either turbidity or colored products of substrate metabolism. Calculations are performed on raw data and compared to thresholds to determine reactions for each test. The change in transmission of light is compared with a preset threshold value for each well. Values greater than or equal to the threshold value are considered to be positive reactions, whereas values less than the threshold are considered to be negative until the next reading.

The VITEK® also can be used for antibiotic susceptibility testing for gram-positive and gram-negative organisms. A gram-positive or gram-negative susceptibility card is inoculated, and the reader measures the amount of light passing through each well hourly for 15 hours. As the organism grows, the amount of light transmitted decreases. Increased turbidity and resulting decreased transmission of light usually indicate the organism is resistant to the antibiotic. A growth curve is developed based on the decline of the percentage of transmission. MICs can be determined based on the growth curve and slope of the curve.

The MicroScan WalkAway® (Siemens Medical Solutions Diagnostics, formerly available from Dade Behring) is a fully automated computer-controlled system that uses both colorimetric and fluorometric principles for the identification and susceptibility testing of microorganisms. This system offers simultaneous automation of overnight, rapid, and specialty panels that test for both gram-negative

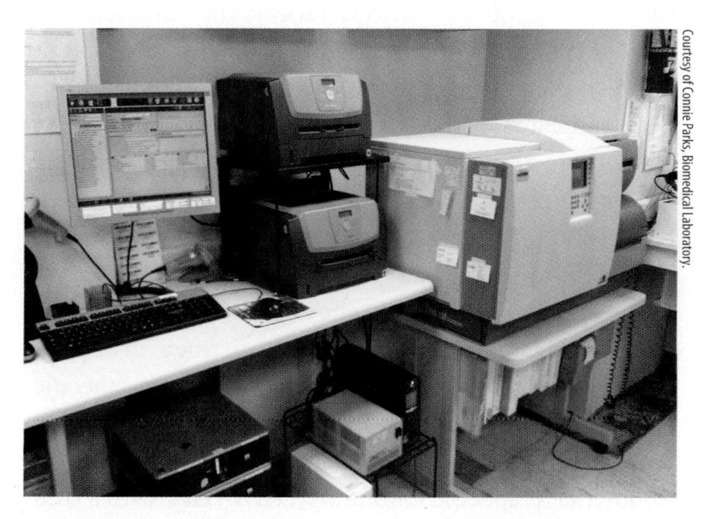

Courtesy of Connie Parks, Biomedical Laboratory.

FIGURE 5-5 VITEK® System.

and gram-positive bacteria. There are two new instrument models—a 40-panel-capacity model for medium-volume laboratories and a 96-panel-capacity model for high-volume laboratories. These instruments have been designed to replace the current WalkAway SI 40 and 96 Systems.

The higher volume instrument can incubate up to 96 conventional panels or MicroScan® panels. Reagents are added automatically to the panels as needed, and the panels are read and interpreted and results printed. The incorporation of fluorescent labels into some of the substrates provides for bacterial identification within 2 hours. Each fluorescent substrate has a fluorophore attached to a phosphate, sugar, or amino acid compound. In fluorogenic reactions, if the enzyme is produced by the organism, it cleaves the fluorescent compound, releasing the fluorophore, and fluorescent is emitted. In fluorometric reactions, if the organism uses the substrate, the pH drops, and there is a decrease in fluorescence.

Results of the reactions are converted into 15-digit codes, which are interpreted by the computer. The fluorogenic 2-hour Rapid Negative Identification Panel uses 36 tests and can identify up to 150 species. Currently, identification systems are available for gram-positive bacteria, gram-negative bacteria, yeast, anaerobes, *Haemophilus*, and *Neisseria*. Susceptibility testing is available for gram-negative and gram-positive bacteria. The fluorometric system allows for rapid identification results within 2 hours for certain bacteria. The rapid colorimetric system can identify other microorganisms within 4 hours, and susceptibility results are available in 4 to 7 hours. The system uses microtiter trays that contain fluorescent-labeled substrates containing a synthetic and metabolic component. A halogen quartz incandescent lamp is focused on the trays. If the organism produces the enzyme to act on a substrate, the synthetic moiety is released, which enables it to fluoresce. The degree of fluorescence is measured using a fluorometer. Some of the substrates contain fluorescent pH indicators, which emit or fail to emit fluorescence when the pH changes. The colorimetric tests are read spectrophotometrically for a color change. For antibiotic susceptibility testing, the microtiter wells contain a growth medium, a fluorogenic substrate, and various concentrations of antibiotics. The wells are inoculated and incubated, and the amount of fluorescence in each test well is compared with that in a control well with no antibiotic present. If growth is inhibited, less fluorescence occurs, indicating susceptibility. If more fluorescence occurs, indicating the presence of bacterial growth, resistance may be indicated.

Immunochemical Methods

There are several types of immunochemical methods used in clinical microbiology that may detect either antigen or antibody. Each immunochemical method has both advantages and limitations. These techniques use different markers to visualize reactions and have specific applications in clinical microbiology.

ANTIGENS AND ANTIBODIES

Immunochemical methods in clinical microbiology rely on the principles of antigen and antibody reactions to detect microorganisms when the infectious agent cannot be cultured on artificial media. They are also useful to identify specific antigens or products of the infectious agent when long incubation periods are needed. Immunochemical methods can be used directly on a clinical specimen to detect an infectious agent. These methods also are used to identify microorganisms once they have been grown and isolated on laboratory media.

Antigens are foreign compounds that stimulate an immune response, leading to the formation of proteins, known as antibodies. Antigens are of high molecular weight and may consist of a part of the organism's cell wall, a protein, or toxin produced by the infectious agent. Antibody **affinity** is the strength of the reaction between a single antigenic determinant and a single combining site on the antibody. Affinity reflects the cumulative effects of the forces of attraction and repulsion that occur between the antigen and the antibody. Antibody **avidity** is an indicator of the strength of binding of an antigen with many antigenic determinants and many antibody binding sites. Avidity reflects the sum total of all binding between antigen and antibody in a solution. The specific part of the antibody that reacts with the antigen is known as the **epitope**, or the antigenic determinant. **Specificity** refers to the ability of an antibody to distinguish between antigens that have very small differences. Thus, specificity is a measure of the antibody to differentiate between epitopes. **Cross-reactivity** measures the ability of an antibody that is specific for one antigen to react with a similar, yet not related, antigen. Cross-reactivity occurs when the cross-reacting antigen shares a common epitope with the immunizing antigen or when the two antigens share a very similar structure. Antibodies with low specificity may be associated with false-positive reactions; thus, high specificity is a desired antibody property. **Sensitivity** refers to the ability of the system to detect small amounts of antigen or antibody. Therefore, test systems with high sensitivity levels are better able to detect small quantities of the substance being analyzed. Sensitivity and specificity are inversely proportional, and test systems rely on a balance of sensitivity and specificity. **TABLE 5-1** summarizes the relationship between sensitivity and specificity.

The use of **monoclonal antibodies** has provided a mechanism for the production of vast amounts of homogeneous antibody. When animals, such as rabbits, sheep, and goats, are injected with an antigen, heterogeneous antibody production results in the production of **polyclonal antibodies**. Polyclonal antibodies contain a variety of binding sites and must be isolated and purified. However, they still may contain several binding sites, which affect their affinity and avidity. Monoclonal antibody production permits the development of an immortal cell line that can produce large amounts of a highly specific antibody. The purified antibodies are cloned from a single hybrid cell.

In the technique, an animal, usually a mouse, is immunized with several doses of a specific antigen. The animal responds by producing antibody to the antigen injected. Next, the animal's spleen, which contains the antibody-producing cells, is removed and emulsified. The antibody-producing cells are removed. These cells cannot survive or multiply in tissue culture. Therefore, they are fused with immortal mouse myeloma cells, which are able to survive. These "hybrid cells" are next placed in HAT medium (hypoxanthine, aminopterin, thymidine), which permits the formation of 300 to 500 hybrids from a single clone. The hybrids are able to produce large quantities of the antibody.

Monoclonal antibodies have been used in the analysis of tissue and erythrocyte membranes and in leukocyte typing. Monoclonal antibodies can be bound to latex beads, a fluorescent dye, or enzyme conjugates to detect bacterial or viral antigen in specimens, and they offer several advantages over traditional detection methods. Kits are available from manufacturers for the detection of *Neisseria meningitidis* type b capsule, *Chlamydia*, and several viruses such as rotavirus. Nonspecific agglutination is avoided; the methods are usually very sensitive, resulting from the high affinity of the antigen for the monoclonal antibody, and very specific.

TABLE 5-1 Sensitivity and Specificity in Antigen Detection

	Antigen present	Antigen absent
Test positive	True positive (TP)	False positive (FP)
Test negative	False negative (FN)	True negative (TN)
	Sensitivity: TP/TP + FN	Specificity: TN/FP + TN

IMMUNOCHEMICAL METHODS TO DETECT MICROORGANISMS

There are several immunochemical methods to detect microorganisms in specimens and after the microorganism has been grown in culture. These methods are listed in BOX 5-1, and some of the more commonly used methods are discussed in the sections below.

Precipitin Tests

Precipitin tests detect soluble antigen in solution. The classic precipitin test is **double immunoelectrophoresis**, or the Ouchterlony technique. In this method, wells are cut in agar or agarose, and patient specimen that contains the antigen is added to one well. Antibody specific for the

BOX 5-1 **Immunochemical Methods to Detect Microorganisms**

- Precipitin tests
    - Double immunoelectrophoresis
    - Counterimmunoelectrophoresis
    - Nephelometry
- Agglutination
    - Particle Agglutination
    - Latex agglutination
    - Hemagglutination
    - Coagglutination
    - Liposome-enhanced agglutination
- Immunofluorescence
- Enzyme immunoassay
    - Solid-phase immunoassay
    - Membrane-bound solid-phase immunoassay

target antigen is added to an adjacent well. The antigen and antibody diffuse toward one another and meet at the zone of equivalent, where a precipitin band forms. This method is no longer practical, and its use is limited for the detection of exoantigens found in fungi, such as *Blastomyces*, *Histoplasma*, and *Coccidioides*.

Counterimmunoelectrophoresis is useful to detect small amounts of antibody and utilizes the principle of immunoelectrophoresis combined with an electrical current to decrease the reaction time. In this technique, solutions of antibody and sample are placed in small wells cut into agarose. A paper wick connects the two sides of the agarose to trays of buffer. An electrical current is applied through the buffer. The negatively charged bacterial antigens migrate to the positive electrode, while the neutral antibodies are carried by the weakly alkaline buffer to the negative electrode. At the zone of equivalence, antigen and antibody form a complex, and a visible band of precipitin forms. This method also has limited use because of its cost and is somewhat less sensitive than other methods, such as agglutination.

Nephelometry is used to measure the amount of serum antibody through the principle of light scattered from the formation of a precipitin between the antibody and corresponding antigen. The antigen is mixed with patient serum in an optically clear test tube or cuvette. This system uses light rays produced from a high-intensity light source, such as a laser, which are collected onto a focusing lens and then passed through the sample tube. If the patient has the antibody, a precipitin forms with the antigen; this complex reflects the transmitted light. The amount of light scattered at a 70° angle is measured and corresponds to the concentration of the antibody present in the patient specimen.

Particle Agglutination

Agglutination refers to the clumping or aggregation of cells, bacteria, or other particles coated with antigen or antibody with their corresponding antibody or antigen. The antigens or antibodies are attached to the surface of the particle by covalent bonds or electrical forces. In agglutination an aggregation of antibodies and antigens forms a visible framework. There are two stages to agglutination. In the first stage, known as sensitization, antigen combines with antibody. This reaction is not visible. In the second, or visible, reaction, a lattice forms between the antibody-coated particles.

There are several types of agglutination reactions, including direct agglutination, indirect or passive agglutination, and coagglutination. If the test system utilizes an antigen bound to an inert surface, such as latex, the presence of antibody can be detected in a specimen or isolate. Conversely, if the test system utilizes an antibody bound to an inert surface, the presence of antigen can be detected. Various markers to visualize identification can be used, including latex beads, erythrocytes, fluorescent markers, and enzyme conjugates. Several of these methods are described in the next sections.

Agglutination reactions are very sensitive, and either antigen or antibody can be detected depending on which is bound to the carrier. Bacterial antigens, capsular antigens, and bacterial toxins can be detected. Direct agglutination refers to the detection of bacterial or viral antigens through reaction with the corresponding antibody. A common application of antigen detection is the direct detection of group A streptococcal antigen in throat swabs. The group A streptococcal antigen is extracted and then reacted with latex beads that have been coated with antigroup A streptococcal antibodies. The detection of patient antibodies in patient serum is an application of indirect agglutination. For example, rubella antibodies in an individual's serum can be detected through reaction with latex beads that are coated with antigens of the rubella virus.

Hemagglutination reactions use the aggregation of erythrocytes as a positive indicator.

Latex Agglutination

Latex is a frequently used carrier molecule for agglutination reactions because the molecule is stable and readily covalently bonds with proteins. The latex particle can hold many antibody-binding sites. Antigen present in the patient specimen combines with the binding site of the antibody, which has been bound to the latex particle. Cross-linked aggregates of latex beads with antigen are observed in positive reaction. Latex agglutination is dependent on the proper pH, ionic strength of the reaction solution, and osmolarity. There may be false-positive reactions because of nonspecific antibodies or antibody-like compounds. Latex agglutination reactions are performed on cardboard slides or glass surfaces and are graded from 1+ to 4+. In addition to direct specimen testing, latex agglutination may be performed on bacteria isolated from cultures. Latex agglutination methods are rapid and are not labor intensive.

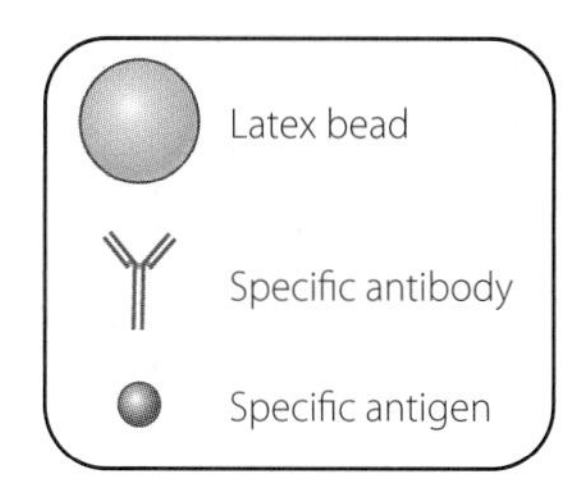

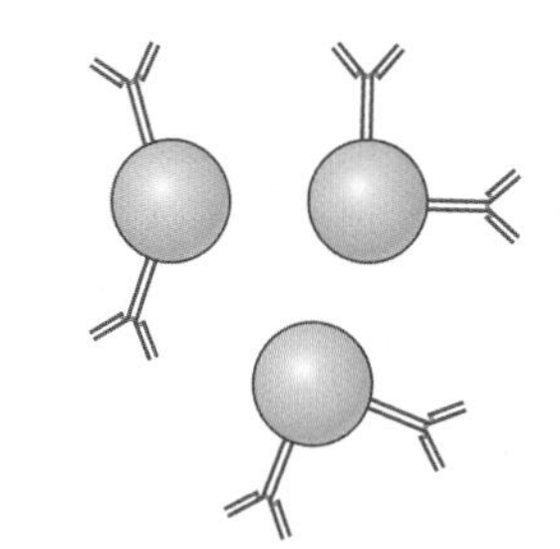
Specific antibody bound to latex beads

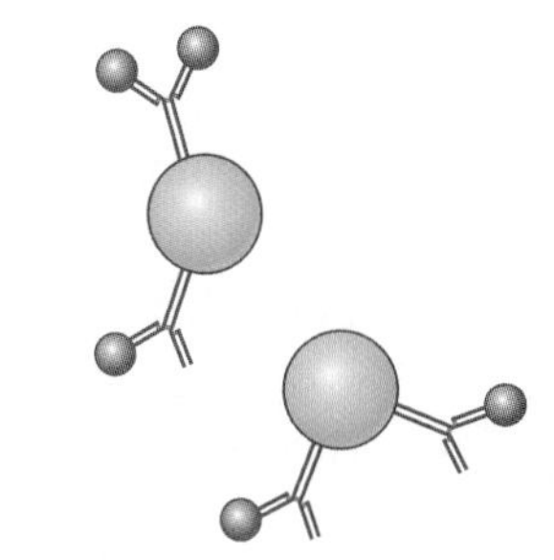
Add specimen (e.g. serum, cerebrospinal fluid).
If antigen is present, it will bind to antibody.

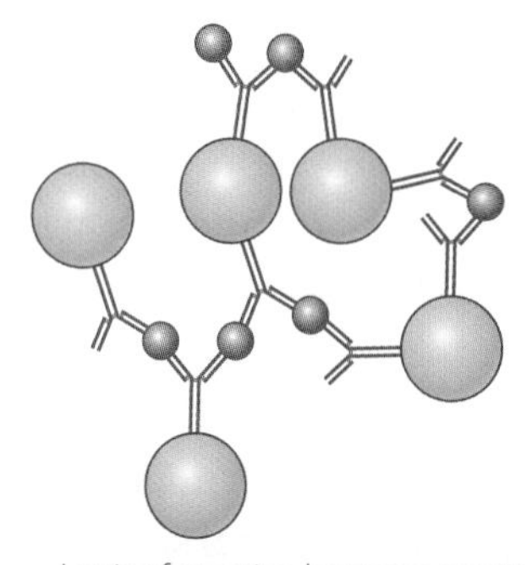
Lattice formation between sensitized
cells results in agglutination.

FIGURE 5-6 Latex agglutination (or Direct agglutination).

In **direct agglutination** (**FIGURE 5-6**), bacterial antigens aggregate in the presence of the corresponding antibody. In direct bacterial agglutination, antibodies produced by the host to antigens present on the surface of the bacterium are detected. An example of this technique is **febrile agglutinins,** which detect host antibody to *Salmonella* O antigens of groups A, B, and D and flagellar a, b, and d antigens; *Brucella abortus* antigen; *Proteus* OX-19, OX-2, and OX-K antigens; and *Francisella tularensis* antigen. These tests are helpful diagnostic tools for these microorganisms, which are difficult to culture on traditional media. Some of these procedures, such as the Widal test to detect typhoid fever agglutinins caused by *Salmonella*, are no longer suitable because of cross-reacting antibodies. The **Weil-Felix test** detects the cross-reacting antibodies of rickettsial infections, which also agglutinate *Proteus* bacteria.

In **indirect**, or **passive, agglutination**, soluble antigen is extracted from a microorganism and attached to a **carrier** particle. The carrier particle is inert and can be red blood cells, charcoal particles, or white or colored latex beads. Patient serum is then reacted with the carrier, which has been coated with antigen. In a positive reaction the patient's antibody binds to the antigen and agglutination occurs. Applications of this technique include the detection of antibody to several viruses, including cytomegalovirus and varicella-zoster virus, as well as the detection of antibodies against *Mycoplasma*.

Indirect, or passive, hemagglutination techniques utilize specific antigens that are bound to red blood cells. One application is the microhemagglutination test for *Treponema pallidum*, which detects patient antibody to the organism. In a positive reaction, hemagglutination occurs.

In hemagglutination inhibition, the ability of a soluble antigen to inhibit the agglutination of antigen-coated red cells by antibodies is determined. In this method, antibodies are bound to red cells that have been coated with antigens. If the patient's specimen contains the corresponding antigen, the soluble antigen will compete with the antigen coated on the red cells for antibody-binding sites. Thus, the agglutination of red cells is inhibited in a positive reaction. This technique also is used to semiquantitate the amount of antibodies in patient serum against the influenza virus. Influenza virus has a hemagglutinin antigen, which causes the agglutination of red cells. Patient antibody to the hemagglutinin antigen will prevent red cell agglutination.

Coagglutination

In **coagglutination** (**FIGURE 5-7**), antibody is bound to a particle to improve the visibility of the reaction. Labile *Staphylococcus aureus* (the Cowan 1 strain) contains large amounts of protein A, an antibody-binding protein, in its cell wall. Protein A has the unusual property of binding antibody not in the classical antigen–antibody reaction but through the antibody's Fc portion. This allows the specific antigen-binding site of the antibody molecule, the Fab portion, to be free to react with the homologous antigen. The

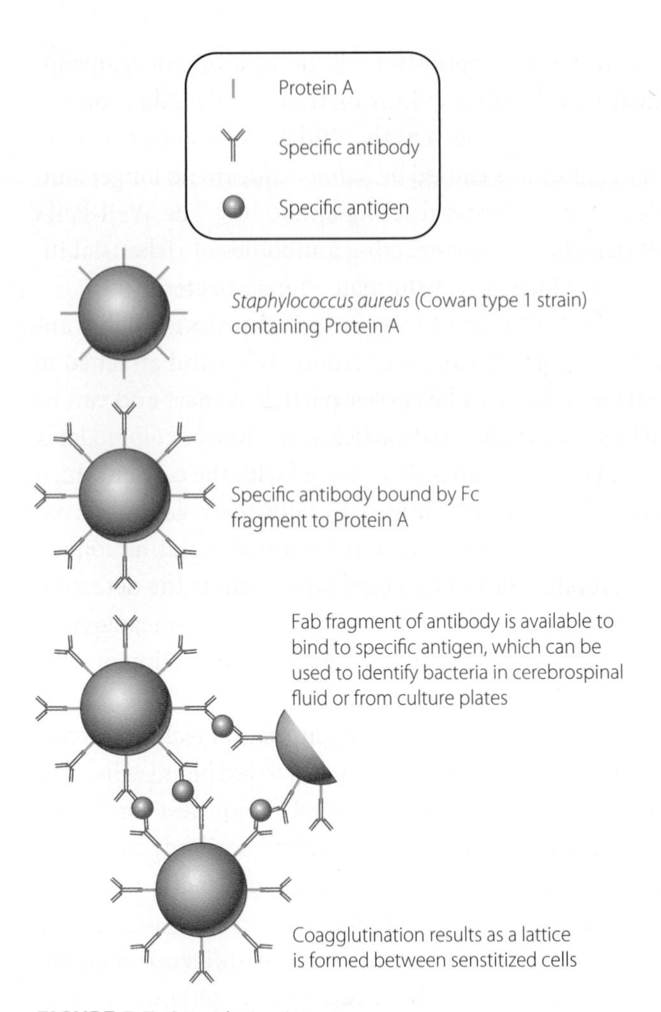

FIGURE 5-7 Coagglutination.

Staphylococcus coagglutination principle has been applied to the detection of soluble antigens in acute and chronic meningitis to identify organisms such as *Haemophilus influenzae*, *Escherichia coli*, *Streptococcus pneumoniae*, *Streptococcus agalactiae*, and *Cryptococcus neoformans* in cerebrospinal fluid. Lancefield antigens A, B, C, D, F, G, and N, as well as *H. influenzae* serotypes A through F, can be identified through coagglutination.

NEUTRALIZATION

In **neutralization tests**, the production of an antibody that blocks the actions of a virus or bacterium can be detected. Streptolysin O is an extracellular product produced by *Streptococcus pyogenes*. The production of antistreptolysin O is an indicator of prior infections with the organism.

Enzyme-Linked Immunosorbent Assay

In **enzyme-linked immunosorbent assays (ELISA)**, antibody or antigen is bound to an enzyme that is able to catalyze a reaction. The antibody-binding site remains free to react with antigen, and the enzyme catalyst remains unaltered during the reaction. The colored end product is then measured spectrophotometrically. The incorporation of monoclonal antibodies into ELISA methods has enhanced its specificity. Antigen can be detected using competitive ELISA techniques or noncompetitive techniques. Noncompetitive, or "sandwich," techniques are used more often than competitive techniques and also can be used to detect antibody. ELISA methods are sensitive and economical, are not labor intensive, and do not require expensive instrumentation.

In solid-phase immunosorbent assay (SPIA), antibody or antigen is fixed to a solid phase. The solid phase can be the polystyrene wells of a microtiter tray, plastic beads, filter pads, or ferrous metal beads. Serum or another body fluid is added to the solid phase. If the corresponding antigen or antibody is present, a complex will form. Next, the reaction is washed to remove any unbound, unspecific antibodies. A second antibody that has been complexed to an enzyme is added. The second antibody is usually an antiglobulin conjugate, either horseradish peroxidase or alkaline phosphatase enzyme. If initial binding between the antibody and antigen has occurred, this complex will bind the second antibody, which forms a sandwich with the antigen in the middle. The reaction is washed again to remove any unlabeled antibody, and an enzyme substrate is added. Typical substrates are orthophenylenediamine for horseradish peroxidase and nitrophenyl phosphate for alkaline phosphatase. In a positive reaction the enzyme complex will act on the substrate, converting it to a colored end product. The intensity of the color, which is read spectrophotometrically, is proportional to the amount of antibody or antigen in the original sample.

Several commercial applications of ELISA are available. For example, kits are available for the detection of antigens of *Giardia*, *Cryptosporidium*, *Chlamydia*, *Neisseria gonorrhoeae*, and several viral antigens. Antibodies to *Legionella*, *Mycoplasma*, rubella virus, varicella virus, *Borrelia burgdorferi* (Lyme disease), and several other pathogens can be detected through indirect ELISA techniques.

In membrane-bound SPIA, nitrocellulose or nylon membranes are used to enhance the speed and sensitivity of the reaction. An absorbent material below the membrane pulls reactants through and separates the antigen–antibody complexes from other nonspecific reactants. This principle has been used in rapid methods that detect group

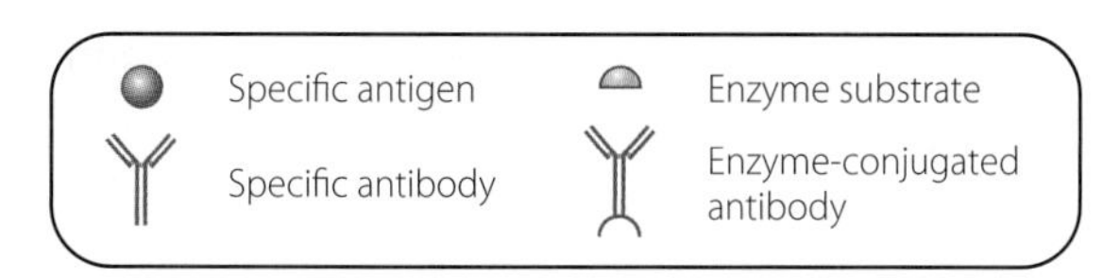

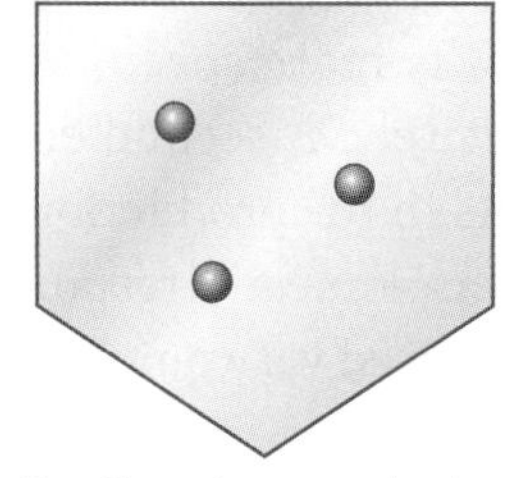
Specific antigens attached to solid phase (latex beads, walls of microtiter plates).

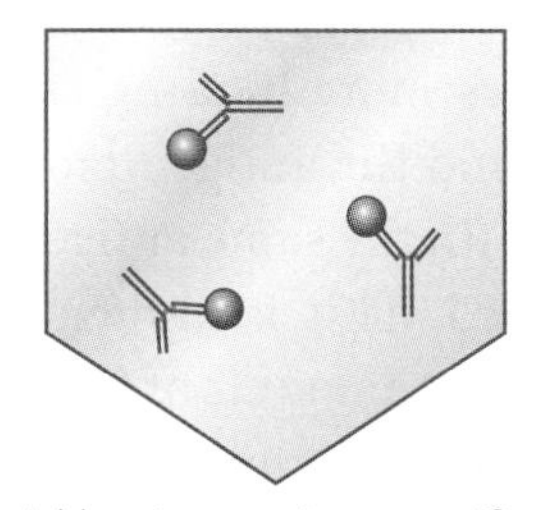
Add patient specimen; specific antibody binds to antigen. Nonspecific antibody does not bind and is washed away.

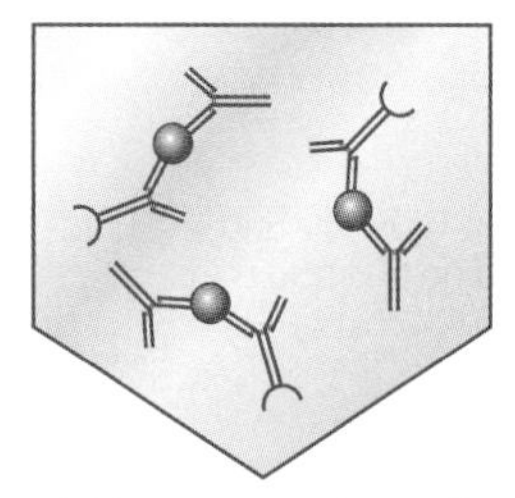
Add enzyme-conjugated antibody (immunoglobulin), which binds to the antigen antibody complex if present. Wash away excess enzyme conjugate.

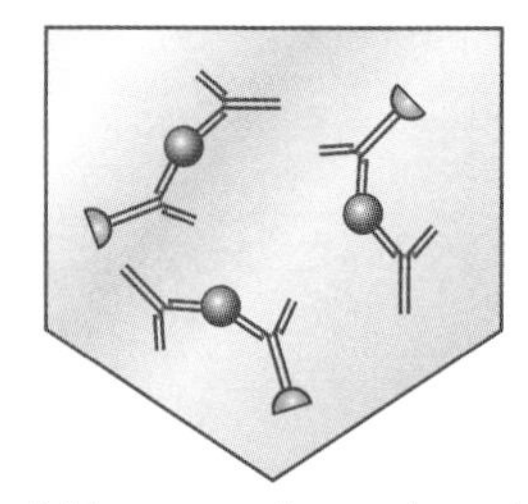
Add enzyme substrate, bound enzyme substrate initiates hydrolytic reaction, forming colored end product. Intensity of color is proportional to amount of antibody in specimen.

FIGURE 5-8 ELISA for detection of antibody.

A streptococcal antigen in throat swabs and group B streptococcal antigen in vaginal swabs. The ELISA principle is summarized in **FIGURE 5-8**.

Immunofluorescence

Fluorescence is based on the ability of fluorochrome dyes to absorb energy in the ultraviolet range and convert this energy into light at a visible wavelength. The most commonly used fluorescent dye is fluorescein isothiocyanate (FITC), which fluoresces apple green; counterstaining with rhodamine, which is a red fluorescent dye, provides contrast. In immunofluorescence, antibodies are labeled with fluorescent dyes to detect antigen in a sample. Conversely, antigen can be labeled with the dye to detect antibody. After the formation of the antigen–antibody complex, unreacted proteins and unbound antibodies are washed away. In fluorescent microscopy, the antigen–antibody complex is detected with a fluorescent microscope, which uses a mercury vapor lamp.

In **direct immunofluorescence**, or direct fluorescent antibody (DFA) techniques, the specimen is added to a microscopic slide. Next, fluoroscein-conjugated antibody is added to the slide. The specimen is incubated with the labeled antibody, at which time the antigen and antibody form a complex. Washing removes unbound antibody, and the excited fluorochromes emit visible light. DFA techniques detect only antigen. Applications include the detection of chlamydial antigen in urogenital specimens and the detection of *Bordetella pertussis* antigen in nasopharyngeal specimens.

Indirect immunofluorescence, or indirect fluorescent antibody (IFA) techniques, can detect either antigen or antibody. To detect antigen, specimen or tissue is fixed on a microscopic slide. Next, an excess of unlabeled antibody directed against the organism to be detected is added to the slide and permitted to react with the antigen present in the specimen. Incubation for 30 to 45 minutes at 35°C to 37°C permits the complexing of antigen to antibody. Unbound antibody is removed by washing. Next, a second antibody, such as fluoroscein-labeled immunoglobulin, is added. If the first antibody has formed a complex with the antigen, the second labeled antibody will now bind to the complex. After a second wash to remove unbound antibody, fluorescence is detected using a fluorescent microscope.

IFA to detect antibody usually involves the detection of antibody present in the specimen to antigens that are fixed on a microscopic slide. The microscopic slide contains wells that hold viral- or bacterial-infected tissue culture cells. Patient serum is serially diluted and added to the wells. After incubation and washing to remove unbound antibody, a fluorescein-labeled conjugate is added to each slide area. After a second washing, the slide is examined microscopically for fluorescence. Because the patient's serum is serially diluted, the amount of antibody present can be quantitated. The end point of the reaction or titer of antibody is the highest dilution showing positive fluorescence.

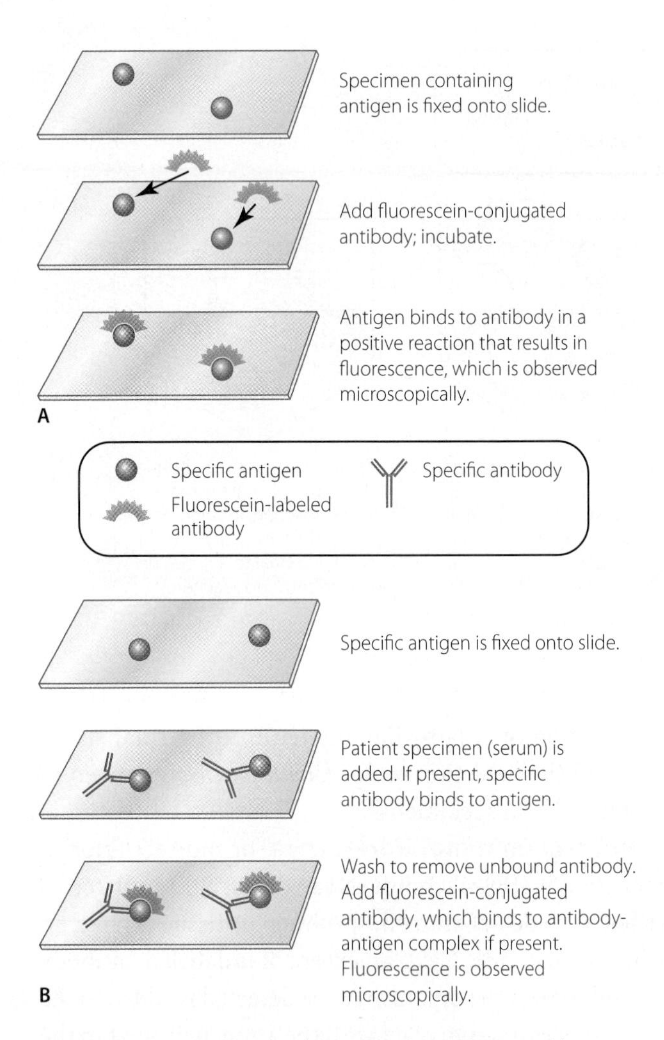

FIGURE 5-9 Immunofluorescence illustrating (A) direct fluorescent antibody (DFA) for detection of antigen and (B) indirect fluorescent antibody (IFA) for detection of antibody.

Fluorescent techniques are labor intensive but very sensitive. The indirect method is considered to be more sensitive and offers the advantage of using a single fluorescent conjugate for the detection of several antibodies. In DFA, a specifically labeled fluorescent conjugate is required for each antigen to be detected.

Immunofluorescent techniques are shown in **FIGURE 5-9**.

Immunoserological Techniques

Immunoserological techniques also can be used to detect an individual's humoral immune response to a particular pathogen. On primary exposure to an antigen, the majority of the immune response is in the form of immunoglobulin M (IgM). Eventually, IgG will replace some of the IgM produced. Although IgM can bind more antigens because it is a larger molecule and has more binding sites, IgG is more specific and can bind the antigen more effectively. A second encounter with the same antigen results in the production of only IgG. This is known as the anamnestic response, and large amounts of IgG are produced very quickly because type B lymphocytes have retained memory of the first exposure with the antigen.

ACUTE AND CONVALESCENT PHASE SPECIMENS

Serum to detect patient antibody production to a particular pathogen should be collected when the disease is first suspected. This sample is known as the **acute phase specimen**. The **antibody titer** is the reciprocal of the highest dilution of the patient's serum in which antibody is detected. The antibody titer in the acute phase specimen is usually very low or absent, assuming this is the patient's first contact with the organism. A second specimen, or **convalescent phase specimen**, is collected while the patient is recovering or convalescing. This specimen is usually drawn 2 weeks after the acute phase specimen, although the time may vary depending on the microorganism. In a current infection, the antibody titer in the convalescent phase specimen will show an increase in titer compared with the acute phase. For the test to be diagnostic, a fourfold increase, or two doubling dilutions in the patient's antibody titer in the two specimens, is required. For example, if the acute specimen showed positive in a 1:4 dilution, the convalescent specimen must show positive results in at least a 1:16 dilution.

Because individuals may develop antibody to a particular pathogen without having the infectious disease, paired sera are recommended to diagnose current disease. For example, an individual may have an antibody titer to a virus from being an asymptomatic carrier, having a prior infection, or having a subclinical infection. Although the antibody titer may be positive, it simply indicates prior exposure and may not indicate a current infectious disease. Thus, it is important to collect the acute and convalescent sera at the correct time in the physiology of the disease so that results can be compared.

To determine whether an individual has been exposed to a particular agent, a single serum sample can be used.

For example, to determine whether an individual has been immunized to varicella-zoster, the viral agent in chickenpox, a serum sample can be collected to determine whether the individual has antibodies to the viral antigens.

IMMUNOSEROLOGICAL APPLICATIONS

Many of the immunochemical techniques previously described also are applied to immunoserological testing. **Precipitin tests** detect the formation of a fine precipitate that denotes the reaction of soluble antigen with antibody. An example is the **flocculation test**, known as the **Venereal Disease Research Laboratories, or VDRL**, test, which detects the compound **reagin**, an antibody-like compound that binds to the antigen (cardiolipin-lecithin-coated cholesterol). The VDRL was used in the past as a screening test for syphilis but has been replaced in most instances by the **rapid plasma reagin, or RPR**. The VDRL remains the method of choice to detect neurosyphilis. The RPR uses a reaction card and cardiolipin-lecithin-coated cholesterol with choline chloride and visible charcoal particles to aid in identification of flocculation. Both tests can produce biological false-positives as a result of cross-reacting antibodies, as may be produced in autoimmune diseases and other infectious diseases.

Direct whole particle agglutination can be used to detect antibody in an individual's serum. The antigen is attached to a particle, such as a latex bead, and the serum antibody will agglutinate in a positive reaction. Red blood cells also can be used as the carrier for the antigen. The microhemagglutination test for *Treponema pallidum* uses red blood cells coated with antigens from an organism. In a positive reaction, the patient's antibodies bind to the bacterial antigens, as evidenced by hemagglutination.

Counterimmunelectrophoresis may be used to detect small amounts of antibody; patient serum and the antigen of interest are placed in adjacent wells in an agarose plate. After application of an electric current, a positive reaction is noted by a precipitin band at the zone of equivalence. In neutralization tests, the presence of an antibody that blocks the actions of a virus or bacterium is detected. Streptolysin O is an extracellular product produced by *Streptococcus pyogenes*. The production of antistreptolysin O is an indicator of prior infection with this organism.

ELISA techniques also are useful in detecting the presence of specific antibody to a variety of infectious agents, especially viruses. There are commercially available methods to identify serum antibodies to the hepatitis viruses, herpes simplex viruses types 1 and 2, respiratory syncytial virus, cytomegalovirus, human immunodeficiency virus, rubella virus, *Mycoplasma*, and other infectious agents. ELISA methods have been adapted to detect only IgM-type antibody and separate it from IgG from the same infectious agent.

Membrane-bound ELISA offers increased sensitivity. The slot blot and dot blot modifications force the target antigen through a membrane filter. After adding the patient's serum, the antibody will bind to the antigen on the dot or slot. The second labeled antibody is added and binds to the antigen–antibody complex in a positive reaction. A particle chromogenic pattern develops on the slot or dot, which facilitates interpretation. Many of these methods have incorporated positive and negative controls within the system. There are many membrane-bound ELISA methods that use a cassette framework in which single specimens can be tested.

Immunofluorescent assays to detect patient antibody use antigens that are fixed onto a glass slide. If the patient has the corresponding antibody, it will bind to the specific antigen. Washing removes any unbound antibody, and a conjugate and antihuman globulin are added. The globulin may be specific for IgG or IgM and is labeled with a fluorescent dye. A positive reaction is indicated by fluorescence. These assays are available for *Legionella*, *Borrelia burgdorferi*, *Toxoplasma gondii*, varicella-zoster virus, cytomegalovirus, and herpes simplex viruses types 1 and 2. Another application is the fluorescent treponemal antibody-absorbtion (FTA-ABS) test, which detects antibody to *Treponema pallidum*.

Very specific antibody proteins can be detected using the **Western blot** technique. Endonuclease is used to cleave the DNA or RNA of an organism. The proteins are separated using agarose gel electrophoresis and blotted onto a nitrocellulose gel. Next, serum suspected of containing a specific antibody is reacted with the gel. If the antibody is present, it will bind to the specific viral nucleic acids. Enzyme-labeled or fluorescent-labeled probes are used to visualize the reaction. Western blot thus uses a protein sample with an immunoglobulin detector.

Even though Western blot methods are very specific, they are very cumbersome techniques to perform in the routine clinical microbiology laboratory. The techniques are used in reference and research laboratories. The confirmatory test for human immunodeficiency virus (HIV), which identifies specific protein (p) or glycoprotein (gp) bands (p24, gp41, and gp120/160), is one application of Western blot.

Introduction to Molecular Techniques

Molecular techniques have added a new dimension to clinical microbiology and are useful when traditional phenotypic methods are not available or not practical. These methods offer sensitivity and rapid identification in specific circumstances. For example, certain microorganisms, such as viruses, cannot be cultivated on traditional culture media. Other infectious agents, such as *Mycobacterium tuberculosis*, require long incubation periods to grow and perform and interpret phenotypical reactions. For other microorganisms, such as for chlamydia, there may be no practical traditional method of identification. In other cases, such as with *Bacillus anthracis*, culturing the organism may present an extreme biohazard for the microbiologist. Molecular testing is particularly useful in the identification of viruses and the determination of the viral load. Molecular techniques may be used as a supplement to or instead of traditional methods of culture and identification.

NUCLEIC ACID PROBES

Nucleic acid, or **genetic, probes** are short, specific sequences of single-stranded deoxyribonucleic acid (DNA) or ribonucleic acid (RNA). Their purpose is to identify one or more sequences of interest within the nucleic acid. Probes form strong covalent bonds with the specific complementary nucleic acid strand. Probes contain the known, labeled sequence of DNA or RNA and are used to detect complementary sequences in target nucleotides. The target nucleic acid is the sequence of interest to be identified in a clinical specimen or culture. Most nucleic acid probes are synthetic oligonucleotides that range in size from 15 to 1,000 nucleotides; most probes contain approximately 20 to 50 bases. Probes permit identification at the taxonomic level directly in the clinical specimen or following isolation through culture. There are several formats, which include liquid phase, solid phase, and in situ hybridization. Liquid phase hybridization, which is used by Gen-Probe, Inc., is most commonly used.

Production of Probe Nucleic Acid

The nucleic acid probe must be produced and labeled first; the composition of the probe depends on the desired target nucleic acid and also on the level of identification needed. For example, should the probe be produced to identify to the genus or species level? Early probes were produced by using recombinant DNA and cloning techniques that incorporated the nucleic acid sequence. The organism was lysed, freeing the DNA. The DNA was treated with bacterial endonuclease enzymes that broke the viral DNA into small segments. Restriction endonuclease enzymes that recognized small sequences of DNA and cleaved the DNA near the restriction site were used. These small segments were then inserted into the DNA of a plasmid vector. The plasmid was a small, circular, self-replicating DNA molecule present in bacteria. Foreign genetic material was introduced into the plasmid and amplified as the plasmid replicated. Thus the plasmid multiplied in the bacterial host. The plasmids were released from the host and isolated based on molecular weight and charge. The DNA fragment, or probe, that matched the original sequence was isolated, purified, and labeled with a radioactive tag, the drug digoxigenin, or biotin.

Today, nucleic acid probes are chemically synthesized with instrumentation and are commercially available. By providing the manufacturer with the needed base sequence, the probe can be produced. Online directories that provide nucleotide base sequences for probes are also available.

Detection of Hybridization with Labels or Reporter Molecules

To detect hybridization, a labeled molecule or reporter molecule is used to visualize the probe and detect the reaction. This molecule forms a chemical complex with the single-stranded probe DNA. Probes may be labeled with biotin-avidin, digoxigenin, radioactive labels, or chemiluminescent markers. Radioactive reporters use ^{32}P, ^{125}I, and ^{35}S labels; X-ray film is placed in contact with the labeled hybridized duplex. Black areas on the film are found where radioactivity is emitted from the probe that has bound to the target. The result is read using autoradiography. Although radioactive labels are very sensitive, disadvantages include expense, a short half-life, and safety and disposal problems.

Biotinylation uses a biotin-labeled probe and the protein avidin, which has been conjugated to the enzyme horseradish peroxidase. After the biotin-labeled probe forms a hybridized duplex with the target nucleic acid, the avidin-enzyme complex is added and binds to the hybridized duplex. Next a chromogenic substrate is added, which is hydrolyzed by the biotin-avidin-enzyme complex. A positive hybridization is detected colorimetrically and read in a spectrophotometer.

Digoxigenin-labeled probes use antidigoxigenin antibodies that have been bound to an enzyme. If a hybrid duplex forms, the enzyme acts on a chromogenic substrate, leading to the production of color. Fluorescent tags also can be used instead of enzymes in digoxigenin-labeled assays.

Chemiluminescent labels measure light emission. The probe is labeled with acidium, and if it forms a hybridized duplex with the target nucleic acid, light is emitted. The light is measured with a luminometer. This is the technology used by Gen-Probe.

Preparation of Target Nucleic Acid

The target nucleic acid must be single stranded, yet the base sequence and integrity must be maintained. Preparation involves enzymatic or chemical treatment of the cell wall to release the target nucleic acid and stabilization to maintain the integrity of the nucleic acid. DNA targets must be denatured to single-stranded DNA so that it can bind to the complementary probe. RNA targets can remain as double-stranded nucleic acids.

Hybridization of Target and Probe

Hybridization is the interaction between two single-stranded nucleic acid molecules to form a double-stranded molecule. The degree of hybridization between the target and the probe depends on the degree of base sequence homology and the environmental reaction conditions. These two factors determine the stringency of the reaction. Stringency is the combination of conditions in which the target is exposed to the probe. Environmental conditions that can affect stringency include the salt concentration, temperature, and concentration of destabilizing agents. A high degree of stringency would require a high degree of base pair complements between the target and probe, whereas a lesser degree of stringency would tolerate fewer base pairings. The desired stringency depends on the purpose of the assay; for example, a higher stringency is needed to detect at the species level compared to the genus level. If a stringency is set too high, more exact target to probe binding is needed; if the stringency is set too low, there may be nonspecific binding of the target to the probe.

Detection of Hybridization and Reaction Formats

Detection of hybridization depends on the type of label reporter molecule used to label the nucleic acid and the type of hybridization format. Autoradiography is used to measure radioisotope labels. Colorimetry is measured with the spectrophotometer; fluorescence, with a fluorometer; and chemiluminescence, with a luminometer.

There are also various formats in which the reaction can take place. In the solution format, the probe and target are mixed in a liquid reaction media. This facilitates quick binding, but the nonhybridized probe must be separated from the hybridized probe *before* detection of hybridization.

Solid support formats include filter hybridization, southern hybridization, sandwich, in situ, and peptide nucleic acid (PNA) probes. In filter hybridization, the sample is fixed onto a nitrocellulose or nylon membrane. The target nucleic acid is released and denatured to single-stranded DNA. The labeled probe is added, and after incubation, hybrids form. The membrane is washed to remove unbound probe, and the membrane is processed to detect the hybrid duplexes. Southern hybridization also uses a membrane format, but the nucleic acid target first has been purified from the microorganism and digested with enzymes to produce nucleic acid fragments, which are stained with the fluorescent dye ethidium bromide. These target fragments are separated by gel electrophoresis and transferred to a membrane where they are denatured to single strands. A labeled probe is added, and hybridization with the target fragment occurs, which is detected by the reporter molecule.

In the sandwich method, two probes are used. The first probe, which is not labeled, attaches to a solid-support medium where it hybridizes and captures target nucleic acid from the sample, forming a duplex. The second probe, which is specific for another portion of the target sequence, detects the duplex, forming a "sandwich" of the target between the two probes. Sandwich techniques increase specificity but require additional processing and washing steps. The usual solid-support system consists of plastic microtiter wells that are coated with probes that can accommodate multiple specimens and facilitate the washing and processing steps.

In situ hybridization uses patient cells or tissues as solid support. Formalin-fixed or paraffin-embedded tissues contain the infectious agent that is processed to release the nucleic acid while maintaining the integrity of the cells and tissue. A histopathology examination also can be performed on in situ hybridization slides; however, the method is complex to perform.

Peptide nucleic acid (PNA) probes use synthetic pieces of DNA that have a neutral polyamide structure instead of a negatively charged sugar–phosphate chain. The repetitive units of polyamide attach to nucleotide bases rapidly and then can be used as probes to hybridize to the nucleic acid target molecules. PNA probes are very specific and attach with more speed than do other nucleic acid probes; they are not denatured by enzymes and do not expire as quickly as nucleic acid probes. Applications of PNA probes include the identification of bacteria in blood cultures within 2 to 3 hours through the fluorescent in situ hybridization technique.

AMPLIFICATION METHODS

Polymerase chain reaction was first developed in 1985 and was heralded as the new gold standard in clinical microbiology. Because a single copy of a nucleic acid may go undetected, a practical method to amplify the nucleic acid to improve sensitivity was developed. The most widely used method to amplify the target nucleic acid is polymerase chain reaction. The nucleic acid or target may be amplified.

Amplification of Nucleic Acids

In signal amplification, there is an increased concentration of labeled molecule attached to target nucleic acid but no increase in the concentration of the probe or the target. Signal amplification uses multiple enzymes and many layers of probes, which reduce background noise and enhance detection. The amount of target is not alerted, so the signal is directly proportional to the amount of target sequence present in the clinical specimen. Signal amplification is not affected by enzyme inhibitors in specimens. Another advantage is the use of simple extraction methods.

Branched DNA (bDNA) is solid-phase sandwich hybridization that uses multiple sets of synthetic probes. This methodology uses an amplifier molecule, which is a bDNA molecule with 15 identical branches, each able to bind to three labeled probes. Applications include the Siemens Healthcare Diagnostics bDNA assays for human immunodeficiency virus type 1 (HIV-1) RNA, hepatitis B virus (HBV) DNA, and hepatitis C virus (HCV) RNA. These reactions are read automatically in instruments, which are the System 340 and 440 analyzers.

Hybrid capture assays are a solution hybridization antibody capture method with chemiluminescence detection of the hybrid molecules. Target DNA specimen is denatured and then hybridized with a specific RNA probe. The DNA–RNA hybrids are "captured" by antihybrid antibodies, which are coated to the surface of a tube. Alkaline–phosphatase conjugated antihybrid antibodies bind to the DNA–RNA hybrids. Bound antibody is detected with chemiluminescent substrate, and light is measured with a luminometer. The signal is amplified because multiple alkaline phosphatase conjugates bind to each hybrid molecule. Applications of hybrid capture assays from Qiagen include the identification of *Neisseria gonorrhoeae*, *Chlamydia trachomatis*, human papillomavirus (HPV), and *Cytomegalovirus* (CMV) in clinical specimens.

Target Amplification

In target amplification, an enzyme or multiple enzymes produce copies of the target nucleic acid. The amplification products are detected by two oligonucleotide primers that bind to complementary sequences on opposite strands of double-stranded targets. Target amplification leads to the production of millions of copies of the targeted sequence in a few hours. These products then act as templates for subsequent amplification cycles. Cross-contamination can occur, which leads to false-positives; thus, laboratory designs to minimize contamination must be established.

In polymerase chain reaction (PCR), millions of copies of the desired nucleic acid sequence are produced. This process involves cycling at one temperature to first separate or denature the double-stranded nucleic acid into single strands so that it can be replicated. Heating the sample to 94°C to 96°C disrupts the microorganism, which releases the target nucleic acid and denatures the target DNA into single strands.

Primers are short sequences of nucleic acid (20–30 nucleotides in length), which are selected to anneal or hybridize to a particular nucleic acid target. The primer is selected based on the purpose of the technique. For example, is this a genus- or species-specific probe, or is the purpose to identify virulence genes or antibiotic-resistant genes?

The next step in the process is annealing. The extracted target and primers are added to covalent ions, buffers, and enzymes in the reaction mixture. The thermal cycler holds the reaction vessel and carries the PCR reaction through each step, including amplification. With the use of heat-stable enzymes, thermal cyclers can be used that move the reaction mix quickly through each required incubation temperature.

The target nucleic acid must be single stranded for annealing to occur. For RNA, however, the target nucleic acid does not need to be single stranded. Cooling to 50°C to 70°C enables the primers to anneal to the target DNA. During annealing, the primers pair with the denatured DNA: one primer anneals to the specific site at one end of the target sequence of one target strand, and the other primer anneals to the specific site at the opposite end of the other complementary target strand. The duplexes form in the last step of the cycle, mimicking DNA replication. The primer–target duplex is extended as primers anneal to the targets, forming a template.

The third step in the process is primer extension. DNA synthesis occurs by forming a copy of the template DNA by adding nucleotides to the hybridized probe. DNA polymerase can add nucleotides to the 3' end of each primer, producing an extension of the sequence complementary to the target template. *Taq* polymerase, which is an enzyme produced by thermophilic bacteria, catalyzes the extension of primers at 68°C to 72°C. All of the required components (target nucleic acid, primers, buffers, DNAs) are placed in a reaction tube, where denaturation, annealing, and extension occur. The primer extension products are dissociated from the target DNA by heating. Now, each extension product and the original target act as templates for subsequent cycles of annealing and extension.

Each target in the original mixtures produces two double-stranded fragments, which double with each cycle. For example, in the second cycle, the denatured DNA now produces four templates to which primers anneal, so at the end of the second cycle, there are four double-stranded fragments. Therefore, after each cycle the target nucleic acid doubles, and within 30 to 40 cycles, there are between 10^7 to 10^9 copies in the reaction vessel. The product is detected using colorimetric, fluorometric, chemiluminescent, or radioactive signals to detect a probe hybridized with the **amplicon**, or amplified target nucleic acid.

Applications of PCR

Reverse transcriptase PCR (RT-PCR) is used to amplify RNA targets. In this method, cDNA is formed from RNA targets using reverse transcription followed by amplification of the cDNA using PCR. Thermostable DNA polymerase from thermophilic bacteria can be used as both an RT and a DNA polymerase. Earlier RT-PCR used two separate enzymes, which led to nonspecific primer annealing and poor primer extension.

Nested PCR uses two pairs of amplification primers. The first primer pair is used for the first 15 to 30 cycles. It produces an amplicon that is used as a target sequence for the second amplification, which uses the second set of primers. Nested PCR has a high sensitivity as a result of the high total cycle number and high specificity because of the annealing of the second primer set to sequences found in the first set of products. The second amplicon confirms the accuracy of the first DNA manipulation. This system may be prone to contamination, which may occur during transfer of first-round products to tubes for second amplification.

Multiplex testing uses two or more primer pairs to amplify different targets in the same reaction mixture. The first primer pair is the control, or general primer, and is directed toward many sequences, and the second primer can be directed at a specific gene. In multiplex testing, many different targets can be used within one reaction. For example, respiratory infections caused by a panel of bacterial and viral respiratory pathogens that produce similar symptoms in the patient can be tested within one assay. For instance, a multiplex system with RT-PCR can detect influenza A, influenza B, respiratory syncytial virus A and B, parainfluenza virus, rhinovirus, enterovirus, and coronavirus.

Real-time PCR is based on PCR technology and utilizes small automated systems that combine target nucleic acid amplification with the qualitative or quantitative measurement of amplified product. These systems use instruments or platforms that utilize amplification with real-time detection of the product. Real-time PCR has many advantages, which include the ability to detect the amplified target nucleic acid by fluorescent-labeled probes as the hybrids form. Cross-contamination between samples is lessened because amplification and product detection occur in one reaction vessel. Real-time PCR methods also can measure the amount of amplicon and, thus, can quantify the number of copies of target nucleic acid in the original specimen. Real-time PCR requires less time than does conventional PCR because of the use of fluorescent probes and their very rapid thermal cycling.

Restriction Fragment Length Polymorphisms

Restriction fragment length polymorphisms (RFLPs) involve the use of restriction endonuclease enzymes, followed by electrophoresis of the DNA segments. This identification method has high specificity but not to the degree provided by nucleic acid sequencing. An endonuclease enzyme recognizes a specific nucleotide sequence and then catalyzes the digestion of the nucleic acid, which forms a break in the sequence. The endonuclease enzymes selected have only a few restriction sites; each DNA molecule produces 10 to 20 DNA fragments that are 10 to 1,000 kilobases in size. The resulting fragments are separated on agarose gel, using pulsed-field electrophoresis, whereby the DNA pieces separate according to size, with the smaller fragments migrating faster and to a greater distance. By varying the voltage and time, the fragments are separated out into bands. The resulting nucleic acid bands are stained with ethidium blue, a fluorescent dye that binds to the nucleic acid bands. These bands can be photographed and maintained; the particular pattern is known as a restriction pattern. The differences between the restriction patterns of microorganisms are known as restriction fragment length polymorphisms.

RFLPs are indicators of the differences or likenesses in nucleotide sequences and thus can be used to identify organisms and determine strain relatedness between species. One application is the APTIMA Combo 2® Assay for *Neisseria gonorrhoeae*, which is a target amplification nucleic acid probe test that utilizes target capture for the in vitro qualitative detection of ribosomal RNA (rRNA) from *Neisseria gonorrhoeae.* The reaction can be read using the TIGRIS® DTS® Automated Analyzer or semiautomated instrumentation.

NUCLEIC ACID SEQUENCING

Nucleic acid sequencing is used to determine the nucleotide sequence of a nucleic acid segment from an infectious agent. The exact nucleotide sequence from a microorganism can be identified in a clinical specimen or a culture. An amplified target from the microorganism and an automated DNA sequence analyzer are used. Today, several commercially available automated systems exist for automated sequencing.

Nucleic acid sequencing may be used to identify an organism in a clinical specimen or from an organism grown in culture. These methods have high sensitivity when combined with target or signal amplification. They are particularly useful in cases where the organism cannot be grown on traditional culture media. They also are useful for those pathogens that do not require antimicrobial susceptibility testing to be performed.

Nucleic acid sequencing also is used to determine strain relatedness, which is used in the investigation of health care–associated infections. It is used to identify a common source of isolates in an outbreak, when the need exists to identify beyond the species level. Molecular methods compare nucleotide sequences between strains or find similar sequences in nucleotide sequences in the outbreak isolate. These are used in following antimicrobial resistance in health care–associated infections, such as in methicillin-resistant *Staphylococcus aureus* and vancomycin-resistant *Enterococcus*, *Escherichia coli*, *Klebsiella*, and *Enterobacter.* Nucleic acid sequencing is used as an adjunct to traditional phenotypic methods to detect antibiotic resistance. PCR can be used to detect certain resistance profiles, such as the *van* genes that mediate resistance to vancomycin in *Enterococcus* and the *mec* gene for β-lactam resistance in *Staphylococcus.* Applications of molecular based methods used in microbiology are summarized in BOX 5-2.

BOX 5-3 shows a partial list of current applications of molecular diagnostics in clinical microbiology.

BOX 5-2 **Applications of Molecular-Based Methods in Microbiology**

1. Direct detection of organisms in clinical specimens

   Nucleic acid hybridization

   Target and probe amplification

   Benefits:

   - Specificity: positive assay shows presence and identification of microorganism and follow-up culture may not be needed.
   - For certain microorganisms, there is no need to do antimicrobial susceptibility testing.
   - Existing reliable tests are slow or not available.
   - Need to quantify viral load (HIV in AIDS).

   Limitations:

   - High specificity limits that can be detected, especially in mixed infections.
   - Sensitivity may be low if there are small amounts of organism in patient specimen; amplification increases sensitivity.
   - Also may need antibiotic resistance testing for certain microorganisms.

2. Identification of microorganisms in culture

   Apply hybridization, amplification, or RFLP to organism grown in culture.

   Benefits:

   - Sensitivity not a problem because high concentration of organism's nucleic acid is available.
   - Reduced time to identify compared to that of traditional phenotypic methods.

   Comments:

   - Some methods are labor intensive, while others provide quicker results.

3. Additional characteristics of microorganisms

   - Strain relatedness: used in health care–associated infection to identify common source of isolates in an outbreak.
   - Uses RFLPs and pulsed-field gel electrophoresis (PFGE): methicillin-resistant *Staphylococcus aureus*, vancomycin-resistant *Enterococcus* and gram-negative bacilli (*E. coli*, *Klebsiella*, *Enterobacter*)
   - Recurrent infection in same patient: Is it the same strain or one that has developed resistance?
   - Antimicrobial resistance: use as adjunct to traditional phenotypic methods to detect resistance. PCR can be used to detect certain resistance profiles, such as the *van* genes, which mediate resistance to vancomycin in *Enterococcus*, and the *mec* gene for β-lactam resistance in *Staphylococcus*.

BOX 5-3 **Examples of Current Technologies of Molecular Diagnostics**

Gen-Probe

- **AMPLIFIED MTD® (Mycobacterium Tuberculosis Direct) Test** detects *Mycobacterium tuberculosis* rRNA directly. The test is specific for *Mycobacterium tuberculosis* complex.
- **APTIMA Combo 2® Assay** is a target amplification nucleic acid probe test that utilizes target capture for the in vitro qualitative detection and differentiation of ribosomal RNA (rRNA) from *Chlamydia trachomatis* (CT) and/or *Neisseria gonorrhoeae* (GC).
- **APTIMA® HPV Assay** is an in vitro nucleic acid amplification test for the qualitative detection of E6/E7 viral messenger RNA (mRNA) from 14 high-risk types of human papillomavirus (HPV) in cervical specimens. The high-risk HPV types detected by the assay include 16, 18, 31, 33, 35, 39, 45, 51, 52, 56, 58, 59, 66, and 68.
- **APTIMA® Trichomonas vaginalis Assay** is a nucleic acid amplification test (NAAT) for the detection of *T. vaginalis*.
- **GASDirect® Test for Group A Streptococcus** is a DNA probe assay that uses nucleic acid hybridization for the qualitative detection of group A streptococcal RNA directly from throat swabs.
- **ACCUPROBE® Group B Streptococcus Assay** is a rapid DNA probe test that utilizes the techniques of nucleic acid hybridization for the identification of group B streptococcus from cultures based on the detection of specific ribosomal RNA sequences that are unique to *Streptococcus agalactiae*.
- **Prodesse® ProFlu™+** is a real-time multiplex RT-PCR kit for detection and differentiation of influenza A, influenza B, and respiratory syncytial virus. There is also a real-time multiplex RT-PCR kit for detection and differentiation of parainfluenza 1, 2, and 3 viruses (Prodesse® ProParaflu®+).
- **APTIMA® HIV-1 RNA Qualitative Assay** is an in vitro nucleic acid assay system for the detection of human immunodeficiency virus (HIV-1) in human plasma and serum (HIV and HIV-1 screening).
- **APTIMA® HCV Assay** is an in vitro nucleic acid amplification assay for the detection of HCV RNA in human plasma or serum (HCV screening). Detection of HCV RNA is evidence of active HCV infection.
- **Prodesse® ProGastro® Cd Assay** is a real-time PCR kit for detection of toxigenic strains of *Clostridium difficile*.

Neogen (formerly Gene-Trak)

- **GeneQuence®** are rapid pathogen detection assays that utilize DNA hybridization technology in a microwell format to detect *Salmonella*, *Listeria*, or *Listeria monocytogenes*.
- **NeoSEEK™** is a pathogen detection and identification technology that provides next-day, DNA-specific test results for pathogenic STEC *E. coli* strains.

AvanDx

- **PNA FISH®**

  Once a blood culture turns positive, a Gram stain is performed, and based on the results the appropriate PNA FISH test is selected, which is a qualitative nucleic acid hybridization assay. Identification results are available within just a few hours.

  Applications of **PNA FISH®** include Group B Streptococcus, Gram Negative Rods—*E. coli/P. aeruginosa*,a and *Candida. albicans*

Abbott Molecular

- **RealTime CT/NG assay** is an in vitro polymerase chain reaction (PCR) assay for the direct, qualitative detection of the plasmid DNA of *Chlamydia trachomatis* and the genomic DNA of *Neisseria gonorrhoeae*. The method is a multiplex, homogeneous real-time PCR assay.
- **RealTime HCV assay** is an in vitro reverse transcription-polymerase chain reaction (RT-PCR) assay for the quantitation of hepatitis C virus (HCV) RNA in human serum or plasma (EDTA) from HCV-infected individuals.
- **RealTime HIV-1 assay** is an in vitro reverse transcription-polymerase chain reaction (RT-PCR) assay for the quantitation of human immunodeficiency virus type 1 (HIV-1).

- **RealTime HBV assay** is an in vitro polymerase chain reaction (PCR) assay for the quantitation of hepatitis B virus (HBV) DNA.
- **ViroSeq® HIV-1 Genotyping System** is intended for use in detecting HIV genomic mutations that confer resistance to specific types of antiretroviral drugs, as an aid in monitoring and treating HIV infection.

Luminex Corporation

- **xTAG® Respiratory Viral Panel (RVP)** is a qualitative nucleic acid multiplex test intended for the simultaneous detection and identification of multiple respiratory virus nucleic acids in nasopharyngeal swabs from individuals suspected of respiratory tract infections. The following virus types and subtypes are identified using RVP: influenza A; influenza A subtype H1; influenza A subtype H3; influenza B; respiratory syncytial virus subtype A; respiratory syncytial virus subtype B; parainfluenza 1, 2, and 3 virus; human metapneumovirus; rhinovirus; and adenovirus.

Roche Molecular Diagnostics

- **AMPLICOR® CT/NG Test** is a qualitative in vitro test for the detection of *Chlamydia trachomatis* and/or *Neisseria gonorrhoea* with the polymerase chain reaction (PCR) nucleic acid amplification technique and nucleic acid hybridization for the detection of CT and/or NG.
- **COBAS® AMPLICOR CMV MONITOR Test** (automated cytomegalovirus (CMV) viral load quantification) is an in vitro nucleic acid amplification test for the quantification of human CMV DNA.
- **COBAS® AmpliPrep/COBAS® AMPLICOR HCV Test, v2.0. Hepatitis C Virus (HCV) detection**; in vitro diagnostic nucleic acid amplification test for the qualitative detection of HCV RNA.
- **COBAS® AmpliPrep/COBAS® TaqMan® CMV Test** is an in vitro nucleic acid amplification test for the quantitation of cytomegalovirus DNA. The test can quantitate CMV DNA over a range of 150 to 10,000,000 copies/ml.
- **COBAS® AmpliScreen HBV Test** is a qualitative in vitro test for the direct detection of hepatitis B virus (HBV) DNA.
- **LightCycler® MRSA Advanced Test** is a qualitative in vitro diagnostic test for the direct detection of nasal colonization with methicillin-resistant *Staphylococcus aureus* (MRSA). Uses polymerase chain reaction (PCR) for the amplification of MRSA DNA and fluorogenic target-specific hybridization probes for the detection of the amplified DNA.
- **LightCycler® CMV Quantitative Kit** is an in vitro diagnostic assay used for the rapid quantitative detection of cytomegalovirus (CMV) DNA utilizing real-time polymerase chain reaction (PCR) technology.
- **LightCycler® EBV Quantitative Kit** is an in vitro diagnostic assay used for the rapid quantitative detection of Epstein-Barr virus (EBV) DNA utilizing real-time polymerase chain reaction (PCR) technology.
- **LightCycler® HSV 1/2 Qualitative Kit** is intended for detection of HSV DNA and differentiation between HSV-1 and HSV-2 in human cerebrospinal fluid (CSF) samples or vesicle material. It is an in vitro diagnostic assay that utilizes real-time PCR amplification of nucleic acids for detection of HSV DNA.
- **COBAS® AmpliScreen HCV Test** is a PCR test that detects the presence of HCV RNA in plasma of blood, organ, and tissue donors.
- **COBAS® HPV Test** is a qualitative multiplex assay that provides specific genotyping information for HPV types 16 and 18 while concurrently detecting the other 12 high-risk HPV types in a pooled result.
- **COBAS® TaqMan® MTB Test** uses real-time PCR nucleic acid amplification and hydrolysis probes for qualitative detection of *Mycobacterium tuberculosis* (MTB) complex DNA in liquefied, decontaminated, and concentrated human respiratory specimens, including expectorated and induced sputum and bronchoalveolar lavages (BAL).
- **LightCycler® VZV Qualitative Kit** is an in vitro diagnostic assay used for the rapid detection of varicella-zoster virus (VZV) DNA utilizing real-time polymerase chain reaction (PCR) technology.
- **LINEAR ARRAY Hepatitis C Virus Genotyping Test** is an in vitro test to be used for determining the genotype of the hepatitis C virus. The test detects six major hepatitis C virus genotypes: 1, 2, 3, 4, 5, and 6.

Sources: Gen-Probe, Inc., San Diego, CA; Neogen Corp., Lansing, MI; AdvanDx, Woburn, MA; Abbott Laboratories, Abbott Park, IL; Luminex Corp., Austin, TX; and Roche Molecular Diagnostics, Pleasanton, CA.

Review Questions

Multiple Choice

1. The automated principle that utilizes a spectrophotometer to detect changes in color is:
   a. Colorimetry
   b. Nephelometry
   c. Turbimetry
   d. Fluorometry
2. Which of the following is *not* a fully automated identification system for microbiology?
   a. MicroScan
   b. VITEK
   c. Enterotube
   d. Phoenix
3. Which of the following systems uses nephelometry for the identification of microorganisms?
   a. Phoenix
   b. VITEK
   c. MicroScan
   d. None of the above
4. To detect antibody production to a particular infectious agent, the acute phase specimen should be collected:
   a. When the disease is first suspected
   b. When the disease is first diagnosed
   c. While the patient is recovering
   d. While the patient is relapsing
5. An acute phase specimen for the detection of antibody to cytomegalovirus yielded a titer of 1:8. The convalescent phase specimen yielded a titer of 1:32. This is diagnostic for a current infection of cytomegalovirus.
   a. True
   b. False
6. Febrile agglutinins are an example of ________, in which bacterial antigens aggregate in the presence of the corresponding antibody.
   a. Coagglutination
   b. Direct agglutination
   c. Indirect agglutination
   d. Flocculation
7. The procedure that detects the production of antibody blocking the actions of a microorganism is:
   a. Coagglutination
   b. Counterimmunoelectrophoresis
   c. Enzyme-linked immunosorbent assay
   d. Neutralization
8. In enzyme-linked immunosorbent assay:
   a. Antibody or antigen is bound to an enzyme, which catalyzes a reaction
   b. Noncompetitive techniques can detect antigen or antibody
   c. Substrates for reaction include horseradish peroxidase and nitrophenyl phosphate
   d. All the above
9. Indirect fluorescent antibody techniques:
   a. Can detect only antigen
   b. Use both an unlabeled antibody and labeled antibody
   c. Are not very sensitive detection methods
   d. Cannot be quantitated
10. The interaction between single-stranded nucleic acid molecules to form a double-stranded molecule is known as:
    a. Blotting
    b. Hybridization
    c. Denaturation
    d. A DNA probe
11. The molecular method that involves the synthetic amplification of a known DNA sequence using several denaturation and polymerization cycles is known as:
    a. Southern blot
    b. DNA hybridization
    c. Polymerase chain reaction
    d. DNA cloning
12. An example of a particle agglutination test is:
    a. Latex agglutination
    b. Enzyme linked immunoassay
    c. Nephelometry
    d. Double immunoelectrophoresis
13. The first step in polymerase chain reaction is:
    a. Extension of the primer
    b. Denaturation of the nucleic acid
    c. Annealing
    d. None of the above
14. Which of the following uses two or more primer pairs that amplify different targets in the same reaction mix?
    a. Nested PCR
    b. Reverse transcriptase PCR
    c. Multiplex PCR
    d. Real-time PCR
15. In ________, amplification and product detection occur in the same reaction vessel, and target nucleic acid is detected by fluorescent probes as the hybrids form.
    a. Nested PCR
    b. Reverse transcriptase PCR
    c. Multiplex PCR
    d. Real-time PCR

Bibliography

BD Phoenix™ System—The New Choice in Automated Microbiology. (2008). Available at http://www.bd.com/ds/learningCenter/labo/nl_labo_222728.pdf

Buckingham, L., & Flaws, M. L. (2007). Nucleic acid amplification. In *Molecular diagnostics: Fundamentals, methods and clinical applications.* Philadelphia, PA: F.A. Davis Company.

Carroll, K. C., Glanz, B. D., Borek, A. P., Burger, C., Bhally, H. S., Henciak, S., & Flayhart, D. (2006). Evaluation of the BD Phoenix automated system for identification and susceptibility testing of *Enterobacteriaceae. Journal of Clinical Microbiology, 44,* 3506–3509.

Dallas, S. D., Avery, A. L., Pekarek, P. M., Mills, T. J., Neal, W. J., Smallbrook, A. G., & Hejna, J. (2005). Comparison of BD Phoenix to Biomerieux Vitek for the identification and susceptibility testing of common bacterial isolates. White paper presented at the 105th General Meeting of the American Society for Microbiology. Available at http://www.bd.com/ds/technicalCenter/whitepapers/lr905.pdf

Espy, M. J., Uhl, J. R., Sloan, L. M., Buckwalter, S. P., Jones, M. F., Vetter, E. A., . . . Smith, T. F. (2006). Real-time PCR in clinical microbiology: Applications for routine laboratory testing. *Clinical Microbiology Review, 19,* 165–256.

Forbes, B. A., Sahm, D. F., & Weissfeld, A. S. (2007). Immunochemical methods used for organism detection. In *Bailey and Scott's diagnostic microbiology,* 12th ed., St. Louis, MO: Mosby.

James, K. (1990). Immunoserology of infectious disease. *Clinical Microbiology Review, 3,* 132–152.

Mahony, J. B. (2008). Detection of respiratory viruses by molecular methods. *Clinical Microbiology Review, 21,* 716–747.

Miller, M. B., & Tank, Y. W. (2009). Basic concepts of microarrays and potential applications in clinical microbiology. *Clinical Microbiology Review, 22,* 611–633.

Muthukumar, A., Zitterkoopf, N. L., & Payne, D. (2008). Molecular tools for the detection and characterization of bacterial infections: A review. *Laboratory Medicine, 39,* 430–436.

Nolte, F. S., & Caliendo, A. M. (2011). Molecular microbiology. In J. Versalovic (Ed.), *Manual of clinical microbiology,* 10th ed. Washington, DC: ASM Press.

Payne, W. J., Marshal, D. L., Shockley, R. K., & Martin, W. J. (1988). Clinical applications of monoclonal antibodies. *Clinical Microbiology Review, 1,* 313–329.

Persing, D. H. (1991). Polymerase chain reaction: Trenches to benches. *Journal of Clinical Microbiology, 29,* 1281–1285.

Pincus, D. H. (2006). Microbial identification using the bioMéreiux VITEK 2 system. In M. J. Miller (Ed.), *Encyclopedia of rapid microbiological methods,* vol. II. PDA/DHI. Available at https://store.pda.org/TableOfContents/ERMM_V2_Ch01.pdf

Sellenriek, P., Holmes, J., Ferrett, R., Drury, R., & Storch, G. A. (2005). Comparison of MicroScan Walk-Away®, Phoenix™, and VITEK-TWO® microbiology systems used in the identification and susceptibility testing of bacteria. White paper presented at the 105th General Meeting of the American Society for Microbiology. Available at http://www.bd.com/ds/technicalCenter/whitepapers/lr900.pdf

Stager, C. E., & Davis, J. R. (1992). Automated systems for identification of microorganisms. *Clinical Microbiology Review, 5,* 302–327.

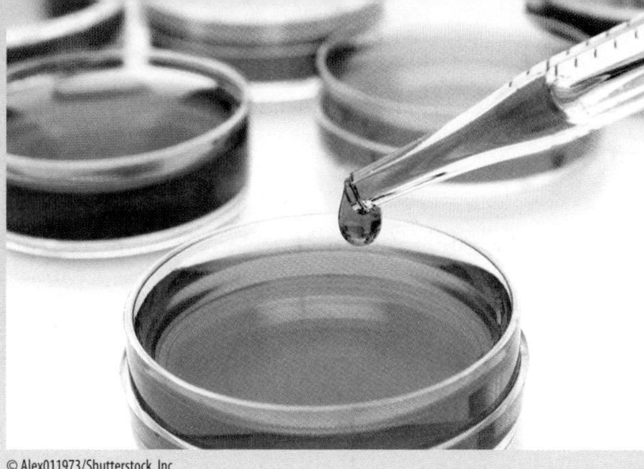

CHAPTER 6

Antimicrobial Susceptibility Testing

CHAPTER OUTLINE

Overview of Antibiotic Susceptibility Testing
Resistance to Antimicrobial Agents
Laboratory Methods for Susceptibility Testing

KEY TERMS

Acquired resistance
Additive
Antagonistic
Antibacterial agents
Antibiograms
Antibiotics
Antifungal agents
Antimicrobial agents
Antiviral agents
Autonomous
β-lactamases
Bacteriocidal agents
Bacteriostatic agents
Broad-spectrum antibiotics
Extended spectrum β-lactamase (ESBL)
Intrinsic resistance
Minimal bacteriocidal concentration
Minimal inhibitory concentration
Narrow-spectrum antibiotics
Peak and trough specimens
Plasmids
Resistant
Serum bacteriocidal test
Superinfection
Susceptible
Synergistic
Transposons

LEARNING OBJECTIVES

1. Define the following terms:
   a. Antibiotic
   b. Antimicrobial agent
   c. Bacteriocidal
   d. Bacteriostatic
2. Differentiate narrow-spectrum from broad-spectrum antibiotics.
3. Describe the factors that are considered in the selection of an antimicrobial agent.
4. State the mode of activity, give examples, and describe the spectrum for the major antibiotics and antibiotic classes including:
   a. β-lactam antibiotics (cell wall inhibitors)
   b. Alteration of cell membrane
   c. Inhibitors of protein synthesis
   d. Folic acid antimetabolites
   e. Inhibitors of DNA gyrase
5. List the important antimycobacterial agents.

6. List antiviral agents used to treat HIV and other viral infections.
7. List and describe the antifungal agents.
8. Describe acquired resistance and differentiate from intrinsic resistance.
9. Discuss the role of plasmids and transposons in antibiotic resistance.
10. Describe and give examples of the following mechanisms of resistance.
    a. Modification of target site
    b. Plasmid- or transposon-mediated resistance of target site
    c. Inactivation of antimicrobial agent by enzymes
    d. Efflux
11. Define and identify the following:
    a. Susceptible
    b. Resistant
    c. Synergistic
    d. Antagonistic
12. Describe the important test characteristics in antibiotic disk diffusion susceptibility testing that must be met to obtain consistent results.
13. Explain how the results of disk diffusion testing are affected when:
    a. Inoculum is too dense
    b. Inoculum is too light
    c. pH is too acidic
    d. Disks are placed too close together
    e. Plates are incubated in increased carbon dioxide
14. Describe how to interpret the following in disk diffusion testing:
    a. Colonies within zone of inhibition
    b. Zone overlapping
    c. Zone within a zone
    d. *Proteus* swarming into a zone of inhibition
15. Perform a minimum of five disk diffusion susceptibility tests, using the correct quality-control strains. Interpret all results without error.
16. State the principle and purpose of quantitative dilution susceptibility testing.
    a. Define minimal inhibitory concentration (MIC).
    b. Define minimal bacteriocidal concentration (MBC).
17. When given the volumes of broth, concentration and volume of antibiotic, and concentration and volume of inoculum, determine the antibiotic concentration in each dilution of a macrotube dilution susceptibility test.
18. Perform one macrobroth dilution susceptibility test, determining the MIC and MBC.
19. Perform and interpret at least four microbroth dilution susceptibility tests.
20. Explain gradient diffusion testing.
21. List the three types of procedures available for detection of β-lactamase.
22. Perform and interpret at least three β-lactamase determinations.
23. Describe the serum bacteriocidal test (SBT).
24. Explain how methicillin-resistant *Staphylococcus aureus* is detected using the oxacillin agar screen, cefoxitin disk screen, and chromogenic media.
25. Discuss how vancomycin resistance in enterococci and staphylococci is detected.
26. List and describe the major mechanisms of β-lactamase resistance.
27. Describe extended spectrum β-lactamases (ESBL), AmpC, and carbapenemase as related to resistance in gram-negative bacilli.
28. Explain how a predictor antibiotic is used in susceptibility testing.
29. Define *peak* and *trough* and relate these terms to drug assays.
30. Give the purpose of an antibiogram.

Overview of Antibiotic Susceptibility Testing

Proper selection of antimicrobial agents to treat an infection first requires the isolation and identification of the causative agent. Next, the susceptibility and resistance of the organism to several antimicrobial agents is determined. There are a variety of methods used to determine the in vitro susceptibility of microorganisms to antibiotics. There are manual and automated methods, as well as tests to determine zone diameters, and methods to identify the minimal inhibitory concentration of an antibiotic. Based on these results and other important factors, the appropriate therapy for the patient is determined and prescribed.

Antibiotics are chemical substances produced by microorganisms that inhibit the growth of other microorganisms. Some antibiotics are chemically modified. **Antimicrobial agents** are agents that destroy microorganisms through inhibiting their development or pathogenic action. Such agents may be obtained either from microorganisms or synthetically in the laboratory. More specifically, **antibacterial agents** are destructive to or inhibit the action of bacteria, **antiviral agents** inhibit or weaken the action of viruses, and **antifungal agents** inhibit the action of fungi.

Antimicrobial agents may be classified as bacteriocidal (bactericidal) or bacteriostatic. **Bacteriocidal agents** kill the microbe, resulting in cell lysis. Most often these agents are used for more serious or life-threatening infections and for infections in immunosuppressed hosts. Examples of bacteriocidal antibiotics include the penicillins and cephalosporins and vancomycin. **Bacteriostatic agents** inhibit the growth of the microorganism but rely on the host's cellular and humoral immune system to kill the microorganism. Some examples of bacteriostatic agents include tetracycline, the sulfonamides, and erythromycin. The categories may overlap, and classification of an agent as bacteriostatic or bacteriocidal also depends on the dosage, route of administration, and site of infection.

Those antimicrobial agents with a limited spectrum of action are known as **narrow-spectrum antibiotics**. For example, penicillin G is primarily effective against only gram-positive bacteria. **Broad-spectrum antibiotics** have action against both gram-positive and gram-negative bacteria. An example of a broad-spectrum antibiotic is tetracycline. A disadvantage of broad-spectrum antibiotics is the inhibition or destruction of the normal flora of the patient. A new infection, known as a secondary infection, or **superinfection**, may appear as a result of treatment of the primary infection. A superinfection follows a previous infection, especially when caused by microorganisms that have become resistant to the antibiotics used earlier. These infections occur during or after treatment of another pre-existing infection. This secondary infection, or superinfection, may result from the treatment itself or from changes in the host's immune system. For example, a vaginal yeast infection that occurs after antibiotic treatment of a bacterial infection is a secondary infection. Bacterial pneumonia after a viral upper respiratory infection is another example. Superinfections frequently involve the mouth, respiratory tract, and genitourinary tract and are often difficult to treat. Examples of organisms associated with superinfections include *Pseudomonas aeruginosa*, *Candida albicans*, and *Staphylococcus aureus*.

SELECTION OF ANTIBIOTICS

Selection of the appropriate antimicrobial agent depends on several factors. BOX 6-1 summarizes some of these important considerations.

BOX 6-1 Selection of Antimicrobial Agents

- Does the antimicrobial agent have strong lethal effects and activity against the microorganism?
- Does the agent have low toxicity toward the host?
- Is the agent least toxic toward normal flora of the host? Narrow-spectrum antibiotics should be used when possible.
- Are the appropriate pharmacological properties or mode of activity of the antibiotic effective against the microorganism?
- What is the status of the host's immune system, and what are other medical considerations, such as use of corticosteroids, prolonged antibiotic therapy, and chemotherapy?
- What is the host's organ function? Consideration should be made for renal function for drug elimination and hepatic function for biotransformation.
- Is the antimicrobial agent water soluble, and can it be distributed readily through the blood?
- Is there underlying medical disease in the host, including circulatory problems? Can the medication reach the infected site?
- What is the age of the patient? Certain agents are toxic to very young patients and may affect geriatric patients in an atypical manner.
- What is the site of infection?

(*continues*)

BOX 6-1 **Selection of Antimicrobial Agents (Continued)**

- Can effective blood or tissue levels be achieved? For example, a large polar molecular, such as vancomycin, is highly water soluble, so its major site of action is in the blood. It is not distributed very well in several other tissues. The sulfonamides, such as Bactrim and rifampin, are nonpolar; they are distributed well and can attain high concentrations in tissues other than blood.
- What is the route of administration?
- Does the antibiotic cross the placenta, which may be toxic to the fetus?
- Does the antibiotic penetrate the blood-brain barrier, which is necessary in central nervous system infections?
- Is surgical intervention a part of the treatment, such as drainage or debridement for anaerobic infections?
- How cost effective is the treatment?
- Is the host allergic or hypersensitive to the agent? Mild allergic reactions include skin rashes, hives, and urticaria, whereas more severe reactions include life-threatening anaphylaxis, which is associated with vasodilation, edema, and bronchoconstriction.

CATEGORIES AND TYPES OF ANTIBIOTICS

The mode of activity of the antibiotic is an important consideration. For example, the β-lactam antibiotics function by inhibition of cell wall synthesis. When treated with an antibiotic that inhibits cell wall synthesis, nucleotide intermediates accumulate in the cell wall, which results in cell lysis and death. Other examples of cell wall–inhibiting antibiotics include vancomycin and the cephalosporins. β-lactam antibiotics are summarized in BOX 6-2.

Other antibiotics, such as bacitracin, function by altering the bacterial cell membrane. These are summarized in BOX 6-3.

Another large group of antibiotics function by inhibition of protein synthesis. The aminoglycosides, such as tobramycin and gentamycin, interfere with the protein synthesis at the 30S ribosomal subunit. This also is the mechanism for tetracycline. Clindamycin and erythromycin inhibit protein synthesis by binding to the 50S ribosomal subunit. BOX 6-4 summarizes those antibiotics that inhibit protein synthesis.

BOX 6-2 **β-Lactam Antibiotics**

Important Facts

- All β-lactam antibiotics contain the β-lactam ring.
- Mode of activity: inhibition of cell wall synthesis by inhibition of enzymes needed for peptidoglycan formation.
- It is estimated that up to 10% of the population is hypersensitive or allergic to penicillin.

1. **Penicillins**

   A. Natural penicillins: penicillin G and penicillin V

   Source: the mold *Penicillium notatum*

   Spectrum: gram-positive spectrum other than *Staphylococcus*

   Major indication is for *Streptococcus* infections, other than *Enterococcus*

   Most *Staphylococcus* species are resistant.

   Limited gram-negative bacteria such as *Neisseria meningitidis* and *Pasteurella*, β-lactamase–negative anaerobes, and *Treponema pallidum*

   B. Penicillinase-resistant penicillins: methicillin, nafcillin, oxacillin, cloxacillin, and dicloxacillin

Various side chains added to the penicillin molecule confer resistance to penicillinase.

Spectrum: gram-positive spectrum, including *Streptococcus* and methicillin-susceptible *Staphylococcus aureus*

Active against penicillinase-producing *Staphylococcus*, although there is increased resistance to some of these agents.

C. Extended-spectrum penicillins

Chemically modified and semisynthetic

i. Aminopenicillins: ampicillin, amoxicillin, and bacampicillin

Have α-amino group added to side chain

Spectrum: extended spectrum of gram-positive and gram-negative bacteria, including *Escherichia coli, Proteus mirabilis, Haemophilus influenzae, Salmonella*, and *Shigella*. They are less active than penicillin G against *Streptococcus pneumoniae, Streptococcus pyogenes, Enterococcus*, and other gram-positive cocci.

Can penetrate outer membrane of gram-negative bacteria

ii. Carboxypenicillins: carbenicillin and ticarcillin

Have α-carboxy group added to side chain

Spectrum: primarily a gram-negative spectrum; used in treatment of serious gram-negative Enterobacteriaceae infections and *Pseudomonas aeruginosa*; may be used in combination with an aminoglycoside. *Klebsiella* species are resistant.

Can penetrate outer membrane of gram-negative bacteria

iii. Acyclaminopenicillins: azlocillin, mezlocillin, and piperacillin

Spectrum: primarily a gram-negative spectrum; greater activity against enteric bacteria and *P. aeruginosa*; also active against *H. influenzae, Serratia*, and *Bacteroides fragilis*. Synergistic activity occurs with the aminoglycosides.

iv. Ureidopenicillins: ureido or piperazine ring

Spectrum: similar to carboxypenicillins; also useful for *P. aeruginosa* and anaerobes

D. Penicillin codrugs

Combination of a β-lactam with β-lactamase inhibitor. The inhibitor binds to β-lactamase, inactivating the enzyme.

Augmentin: amoxicillin with clavulanate potassium (clavulanic acid)

Timetin: ticarcillin with clavulanate potassium (clavulanic acid)

Piperacillen/Tazobactam

Ampicillin/sulbactam: gram-negative and gram-positive spectrums. They also exhibit activity against β-lactamase–producing *Staphylococcus, H. influenzae, Bacteroides*, and other anaerobes and some enteric bacteria.

2. **Cephalosporins**

Source: fungus *Acremonium* (metabolic by-products)

The cephalosporins are structurally similar to penicillin but are better able to withstand the action of β-lactamase and are more modifiable. Original cephalosporin was cephalosporin C, which was modified to aminocephalosporanic acid, which has been further modified into first-, second-, third-, fourth-, and fifth-generation cephalosporins.

A. First-generation cephalosporins

Cephalothin, cephapirin, cefazolin, cephalexin, cefadroxil, and cephradine

Spectrum: active against gram-positive cocci, other than *Enterococcus* and methicillin-resistant *Staphylococcus aureus* (MRSA) and active against enteric bacteria, such as *E. coli, P. mirabilis*, and *Klebsiella* and anaerobes other than *Bacteroides fragilis*.

First-generation cephalosporins may be inactivated by β-lactamase.

(*continues*)

BOX 6-2 **β-Lactam Antibiotics (Continued)**

B. Second-generation cephalosporins

Cefamandole, cefoxitin, cefuroxime, cefonicid, ceforanide, cefotetan, cefaclor, and cefuroxime

Spectrum: slightly more active than first-generation cephalosporins against Enterobacteriaceae and other gram-negative bacteria but less active against *Staphylococcus*; also active against *H. influenzae* and *Moraxella*. Cefaclor is active against anaerobes.

More resistant to effects of β-lactamase than were the first-generation cephalosporins.

C. Third-generation cephalosporins

Cefoperazone, cefotaxime, ceftriaxone, moxalactam, ceftizoxime, ceftazidime, and cefixime

Spectrum: greatly increased activity against gram-negative bacilli and less active against gram-positive cocci when compared with other cephalosporins; useful in nosocomial and multidrug-resistant gram-negative infections. Cefotaxime is useful for *E. coli*, *Serratia*, and *Klebsiella* infections, whereas ceftriaxone has activity against *Neisseria gonorrhoeae*. Several third-generation cephalosporins are active against *P. aeruginosa* and most anaerobes.

Third-generation cephalosporins have increased stability against β-lactamase.

D. Fourth-generation cephalosporin

Cefepime

Spectrum: useful for gram-negative bacilli that are resistant to third-generation cephalosporins

E. Fifth-generation cephalosporin

Ceftobiprole

Spectrum: useful for *P. aeruginosa*, MRSA, and penicillin-resistant *S. pneumoniae*

3. **Monobactams: Aztreonam**

Originally made from *Chromobacterium violaceum* (now produced from a synthetic source)

Spectrum: *P. aeruginosa* and other gram-negative bacteria; low activity against gram-positive bacteria and anaerobes

4. **Miscellaneous β-Lactams**

Carbapenems: imipenem, meropenem, doripenem, and ertapenem

Spectrum: activity similar to third-generation cephalosporins, with slightly greater activity toward Enterobacteriaceae, *P. aeruginosa*, and anaerobes. They are also active against gram-positive cocci but are not effective for MRSA or vancomycin-resistant enterococcus (VRE).

5. **Glycopeptides**

Mode of activity: inhibition of cell wall formation through inhibition of peptidoglycan synthesis; interferes with cross-linking in peptidoglycan chains

Vancomycin: first isolated in 1953 by Edmund Kornfeld, an organic chemist working at Eli Lilly from a soil sample collected deep in the interior jungles of Borneo. Soil sample showed activity against *Staphylococcus aureus* and was found to contain an organism, which was subsequently named *Streptomyces* (*Amycolatopsis*) *orientalis*. The compound was originally named "compound 05865" but later was given the name vancomycin, derived from the term "vanquish."

Spectrum: primarily gram-positive spectrum; used for MRSA and nosocomial infections from coagulase-negative *Staphylococcus*. It is also used for *Clostridium difficile* colitis and as a penicillin alternative to treat endocarditis from viridans streptococcus. Vancomycin is also useful for *Listeria*, *Bacillus*, and other *Clostridium* infections. Vancomycin is a large molecule that is highly concentrated in the stool, which makes it useful in the treatment of *Clostridium difficile* colitis. Resistance is a concern, especially VRE, which emerged in the middle 1980s. There have also been concerns of vancomycin-intermediate *S. aureus* (VISA) and vancomycin-resistant *S. aureus* (VRSA), which first emerged in the 1990s.

BOX 6-3 **Antibiotics That Alter Bacterial Cell Membranes**

Bind to outer surface of cell membrane and alter phospholipids, which damage and disrupt the cell membrane, causing increased permeability and leakage.

1. **Bacitracin**

   Source: *Bacillus licheniformis*

   Indications: topical agent for skin and mucous membrane infections, cuts, burns, and ear and eye infections

   Too toxic for internal use

   Primarily gram-positive spectrum, including *Staphylococcus* and some gram-negative infections

2. **Polymyxins B and E (Colistin)**

   Gram-negative spectrum; used as topical agents in combination with other antibiotics to treat skin, burns, and wound infections

BOX 6-4 **Antibiotics That Inhibit Protein Synthesis**

Important Facts

Protein subunits of prokaryotes are 50S (Svedberg units) and 30S, which form a 70S ribosome. Eukaryotes have 60S and 40S subunits, which form an 80S ribosome, a ribosome that is larger than that of the prokaryote. Svedberg units are sedimentation rates when the ribosomes are centrifuged. This difference in the subunits of the ribosomes permits development of antibiotics that can be selectively toxic on the prokaryotic cell.

1. **Aminoglycosides**

   Mode of activity: interference with protein synthesis at 30S ribosomal subunit, which prevents translation of messenger RNA.

   Structure consists of two or more amino carbohydrates linked with an aminocytocyclitol ring; very water soluble, poorly absorbed in the gastrointestinal tract, and concentrated and excreted in the kidney

   Route is intravenous, intramuscular, or topical because of poor GI absorption and toxicity

   Narrow therapeutic index requires monitoring through peak and trough blood levels

   Spectrum: most are bacteriocidal gram-positive and gram-negative spectrum; not effective against anaerobes

   Used in combination therapy with β-lactams or vancomycin

   Side effects include ototoxicity, which can result in permanent hearing loss from damage to the auditory nerve, and nephrotoxicity.

   Dosage should be monitored using peak and trough values to avoid toxic effects.

   Streptomycin, gentamycin, tobramycin, kanamycin, and neomycin are natural aminoglycosides, and netilomycin and amikacin are semisynthetic aminoglycosides.

Streptomycin:

   Oldest aminoglycoside, dating back to the 1940s

   Derived from *Streptomyces griseus*

   May be used in combination therapy for tuberculosis and with a β-lactam for enterococcal infections

Gentamycin:

   Derived from fermentation metabolites of *Micromonospora purpurea*

(continues)

BOX 6-4 **Antibiotics That Inhibit Protein Synthesis (Continued)**

Bacteriocidal; used to treat health care–associated infections caused by gram-negative bacilli; often used synergistically with β-lactam drugs to treat severe systemic infections because the β-lactam facilitates the penetration of gentamycin through the cell wall

Is the most cost-effective aminoglycoside

Tobramycin:

Derived from *Streptomyces fradiae*

Similar to gentamycin with increased activity against *P. aeruginosa* and *Acinetobacter*

Recommended when microorganism shows resistance to gentamycin

Amikacin:

Similar to gentamycin and tobramycin; used to treat gram-negative bacilli that are resistant to both gentamycin and tobramycin; also has activity against *Nocardia asteroides* and *Mycobacterium avium-intracellulare* complex

Netilmicin:

Similar to gentamycin and tobramycin; slightly less active against *P. aeruginosa* and *Serratia*

Semisynthetic—derived from sisomicin, which is derived from *Micromonspora*

Neomycin: oral and topical antibacterial agent, derived from *Streptomyces fradiae*

Spectinomycin: Used only for treatment of gonorrhea, although the organism has shown resistance

2. **Tetracyclines**

Mode of activity: Interference with protein synthesis at 30S ribosomal subunit, which prevents transfer RNA from attaching

The tetracycline molecule contains four fused rings with a hydronaphthacene nucleus; various side chains are added, which form the specific antibiotics.

Minocycline, doxycycline, chlortetracycline, oxytetracycline, demeclocycline, and methacycline

Bacteriostatic, broad-spectrum with activity against gram-positive and gram-negative bacteria; also useful for intracellular microorganisms, *Mycoplasma* and chlamydia/*Chlamydophila*, *Brucella*, *Rickettsia*, *Ehrlichia*, *Shigella*, and spirochetes; also may be used for VRE, MRSA, and *Acinetobacter baumanni*.

Many tetracyclines are used in topical acne medications.

Growing plasmid-mediated resistance, especially in β-hemolytic streptococci

Side effects include suppression of normal flora, secondary infections, such as *Candida* infections and pseudomembranous colitis, and photosensitivity; contraindicated for children and pregnant women because of deposits in bones and teeth.

Tetracyclines are amphoteric and show decreased absorption when taken with foods or medications containing calcium, aluminum, magnesium, or iron.

Glycylcycline (tigecycline) has a tetracycline core with various substitutions; it is not affected by the most common tetracycline-resistance mechanisms and can be used to treat tetracycline-resistant infections, such as MRSA, VRE, and antibiotic-resistant *P. aeruginosa* and enterococcal infections.

3. **Macrolides and Lincosamides**

Mode of activity: inhibition of protein synthesis by binding to 50S ribosomal subunit inhibiting transfer RNA.

Macrocytic lactones that have a macrolide ring and two carbohydrates; specific antibiotics differ in substitutions and side chains

Macrolides can penetrate white blood cells and are concentrated in phagocytes, which makes them useful for intracellular pathogens.

Erythromycin: gram-positive spectrum; respiratory infections from *S. pyogenes* and *S. pneumoniae* in penicillin-allergic patients; it also is effective for *Mycoplasma pneumoniae, Legionella* infections, spirochetes, *Neisseria*, and *Haemophilus*.

Oleandomycin and spiramycin are naturally occurring macrolides, and azithromycin, clarithromycin, and dirithromcyin are semisynthetic macrolides. Telithromycin is a ketolide that has activity against most macrolide-resistant gram-positive bacteria; telithromycin does not induce the common macrolide-resistance mechanism.

The older macrolides mainly have a gram-positive activity and are not effective against gram-negative bacteria, whereas the newer ones also have some gram-negative activity.

Macrolides also are used to treat some anaerobic infections, atypical mycobacteria (including *Mycobacterium avium*-intracellular complex), *Bordetella pertussis*, mycoplasma, legionella, rickettsii, and chlamydial/ *Chlamydophila* infections.

Oxaolidinoses (linezolid): a synthetic agent that also inhibits protein synthesis

Clindamycin: gram-positive spectrum. It is active against most aerobic gram-positive cocci other than MRSA and *Enterococcus*, as well as against most anaerobes, including *B. fragilis*, although resistance has been noted.

4. **Chloroamphenicol**

Mode of activity: interference with protein synthesis by binding to 50S ribosomal subunit, preventing attachment of the amino acids

It has activity against many gram-positive and gram-negative infections; however, because of serious side effects and the availability of other, safer antibiotics, its use has been much diminished. It is reserved for serious gram-negative infections, such as typhoid fever and salmonellosis; one severe side effect is bone marrow aplasia.

The sulfonamides function by competitive inhibition of folic acid formation, whereas the quinolones inhibit deoxyribonucleic acid (DNA) gyrase activity. BOX 6-5 summarizes the sulfonamides, quinolones, and other antibiotics.

In general, erythromycin, vancomycin, and the cephalosporins and penicillins can be used for infections involving gram-positive bacilli and *Staphylococcus*. There are increasing numbers of strains of *Staphylococcus aureus* that are resistant to penicillin, including the penicillinase-resistant penicillins. An increased resistance to methicillin has been identified, and methicillin-resistant *S. aureus* (MRSA) has become a serious concern both in hospital- and community-acquired infections. Serious *Enterococcus* infections, such as endocarditis, are treated with a combination therapy of penicillin and an aminoglycoside or vancomycin. The emergence of VRE presents an additional concern in the treatment of these infections. Less serious enterococcal infections usually respond to penicillin or ampicillin. Nonenterococcal streptococci generally respond well to the penicillins. Group A *Streptococcus* is universally susceptible to penicillin, and there is usually no need for susceptibility testing in most patients. Groups B, C, F, and G are likewise generally susceptible to penicillin. Erythromycin can be substituted in individuals who are hypersensitive or allergic to penicillin. The viridans streptococci have shown an increased resistance to penicillin, and infections are usually treated with a combination therapy of a penicillin with an aminoglycoside. *Streptococcus pneumoniae*, once universally susceptible to penicillin, also has shown increased resistance to penicillin.

Gram-negative bacteria other than *P. aeruginosa* can be treated with aminoglycosides, extended-spectrum penicillins, cephalosporins, quinolones, and imipenem. *P. aeruginosa* can be treated with the aminoglycosides, extended-spectrum penicillins, third-generation cephalosporins, and imipenem. *Haemophilus influenzae* is generally resistant to the first-generation cephalosporins; some strains also are resistant to ampicillin and may be treated with third-generation cephalosporins. *Neisseria gonorrhoeae* was susceptible to penicillin until the 1970s, when penicillinase-producing *N. gonorrhoeae* (PPNG) was detected. An increase in resistance to tetracycline has also occurred. Today the recommended therapy for this pathogen is ceftriaxone with doxycycline (a tetracycline). *Neisseria meningitidis* has remained susceptible to penicillin but has developed some resistance to the sulfonamides and rifampin, used for prophylactic contacts.

BOX 6-5 **Sulfonamides, Quinolones, and Other Antibiotics**

1. **Sulfonamides**

   Mode of activity: competitive inhibition of folic acid synthesis. Sulfonamides bind to dihydropteroate synthase–inhibiting folic acid metabolism; all have a para-amino sulfonamide group, which acts as an antimetabolite of para-aminobenzoic acid, forming a nonfunctional analogue of folic acid.

   Sulfamethoxazole: used primarily for acute urinary tract infections

   Trimethoprim: also targets the folic acid pathway, inhibiting the enzyme dihydrofolate reductase

   Trimethoprim-sulfamethoxazole: used for treatment of chronic UTIs and Enterobacteriaceae infections, especially *E. coli, H. influenzae, Moraxella catarrhalis, and Pseudomonas cepacia*. Anaerobes are resistant.

   Combination attacks folic acid metabolism in two sites.

2. **Quinolones**

   Mode of activity: inhibition of DNA gyrase activity, which interferes with the synthesis of DNA

   Nalidixic acid: first quinolone; used to treat urinary tract infections

   Fluoroquinolones, such as ciprofloxacin, are derivatives of the quinolones and have a broader spectrum. They are used to treat serious infections, such as complicated urinary tract infections and invasive ear infections from Enterobacteriaceae, *Pseudomonas, Neisseria meningitidis, M. catarrhalis,* and *H. influenzae*. They have decreased activity against *Streptococcus* and *Enterococcus* and are effective against *Staphylococcus* other than MRSA. The fluoroquinolones also have activity against *Legionella pneumophlia*, *Mycoplasma*, and chlamydia/*Chlamydophila* spp.

   Norfloxacin is very useful in treating urinary tract infections because it is excreted and concentrated in the urine. It is effective against *E. coli, Klebsiella, Enterobacter,* and *Proteus*, but is not active against gram-positive cocci or *Pseudomonas*.

3. **Nitrofurantoin**

   Mode of activity: inhibition of bacterial enzymes or protein synthesis

   Used in treatment of urinary tract infections; active against most gram-positive and some gram-negative bacteria, such as *E. coli* and *Klebsiella*; not effective against *P. aeruginosa, Serratia,* or *Proteus*

4. **Rifampin**

   Mode of activity: inhibition of DNA-dependent ribonucleic acid (RNA) polymerase

   Semisynthetic derivatives of rifamycin, which are obtained from *Streptomyces mediterranei*

   Used in the treatment of tuberculosis and as a prophylaxis for *Neisseria meningitidis* carriers and asymptomatic contacts of those with meningococcal disease

   Concentrated within cells, which makes it useful for intracellular pathogens; also used in combination therapy for MRSA, *Campylobacter*, and *Haemophilus* infections

5. **Metronidazole**

   Mode of activity: Reduction products of metronidazole cause altered DNA synthesis, resulting in bacteriocidal effect. It is activated under anaerobic conditions, which makes metronidazole useful for treatment of most anaerobes; it also is used to treat *Gardnerella* vaginosis and pseudomembranous colitis resulting from *C. difficile.* It also has activity against parasitic amoeba and flagellates, including *Trichomonas vaginalis*. It has no activity against most aerobes.

Most anaerobic infections can be treated with extended-spectrum penicillins, β-lactam drugs that are resistant to β-lactamase, cefoxitin, chloramphenicol, imipenem, or metronidazole.

ANTIMYCOBACTERIAL AGENTS

Mycobacterial infections require combination therapy and are long-term therapies; this is necessary to reduce the possibility of antibiotic resistance and because mycobacteria

BOX 6-6 Antimycobacterial Agents

Multiple drugs are used to minimize the incidence of drug-resistant *Mycobacterium tuberculosis*. Some of these agents function by inhibiting mycolic acid formation in the cell wall, whereas others inhibit DNA-dependent RNA polymerase.

Rifampin: inhibits DNA-dependent RNA polymerase

Isoniazid (INH): possibly interferes with formation of mycolic acid in acid wall of mycobacteria; used in combination therapy; bacteriocidal to growing cells

Pyrazinamide (PZA): bacteriocidal

Ethambutol: bacteriostatic; inhibits mycolic acid

Streptomycin: an aminoglycoside; generally used as a second-line drug

Other antibiotics, such as quinolones and aminoglycosides, are used in combination therapy to treat multiple drug–resistant *Mycobacterium tuberculosis* (MDRTB), although these are not as effective as the other agents listed.

have a slow doubling time. Antimycobacterial agents are summarized in BOX 6-6.

ANTIFUNGAL AGENTS

Antifungal agents are summarized in BOX 6-7; systemic fungal infections are treated with amphotericin B or imidazoles.

ANTIVIRAL AGENTS

There are antiviral agents available for human immunodeficiency virus (HIV); herpes simplex virus (HSV); varicella-zoster virus (VZV), the agent of chicken pox; herpes zoster (shingles); cytomegalovirus (CMV); influenza A and B; and respiratory syncytial virus (RSV). These agents are summarized in BOX 6-8.

Antibiotics may be prescribed singly or in combination therapy. It is important to know the interactions between antibiotics so that their effects are not diminished when prescribed together. BOX 6-9 summarizes the interactions that can occur when two or more antibiotics are given together.

BOX 6-7 Antifungal Agents

Amphotericin B: attacks sterols in fungal cell wall, especially ergosterols; alters cell membrane of yeast

Used in treatment of invasive and systemic fungal infections, including invasive *Cryptococcus* and *Candida* infections; toxic to kidneys

5-Fluorocytosine (5-FC): inhibits RNA transcription and DNA synthesis in yeasts; used to treat *Cryptococcus* and *Candida* infections; given with amphotericin B for cryptococcal meningitis; toxic to kidneys, bone marrow, and liver

Imidazoles

Prevent sterol synthesis affecting cell membrane, which becomes leaky

Used to treat *Candida*, *Cryptococcus*, *Coccidioides*, *Histoplasma*, *Paracoccidiodes*, and *Blastomyces* infections

Clotrimazole: used to treat dermatophytic, yeast, and superficial fungal infections

Ketoconazole: fungistatic; used to treat non-life-threatening histoplasmosis and blastomycosis

Fluconazole: used to treat severe or disseminated candidiasis and cryptococcus infections; can penetrate into cerebrospinal fluid

Miconazole: used as a topical agent for cutaneous and subcutaneous candidiasis

Itraconazole: used to treat aspergillosis and *Sporothrix* infections

Griseofulvin: binds to keratin in hair and nails; used to treat dermatophytic infections, *Microsporum*, *Trichophyton*, and *Epidermophyton*

Nystatin

Binds to ergosterol in fungal cell membrane; source is *Streptomyces noursei*

Used as oral and topical agents; too toxic for injection; used to treat superficial skin and mucous membrane infections caused by yeast and dermatophytes.

BOX 6-8 **Viruses with Associated Antiviral Agents**

Human Immunodeficiency Virus (HIV)

Nevirapine: nonnucleoside reverse transcriptase inhibitors (NNRTIs); inhibit the reverse transcriptase enzyme, which transcribes viral RNA into DNA

Zidovudine (INN), azidothymidine (AZT), and tenofovir disoproxil fumarate: nucleoside analogue reverse-transcriptase inhibitors (NRTIs) or nucleoside/nucleotide analogues resemble nucleotides and produce nonfunctional DNA when incorporated into the HIV molecule, thereby inhibiting replication.

Saquinavir: Protease inhibitors inhibit enzymes that cleave viral polyproteins into functional HIV proteins that are needed to assemble the virion particle.

Enfuvirtide: Fusion inhibitors block merging of viral envelope with cell membrane so that virus cannot enter host's cells and host's proteins and metabolic compounds cannot be used by the virus.

Influenza A

Amantadine and rimantadine inhibit penetration and uncoating of virus, preventing attachment to host's cell membrane.

Influenza A and B

Oseltamivir (Tamiflu): a neuraminidase inhibitor that blocks the activity of the viral neuraminidase (NA) enzyme and prevents new viral particles from being released by infected cells

Zanamivir: a neuraminidase inhibitor used in the treatment and prophylaxis of influenza A and B viral infections

Hepatitis B virus (HBV)

Lamivudine: an analogue of cytidine that inhibits reverse transcriptase in HBV. It also can inhibit HIV reverse transcriptase.

Adefovir dipivoxil (Adefovir): a nucleotide reverse-transcriptase inhibitor that works by blocking reverse transcriptase in HBV

Herpes simplex viruses (HSV-1 and HSV-2)

Acyclovir and ganciclovir: nucleoside analogues that target viral DNA; also useful in CMV infections

Valacyclovir (Valtrex): inhibits DNA polymerase; also used for herpes zoster or singles; is a prodrug and converted to acyclovir

Vidarabine: interferes with the synthesis of viral DNA as a nucleoside analogue; also used for herpes zoster, or shingles

Foscarnet (PFA): a DNA polymerase inhibitor used for acyclovir-resistant HSV infections, herpes zoster (varicella zoster) shingles, and CMV retinitis

Tromantadine: a derivate of amantadine; functions by altering the host cell's glycoproteins so that the virus cannot be absorbed. Penetration of the virus into the host cell is inhibited, and it also affects the uncoating of the virus particle.

Docosanol (Abreva): believed to inhibit the fusion of the host cell with the HSV viral envelope, thus preventing replication. It is used to reduce the duration of HSV fever blisters.

Cytomegalovirus (CMV)

Foscarnet (PFA): a DNA polymerase inhibitor that is used for CMV retinitis, an eye infection that can cause blindness, and as a clinical agent for herpes viruses

Valganciclovir: used for CMV retinitis and CMV disease in those who have received organ or bone marrow transplants and those at risk for CMV disease

Respiratory syncytial virus (RSV)

Ribavirin: used for severe RSV infection and also with α-interferon for hepatitis C infection. It is a prodrug and when metabolized forms a compound that resembles the purine RNA nucleotides. It affects the viral RNA and inhibits its expression and the synthesis of viral proteins.

BOX 6-9 **Possible Antibiotic Interactions**

Autonomous: Indifferent; the antibiotics have no effect on each other.

Result obtained with two drugs is equal to result with most effective drug by itself.

Antagonistic: Result with two drugs is significantly less than the autonomous result.

Additive: Result with two drugs is equal to combined action of each of the drugs used separately.

Synergistic: Result with two drugs is significantly greater than additive response. The antibiotics may have different modes of action or function at different sites. One member of the combination may be resistant to β-lactamase. The uptake of aminoglycosides into the bacterial cell is enhanced by β-lactam drugs. For example, a penicillin derivative with an aminoglycoside shows synergistic action and is used to treat enterococcal endocarditis.

Resistance to Antimicrobial Agents

Bacteria have become resistant to and continue to develop resistance to antibiotics. There are several mechanisms by which microorganisms can become resistant to antibiotics. When a microorganism becomes resistant to an antimicrobial agent, that drug is no longer considered to be effective in the treatment of that infectious agent. However, in some cases, the antibiotic can be given in a higher dose or in a combination therapy to address the resistance. Yet, in other situations, alternative therapies must be given. These antibiotics may be more costly or produce toxic side effects. Of course, there is no guarantee that the resistant organism will not, in turn, develop resistance to the alternative treatments. Therefore, consideration of bacterial resistance to an antibiotic or group of antibiotics is another important factor in antimicrobial susceptibility testing and the treatment of the infection.

INTRINSIC RESISTANCE

Intrinsic resistance, also known as inherent resistance, is a natural resistance of the bacteria to an antibiotic before the antibiotic has been used. Examples include the intrinsic resistance of *Staphylococcus saprophyticus* to novobiocin. Most other members of the Enterobacteriaceae are susceptible to the polymyxins B and E (colistin); however, *Proteus*, *Providencia*, *Morganella*, and *Edwardsiella* are intrinsically resistant to the polymyxins. The polymyxins cannot bind to the membranes of *Proteus*, *Providencia*, *Morganella*, and *Edwardsiella*, rendering them ineffective. Another example of intrinsic resistance includes the resistance of *Pseudomonas aeruginosa* to trimethoprim-sulfamethoxazole and to tetracycline, which are pumped out of the bacteria cell by an inherent mechanism. Intrinsic resistance may be useful for identification of an organism, as is the case in the identification of *S. saprophyticus* by its resistance to novobiocin.

ACQUIRED RESISTANCE

Acquired resistance occurs as a result of prior exposure of the microorganism to the antimicrobial agent. Organisms that were once susceptible are now resistant, following exposure to the antibiotic. Acquired resistance may result from chromosomal mutations or from plasmids. In chromosomal mutations the antibiotic exerts selective pressure on the susceptible strain of the organism. The resistant mutant strain overgrows the susceptible cells, and a new population of resistant cells emerges. Plasmids are small pieces of extrachromosomal DNA that are associated with virulence and antibiotic resistance. Plasmids act independently from the chromosome, and the resistance genes may be transferred from chromosome to plasmid or from plasmid to chromosome. DNA-resistant plasmids are released by the microorganism or acquired by another microorganism that may or may not be of the same genus or species of the original organism.

Transformation occurs when bacteria die and release their DNA. The free DNA can be incorporated into another microorganism, which may transfer resistance. Conjugation occurs when bacterial cells transfer DNA to other bacterial cells. Bacteriophages are viruses that can insert their DNA into bacteria.

Transposons, commonly known as "jumping genes," can insert pieces of DNA into another microorganism, even if no homology exists. Thus, the host range is much broader when compared with plasmids. Transposons can carry part of plasmids or pieces of chromosomes to other bacteria or to other plasmids. Therefore, the DNA can be transferred from plasmid to plasmid, as well as from plasmid to chromosome and chromosome to plasmid.

Target-Site Modification

In these types of resistance, the target site for the antibiotic is altered by either mutation or enzymatic modification; the result is that the antibiotic cannot bind to the intended site. Without binding, the antibiotic cannot inhibit protein synthesis or interfere with cell wall formation. Modifications of the target site may occur because of chromosomal mutations, plasmids, or transposons. The specific mechanisms of resistance include modification of the target site. The antibiotic's ability to bind to the cell wall or ribosome is altered, and the binding affinity of the antibiotic is decreased or nonexistent. This mechanism is seen in the β-lactams, macrolides, tetracyclines, aminoglycosides, vancomycin, and trimethoprim. β-lactams bind to penicillin-binding proteins in the cell wall. Resistance to these agents usually involves interference with the penicillin-binding proteins. One example is the alteration of penicillin-binding protein (PBP), which confers bacterial resistance to penicillins and cephalosporins. This is the mechanism of methicillin-resistant *Staphylococcus aureus* (MRSA), vancomycin-resistant enterococcus (VRE), and penicillin-resistant *Streptococcus pneumoniae.* Other examples of target-site modifications for antibiotic resistance are summarized in BOX 6-10.

Mechanisms of resistance resulting from plasmid- or transposon-mediated effects of the target site are shown in BOX 6-11.

A second mechanism for resistance is inactivation of the antimicrobial agent. In this case, bacterial enzymes convert the active drug into an inactive form. The **β-lactamases (penicillinases)** are a group of enzymes that convert the β-lactam ring of the penicillins and cephalosporins and imipenem into inactive forms. This resistance may be plasmid mediated or chromosomally mediated. β-lactamase

BOX 6-10 Modifications of Target Site

Penicillin-binding protein altered

Affects penicillins and cephalosporins

β-lactam antibiotics cannot bind to altered penicillin-binding site

Examples: MRSA and penicillin-resistant *Streptococcus pneumoniae*

Porins altered in outer-membrane proteins

Decreased permeability and decreased uptake of antibiotic into bacterial cell

Antibiotic doesn't accumulate in sufficient amounts in bacterial cell

Altered DNA gyrase enzymes

Affects quinolone (fluoroquinolone) antibiotics, which function by inhibition of bacterial DNA gyrase

Altered RNA polymerase

Affects rifampin, which functions by interfering with RNA polymerase

Altered ribosomal subunits

Affects streptomycin, which can't bind to the altered ribosomes

Exhibited by *E. coli, S. aureus, Pseudomonas aeruginosa, Enterococcus faecalis,* and *Mycobacterium tuberculosis*

BOX 6-11 Plasmid- or Transposon-Mediated Resistance of Target Site

Transposon-mediated methicillin resistance in *Staphylococcus aureus* (MRSA)

The *mecA* gene encodes for a penicillin-binding protein, which is a β-lactamase–resistant transpeptidase. This protein has a low affinity for methicillin and most other β-lactam antibiotics; the β-lactam ring cannot bind well to methicillin.

- Transposon-mediated vancomycin resistance in *Enterococcus* (VRE); possible transfer of vancomycin resistance to *S. aureus*, resulting in vancomycin-intermediate *S. aureus* (VISA) and vancomycin-resistant *S. aureus* (VRSA)
- Resistance to macrolides, such as erythromycin; enzyme adds a methyl group to the 50S ribosomal subunit; antibiotic can no longer bind to the bacterial 50S subunit
- Plasmid-mediated resistance to trimethoprim resulting from production of enzyme dihydrofolate reductase, which interferes with the folic acid pathway
- Plasmid-mediated resistance to sulfonamide resulting from production of dihydropteroate synthetase, which interferes with the folic acid pathway

production was first directed against the natural penicillins, but now there are many types of β-lactamase enzymes with resistance directed against broad-spectrum penicillins and some cephalosporins. When the β-lactam ring is destroyed, the antibiotic cannot bind to the penicillin-binding proteins, which must occur for the antibiotic to be effective. β-lactamase production exhibited by *S. aureus*, *Hemophilus influenzae*, *Neisseria gonorrhoeae*, *Moraxella catarrhalis*, and some gram-negative anaerobes results in the release of the enzyme into the bacterial environment. In these cases, the β-lactamase can be detected using procedures such as Cefinase, which detects the extracellular product. For the gram-negative bacteria, such as *E. coli*, *Klebsiella*, and *Stenotrophomonas maltophilia*, the β-lactamase remains in the periplasmic space. This β-lactamase is not detected using methods that detect the extracellular enzyme.

Examples of inactivation of the antimicrobial agent are shown in BOX 6-12.

Another mechanism for resistance includes decreased permeability of the bacterial cell wall, which results in poor entry of the antibiotic into the bacterial cell. This is seen in gram-negative bacteria, whose outer lipid membrane renders them impermeable to certain antibiotics. For example, vancomycin is too large of a molecule to penetrate the outer lipid membrane of the gram-negative bacteria.

Other bacteria can prevent the accumulation of the antibiotic through a pumping mechanism, known as efflux. Efflux is a type of active transport, and the antibiotic cannot reach high enough levels to be effective. Examples of efflux-resistant mechanisms include the low-level resistance of *Pseudomonas aeruginosa* to many antibiotics. Another example of efflux is the production of the *msrA* gene by *S. aureus* and the *Enterococcus* against the macrolides. Macrolide resistance efflux by *Streptococcus agalactiae* by production of the *mreA* gene is another example.

Alteration of porin channels is another type of resistance that affects the permeability of the bacterial cell wall. These water-filled channels permit diffusion of molecules across the gram-negative outer membrane. When the porins are altered, some antibiotics cannot travel through the channels. Therefore, they cannot reach the ribosomes or penicillin-binding proteins. An example is the production of OmpF and OmpC by *E. coli*, which affects the permeability of the cell wall to the β-lactam antibiotics.

These various mechanisms of resistance may occur singly or in combinations by certain bacteria. When the mechanisms coexist in the same host, multidrug resistance occurs.

BOX 6-12 Inactivation of Antimicrobial Agent

- Production of β-lactamase by *Staphylococcus aureus* and other bacteria that destroy the β-lactam ring
- Production of cephalosporinase by gram-negative bacteria; chromosomal-mediated resistance, known as AmpC, by most Enterobacteriaceae and some *Pseudomonas aeruginosa*
- Production of imipenemase by *Enterobacter cloacae* and *Serratia marcescens*, thus rendering them resistant to imipenem
- Plasmid-mediated production of β-lactamase enzymes by gram-negative bacteria with accumulation in periplasmic space. This is known as TEM-1 resistance to ampicillin, carbenicillin, piperacillin, ticarcillen, and some first-generation cephalosporins, such as cephalothin. Resistance now includes plasmid-mediated resistance to broader spectrum cephalosporins, such as cefamandole, cefotaxime, and ceftriaxone
- Plasmid-mediated resistance to chloroamphenicol resulting from the production of an acetyltransferase enzyme from *E. coli*; plasmid-mediated resistance transferred to many other gram-negative and gram-positive bacteria and anaerobes

Laboratory Methods for Susceptibility Testing

Selection of the specific type of susceptibility test to be performed and selection of specific antibiotics to be tested should be determined jointly by the director of microbiology, the infectious disease department, and the medical staff. The pharmacy department also may have input into the selection of specific antibiotics because this department may be responsible for the delivery and supply of the antimicrobial agents.

Various susceptibility testing methods are currently available, and each has its advantages and disadvantages. There are manual and automated methods; there are diffusion tests that determine zone diameters and those that determine quantitative parameters, such as the minimal inhibitory concentration (MIC). There are agar and broth methods and gradient diffusion methods, including the Etest® (bioMérieux) and MIC Evaluator (Oxoid). Automated systems (discussed in Chapter 5) include the MicroScan (Siemens Health Care Diagnostics), VITEK (bioMérieux), BD Phoenix, and Sensititre (Trek Diagnostics). The particular methods used by a microbiology laboratory depend on the facility's volume of testing and specific needs.

DISK DIFFUSION SUSCEPTIBILITY TESTING

Disk diffusion susceptibility testing, or the **Kirby-Bauer disk diffusion test**, is performed by inoculating a standardized suspension of bacteria onto Mueller-Hinton agar. Paper disks impregnated with specific antibiotics are placed on the agar and incubated under well-defined conditions. The antibiotics diffuse into the surrounding medium. The presence of a clear zone indicates the lack of growth of the microorganism in the presence of the antibiotic; this is known as the zone of inhibition. After overnight incubation, the zones of inhibition around each antibiotic are measured and compared with established interpretative values. The diameter of the zone of inhibition is an indicator of the relative susceptibility of the organism to the antibiotic. Results are reported as **susceptible**, **intermediate**, or **resistant**.

Susceptible (also referred to as sensitive) results indicate that the antibiotic appears to be effective against the bacteria because growth is inhibited in vitro. Resistant results indicate the antibiotic appears to be ineffective against the bacteria tested. In vivo activity of the antibiotic against the microbe also depends on host factors, the site of infection, the specific antibiotic used, and specific properties of the microorganism. The Clinical and Laboratory Standards Institute (CLSI) is one of the organizations that establishes standards for generic test methods, including the disk diffusion susceptibility test.

The principle of the disk diffusion test is based on the inverse linear relationship between the diameter of the zone of inhibited growth around the antibiotic disk and the logarithm of the **minimal inhibitory concentration** (MIC) of the antibiotic. The MIC is the lowest concentration of antibiotic that inhibits in vitro bacterial growth. Thus the diameter of the zone of inhibition is proportional to the susceptibility of the organism to the antibiotic tested. As the MIC increases, the zone diameter decreases. The interpretative tables used to classify bacteria as susceptible, intermediate, or resistant are developed with consideration of the antibiotic's diffusion coefficient and the organism's rate of replication and antibiotic susceptibility. The diffusion coefficient is influenced by the composition of the medium and the antibiotic's biochemical properties. If two bacteria have the same susceptibility to a particular antibiotic, the organism with a quicker replication rate will produce smaller zones of inhibition. The zone of inhibition is affected by the organism's lag phase and exponential phase of growth.

For disk diffusion testing to be accurate and reproducible, several testing parameters must be constant. The medium must have a well-defined chemical composition, support the growth of those bacteria most frequently isolated from clinical cultures, be buffered to prevent pH changes during incubation, not antagonize antibiotic activity, and have a composition that is reproducible and constant. The recommended testing medium is Mueller-Hinton agar, which has most of these properties. Mueller-Hinton agar contains beef infusions, nucleic acids, vitamins, casein hydrolysate as a peptone source, cornstarch to neutralize fatty acids, and agar as a solidifying agent. This medium supports the growth of most bacteria and can be supplemented with blood to grow fastidious bacteria such as *S. pneumoniae*.

Increased concentrations of calcium and magnesium ions in the agar may lead to a decreased activity of the aminoglycosides against *P. aeruginosa* and decreased activity of the tetracyclines against all bacteria. Decreased concentrations of magnesium and calcium salts lead to increased activity against these agents. Thus the medium must have acceptable levels of these cations. This can be monitored through quality-control organisms to ensure acceptable zone diameters. Increased levels of thymidine or thymine may lead to decreased activity of the sulfonamides, trimethoprim, and trimethoprim-sulfamethoxazole. This also can be monitored through using appropriate quality-control measures.

The pH of the test medium must be 7.2 to 7.4. Increased pH levels lead to increased activity against the aminoglycosides, erythromycin, and clindamycin. Thus, if the pH is greater than 7.4, results may be obtained that indicate susceptibility of the organism, when in reality the organism may be resistant. Also, an increased pH may lead to decreased activity of tetracycline, with incorrect results indicating resistance to the antibiotic. Decreased pH levels lead to the opposite results, that is, decreased activity against the aminoglycosides, erythromycin, and clindamycin and increased activity against the tetracyclines.

The agar depth for disk diffusion testing must be held constant at 4 mm. Plates poured to a thicker depth lead to smaller zones of inhibition and possible false-resistant results, whereas thinner plates may lead to larger zones of inhibition and false-susceptible results.

The most important variable in controlling reproducibility of the test is the density of the inoculum. Only pure cultures can be tested, and it is essential that the inoculum be adjusted to the concentration of a 0.5 McFarland standard, which is approximately equal to 1.5×10^8 CFU/ml. False-susceptible results may be seen in inoculums that are too light, whereas false-resistant results may be seen in inoculums that are too heavy. In addition, only overnight colonies less than 24 hours old should be tested. The use of older cultures may result in false-susceptible results since many of the colonies may be nonviable. The plate is swabbed in three directions so that there is complete and uniform inoculation of the plate, producing a lawn of growth. The inoculum is permitted to absorb onto the agar surface for up to 15 minutes.

Antibiotic disks used in the testing must be stored according to the manufacturer's directions. The use of frost-free refrigerators or freezers is recommended. Antibiotic disks must be stored with a desiccant at –20°C ± 8°C to prevent deterioration according to the manufacturer's specifications. Disks should be permitted to adjust to room temperature before use so that condensation can be minimized. Disks are held for up to only one week in the refrigerator. Disk dispensers are used to apply the antibiotics to the agar plates. This ensures that the disks are evenly distributed and applied flat onto the surface of the agar. The disk dispenser also should be stored with a desiccant and should have tightly fitting lids. Antibiotics should be applied within 15 minutes of inoculating the plate.

Incubation is usually at 35°C ± 2°C for 16 to 18 hours in ambient air for disk diffusion testing. Lower temperatures lead to larger zones of inhibition since the growth rate of most bacteria is prolonged and antibiotics diffuse more slowly. Plates should not be stacked more than five high since the required temperature may not be obtained in those plates located in the center of larger stacks. At temperatures greater than 35°C, MRSA may not be detected. Incubation under increased carbon dioxide (CO_2) is to be used for only fastidious bacteria that need increased CO_2 for growth. CO_2 incubation leads to a decreased pH, which can alter the activity of some antibiotics.

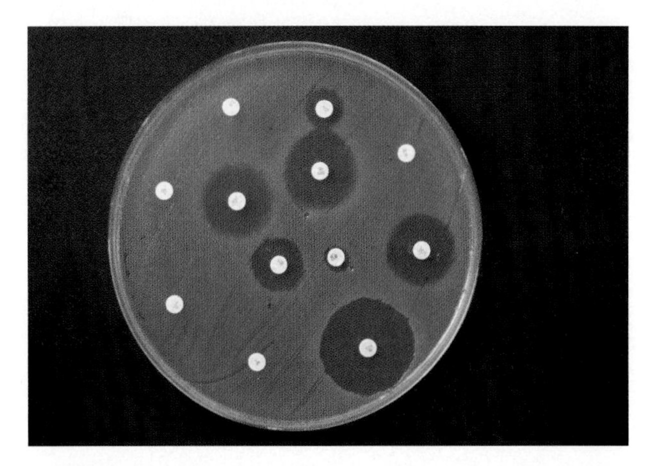

FIGURE 6-1 Kirby-Bauer susceptibility test showing proper disk placement on Mueller-Hinton agar. Disks should be placed so that interpretive zones do not overlap.

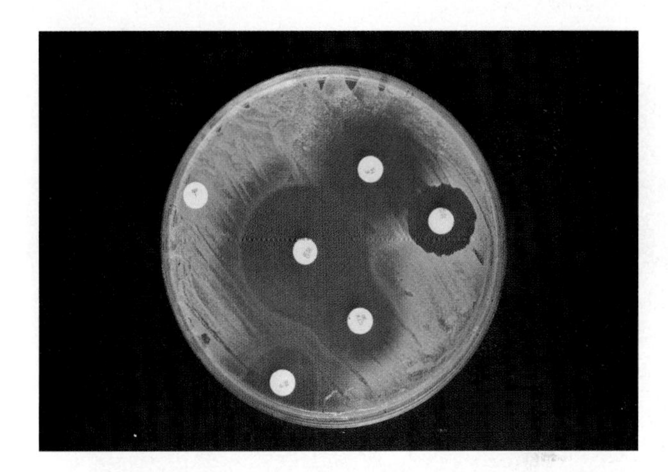

FIGURE 6-2 Kirby-Bauer susceptibility test showing poor disk placement, which has resulted in overlapping of zones.

Zone diameters are reliable only when a confluent lawn of growth is obtained. **FIGURE 6-1** illustrates proper disk placement, whereas **FIGURE 6-2** illustrates poor disk placement, which has resulted in an overlapping of zone diameters. Mueller-Hinton plates are read most accurately from the bottom when held over a black surface and illuminated with a reflected light. When using plates containing blood, the lid of the plate is removed and the zones measured when illuminated with a reflected light. **FIGURE 6-3** illustrates Mueller-Hinton agar supplemented with sheep blood. The plate has been inoculated with *S. pneumoniae*, which requires supplementation with blood for growth. **FIGURE 6-4** illustrates a poorly streaked plate since gaps in the growth hamper proper interpretation of results.

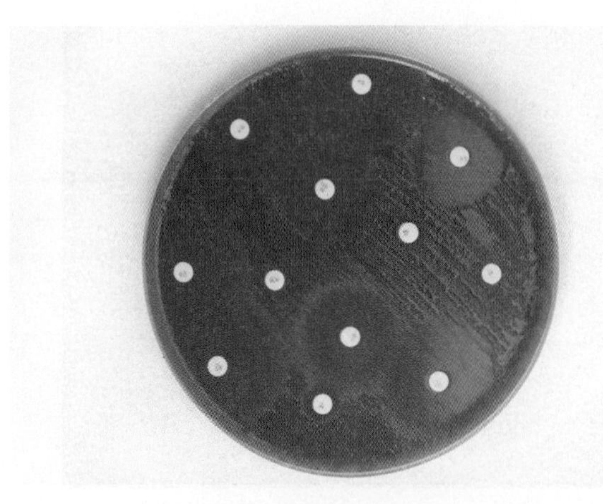

FIGURE 6-3 Kirby-Bauer susceptibility test showing Mueller-Hinton agar that has been supplemented with sheep blood. The organism is *Streptococcus pneumoniae*, which requires sheep blood for growth.

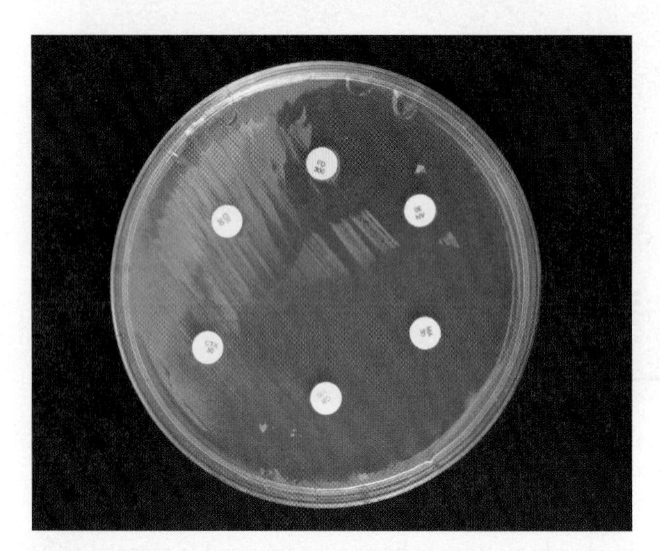

FIGURE 6-4 Kirby-Bauer susceptibility test showing a poorly streaked plate, which has resulted in gaps in the growth, causing inaccurate interpretation of the zone diameters.

One should ignore any slight growth for the sulfonamides and measure only the zone of heavy growth. Likewise, the swarming of *Proteus* should be ignored when measuring the zones (**FIGURE 6-5**). Any tiny colonies growing within the zone of inhibition should be ignored; however, any large mutant colonies should be isolated, identified, and retested.

The procedure for the Kirby-Bauer disk diffusion test is described later in this chapter. **TABLE 6-1** is an example of an interpretative chart for the disk diffusion method for aerobic bacteria. **TABLE 6-2** shows quality-control limits for aerobic bacteria.

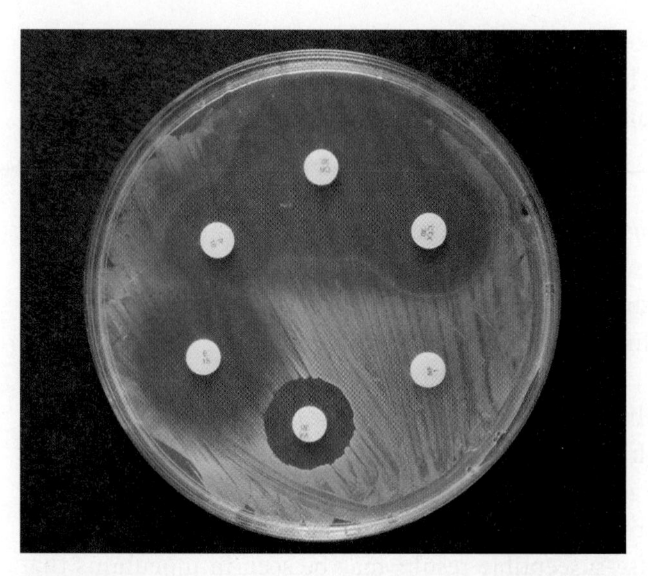

FIGURE 6-5 Swarming of *Proteus mirabilis* on Mueller-Hinton agar. Swarming should be ignored when interpreting zone diameters.

Selection of Antibiotics for Testing

Antibiotics selected for testing should provide information so that the physician can appropriately treat the patient's infection. Antibiotics that are not effective against a particular pathogen or within a particular body site should not be tested. Those tested should be relevant and not redundant. Typical antibiotic selections for bacteria are shown in **TABLE 6-3**.

QUANTITATIVE DILUTION SUSCEPTIBILITY TESTING

Dilution susceptibility tests are used to quantitate the in vitro activity of an antimicrobial agent against a microorganism. Varying concentrations of the antimicrobial agent are tested with the organism. Usually, serial twofold dilutions of the antibiotic are used. After overnight incubation the tubes or plates are examined for visual bacterial growth. Either broth or agar dilution tests can be performed. The broth dilution test can be performed using test tubes (macrobroth dilution) or multiwell microdilution trays (microbroth dilution). The macrobroth dilution method using broth is a reference method for antibiotic susceptibility testing. Quantitative dilution techniques are used to determine the MIC. Thus the first tube or well in the serial dilution showing no visible bacterial growth is the MIC. If the macrotube dilution method is used, all broths with no visible macroscopic growth are

TABLE 6-1 Interpretative Guidelines for Aerobic Bacteria: Zone Diameter Interpretative Standards*

Antimicrobial agent	Code	Disk content	R	I	S
Amdinocillin	AMD-10	10 µg			
Enterobacteriaceae			≤15		≥16
Amikacin	AN-30	30 µg			
Enterobacteriaceae, *P. aeruginosa*, *Acinetobacter*, staphylococci			≤14	15–16	≥17
Amoxicillin/Clavulanic Acid	Amc-30	20/10 µg			
Enterobacteriaceae			≤13	14–17	≥18
Staphylococcus spp.			≤19		≥20
Haemophilus spp.			≤19		≥20
Ampicillin	AM-10	10 µg			
Enterobacteriaceae and *V. cholerae*			≤13	14–16	≥17
Staphylococcus			≤28		≥29
Enterococcus			≤16		≥17
Listeria monocytogenes			≤19		≥20
Haemophilus spp.			≤18	19–21	≥22
Streptococcus (not *S. pneumoniae*, only β-hemolytic streptococci)					≥24
Ampicillin/Sulbactam	SAM20	10/10 µg			
Enterobacteriaceae, *P. aeruginosa*, *Acinetobacter*, and staphylococci			≤11	12–14	≥15
Haemophilus			≤19		≥20
Azithromycin	AZM-15	15 µg			
Staphylococcus spp.			≤13	14–17	≥18
Haemophilus spp.					≥12
Streptococcus pneumoniae and other streptococci			≤13	14–17	≥18
Azlocillin	AZ-75	75 µg			
P. aeruginosa			≤17	—	≥18
Aztreonam	ATM-30	30 µg			
Enterobacteriaceae, *P. aeruginosa*, and *Acinetobacter*			≤15	16–21	≥22
Haemophilus spp.					≥26
Bacitracin	B-10	10 U	≤8	9–12	≥13
Carbenicillin	CB-100	100 µg			
Enterobacteriaceae and *Acinetobacter*			≤19	20–22	≥23
P. aeruginosa			≤13	14–16	≥17
Cefaclor	CEC-30	30 µg			
Enterobacteriaceae and *Staphylococcus*			≤14	15–17	≥18
Haemophilus spp.			≤16	17–19	≥20
Cefamandole	MA-30	30 µg			
Enterobacteriaceae and *Staphylococcus*			≤14	15–17	≥18
Cefazolin	CZ-30	30 µg			
Enterobacteriaceae and *Staphylococcus*			≤14	15–17	≥18

(*continues*)

TABLE 6-1 Interpretative Guidelines for Aerobic Bacteria: Zone Diameter Interpretative Standards* (Continued)

Antimicrobial agent	Code	Disk content	R	I	S
Cefdinir	CDR-5	5 µg			
Enterobacteriaceae and methicillin-susceptible *Staphylococcus*			≤16	17–19	≥20
Haemophilus spp.					≥20
Cefepime	FEP-30	30 µg			
Enterobacteriaceae, *P. aeruginosa*, *Acinetobacter*, and staphylococci			≤14	15–17	≥18
Haemophilus spp.					≥26
Neisseria gonorrhoeae					≥31
Viridans streptococci (not *S. pneumoniae*)			≤21	22–23	≥24
Streptococcus (not *S. pneumoniae*, only β-hemolytic streptococci)					≥24
Cefixime	CFM-5	5 µg			
Enterobacteriaceae			≤15	16–18	≥19
Haemophilus spp.					≥21
N. gonorrhoeae					≥31
Cefmetazole	CMZ-30	30 µg			
Enterobacteriaceae and *Staphylococcus*			≤12	13–15	≥16
N. gonorrhoeae			≤27	28–32	≥33
Cefonicid	CID-30	30 µg			
Enterobacteriaceae and *Staphylococcus*			≤14	15–17	≥18
Haemophilus spp.			≤16	17–19	≥20
Cefoperazone	CFP-75	75 µg			
Enterobacteriaceae, *P. aeruginosa*, *Acinetobacter*, and staphylococci			≤15	16–20	≥21
Cefotaxime	CTX-30	30 µg			
Enterobacteriaceae, *P. aeruginosa*, *Acinetobacter*, and staphylococci			≤14	15–22	≥23
Haemophilus spp.					≥26
N. gonorrhoeae					≥31
Viridans streptococci (not *S. pneumoniae*)			≤25	26–27	≥28
Streptococcus (not *S. pneumoniae*, only β-hemolytic streptococci)					≥24
Cefotetan	CTT-30	30 µg			
Enterobacteriaceae and *Staphylococcus*			≤12	13–15	≥16
N. gonorrhoeae			≤19	20–25	≥25
Cefoxitin	FOX-30	30 µg			
Enterobacteriaceae and *Staphylococcus*			≤14	15–17	≥18
N. gonorrhoeae			≤19	20–25	≥25
Cefpodoxime	CPD-10	10 µg			
Enterobacteriaceae and *Staphylococcus*			≤17	18–20	≥21
Haemophilus spp.					≥21
N. gonorrhoeae					≥29
Cefprozil	CPR-30	30 µg			
Enterobacteriaceae and *Staphylococcus*			≤14	15–17	≥18
Haemophilus spp.			≤14	15–17	≥18

TABLE 6-1 Interpretative Guidelines for Aerobic Bacteria: Zone Diameter Interpretative Standards* (Continued)

Antimicrobial agent	Code	Disk content	R	I	S
Ceftazidime	CAZ-30	30 µg			
Enterobacteriaceae, *P. aeruginosa, Acinetobacter*, and staphylococci			≤14	15–17	≥18
Haemophilus spp.					≥26
N. gonorrhoeae					≥31
Ceftibuten	CTB-30	30 µg			
Enterobacteriaceae			≤17	18–20	≥21
Haemophilus spp.					≥28
Ceftizoxime	ZOX-30	30 µg			
Enterobacteriaceae, *P. aeruginosa, Acinetobacter*, and staphylococci			≤14	15–19	≥20
Haemophilus spp.					≥26
N. gonorrhoeae					≥38
Ceftriaxone	CRO-30	30 µg			
Enterobacteriaceae, *P. aeruginosa, Acinetobacter*, and staphylococci			≤13	14–20	≥21
Haemophilus spp.					≥26
N. gonorrhoeae					≥35
Viridans streptococci (not *S. pneumoniae*)					≥27
Streptococcus (not *S. pneumoniae*, only β-hemolytic streptococci)					≥24
Cefuroxime	CXM-30	30 µg			
Enterobacteriaceae and *Staphylococcus* (parenteral)			≤14	15–17	≥18
Haemophilus spp.			≤16	17–19	≥20
N. gonorrhoeae			≤25	26–30	≥31
Cephalothin	CF-30	30 µg			
Enterobacteriaceae and *Staphylococcus*			≤14	15–17	≥18
Chloramphenicol	C-30	30 µg			
Enterobacteriaceae, *P. aeruginosa, Acinetobacter*, staphylococci, enterococci, and *V. cholerae*			≤12	13–17	≥18
Haemophilus spp.			≤25	26–28	≥29
S. pneumoniae			≤20		≥21
Streptococcus (not *S. pneumoniae*)			≤17	18–20	≥21
Cinoxacin	CIN-100	100 µg			
Enterobacteriaceae			≤14	15–18	≥19
Ciprofloxacin	CIP-5	5µg			
Enterobacteriaceae, *P. aeruginosa, Acinetobacter*, staphylococci, and enterococci			≤15	16–20	≥21
Haemophilus spp.					≥21
N. gonorrhoeae			≤27	28–40	≥41
Clarithromycin	CLR-15	15 µg			
Staphylococcus spp.			≤13	14–17	≥18
Haemophilus spp.			≤10	11–12	≥13
S. pneumoniae and other streptococci			≤16	17–20	≥21

(*continues*)

TABLE 6-1 Interpretative Guidelines for Aerobic Bacteria: Zone Diameter Interpretative Standards* (Continued)

Antimicrobial agent	Code	Disk content	R	I	S
Clindamycin	CC-2	2μg			
Staphylococcus spp.			≤14	15–20	≥21
S. pneumoniae and other streptococci			≤15	16–18	≥19
Colistin	CL-10	10 μg	≤8	9–10	≥11
Doxycycline	D-30	30 μg			
Enterobacteriaceae, *P. aeruginosa, Acinetobacter,* staphylococci, and enterococci			≤12	13–15	≥16
Enoxacin	ENX-10	10 μg			
Enterobacteriaceae and staphylococci			≤14	15–17	≥18
N. gonorrhoeae			≤31	32–35	≥36
Ertapenem	ETP-10	10 μg			
Enterobacteriaceae and staphylococci			≤15	16–18	≥19
Haemophilus spp.			—	—	≥19
Erythromycin	E-15	15 μg			
Staphylococcus spp. and enterococci			≤13	14–22	≥23
S. pneumoniae and other streptococci			≤15	16–20	≥21
Fosfomycin	FOS-200	200 μg			
E. coli and *E. faecalis* only			≤12	13–15	≥16
Gatifloxacin	GAT-5	5 μg			
Enterobacteriaceae and *Staphylococcus* spp.			≤14	15–17	≥18
P. aeruginosa, Acinetobacter spp., and enterococci			≤14	15–17	≥18
H. influenzae and *H. parainfluenzae*			—	—	≥18
N. gonorrhoeae			≤33	34–37	≥38
S. pneumoniae and other streptococci (non-*S. pneumoniae,* β-hemolytic only)			≤17	18–20	≥38
Gemifloxacin	GEM-5	5 μg			
Enterobacteriaceae			≤15	16–19	≥20
H. influenzae and *H. parainfluenzae*			—	—	≥18
S. pneumonia			≤19	20–22	≥23
Gentamycin	GM-10	10 μg			
Enterobacteriaceae, *Staphylococcus* spp., *P. aeruginosa*, and *Acinetobacter* spp.			≤12	13–14	≥15
Enterococci for high-level resistance	GM-120	120 μg	≤6	7–9	≥10
Imipenem	IPM-10	10 μg			
Enterobacteriaceae, *Staphylococcus* spp., *P. aeruginosa*, and *Acinetobacter* spp.			≤13	14–15	≥16
Haemophilus spp.			—	—	≥16
Kanamycin	K-30	30 μg			
Enterobacteriaceae and *Staphylococcus* spp.			≤13	14–17	≥ 18

TABLE 6-1 Interpretative Guidelines for Aerobic Bacteria: Zone Diameter Interpretative Standards* (Continued)

Antimicrobial agent	Code	Disk content	R	I	S
Levofloxacin	LVX-5	5 µg			
Enterobacteriaceae, *Staphylococcus* spp., *P. aeruginosa, Acinetobacter* spp., and enterococci			≤13	14–16	≥17
Haemophilus spp.			—	—	≥17
S. pneumoniae and other streptococci (non-*S. pneumoniae,* β-hemolytic only)			≤13	14–16	≥17
Linezolid	LZD-30	30 µg			
Staphylococcus spp.			—	—	≥21
Enterococcus spp.			≤20	21–22	≥23
S. pneumoniae and other streptococci			—	—	≥21
Lomefloxacin	LOM-10	10 µg			
Enterobacteriaceae, *Staphylococcus* spp., *P. aeruginosa*, and *Acinetobacter* spp.			≤18	19–21	≥22
Haemophilus spp.			—	—	≥22
N. gonorrhoeae			≤26	27–37	≥38
Loracarbef	LOR-30	30 µg			
Enterobacteriaceae and *Staphylococcus* spp.			≤14	15–17	≥18
Haemophilus spp.			≤15	16–18	≥19
Meropenem	MEM-10	10 µg			
Enterobacteriaceae, *Staphylococcus* spp., *P. aeruginosa*, and *Acinetobacter* spp.			≤13	14–15	≥16
Haemophilus spp.			—	—	≥20
Mezlocillin	MZ-75	75 µg			
Enterobacteriaceae and *Acinetobacter* spp.			≤17	18–20	≥21
P. aeruginosa			≤15	—	≥16
Minocycline	MI-30	30 µg			
Enterobacteriaceae, *P. aeruginosa, Acinetobacter* spp., staphylococci, and enterococci			≤14	15–18	≥19
Moxalactam	MOX-30	30 µg			
Enterobacteriaceae, *P. aeruginosa, Acinetobacter* spp., and staphylococci			≤14	15–22	≥23
Moxifloxacin	MXF-5	5 µg			
Enterobacteriaceae and *Staphylococcus* spp.			≤15	16–18	≥19
H. influenzae and *H. parainfluenzae*			—	—	≥18
S. pneumonia			≤14	15–17	≥18
Nafcillin	NF-1	1 µg			
S. aureus			≤10	11–12	≥13
Nalidixic Acid	NA-30	30 µg			
Enterobacteriaceae			≤13	14–18	≥19
Neomycin	N-30	30 µg	≤12	13–16	≥17
Netilmicin	NET-30	30 µg			
Enterobacteriaceae, *P. aeruginosa, Acinetobacter* spp., and staphylococci			≤12	13–14	≥15

(*continues*)

TABLE 6-1 Interpretative Guidelines for Aerobic Bacteria: Zone Diameter Interpretative Standards* (Continued)

Antimicrobial agent	Code	Disk content	R	I	S
Nitrofurantoin	F/M 300	300 µg			
Enterobacteriaceae, staphylococci, and enterococci			≤14	15–16	≥17
Norfloxacin	NOR-10	10 µg			
Enterobacteriaceae, *P. aeruginosa, Acinetobacter* spp., staphylococci, and enterococci			≤12	13–16	≥17
Novobiocin (veterinarian use only)	NB-30	30 µg	≤17	18–21	≥22
Ofloxacin	OFX-5	5 µg			
Enterobacteriaceae, *P. aeruginosa, Acinetobacter* spp., and staphylococci			≤12	13–15	≥16
Haemophilus spp.					≥16
N. gonorrhoeae			≤24	25–30	≥31
S. pneumoniae and other streptococci (non-*S. pneumoniae*, β-hemolytic only)			≤12	13–15	≥16
Oxacillin	OX-1	1 µg			
S. aureus			≤10	11–12	≥13
Staphylococcus, coagulase negative			≤17	—	≥18
S. pneumoniae (for penicillin G susceptibility)			—	—	≥20
Oxolinic Acid	OA-2	2 µg	≤10	—	≥11
Penicillin	P-10	10 U			
Staphylococcus spp.			≤28	—	≥29
Enterococcus spp.			≤14	—	≥15
L. monocytogenes			≤19	20–27	≥28
N. gonorrhoeae			≤26	27–46	≥47
S. pneumoniae (non-*S. pneumoniae,* β-hemolytic only)			—	—	≥24
Piperacillin	PIP-100	100 µg			
Enterobacteriaceae and *Acinetobacter* spp.			≤17	18–20	≥21
P. aeruginosa			≤17	—	≥18
Piperacillin/Tazobactam	TZP-100	100/10 µg			
Enterobacteriaceae and *Acinetobacter* spp.			≤17	18–20	≥21
Staphylococcus spp. and *P. aeruginosa*			≤17	—	≥18
Polymyxin B	PB-300	300 U	≤8	9–11	≥12
Quinupristin/Dalfopristin	SYN-15	4.5/10.5 µg			
Staphylococcus spp., *Enterococcus faecium*, and *Streptococcus pyogenes* only			≤15	16–18	≥19
Rifampin	RA-5	5 µg			
Staphylococcus spp. and *Enterococcus* spp.			≤16	17–19	≥20
Haemophilus spp.			≤16	17–19	≥20
S. pneumonia			≤16	17–18	≥19
Sparfloxacin	SPX-5	5 µg			
Staphylococcus spp.			≤15	16–18	≥19
S. pneumonia			≤15	16–18	≥19
Spectinomycin	SPT-100	100 µg			
N. gonorrhoeae			≤14	15–17	≥18

TABLE 6-1 Interpretative Guidelines for Aerobic Bacteria: Zone Diameter Interpretative Standards* (Continued)

Antimicrobial agent	Code	Disk content	R	I	S
Streptomycin					
Enterobacteriaceae	S-10	10 µg	≤11	12–14	≥15
Enterococci for high-level resistance	S-300	300 µg	≤6	7–9	≥10
Sulfisoxazole	G-.25	250 µg			
Enterobacteriaceae, *P. aeruginosa, Acinetobacter,* staphylococci, and *V. cholerae*			≤12	13–16	≥17
Telithromycin	TEL-15	15 µg			
S. aureus			—	—	≥22
Haemophilus spp.			≤11	12–14	≥15
S. pneumonia			≤15	16–18	≥19
Tetracycline	Te-30	30 µg			
Enterobacteriaceae, *P. aeruginosa, Acinetobacter,* staphylococci, enterococci, and *V. cholerae*			≤14	15–18	≥19
Haemophilus spp.			≤25	26–28	≥29
N. gonorrhoeae			≤30	31–37	≥38
S. pneumoniae and other streptococci			≤18	19–22	≥23
Ticarcillin	TIC-75	75 µg			
Enterobacteriaceae and *Acinetobacter*			≤14	15–19	≥20
P. aeruginosa			≤14	—	≥15
Ticarcillin-clavulanic acid	TIM-85	75/10 µg			
Enterobacteriaceae and *Acinetobacter*			≤14	15–19	≥20
P. aeruginosa			≤14	—	≥15
Staphylococcus spp.			≤22		≥23
Tigecycline	TGC-15	15 µg			
Enterobacteriaceae			≤14	15–19	≥20
S. aureus (including MRSA)			—	—	≥19
E. faecalis (vancomycin-susceptible isolates only)			—	—	≥19
Streptococcus spp. (other than *S. pneumoniae*)			—	—	≥19
Tobramycin	NN-10	10 µg			
Enterobacteriaceae, *P. aeruginosa, Acinetobacter,* and staphylococci			≤12	13–14	≥15
Trimethoprim	TMP-5	5 µg			
Enterobacteriaceae and staphylococci			≤10	11–15	≥16
Trimethoprim/sulfamethoxazole	SXT	1.25/			
Enterobacteriaceae, *P. aeruginosa, Acinetobacter,* staphylococci, and *V. cholerae*		23.75 µg	≤10	11–15	≥16
Haemophilus spp.			≤10	11–15	≥16
S. pneumonia			≤15	16–18	≥19
Vancomycin	Va-30	30 µg			
Staphylococcus spp.			—	—	≥15
Enterococcus spp.			≤14	15–16	≥17
S. pneumoniae and other streptococci			—	—	≥17

*R, resistant; I, intermediate; S, susceptible

TABLE 6-2 Quality-Control Limits for Monitoring Antimicrobial Disk Susceptibility Tests

		E. coli	*S. aureus*	*P. aeruginosa*	*H. influenzae*	*N. gonorrhoeae*	*S. pneumoniae*
Antimicrobial agent	**Code/Disk content**	**ATCC 25922**	**ATCC 25923**	**ATCC 25853**	**ATCC 49247**	**ATCC 48226**	**ATCC 49719**
		Zone diameter (mm)					
Amdinocillin	AMD-10 10 µg	23–29	—	—	—	—	—
Amikacin	AN-30 30 µg	19–26	20–26	18–26	15–23	—	—
Amoxicillin/ clavulanic acid	AMC-30 20/10 µg	18–24	28–36	—	1–23		
Ampicillin	AM-10 10 µg	16–22	27–35	—	13–21	—	30–36
Ampicillin/ sulbactam	SAM 20 10/10 µg	19–24	29–37	—	14–22	—	30–36
Azithromycin	AZM-15 15 µg	—	21–26	—	13–21		19–25
Azlocillin	AZ-75 75 µg	—	—	24–30	—	—	—
Aztreonam	ATM-30 30 µg	28–36	—	23–29	30–38	—	—
Bacitracin	B-10 10 U	—	12–22	—	—	—	—
Carbenicillin	CB-100 100 µg	23–29	—	18–24	—	—	—
Cefaclor	CEC-100 100 µg	—	23–27	27–31	25–31*	—	—
Cefamandole	MA-30 30 µg	26–32	26–34	—	—	—	—
Cefazolin	CZ-30 30 µg	21–27	29–35	—	—	—	—
Cefdinir	CPR-5 5 µg	24–28	25–32	—	24–32*	—	—
Cefepime	FEP-30 30 µg	31–37	23–29	24–30	25–31	37–46	28–35
Cefixime	CFH-5 5 µg	23–27	—	—	25–33	37–45	—
Cefmetazole	CMZ-30 30 µg	26–32	25–34	—	—	31–36	—
Cefonicid	CID-30 30 µg	25–29	22–28	—	30–38	—	—
Cefoperazone	CFP-75 75 µg	28–34	24–33	23–29	—	—	—
Cefotaxime	CTX-30 30 µg	29–35	25–31	18–22	31–39	38–48	31–39
Cefotetan	CTT-30 30 µg	28–34	17–23	—	—	30–36	—

TABLE 6-2 Quality-Control Limits for Monitoring Antimicrobial Disk Susceptibility Tests (Continued)

		E. coli	*S. aureus*	*P. aeruginosa*	*H. influenzae*	*N. gonorrhoeae*	*S. pneumoniae*
Antimicrobial agent	**Code/Disk content**	**ATCC 25922**	**ATCC 25923**	**ATCC 25853**	**ATCC 49247**	**ATCC 48226**	**ATCC 49719**
Cefoxitin	FOX-30 30 μg	23–29	23–29	—	—	—	33–41
Cefpodoxime	CPD-10 10 μg	23–28	19–25	—	25–31	35–43	—
Cefprozil	CPR-10 10 μg	21–27	27–33	—	20–27*	—	—
Ceftazidime	CAZ-30 30 μg	25–32	16–20	22–29	27–33	35–43	—
Ceftibuten	CTB-30 30 μg	27–35	—	—	29–36	—	—
Ceftizoxime	ZOX-30 30 μg	30–36	27–35	12–17	—	—	—
Ceftriaxone	CRO-30 30 μg	27–35	22–28	17–23	31–39	39–51	30–35
Cefuroxime	CXM-30 30 μg	20–26	27–35	—	28–36*	33–41	—
Cephalothin	CR-30 30 μg	15–21	29–37	—	—	—	—
Chloramphenicol	C-30 30 μg	21–27	19–26	—	31–40	48–58	—
Cinoxacin	CIN-100 100 μg	26–32	—	—	—	—	—
Ciprofloxacin	CIP-5 5 μg	30–40	22–30	25–33	34–42	48–52	25–31
Clarithromycin	CLR-15 15 μg	—	26–32	—	11–17	—	25–31
Clindamycin	CC-2 2μg	—	24–30	—	—	—	19–25
Colistin	CL-10 10 μg	11–15	—	—	—	—	19–25
Doxycycline	D-30 30 μg	18–24	23–29	—	—	—	—
Enoxacin	ENX-10 10 μg	28–36	22–28	22–28	—	43–51	28–35
Ertapenem	ETP-10 10 μg	29–36	24–31	13–21	20–28	—	25–30
Erythromycin	E-15 15 μg	—	22–30	—	—	—	25–30
Fosfomycin	FOS-200 200 μg	22–30	25–33	—	—	—	—
Gatifloxacin	GAT-5 5 μg	30–37	27–33	20–28	33–41	45–56	24–31
Gemifloxacin	GEM-5 5 μg	29–36	27–33	19–25	30–37	—	28–34

(*continues*)

TABLE 6-2 Quality-Control Limits for Monitoring Antimicrobial Disk Susceptibility Tests (Continued)

		E. coli	*S. aureus*	*P. aeruginosa*	*H. influenzae*	*N. gonorrhoeae*	*S. pneumoniae*
Antimicrobial agent	**Code/Disk content**	**ATCC 25922**	**ATCC 25923**	**ATCC 25853**	**ATCC 49247**	**ATCC 48226**	**ATCC 49719**
Gentamycin	GM-10 10 µg	19–26	19–27	16–21	—	—	—
Imipenem	IPM-10 10 µg	26–32	—	20–28	21–29	—	—
Kanamycin	K-30 30 µg	17–25	19–26	—	—	—	—
Linezolid	LZD-30 30 µg	—	25–32	—	—	—	25–34
Lomefloxacin	LOM-10 10 µg	27–33	23–29	22–28	33–41	45–54	—
Loracarbef	LOR-30 30 µg	23–29	23–31	—	26–32*	—	—
Lovofloxacin	LVX-5 5 µg	29–37	25–30	19–26	32–40	—	20–25
Mezlocillin	MZ-75 75 µg	23–29	—	19–25	—	—	—
Minocycline	MI-30 30 µg	19–25	25–30	—	—	—	—
Moxalactam	MOX-30 30 µg	28–35	18–24	17–25	—	—	—
Moxifloxacin	MXF-5 5 µg	28–35	28–35	—	31–39	—	25–31
Nafcillin	NF-1 1 µg	—	16–22	—	—	—	—
Nalidixic acid	NA-30 30 µg	22–28	—	—	—	—	—
Neomycin	N-30 30 µg	17–23	18–26	—	—	—	—
Netilmicin	NET-30 30 µg	22–30	22–31	17–23	—	—	—
Nitrofurantoin	F/M 300 300 µg	20–25	18–22	—	—	—	—
Norfloxacin	NOR-10 10 µg	28–35	17–28	22–29	—	—	—
Novobiocin (veterinarian use only)	NB-30 30 µg	—	22–31	—	—	—	—
Ofloxacin	OFX-5 5 µg	29–33	24–28	17–21	31–40	43–51	16–21
Oxacillin	OX-1 1 µg	—	18–24	—	—	—	— <12

TABLE 6-2 Quality-Control Limits for Monitoring Antimicrobial Disk Susceptibility Tests (Continued)

		E. coli	*S. aureus*	*P. aeruginosa*	*H. influenzae*	*N. gonorrhoeae*	*S. pneumoniae*
Antimicrobial agent	**Code/Disk content**	**ATCC 25922**	**ATCC 25923**	**ATCC 25853**	**ATCC 49247**	**ATCC 48226**	**ATCC 49719**
Oxolinic acid	OA-2 2 μg	20–24	10–13	—	—	—	—
Penicillin	P-10 10 U	—	26–37	—	—	26–34	24–30
Piperacillin	PIP-100 100 μg	24–30	—	25–33	—	—	—
Piperacillin/ Tazobactam	TZP-110 100/10 μg	24–30	27–36	25–33	—	—	—
Polymyxin B	PB-300 300 μg	12–16	—	—	—	—	—
Quinupristin/ Dalfopristin	SYN-15 4.5/10.5 μg	—	21–28	—	—	—	19–24
Rifampin	RA-5 5 μg	8–10	26–34	—	22–30	—	25–30
Sparfloxacin	SPX-5 5 μg	30–38	27–33	21–29	—	—	21–27
Spectinomycin	SPT-100	—	—	—	—	23–29	—
Streptomycin	S-10 10 μg	12–20	14–22	—	—	—	—
Sulfisoxazole	G-0.25 250 μg	15–23	24–34	—	—	—	—
Telithromycin	TEL-15 15 μg	—	24–30	—	—	—	—
Tetracycline	Te-30 30 μg	18–25	24–30	14–22	30–42	27–31	—
Ticarcillin	TIC-75 75 μg	24–30	—	21–27	—	—	—
Ticarcillin/ clavulanic acid	TIM-85 75/10 μg	24–30	29–37	20–28	—	—	—
Tigecycline	TGC-15 15 μg	20–27	20–25	9–13	23–31	30–40	23–29
Tobramycin	NN-10 10 μg	18–26	19–29	19–25	—	—	—
Trimethoprim	TMP-5 5 μg	21–28	19–26	—	—	—	—
Trimethoprim/ sulfamethoxazole	SXT 1.25/23.75 μg	23–29	24–32	—	—	—	20–28
Vancomycin	Va-30 30 μg	—	17–21	—	—	—	20–27

*R, resistant; I, intermediate; S, susceptible

TABLE 6-3 Selection of Antimicrobial Agents

Antimicrobial agents	Enterobacteriaceae	*Staphylococcus*	*Pseudomonas aeruginosa*	*Enterococcus*	*Streptococcus pneumoniae*
Penicillins	Ampicillin Piperacillin/ tazbactam	Penicillin Oxacillin	Piperacillin/ tazbactam	Ampicillin	Penicillin
Cephalosporins	Cefazolin Cefotetan Ceftrixone Cefotaxime Ceftazidime		Ceftazidime		Ceftrixone Cefotaxime
Other β-lactams	Aztreonam Imipenem		Aztreonam Imipenem		Imipenem
Aminoglycosides	Gentamycin Tobramycin Amikacin		Gentamycin Tobramycin Amikacin	Gentamycin (high level)	
Quinolones	Ciprofloxacin Levofloxacin	Ciprofloxacin Levofloxacin	Ciprofloxacin Levofloxacin		Ciprofloxacin Levofloxacin
Others	Trimethoprim Sulfamethoxazole Tigecycline	Vancomycin Erythromycin Clindamycin Trimethoprim Sulfamethoxazole Tigecycline Daptomycin Linezolid Telithromycin		Vancomycin Tigecycline Daptomycin Linezolid	Vancomycin Erythromycin Clindamycin Trimethoprim Sulfamethoxazole Telithromycin

subcultured onto a suitable medium. After incubation for 24 to 48 hours, the plates are read for growth. The lowest concentration of the antibiotic that killed the bacterium is the **minimal bacteriocidal concentration** (MBC). The MBC is defined as the lowest concentration of antibiotic that totally kills 99.9% of the standardized inoculum.

Agar Dilution Susceptibility Testing

Agar dilution MIC tests involve the addition of various concentrations of antimicrobial agents into agar that is heated and not solidified. A separate plate is needed for each antibiotic concentration tested. After the agar has hardened, a standard inoculum of bacteria is spot-inoculated onto the agars containing antimicrobial agents. The plates are incubated overnight and examined for visible growth. The lowest antibiotic concentration that inhibits in vitro visible growth is the MIC.

Agar dilution tests have been modified and can be performed on agar plates with wells that contain different concentrations of the antibiotic to be tested. The wells can be inoculated with a multipronged diluter and read for the presence or absence of growth. This method, although accurate, is cumbersome for a routine microbiology laboratory. Its routine use has been in anaerobic susceptibility testing and in research facilities.

Macrobroth Dilution Susceptibility Testing

The macrobroth dilution (or macrodilution broth) test uses Mueller-Hinton broth with calcium and magnesium ions (Ca^{2+} and Mg^{2+}) added. The medium supports the growth of most bacteria. When testing *Staphylococcus* with methicillin, oxacillin, or nafcillin, the medium should be supplemented with 2% sodium chloride (NaCl). In this method, 13 tubes are labeled and 1.0 ml of Mueller-Hinton broth is pipetted into tubes 2 through 10, 11, and 13. Next, 2.0 ml of broth is pipetted into tube 12. Tubes 1, 2, and 13 receive 1.0 ml of the working antibiotic solution. Twofold serial dilutions in 1.0 ml amounts in tubes 2 through 10 are performed. Then 1.0 ml of the standardized inoculum is pipetted to tubes 1 through 11. The tubes are mixed and incubated at 35°C for 18 to 24 hours. After incubation the first tube showing no visible growth is considered to be the MIC. One should subculture all tubes showing no growth to media, incubate, and note the lowest antibiotic concentration that has resulted in 99.9% killing. This is the MBC. The MBC should be performed on immunosuppressed patients or those with diminished immunity and serious infections, such as endocarditis. Agents that are bacteriocidal usually produce MBCs within one or two dilutions of the MIC. **FIGURE 6-6** depicts a typical broth dilution test, showing determination of the MIC and MBC.

The macrobroth method also provides excellent practice on performing and interpreting dilutions. Furthermore, the concepts of the MIC and MBC are clearly elucidated using this method.

Microbroth Dilution Susceptibility Testing

The macrobroth dilution test is useful for laboratories testing a few antibiotics with a few organisms. It is cumbersome to perform in laboratories where large volumes of organisms and large numbers of antibiotics must be tested. The microbroth dilution method was developed from the

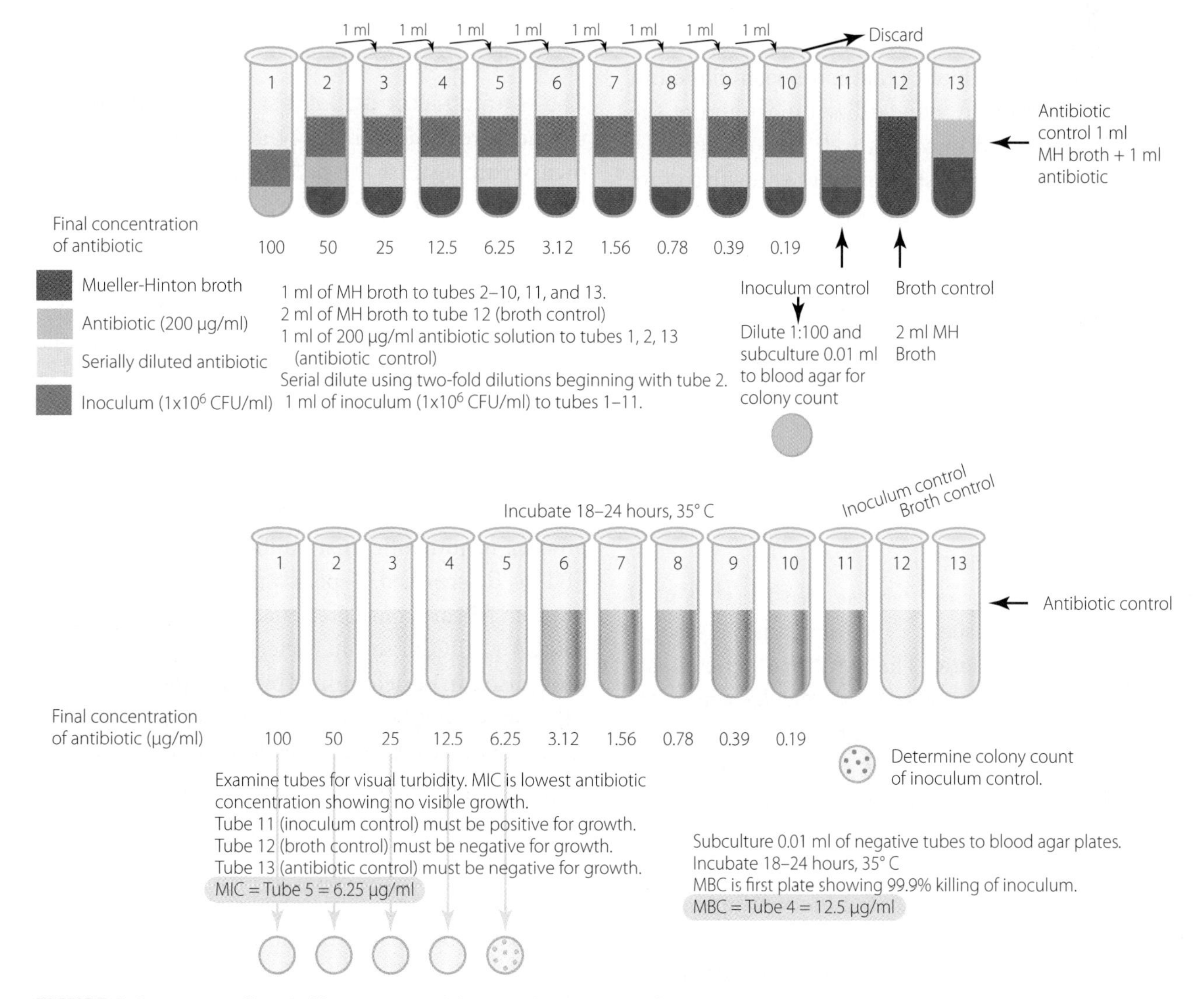

FIGURE 6-6 Diagram of broth dilution susceptibility test showing procedure setup and determination of MIC and MBC.

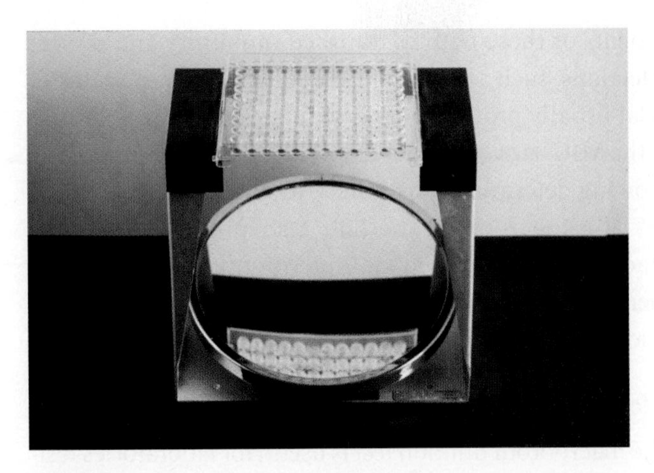

FIGURE 6-7 Microdilution tray with viewing mirror used to observe for the presence or absence of growth in each well.

macrobroth method and is more practical in such cases. In this technique, plastic trays with approximately 80 wells are filled with minute volumes (50 µl to 100 µl) of serial twofold dilutions of several antibiotics that have been diluted in Mueller-Hinton broth. A standardized inoculum of the organism is inoculated into each well through use of a multipronged dilutor. The system includes a growth control and purity control. The plastic trays are commercially available from a number of manufacturers, and the user also may select the battery of antimicrobial agents to be included. The antibiotics are either frozen or lyophilized when obtained from the manufacturer. With the advent of automation, the plates can be automatically inoculated and read with an instrument. The method for the microdilution broth susceptibility test is described later in this chapter. **FIGURE 6-7** shows a typical microtiter dilution tray.

Gradient Diffusion Testing

The Epsilometer test (usually abbreviated Etest®) is used to determine whether a specific microorganism is susceptible to a specific antibiotic. The Etest® (bioMérieux) is a variation to the disk diffusion test and provides a quantitative value and also can identify the presence of antimicrobial resistance. This test consists of a predefined gradient of antibiotic concentrations on a plastic strip and is used to determine the MIC of antibiotics, antifungal agents, and antimycobacterial agents. An interpretation scale is printed on one side of the strip. After inoculating the agar plate, the Etest® strips are placed on the agar surface; multiple strips can be placed on one agar plate, forming a pattern that resembles spokes of a wheel. After incubation, the result is an elliptical zone of inhibition relative to the antibiotic concentration. The MIC is that place on the scale where the zone of inhibition intersects the strip. The Etest® can determine the MIC across 15 antibiotic dilutions; there are currently over 100 antibiotics available to test for aerobic bacteria and fastidious organisms, such as *S. pneumoniae*, *Haemophilus* spp., *Helicobacter pylori*, *Neisseria meningitidis*, and *N. gonorrhoeae* and anaerobes, fungi, and mycobacteria. The MIC is clearly determined by reading the value from the visible MIC gradient scale on each plastic strip. Resistance mechanisms also can be detected using the Etest®, including ESBL and AmpC.

The M.I.C. Evaluator (M.I.C.E.™) strips from Oxoid also use the gradient format to determine the MIC. There are strips available for a variety of microorganisms, which have a distinct scale that conforms to international standards.

Serum Bacteriocidal Test

The **serum bacteriocidal test** (SBT), or **Schlichter test**, is a measure of the activity of the antibiotic in the patient's own serum against the pathogen. It is used as a guideline to determine whether the patient is receiving effective therapy for a serious infection, such as meningitis, endocarditis, or osteomyelitis. The SBT is defined as the lowest dilution of the patient's serum that kills a standardized inoculum of bacteria. A **trough specimen** is collected within 15 minutes before the next antibiotic dose, and a **peak specimen** is collected approximately 30 to 60 minutes after the antibiotic is given. Twofold serial dilutions of the patient's serum samples are then tested against the standardized inoculum. The highest dilution (or lowest amount of antibiotic) that inhibits the organism (MIC for SBT) is determined. A peak value of >1:64 and a trough level of >1:32 are considered effective for bacterial endocarditis. An MBC, or serum bacteriocidal titer for the procedure, also can be determined by following the macrobroth dilution susceptibility procedure. Because more effective laboratory methods are available, the SBT test is no longer frequently performed.

Peak and Trough Assays

Assays of specific antimicrobial agents may be indicated for those drugs that have a low therapeutic index. Such drugs have a small window between a level that is therapeutic and a level that is toxic to the host. Agents that may require assays include the aminoglycosides (tobramycin, gentamycin), vancomycin, and chloramphenicol. Often the assays are requested to determine the amount of antibiotic that is in the patient's circulation or that has reached a particular body fluid, such as cerebrospinal fluid. This level may be affected by the biotransformation of the agent as affected by hepatic function, the elimination of the agent as related to renal function, and other host factors. The assays require the collection and analysis of a peak and a trough specimen. The **peak specimen** is collected 30 minutes after the agent is administered through the intravenous route and approximately 60 minutes when given intramuscularly. The peak specimen represents the highest level of antibiotic that has reached the blood. The **trough specimen** should be collected 15 minutes before the next dose. At least one dose of the antibiotic must have been given to collect a valid trough specimen.

SPECIFIC METHODS TO DETERMINE BACTERIAL RESISTANCE

Bacterial isolates also can be tested for the presence of resistance to an antibiotic or to a group of antibiotics. This section discusses some of the more significant tests for antibiotic resistance.

β-Lactamase and Cefinase

The β-lactamase enzymes cleave the β-lactam ring of penicillins and cephalosporins. Both gram-negative and gram-positive organisms are known to produce β-lactamases. Bacteria that most often produce β-lactamase are *Staphylococcus* species, *H. influenzae*, *N. gonorrhoeae*, *Moraxella catarrhalis*, and *Enterococcus* species. The substrate to detect β-lactamase may be a penicillin or a cephalosporin, and the principles that may be used include iodometric, acidometric, and chromogenic techniques. In iodometric methods, the end products of the activity of β-lactamase on the penicillin substrate reduce iodine, which is bound to starch. A positive reaction is indicated by the disappearance in color as the starch–iodine complex is degraded. In acidometric methods, penicillin is hydrolyzed into acidic end products in the presence of β-lactamase. An indicator that changes color in the presence of acid is used to visualize the reaction. The most sensitive method and the method that has been effective in detecting many types of β-lactamase is the one using the chromogenic cephalosporin Nitrocefin. In the presence of β-lactamase the amide bond in the β-lactam ring is hydrolyzed. This results in a color change of the chromogen from yellow to red. One type of test that can be commercially obtained is the Cefinase procedure (BD BBL™), which uses filter paper disks impregnated with Nitrocefin. This method will detect only those β-lactamase enzymes that are present in the external environment, such as those produced by *Staphylococcus* species, *H. influenzae*, *N. gonorrhoeae*, and *Moraxella catarrhalis* and not those that remain in the periplasmic space that are produced by the gram-negative bacilli. The Cefinase procedure is described later in this chapter and is illustrated in **FIGURE 6-8**.

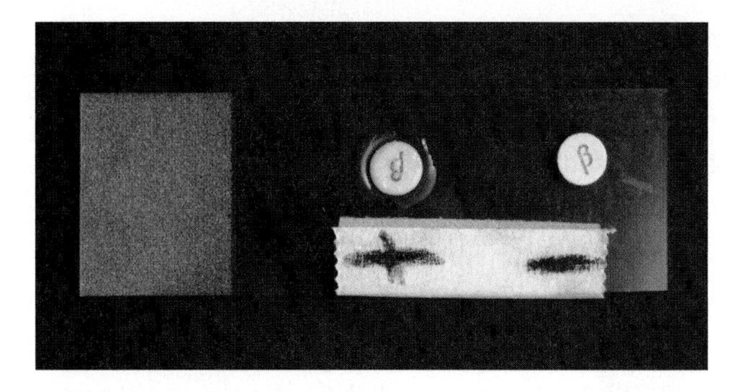

FIGURE 6-8 Cefinase procedure for determination of β-lactamase activity.

Laboratory Detection of Oxacillin-/Methicillin-Resistant *Staphylococcus aureus*

Resistance to penicillin by *S. aureus* was observed soon after the introduction of penicillin in the 1940s. There were strains of *S. aureus* resistant to methicillin/oxacillin by the late 1960s.

Today, approximately 10% of *S. aureus* isolates in the United States remain susceptible to penicillin, according to the CDC. Some of these penicillin-resistant strains remain susceptible to penicillinase-stable penicillin, such as oxacillin and methicillin. Those strains that are resistant to oxacillin and methicillin are known as methicillin-resistant *S. aureus* (MRSA). When resistance was first described in the 1960s, methicillin was used to test and treat *S. aureus* infections. Oxacillin was later used as the agent of choice to treat staphylococcal infections in the 1990s. The acronym, MRSA, is still used to describe these isolates that are resistant to methicillin/oxacillin. These strains also are usually resistant to all β-lactam antibiotics, including the cephalosporins and carbapenems. Strains of MRSA acquired in the health care setting are generally resistant to multiple antibiotics, including erythromycin, tetracycline, and clindamycin. Community-acquired MRSA seems to be resistant to only other β-lactams or erythromycin. An additional concern is that MRSA strains with decreased susceptibility to vancomycin have been reported.

There are three mechanisms for resistance to the β-lactam antibiotics in *S. aureus*:

1. Production of supplemental penicillin-binding protein (PBP) that is encoded for by the *mecA* gene. This is the classic type of resistance, and strains that have the *mecA* gene are either homogeneous or heterogeneous in resistance expression. In homozygous expression, almost all of the cells show resistance when tested by in vitro methods; in heterozygous expression, some of the cells are susceptible, and some show resistance in laboratory tests. Because there may be as few as one in 1,000 or one in 100 million resistant cells, heterozygous strains may show a borderline MIC of 2 μg/ml to 8 μg/ml, which may be reported incorrectly as susceptible. Thus, additonal tests are needed to identify this type of resistance. This classic resistance pattern also usually shows resistance to other antibiotics, such as clindamycin, erythromycin, chloroamphenicol, tetracycline, trimethoprim sulfamethoxazole, some of the aminoglycosides, and older fluoroquinolones.
2. Hyper β-lactamase production also may show borderline resistance, but it is generally not resistant to multiple antibiotics.
3. Production of modified PBPs that reduce the organism's affinity for β-lactam antibiotics may also produce borderline resistance.

Methicillin resistance can be detected using the cefoxitin disk screen test, latex agglutination for PBB2a, or Mueller-Hinton agar supplemented with NaCl and 6 μg/ml of oxacillin according to the Clinical and Laboratory Standards Institute (CLSI). In the oxacillin/methicillin agar screen method, Mueller-Hinton agar is supplemented with sodium chloride to enhance the growth of the PRP-resistant subpopulations. The medium contains oxacillin, which is preferred for detection of PRP resistance. Oxacillin is used in the test instead of methicillin because methicillin is no longer commercially available in the United States. Also, oxacillin maintains its activity better when stored and is more likely to detect heteroresistant strains. Growth on the plate indicates resistance to methicillin/oxacillin. This method is found in the laboratory exercises at the end of the chapter.

Cefoxitin is an even superior inducer of the *mecA* gene, and disk diffusion tests that use cefoxitin give clearer end points and may be preferred to the oxacillin method. The method is also found at the end of this chapter.

There are also chromogenic agars commercially available that can detect MRSA. BBL™ CHROMagar™ MRSA is a selective and differential medium that can detect nasal colonization by methicillin-resistant *Staphylococcus aureus*. The test is useful in the identification of carriers of MRSA and is performed by swabbing the anterior nares of patients and health care workers to screen for colonization. This agar uses specific chromogenic substrates and cefoxitin. MRSA strains will grow in the presence of cefoxitin and produce mauve-colored colonies resulting from hydrolysis of the chromogenic substrate. There are other agents in the medium that suppress the growth of gram-negative organisms, yeast, and some gram-positive cocci. Bacteria other than MRSA may utilize other chromogenic substrates in the medium, resulting in blue- to blue-green–colored colonies, or if no chromogenic substrates are utilized, the colonies appear as white or colorless.

The chromogen in Oxoid Chromogenic MRSA Agar detects phosphatase activity, which is present in MRSA strains, producing distinct, easily visible, denim-blue colonies. Antimicrobial compounds within the medium, including cefoxitin, inhibit the growth of other organisms, which enhances the ability to identify MRSA. Oxoid Chromogenic MRSA Agar may be inoculated directly from swabs or from isolates or culture suspensions. The plate is examined for MRSA colonies after an 18-hour incubation.

Inducible Resistance to Clindamycin

Health care–associated infections (HAI) from MRSA are also usually resistant to erythromycin and clindamycin, whereas community-acquired (CA) MRSA infections are usually susceptible to clindamycin. The erythromycin resistance is a result of the *msrA* gene, which promotes the efflux of the antibiotic out of the bacterial cell. The *erm* gene activates the resistance to clindamycin. The D test can be used to determine inducible resistance to clindamycin. In this method, the suspension of the organism is streaked onto Mueller-Hinton agar. The erythromycin disk is placed so that its edge is 15 mm to 26 mm from the edge of the clindamycin disk. In the presence of inducible clindamycin resistance, there is a flattened zone observed between the two discs. The zone around the clindamycin disk resembles the letter "D," a pattern that occurs with antagonistic antibiotics. This indicates that the *erm* gene has been triggered for clindamycin in the organism.

Vancomycin Resistance in Staphylococcus

Vancomycin-resistant *Staphylococcus aureus* (VRSA) and vancomycin-intermediate *Staphylococcus aureus* (VISA) have been identified. Therefore, it is necessary to separate VRSA and VISA from strains of *S. aureus* that are susceptible to vancomycin. Those *S. aureus* with reduced susceptibility to vancomycin have MICs of 4 μg/ml to 16 μg/ml. The disk diffusion susceptibility test can make this differentiation; thus other test methods such as broth dilution or gradient diffusion tests are needed to determine the MIC. An agar screen method that uses brain-heart infusion agar with 6 μg of vancomycin also can be used. Growth indicates resistance, whereas no growth indicates susceptibility.

Vancomycin Resistance in Enterococcus

Enterococcus has shown resistance to vancomycin since the 1980s. This is a plasmid-mediated resistance mechanism that alters the target molecule. There are six types of vancomycin resistance based on genetic and phenotypic characteristics. The VanA phenotype is encoded by the *vanA* gene and shows inducible high-level resistance to vancomycin and teicoplanin. The VanB phenotype, encoded by the *vanB* gene, shows a variable amount of resistance to vancomycin alone. Both the VanA and VanB phenotypes can be transferred via plasmids; these are the two most common phenotypes. The VanC phenotype is associated with noninducible low-level resistance to vancomycin and is coded for by the intrinsic *vanC* genes; it cannot be transferred through plasmids. The VanD phenotype shows variable resistance to both vancomycin and teicoplanin, and VanE and VanG phenotypes show low-level resistance to vancomycin and are susceptible to teicoplanin. VanC, D, E, and G are found on the chromosomes. *E. faecalis* makes up approximately 80% of all enterococcal isolates, and *E. faecium* makes up about 15% of all clinical isolates. These two species can acquire and transfer vancomycin resistance. VanC is most commonly found in *E. casseliflavis*, *E. gallinarum*, and *E. flavescens*, which cannot transfer resistance.

Vancomycin screen agar with 6 μg of vancomycin in brain-heart infusion agar is used to detect VRE. A 0.5 McFarland suspension of the organism is spotted onto the agar, incubated for a full 24 hours at 35°C. Any growth indicates resistance, which should be investigated further by determining the MIC.

Vancomycin-dependent enterococci (VDE) actually uses vancomycin for cell wall synthesis. In the disk diffusion test, VDE grows in the area around the vancomycin disk since the antibiotic stimulates their growth.

High-Level Aminoglycoside Resistance

Enterococci are intrinsically resistant to aminoglycosides; a combination therapy using an aminoglycoside with vancomycin has been known to increase the effectiveness of the aminoglycoside. It is important to identify this high-level aminoglycoside resistance (HLAR) to provide appropriate therapy. Conventional disk diffusion methods do not detect HLAR. Brain-heart infusion agar is inoculated with a 0.5 McFarland suspension of the organism. Next, a 120 mg/ml gentamycin disk and a 300 μg/ml streptomycin disk are placed onto the inoculated agar. After incubation for a full 24 hours at 35°C, the zones are measured. Zones greater than 10 mm indicate susceptibility, whereas zones less than 6 mm indicate resistance. Zones of 7 mm to 9 mm are reported as inconclusive. Alternatively, commercially available agar (Remel, BBL) containing gentamycin (500 μg/ml) and streptomycin (1,000 μg/ml) can be used. Growth indicates resistance, whereas no growth indicates the organism is susceptible.

Penicillin Resistance in Streptococcus pneumoniae

With penicillin resistance emerging in *Streptococcus pneumoniae*, the disk diffusion test was no longer able to detect changes in susceptibility that may indicate resistance. The oxacillin screen test can be used to detect resistance to penicillin. In this method, Mueller-Hinton agar supplemented with sheep blood is inoculated. A 1 μg/ml oxacillin disc is placed onto the inoculated agar and incubated for 20 to 24 hours at 35°C under increased CO_2. Susceptibility is indicated by zones of inhibition ≥20 mm. Zones that are <20 mm may be penicillin resistant or intermediate but must be confirmed with an MIC or diffusion gradient test.

β-Lactamases in Gram-Negative Bacilli

There are many types of β-lactamase enzymes in gram-negative bacilli, which has resulted in multiple resistance. These mechanisms may be chromosomal or plasmid mediated; some organisms may have more than one mechanism. The β-lactamase resistance mechanisms are summarized in **TABLE 6-4**.

TABLE 6-4 Mechanisms of β-Lactamase Resistance

Class	Function
A	Hydrolyze aminopenicillin and penicillinase-stable penicillins
	Can be inhibited by clavulanic acid
	Plasmid mediated and transferred between different genera
	Found in *Staphylococcus* and *Enterococcus*
	Include some extended-spectrum β-lactamases (ESBLs)
B	Need metal ion, such as zinc, to hydrolyze β-lactam ring
	Not inhibited by clavulanic acid
	Plasmid mediated
	First found in *Stenotrophomonas maltophilia* and transferred to *Pseudomonas aeruginosa, Acinetobacter* spp., and some Enterobacteriaceae
	Resistant to aminoglycosides and fluoroquinolones
C	Cephalosporinase AmpC
	Chromosomal mediated
	Require prior exposure to β-lactam
	Not inhibited by clavulanic acid
	Resistant to imipenem
	Found in most Enterobacteriaceae
D	Least common β-lactamase mechanism
	Not inhibited by clavulanic acid
	Active against carbapenems, cephalosporins, penicillins, and oxacillin
	Found in *Pseudomonas aeruginosa, Acinetobacter* spp., and a few Enterobacteriaceae

Extended-Spectrum β-Lactamases (ESBLs)

This is a plasmid-mediated mechanism involving genes that code for β-lactamases, which were first discovered in Western Europe in the middle 1980s and later in the United States in the late 1980s. These include TEM-1, SHV-1, and OXA-1 in the Enterobacteriaceae. Multidrug resistance also is likely because most plasmids that carry ESBLs also are likely to carry resistance genes to other non–β-lactam antibiotics. The resistance can be transferred between different genera. First found in *E. coli* and *Klebsiella*, ESBLs now are found in *Proteus*, *Morganella*, *Serratia marcescens*, *Enterobacter*, and *Pseduomonas aeruginosa*. These mechanisms result in resistance to the carboxypenicillins (ticarcillin and carbenicillin), the ureidopenicillins (piperacillin and mezlocillin), aztreonam, and the cephalosporins other than cefoxitin. Organisms with ESBLs usually remain susceptible to the carbapenems (imipenem, meropenem, doripene, and ertapenem), cefoxitin, and β-lactamase inhibitors with clavulanic acid (tazobactams and sulbactams).

In an ESBL screen, indicator antibiotics are used to determine resistance. For example, ceftazidime or cefotaxime are tested using the disk diffusion method alone and with clavulanic acid. ESBL is identified if the zone diameter increases over 5 mm with clavulanic acid present compared to testing the antibiotic alone. The resistance is confirmed using an MIC procedure; a threefold increase in the MIC with clavulanic acid confirms the ESBL.

AmpC

The production of cephalosporinase is a chromosomal-mediated resistance. It is inducible, and the organism must have been exposed to the antibiotic before the enzyme was produced. Cephalosporinase enzymes act on first-, second-, and third-generation cephalosporins, penicillins, and aztreonam but are not active against carbapenems or cefipime (a fourth-generation cephalosporin). AmpC is induced by cefoxitin, imipenem, and ampicillin. It is found in *Serratia* spp., *Providencia*, *Aeromonas*, *Citrobacter freundii*, *Enterobacter* spp., *Morganella morganii*, and *Pseudomonas aeruginosa*. In a disk diffusion test, organisms with AmpC are resistant to cefoxitin and susceptible to cefepime. A D test using cefoxitin as an inducer and ceftazidine as a detector antibiotic can be used. There will be no zone around the cefoxitin and a D-shaped, flattened zone around the ceftaxidime.

Carbapenemase

Carbapenemase was first found in *Klebsiella pneumoniae* (KPC) but is now found in other Enterobacteriaceae, which are known as carbapenem-resistant Enterobacteriaceae (CRE). This is a plasmid-mediated mechanism that inhibits β-lactamase–resistant penicillins, clavulanic acid, and tazobactam. These infections usually must be treated with tigecycline. In the modified Hodge test, *E. coli* is plated onto Mueller-Hinton agar, and either an ertapenem or a meropenem disk is placed in the center of the plate. Next, three to five colonies of the test organism are streaked over the *E. coli* in lines extending from the edge of the antibiotic disk to the edge of the plate. If carbapenemase is present, the antibiotic will be hydrolyzed, and the *E. coli* will be able to grow up to the disk. In a negative test, the *E. coli* will remain susceptible to the antibiotic, and there will be no growth near the disk.

Predictor Drugs

In some cases, predictor agents can be used in the test batteries. The predictor drug is the most sensitive indicator of resistance for a certain group of antimicrobial agents. The susceptibility report is based on the likelihood that the resistance mechanisms might have an effect on the antibiotics considered to treat the patient. For example, high-level gentamycin resistance in enterococci predicts resistance to all other currently available aminoglycosides, including tobramycin, amikacin, netilmicin, and kanamycin. Staphylococcal resistance to oxacillin is used to predict resistance to all currently available β-lactams (penicillins, cephalosporins, and carbapenems). Use of a predictor antimicrobial agent can assist the laboratory in determining which antibiotics to test and also assist the clinician in the selection of suitable therapeutic agents.

Molecular methods to detect antibiotic resistance were previously discussed in Chapter 5.

Antibiograms

Antibiograms can be used to compare the susceptibility of a particular bacterial isolate to several antibiotics with the standard predictable pattern of that microorganism. In doing so, the development of resistance to a certain agent can be detected. In addition, an antibiogram can alert the clinician to verify and investigate any unusual resistant patterns.

Laboratory Procedures

Procedure

β-lactamase (Cefinase)

Purpose

Cefinase disks are used to detect β-lactamase production by testing isolated colonies of *Staphylococcus* species, *Haemophilus influenzae, Neisseria gonorrhoeae,* and anaerobic bacteria. Isolates containing these organisms should be routinely tested for β-lactamase activity.

Principle

The Cefinase disk is impregnated with the chromogenic cephalosporin Nitrocefin. A rapid color change from yellow to red occurs when the amide bond in the β-lactam ring is hydrolyzed by β-lactamase.

Materials

Cefinase disks (available through Becton Dickinson Microbiology Systems)
Microscope slides or petri plates
Sterile loop or application sticks

Procedure

1. Dispense a Cefinase disk from the dispenser or remove one disk from the vial using sterile forceps and place on a microscope slide or empty petri plate.
2. Moisten each disk with one drop of purified water.
3. Using a sterile loop or applicator stick, select several well-isolated colonies and smear onto the moistened disk surface.
4. Observe disk for color change.
5. Alternatively, using forceps, moisten disk with one drop of purified water and wipe across surface of colony.

Results

Positive: color change from yellow to red. Color change usually does not occur over entire disk. Most bacterial strains develop a positive result within 5 minutes. Positive reactions for some strains of *Staphylococcus* may take up to 1 hour to develop.
Negative: Color change does not occur on the disk.

Quality Control

Positive: *Staphylococcus aureus* ATCC 29213: color change from yellow to red
Negative: *Haemophilus influenzae* ATCC 10211: no color change

Procedure

Macrodilution broth susceptibility test

Purpose

The minimal inhibitory concentration (MIC) and minimal bacteriocidal concentration (MBC) of a particular antibiotic are determined through serially diluting an antibiotic.

Principle

Dilutions of an antibiotic are added to Mueller-Hinton broth and a standard concentration of the inoculum. The tubes are incubated overnight and read visually for turbidity. The lowest concentration showing no visible growth or macroscopic inhibition is the MIC. Broth cultures showing no visible growth are subcultured onto appropriate agar and incubated to determine whether the organism has been killed. The lowest concentration of antibiotic that exhibits at least 99.9% killing on the subculture is the MBC.

Materials

Antibiotic standard: For penicillin, use a working solution of 20 U of activity/ml; for other antibiotics, use a 200 mg/ml working solution.

Subculture of organism to be tested: An overnight culture grown at 35°C on blood agar is recommended.

Inoculate a trypticase soy broth with the overnight culture.

Mueller-Hinton broth

Sterile 13 mm × 100 mm test tubes with screw caps

Procedure

1. Set up 13 sterile 13 × 100 mm test tubes with caps and label 1 through 13.
   Tube 11 will be the inoculum control.
   Tube 12 will be the broth control.
   Tube 13 will be the antibiotic control.
2. Pipette 1.0 ml of Mueller-Hinton broth into tubes 2 through 10, tube 11, and tube 13. Pipette 2.0 ml of Mueller-Hinton broth into tube 12.
3. Pipette 1.0 ml of the working antibiotic solution into tubes 1, 2, and 13.
4. Make twofold dilutions in 1.0 ml amounts in tubes 2 through 10. Mix and change pipettes at each dilution. This is done by mixing tube 2 and transferring 1.0 ml of its contents to tube 3. The process is continued to tube 10. Discard 1.0 ml from tube 10.
5. Standardize the inoculum to a 0.5 McFarland standard. Then further adjust the inoculum by adding 0.1 ml of the inoculum to 19.9 ml of Mueller-Hinton broth. This is a 1:200 dilution. The final concentration of bacteria is approximately 1×10^5 to 1×10^6 CFU/ml.
6. Pipette 1.0 ml of the standardized inoculum into tubes 1 through 11. Mix each tube well and incubate at 35°C for 18 to 24 hours. Do not incubate under increased CO_2 unless this is required for growth.
7. Prepare plate for colony count. This is done by preparing a 1:100 dilution of the inoculum and plating 0.01 ml of the dilution onto a blood agar plate. Incubate at 35°C for 18 to 24 hours. Do not incubate under increased CO_2 unless this is required for growth.

Interpretation

Determination of MIC: The tube with the lowest antibiotic concentration showing no visible growth is considered to be the MIC.

Inoculum control (tube 11): must show visible growth for test to be valid

Broth control (tube 12): must show no visible growth for test to be valid

Antibiotic control (tube 13): must show no visible growth for test to be valid

Determination of MBC

1. Subculture 0.01 ml from each tube showing no visible growth and the first tube with visible growth onto a blood agar plate. Streak the inoculum in several directions to maximally dilute the antibiotic.
2. Incubate the plates for 18 to 24 hours at 35°C. Do not incubate under increased CO_2 unless required for growth.
3. The MBC is the lowest antibiotic concentration that results in 99.9% killing. This is illustrated by the lowest antibiotic concentration permitting no survival of the organism.

Procedure

Kirby-Bauer disk diffusion test

Purpose

The Kirby-Bauer test is routinely used to determine the susceptibility or resistance of a pathogenic organism to various antimicrobial agents.

Principle

A standardized suspension of organisms is inoculated onto Mueller-Hinton agar. Paper disks impregnated with specific antibiotic concentrations are placed onto the agar. After 18 to 24 hours of incubation, the diameters of the zones of growth are measured. The results are compared with established values to determine the organism's susceptibility or resistance to each antibiotic.

Reagents and Materials

Mueller-Hinton Medium

1. Prepare and autoclave Mueller-Hinton medium according to the manufacturer's directions.
2. Cool in a 45°C to 50°C water bath to avoid the collection of moisture on the agar surface. Pour 25 ml to 30 ml into 100 mm plates or 60 ml to 70 ml into 150 mm plates on a level surface to a uniform depth of 4 mm. Allow medium to harden.
3. Leave top of plate slightly ajar until medium solidifies to minimize moisture collection on the surface of the medium. If moisture does collect, incubate plates at 35°C for 10 to 30 minutes or at room temperature for 1 hour before use. The final pH of the medium must be 7.2 to 7.4.
4. Incubate sample plates at 30°C to 35°C overnight to check sterility. Discard the sample plates.

5. Use plates immediately or refrigerate and use within 7 days if medium shows no signs of dehydration. If precautions are adequate to decrease dehydration and if quality control has been met, the shelf life can be extended.

Susceptibility Disks

1. Maintain anhydrous storage conditions at –20°C ± 8°C for maximum stability. When indicator changes color, replace the desiccant.
2. Remove disks from refrigerator to room temperature 1 to 2 hours before use to minimize possibility of condensation. Disks should be held in the refrigerator for up to only one week.
3. Do not use disks that have passed their expiration date.

Turbidity Standard

1. Prepare a 0.5 McFarland turbidity standard to measure inoculum density. Add 0.5 ml of 0.048 *N* $BaCl_2$ (or 0.5 ml of 1.175% $BaCl_2$-$2H_2O$) to 99.5 ml of 0.36 A/H_2SO_4(1% v/v).
2. Verify density of standard. The absorbance of a 0.5 McFarland turbidity standard at 625 nm should be 0.08 to 0.1 with a 1 cm pathway, using matched cuvettes in the spectrophotometer.
3. Distribute 4 ml to 6 ml amounts into screw-cap tubes of the same size as those being used to grow the broth culture inoculum.
4. Seal tubes tightly and store at room temperature in the dark.
5. Vigorously agitate the turbidity standard using a vortex before each use.
6. Prepare new standards at least every 3 to 6 months.

Procedure

1. Inoculate test plates by transferring four or five colonies from the primary isolation medium into approximately 5 ml trypticase soy broth (soybean-casein digest broth) by touching the top of the colonies with a sterilized cooled wire loop or disposable loop.
2. If the resting culture suspension is less turbid than the 0.5 McFarland turbidity standard when read using adequate light against a white background with black lines, incubate the culture at 35°C for 2 to 8 hours until the turbidity equals or exceeds that of the standard. The inoculum should contain approximately $1\text{–}2 \times 10^8$ CFU/ml. Dilute the culture suspension with sterile saline if necessary. Proceed without incubation if the turbidity of the inoculated suspension is comparable to that of the standard. Do not use overnight broth cultures for this procedure.
3. Within 15 minutes of standardization, dip a sterile cotton swab into the standardized culture suspension, and express excess fluid by rotating the swab firmly against the inside wall of the test tube. Refrigerate tubes if inoculation is delayed more than 15 minutes.
4. Inoculate the entire agar surface, streaking in three different directions by rotating the plate at 60° angles after each streak. If the plate is properly streaked, a confluent lawn of growth will develop. Avoid extremes of inoculum density.
5. Allow inoculum to dry 3 to 15 minutes. The lid may be left ajar for 3 to 5 minutes and no more than 15 minutes to permit surface moisture to be absorbed before applying the antibiotic disks.
6. Apply appropriate susceptibility disks manually or with a dispenser onto the inoculated agar surface. Gently press each disk down with sterile forceps; flame and cool between each disk to ensure complete contact with the agar. A minimum spacing of 24 mm from disk center to center to avoid overlapping inhibition zones should be observed. Do not move a disk once it has contacted the agar because the antibiotic diffuses almost instantaneously.
   Penicillin and cephalosporin should be placed no less than 10 mm from the edge of the petri plate, with centers at least 30 mm apart. These disks should not be placed next to each other. When testing *Haemophilus influenzae*, *Neisseria gonorrhoeae*, and *Streptococcus pneumoniae*, use no more than four disks for a 100 mm plate and no more than nine disks for a 150 mm plate.
7. Within 15 minutes of applying disks, aerobically incubate the inverted plates at 35°C ± 2°C for 16 to 18 hours. For *Haemophilus influenzae*, *Neisseria gonorrhoeae*, and *Streptococcus pneumoniae*, incubate plates for 20 to 24 hours. For MRSA, VRSA, and VRE, incubate plates for a full 24 hours. Temperatures over 35°C may not detect methicillin-resistant *S. aureus*.
8. Examine plates with the unaided eye using reflected light against a nonreflecting black background. Measure diameters of complete inhibition to the nearest whole millimeter using a caliper or ruler. On blood agar, remove the cover and measure inhibition zones from the surface illuminated with reflected light. Observe the following:
   a. Ignore the haze produced by the swarming of *Proteus* if zones of inhibition are clearly outlined.

b. Measure sulfonamide zones at the margin of heavy growth. Sulfonamides may not inhibit organisms for several generations, so slight growth or haze within the inhibition zones may be disregarded.
c. The *end point* is defined as that area showing no visible growth when observed with the unaided eye. An occasional culture may produce a mutant colony, which is visible within the inhibition zones with transmitted or assisted vision. Disregard such growth.
d. Subculture, isolate, identify, and retest large numbers of colonies or large-sized colonies growing with a clear zone of inhibition. These may be a second organism or another strain of the same organism.

9. Interpret the sizes of zones of inhibition by referring to Table 6-1.
10. Report the result of each antibiotic as susceptible, intermediate, or resistant.

Quality Control

Quality control should be performed daily and when new antibiotics or media are used.
Escherichia coli ATCC 25922: gram-negative drugs
Staphylococcus aureus ATCC 25923: gram-positive drugs
Pseudomonas aeruginosa ATCC 27853: aminoglycosides and other gram-negative drugs
Haemophilus influenzae ATCC 49247 and ATCC 49766
Neisseria gonorrhoeae ATCC 48226
Streptococcus pneumoniae ATCC 49719
Compare results with control limits for these quality-control limits found in Table 6-2.

Interpretation

Susceptible implies infection because the strain may be appropriately treated with a dosage of antimicrobial agent recommended for that type of infection unless otherwise contraindicated.

Intermediate implies strains that may be inhibited by attainable concentrations of certain antibiotics, provided higher dosages are used, or inhibited in body sites (such as urine) where the drugs are physiologically concentrated. This category also prevents small, technical factors from causing major discrepancies in the interpretation. This includes species that should have few or no end points in this range, drugs affected by media variation, or drugs with narrow pharmacotoxic margins. For drugs with zones falling in this range, the results are considered equivocal. If the organism is not fully susceptible to alternative antibiotics, the test should be repeated or compared with a dilution test. Intermediate antibiotics may be effective but less effective when compared to susceptible drugs.

Resistant implies the strain is not inhibited by the usually achievable systemic concentration of the agent with normal dosage. Specific microbial-resistance mechanisms may be likely, such as β-lactamases. These antibiotics are not appropriate choices because the microorganism is not inhibited by the antibiotic.

Reference: BBL™ Sensi-Disc™ Antimicrobial Susceptibility Test Disc package insert; Becton, Dickinson and Company, Sparks, Maryland

Procedure

Microdilution broth susceptibility test

Purpose

Various concentrations of several antibiotics are tested against an inoculum. The minimal inhibitory concentration (MIC), which is the lowest concentration of antibiotic that inhibits growth of the organism, is determined.

Principle

A standard inoculum of the isolate is tested with serial dilutions of each antimicrobial agent. Each well is visually examined for the presence or absence of growth. The concentration of the agent that inhibits bacterial growth is determined.

Reagents

Nutrient broth (soybean-casein digest broth)
0.5 McFarland turbidity standard
Frozen or lyophilized microtiter plates containing antibiotics
Inoculator (multipronged if available) to deliver 50 μl standardized inoculum
Viewing mirror
Sterile saline
10 ml serological pipette

Procedure

1. Using a sterile applicator stick, select at least five colonies from a pure plate culture that has been incubated at 35°C for 18 to 24 hours.
2. Suspend the colonies in nutrient broth, and standardize the suspension to that of the 0.5 McFarland turbidity standard.

3. Prepare a 100-fold dilution of the inoculum using sterile saline. The final concentration of the inoculum is approximately 1×10^6 CFU/ml. The inoculum must be used within 15 minutes of preparation.
4. Pour the inoculum into a seed tray if using one. Set multipronged inoculator into inoculum and carefully draw up the prescribed volume. Avoid drawing up air bubbles.
5. Carefully dispense 50 μl into each well of the microtiter plate using the multipronged inoculator or a micropipette set to deliver 50 μl.
6. One well must contain bacteria without antibiotic (growth control), and one well must contain broth only (sterility control).
7. Seal tray with plastic lids provided or use a plastic bag or plastic tape. This is necessary to prevent dehydration.
8. Inoculate a nonselective medium, such as nutrient agar or blood agar, to check for purity of the inoculum.
9. Incubate for 18 to 24 hours at 35°C in ambient air. Trays should not be stacked more than five high in the incubator.

Interpretation

After incubation, trays are read for the ability of the microorganism to grow in the presence of the antimicrobial agents. Growth can appear as dense or hazy turbidity that is uniformly distributed through the well or as concentrated or diffuse buttons of growth at the bottom of the well. The absence of turbidity is considered to be no growth.

1. Trays should be read for growth by viewing each well through the bottom using a magnifying mirror reader. An overhead light source adjusted to give good contrast is recommended.
2. First, read the positive growth control well. The absence of growth in this well invalidates all results.
3. Next, read the sterility control well. The presence of growth in this well invalidates all results.
4. Check the agar plate for purity. Perform a Gram stain for any questionable growth that may indicate contamination. Repeat the procedure if contamination is present.
5. Record results starting with the first antimicrobial agent, reading all concentrations of the agent. Read all agents in a similar manner.
6. The lowest concentration of each antibiotic showing complete inhibition of growth is recorded as the MIC. Always read from left to right or from lowest concentration to highest concentration of the agent. The MIC is the first clear well.
7. If all dilutions for an antimicrobial agent show growth, the end point is recorded as greater than the highest concentration tested.
8. If all dilutions for an antimicrobial agent show inhibition of growth, the end point is recorded as less than or equal to the lowest concentration tested.
9. One clear well within a series of wells that contain growth may indicate a skipped well and can be ignored. If two or more skips are found, discard the results and repeat the test.

Effective antimicrobial activity usually requires a drug concentration at the site of infection that is two to four times the in vitro MIC. Results must be interpreted with guidelines established through the Clinical and Laboratory Standards Institute and the individual microbiology laboratory. Table 6-3 serves as a sample interpretation for student use. The categories of susceptible, moderately susceptible, and resistant depend on several factors, including host factors, pharmacokinetics of the agent, and the particular pathogen involved. These categories are defined as follows:

Susceptible: infecting organism is inhibited by levels of antimicrobial agent attained in the blood or tissue on usual dosage

Resistant: infecting organism is resistant to usually achievable levels of antimicrobial agent

Procedure

Oxacillin screen agar

Purpose

Oxacillin screen agar was originally known as MRSA screen agar and was developed to detect methicillin-resistant *Staphylococcus aureus* (MRSA). These bacterial strains are resistant to penicillinase-resistant penicillins (PRPs), such as methicillin, oxacillin, and nafcillin. This method uses the same inoculate (0.5 McFarland standard) as the disk diffusion antimicrobial susceptibility procedure.

Principle

Mueller-Hinton agar with 6 μg/ml of oxacillin supplemented with 4% w/v (0.68 mol/l) NaCl is inoculated with an 18- to 24-hour isolate of *S. aureus* adjusted to a 0.5 McFarland standard. Growth indicates resistance to β-lactam antimicrobial agents.

Procedure

1. Suspend several well-isolated colonies of the *S. aureus* test isolate from an 18- to 24-hour plate culture into a broth medium, such as trypticase soy broth. Adjust turbidity to match that of a 0.5 McFarland turbidity standard.
2. Spot inoculate the plate with 10 μl of the test suspension using a micropipette. Alternatively, saturate a cotton swab with the test suspension and express out the excess fluid in the test tube. Streak plate by drawing the swab over a 1 inch area.
3. Inoculate a sheep blood agar plate to serve as the growth control.
4. Incubate plates at 30°C to 35°C for a full 24 hours. Do not incubate above 35°C.
5. Observe plates for growth.

Interpretation

Any growth, even a single colony, indicates that the isolate is methicillin/oxacillin resistant.

No growth indicates that the isolate is susceptible to penicillinase-resistant penicillins, such as methicillin, oxacillin, and nafcillin.

Notes

1. The oxacillin agar plate and blood agar plate can be divided into several wedges to test several isolates on the plates at one time.
2. Isolates that grow on oxacillin screen agar should be reported as resistant to all β-lactam antimicrobial agents, including β-lactam/β-lactamase inhibitor combinations and cephalosporins.
3. Test any isolate growing on oxacillin screen agar by broth or agar dilution to confirm resistance to oxacillin and resistance to other antimicrobial agents, such as chloroamphenicol, clindamycin, erythromycin, gentamycin, and tetracycline.
4. This method is not recommended for detection of methicillin/oxacillin resistance in coagulase-negative staphylococci.
5. Confirm results with method to determine MIC.

Reference: Oxacillin Screen Agar in *Difco & BBL Manual of Microbiological Culture Media*, 2nd edition, Becton, Dickinson and Company, 2009, Sparks, Maryland

Procedure

Cefoxitin disk diffusion test

Purpose

Cefoxitin is a potent inducer of the *mecA* gene system and can be used to detect methicillin resistance in *S. aureus*. These bacterial strains are resistant to penicillinase-resistant penicillins, such as methicillin, oxacillin, and nafcillin. This method uses the same inoculate (0.5 McFarland standard) as the disk diffusion antimicrobial susceptibility procedure.

Principle

Cefoxitin is used as a surrogate marker for the detection of the *mecA* gene–mediated methicillin resistance. The test is performed using a 30 μg cefoxitin disk and Mueller-Hinton agar.

Heteroresistance may be determined using this method; these colonies appear within the ring of inhibition.

Procedure

1. Suspend several well-isolated colonies of the *S. aureus* test isolate from an 18- to 24-hour plate culture into a broth medium, such as trypticase soy broth. Adjust turbidity to match that of a 0.5 McFarland turbidity standard.
2. Saturate a cotton swab with the test suspension and streak the Mueller-Hinton plate in three directions to obtain a lawn culture of growth.
3. Within 15 minutes of inoculating the plate, apply a 30 μg cefoxitin disk to the center of the growth.
4. Incubate plates at 30°C to 35°C for a full 24 hours. Do not incubate above 35°C.
5. Observe plates for zones of inhibition.
6. For *S. aureus*, zones of ≥22 mm are reported as susceptible and zones of ≤21 mm are reported as resistant. For coagulase-negative staphylococci, zones of ≥25 mm are reported as susceptible and zones of ≤24 mm are reported as resistant.

Laboratory Exercises

1. Perform the disk diffusion susceptibility test on each organism listed. Select the appropriate antibiotic panel. Interpret your results by consulting Table 6-1 after 18 to 24 hours of incubation, and report each antibiotic as resistant (R), susceptible (S), or intermediate (I) by checking the appropriate column. Consult Table 6-2 to interpret quality control.

Organism	Antimicrobial agent Code/content	Zone diameter (mm)	S	I	R
Staphylococcus aureus					

Organism	Antimicrobial agent Code/content	Zone diameter (mm)	S	I	R
Enterococcus faecalis					

Organism	Antimicrobial agent Code/content	Zone diameter (mm)	S	I	R
E. coli					

Organism	Antimicrobial agent Code/content	Zone diameter (mm)	S	I	R
Proteus mirabilis					

Organism	Antimicrobial agent Code/content	Zone diameter (mm)	S	I	R
Pseudomonas aeruginosa					

Quality Control

Organism	Antimicrobial agent Code/content	Zone diameter (mm)
E. coli ATCC 25922		

Are all results within acceptable limits? ____________

____

Explain any results not within the quality-control limits. ____________________________________

____

____

Organism	Antimicrobial agent Code/content	Zone diameter (mm)
S. aureus ATCC 25923		

Are all results within acceptable limits? ____________

____

Explain any results not within the quality-control limits. ____________________________________

____

____

Organism	Antimicrobial agent Code/content	Zone diameter (mm)
P. aeruginosa ATCC 27853		

Are all results within acceptable limits?____________

____

Explain any results not within the quality-control limits.______________________________

____

2. Perform the macrotube (macrobroth) dilution test for *E. coli*, using ampicillin as the antibiotic. For each tube, calculate and list the antibiotic concentration.

   Tube 1: ______ Tube 8: ______
   Tube 2: ______ Tube 9: ______
   Tube 3: ______ Tube 10: ______
   Tube 4: ______ Tube 11: inoculum (growth) control ______
   Tube 5: ______
   Tube 6: ______ Tube 12: broth control ______
   Tube 7: ______ Tube 13: antibiotic control ______

   Mark the dilution that is the MIC and the dilution that is the MBC.

   Define MIC: ______________________________

   Define MBC: ______________________________

   Based on the results for tubes 11, 12, and 13, indicate whether this is a valid test: ______________________________

   Explain your reasoning: ______________________________

   ____

3. Perform the microtube (microbroth) dilution procedure on the organisms indicated. Interpret the plates using a viewing mirror, and indicate the MIC of each antibiotic for each organism.

Organism	Antimicrobial agent Code/content	MIC (µg/ml)	S	I	R
E. coli					

Organism	Antimicrobial agent Code/content	MIC (µg/ml)	S	I	R
S. aureus					

Organism	Antimicrobial agent Code/content	MIC (µg/ml)	S	I	R
P. aeruginosa					

4. Perform the β-lactamase procedure on the following organisms. Describe your observations and interpret your results.

Organism	Observations	Interpretation
S. aureus		
M. catarrhalis		
H. influenzae		

   State the principle of this procedure: ______________________________

   ____

   Does this method detect all types of β-lactamase enzymes?______________________________

   Explain:______________________________

   ____

5. Perform the oxacillin screen on *Staphylococcus aureus*. Record your observations and results.______________

   What do your results indicate?______________

   Why is oxacillin agar and not methicillin agar used?

   ____

6. Perform the cefoxitin screen on *Staphylococcus aureus*. Record your observations and results. ______________

   What do your results indicate?______________

   What are the advantages of using cefoxitin to screen for MRSA?______________________________

Review Questions

Matching

Match the antibiotic with its most correct description:

1. Penicillin G
2. Ampicillin
3. Erythromycin
4. Amoxicillin/clavulanate potassium
5. Cephalothin
6. Cefotaxime
7. Tobramycin
8. Tetracycline
9. Trimethoprim/sulfamethoxazole
   a. Extended-spectrum penicillin with no activity against β-lactamase producers
   b. Penicillin codrug with broad-spectrum activity and resistance to β-lactamase
   c. Third-generation cephalosporin with enhanced activity against gram-negative bacteria
   d. Used for gram-positive infections, in particular nonenterococcal *Streptococcus* infections
   e. Aminoglycoside used to treat serious gram-negative infections, including *Pseudomonas*
   f. Folic acid inhibitor used to treat chronic urinary tract infections
   g. Gram-positive spectrum, used to treat streptococcal infections in penicillin-allergic patients
   h. First-generation cephalosporin with primarily a gram-positive spectrum
   i. Broad-spectrum antibiotic with activity against gram-positive and gram-negative bacteria, mycoplasmas, and chlamydia

Multiple Choice

For questions 10 to 15, mark "A" if the antimicrobial agent functions by inhibition of cell wall synthesis, and mark "B" if the agent functions by inhibition of protein synthesis:

10. Penicillin G
11. Cephalosporins
12. Ampicillin
13. Tetracycline
14. Erythromycin
15. Chloramphenicol

16. Antimicrobial agents that kill the microbe, leading to cell lysis, are categorized as:
    a. Bacteriostatic
    b. Bacteriocidal
    c. Narrow-spectrum antibiotics
    d. Super antibiotics
17. Which of the following is an antiviral agent?
    a. Amphotericin B
    b. Acyclovir
    c. Isoniazid
    d. Nystatin
18. If the interaction of two antibiotics results in activity that is significantly greater than the response from the combined action of each drug used separately, the response is termed:
    a. Autonomous
    b. Antagonistic
    c. Additive
    d. Synergistic

For questions 19 through 23, consider each of the following parameters in performing a Kirby-Bauer disk susceptibility test. Indicate if the parameter is correct (C) or incorrect (I):

19. Depth of media: 6.0 mm
20. pH of media: 7.2 to 8.4
21. Type of media: trypticase soy agar
22. Inoculum concentration: 0.5 McFarland turbidity standard
23. Incubation at 35°C at increased CO_2 for 18 to 24 hours
24. In a Kirby-Bauer disk susceptibility test, the zones of inhibition are too large. Which of the following is a possible cause of this result?
    a. Inoculum too dense
    b. Agar depth too thick
    c. Incubation temperature too low
    d. Antibiotic not stored at proper temperature without desiccant

Use the following information for questions 25 to 27:
In a macrotube (macrobroth) dilution susceptibility test, 1.0 ml of Mueller-Hinton (MH) broth is pipetted into tubes 2 through 10, tube 11, and tube 13. Two milliliters of MH broth is pipetted into tube 12; 1.0 ml of 200 mg/dl ampicillin is added to tubes 1, 2, and 13. A twofold serial dilution is performed in 1.0 ml amounts in tubes 2 through 10. The standardized inoculum is diluted 1:200, and 1.0 ml is added to tubes 1 through 11. The tubes are incubated for 20 hours at 35°C. After this time the tubes are examined for visual growth. Tubes 6 through 7 are visibly turbid, while tubes 1 through 5 show no signs of growth. Tubes 1 through 5 are plated on blood agar, incubated overnight at 35°C, and read for growth. Plates 1 through 4 show no growth, while several colonies are observed on plate 5.

25. The MIC is:
    a. 25 μg/ml
    b. 12.5 μg/ml
    c. 6.25 μg/ml
    d. 3.12 μg/ml
    e. None of the above
26. The MBC is:
    a. 25 μg/ml
    b. 12.5 μg/ml

c. 6.25 μg/ml
d. 3.12 μg/ml
e. None of the above

27. Which of the following criteria must be met for the test to be valid?

	Control	Antibiotic Control	Broth Control
a.	Positive	Negative	Positive
b.	Positive	Positive	Negative
c.	Positive	Negative	Negative
d.	Negative	Positive	Positive

28. For antibiotics given through the intravenous route, the peak specimen should be drawn:
a. Immediately before the next dose
b. 30 minutes after the dose
c. 60 minutes after the dose
d. 90 minutes after the dose

29. The lowest amount of antibiotic that results in 99.9% in vitro killing of the organism is the:
a. Minimal bacteriostatic concentration
b. Serum bacteriocidal level
c. Serum peak level
d. Minimal bacteriocidal concentration

30. A measure of the activity of the antibiotic in the patient's own serum against an infecting organism is determined in the:
a. Microbroth dilution susceptibility test
b. Cefinase procedure
c. Serum bacteriocidal test
d. Antibiogram

31. Oxacillin/methicillin resistance in *S. aureus* can be detected by all of the following *except*:
a. Cefoxitin disk screen test
b. Oxacillin agar screen
c. Chromogenic agar
d. D test

32. ESBLs
a. are chromosomal mediated.
b. are also known as AmpC resistance.
c. confer resistance to vancomycin and penicillin.
d. were first found in *Klebsiella* and *E. coli.*

Bibliography

Barry, A. L., Coyle, M. B., Thornsberry, C. R., Gerlach, E. H., & Hawkinson, R. W. (1979). Methods of measuring zones of inhibition with the Bauer-Kirby disk susceptibility test. *Journal of Clinical Microbiology, 10,* 885–889.

Bauer, A. W., Kirby, W. M., Sherris, J. C., & Turck, M. (1966). Antibiotic susceptibility testing by a standardized single disk method. *American Journal of Clinical Pathology, 45,* 493.

Bradford, P. A. (2001). Extended-spectrum β-lactamases in the 21st century: Characterization, epidemiology, and detection of this important resistance threat. *Clinical Microbiology Reviews, 14,* 933–951.

Cetinkaya, Y., Falk, P., & Mayhall C. G. (2000). Vancomycin-resistant enterococci. *Clinical Microbiology Reviews, 13,* 686–707.

Chambers, H. F. (1997). Methicillin resistance in staphylococci: Molecular and biochemical basis and clinical implications. *Clinical Microbiology Reviews, 10,* 781–791.

Clinical and Laboratory Standards Institute. (2008). Development of in vitro susceptibility testing criteria and quality control parameters; approved guideline. Third ed. CLSI document M23–A3. Wayne, PA.

Clinical and Laboratory Standards Institute. (2009). Performance standards for antimicrobial disk susceptibility tests. Approved standard M2–A10. Wayne, PA.

Clinical and Laboratory Standards Institute. (2009). Performance standards for antimicrobial susceptibility testing. Nineteenth informational supplement M100–S19. Wayne, PA.

Depardieu, F., Podglajen, I., Leclercq, R., Collatz, E., & Courvalin, P. (2007). Modes and modulations of antibiotic resistance gene expression. *Clinical Microbiology Reviews, 20,* 79–114.

Drawz, S. M., & Bonomo, R. A. (2010). Three decades of β-lactamase inhibitors. *Clinical Microbiology Reviews, 23,* 160–201.

Gootz, T. D. (1990). Discovery and development of new antimicrobial agents. *Clinical Microbiology Reviews, 3,* 13–31.

Howden, B. P., Davies, J. K., Johnson, P. D., Stinear, T. P., & Grayson, M. L. (2010). Reduced vancomycin susceptibility in *Staphylococcus aureus*, including vancomycin-intermediate and heterogeneous vancomycin-intermediate strains: Resistance mechanisms, laboratory detection, and clinical implications. *Clinical Microbiology Reviews, 23,* 99–139.

Jorgensen, J. H. and Ferraro, M. J. (2009). Antimicrobial susceptibility testing: a review of general principles and contemporary practices. *Clinical Infectious Diseases, 49,* 1749–1755.

Klugman, K. P. (1990). Pneumococcal resistance to antibiotics. *Clinical Microbiology Reviews, 3,* 171–196.

Moellering, R. C. (2006). Vancomycin: A 50-year reassessment. *Clinical Infectious Diseases, 42,* S3–S4.

Patel, J. B., Tenover, F. C., Turnidge, J. D., & Jorgensen, J. H. (2007). Susceptibility testing methods: Diffusion and disk diffusion methods. In P. R. Murray, E. J. Baron, J. H. Jorgensen, M. L. Landry, & M. A. Pfaller (Eds.), *Manual of clinical microbiology*, 9th ed. Washington, DC: American Society for Microbiology.

Paterson, D. L., & Bonomo, R. A. (2005). Extended-spectrum β-lactamases: A clinical update. *Clinical Microbiology Reviews, 18,* 657–686.

Piddock, L. V. (2006). Clinically relevant chromosomally encoded multidrug resistance efflux pumps in bacteria. *Clinical Microbiology Reviews, 19,* 382–402.

Sanford, J. P. (1993). Guide to antimicrobial therapy. Sperryville, VA: Antimicrobial Therapy, Inc.

Speer, B. S., Shoemaker, N. B., & Salyers, A. A. (1992). Bacterial resistance to tetracycline: Mechanisms, transfer, and clinical significance. *Clinical Microbiology Reviews, 5,* 387–399.

Srinivasan, A., Dick, J. D., & Perl, T. M. (2002). Vancomycin resistance in staphylococci. *Clinical Microbiology Reviews, 15,* 430–438.

Turnidge, J., & Paterson, D. L. (2007). Setting and revising antibacterial susceptibility breakpoints. *Clinical Microbiology Reviews, 20,* 391–408.

Vakulenko, S. B., & Mobashery, S. (2003). Versatility of aminoglycosides and prospects for their future. *Clinical Microbiology Reviews, 16,* 430–450.

Wilson, F. (2001). Battling bacterial resistance. *Lab Medicine, 32,* 73–76.

Winn, Jr., W., Allen, S., Janda, W., Konemen, E., Procop, G., Schreckenberger, P., & Woods, G. (Eds.). (2005). Antimicrobial susceptibility testing. In *Koneman's color atlas and textbook of diagnostic microbiology,* 6th ed. Philadelphia, PA: Lippincott Williams & Wilkins.

Woodford, N., Johnson, A. P., Morrison, D., & Speller, D. C. (1995). Current perspectives on glycopeptide resistance. *Clinical Microbiology Reviews, 8,* 585–615.

CHAPTER 7

Staphylococci and Other Catalase-Positive Gram-Positive Cocci

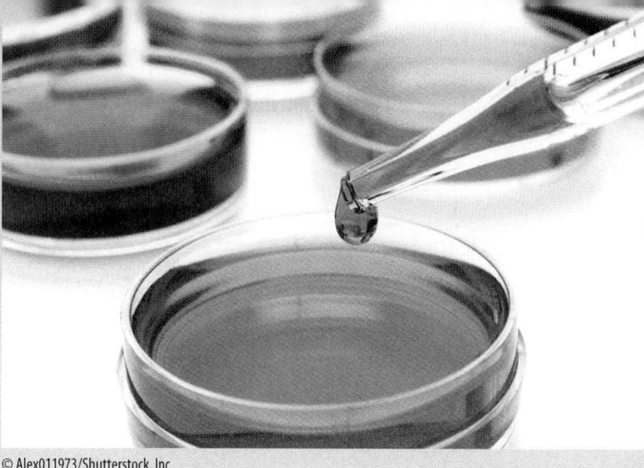

CHAPTER OUTLINE

Gram-Positive Cocci
Staphylococcus
Coagulase-Negative Staphylococci

KEY TERMS

β-lactamase
Bound coagulase
Coagulase-negative staphylococci
Enterotoxins
Fibrinolysin
Free coagulase
Hemolysins
Leukocidin
Methicillin-resistant *Staphylococcus aureus* (MRSA)
Osteomyelitis
Pyogenic
Staphylococcal toxic shock syndrome
Vancomycin-intermediate *Staphylococcus aureus* (VISA)
Vancomycin-resistant *Staphyloccus aureus* (VRSA)

LEARNING OBJECTIVES

1. Discuss the classification of the catalase-positive gram-positive cocci.
2. Differentiate *Staphylococcus* from *Micrococcus.*
3. List and describe the media on which *Staphylococcus* can be isolated.
4. List and describe methods to differentiate *Staphylococcus* from *Streptococcus* to include:
   a. Gram stain
   b. Colonial morphology
   c. Catalase reaction
5. Differentiate *Staphylococcus* from *Streptococcus* when given an unknown culture.
6. State the principle and purpose of the catalase reaction. Perform and interpret the catalase test without error.
7. State the principle and purpose of the coagulase test.
   a. Perform the slide and tube coagulase tests without error.
   b. Differentiate bound from free coagulase and name the tests used to detect each.
   c. Discuss sources of error and limitations of each procedure.
8. Give the principle and purpose of the following media. Inoculate and interpret each reaction without error.
   a. Mannitol salt agar
   b. DNase medium
9. Differentiate *Staphylococcus aureus* from coagulase-negative staphylococci.
10. Describe each of the following compounds and the role each plays in infections caused by *Staphylococcus aureus:*
    a. Protein A
    b. Capsular polysaccharide
    c. Peptidoglycan and teichoic acids
    d. Coagulase
    e. Enterotoxins

f. Hemolysins
g. Leukocidin
h. Exfoliatin
i. Hyaluronidase
j. Staphylokinase
k. Superantigens
l. Toxic shock syndrome toxin (TSST)
m. β-lactamase (penicillinase)

11. List and describe the more *common* infections caused by *Staphylococcus aureus.*
12. List and describe the more *serious* infections caused by *Staphylococcus aureus.*
13. Describe the carrier state and its relationship to transmission of staphylococcal infection.
14. Describe β-lactamase and its role in infection and antibiotic treatment of *Staphylococcus aureus* infections.
15. Indicate what the following acronyms mean and describe the significance of each:
    a. MRSA
    b. VRSA
    c. VISA
16. Explain how latex agglutination is used to identify *S. aureus.*
17. Explain how methicillin resistance can be determined.
18. List medically significant species classified as coagulase-negative staphylococci (CoNS) and describe infections attributed to these organisms.
19. Describe the identification of *Staphylococcus epidermidis.* Identify *Staphylococcus epidermidis* from an unknown culture without error.
20. Discuss the clinical relevance of *Staphylococcus epidermidis, Staphylococcus saprophyticus,* and the other CoNS.
21. State the purpose and principle of the novobiocin test. Perform and interpret this test without error.
22. Identify *Staphylococcus saprophyticus* from an unknown culture without error.

Gram-Positive Cocci

The medically significant gram-positive cocci include *Staphylococcus, Streptococcus, Enterococcus,* and other less frequently isolated bacteria. The gram-positive cocci all contain a high content of peptidoglycan and a low level of lipid in the cell wall. This accounts for the fact that alcohols and other solvents do not penetrate the gram-positive cell wall but instead cause the cell wall to tighten, shrink, or crenate. This is why gram-positive organisms retain the primary stain, crystal violet, in the Gram stain procedure. The decolorizer, acetone/alcohol, causes the gram-positive cell wall to seal tightly, trapping the crystal violet within.

The gram-positive cocci are natural habitants of skin and mucous membranes in humans and can be ubiquitous in the environment. Gram-positive infections are spread through direct contact with infected individuals or contaminated objects. Such infections are termed **pyogenic**, resulting from the accumulation of neutrophils, bacterial cells, and fluids at the infection site.

Analysis based on DNA ribosomal RNA hybridization of the gram-positive cocci has resulted in the reclassification of several of these organisms. According to *Bergey's Manual of Systematic Bacteriology,* published in 1996, the family Micrococcaceae included four genera: *Micrococcus, Staphylococcus, Planococcus,* and *Stomatococcus.* In a more recent edition of *Bergey's Manual,* the following changes have occurred. Genus *Staphylococcus,* as well as *Gemella, Macrococcus,* and *Salinicoccus,* is now classified in the family Staphylococcaceae. The major human pathogens in this family are *Staphylococcus,* which has a characteristic colony size of 1.0 μm to 2.0 μm. *Macrococcus* is a new genus that is characterized by larger colonies of 1.0 μm to 2.5 μm, with no human infections yet attributed to this organism. The family Micrococcaceae now includes *Micrococcus, Arthrobacteria,* and *Kocuria. Micrococcus* typically arrange in tetrads but may also appear in pairs and clusters and produce colonies that measure 0.5 μm to 1.5 μm in diameter. The *Micrococcus* organisms may colonize human skin but rarely are infectious, and thus they are identified to the genus level by most microbiology laboratories. *Stomatococcus mucilaginosus,* the only member of *Stomatococcus,* is classified in the genus *Rothia. R. mucilaginosus* is found as normal flora in the human upper respiratory tract. The organism has been rarely

TABLE 7-1 Differentiation of *Staphylococcus* from *Micrococcus**

	Staphylococcus	*Micrococcus*
Catalase	+	+
Aerobic growth	+	+
Anaerobic growth	+	–
Glucose utilization (of media)	Fermentative	Oxidative or nonsaccharolytic
Modified oxidase	–	+
Benzidine	–	+
Resistant to lysostaphin (200 µg/ml)	–	+
Resistant to bacitracin (0.04 U)	+	–

*+ = plus; – = negative

isolated from blood cultures as the agent of endocarditis and bacteremia. *Stomatococcus* cannot grow in the presence of 5% NaCl as can *Staphylococcus* and *Micrococcus*. The organism also has a capsule and is coagulase negative and weakly catalase positive.

It is sometimes necessary to differentiate *Staphylococcus* from *Micrococcus*. Staphylococci are facultative anaerobes and ferment glucose anaerobically, whereas micrococci are strict aerobes, which utilize glucose oxidatively or are nonsaccharolytic. Micrococci are resistant to 200 µg/ml of lysostaphin and modified oxidase positive, whereas staphylococci are susceptible to lysostaphin and modified oxidase negative. Lysostaphin is a peptidase that breaks the glycine peptide linkages in the cell wall of the staphylococci. In addition, *Staphylococcus* is resistant to 0.04 unit of bacitracin, whereas *Micrococcus* is susceptible. **TABLE 7-1** lists characteristics for the differentiation of *Micrococcus* from *Staphylococcus*.

Staphylococcus

The genus *Staphylococcus* is composed of several species, which are found in humans, other animals, and the environment. These organisms may be found on the skin and mucous membranes of humans and are associated with human colonization or infection. Significant human species include *Staphylococcus aureus*, *S. epidermidis*, *S. saprophyticus*, *S. hominis*, *S. hemolyticus*, and *S. warneri*. Coagulase is an enzyme that converts fibrinogen to fibrin and is produced by the pathogenic species, notably *S. aureus*. Those species such as *S. epidermidis* and *S. saprophyticus* do not produce coagulase and are known as coagulase-negative staphylococci (CoNS).

Staphylococci are gram-positive cocci most often arranged in tetrads or clusters that are nonmotile and nonspore forming. Most species are facultative anaerobes. Staphylococci produce medium-sized, raised, creamy colonies on blood agar or colistin-nalidixic acid (CNA) with white, cream, or golden pigmentation. These bacteria are catalase positive, modified oxidase negative, and lysostaphin susceptible and bacitracin resistant, and reduce nitrates to nitrites. Staphylococci are salt tolerant and, thus, able to grow in 7.5% to 10% NaCl. These criteria are very important in differentiating *Staphylococcus* from *Streptococcus* species, which are typically arranged in pairs or chains and are pinpoint, flat, colorless colonies with wide zones of hemolysis. Streptococci are typically catalase negative. **FIGURE 7-1** illustrates positive and negative catalase reactions.

FIGURE 7-1 Catalase negative (left) and positive (right).

Staphylococci are easily isolated on blood agar, colistin-nalidixic acid (CNA), or mannitol salt agar (MSA). On blood agar, colonies are medium convex, creamy, and dome shaped. The pigment varies from white to golden yellow. **FIGURES 7-2**, **7-3**, and **7-4** illustrate staphylococcal species on sheep blood agar. CNA is a selective medium with a blood agar base that contains the antibiotics colistin and nalidixic acid. The medium is selective for gram-positive cocci, inhibiting the growth of gram-negative bacilli.

MSA contains 7.5% to 10% sodium chloride (NaCl), the carbohydrate-alcohol mannitol, and phenol red indicator.

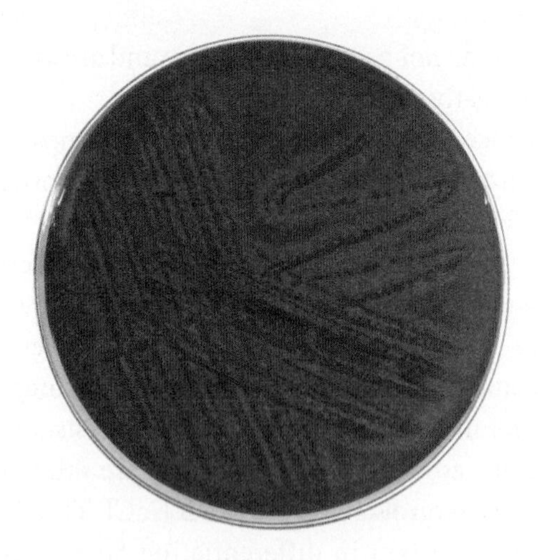

FIGURE 7-2 *S. aureus* on sheep blood agar.

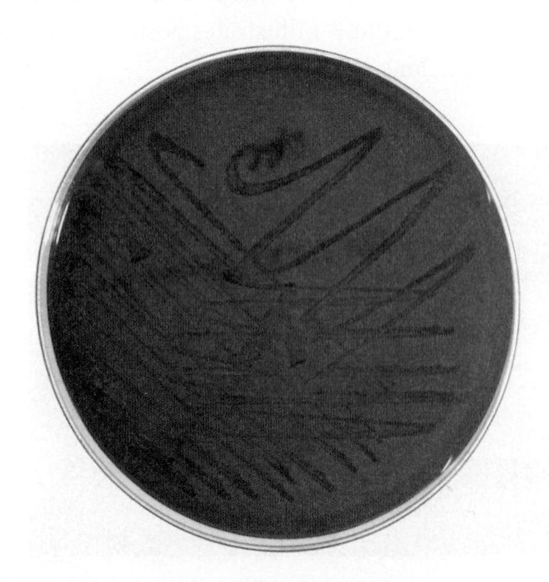

FIGURE 7-3 *S. epidermidis* on sheep blood agar.

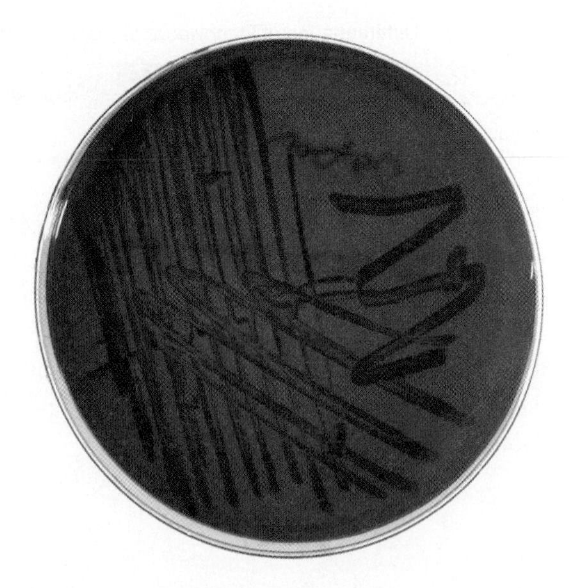

FIGURE 7-4 *S. saprophyticus* on sheep blood agar.

The medium is typically used for the selective isolation of *Staphylococcus* because most other bacteria cannot sustain the high salt concentration. The plate is read for growth and fermentation of mannitol, which is characterized by a yellowing of the medium, as the phenol red indicator takes on its acidic color. Positive fermentation of MSA is illustrated in **FIGURE 7-5**, and negative fermentation is illustrated in **FIGURE 7-6**.

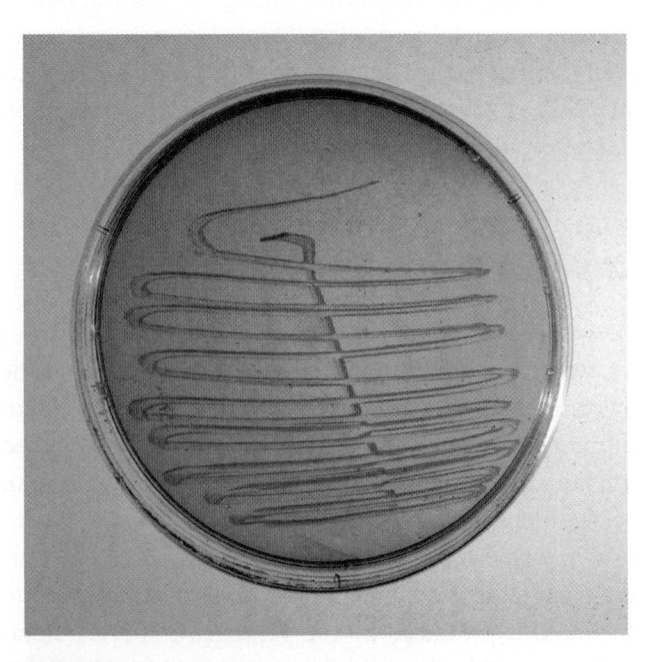

FIGURE 7-5 MSA *S. aureus*.

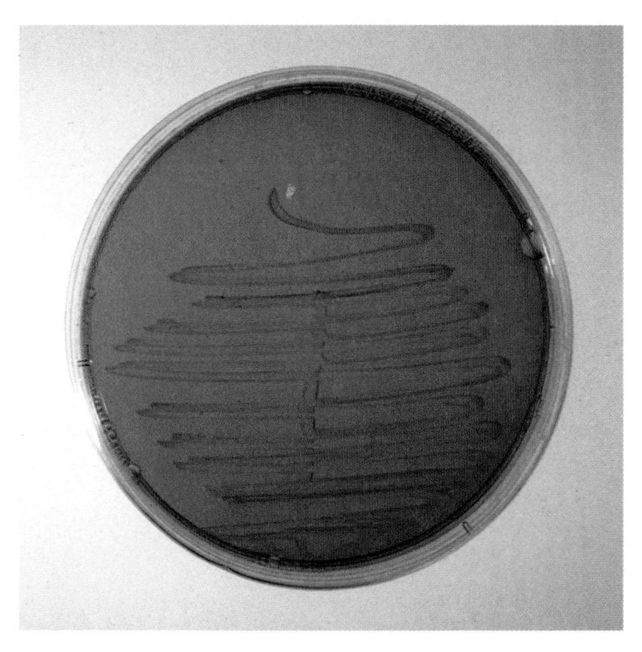

FIGURE 7-6 MSA *S. epidermidis.*

STAPHYLOCOCCUS AUREUS

Identification

Most strains of *Staphylococcus aureus* appear as medium to large colonies, 1.0 μm to 2.0 μm in diameter after 24 hours of incubation. Colonies show a smooth, butyrous, creamy appearance. The edge is entire, and the colonies may be pigmented white to golden yellow. Most strains of *S. aureus* exhibit a narrow zone of β-hemolysis, whereas some strains are nonhemolytic. Hemolysis and pigmentation are more evident after incubation of 2 to 3 days, at room temperature. Similar colonies are observed on CNA.

To differentiate *S. aureus* from other *Staphylococcus* species, the coagulase test is the most reliable method. There are two types of coagulase: bound coagulase, or clumping factor, and free coagulase. *S. aureus* is the only staphylococcal species pathogenic to humans that produces coagulase. **Bound coagulase**, or clumping factor, is detected in the slide coagulase test; most strains of *S. aureus* produce bound coagulase. In this method, the bacterial colony is mixed with rabbit plasma. In a positive reaction, agglutination occurs within 1 minute, which is noted by the appearance of white fibrin clots. This indicates the conversion of **fibrinogen** to **fibrin**. (**FIGURE 7-7**).

If the slide test is negative, the tube coagulase test must be performed to determine whether **free coagulase** is present. Free coagulase is an extracellular toxin that reacts

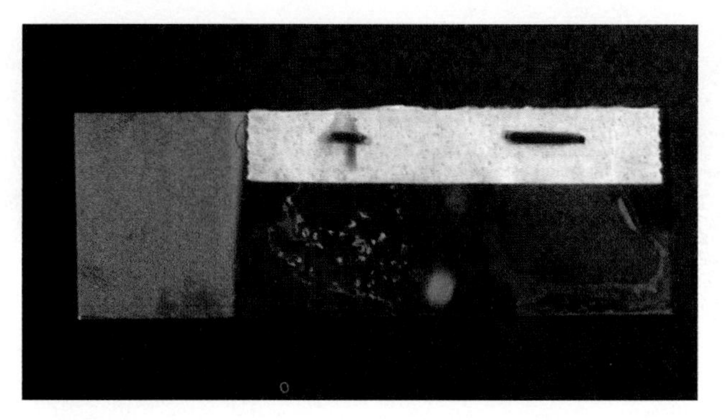

FIGURE 7-7 Coagulase slide.

in the presence of coagulase-reacting factor (CRF), a compound normally found in plasma to form coagulase–CRF complex. This complex resembles thrombin and converts fibrinogen to fibrin. In the coagulase tube test, 0.5 ml of rabbit plasma is inoculated with the organism and incubated in a 35°C to 37°C water bath and read for partial or complete clot formation at 30 minute intervals for up to 4 hours. Because some strains of *S. aureus* produce a **fibrinolysin** (staphylokinase), clot lysis may occur, resulting in a false-negative result. Tests that are negative for fibrin clot formation at 4 hours should be incubated at room temperature overnight for 16 to 18 hours to detect slower coagulase producers (**FIGURE 7-8**).

Some species of *Staphylococcus* (*S. lugdunensis* and *S. scheiferi*) may produce clumping factor and must be differentiated from *S. aureus.*

Coagulase activity also can be detected using agglutination or passive agglutination methods that are commercially available. These methods generally provide for a

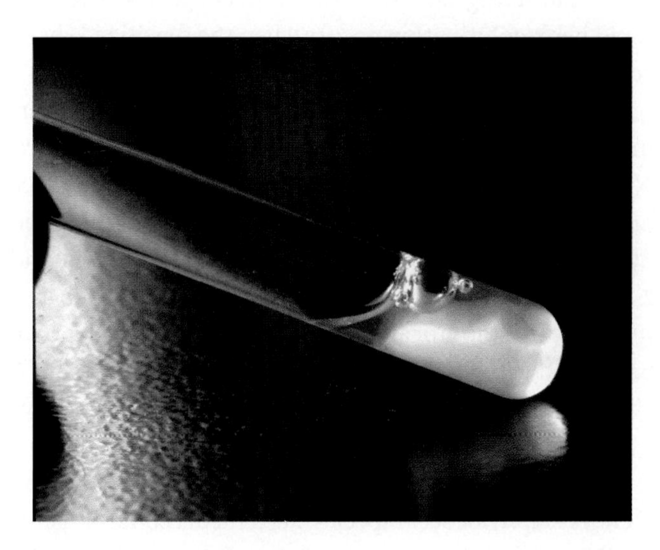

FIGURE 7-8 Coagulase tube.

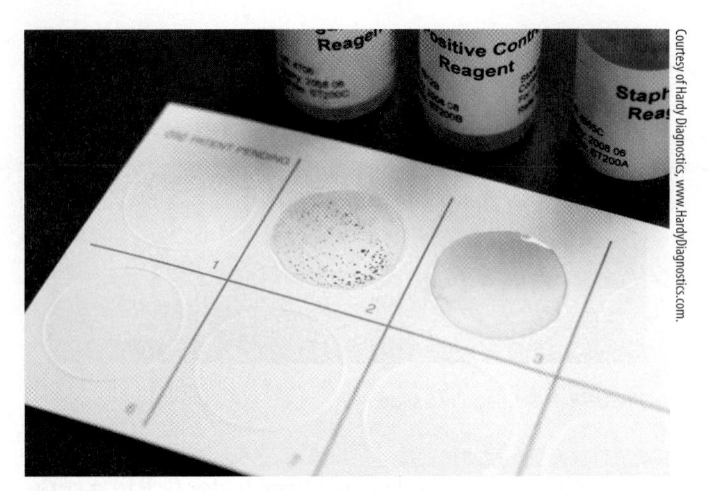

Courtesy of Hardy Diagnostics, www.HardyDiagnostics.com.

FIGURE 7-9 StaphTEX™ Blue procedure.

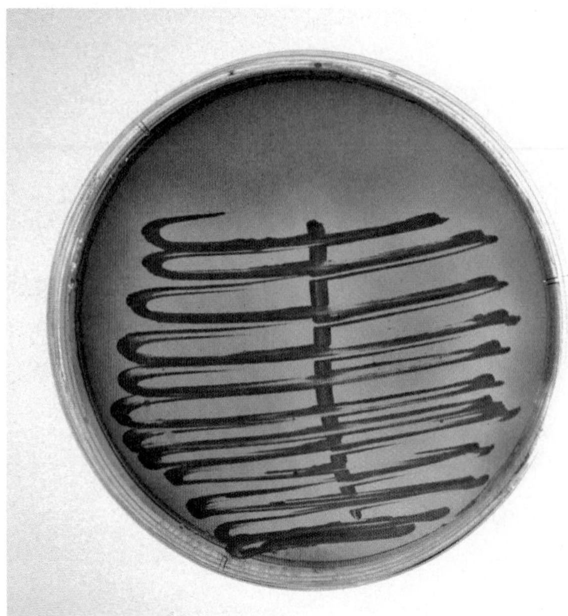

FIGURE 7-10 DNAse clearing.

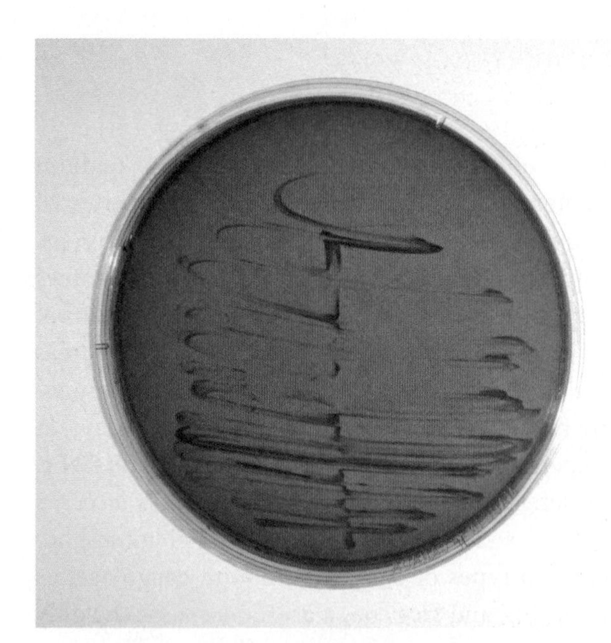

FIGURE 7-11 DNAse not clearing.

more rapid detection of coagulase and thus, a more timely identification of *S. aureus*. In latex agglutination techniques, such as the BBL™ Staphyloslide™, Wampole Staph Latex Test, and Staphaurex® (Remel), latex particles are coated with human plasma fibrinogen and immunoglobulin G (IgG), which will react with clumping factor and protein A of *S. aureus*. The BBL Staphyloslide Latex Test consists of blue latex particles coated with human fibrinogen and IgG. On mixing the latex reagent with colonies of staphylococci that have clumping factor or protein A present, cross-linking will occur, giving visible agglutination of the latex particles. The StaphTEX™ Blue procedure (Hardy Diagnostics) tests for both the clumping factor and protein A found in *S. aureus* (**FIGURE 7-9**). Hemagglutination uses sheep red blood cells coated with fibrinogen, which will detect clumping factor. In the Hemastaph test (Remel), rapid hemagglutination occurs when the sensitized sheep cells react with clumping factor.

Other tests to identify *S. aureus* include growth and fermentation of MSA. The organism can grow in 6.5% to 10% NaCl and ferment the carbohydrate alcohol mannitol. *S. aureus* also gives a positive DNase test reaction, as indicated by a clearing of the dye toluidine blue (**FIGURES 7-10** and **7-11**), which is incorporated into the nutrient agar–based medium. In a modification of the DNase test, the plate can be flooded with dilute hydrochloric acid after incubation. A change in color from blue-green to pink indicates a positive hydrolysis of deoxyribonucleic acid (DNA).

Chromogenic agars also can be used to isolate and identify staphylococcal species. Such media contain agents inhibitory to gram-negative bacteria, yeast, and some gram-positive bacteria and a nutrient source, peptones. Chromogens or artificial substrates are incorporated into the media and are utilized by specific bacterial enzymes that result in the formation of colored compounds. When using HardyCHROM™ Staph aureus agar, *S.aureus* appears as deep pink– to fuchsia-colored colonies, whereas *S. epidermidis* may be partially or totally inhibited and *S. saphrophyticus* appears as turquoise-colored colonies

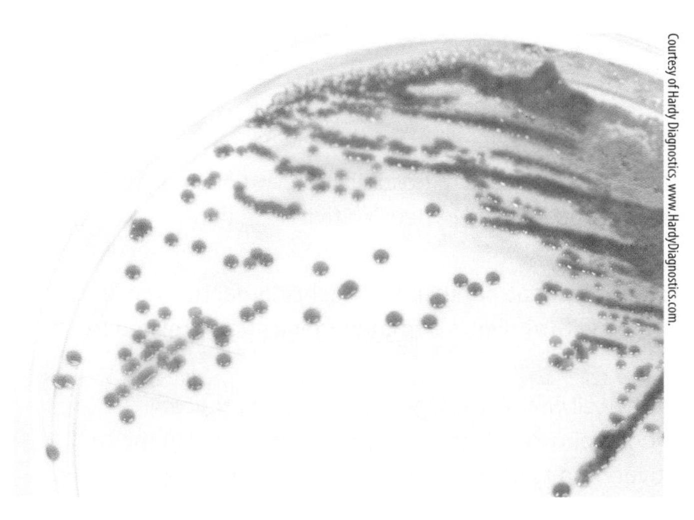

FIGURE 7-12 HardyCHROM™ *S. aureus.*

within 24 hours. **FIGURE 7-12** shows *S. aureus* on Hardy-CHROM™ Staph aureus agar.

S. aureus is also thermostable nuclease positive. This enzyme is detected by boring small wells into DNase agar. The wells are then filled with a broth culture of the organism, which has been boiled in a water bath for 15 minutes. A positive reaction is indicated by the presence of pink halos surrounding the wells. BOX 7-1 summarizes some of the important characteristics of S. aureus.

SPECIMEN COLLECTION

Specimens suspected of containing *Staphylococcus* species should be plated onto sheep blood agar and CNA. Staphylococcal species are associated with infections from many specimen sites, including wounds, sputum, blood, and urine. Gram stains prepared directly from these sites are examined for the presence of gram-positive cocci, and neutrophils are noted.

BOX 7-1 Important Characteristics of *S. aureus*

Medium to large, raised colonies on blood agar and CNA with cream to golden yellow pigmentation

Gram stain: Gram-positive cocci arranged in clusters

β-hemolytic on sheep blood agar

Bound coagulase (clumping factor): Positive

Free coagulase: Positive

MSA: Growth and fermentation

DNase: Positive

Thermostable nuclease: Positive

INFECTIOUS PROCESSES

Staphylococcus aureus is a very common bacterial pathogen and is the cause of many infections of the skin and soft tissue as well as the cause of more invasive, serious diseases. It also is associated with pneumonia, osteomyelitis, septicemia, endocarditis, food-borne disease, and toxic shock syndrome. *S. aureus* liberates a number of extracellular toxins and compounds, which contribute to its frequency and diversity in infections. The organism is ubiquitous and may be a part of the normal human flora in the axillae, inguinal, and perineal areas; the skin, and anterior nares. Approximately 10% to 30% of adults are colonized with the organism and carry it asymptomatically in the anterior nares or on the skin. The carrier rate is even higher in the health care setting, and colonization serves as a possible source of infection in the community and in health care settings. *S. aureus* is also an opportunistic pathogen, and those with chronic diseases, skin trauma, viral infections, prosthetic devices, intravenous lines, leukemia, and other underlying disorders may be at greater risk for these infections.

S. aureus causes disease by invading tissues and producing toxins. The organisms may be spread from the site of carriage to the site of infection by breaks in the skin, including surgical wounds or skin abrasions. Abscesses composed of bacteria and leukocytes enclosed by tissue and fibrin are characteristic of staphylococcal infection. The organism may then be spread through the blood to the lungs, bones, liver, brain, or heart. *S. aureus* produces many extracellular toxins and enzymes, which are associated with specific types of infections. These exotoxins are released from living cells into the extracellular environment. For example, the **enterotoxin** of S. aureus is associated with food borne disease or gastroenteritis. **Hemolysin** can lyse red blood cells and **leukocidan** can inhibit white blood cells. Some of the more significant examples of such toxins and enzymes are listed in BOX 7-2, as are several surface characteristics that play a role in the establishment and course of infection.

Infections caused by *S. aureus* are characteristically pyogenic in nature. These infections are accompanied by swelling, redness, increase in temperature to the affected area, and accumulation of leukocytes. Many infections are nosocomial, including surgical wound infections

BOX 7-2 ***Staphylococus aureus*** **Virulence Factors**

Factor Function

Protein A: Binds to the Fc fraction of most IgG antibody molecules; interferes with opsonization and phagocytosis from neutrophils and activation of complement; affects immediate and delayed hypersensitivity reactions; immunogenic

Capsular polysaccharide: Enables organism to resist phagocytosis by neutrophils; may enhance organism's ability to bind to host cells and prosthetics; specific types may be associated with virulence and pathogenicity and related to septicemia and toxin production

Peptidoglycan and teichoic acids: Compounds that support the cell wall. Peptidoglycan consists of N-acetyl-glucosamine and N-acetyl-muramic acid, and techoic acid is ribotal phosphate polymers. These are found in the cell wall and give the cell wall firmness. These compounds can activate complement; enhance neutrophils, chemotaxis, and formation of opsonins; aid in the organism's attachment to mucous membranes; and enable organism to resist unfavorable environmental conditions. Peptidoglycan incorporates other proteins, such as clumping factor, adhesions, and collagen-binding proteins

Extracellular Enzymes

Catalase: Inactivate hydrogen peroxide formed in neutrophils as they ingest and destroy bacteria with myeloperoxidase enzymes

Clumping factor or Bound Coagulase: Conversion of fibrinogen to fibrin; fibrin may coat neutrophils, which protects organism from phagocytosis

Staphylokinase (fibrinolysin): Dissolves fibrin clots and may enable infection to spread once clot has been dissolved

Hyaluronidase: Hydrolysis of hyaluronic acid present in connective tissue, which can result in the spread of infection

Lipase: Hydrolyzes lipids in plasma and skin; enables staphylococci to colonize certain body areas; is associated with initiation of skin infections, such as boils, carbuncles, and furuncles

Nucleases: Deoxyribonuclease (DNase): degradation of DNA

β-lactamase (penicillinase): Hydrolysis and inactivation of penicillin antibiotics through breakdown of β-lactam ring in penicillin molecule; resistance to ampicillin and other antibiotics

Hemolysins: Group of α-, β-, γ-, and Δ-hemolysins that lyse erythrocytes. In addition, α-, γ-, and Δ-hemolysins may be toxic to leukocytes

Toxins

Exfoliatins: Proteolytic and hydrolyzed tissue through cleavage of stratum granulosum; associated with staphylococcal scalded skin syndrome

Enterotoxins: Group of seven heat-stable proteins—A, B, C, D, E, H, and I. Most staphylococcal-related food poisonings are associated with enterotoxins A and B.

Superantigens: Enterotoxins are included in pyrogenic toxin superantigens that include toxic shock syndrome toxin-1 (TSST-1), as well as several streptococcal pyrogenic exotoxins. TSST-1 promotes cytokine release and rapid progression of toxic shock syndrome.

Leukocidins: Lysis of neutrophils and macrophages; inhibit phagocytosis

and those involving prosthetic devices. Pneumonia in infants, immunosuppression in patients, and ventilator-associated pneumonia also are associated with *S. aureus*. Bacteremia and septicemia from *S. aureus* also occur in patients with cardiovascular disease, diabetes mellitus, and immunosuppressive conditions and in those with prosthetic devices. Many cases of bacteremia are nosocomial, and complications include endocarditis.

The most common staphylococcal infections include those of the skin and soft tissues, such as folliculitis, an infection of the hair follicle; boils; furuncles; and carbuncles. Furuncles are small abscesses of the skin and subcutaneous tissue generally found in the neck and axillae. Carbuncles consist of a group of furnuncles and may involve deeper tissue. Impetigo is a superficial skin infection that begins as a reddening of the skin and soft tissue that then develops into fluid-filled lesions. It is found in newborns, infants, and young children. Scalded skin syndrome, generally seen in newborns and young children, occurs from exfoliation. Blisters form and burst, and the epidermis peels away, leaving a red, moist area. Acne and postoperative surgical wound infections are also associated with *S. aureus*. Skin infections can be self-limiting but may also spread through the blood, causing septicemia.

S. aureus is considered to be the most common cause of food-borne illness in the United States. Strains of *S. aureus* that produce enterotoxins A–E, H, and I are associated with the symptoms of food poisoning. The preformed enterotoxin is ingested in contaminated foods, such as custards, cream puffs, eggs, potato salad, chicken salad, and processed meats. The toxin is produced at room temperature but is inactive at refrigerated temperatures. Symptoms include the rapid onset of nausea and vomiting approximately 2 to 6 hours after ingestion of the enterotoxin. The condition is usually self-limiting, and recovery occurs within 8 to 12 hours in most individuals.

Osteomyelitis, or bone infections, is seen in children as a complication in patients with diabetes mellitus or atherosclerosis and as a result of trauma or surgery.

Toxic shock syndrome (TSS), a clinical syndrome characterized by hypotension, fever, desquamation of the palms and soles, fever, chills, headache, and vomiting, was first characterized by Todd in 1978. Described as affecting women during menstruation using high-absorbency tampons, the syndrome is known to occur in a variety of individuals, including men, children, and nonmenstruating women. This multisystemic disease is attributed to strains of *S. aureus* that produce toxic shock syndrome toxin-1. Symptoms of **Staphylococcal toxic shock syndrome** include a rapid onset of fever; headache; chills; diffuse erythema; hypotension; vomiting; diarrhea; severe myalgia; and renal, hepatic, and hematologic involvement. TSS may occur following staphylococcal wound infections, pneumonia, or abscesses.

Because many *S. aureus* isolates produce **β-lactamase** and are resistant to penicillin, penicillinase-resistant drugs are the drugs of choice in the treatment of most staphylococcal infections. Examples of penicillinase-resistant penicillins include oxacillin, cloxacillin, and methicillin. **Methicillin-resistant *Staphylococcus aureus*** (MRSA) strains are resistant to antibiotics known as β-lactams. These antibiotics include penicillin, oxacillin, and amoxicillin as well as other β-lactam drugs, including the cephalosporins. MRSA was first documented in the United States over 40 years ago in the hospital setting and then emerged as a significant nosocomial pathogen. Risk factors for MRSA include hospitalization—especially in an intensive care unit—surgical wounds; an indwelling line or catheter; malignancy; recent antibiotic use; and chronic lung, liver, or vascular disease. Within the health care setting, MRSA causes very serious infections, such as septicemia, infections of surgical wound sites, and pneumonia. Beginning in the 1990s, MRSA infections were also identified in the outpatient population in individuals who did not have the recognized MRSA-associated risk factors. Community-acquired MRSA (CA-MRSA) refers to a methicillin-resistant *S. aureus* that is acquired within the community or in a non–health care setting. CA-MRSA most frequently involves infections of the skin, which are red and swollen and contain pus. Often, CA-MRSA may occur following cuts and abrasions to the skin.

S. aureus also has shown resistance to the antimicrobial agent vancomycin. While most isolates of *S. aureus* remain susceptible to vancomycin, with an MIC of 0.5 μg/ml to 2.0 μg/ml, some degree of resistance has developed, and this is evidenced by a higher MIC. Those *S. aureus* that have a minimal inhibitory concentration (MIC) of 4 μg/ml to 8 μg/ml are known as **vancomycin-intermediate *S. aureus*** (VISA), and if the MIC is ≥16 μg/ml, the isolate is classified as **vancomycin-resistant *S. aureus*** (VRSA).

DETECTION OF ANTIBIOTIC-RESISTANT *STAPHYLOCOCCUS AUREUS*

It is important to identify strains of *S. aureus* that are resistant to penicillin and other β-lactam antibiotics, especially methicillin. The production of β-lactamase by bacteria, including *S. aureus*, can be detected using iodometric, acidometric, and chromogenic substrates. Chromogenic substrates are commercially available and include the chromogenic cephalosporin, Nitrocefin (BBL), which generally can detect all known β-lactamases including the staphylococcal penicillinases.

Methicillin resistance can be detected using the cefoxitin disk screen test, latex agglutination for PBB2a, or

Mueller-Hinton agar supplemented with NaCl with 6 μg/ml of oxacillin according to the Clinical and Laboratory Standards Institute. These methods are outlined in Chapter 6. In addition, agars have been developed that detect and identify MRSA through the incorporation of specific chromogenic substrates and cefoxitin. One example is BBL™ CHROMagar™ MRSA, on which MRSA strains will grow in the presence of cefoxitin and produce mauve-colored colonies. Bacteria other than MRSA may utilize other chromogenic substrates in the medium, resulting in blue to blue-green–colored colonies, or if no chromogenic substrates are utilized, the colonies appear as white or colorless.

Detecting the gene that codes for methicillin resistance (*mecA*) or its product, penicillin-binding protein 2' (2a) or PBP2 (PBP2a), which is found in the cell walls of the organism, provides another method to identify MRSA. The gene can be detected through nucleic acid hybridization and DNA amplification methods, such as polymerase chain reaction. MRSA screens utilizing a latex reagent sensitized with monoclonal antibody against PBP2 also have been developed to identify MRSA. The gene is extracted from the organism's cell membrane, and a presumptive positive reaction is evidenced by visible clumping with the latex reagent, as seen in the MRSA Latex Test for PBP2 (Hardy Diagnostics) in **FIGURE 7-13**.

Coagulase-Negative Staphylococci

In the past, the **coagulase-negative staphylococci** (CoNS) were considered to be contaminants with little clinical relevance. However, these bacteria have been isolated with increasing frequency as agents of infection in recent decades. These bacteria are important causes of blood infections, infections involving prosthetic devices, and urinary tract infections. Because these bacteria are found in large numbers as normal flora on the skin and mucous membranes, it is difficult to distinguish contaminants and commensal isolates from clinically relevant pathogens. Those at highest risk of CoNS infections include hospitalized patients, especially premature newborns, the elderly, those immunocompromised, and those with other medical complications. There are several species of CoNS isolated from humans, of which *S. epidermidis* and *S. saprophyticus* are most significant.

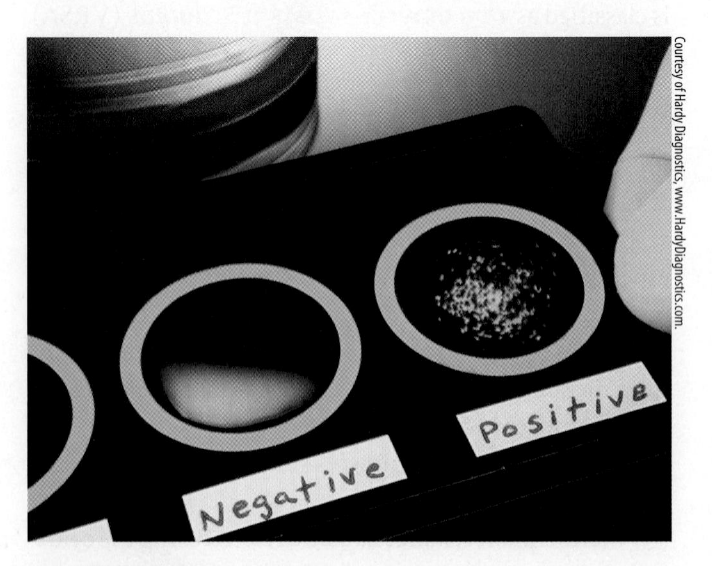

Courtesy of Hardy Diagnostics, www.HardyDiagnostics.com.

FIGURE 7-13 MRSA Latex PBP2.

STAPHYLOCOCCUS EPIDERMIDIS

Staphylococcus epidermidis resembles *S. aureus* in the Gram stain preparation. Colonial morphology typically shows white, creamy colonies that are nonhemolytic. More than 50% of all clinical isolates of CoNS are *S. epidermidis*. Identifying characteristics of *S. epidermidis* are shown in BOX 7-3.

The coagulase test is used to differentiate *S. epidermidis* from *S. aureus*. For both the slide and tube coagulase tests, *S. epidermidis* gives negative reactions. In addition, the organism cannot ferment mannitol and is DNase negative.

S. epidermidis is normal flora of the skin and mucous membranes of humans and other animals. *S. epidermidis* is associated with prosthetic valve endocarditis and also can colonize prosthetic devices, including central nervous system shunts, intravascular catheters, and prosthetic

BOX 7-3 Identifying Characteristics of *S. epidermidis*

- Gram-positive cocci in clusters
- White, creamy, raised growth on blood agar
- Nonhemolytic on blood agar
- Positive growth on CNA
- Growth, but lack of fermentation of MSA
- Coagulase negative
- DNase negative
- Susceptible to novobiocin

orthopedic devices, resulting in infections such as bacteremia and septicemia. In addition, the organism has been found to cause urinary tract infections and cutaneous infections and has been implicated in dialysis-associated catheter infections. Infections of *S. epidermidis* and other CoNS often occur in the immunocompromised hosts, including individuals with malignancies or severe burns or in transplant patients. A great majority of *S. epidermidis* infections are acquired in the health care setting.

Virulence factors of *S. epidermidis* include its ability to form biofilms through the production of cell surface and extracelluar compounds that promote the bacteria to adhere to plastic surfaces of prosthetic devices. One such compound is Ps/A, which assists the organism in its ability to adhere to surfaces and also to resist phagocytosis.

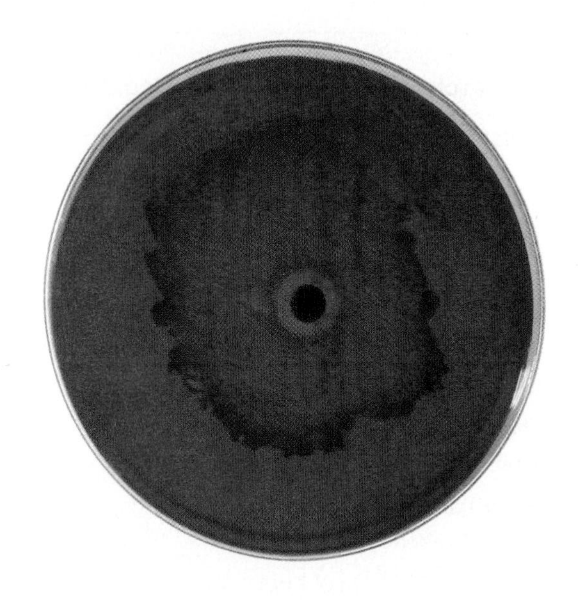

FIGURE 7-14 Novobiocin susceptible showing zone of inhibition.

STAPHYLOCOCCUS SAPROPHYTICUS

Staphylococcus saprophyticus is an important cause of urinary tract infections, such as pyelonephritis and cystitis, especially in sexually active young women. It also is the cause of catheter-associated urinary tract infections in men and women. Virulence factors associated with *S. saprophyticus* include its ability to adhere to epithelial cells in the urinary tract and to urethral cells.

The organism is coagulase negative, DNase negative, and nonhemolytic on blood agar. Fermentation of mannitol is variable. Initial colony counts to confirm the urinary tract infection are usually less than 1.0×10^5/ml. *S. saprophyticus* is resistant to novobiocin, and this principle is used to differentiate the organism from *S. epidermidis* and other clinically significant CoNS that are susceptible to novobiocin. A 0.5 McFarland standard of the suspect organism is prepared and streaked on a blood agar plate, and a 5 μg novobiocin disk is applied. The plate is then incubated for 18 to 24 hours overnight at 35°C. *S. saprophyticus* will exhibit zone sizes of 6 mm to 12 mm, indicating resistance, while other CoNS will exhibit zone sizes of at least 16 mm. **FIGURES 7-14** and **7-15** illustrate examples of novobiocin susceptibility and resistance. BOX 7-4 lists other CoNS that are more rarely isolated.

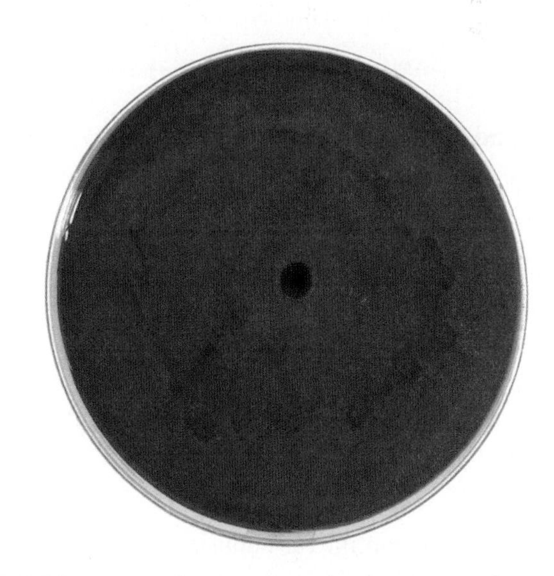

FIGURE 7-15 Novobiocin resistant showing no zone of inhibition.

Laboratory Procedures

Procedure
Catalase

Purpose
Catalase enzymatically converts hydrogen peroxide into water and oxygen. Most aerobes and facultative anaerobes possess the enzyme. The test is useful in the differentiation of gram-positive cocci. *Staphylococcus* are catalase positive, and *Streptococcus* are catalase negative.

Principle
Catalase converts hydrogen peroxide (H_2O_2) into water and oxygen. A positive reaction is indicated by rapid and continuous bubble formation.

BOX 7-4 Rarely Isolated Coagulase-Negative *Staphylococcus* Found in Humans

S. auriculoris: Normal flora of human external ear canal; rare pathogen

S. capitis: Normal flora of human scalp; rare pathogen in sepsis and prosthetic valve endocarditis

S. cohnii: Normal flora of human skin; rare opportunistic pathogen in community-acquired pneumonia and sepsis

S. haemolyticus: Normal flora of human skin; etiologic agent in endocarditis, septicemia, and peritonitis

S. hominis: Normal flora of human skin; rare pathogen-causing septicemia in immunocompromised hosts

S. lugdunerisis: Opportunistic pathogen in septicemia, wound and skin infections, and endocarditis in those with prosthetic valves, osteomyelitis, and urinary tract infections

S. saccharolyticus: Normal flora of human mucous membranes; rare cause of endocarditis; formerly known as the anaerobic species *Peptococcus saccharolyticus*

S. schleiferi: Rare human pathogen in wound infections and bacteremia, prosthetic valve endocarditis, and nosocomial urinary tract infections

S. simuloris: Normal flora of human mucous membranes; rare cause of septicemia and osteomyelitis

S. warneri: Normal flora of human skin; usually nonpathogenic but has been found to be associated with bacteremia and endocarditis

S. xylosus: Normal flora of humans; rare cause of urinary tract infections

Reagents and Materials

3% hydrogen peroxide (store in a dark bottle in refrigerator)
Microscope slides

Procedure

1. Transfer a small portion of a well-isolated colony that is 18 to 24 hours old onto a clean microscope slide.
2. Add one to two drops of 3% hydrogen peroxide.
3. Observe for the formation of rapid and continuous bubbles.

Interpretation

Positive: Rapid and continuous bubbles
Negative: Lack of bubble formation 30 seconds later

Quality Control

Staphylococcus epidermidis: Positive—bubbling
Streptococcus pyogenes: Negative—no bubbling

Notes

1. The order in the procedure should not be reversed. Do not add the organism to the reagent. This may lead to a false-positive reaction.
2. Because red blood cells also contain catalase, avoid inclusion of red cells from the medium into the test reaction. This may lead to false-positive reactions.

Procedure

Modified oxidase

Purpose

Micrococcus organisms possess cytochrome C in the cytochrome-oxidase system, whereas most *Staphylococcus* organisms do not. The procedure can be combined with other procedures, such as bacitracin susceptibility, to differentiate *Micrococcus* from *Staphylococcus*.

Principle

Those bacteria that possess cytochrome C produce a dark-blue end product when reacted with modified oxidase reagent (6% tetramethylphenylenediamine hydrochloride in dimethyl sulfoxide).

Reagents and Materials

Modified oxidase reagent and filter paper or Microdase Disks (filter paper disks impregnated with modified oxidase reagent; available from Remel Laboratories)

Procedure

1. Smear the suspected 18- to 24-hour colony onto filter paper.
2. Add one drop of modified oxidase reagent.
3. Observe for a dark-blue color.

If using Microdase Disks, smear colony onto disk and observe for dark-blue color.

Interpretation

Positive reaction: dark-blue color
Negative reaction: No color change

Quality Control

Micrococcus luteus: Positive—dark-blue color

Staphylococcus epidermidis: Negative—no color change

Notes

All *Micrococcus* species are modified oxidase positive, whereas all *Staphylococcus* species are oxidase negative except the rare isolate *S. sciuri.*

Procedure

Bacitracin susceptibility

Purpose

Micrococcus and *Rothia* are susceptible to 0.04 unit of bacitracin, whereas *Staphylococcus* species are resistant. The test can be used to differentiate *Micrococcus* and *Rothia* from *Staphylococcus* when combined with other procedures, such as the modified oxidase.

Principle

Bacitracin inhibits the growth of *Micrococcus* and *Rothia*, while having no effect on *Staphylococcus*, which is resistant.

Reagents and Materials

Trypticase soy broth

Mueller-Hinton agar or trypticase soy agar

Bacitracin disks (0.04 U)

Procedure

1. Inoculate a trypticase soy broth with sufficient isolate to match the turbidity of a 0.5 McFarland standard.
2. Saturate a swab in this solution and streak the Mueller-Hinton or trypticase soy agar in three directions to form a lawn of growth.
3. Place a 0.04 U bacitracin disk in the center of the streak.
4. Incubate at 35°C for 18 to 24 hours.
5. Interpret for zone of inhibition.

Interpretation

Zones greater than 10 mm indicate susceptibility and are typical of *Micrococcus.*

Staphylococcus organisms typically produce no zone of inhibition and are considered resistant.

Quality Control

Micrococcus luteus: Susceptible—zone diameter greater than 10 mm

Staphylococcus epidermidis: Resistant—no zone of inhibition

Procedure

Coagulase

Purpose

Coagulase is an enzyme that converts soluble fibrinogen into soluble fibrin. *Staphylococcus aureus* is the only pathogenic species of *Staphylococcus* that possesses the coagulase enzymes and, thus, coagulates plasma. Staphylococci that do not possess the enzymes are termed coagulase-negative *Staphylococcus* (CoNS) and include *S. epidermidis* and *S. saprophyticus.*

Principle

In the presence of coagulase, fibrinogen is converted to fibrin. There are two forms of coagulase: bound coagulase, or clumping factor, and free coagulase. Bound coagulase remains attached to the organism's cell wall and is detected in the coagulase slide test. Free coagulase is an extracellular enzyme produced in broth culture and is detected in the coagulase tube test.

Reagents and Materials

Rabbit plasma (anticoagulated with EDTA)

Microscope slides 12 mm × 75 mm test tubes

Pipette to deliver 0.5 ml

Coagulase slide test

Procedure

1. Place a drop of rabbit plasma on a clean microscope slide.
2. Place a drop of sterile saline or distilled water on a separate area of the slide.
3. Using a sterile inoculating loop, emulsify a suspension of the organism in the saline or water. This is the negative control.
4. Emulsify a suspension of the organism in the plasma. Try to form a smooth suspension.
5. Slide back and forth for 1 minute.
6. Interpret slide for agglutination.

Interpretation

Positive: White fibrin clots in plasma

Negative: Smooth suspension

Quality Control

Staphylococcus aureus: Positive—immediate agglutination in the slide test with complete clearing of background

Staphylococcus epidermidis: Negative—smooth, milky suspension

Notes

1. Agglutination in the test and in the negative control indicates autoagglutination and an invalid test.

2. All negative coagulase slide tests must be confirmed by the tube test.
3. Results must be read within 10 seconds, or false-positive results may occur.
4. The slide coagulase test is not reliable in detecting bound coagulase in some oxacillin-resistant *S. aureus*.
5. Autoagglutination may occur if colonies from media with a high salt concentration, such as mannitol salt agar, are used.

Procedure

Coagulase tube test

1. Add 0.5 ml of rehydrated rabbit plasma to a sterile test tube.
2. Add either one loopful, two to four colonies from a noninhibitory agar plate of the organism to be tested, or 0.1 ml of a pure broth culture to the tube of plasma.
3. Incubate in a 35°C to 37°C water bath or heating block. Observe for clot formation by gently tipping the tube at intervals of 30 minutes for the first 4 hours of incubation. Care should be taken not to disrupt the clot.
4. Tubes that are negative after 4 hours should be incubated at room temperature and examined at 18 to 24 hours.

Interpretation

Positive: Any degree of clot formation
Negative: No clot formation

Quality Control

Staphylococcus aureus: Positive—clot formation
Staphylococcus epidermidis: Negative—no clot formation

Notes

1. Tubes should be checked for clot formation at intervals because of the possible production of fibrinolysin (staphylokinase), which may lyse the fibrin clot and be interpreted as a false-negative reaction.
2. False-positive clot formation may occur if citrated plasma is used because some bacteria use citrate in their metabolism.

Procedure

Novobiocin susceptibility

Purpose

The novobiocin susceptibility test differentiates *Staphylococcus saprophyticus*, which is resistant to novobiocin, from other coagulase-negative staphylococci (CoNS), which are susceptible to novobiocin.

Principle

S. saprophyticus is resistant to 5 μg of novobiocin, whereas other CoNS, such as *S. epidermidis,* are susceptible to novobiocin.

Materials

Sheep blood agar or Mueller-Hinton agar
5 μg novobiocin disks

Procedure

1. Streak the organism in three directions to form a lawn of growth on the sheep blood (or Mueller-Hinton) agar plate.
2. Place a 5 μg novobiocin disk in the center of the inoculum.
3. Incubate at 35°C to 37°C for 18 to 24 hours.
4. Examine the plate for inhibition around the disk. Measure the zone diameter in millimeters.

Interpretation

Susceptible: Zone diameter >16 mm
Resistant: Zone diameter ≤16 mm

Quality Control

S. epidermidis: Susceptible—zone diameter greater than 16 mm
S. saprophyticus: Resistant—zone diameter less than or equal to 16 mm

Procedure

Deoxyribonuclease (DNase) test

Purpose

DNase test agar is used to detect DNase activity in species of aerobic bacteria, including *Staphylococcus aureus* and *Serratia marcescens.* Toluidine blue and methyl green are metachromatic dyes, which can be used to detect DNase activity. When toluidine blue is bound to DNA, the dye appears blue. When DNase activity occurs and DNA is degraded to oligonucleotides, the dye appears rose pink in the area of the medium where degradation occurred. Methyl green is green when bound to DNA, but when DNA is degraded, the methyl green is released and becomes colorless. Toluidine blue is toxic to many gram-positive bacteria.

Principle

In this procedure, DNase medium using methyl green becomes colorless in the presence of DNase.

Materials

DNase agar

Procedure

1. Streak DNase plate with a heavy inoculum.
2. Incubate 35°C to 37°C for 18 to 24 hours and up to 48 hours.
3. Interpret plate for growth and clearing of dye.

Interpretation

Positive: Hydrolysis of the surrounding medium, resulting in a clear zone
Negative: No clearing is observed

Quality Control

Serratia marcescens and *Staphylococcus aureus:* Positive—clear zone
Enterobacter cloacae and *Staphylococcus epidermidis:* Negative—no clearing

Procedure

Mannitol salt agar

Purpose

Mannitol salt agar (MSA) is a selective and differential medium useful for isolation and differentiation of *Staphylococcus* species. MSA contains high levels of sodium chloride (7.5%). *Staphylococcus* species (and some salt-tolerant strains of *Micrococcus* and *Enterococcus*) are able to grow in this concentration of NaCl, whereas most gram-negative organisms and other gram-positive organisms cannot.

Principle

MSA contains beef extract, NaCl, D-mannitol, and phenol red indicator. *Staphylococcus aureus* grows on MSA and ferments mannitol, producing yellow colonies. Most coagulase-negative strains of *Staphylococcus* do not ferment mannitol and grow as small red colonies surrounded by red or purple zones. The differential colors are caused by the reactivity of phenol red indicator, which is red at pH 8.4 and yellow at pH 6.8.

Materials

Mannitol salt agar

Procedure

1. Inoculate specimen onto medium for primary isolation, or inoculate isolated colonies for differentiation.
2. Incubate at 35°C to 37°C for 18 to 24 hours.
3. Interpret plates for growth and fermentation.
4. Record results.

Interpretation

Staphylococcus and other salt-tolerant bacteria will grow.
Growth without fermentation: Plate remains pink to red, with no yellow halo surrounding growth
Growth and fermentation: Yellow halos surrounding growth

Quality Control

S. aureus: Growth, yellow zone around colonies
S. epidermidis: Growth, red zone around colonies

Case Studies

1. A hospital patient recovering from hip replacement surgery develops redness and tenderness at the site of incision. Clinical signs reveal a temperature of 101°F and a blood pressure of 170/90. Anaerobic and aerobic cultures are requested on the incision site. The Gram stain of the incision site reveals numerous gram-positive cocci in clusters with a moderate number of neutrophils. In the space below, indicate which agar plates you would inoculate and what biochemical tests you would perform to identify this organism.
   Media inoculated: ______________________
   Biochemical tests: ______________________
2. A urine culture is received in the laboratory from a 25-year-old female. She has experienced painful urination and developed a low-grade fever. The culture was plated using a 1 μl calibrated inoculating loop on sheep blood agar, as well as on MacConkey agar. About 75 medium, creamy white colonies grew on the blood agar at 24 hours, while no growth was evident on the MacConkey plate. The following tests were performed with the results shown:
   Catalase: Positive
   Slide coagulase: Negative
   Tube coagulase: Negative
   Novobiocin: 7 mm zone
   Identify the organism and determine the colony count:
   ____
   ____

Laboratory Exercises

1. Prepare a Gram stain of *Staphylococcus epidermidis.* Describe your observations.
   ____
   ____
2. Inoculate a blood agar or colistin-nalidixic acid plate with each of the following organisms. After

appropriate incubation, describe the colonial morphology and hemolytic reactions of each.
Colonial morphology hemolysis: ______
Staphylococcus epidermidis: ______
Staphylococcus aureus: ______
Staphylococcus saprophyticus: ______
Micrococcus luteus: ______

3. Inoculate mannitol salt agar with the following organisms. After appropriate incubation, describe your observations and record your results.
Observations/Results
S. epidermidis: ______
S. aureus: ______
State the principle of MSA: ______
______

4. Inoculate DNase agar with the following organisms. After appropriate incubation, describe your observations and record your results.
Observations/Results
S. epidermidis: ______
S. aureus: ______
State the principle of DNase. ______

5. Perform the coagulase slide test on the following organisms. Record your observations and interpret your results.
Observations/Results
S. epidermidis: ______
S. aureus: ______
S. saprophyticus: ______
Explain why it is necessary to perform the coagulase tube test on those bacteria that give a negative slide test. ______
______
Perform the coagulase tube test on all organisms that gave a negative slide test. Record your observations and results.
Organism Observations/Results
______
______
Why is it important to check the tube for clots periodically during incubation?
______
______

6. Differentiate an unknown catalase-positive gram-positive coccus by performing the modified oxidase and bacitracin susceptibility tests. Record your observations and results. Indicate whether the organism belongs to the genus *Staphylococcus* or *Micrococcus*.
Unknown number:

	Observation	Result
Modified oxidase		
Bacitracin susceptibility		
Identification and explanation		

7. Identify an unknown member of the genus *Staphylococcus*. Inoculate appropriate media and perform necessary tests. Record your observations and results, and identify the unknown.
Unknown number:

Media inoculated	Observation	Result
Procedures performed	**Observation**	**Result**
Identification and explanation		

Review Questions

Matching

Match the staphylococcal toxin or extracellular product with its effect or description.

1. Enterotoxins
2. Hemolysins
3. Leukocidin
4. Staphylokinase
5. Exfoliation
   a. Fibrin clot lysis
   b. Scalded skin syndrome
   c. Food poisoning
   d. Inhibition of leukocytes
   e. Breakdown of red blood cells

Multiple Choice

6. Which of the following indicates the correct biochemical reactions for *Micrococcus*?

	Aerobic Growth	Glucose Utilization	Modified Oxidase	Lysostaphin Resistance
a	Negative	Fermentative	+	+
b	Positive	Oxidative	+	+
c	Positive	Oxidative	–	–
d	Positive	Fermentative	–	–

7. Which of the following correctly describes the genus *Staphylococcus*?
   a. Susceptible to 0.04 unit of bacitracin
   b. Catalase positive
   c. Gram-negative cocci in clusters
   d. Motile
8. Which of the following best describes the colonial morphology of *Staphylococcus aureus* on blood agar?
   a. Small, pinpoint, nonhemolytic
   b. Medium, creamy, usually β-hemolytic
   c. Flat, clear, α-hemolytic
   d. Pinpoint, white, usually β-hemolytic
9. A *Staphylococcus* produced a fibrin clot in the tube coagulase test but not in the slide coagulase test. This organism:
   a. Produces only free coagulase and is most likely *S. aureus*
   b. Produces only bound coagulase and is most likely *S. aureus*
   c. Is most likely *S. epidermidis* because of the negative slide test
   d. Is most likely *S. epidermidis* because the slide test is unreliable
10. Which statement is incorrect for *Staphylococcus epidermidis*?
    a. Is coagulase negative
    b. Fails to grow on mannitol salt agar
    c. Is DNase negative
    d. Susceptible to novobiocin
11. Growth surrounded by yellow halos on mannitol salt agar indicates:
    a. The organism cannot ferment mannitol
    b. The organism cannot tolerate high salt concentrations
    c. The organism can sustain high salt concentrations and ferment mannitol
    d. None of the above
12. Which of the following infections can be attributed to *Staphylococcus aureus*?
    a. Skin and wound infections
    b. Toxic shock syndrome and bacteremia
    c. Osteomyelitis and food poisoning
    d. All the above
13. Most cases of community-acquired MRSA infections
    a. involve the blood.
    b. are urinary tract infections.
    c. involve the skin.
    d. include pneumonia.

Bibliography

Baker, J. S. (1984). Comparison of various methods for differentiation of staphylococci and micrococci. *Journal of Clinical Microbiology, 19,* 875–879.

Bannerman, T. L., & Peacock, S. J. (2007). *Staphylococcus, Micrococcus,* and other catalase positive cocci. In P. R. Murray, E. J. Baron, J. H. Jorgensen, M. L. Landry, & M. A. Pfaller (Eds.), *Manual of clinical microbiology,* 9th ed. Washington, DC: American Society for Microbiology.

Centers for Disease Control and Prevention. (2000). *Staphylococcus aureus* with reduced susceptibility to vancomycin—Illinois, 1999. *Morbidity and Mortality Weekly Report, 48,* 1165–1167.

Centers for Disease Control and Prevention. (2010). Laboratory detection of oxacillin/methicillin-resistant *Staphylococcus aureus.* Retrieved from http://www.cdc.gov/mrsa/lab/lab-detection.html

Centers for Disease Control and Prevention. (2010). MRSA infections. Retrieved from http://www.cdc.gov/mrsa/index.html

Chambers, H. F. (1988). Methicillin resistant staphylococci. *Clinical Microbiology Reviews, 1,* 173–186.

David, M. Z., & Daum, R. S. (2010). Community associated methicillin resistant *Staphylococcus aureus*: Epidemiology and clinical consequences of an emerging epidemic. *Clinical Microbiology Reviews, 23,* 616–687.

Deresinski S. (2005). Methicillin-resistant *Staphylococcus aureus:* an evolutionary, epidemiologic, and therapeutic odyssey. *Clinical Infectious Diseases, 40,* 562–573.

Dinges, M. M., Orwin, P. M., & Schlievert, P. M. (2010). Exotoxins of *Staphylococcus aureus. Clinical Microbiology Reviews, 13,* 16–34.

Fuchs, D. C., & Smith, L. (1985). Novobiocin susceptibility as a test for presumptive identification of *Staphylococcus saprophyticus. Laboratory Medicine, 16,* 422.

Garrity, G., & Holt, J. G. (2000). *Bergey's manual of systematic bacteriology: An overview of the road map to the manual.* New York, NY: Bergey's Manual Trust.

Hageman, J., Patel, J. B, Carey, R. C., Tenover, F. C., & Mcdonald, L. C. (2006). Investigation and control of vancomycin-intermediate and -resistant *Staphylococcus aureus*: A guide for health departments and infection control personnel. Available at http://www.cdc.gov/HAI/organisms/visa_vrsa/visa_vrsa.html

Howden, B. P., Davies, J. K., Johnson, P. D. R., Stinear, T. P., & Grayson, M. L. (2010). Reduced vancomycin susceptibility in *Staphylococcus aureus*, including vancomycin-intermediate and heterogeneous vancomycin-intermediate strains: Resistance mechanisms, laboratory detection, and clinical implications. *Clinical Microbiology Reviews, 23,* 99–139.

Klein, J. O. (1990). From harmless commensal to invasive pathogen: Coagulase negative staphylococci. *New England Journal of Medicine, 323,* 323–339.

Kloos, W. E., & Bannerman, T. L. (1994). Update on clinical significance of coagulase-negative staphylococci. *Clinical Microbiology Reviews, 7,* 117–140.

McDowell, B., & Papasian, C. J. (1991). *Staphylococcus aureus* identification: Thermonuclease agar for direct testing of blood isolates and a new slide agglutination test. *Clinical Laboratory Science, 4,* 299.

MRSA Latex Test for PMP2'. (2011). Hardy Diagnostics.

Srinivasan, A., Dick, J. D., & Perl, T. M. (2002). Vancomycin resistance in staphylococci. *Clinical Microbiology Reviews, 15,* 521 –540.

Todd, J. K. (1988). Toxic shock syndrome. *Clinical Microbiology Reviews, 1,* 132.

Winn, Jr., W., Allen, S., Janda, W., Konemen, E., Procop, G., Schreckenberger, P., & Woods, G. (Eds.). (2005). Staphylococci and related gram-positive cocci. In *Koneman's color atlas and textbook of diagnostic microbiology,* 6th ed. Philadelphia, PA: Lippincott Williams & Wilkins.

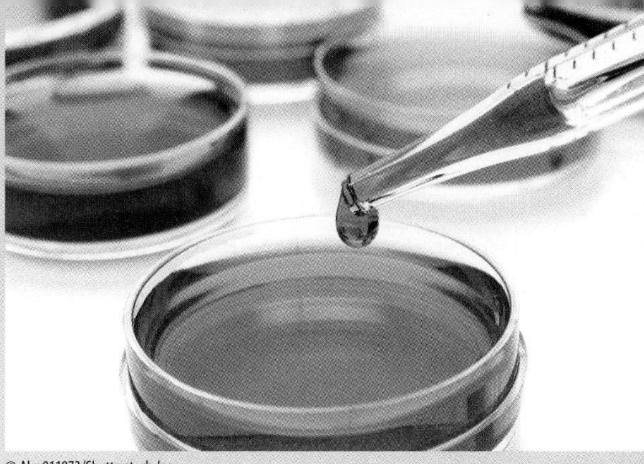

CHAPTER 8

Streptococcus, *Enterococcus*, and Related Organisms

CHAPTER OUTLINE

Streptococcus

Enterococcus

KEY TERMS

Bacitracin test
Bile esculin
Brown's classification
CAMP reaction
M (*emm*) protein
Lancefield antigen grouping
Optochin test
Pneumolysin
Pyogenic exotoxins A, B, and C
PYR reaction
Salt tolerant
Streptokinase
Streptococcal toxic shock-like syndrome
Streptolysin O
Streptolysin S
Superantigens
SXT
Viridans streptococci

LEARNING OBJECTIVES

1. Describe characteristics of the genus *Streptococcus.*
2. List the media typically used to isolate streptococci.
3. List, recognize, and describe the types of hemolysis.
4. Differentiate between streptolysin S and streptolysin O.
5. Give the Lancefield group and preliminary tests used to identify each of the following streptococcal species:
   a. *S. pyogenes*
   b. *S. agalactiae*
   c. *Enterococcus*
   d. *Streptococcus bovis* group
6. List the primary infections caused by group A *Streptococcus.*
7. Discuss the invasive Group A Streptococcal infections and list the associated virulence factors.
8. Describe the M (*emm*) protein and relate its role to GAS infections.
9. Discuss the role of group B streptococcus as a neonatal pathogen.
10. Briefly discuss the significance of the Lancefield groups C, F, and G streptococci.
11. Discuss how the viridans streptococci are classified and list the significant species and their clinical relevance.
12. Describe and recognize the appearance of *Streptococcus pneumoniae* on:
    a. Gram-stained smear
    b. Blood agar at 24-hour and 48-hour incubations
13. Differentiate between viridans streptococcus and *Streptococcus pneumoniae.*
14. State the principle of and perform and interpret the optochin test without error.

15. Describe the principle and use of the following in the identification of *Streptococcus pneumoniae*:
    a. Neufeld (Quellung) reaction
    b. Latex agglutination
16. List and describe infections associated with *Streptococcus pneumoniae.*
17. Differentiate between the *Enterococcus* and *Streptococcus bovis* group.
18. Discuss the infections attributed to viridans streptococcus.
19. Describe the infections associated with the *Enterococcus.*
20. Discuss intrinsic and acquired antibiotic resistance in the *Enterococcus.*
21. Discuss the significance of vancomycin-resistant *Enterococcus.*
22. State the principle and purpose of the following tests. Perform and interpret each test without error.
    a. Bacitracin (A disk)
    b. SXT
    c. CAMP reaction
    d. Bile-esculin
    e. 6.5% salt broth
    f. PYRase
23. Describe the principle and purpose of rapid tests for group A streptococci.
24. List antibiotics effective in the treatment of streptococcal infections.
25. List the names of those bacteria classified as nutritionally variant streptococci and describe their important characteristics.

The focus of this chapter is on *Streptococcus* and *Enterococcus*, members of the family Streptococcaceae, which are frequently associated with a variety of human infections. Streptococci have been classified by a number of criteria. Within the past several years, the taxonomy has been revised based on molecular biology techniques, including 16S rRNA and DNA–DNA reassociation techniques. The *Enterococcus* species were previously classified in the genus *Streptococcus* and have been elevated to the genus level of *Enterococcus.* The genus *Streptococcus* was divided into three genera, which are *Streptococcus, Enterococcus*, and *Lactococcus* according to *Bergey's Manual of Determinative Bacteriology.*

Other microorganisms that resemble the streptococcus include *Aerococcus, Gemella, Leuconostoc, and Pediococcus.*

Streptococcus

The genus *Streptococcus* contains a variety of species; some are nonpathogenic and normal flora for humans, whereas others are important human pathogens. Streptococci are widely distributed in the environment, in dairy products and as normal flora of the human gastrointestinal tract.

Streptococci are typically gram-positive cocci and are arranged in pairs or chains because cell division occurs in one plane. An important biochemical distinction from *Staphylococcus* is the catalase reaction; *Streptococcus* species are catalase negative.

Most strains of *Streptococcus* are fastidious, and isolation is best achieved through enriched media, such as blood agar, Todd-Hewitt broth, or chocolate agar. Colonies are typically small (0.5 to 2.0 μm in diameter), pinpoint, and translucent or clear. Frequently, large hemolytic zones are observed. Growth is enhanced when the blood agar plates are incubated under increased (5% to 10%) carbon dioxide. Because streptococci are facultative anaerobes, growth may be observed both aerobically and anaerobically. The streptococci are nonmotile. Important characteristics of the genus *Streptococcus* are shown in BOX 8-1.

BOX 8-1 Characteristics of *Streptococcus*

Gram-positive cocci 0.5 to 2.0 μm in diameter that occur in pairs or chains

Nonmotile

Nonspore forming

Facultative anaerobes

Some species show enhanced growth under increased (5%–10%) CO_2

Require supportive or enriched media, such as blood agar, for growth

Catalase negative

Enhanced recovery of β-hemolytic streptococci from clinical specimens may be accomplished through use of a selective blood agar medium that is inhibitory to other bacteria, including staphylococci and gram-negative bacilli. Blood agar containing the antibiotics trimethoprim and sulfamethoxazole is one example of a medium available to facilitate the isolation of β-hemolytic streptococci.

CLASSIFICATION

Streptococci may be classified according to the type and pattern of hemolysis, physiologic divisions, and antigenic character of a group-specific cell wall polysaccharide known as the **Lancefield antigen grouping**. Classification based on hemolysis was first described by J. H. Brown in 1919. This is an important phenotypic characteristic in the identification process. Types of hemolysis are affected by the source of red blood cells incorporated into the medium and also the incubation atmosphere. Because hemolysis varies with the animal source of the red blood cells used in the production of the blood agar, it is important to know the source of the red blood cells. Sheep blood agar is used most often in microbiology laboratories in the United States; however, other sources also are used for specific methods. Other types of blood agar include horse, rabbit, and human blood agars. Traditional classifications of hemolytic patterns largely have been established on 5% sheep blood agar, with a trypticase soy agar base. Hemolysis is determined by holding the plate directly in front of a light source. BOX 8-2 presents the hemolytic patterns known as **Brown's classification**. β-hemolysis results from the production of two hemolysins, streptolysin S and streptolysin O. **Streptolysin O** is antigenic, oxygen labile, and produced mainly by group A streptococci. Recent group A streptococcal infections can be diagnosed through the detection of **antistreptolysin O**, an antibody in the patient's serum. **Streptolysin S** is nonantigenic and oxygen stable and thus noted as surface hemolysis. To demonstrate streptolysin O, the blood agar should be cut or stabbed several times to force some of the organism to grow in the reduced oxygen content. Stabs made approximately half the depth of the agar with the inoculating loop while streaking the culture will allow for the detection of streptolysin O.

In 1933, Rebecca Lancefield identified several distinct β-hemolytic streptococcal groups based on specific carbohydrate group antigens. She named the first five groups A, B, C, D, and E. Today, there are numerous Lancefield groups; those that are clinically significant include groups A, B, C, D, F, and G. Serological methods are available whereby the cell wall antigen can be extracted and the organism serotyped by reacting with type-specific antisera.

In 1937, Sherman classified the *Streptococcus* into four physiologic divisions: pyogenic, viridans, lactic, and the *Enterococcus*. He based these divisions on hemolytic reactions, carbohydrate antigens, and phenotype tests. The pyogenic division included the β-hemolytic strains, A, B, C, E, F, and G, and the viridans division included those streptococcus that were not β-hemolytic and not salt tolerant or able to grow at a high pH. The *Enterococcus* division included those streptococci that were salt tolerant and able to grow at a high pH and at a temperature range of 10°C to 45°C. The lactic division included streptococcus that were not clinically significant and were associated with the dairy industry.

BOX 8-2 Brown's Classification of Hemolysis

Alpha (α): Incomplete or partial hemolysis; green or brown color surrounding the colony. This pattern is seen with the viridans streptococci, which are the major normal flora of the oropharynx and *Streptococcus pneumoniae*, an important cause of bacterial pneumonia. α-hemolysis occurs as a result of hydrogen peroxide production by the organism, which destroys the red cells and releases hemoglobin.*

Beta (β): Complete hemolysis of red blood cells; clearing or colorless zone around colony. An example of this type of hemolysis is exhibited by *Streptococcus pyogenes*, the agent of streptococcal pharyngitis.

Nonhemolytic: Lack of hemolysis; no apparent change in color of area surrounding colony; has been referred to as gamma (γ) hemolytic. Most *Enterococcus* species of Lancefield group D are nonhemolytic.

Alpha prime (α'): A small zone of α-hemolysis surrounds the colony. A small zone of β-hemolysis surrounds the zone of α-hemolysis.

*Alpha hemolysis requires the presence of oxygen and appears as nonhemolytic when there is no oxygen in the system.

β-HEMOLYTIC *STREPTOCOCCUS*

Currently, 11 species and four subspecies of β-hemolytic streptococci are recognized. Some are found in animals other than humans and are not pathogenic in humans. Those that are associated with human infection include *S. pyogenes* (Lancefield group A), *S. agalactiae* (Lancefield group B), *S. dysgalactiae* (Lancefield groups C and G), *S. equi* (Lancefield groups C and G), and *S. anginosus* (Lancefield groups A, C, F, and G). The identification of these organisms is summarized in **TABLE 8-1**.

STREPTOCOCCUS PYOGENES (GROUP A *STREPTOCOCCUS*)

Streptococcus pyogenes, or Group A *Streptococcus* (GAS), causes bacterial pharyngitis, skin infections, and other invasive diseases. It also is associated with complications or sequelae such as rheumatic heart disease and acute glomerulonephritis. GAS is not considered to be normal flora, and may be found on the skin and upper respiratory tract of humans on the nasal and pharyngeal mucosa. Infections are spread through direct person-to-person contact or indirectly in aerosol droplets from coughing or sneezing.

S. pyogenes is isolated on blood agar, and the incorporation of trimethoprim and sulfamethoxazole (**SXT**) to the blood agar will enhance its recovery from highly contaminated specimens. After 18 to 24 hours of incubation at 35°C to 37°C, growth is typically pinpoint (0.5 to 1.0 μm in diameter) and translucent, opalescent, or clear in appearance and white to gray in color. The colonies are surrounded by a wide zone of β-hemolysis. **FIGURE 8-1** illustrates group A *Streptococcus* on sheep blood agar.

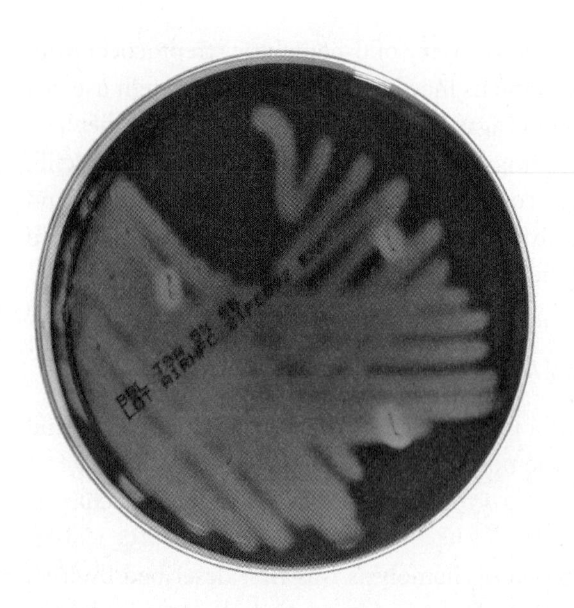

FIGURE 8-1 Group A *Streptococcus* on sheep blood agar.

Group A streptococcal colonies may appear either smooth and glossy or round and mucoid, which indicates the presence of **M (*emm*) protein**. M protein contains hyaluronic acid and is a surface protein found in encapsulated strains of *S. pyogenes*; its presence is associated with virulence. M protein holds antiphagocytic properties and permits the bacterium to survive within the host. Therefore infection can be established in the absence of type-specific antibody. M protein has been serologically typed by using a capillary precipitin test to subtype the organism. More recently, the *emm* typing system, which sequences the gene that codes for the hypervariable region of the M protein, has

TABLE 8-1 Identification of β-Hemolytic *Streptococcus*

Species	Lancefield antigen	Bacitracin	PYR	CAMP	Hippurate	Bile esculin	Voges-Proskauer
S. pyogenes	A	Susc	+	–	–	–	–
S. agalactiae	B	Res	–	+	+	–	–
S. dysgalactiae subsp. *dysgalactiae* and subsp. *equisimilis*	, C and G	Res	–	–	–	V	–
S. equi subsp. *equi* and subsp. *zooepidemicus*	C and G	Res	–	–	–	–	–
S. anginosus	A, C, F, G	Res	–	–	–	+	+

Key:
Susc: Organism is susceptible or sensitive (+)
Res: Organism is resistant (–)
+: Most are positive for the reaction
–: Most are negative for the reaction
V: Reaction is variable

been used for this purpose. There are over 80 *emm* types according to the CDC. Specific serogroups of M protein are associated with throat infection, rheumatic fever, acute glomerular nephritis skin infections, and invasive diseases.

Presumptive identification of *S. pyogenes* is through the **bacitracin test** and the **pyrrolidonyl arylamidase (PYR) test**. *S. pyogenes* is susceptible to 0.02 to 0.04 unit of bacitracin and is PYR positive. When performing the bacitracin test, the isolate tested must be in pure culture. The bacitracin disk never should be directly placed on a primary isolation plate from the specimen site. Bacitracin results are illustrated in **FIGURES 8-2** (susceptible or inhibited) and **8-3** (resistant). Any zone of inhibition is reported as susceptible or as a positive reaction.

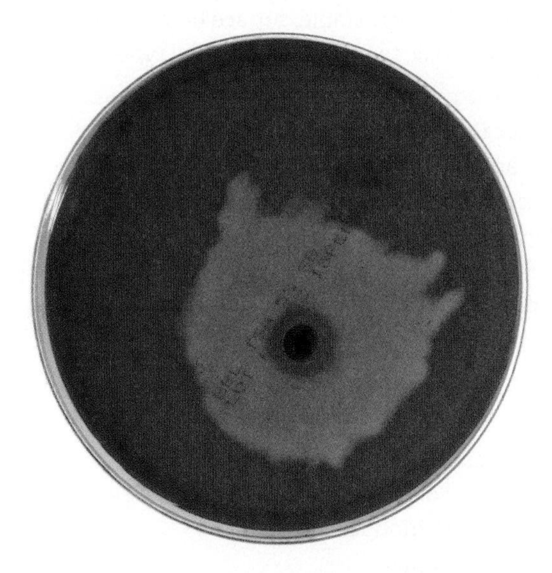

FIGURE 8-2 Bacitracin susceptible or inhibited.

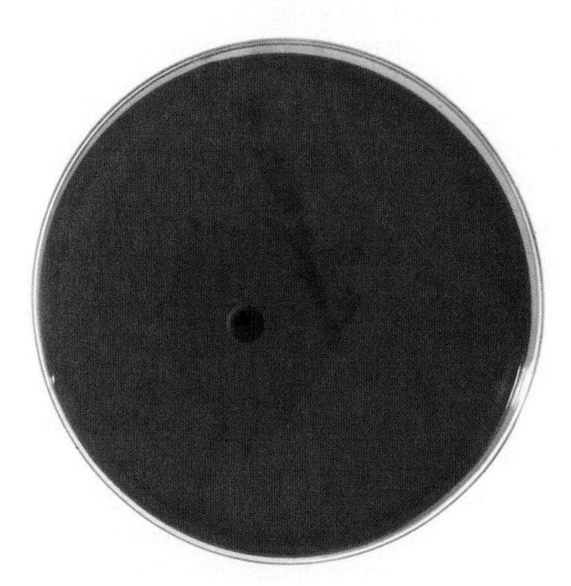

FIGURE 8-3 Bacitracin resistant.

Because a small percentage of other β-hemolytic streptococci (groups B, C, and G) may also exhibit zones of inhibition when grown in the presence of 0.02 to 0.04 unit of bacitracin, other techniques are needed to identify group A *Streptococcus*. Additional testing may include the **PYR reaction**, performing the bacitracin on SXT blood agar or with an SXT disk, and antigen typing for the group A antigen. Group A streptococci, as are the *Enterococcus*, discussed later in this chapter, are PYR positive. PYR can be detected using commercially available PYR disks that are impregnated with the substrate L-pyrrolidonyl-β-naphthylamide. Combined with the bacitracin test, PYR is useful in identifying *S. pyogenes*, which is the only β-hemolytic streptococcus that is susceptible to bacitracin and PYR positive. The PYR test is also used to differentiate the *Enterococcus* species, which are PYR positive, from the non-*Enterococcus* species, which are PYR negative. Organisms resistant to SXT but susceptible to bacitracin can be presumptively identified as group A streptococci. If resistant to both disks, the organism is most likely a group B streptococcus. **FIGURES 8-4** and **8-5** illustrate typical reactions for group A and group B streptococci for SXT and bacitracin. Groups C, F, and G are susceptible to SXT and resistant to bacitracin.

Direct antigen testing of throat swabs for rapid screening of group A *Streptococcus* is a common diagnostic procedure. Direct antigen testing can provide an early diagnosis of group A pharyngitis, and appropriate antibiotic therapy

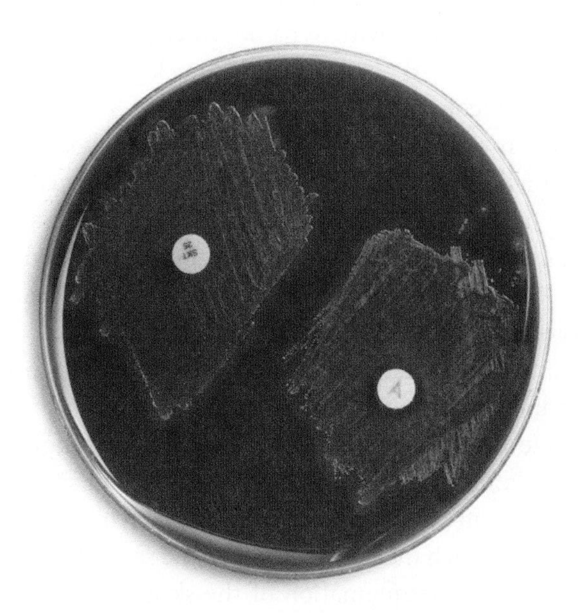

FIGURE 8-4 SXT and bacitracin susceptible.

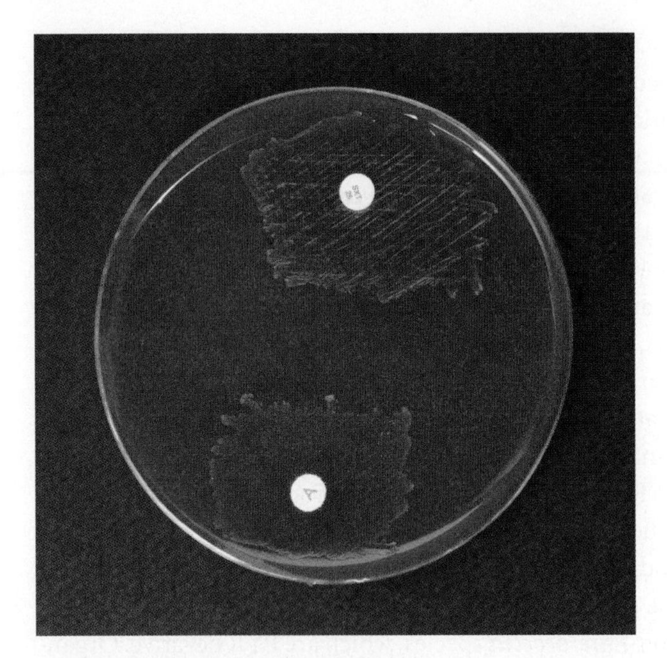

FIGURE 8-5 SXT and bacitracin resistant.

can be initiated. The specific group A streptococcal antigen is extracted using nitrous acid or enzymatic methods directly from a throat swab. Once extracted, the group A antigen is detected immunologically using slide agglutination, ELISA (enzyme linked immuosorbent assay), or other optical methods. The sensitivity varies on the test method and amount of antigen present in the specimen. Thus, to avoid a false-negative, all negative direct antigen tests are confirmed with a throat culture and appropriate testing as discussed above.

Group A *Streptococcus* produces a variety of extracellular products associated with its pathogenicity, which are summarized in BOX 8-3. BOX 8-4 provides quick facts about Group A Streptococcus.

Primary infections caused by group A *Streptococcus* (GAS) include pharyngitis, tonsillitis, or strep throat. GAS is the most common cause of bacterial pharyngitis. Although strep throat is primarily an infection of children aged 5 to 15 years, the infection also is readily spread in crowded conditions, such as those in schools and on military bases. Streptococcal pharyngitis occurs more often in the fall and winter.

Scarlet fever may occur after streptococcal pharyngitis, as well as after other GAS infections at different sites. The pyogenic exotoxins are associated with the symptoms of scarlet fever, which include a characteristic rash, strawberry tongue, and desquamation of the skin. The skin rash typically first appears on the upper chest and spreads to the trunk, neck, arms, and legs. The tongue becomes yellow-white, with red papillae; hence, it's description as a "strawberry tongue."

Skin infections, or pyoderma, are also common group A streptococcal infections. These include impetigo, cellulitis, wound infections, and erysipelas. Whereas impetigo is a superficial skin infection, GAS may also penetrate the

BOX 8-3 Extracellular Products and Other Virulence Factors of *Streptococcus pyogenes*

Extracellular Products

Streptolysin O: Toxic to red and white blood cells; subsurface hemolysin; suppression of neutrophils; induces an antibody response known as antistreptolysin O (ASO). ASO prevents red cell hemolysis and is a serological test used to diagnose recent group A infections, especially in complicated cases. An ASO antibody titer of ≥166 Todd units is usually indicative of group A *Streptococcus* infection. Streptolysin O also is produced by Lancefield groups C and G.

Streptolysin S: Oxygen-stable, surface hemolysin; antiphagocytic; toxic to various human cell types

Pyogenic exotoxins A, B, or C or Superantigens:
Streptococcal toxic shock syndrome—invasion of soft tissue and necrotizing fasciitis fever, alteration of blood-brain barrier; may be associated with organ damage and skin rash of scarlet fever and induce fever and shock. Superantigens stimulate T cell responses by producing cytokines that mediate shock and tissue damage.

Streptokinase: Fibrinolysin that lyses blood clots, prevents fibrin barrier, and allows spread of infection

Streptodornase: Group of four enzymes with nuclease activity; degrade host deoxyribonucleic acid (DNA) and/or ribonucleic acid (RNA)

Cell Surface Antigens

M protein: Associated with virulence; antiphagocytic; interferes with complement activity. Strains lacking M protein are avirulent. Eighty types of M protein have been identified. Immunity depends on development of antibody to type-specific M protein.

Hyaluronic acid: Mucoid strains; present in capsule; antiphagocytic epidermis through abrasions and invade the subcutaneous tissues, causing cellulitis. Erysipelas, one type of cellulitis, is characterized by erythematous lesions of the skin, with edema, most commonly on the face or legs. Pyoderma occurs most frequently in the summer. These skin infections also may become associated with acute glomerulonephritis. Other infections associated with the organism include otitis media, pneumonia, and bacteremia.

Sequelae of GAS infections include rheumatic heart disease, acute rheumatic fever (ARF), and acute glomeruloneprhritis. These sequelae are believed to result from a cross-reacting antibody that attacks cardiac or renal tissue while attempting to destroy streptococcal antigens. Rheumatic fever arises as a delayed sequel to group A streptococcal pharyngitis and may occur 1 to 5 weeks after pharyngitis. During this time, it is believed that the host produces antibody, which attacks the tissues of the affected organs. Symptoms include inflammation of the heart, joints, skin, and nervous system. Rheumatic fever was once a common cause of heart disease in children in the United States. Today, its incidence has declined in the United States but remains a major worldwide health care concern in underdeveloped countries. Specific *emm* protein types and host susceptibility factors contribute to the development of rheumatic fever. The most common expression of rheumatic fever is arthritis, while carditis is its most serious manifestation. Carditis may lead to chronic rheumatic heart disease and progressive degeneration of the heart valves. Increased antibodies against streptolysin O and anti-DNase B antibody levels are observed in rheumatic fever.

Acute glomerulonephritis (AGN) may be observed in patients following streptococcal pharyngitis or skin infections. AGN is observed more often in children and young adults and is more frequently found in males. AGN is characterized by edema of the extremities and face, hypertension, hematuria, proteinuria, and red blood cell casts in the urine. There is a latency period of 1 to 2 weeks following GAS pharyngitis, and the ASO titers are elevated in AGN, resulting from pharyngitis. For AGN resulting from skin infection, there is a longer latency period of 3 to 6 weeks and the ASO titers may be low. Specific M protein serogroups are associated with AGN.

Streptococcus pyogenes strains that produce pyogenic exotoxins and other virulence factors are associated with invasive infections, including streptococcal toxic shock syndrome and necrotizing fasciitis. Virulence factors of these invasive diseases include pyogenic exotoxins A, B, and C, as well as superantigen exotoxin F and streptococcal superantigen. These infections are most frequently found in individuals with underlying medical conditions, including surgery, skin trauma, burns, and disruptions to the skin barrier. The syndrome known as **streptococcal toxic shock-like syndrome** (TSLS) is a toxin-mediated disease that causes hypotension and multiple organ failure. Other symptoms of TSLS include fever, erythema, swelling, tachycardia, acute respiratory distress, renal impairment, and shock. There also may be severe pain and rapid necrosis of skin and cutaneous tissues; the mortality rate has been estimated to be as high as 50%. Specific M protein serotypes have been associated with these syndromes.

BOX 8-4 Group A *Streptococcus* Quick Facts

Wide-zone β-hemolytic
Bacitracin susceptible
PYRase positive
SXT resistant
CAMP negative

Puerperal sepsis, a once common infection, is infrequently attributed to group A *Streptococcus* today.

S. pyogenes is generally treated with penicillin, macrolides such as erythromycin, and certain cephalosporins.

STREPTOCOCCUS AGALACTIAE (GROUP B *STREPTOCOCCUS*)

Streptococcus agalactiae, group B *Streptococcus* (GBS), is isolated on sheep blood agar. Colonies are medium in size, flat, and translucent or opaque. Most often, the colonies show narrow-zone β-hemolysis (95% to 99% of clinical isolates); however, nonhemolytic colonies also rarely may be observed. **FIGURE 8-6** shows *Streptococcus agalactiae* on sheep blood agar.

The **CAMP reaction** is an acronym for Christie, Atkins, and Munch-Petersen, those individuals who first identified the synergistic hemolysis between group B *Streptococcus* and β-hemolytic *Staphylococcus aureus*. In this reaction, an arrowhead-shaped zone of hemolysis forms when group B *Streptococcus* is streaked perpendicularly to a β-hemolytic strain of *Staphylococcus aureus* (**FIGURE 8-7**). The CAMP factor is an extracellular, thermostable, antigenic protein produced by group B *Streptococcus*. A small percentage of

FIGURE 8-6 *S. agalactiae* on sheep blood agar.

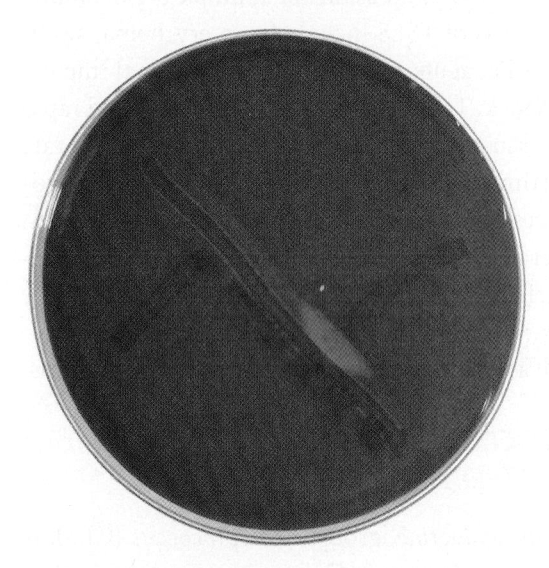

FIGURE 8-7 CAMP reaction.

group A *Streptococcus* also may give a positive reaction. Thus, to differentiate group A from group B *Streptococcus* and other β-hemolytic *Streptococcus*, the bacitracin, CAMP, PYRase, and SXT reactions may be used.

The **hippurate reaction** also may be used to identify group B *Streptococcus*. In this reaction, group B *Streptococcus* hydrolyzes sodium hippurate to benzoic acid and glycine. Benzoic acid is detected with ferric chloride. Alternatively, glycine may be detected with ninhydrin reagent.

Group B streptococci are resistant to bacitracin and SXT and are bile-esculin negative. BOX 8-5 provides quick facts for Group B Streptococcus.

BOX 8-5 **Group B *Streptococcus* Quick Facts**

β-hemolytic (narrow zone) or nonhemolytic
CAMP positive
Hippurate positive
Bactitracin resistant
SXT resistant
PYRase negative
Bile-esculin hydrolysis negative

Group B *Streptococcus* is normal flora of the gastrointestinal tract, and vaginal tract. The organism may colonize the mucous membranes of the genitourinary, upper respiratory tract, and gastrointestinal systems. GBS is an important cause of neonatal infections, including pneumonia, meningitis, and sepsis. Mothers colonized with GBS may transmit the organism through the amniotic fluid during pregnancy or labor. The infant may aspirate the organism into the lungs. GBS also may invade the blood or central nervous system, causing bacteremia and meningitis. Infections acquired within the first week of life are termed early onset, while those acquired 1 week to 3 months after birth are known as late onset. Currently, the CDC recommends screening all pregnant women for vaginal and rectal colonization between 35 and 37 weeks gestation using an enrichment broth and then subculturing to blood agar. A selective enrichment broth, such as Strep B Carrot Broth™ (Hardy Diagnostics) uses chromogenic pigments and provides enhanced sensitivity and specificity and decreased incubation time. The production of orange, red, or brick-red pigment is unique for β-hemolytic GBS. Appropriate antibiotics then can be administered to prevent infection. Direct antigen testing for the group B antigen also can be performed on the infant's spinal fluid or blood.

Adult group B streptococcal infections include skin and soft tissue infections, pneumonia, septic arthritis, bacteremia, urinary tract infections (UTIs), and endocarditis. These infections are often nosocomial and frequently involve an immunosuppressed host. Infections are generally treated with penicillin and an aminoglycoside.

MISCELLANEOUS β-HEMOLYTIC *STREPTOCOCCUS*

Other clinically significant β-hemolytic streptococci include Lancefield groups C, F, and G. The Lancefield

TABLE 8-2 Phenotypic Categories of Viridans Streptococci

Phenotypic group	Representative or significant species	Important biochemical reactions						Comments
		Arginine	Voges Proskauer	Mannitol	Sorbitol	Esculin	Urea	
Mutans group	*S. mutans* and *S. sorbinus*	–	+	+	+	+	–	
Salivarius group	*S. salivarius, S. vestibularius,* and *S. infantarius*	–	+	–	–	V	V	Related to *S. bovis* group based on rRNA
Anginosus group	*S. anginosus, S. constellatus,* and *S. intermedius*	+	+	–	–	+	–	May be α-, β-, or nonhemolytic; β-strains may have Lancefield antigens A, C, F, or G or none. α-strains are more common.
Sanguinus group	*S. sanguinis, S. parasanguinis,* and *S. gordonii*	+	–	–	V	+	–	Formerly, *S. sanguis. S. sanguinis* is associated with subacute bacterial endocarditis.
Mitis group	*S. mitis, S. oralis, S. cristatus,* and *S. infantis*	–	–	–	–	–	–	Found in oral cavity
Bovis group	*S. equinus*		+	V	–	+	–	*S. bovis* and *S. equinus* are now a single species.

group C antigen is found in the following species of *Streptococcus*: *S. equi* subsp. *zooepidemicus*, *S. equi* subsp. *equi*, and *S. dysagalactiae* subsp. *equisimilis*, *S. dysagalactiae* subsp. *dysagalactiae*. *S. dysagalactiae* causes infections similar to those of group A *Streptococcus*, including pharyngitis, skin and soft tissue infections, and bacteremia. The organism is β-hemolytic and gives negative reactions for the CAMP factor, PYR, and bile-esculin hydrolysis and is susceptible to SXT. *S. dysagalactiae* may alternatively carry the Lancefield group F antigen.

S. anginosus generally carries the Lancefield group F antigen and is usually considered as normal flora in the oropharynx and urogenital tracts. It may be the cause of cellulitis, abscesses, and bacteremia. Particular strains of *S. anginosus* also may have A-, C-, or G-type or no Lancefield antigens. Colonies are typically small, and there may be α-, β- or no hemolysis. It is important to differentiate *S. anginosus* from other streptococcal species.

To identify Lancefield groups C, F, and G, biochemical reactions and antigen testing are required. To identify the group antigen, the organism is first isolated on blood agar, and the cell wall antigen is extracted. The extract is then combined with antisera specific for each Lancefield group, which has been tagged with latex beads to aid visualization. Agglutination should occur with a single antiserum type, thus identifying the specific Lancefield group. Several kits are commercially available for Lancefield group antigen identification.

VIRIDANS STREPTOCOCCI

The **viridans streptococci** are a group of streptococcal species characterized by α-hemolysis on sheep blood agar. There are many classification strategies used for the viridans streptococci, which currently include 26 species and six phenotypic groups. **TABLE 8-2** summarizes one classification system based on phenotypic characteristics. Some species may possess specific Lancefield antigens.

Some of the numerous viridans streptococci species in this group include *S. mutans*, *S. salivarius*, *S. anginosus*, *S. mitis*, *S. sanguinis*, *S. constellatus*, and *S. intermedius*. Most are normal flora of the human oropharynx, gastrointestinal, and female genital tracts. The viridans streptococci are important agents of subacute bacterial endocarditis, especially in those with damaged valvular heart tissue, such as mitral valve prolapse, and also in individuals who have prosthetic heart valves. The organism may transiently enter the blood from the oropharynx following dental or genitourinary procedures. Viridans streptococci may cause bacteremia and septicemia, especially in patients who are immunocompromised, including those who are neutropenic. *S. mutans* produces the enzyme glucosyl tranferase, which breaks down sucrose that then binds to glucose to form the complex polysaccharides glucan and dextran. These facilitate the attachment of *S. mutans* to tooth enamel, thus playing a role in dental caries.

The level of identification of the viridans streptococci depends on the specimen source and immune status of the patient. While it is sometimes acceptable to report viridans streptococci, it may be necessary to identify the specific streptococcal species in other situations. Penicillin resistance is a concern, especially in certain species such as *S. mitis.*

All viridans streptococci are resistant to surface active agents, such as bile, sodium desoxycholate, and optochin. In fact, viridans streptococci are often identified by exclusion, which means that negative results are obtained for most presumptive tests used to identify the other streptococci. The organisms may be grouped phenotypically based on specific biochemical reactions, such as fermentation of mannitol and sorbitol, production of urease, and the VP reaction. Commercially available identification kits are also available, as are automated procedures to identify the viridans streptococci to the species level.

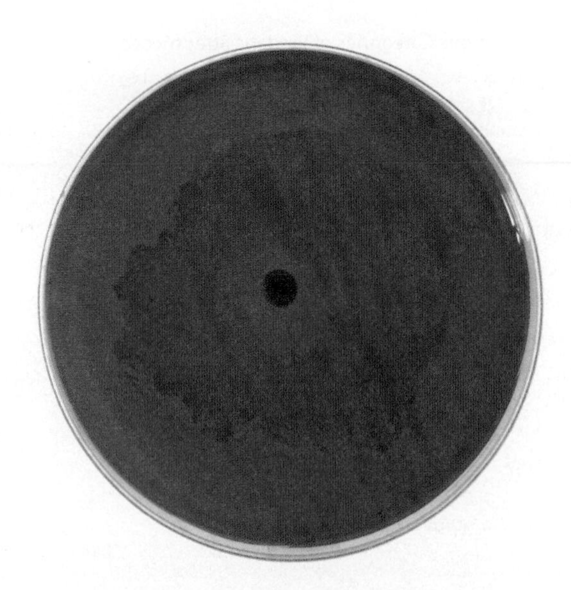

FIGURE 8-8 Optochin (P) disk susceptibility.

STREPTOCOCCUS PNEUMONIAE

Streptococcus pneumoniae differs from other streptococci in its Gram-stain appearance. These gram-positive diplococci are lancet or bullet shaped and form chains. *S. pneumoniae* can be isolated on sheep blood agar and requires 5% to 10% CO_2. Thus primary isolation plates should be incubated in a candle jar or CO_2 chamber. At 24 hours of incubation at 35°C to 37°C, encapsulated strains produce small, round, glistening, dome-shaped colonies that are transparent, with an entire edge. The colonies may run together. Mucoid colonies indicate the presence of a capsule. Colonies show a wide zone of α-hemolysis when incubated aerobically at 24 hours incubation. This α-hemolysis may be attributed to the production of **pneumolysin** by the organism. As the colonies age, **autolysis** occurs, and the colonies collapse and appear umbilicated, leaving an outer elevated margin and a centrally depressed region when observed at 48 hours of incubation.

S. pneumoniae is identified using the **optochin test** (P disk). Optochin contains ethylhydrocupreine hydrochloride and selectively inhibits the growth of *S. pneumoniae* at low levels. A zone of inhibition of at least 14 mm around a 6 μm optochin disk indicates a positive susceptibility test, which identifies *S. pneumoniae.* Other α-hemolytic streptococci, including viridans streptococci and enterococci, are resistant to this concentration of optochin. **FIGURE 8-8** illustrates *S. pneumoniae*'s susceptibility to optochin, and **FIGURE 8-9** illustrates the resistance of viridans streptococci to optochin.

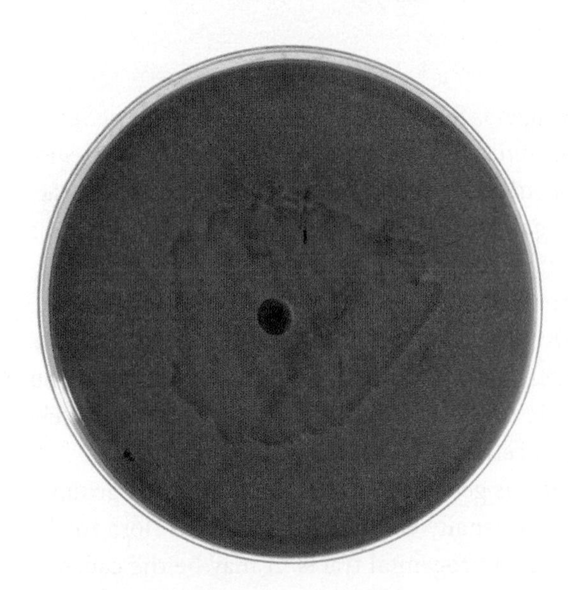

FIGURE 8-9 Optochin (P) disk resistant.

S. pneumoniae also can be identified using **bile solubility tests**. Surface active agents or bile salts, such as sodium desoxycholate and sodium taurocholate, are able to lyse *S. pneumoniae* when grown in culture. On agar, colonies of the organism will lyse or break down when exposed to surface active agents; other α-hemolytic streptococci are resistant to the action of these agents.

The **Quellung reaction**, or **capsular swelling test**, has been used to identify *Streptococcus pneumoniae* directly in body fluids, such as cerebrospinal fluid, synovial fluid, or sputum. The bacteria must be present in large numbers for detection to be accurate. Equal amounts of the specimen are mixed with *S. pneumoniae*–specific capsular antisera. If the reaction is positive, the antisera will bind to the capsular antigen, making the capsule swell, or become more prominent. This principle is utilized in direct antigen testing for pneumococcal capsular polysaccharide in commercially available kits. In such techniques, polyvalent antisera, which reacts with most serogroups of *S. pneumoniae*, is tagged with latex particles. Agglutination will occur in the presence of the corresponding capsular antigen. These tests are rapid and may be used on broth or isolated colonies on agar or directly on blood culture and other clinical specimens.

Extracellular products or antigenic compounds associated with *S. pneumoniae* that contribute to its virulence include capsular polysaccharide antigen, M protein, pneumolysin, and autolysin. These are summarized in BOX 8-6.

Because *S. pneumoniae* may be a part of the normal flora of the upper respiratory tract, it may be difficult to interpret its recovery from sputum and lower respiratory tract cultures. Also, it is sometimes problematic to recover *S. pneumoniae* from clinical specimens, and many patients who are positive for infection may be culture negative. For that reason, the direct Gram stain is an important diagnostic tool. Bartlett's classification scheme, discussed in Chapter 3, can be used to evaluate the suitability of the sputum sample and the presence of infection.

Characteristically, sputum specimens from individuals with neumococcal infections of the lower respiratory tract show a predominance of *S. pneumoniae,* with a decrease or lack of normal oropharyngeal flora. A moderate to large amount of neutrophils also may be present, and the sputum may be rust tinged or bloody.

S. pneumoniae is transmitted from person to person contact through respiratory droplets of asymptomatic carriers or from individuals who are infected with the organism.

Diseases attributed to *S. pneumoniae* include pneumonia, bacteremia, sinusitis, otitis media, and meningitis. There are over 80 serotypes of the organism. The organism is the most common cause of bacterial community-acquired pneumonia. Those at higher risk include the elderly and debilitated, children under 2 years of age, and those with underlying medical conditions, including HIV infection and sickle cell anemia. The pneumococcal vaccine is recommended for the elderly and other high-risk groups.

S. pneumoniae is also a leading cause of otitis media in infants and small children, accounting for numerous middle ear infections. It is also an important cause of bacteremia, septicemia, endocarditis, meningitis, and pericarditis.

S. pneumoniae, once sensitive to penicillin, has exhibited increasing resistance to the penicillins, cephalosporins, and macrolides. Susceptibility testing is used to identify appropriate antibiotics for treatment.

Infection may be prevented through the pneumococcal conjugate vaccine. There is a pneumococcal conjugate vaccine, which is recommended for infants and young children, that protects against 13 types of pneumococci. There is also a 23-valent polysaccharide vaccine, which is recommended for use in all adults who are 65 years of age or older and for those who are 2 years and older and at increased risk of diseases, including sickle cell, HIV, and other immunocompromising conditions.

BOX 8-6 Virulence Compounds of *Streptococcus pneumoniae*

Capsular antigens: Antigenic polysaccharides that enable organism to resist phagocytosis and stimulate antibody production. There are over 80 serogroups based on the capsular antigen.

M protein: Type-specific protein antigens

Pneumolysin: Cytotoxic protein that accumulates in cell and is released upon cell lysis; antiphagocytic and hemolytic and activates complement

Autolysin: Breaks down organism at end of its growth cycle and aids in release of pneumolysis

STREPTOCOCCUS BOVIS GROUP

The *Streptococcus bovis* group has undergone many changes in taxonomy, resulting in four DNA clusters. *S. bovis* and *S.equinus* have been determined to be a single species and are currently known as *S. equinus*. Other important species in this group include *S. gallolyticus*, *S. infantarius*, and *S. alactolyicus*. These streptococci are bile-esculin positive, PYR negative, and unable to grow in 6.5% NaCl broth. They are either α-hemolytic or nonhemolytic on sheep blood agar and have the Lancefield group D antigen. In the past, these bacteria were categorized as group D *Streptococcus*—nonenterococcus. Bacteria in the bovis group are found as agents of bacteremia, septicemia, and endocarditis. There has been an association of the isolation of *S. gallolyticus* subsp. *gallolyticus* with gastrointestinal cancer when found in blood cultures.

Enterococcus

The *Enterococcus* were previously classified in the genus *Streptococcus* and were distinguished by possessing the Lancefield group D antigen and also by their increased resistance to chemical and physical agents. Because of molecular techniques, including DNA–DNA reassociation and rRNA sequencing, these organisms have been classified into the genus *Enterococcus*. This Lancefield group possesses the group D antigen and is characterized by the ability to grow in 40% bile and hydrolyze esculin. **FIGURE 8-10** illustrates positive bile-esculin reactions.

There are many species of *Enterococcus*, which are grouped according to phenotype characteristics. *E. faecalis* causes almost 80% to 90% of human enterococcal infections, followed by *E. faecium*, which is implicated in 5% to 10% of enterococcal infections. Other species include *E. durans*, *E. avium*, *E. casseliflavus*, *E. gallinarum*, *E. dispar*, and *E. canis*.

The enterococci grow as colonies 1 mm to 2 mm in diameter after 24 hours of incubation on sheep blood agar and are either α-hemolytic or nonhemolytic, as shown in **FIGURE 8-11**. These organisms are found throughout the environment in foods, plants, and oil and also in many animals, including birds, reptiles, horses, cattle, and other mammals. In humans, the enterococci are found as normal flora of the gastrointestinal tract and also on the skin and in the oral cavity and genitourinary tract. *E. faecalis* is the most common species found colonizing the human gastrointestinal tract.

FIGURE 8-10 Bile-esculin positive.

FIGURE 8-11 *Enterococcus* on sheep blood agar.

The enterococci are bile-esculin positive and can grow in 6.5% sodium chloride (NaCl) broth (are salt tolerant). To differentiate the *Enterococcus* from the *Streptococcus bovis* group, (formerly non-*Enterococcus*), which also carries the Lancefield group D antigen, 6.5% NaCl or PYR can be used. **FIGURE 8-12** illustrates positive and negative reactions for 6.5% NaCl broth, and **FIGURE 8-13** shows the PYR reaction. These reactions are summarized in **TABLE 8-3**.

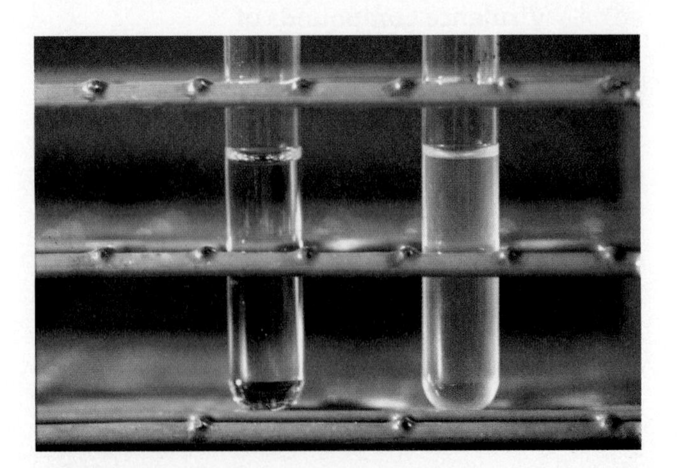

FIGURE 8-12 Positive and negative reactions for 6.5% NaCl broth.

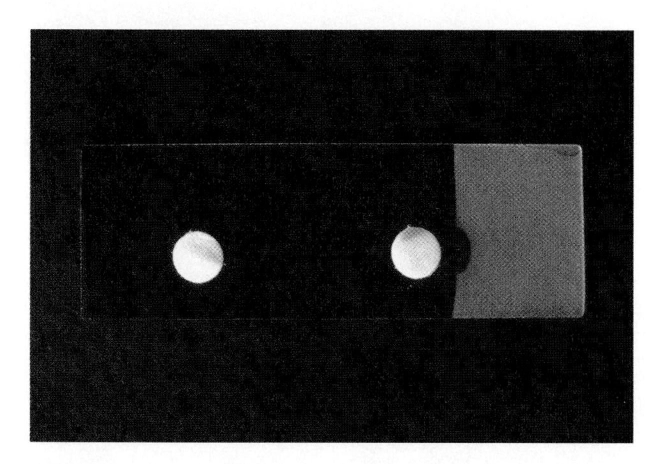

FIGURE 8-13 PYRase reaction: negative on left and positive on right.

Enterococci are opportunistic pathogens and are the agents of nosocomial infections, including urinary tract infections, wound infections, and bacteremia. Infections may be polymicrobic in nature. Intra-abdominal abscesses and endocarditis also are associated with the enterococci. Infections are most frequently seen in individuals with underlying medical disorders, the immunosuppressed, those on prolonged antibiotic therapy, and individuals who have had invasive procedures.

Enterococcal strains are intrinsically resistant to β-lactam antibiotics, including the penicillins and cephalosporins and also to the aminoglycosides. Intrinsic resistance is inherent and coded in the chromosomes of the organism and is found in most enterococci. To overcome this intrinsic resistance, treatment of enterococcal infections has included a combination therapy of a β-lactam (such as penicillin or vancomycin) with an aminoglycoside.

Acquired resistance also is becoming more frequent in the *Enterococcus*, which has shown increased resistance to the aminoglycosides, macrolides, tetracycline, and glycopeptides, especially vancomycin. Acquired resistance occurs as a result of mutations in DNA or plasmids and transposons. Vancomycin-resistant enterococci (VRE) were first reported in 1986, approximately 30 years after vancomycin was used as an antibiotic. VRE continues to increase as a public health issue. There are six types of vancomycin resistance based on genetic and phenotypic characteristics, of which VanA, VanB, and VanC phenotypes are most significant. The VanA phenotype is encoded by the *vanA* gene and shows inducible high-level resistance to vancomycin and teicoplanin. The VanB phenotype, encoded by the *vanB* gene, shows a variable amount of resistance to vancomycin alone. The VanC phenotype is associated with noninducible low-level resistance to vancomyin and is coded for by the *vanC* genes.

TABLE 8-3 Differentiation of Group D Streptococci and Enterococci

	Bile-esculin media	6.5% NaCl broth	PYRase
Group D *Enterococcus*	+	+	+
Streptococcus bovis group Group D non-*Enterococcus*	+	−	−
Not group D	−	−	−

NUTRITIONALLY VARIANT STREPTOCOCCI (NVS): *ABIOTROPHIA* AND *GRANULICATELLA*

Nutritionally variant streptococci are viridans streptococci that require cysteine or pyridoxal (vitamin B_6) for growth. These organisms also are referred to as "satelliting," thiol-requiring or pyridoxal-requiring, or cell wall–deficient streptococci. When in a mixed culture with *Staphylococcus aureus*, NVS "satellite" around the colonies of *S. aureus*, which provide pyridoxal. NVS have been given the new genus status of *Abiotrophia* and *Granulicatella*, of which *A. adjacens*, *A. defectivus*, and *G. adiacens* are important species. The organisms are normal flora of the human oral cavity and have been implicated as endogenous agents in endocarditis.

OTHER CATALASE-NEGATIVE STREPTOCOCCAL-LIKE ORGANISMS

There are other catalase-negative organisms that resemble streptococci that are found as normal flora on the skin and in the gastrointestinal tract or oral cavity. These are generally rare human pathogens but may be associated with infections in immunocompromised hosts. They also may be mistaken for other streptococci. *Aerococcus viridans* is rarely isolated as a cause of endocarditis and meningitis in immunosuppressed individuals. *Leuconostoc* species have been infrequently isolated from several clinical sites, including the blood, and from wounds and abscesses. *Pediococcus* is normal flora of the lower gastrointestinal (GI) tract and has been isolated occasionally from abscesses. *Leuconostoc* and *Pediococcus* both have exhibited resistant to vancomycin. *Lactococcus* and *Gemella* are rare human pathogens, and *Gemella* is a rare isolate of the upper respiratory tract.

The identification of clinically significant streptococci is shown in **FIGURES 8-14** to **8-16**.

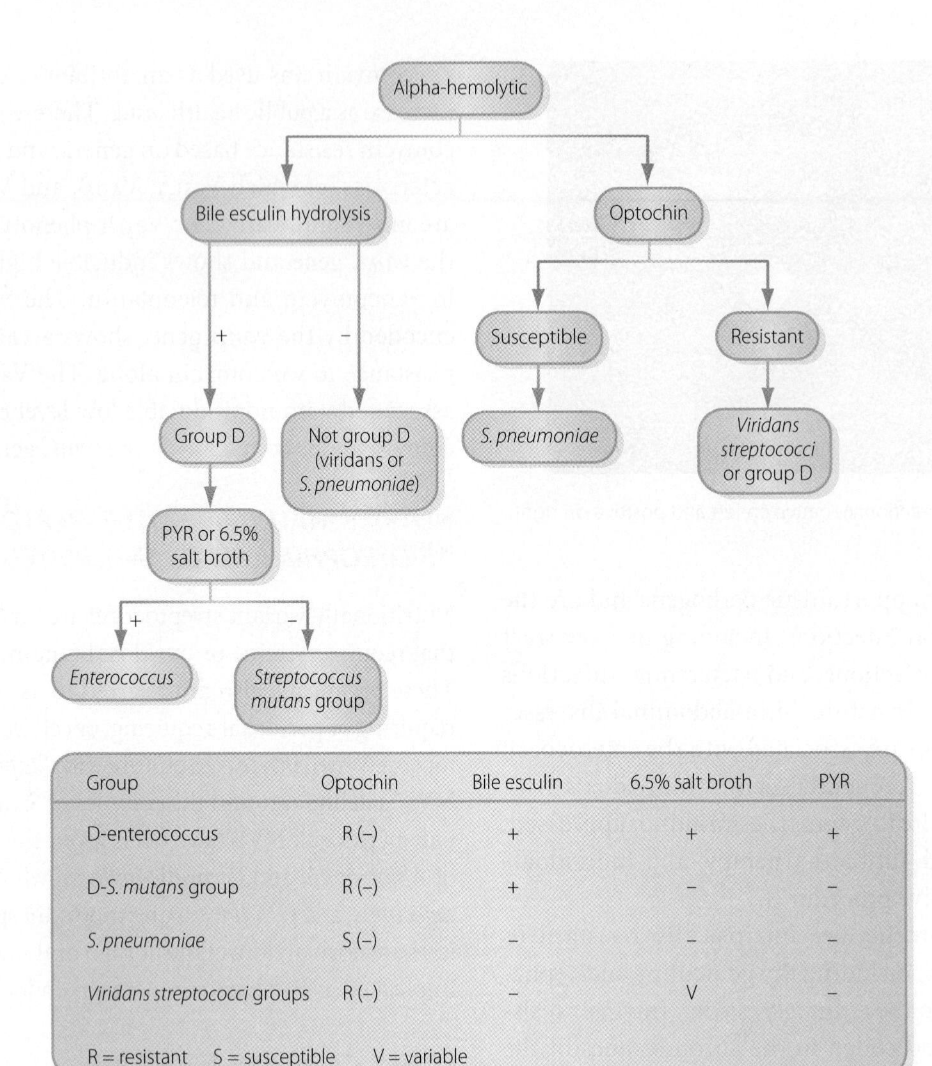

Group	Optochin	Bile esculin	6.5% salt broth	PYR
D-enterococcus	R (–)	+	+	+
D-*S. mutans* group	R (–)	+	–	–
S. pneumoniae	S (–)	–	–	–
Viridans streptococci groups	R (–)	–	V	–

R = resistant S = susceptible V = variable

FIGURE 8-14 Identification of α-hemolytic streptococci.

Laboratory Procedures

Procedure

Bacitracin and sulfamethoxazole-trimethoprim susceptibility tests

Purpose

Tests provide a mechanism to identify group A and group B β-hemolytic streptococci.

Principle

Group A β-hemolytic streptococci (*S. pyogenes*) are susceptible to 0.04 U bacitracin but resistant to 1.25 μg sulfamethoxazole-trimethoprim (SXT). Group B β-hemolytic streptococci are resistant to both bacitracin and SXT.

Reagents and Materials

Blood agar plates
0.04 U bacitracin disks
1.25 μg trimethoprim-sulfamethoxazole disks

Procedure

1. Select a few of the β-hemolytic streptococci to be tested and streak half the plate in three directions to obtain a lawn of growth.
2. Stab agar approximately halfway through its depth, two or three times.
3. Using sterile forceps, place on bacitracin disk and SXT disk in the center of the streak. The disks should be spaced evenly so that zone diameters can be accurately interpreted. Tap gently with forceps.
4. Incubate 18 to 24 hours at 35°C to 37°C.

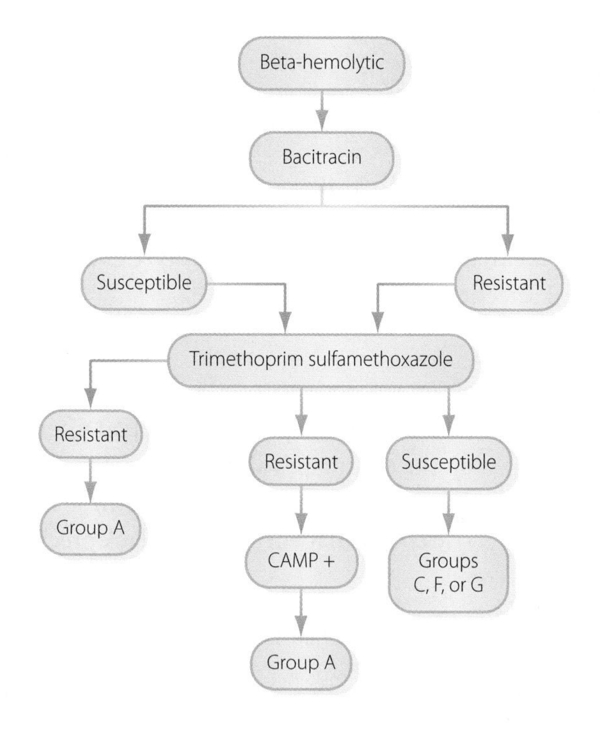

Group	Bacitracin	TS	CAMP	PYRase
A	S (+)	R(–)	–*	+
B	R (–)	R(–)	+	–
C, F, G	R (–)**	S (+)	–	–

TS = Trimethoprim sulfamethoxazole
* A small percentage of Group A give an intermediate CAMP reaction
** A small percentage of Groups C, F, and G are susceptible to bacitracin

FIGURE 8-15 Identification of β-hemolytic streptococci.

Interpretation

Any zone of inhibition around either disk indicates that the organism is susceptible. Growth up to the disk (no zone of inhibition) indicates that the organism is resistant.

Organism	Bacitracin	SXT
Group A	Susceptible	Resistant
Group B	Resistant	Resistant
Not group A or B; possibly group C, F, or G	Resistant	Susceptible

Quality Control

Group A *Streptococcus*: bacitracin susceptible and SXT resistant

Group B *Streptococcus*: bacitracin resistant and SXT resistant

Group C *Streptococcus*: bacitracin resistant and SXT susceptible

Note

A small percentage of Lancefield groups B, C, and F also give a positive bacitracin test; it is advisable also to perform a CAMP reaction and PYR test.

Procedure

CAMP reaction

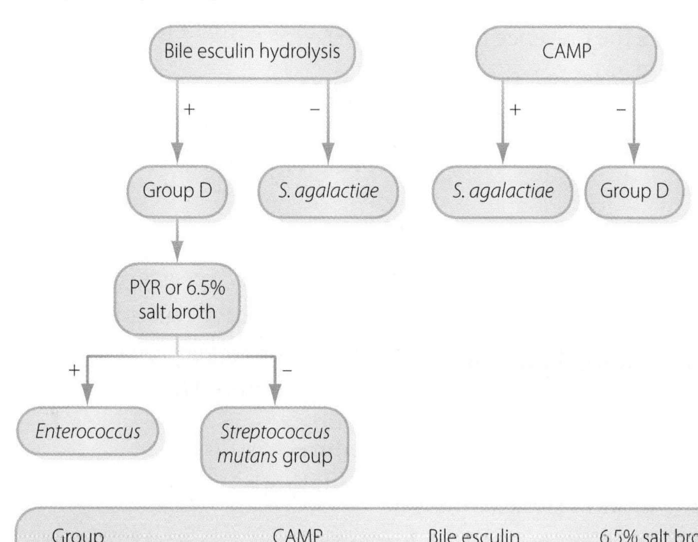

Group	CAMP	Bile esculin	6.5% salt broth	PYR
D-*enterococcus*	–	+	+	+
D-*S. mutans* group	–	+	–	–

FIGURE 8-16 Identification of nonhemolytic streptococci.

Purpose
CAMP is an acronym for those individuals who first described the phenomena of synergistic hemolysis between group B *Streptococcus* and β-hemolytic *Staphylococcus aureus.*

Principle
The CAMP factor is a diffusible, protein-like compound produced by *Streptococcus agalactiae.* A characteristic arrowhead-shaped hemolytic pattern results when the organism is streaked perpendicularly to β-hemolytic *S. aureus.*

Reagents and Materials
5% sheep blood agar
β-hemolytic *S. aureus*

Procedure

1. Streak *S. aureus* down the center of the blood agar plate.
2. At a right angle to the *S. aureus* streak, streak the 18- to 24-hour culture to be tested. The two lines must not touch, even after incubation.
3. Incubate at 35°C to 37°C for 24 hours. Do not incubate anaerobically or under increased CO_2, or false-positive results may occur.

Interpretation
Positive: A zone of enhanced hemolysis given by an arrowhead-shaped appearance at the junction of the *Staphylococcus* and *Streptococcus* indicates the presence of group B *Streptococcus.* Report: "Group B *Streptococcus,* presumptive by CAMP reaction."
Negative: No zone of enhanced hemolysis; not group B *Streptococcus*

Quality Control
Streptococcus agalactiae: Positive—displays enhanced hemolysis in arrowhead-shaped pattern
Streptococcus bovis: Negative—does not show an arrowhead-shaped pattern

Note
Some strains of group A *Streptococcus* will show an intermediate positive reaction for the CAMP test. This is especially seen when incubation is anaerobic or at increased CO_2. Incubation in ambient air is essential for accurate results.

Procedure
Bile-esculin hyrolysis

Purpose
Bile-esculin agar (BEA) is used to distinguish group D *Streptococcus* and *Enterococcus* species. The group D *Streptococcus* can grow in 40% bile and hydrolyze esculin, while other Lancefield groups cannot.

Principle
Esculin is a coumarin derivative of a glycoside that contains a glucose moiety and a glycone moiety. Differentiation is based on the organism's ability to grow in 40% bile and to hydrolyze esculin to produce esculetin. Esculetin reacts with ferric citrate to form a brown-black precipitate.

Materials
Bile-esculin plates or agar slants

Procedure

1. Inoculate the media with two to three well-isolated colonies with a sterile loop and streak BEA plate or slant.
2. Incubate at 35°C to 37°C for 24 to 48 hours.
3. Interpret plates for presence of growth and blackening.

Interpretation
Positive: Growth indicates tolerance to 40% bile (4% oxgall). Blackening indicates hydrolysis of esculin.
Negative: Lack of growth indicates inability of organism to grow in 40% bile, and lack of color change indicates inability of organism to hydrolyze esculin.

Quality Control
Enterococcus faecalis: Growth with black color
Streptococcus pyogenes: No growth and no black color

Note

1. Occasionally, species of viridans streptococci may give a weak positive reaction.
2. Strains of *Lactococcus, Leuconostoc,* and *Pediococcus* may give a positive reaction.

Procedure
6.5% Salt broth

Purpose
Salt (NaCl) broth is useful for classifying bacteria based on their ability to grow in the presence of 6.5% NaCl. The ability to grow in 6.5% NaCl is characteristic of certain

species of gram-positive cocci and gram-negative bacilli. The test is useful for differentiating the Lancefield group D enterococci, which are salt tolerant, from the *Streptococcus bovis* group of streptoccoci, which are intolerant.

Principle

Media containing 6.5% NaCl are used to determine whether bile-esculin positive, catalase negative, gram-positive cocci are salt tolerant. A medium without added salt is tested along with the 6.5% salt broth to serve as a growth control. If growth is equivalent in both media, the organism is tolerant of salt, and a positive result is noted. However, if the growth in the salt-containing medium is very weak or absent when compared to growth in the salt-free medium, a negative result is noted.

An indicator, such as bromcresol purple, can be incorporated into the medium to facilitate interpretation. A positive result is indicated by a change in the color of the indicator from purple to yellow or by the appearance of obvious growth.

Materials

Trypticase soy broth or nutrient broth (control)
6.5% NaCl broth

Procedure

1. Inoculate three to five colonies of the test organism to a tube of 6.5% NaCl and also to a tube of trypticase soy broth (or nutrient broth).
2. Incubate at 35°C to 37°C for 24 to 72 hours.
3. Observe for growth, as evidenced by turbidity.

Interpretation

Compare the degree of turbidity in the 6.5% NaCl tube to the control tube: If growth is equivalent in both media, the organism is salt tolerant, indicating a positive result. If growth is present in the control tube but scant or negative in the salt tube, the organism is salt intolerant, indicating a negative result.

Quality Control

Enterococcus faecalis: Positive—growth in both tubes
Streptococcus bovis: Negative—no growth in NaCl tube, but growth in control tube

Procedure

PYRase

Purpose

PYR tests for the ability of the organism to hydrolyze the substrate L-pyrrolidonyl-β-naphthylamide (PYR). It is a useful test to differentiate the *Enterococcus* species, which are PYR positive, from the *Streptococcus bovis* group, which are PYR negative. In addition, group A streptococci are also PYR positive, which provides a useful method to identify the β-hemolytic streptococci.

Principle

PYR-impregnated disks serve as a substrate for the detection of the enzyme pyrrolidonyl arylamidase. After inoculation of the disk with the test organism, hydrolysis of the substrate occurs, forming β-naphthylamide. This produces a red color with the addition of the color developer *p*-dimethylaminocinnamaldehyde.

Materials

PYR disks
Color developer

Procedure

1. Using sterile water, slightly moisten the PYR disk. Avoid flooding the disk.
2. Pick one or more well-isolated colonies, and rub the inoculum gently over the surface of the moistened disk.
3. Allow the inoculum to incubate with the substrate on the disk for 2 minutes at room temperature.
4. Add one drop of color developer, and observe for development of pink to cherry-red color in 1 minute in inoculated area of disk.

Interpretation

Positive: Pink to cherry-red color after addition of color developer
Negative: No color change in inoculated portion of disk after addition of color developer

Quality Control

Enterococcus: Positive control—pink to cherry-red color
Streptococcus bovis group: Negative control—no color change

Procedure

Optochin

Purpose

The optochin test is used to differentiate *Streptococcus pneumoniae* from other α-hemolytic streptococci.

Principle

In the presence of optochin (ethylhydrocupreine hydrochloride), colonies of *S. pneumoniae* are selectively lysed.

Lysis is indicated by a zone of inhibition after incubation under increased CO_2. Other α-hemolytic streptococci are resistant to optochin and give a negative test.

Materials

Blood agar plates
Optochin disks (P disks) containing ethylhydrocupreine hydrochloride
Candle jar or CO_2 incubator

Procedure

1. Select three or four colonies of the 18- to 24-hour culture to be tested, and streak in three directions to obtain a lawn of growth.
2. Place an optochin disk in the center of each streak. Gently tap with sterile forceps.
3. Incubate in a candle jar for 24 hours at 35°C to 37°C.
4. Measure diameter of the zone and interpret.

Interpretation

Positive (susceptible): Inhibition is indicated by a zone at least 14 mm in diameter when using a 10 μg P disk and at least 10 mm when using a 6 μg P disk. These results indicate the presence of *S. pneumoniae*.
Negative (resistant): Growth up to the disk or a zone of inhibition less than 14 mm with a 10 μg P disk or less than 10 mm with a 6 μg P disk. These results indicate the presence of other α-hemolytic streptococci.

Quality Control

S. pneumoniae: Positive control—zone diameters greater than 14 mm (10 μg disk) or greater than 10 mm (6 μg disk)
Viridans streptococci: Negative control—zone diameters less than 14 mm (10 μg disk) or less than 10 mm (6 μg disk)

Case Studies

1. An ambulatory patient with a temperature of 101°F and painful urination visits her physician, who orders a urine culture. A clean-catch midstream urine sample reveals numerous gram-positive cocci in chains in the Gram stain. The specimen is plated on blood agar and MacConkey. At 24 hours of incubation, flat, gray, nonhemolytic colonies are found on the blood agar. No growth is observed on MacConkey. Further testing revealed that the bile-esculin agar exhibited a black precipitate and the PYRase, a pink color.
   Identify the organism: ____________________
2. Gram-positive diplococci are observed in the Gram stain of a sputum sample of a 72-year-old male patient. Numerous neutrophils are also observed. Sparse growth on blood agar at 24 hours reveals mucoid colonies with a wide zone of α-hemolysis. An optochin test was performed using a 6 μg disk. A 20 mm zone of inhibition was noted.
   This isolate is most likely: ____________________
   ____

Laboratory Exercises

1. Streak blood agar plates for each of the following species of *Streptococcus*. Remember to cut the media. Incubate at 35°C to 37°C for 18 to 24 hours. Record your observations and interpret your results.
   Colonial morphology hemolysis ____________________
   Streptococcus pyogenes ____________________
   Streptococcus agalactiae ____________________
   Enterococcus faecalis ____________________
   Streptococcus bovis ____________________
   Streptococcus pneumoniae ____________________
   Streptococcus mutans ____________________
2. Perform a Gram stain on the following bacteria. Record your observations.
   S. pyogenes ____________________
   E. faecalis ____________________
   S. pneumoniae ____________________
3. Perform the bacitracin and sulfamethoxazole-trimethoprim (SXT) susceptibility tests on the following streptococci. Measure each zone diameter, and interpret your results as susceptible or resistant.
   Bacitracin SXT ____________________
   S. pyogenes ____________________
   S. agalactiae ____________________
   S. equi subsp. *equi* ____________________
4. Perform the bile-esculin, 6.5% salt broth, and PYRase procedures on the following bacteria. Record your observations.
   Bile-esculin 6.5% salt broth PYRase ____________________
   E. faecalis ____________________
   S. bovis ____________________
   S. mutans ____________________
   S. pyogenes ____________________

5. Perform the optochin susceptibility test on the following *Streptococcus* species. Measure the zone diameters, and interpret and record your results.
   S. pneumoniae ______
   S. mutans ______
   E. faecalis ______
6. Design a flow chart to indicate the proper identification scheme for the following:
   a. α-hemolytic streptococci
   b. β-hemolytic streptococci
   c. Nonhemolytic streptococci
   Include names of tests and results in your diagram.
7. Identify an unknown *Streptococcus*. Record all media used, procedures performed, observations, and results.

Media inoculated	Observation	Result
Procedures performed	Observation	Result
Identification and explanation		

Review Questions

Matching

Match the Lancefield group to the correct species:

1. *S. equisimilis*
2. *S. bovis* group
3. *S. agalactiae*
4. *E. faecalis*
5. *S. mutans*
6. *S. pyogenes*
7. *E. faecium*
8. *S. anginosus*
   a. A
   b. B
   c. C
   d. D, *Enterococcus*
   e. D, non-*Enterococcus*
   f. F
   g. G
   h. None of the above

Multiple Choice

9. Lancefield's classification of *Streptococcus* is based on:
   a. Type of hemolysis
   b. Cell wall polysaccharide
   c. Capsular antigens
   d. M protein serotype
10. Streptolysin O is:
   a. Oxygen stable
   b. Antigenic
   c. Observed as surface hemolysis
   d. All the above
11. Which reaction is incorrect for *Enterococcus*?
   a. Positive growth in 6.5% salt broth
   b. Positive hydrolysis of bile-esculin media
   c. Negative catalase reaction
   d. PYR negative
12. Sequelae of group ______ *Streptococcus* infection may lead to acute rheumatic fever of acute glomerulonephritis.
   a. A
   b. B
   c. C
   d. D, *Enterococcus*
13. Colonies of *Streptococcus pneumoniae* at 24 hours are typically:
   a. Mucoid and α-hemolytic
   b. Autolysed and α-hemolytic
   c. Mucoid and β-hemolytic
   d. None of the above
14. β-hemolytic streptococci were isolated from the throat culture of a 15-year-old male. Select the *best* group of tests to identify this organism.
   a. Bacitracin and PYRase
   b. Bacitracin and CAMP
   c. Bile esculin and PYRase
   d. Optochin and CAMP
15. Complete the chart for the expected reactions of the β-hemolytic streptococci. Use "S" for susceptible, indicating a positive reaction, and "R" for resistant, indicating a negative reaction.

Species	Bacitracin	SXT	CAMP
Streptococcus pyogenes			
Streptococcus agalactiae			
Groups C, F, and G			

16. Complete the chart for the expected reactions of α-hemolytic and nonhemolytic streptococci.

Species	Optochin	BEA	6.5% Salt broth	PYRase
Group D *Enterococcus*				
Group D—*S. bovis* group				
Streptococcus pneumoniae				
Viridans streptococci				

17. Identify β-hemolytic streptococci that are PYR negative, CAMP negative, and resistant to bacitracin and susceptible to sulfamethoxazole.
    a. Group A *Streptococcus*
    b. Group B *Streptococcus*
    c. Lancefield group C, F, or G
    d. *Enterococcus*
18. The nutritionally variant streptococci
    a. are classified as Lancefield Group A.
    b. require vitamin B_6 for growth.
    c. are now classified in the genus *Lactococcus.*
    d. do not need pyridoxal for growth.
19. The enterococci
    a. have intrinsic resistance to penicillin and the aminoglycosides.
    b. show acquired resistance to many antibiotics, including vancomycin.
    c. are nosocomial pathogens.
    d. All of the above are correct.

Bibliography

Centers for Disease Control and Prevention. (2010). Licensure of a 13-valent pneumococcal conjugate vaccine (PCV13) and recommendations for use among children. Available at http://www.cdc.gov/mmwr/preview/mmwrhtml/mm5909a2.htm

Centers for Disease Control and Prevention. (2010). Prevention of perinatal group B streptococcal disease. Available at http://www.cdc.gov/mmwr/preview/mmwrhtml/rr5910a1.htm?s_cid=rr5910al_w

Centers for Disease Control and Prevention. (2010). Trends in perinatal group B streptococcal disease. Available at http://www.cdc.gov/mmwr/preview/mmwrhtml/mm5805a2.htm

Cunningham, M. W. (2000). Pathogenesis of group A streptococcal infections. *Clinical Microbiology Reviews, 12,* 470–511.

Carvalho, D. G., Facklam, M. R., Jackson, D., Beall, B., & McGee, L. (2009). Evaluation of three commercial broth media for pigment detection and identification of a group B *Streptococcus* (*Streptococcus agalactiae*). *Journal of Clinical Microbiology, 47,* 4161–4163.

Facklam, R. (2002). What happened to the streptococci: Overview of taxonomic and nomenclature changes. *Clinical Microbiology Reviews, 15,* 613–630.

Gerber, M. A., & Shulman, S. T. (2004). Rapid diagnosis of pharyngitis caused by group A streptococci. *Clinical Microbiology Reviews, 17,* 571–580.

Khan, Z. Z., & Salvaggio, M. R. (2009). Streptococcus group A infections. Available at http://emedicine.medscape.com/article/228936-overview

Spellerberg, B., & Brandt, C. (2007). *Streptococcus.* In P. R. Murray, E. J. Baron, J. H. Jorgensen, M. L. Landry, & M. A. Pfaller (Eds.), *Manual of clinical microbiology,* 9th ed. (pp. 412–429). Washington, DC: American Society for Microbiology.

Rice, L. B. (2001). Emergence of vancomycin-resistant enterococci. *Emerging Infectious Diseases, 7,* 183–187.

Stevens, D. L. (1995). Streptococal toxic-shock syndrome: Spectrum of disease, pathogenesis, and new concepts in treatment. *Emerging Infectious Diseases, 1,* 69–78.

Teixeira, L. M., Siqueira Carvalho, M. D., & Facklam, R. R. (2007): *Enterococcus.* In P. R. Murray, E. J. Baron, J. H. Jorgensen, M. L. Landry, & M. A. Pfaller (Eds.), *Manual of clinical microbiology,* 9th ed. (pp. 430–442). Washington, DC: American Society for Microbiology.

Winn, W., Allen, S., Janda, W., Koneman, E., Procop, G., Schreckenberger, P., & Woods, G. (2006). Gram-positive cocci. Part II: Streptococci, enterococci, and the "Streptococcus-like" bacteria. In *Koneman's Color Atlas and Textbook of Diagnostic Microbiology,* 6th ed. (672–764). Philadelphia, PA: Lippincott Williams & Wilkins.

World Health Organization. (2005). The current evidence for the burden of group A streptococcal disease. Available at http://www.who.int/maternal_child_adolescent/documents/fch_cah_05_07/en/

Yesim, C., Falk, P., & Mayhall, C. G. (2000). Vancomycin-resistant enterococci. *Clinical Microbiology Reviews, 13,* 686–707.

NEWS: INVASIVE GROUP A STREPTOCOCCAL DISEASES

The majority of GAS diseases are self-limited cases of pharyngitis and skin infections and account for over 10 million cases annually in the United States. However, there are also approximately 10,000 cases of invasive streptococcal disease annually, according to the CDC. Worldwide rates of severe invasive disease have increased from the 1980s to the 1990s, while rates have become stable in the United States. Streptococcal toxic shock syndrome (STSS) and necrotizing fasciitis (NF) account for 6% to 7% of these invasive diseases. Invasive GAS diseases have a mortality rate of 10% to 15%, and death occurs in over 35% of those with STSS and in 25% of those with NF. Invasive GAS infections are most commonly associated with M serogroups M 1 and M3, M12, and M18, which produce pyogenic exotoxins A and B. Pyogenic exotoxins cause fever and induce shock by decreasing the threshold to exogenous endotoxin.

Streptococcal toxic shock syndrome is associated with shock and multi-organ failure. Complications include bacteremia, soft tissue infection, shock, acute respiratory distress, and acute renal and hepatic failure. The primary infection site is rarely the pharynx but instead a site of minor local, nonpenetrating skin trauma. In other instances, viral infections, including varicella and influenza, provide the site of entry. The most common clinical sign is severe and rapid onset of pain in an extremity but also may resemble peritonitis, pneumonia, or myocardial infarction. There also may be flu-like symptoms of fever, nausea, vomiting, and diarrhea. Signs of soft tissue infection, such as swelling and erythema, may be observed, which may result in myositis or necrotizing fasciitis.

In STSS, hypotension, or a drop in blood pressure, quickly develops. Laboratory parameters show hemoglobinuria, elevated serum creatinine, and decreased albumin and calcium. The serum creatine kinase is elevated, and there is a mild leukocytosis, with immature white cells seen. Shock quickly may develop, and complications include renal failure, respiratory failure, coagulopathies, and death.

NF is a soft tissue infection with severe necrosis of the fascia, which can be caused by a variety of bacteria, but most commonly GAS. NF occurs when the bacteria invade the subcutaneous tissues and then spread into the superficial and deep fascia. The infection may be polymicrobic or an infection that is associated with many species of bacteria. NF progressively destroys the fascia and fat but not always the skin and muscle. The disease was first described in 1848, was later given the name necrotizing fasciitis, and is sometimes called the "flesh-eating bacteria" because of its rapid and progressive destruction of tissue. There are different types of NF: Type I is a polymicrobic infection, type II is associated with GAS, and type III is known as saltwater NF, which is associated with *Vibrio* bacteria. NF may occur following a variety of medical or surgical procedures. Bacterial toxins and enzymes, host factors such as poor blood circulation and oxygen to the issue, and other host factors such as chronic disease, surgery, and immunosuppression can promote the spread of the disease. Other symptoms of NF include respiratory, renal, and liver failure. *Streptococcus pyogenes* is generally isolated from a normally sterile site.

GAS has been an important human pathogen for hundreds of years. Historians report that there were epidemics of scarlet fever in Europe in the 1600s as well as in the American colonies in 1736. In the 19th century, there were severe epidemics of invasive and severe GAS disease. Outbreaks of rheumatic fever occurred during World War II. In the 1880s, one-fourth of all children with scarlet fever died, yet this figure dropped dramatically to less than 2% by the turn of the century, although this cannot be explained by the use of antibiotics or improved living conditions. Perhaps, this can be attributed to a decreased expression of the virulence factors or improved host immunity within the affected communities. The severity of GAS disease declined from the 1920s until the 1980s, when severe GAS disease seemed to reemerge. The expression of different virulent factors and the lack of immunity to these factors may explain the resurgence of severe GAS infection. These extremely virulent strains (M 1, M3, M12, and M18) have spread globally in this latest occurrence of severe GAS disease.

BIBLIOGRAPHY

Aziz, R. K., & Kotb, M. (2008). Rise and persistence of global M1T1 clone of *Streptococcus pyogenes*. *Emerging Infectious Diseases, 14,* 1511–1517.

Centers for Disease Control and Prevention. (2008). Group A streptococcal (GAS) disease. Retrieved from http://www.cdc.gov/ncidod/dbmd/diseaseinfo/groupastreptococcal_t.htm

Stevens, D. L. (1995). Streptococcal toxic-shock syndrome: Spectrum of disease, pathogenesis, and new concepts in treatment. *Emerging Infectious Diseases, 1,* 69–78.

CHAPTER 9

Neisseria

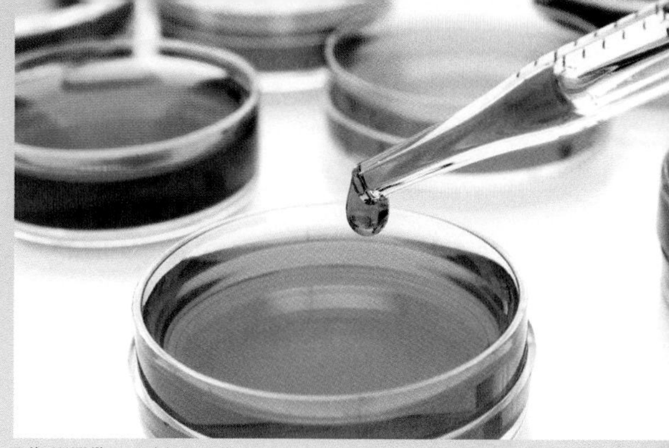

CHAPTER OUTLINE

Characteristics of *Neisseria*
Identification of *Neisseria* Species
Miscellaneous *Neisseria*

KEY TERMS

Auxotype
Capnophilic
Disseminated gonococcal infection
Endocarditis
Gonococcal arthritis
Gonorrhea
Lipooligosaccharide
Meningococcemia
Ophthalmia neonatorum
Outer membrane proteins
Penicillinase Producing *Neisseria gonorrhoeae* (PPNG)
Pili

LEARNING OBJECTIVES

1. Describe the general morphological and biochemical characteristics of *Neisseria*.
2. Explain the significance of pili.
3. List and describe the special growth requirements for the pathogenic *Neisseria*.
4. State the principle and purpose of the cytochrome oxidase reaction. Perform and interpret the reaction without error.
5. List and describe biochemical, chromogenic, and molecular assays used to identify the pathogenic *Neisseria*.
6. List and describe the infections associated with *Neisseria gonorrhoeae*.
7. Identify and explain the correct methods for specimen collection and processing for *N. gonorrhoeae*.
8. List and compare the media selective for isolation of *N. gonorrhoeae*.
9. Describe the use and relevance of the Gram stain in the workup of clinical specimens for *N. gonorrhoeae*.
10. Select, perform, and interpret the necessary media and procedures required to identify *N. gonorrhoeae*.
11. Describe how specimens for *Neisseria meningitidis* are cultured and processed.
12. Explain the infectious process of *N. meningitidis*.
13. Describe how *N. meningitidis* is isolated and identified.
14. Describe the isolation, identification, and clinical relevance of *Moraxella catarrhalis*.
15. Based on growth characteristics and biochemical reactions, differentiate among the following *Neisseria* and *Moraxella* species:
    a. *N. gonorrhoeae*
    b. *N. meningitidis*
    c. *M. catarrhalis*
    d. *N. lactamica*
    e. *N. cinerea*
    f. *N. sicca*
    g. *N. subflava*
    h. *N. flavescens*

BOX 9-1 **Human Species of *Neisseria***

N. gonorrhoeae
N. meningitidis
N. lactamica
N. sicca
N. subflava
N. mucosa
N. flavescens
N. cinerea
N. polysaccharea
N. elongata
N. kochii

The family Neisseriaceae consists of gram-negative aerobic cocci and rods. The family currently is composed of the following genera: *Neisseria, Moraxella, Acinetobacter,* and *Kingella.*

The genus *Neisseria* is composed of 11 species, including the significant human pathogens *Neisseria gonorrhoeae* and *Neisseria meningitidis. N. gonorrhoeae* is the agent of the sexually transmitted disease gonorrhea, which results from infection of the mucous membranes of urogenital sites and the pharynx. *N. meningitidis* may be carried as normal flora in the throat but is an important pathogen that causes bacterial meningitis. Many of the other species are considered to be commensal in the nasopharynx, pharynx, or other areas of the upper respiratory tract. These species are rare causes of opportunistic human infection. For example, *N. subflava* and *N. mucosa* occasionally may be associated with meningitis and endocarditis. *Neisseria* species found in humans are listed in BOX 9-1.

This chapter also discusses *Moraxella catarrhalis* (formerly *Branhamella catarrhalis*), which may be considered as normal flora in the nasopharynx but also may cause respiratory tract infections, such as sinusitis and otitis media.

Characteristics of *Neisseria*

Organisms in the genus *Neisseria* are typically gram-negative diplococci, with adjacent ends flattened, resembling tiny coffee or kidney beans in the Gram stain. Of special note is *N. elongata*, which is the only human species that is rod shaped.

Neisseria species are obligate aerobes but prefer increased carbon dioxide (CO_2) and are thus termed **capnophilic**. A capnophilic environment of 3% to 10% CO_2 can be obtained through a candle jar, the CO_2 Bio-Bag™ Type C (Becton Dickinson Microbiology Systems), the CO_2Gen Compact™ (Oxoid), or a CO_2 incubator. A candle jar is an inexpensive and effective method to obtain an atmosphere with increased CO_2. Agar plates are placed in a large glass jar, and a small wax candle is lit. The lid is secured. When the oxygen in the jar has been used, the candle expires, providing an environment with 3% to 5% CO_2. In addition, the candle jar method also provides a humid environment that prevents the bacteria from drying.

The pathogenic *Neisseria* are very fastidious; *N. gonorrhoeae* requires chocolate agar, and *N. meningitidis* and *M. catarrhalis* require blood agar as the minimal growth standard. Enriched media, such as chocolate agar, provide essential nutrients, including iron; hemin (X factor); and coenzyme I, or nicotinamide adenine dinucleotide (NAD^+, V factor). In addition, *N. gonorrhoeae* requires the amino acid cysteine for growth. Furthermore, these organisms are very sensitive to temperature changes and should be protected from the cold. The pathogenic *Neisseria* grow optimally between 35°C and 37°C. By contrast, most of the commensal *Neisseria* can grow on chocolate or blood agar at room temperature or on nutrient agar at 35°C to 37°C. Media for isolation of the pathogenic *Neisseria* are described in BOX 9-2.

Identification of *Neisseria* Species

All *Neisseria* are **cytochrome oxidase** positive. In this reaction a redox dye such as tetramethyl-*para*-phenylenediamine dihydrochloride is reacted with the organism. The dye is colorless, and if the organism possesses the oxidase enzymes, the dye is oxidized and becomes blue to purple in color (**FIGURE 9-1**). In addition, almost all members of the *Neisseria* are catalase positive, except for *N. elongata*.

Confirmatory tests rely on the ability of *Neisseria* to oxidize various carbohydrates with the production of acids. Traditionally, the cystine trypticase agar (CTA)–based sugars have been used for this purpose. This medium supports the growth of the pathogenic *Neisseria*. The various carbohydrates are added to the agar in a 1% concentration. These carbohydrates include glucose, maltose, lactose, sucrose, and fructose. The tubes are inoculated

> **BOX 9-2 Isolation Media for *Neisseria***
>
> **Modified Thayer-Martin**
>
> Medium consists of a chocolate agar base (heated, defibrinated sheep red blood cells) that contains hemin and nicotinamide adenine dinucleotide (NAD^+).
>
> Vancomycin inhibits gram-positive bacteria.
>
> Colistin inhibits gram-negative bacteria other than *N. gonorrhoeae*.
>
> Nystatin inhibits yeast and mold.
>
> Trimethoprim lactate inhibits swarming of *Proteus*.
>
> **Martin-Lewis**
>
> Medium consists of a chocolate agar base (heated, defibrinated sheep red blood cells) containing hemin and NAD^+.
>
> Vancomycin inhibits gram-positive bacteria.
>
> Colistin inhibits gram-negative bacteria other than *N. gonorrhoeae*.
>
> Anisomycin inhibits yeast and mold.
>
> Trimethoprim lactate inhibits swarming of *Proteus*.
>
> **New York City**
>
> Vancomycin inhibits gram-positive bacteria.
>
> Colistin inhibits gram-negative bacteria other than *N. gonorrhoeae*.
>
> Amphotericin B inhibits yeast and mold.
>
> Trimethoprim lactate inhibits swarming of *Proteus*.
>
> Clear peptone/cornstarch base with horse plasma, 3% hemoglobin, and yeast is added.

with a heavy suspension of the organism and incubated in a non-CO_2 incubator for 24 hours. Tubes are examined for the production of acid, as indicated by a change to yellow in the pH indicator phenol red. Negative tubes are reincubated and examined at 48 and 72 hours. All positive tubes should be Gram stained or subcultured to check for purity of growth because the CTA medium is very rich and supports the growth of many bacteria.

Because acid production by some strains of *Neisseria* is too low to be detected and because of the lengthy incubation time and contamination concerns, the CTA sugars are no longer used in most settings. Contamination may lead to false-positive reactions. However, carbohydrate utilization tests have been commercially developed to identify *Neisseria* species. Newer test systems rely on a heavy concentration of inoculum and a concentrated volume of carbohydrate. The rapid fermentation test (RFT) of Kellogg and Turner was one of the first systems designed for this purpose. Today, numerous test systems exist, including the Minitek™ (Becton Dickinson Microbiological Systems), which is a modification of the CTA medium, with an increased agar and carbohydrate content facilitating acid production and detection through a shift in the phenol red indicator when inoculated with a heavy bacterial inoculum. The CarboFerm™ I, available from Hardy Diagnostics (**FIGURE 9-2**), also provides for the rapid identification of *N. meningitidis*, *N. gonorrhoeae*, and *Moraxella catarrhalis* through acid production from carbohydrates. Results can be read in 2 to 4 hours.

Chromogenic enzyme substrate tests rely on the production of a colored end product following

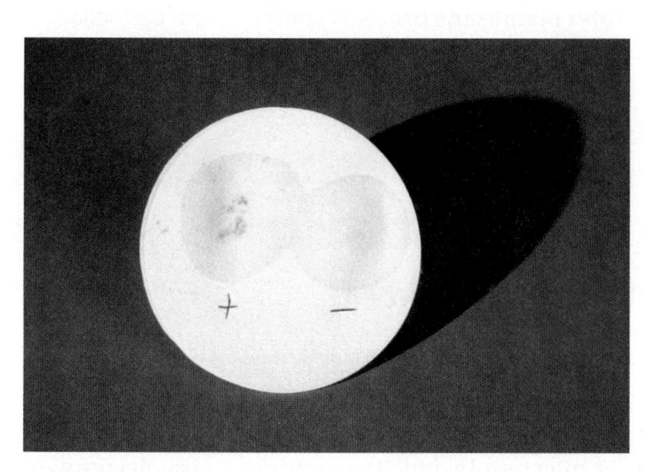

FIGURE 9-1 Oxidase reaction.

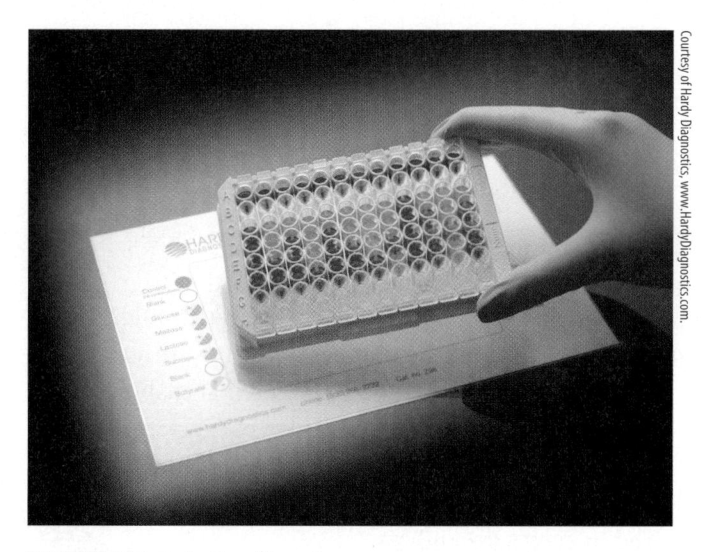

FIGURE 9-2 CarboFerm™ card.

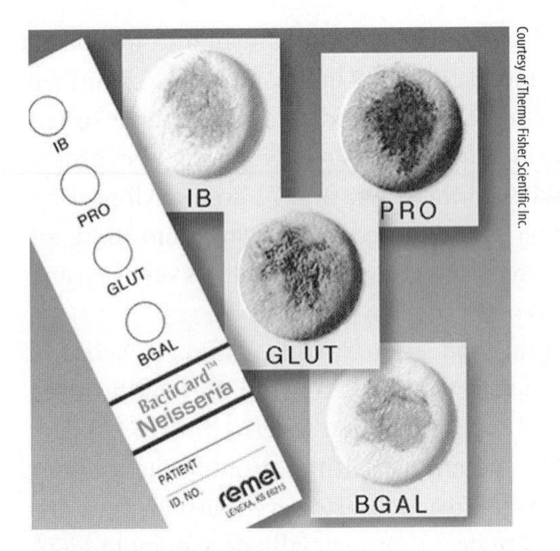

FIGURE 9-3 Bacticard™.

hydrolysis of substrates by specific bacterial enzymes. Enzymes that are detected include β-galactosidase, γ-glutamylaminopeptidase, and hydroxyprolylaminopeptidase. Commerially available products that utilize enzyme reactions include Gonochek II (EY Laboratories) and Bacticard™ Neisseria (Remel Laboratories) (**FIGURE 9-3**).

Multitest identification systems combine carbohydrate utilization with enzymatic reactions. These systems also are useful for identifying other fastidious gram-negative bacilli, such as *Haemophilus*. One example is the RapID™ system (Remel Laboratories). A 4-hour identification is achieved by detecting acid production from carbohydrate utilization, chromogenic substrates, and biochemical reactions, such as urease, indole, and ornithine decarboxylase. This system uses plastic wells impregnated with reagents. The API®-NH system (bioMérieux) is another biochemical system that combines conventional biochemical and substrate reactions.

Immunologic methods, DNA probes, and nucleic acid amplification also can be used to identify pathogenic *Neisseria* species. These are discussed specifically under *Neisseria gonorrhoeae* and *Neisseria meningitidis*.

INFECTIOUS PROCESS

The *Neisseria* organisms establish disease through attachment to the mucous membranes of the host through **pili**, hairlike structures on the bacterial cell that enable the bacteria to bind to human cells. Pili also participate in conjugation and the transfer of genetic material. Other virulence factors of *N. gonorrhoeae* and *N. meningitidis* are summarized in BOXES 9-3 and 9-4.

BOX 9-3 **Virulence Factors of *Neisseria gonorrhoeae***

Pili enable bacteria to bind to human cells.

Fimbriae are used by bacteria to adhere to host's mucosal membranes.

Lipooligosaccharides have an effect on bacterial adherence, inflammatory response, complement activation, and lysis of neutrophils and epithelial cells.

Outer membrane proteins (gonococcal OMP) have many biological effects, such as initiation of humoral and cell-mediated immunity, decreased white blood cell response, and resistance to bacteriocidal effects of serum.

Plasmids have antimicrobial resistance, which includes TEM-1 β-lactamases.

BOX 9-4 **Virulence Factors of *Neisseria meningitidis***

Thirteen types of **capsular polysaccharides** have been identified: serogroups A, B, C, D, H, I, K, L, X, Y, Z, 29E, and W135. They prevent phagocytosis of organisms by white blood cells and promote organism survival in blood and central nervous system.

Lipooligosaccharides have an effect on bacterial adherence, inflammatory response, complement activation, and lysis of neutrophils and epithelial cells.

Pili enable bacteria to bind to human cells.

Fimbriae are used by bacteria to adhere to host's mucosal membranes.

Outer membrane proteins adhere to host epithelial cells and neutrophils and invade endothelial cells.

Plasmids are not common but may be associated with tetracycline resistance.

NEISSERIA GONORRHOEAE

Neisseria gonorrhoeae is the agent of **gonorrhea**, an acute pyogenic infection mainly of the mucous membranes of the endocervix in females and the urethra in males. Other sites of infection include the rectum and oropharynx. In males the acute urethritis is associated with dysuria and a urethral discharge. While generally symptomatic, asymptomatic infections also occur. Long-term effects of gonococcal infections in females may result in scarred fallopian tubes, ectopic pregnancy, and sterility.

Extragenital infections include **ophthalmia neonatorum**, a conjunctivitis acquired by newborns from an infected mother during delivery. The condition may result in blindness if not treated. For this reason, all newborns are prophylactically treated with antibiotic drops or cream to prevent the infection from occurring. In the past, silver nitrate drops were used for this purpose.

N. gonorrhoeae infections can disseminate into the blood, causing **disseminated gonococcal infection (DGI)**, a septicemia characterized by hemorrhagic skin lesions and arthritis. Other complications of DGI include **endocarditis** and **gonococcal arthritis**, which involves the joints of the arms and legs.

Infectious Process

N. gonorrhoeae attaches by pili to susceptible cells of the mucous membranes, which initiates the infection. The pili also inhibit phagocytosis by interfering with the function of neutrophils. The gonococcus also has proteins associated with virulence, including **outer membrane proteins** that impart several biological activities, such as effects on antibody formation, leukocyte response, and cell-mediated immunity. **Lipooligosaccharide** produces endotoxic effects, whereas **protein I** allows for the organism to insert into host cells. **Protein II** is associated with virulence and allows the organism to attach to neutrophils and epithelial cells and to resist the effects of antibodies.

Specimen Collection and Processing

Proper specimen collection is vital to obtain accurate results for the isolation of *N. gonorrhoeae*. Endocervical specimens are recommended for isolation in females, and urethral specimens are recommended for males. Anorectal, oropharyngeal, and conjunctival specimens also may be warranted based on the patient's age, symptoms, and medical history. In patients with suspected DGI, blood or synovial fluid may be cultured.

The use of disinfectants on the patient before collection must be avoided because the organism may be susceptible to these agents. Dacron or Rayon swabs should be used for specimen collection. The use of cotton swabs is discouraged because some types of cotton contain fatty acids that are toxic to the bacterium. However, cotton swabs treated with charcoal to absorb the fatty acids may be used. Also, calcium alginate should be avoided for collection because of possible inhibitory effects on the gonococcus. Because the organism is susceptible to drying, it is essential either to inoculate the appropriate agar immediately or use a transport medium.

Ideally, specimens should be inoculated immediately onto an appropriate medium. The medium recommended is modified Thayer-Martin, Martin-Lewis, or New York City (NYC); all are selective for the isolation of *N. gonorrhoeae* (see descriptions of these media at the end of this chapter). In addition, some facilities prefer to inoculate a chocolate agar plate for those rare strains of *N. gonorrhoeae* that are inhibited on the selective plates.

Because many specimens are collected in physicians' offices or clinics, a transport method may be required. Culture media transport systems are preferred over swab system transport systems. Culture media systems include the **JEMBEC™** plate (an acronym for John E. Martin biological environmental chamber) and the Gono-Pak system (both from Becton Dickinson Microbiological Systems). The JEMBEC™ consists of a flat plastic dish containing a medium selective for gonococcus and a bicarbonate-citric acid pellet, which serves as a CO_2 generator. After inoculation of the agar, the tablet is placed in a well, and the entire dish is placed into a plastic bag. CO_2 is generated as the tablet is activated by moisture in the bag. After incubation for 18 to 24 hours at 35°C, the system is transported to the microbiology laboratory. The plate is observed for growth typical of *N. gonorrhoeae*. Negative plates are re-incubated in a CO_2 incubator or candle jar and examined after an additional 24 hours of incubation.

Identification

The Gram stain is essential in the workup of *N. gonorrhoeae*. By rolling the swab in one direction over the slide, the morphology of the white blood cells and bacteria is better preserved. The Gram stain serves as a presumptive identification in smears prepared from the urethral exudate in male patients and is considered to be highly specific and sensitive in symptomatic males. The sensitivity and specificity are somewhat lower in the diagnosis of gonorrhea in female patients, and thus the Gram stain is somewhat less reliable. This results from the presence of look-alike bacteria that are normally present in the female genital tract. These short gram-negative rods, or coccobacilli, including *Moraxella* and *Acinetobacter*, may be mistaken for *N. gonorrhoeae* in a Gram stained smear from a female patient. Smears are not reliable for the diagnosis of pharyngeal gonorrhea. The Gram stain is used in conjunction with other tests to identify *N. gonorrhoeae* and should not be used as the sole identification method.

On examination of the Gram stain for gonorrhea, one notes the approximate amount of polymorphonuclear neutrophils (PMNs) and the approximate amount of bacteria present. The report contains an estimate of each: "(Few, moderate, or many) gram-negative diplococci occurring (intracellularly or extracellularly) to (few, moderate, or many) PMNs." **FIGURE 9-4** illustrates gram-negative diplococci.

The specimen should be plated immediately both on a plate selective for *N. gonorrhoeae* and on chocolate agar because the vancomycin present in the selective plates may inhibit the gonococcus. Media should not be cold but at room temperature. Plates should be streaked in a Z motion by rolling the swab over the agar surface. Next, the plate is streaked with a loop for isolation. Plates are incubated at 35°C to 37°C in the candle jar CO_2 incubator, providing an atmosphere of 3% to 5% CO_2.

Plates are examined for growth at 24 hours. Plates that are negative for growth should be re-incubated and examined again at 48 hours and also at 72 hours. Colonial appearance is varied because several colonial types are possible. Colonies are typically clear gray to medium gray in color and opaque. Type 1 colonies are small, raised, and moist, whereas type 2 colonies appear small and raised but dry. In addition, both types 1 and 2 are bright and reflective and usually indicate fresher isolates. Also, types 1 and 2 are known to possess pili and are therefore virulent. Types 3, 4, and 5 lack pili and are larger, flatter, and nonreflective; these fail to cause infection in the human urethra. Types 1 and 2 can be converted to types 3, 4, and 5 through nonselective transfer. Atypical, or arginine, hypoxanthine, uracil (AHU), strains are more fastidious and typically smaller in size. AHU strains may require 72 hours for growth. **FIGURE 9-5** illustrates *N. gonorrhoeae* on Martin-Lewis medium.

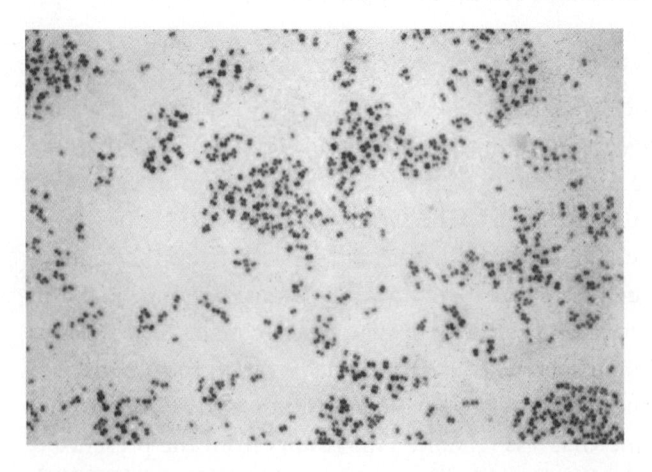

FIGURE 9-4 Gram-negative diplococci typical of *Neisseria* species.

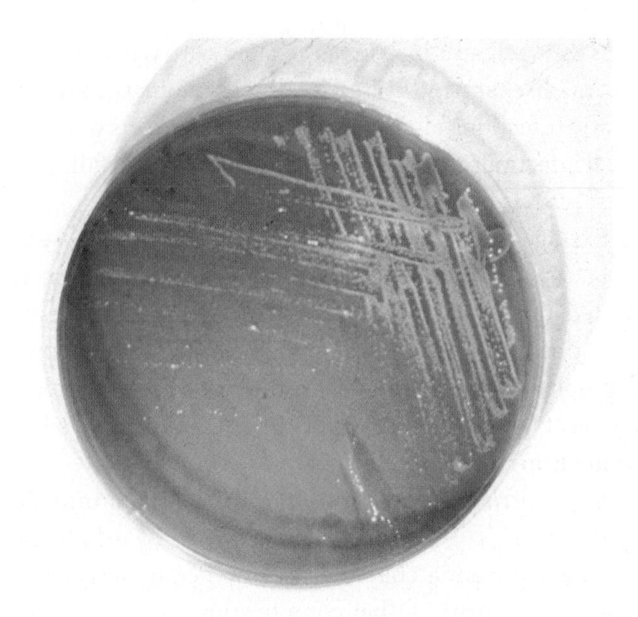

FIGURE 9-5 *N. gonorrhoeae* on Martin-Lewis medium.

The cytochrome oxidase test should be performed on any gram-negative diplococci found growing on media selective for *N. gonorrhoeae*. The previous criteria are useful for placing the organism in the genus *Neisseria* but should not be used for species identification. *N. gonorrhoeae* produces acid from glucose but not from maltose, fructose, lactose, or sucrose in carbohydrate reactions. Characteristics and reactions are summarized in Tables 9-1 and 9-2.

Immunologic methods to confirm the identification of *N. gonorrhoeae* from culture include coagglutination and the direct fluorescent antibody test. In coagglutination, protein A on *Staphylcoccus aureus* cells binds to the Fc region of IgG immunoglobulin. Antibodies to gonorrheal antigens are bound to killed *S. aureus* cells. Agglutination occurs between these antibodies and the gonococcal antigens, which can be visualized through agglutination. Examples of this technique inlude the Phadebact® Monoclonal GC test (MKL Diagnostics) and the GonoGen™ I test (New Horizons Diagnostics). In the GonoGen I test, the monoclonal antibodies are directed against the purified outer membrane proteins (Por) of several serovars of gonococcus. In the GonoGen II test, Por antibodies and monoclonal antibodies are bound to colloidal gold as the detection reagent.

Direct fluorescent antibody (DFA) culture confirmation uses monoclonal antibodies directed against outer membrane proteins. A suspension of the isolated organism is made on the DFA slide and overlaid with DFA reagent and incubated. If present, *N. gonorrhoeae* appears as fluorescent diplococci.

There also are DNA probe procedures for culture confirmation of *N. gonorrhoeae*. Advantages of these systems include increased sensitivity and more rapid turnaround time. Disadvantages include the expense of the assays and testing systems and the need for dedicated laboratory space. Culture is still needed for infections in sites other than the genital tract. The AccuProbe (Gen-Probe) detects species-specific ribosomal RNA sequences. Nucleic acid hybridization tests are based on the ability of complementary nucleic acid strands to align and form stable double-stranded complexes. The AccuProbe uses a single-stranded DNA probe with a chemiluminescent label complementary to the ribosomal RNA *N. gonorrhoeae*. Ribosomal RNA is released from the organism, and the labeled DNA probe combines with the target organism's ribosomal RNA to form a stable DNA:RNA hybrid, which is measured by chemiluminescence.

Nucleic acid hybridization and amplification may be used for the direct detection of *N. gonorrhoeae* in urogenital specimens. The PACE 2 (probe assay chemiluminescence enhanced) nucleic hybridization system from Gen-Probe may be used to identify *N. gonorrhoeae* directly from endocervical and male urethral swab specimens and also to identify the organism when isolated from culture. The ribosomal RNA is released from the gonococcus, and the chemiluminescent-labeled DNA probe hybridizes with copies of gonococcal ribosomal RNA to form DNA:RNA hybrids. The labeled hybrids are separated from the nonhybridized probe and measured in a luminometer for chemiluminescence.

There are also nucleic acid amplification–based assays for direct detection of *N. gonorrhoeae* in clinical specimens. These include the AMPLICOR *N. gonorrhoeae* PCR assay (Roche Diagnostic Systems) and the ProbeTec™ ET System (Becton Dickinson Microbiological Systems). The AMPLICOR test is a qualitative in vitro test for the detection of *C. trachomatis* and/or *N. gonorrhoeae* DNA in urine from males and females, in endocervical swab specimens, and in male urethral swab specimens. The test utilizes the polymerase chain reaction (PCR) nucleic acid amplification technique and nucleic acid hybridization for the detection of *Chlamydia trachomatis* and/or *Neisseria gonorrhoeae* in urogenital specimens. The results are quantitated using the automated COBAS® AMPLICOR analyzers. In the ProbeTec ET System, strand displacement amplification is used for amplification. BOX 9-5 provides quick facts for Neisseria gonorrhoeae.

Antibiotic Susceptibility

Penicillin has been used for over 50 years in the treatment of gonorrhea, with associated resistance. Plasmids that carry genes for β-lactamase resulted in the development of **penicillinase-producing *Neisseria gonorrhoreae***, or PPNG. β-lactamase hydrolyzes the β-lactam ring of the penicillin molecule, enabling the organism to resist the effects of penicillin. Alternative treatments for gonorrhea included spectinomycin and tetracycline, to which the organism also showed resistance. The current CDC-recommended options for treating *Neisseria gonorrhoeae* infections are from a single class of antibiotics, the cephalosporins. Current recommendations from the CDC for uncomplicated gonorrhea include one of five single-dose treatments. These are ceftriaxone, cefixime, ciprofloxacin, ofloxacin, and levofloxacin. Ongoing surveillance of resistant patterns gathered through antibiotic susceptibility testing are important to determine future treatment recommendations.

Nutritionally Variant Strains and Auxotypes

Nutritionally variant strains of *N. gonorrhoeae* exist. The **auxotype** refers to the strains that have different nutritional requirements to promote growth in artificial media. More than 30 auxotypes of the organism are currently

BOX 9-5 *Neisseria gonorrhoeae* Quick Facts

- Etiologic agent of gonorrhea
- Isolate from urethral, endocervical, oropharyngeal, and rectal specimens
- Isolate on selective media, such as modified Thayer-Martin
- Oxidase positive
- Produces acid from glucose

known, based on nutritional requirements of 15 different growth factors. Some of these growth factors include growth requirements for valine, lysine, arginine, proline, hypoxanthine, and uracil. The auxotype also can be used as an aid in determining the potential virulence, degree of invasiveness, and antibiotic resistance of the different strains of *N. gonorrhoeae*. For example, the auxotype AHU, which requires arginine, hypoxanthine, and uracil, is known to be seen frequently in patients with disseminated gonococcal infection who are susceptible to penicillin. Auxotype AHU also is associated with asymptomatic urethritis in males.

NEISSERIA MENINGITIDIS

Neisseria meningitidis is a cause of bacterial meningitis, meningococcemia, and other invasive diseases. The organism is carried by approximately 5% to 10% of the population asymptomatically as normal flora in the ororpharynx or nasopharynx. The carriage rate is higher in adolescents and young adults, especially in military recruits. Protective antibodies against the organism are developed in some carriers. Humans are the only natural host for *N. meningitidis*, and infection is spread through respiratory droplets from individuals who are carriers or who are infected with the organism. Transmission generally requires close contact with the infected salivary secretions of those who are ill with the disease or those who are carriers.

Infectious Process

The main virulence factor is the capsule, which is made of polysaccharide. The capsule protects the organism from phagocytosis and prevents bacteriolysis. There are currently 13 unique polysaccharide capsules serogrouped as A, B, C, D, H, I, K, L, X, Y, Z, 29E, and W135. The predominant serogroups in the United States are B, C, and Y, whereas worldwide, the majority of diseases are caused by serogroups A, B, C, Y, and W135.

Epidemics caused by *N. meningitidis* are less common today, especially in developing countries. The types of serogroups (A, B, C, Y, and W135) vary based on geographic location. Prior to 1996, serogroups B and C were found in most of the cases in Europe and the Americas, and serogroup Y accounted for a small percentage of the cases. However, from 1996 to 2001, the prevalence of serogroup Y has surpassed the others and accounts for 39% of the infections in the United States. The rates of serogroup B (23%) and serogroup C (31%) decreased during this period. Developing countries have increased cases of endemic and epidemic meningococcal disease, which is seen mainly in children. The annual rate is 1 to 3 cases per 100,000 people. Epidemics in Africa and meningococcal cases in Asia are most often associated with *N. meningitidis* serogroup A. In addition, large outbreaks of serogroup W135 have been noted, beginning in 2000 in Saudi Arabia.

Invasive meningococcal disease may occur as meningitis, meningococcemia, and pneumonia; meningitis is the most common type of invasive disease, comprising approximately half of all cases. Disease onset is often abrupt, with rapid progression. In fact, according to the CDC's Meningococcal Diseases and Meningococcal Vaccines Fact Sheet, the case mortality rate is approximately 10% to 14%, with 11% to 19% experiencing serious sequelae, such as loss of limb, neurological disorders, and hearing loss (http://www.cdc.gov/vaccines/hcp/vis/vis-statements/mening.html).

The organism attaches to epithelial cells by pili in the nasopharynx and, in a small number of individuals, may penetrate the mucosa, invade the blood, and cause systemic disease. In the blood, the meningococcus releases endotoxin, which stimulates cytokine production. Cytokines, such as interleukins, are released, which may contribute to increased permeability to the blood-brain barrier and invasion of the cerebrospinal fluid by the meningococcus. **Meningococcemia** refers to the presence of *N. meningitidis* in the blood and can occur as an acute form or a mild, chronic form. **Acute meningococcemia** is very serious, with a mortality rate and serious sequelae. Pili provide a mechanism for the attachment of the organism to the host cell. Eventually, the organism lyses, releasing endotoxin. The release of endotoxin is associated with the formation of a **petechial rash**, tiny hemorrhages into the skin, lower extremities, joints, and lungs. This may result in areas of tissue destruction as a result of **disseminated intravascular coagulation** (DIC), or uncontrollable clotting within the bloodstream. In fulminant meningococcemia, a hemorrhage into the adrenal glands, known as **Waterhouse-Friderichsen syndrome,** may result. The result of DIC is hemorrhage, which may lead to hypovolemic shock and death.

In **chronic meningococcemia** the patient is mildly to moderately ill. This form is characterized by recurrent episodes of meningococcemia, petechiae formation, and eventual development of arthritis.

Meningitis occurs in about half of those with bacteremia and results when the organism crosses the blood-brain barrier and enters the central nervous system. Acute meningococcal meningitis may be characterized by the classic signs of meningitis, such as severe headache, stiff neck, nausea and vomiting, delirium, and a rigid spine. These classic signs are not always exhibited, and there are wide variations in clinical symptoms. The organism is associated with both sporadic and endemic meningitis, although sporadic cases account for over 90% of those reported. Meningococcal meningitis is fatal in about 10% of the cases, yet the mortality rate is approximately 50% in those patients with meningococcemia. The effects of meningococcemia also may be seen in cases of meningitis.

Another invasive disease attributed to *N. meningitidis* is pneumonia. This is generally seen in older adults and most often seen with serogroup Y or W135 infections. Less common invasive infections include arthritis, pericarditis, and otitis media.

There are 1,000 to 2,000 cases of invasive meningococcal disease each year in the United States, with most cases classified as sporadic. In recent years, approximately 20% of all cases of bacterial meningitis in the United States were attributed to *N. meningitidis*.

Specimen Collection and Processing

The choice of specimen collection depends on the stage or type of meningococcal infection suspected. The nasopharynx is cultured to determine whether the carrier state is present. Possible sources for culture include the blood during meningococcemia, skin lesions from the petechial rash if present, cerebrospinal fluid for meningitis, and synovial fluid in cases of suspected septic arthritis.

N. meningitidis is classified as a Biosafety Level 2 organism, which necessitates a biological safety cabinet be used when processing specimens or cultures that may create aerosols by centrifuging, mixing, or other methods.

Identification

Spinal fluid is normally clear and colorless. In cases of meningitis, it may appear slightly cloudy or turbid. All spinal fluids should be cytocentrifuged to concentrate the specimen. The sediment then should be vortexed and plated on chocolate agar and thioglycollate and Gram stained. The appearance of gram-negative diplococci with adjacent ends flattened indicates the presence of *Neisseria*. The presence and number of PMNs and the location of the organisms as intracellular or extracellular to the PMNs should be reported. Because the organism is adversely affected by changes in temperature, spinal fluids should not be refrigerated until the workup is complete.

When culturing a specimen that may be contaminated or contain normal flora, such as a nasopharyngeal specimen, a selective plate also should be inoculated. Modified Thayer-Martin or Martin-Lewis can be used. All plates are incubated at 35°C to 37°C under increased (5% to 10%) CO_2. Unlike *N. gonorrhoeae*, *N. meningitidis* is able to grow on blood agar.

At 24 hours the colonies of *N. meningitidis* are characteristically round, smooth, glistening, and gray in color on chocolate agar. Encapsulated strains may be mucoid. The oxidase test is performed on any growth resembling the organism, and a confirmatory test for carbohydrate utilization is performed. *N. meningitidis* will utilize glucose and maltose in the carbohydrate utilization reactions.

Slide agglutination may be used to presumptively serogroup *N. meningitidis* either directly from cerebrospinal fluid or urine or from culture. The Directogen™ Meningitis Test (Becton Dickinson Microbiological Systems) permits qualitative detection of *N. meningitidis* subgroups A, C, Y, and W135 through reaction with antibody-coated latex beads for these serogroups.

In coagglutination, latex beads or *Staphylococcus aureus* colonies are coated with meningococcal antibodies. In the presence of the organism, binding occurs, as visualized by agglutination. BOX 9-6 provides quick facts for *Neisseria meningitidis*.

Treatment and Prevention

Univalent vaccines are licensed for both groups A and C *N. meningitidis*. A quadrivalent vaccine for groups A, C, Y, and W135, the meningococcal conjugate vaccine (MCV4), was licensed in the United States in 2005 for individuals age 2 to 55 years. Groups at risk for meningococcal disease include college freshmen living in dormitories, military

BOX 9-6 *Neisseria meningitidis* Quick Facts

- Etiologic agent of meningitis and meningococcemia
- May be carried asymptomatically in nasopharynx
- Isolate on sheep blood or chocolate agar
- Oxidase positive
- Produces acid from glucose and maltose

recruits, individuals who travel to or who live in countries where the organism is endemic, those with immune system disorders, and microbiologists who are exposed to isolates of *N. meningitidis*. There currently is no vaccination to protect against serogroup B in the United States.

Antibiotic prophylaxis is provided for close contacts of those with primary meningococcal disease to prevent secondary meningococcemia. Close contacts include household members, day care center contacts, and others who were directly exposed to the oral secretions of the infected individual. Oral rifampin and ciprofloxacin and parenteral ceftriaxone are currently recommended for prophylaxis of meningococcal disease.

Most strains of *N. meningitidis* remain susceptible to penicillin, so penicillin G remains the antibiotic of choice. However, there is concern that some strains are less susceptible to penicillin. Chloroamphenicol may be used in those who are sensitive to penicillin. Also, third-generation cephalosporins, ceftriaxone and cefotaxime, may be administered.

MORAXELLA CATARRHALIS

Although *Moraxella catarrhalis* is similar to other members of the genus *Moraxella* in deoxyribonucleic acid (DNA) composition, it morphologically and biochemically resembles *Neisseria* and is therefore discussed in this chapter.

The organism formerly was considered to be a nonpathogenic member of the normal flora of the upper respiratory tract. It recently has been found to be an increasing cause in infections of the respiratory tract, including otitis media, sinusitis, and pneumonia. In addition, *M. catarrhalis* also has been associated with endocarditis, conjunctivitis, bacteremia, wound infections, and meningitis. Infections are found more frequently in the immunocompromised host, pediatric patients, and others with an underlying medical problem, such as diabetes mellitus or pulmonary problems.

M. catarrhalis will grow on nutrient agar at 35°C to 37°C, unlike *N. meningitidis* and *N. gonorrhoeae*. Some strains will grow on selective media, such as Thayer-Martin, while others may not. The colonies are nonpigmented, opaque, gray, and smooth. When grown on blood agar, the colonies are nonhemolytic. The organism is oxidase positive and fails to produce acid from any carbohydrates in the CTA reactions or using a similar test system. It is DNase positive and often produces β-lactamase. Of note is its positive hydrolysis of tributyrin with the enzyme butyrate esterase.

MISCELLANEOUS *Neisseria*

The following *Neisseria* are considered to be commensals and are rarely associated with human infection. As a general rule, these *Neisseria* are able to grow on trypticase agar at 35°C to 37°C. *N. cinerea* is considered to be saprophytic in the oropharynx and genital tract. It is an occasional cause of bacteremia, conjunctivitis, and nosocomial pneumonia. Because some strains utilize glucose, *N. cinerea* may be confused with *N. gonorrhoeae*. To differentiate the two organisms, *N. cinerea* is able to grow on Mueller-Hinton medium but not on modified Thayer-Martin medium and is susceptible to colistin. *N. gonorrhoeae* is able to grow on modified Thayer-Martin but not on Mueller-Hinton and is resistant to colistin.

N. mucosa is a member of the normal flora of the respiratory tract. It is a rare cause of meningitis, endocarditis, and cellulitis.

N. polysaccharea, another commensal *Neisseria*, utilizes glucose and maltose in carbohydrate testing. A unique property of this species is its ability to produce large amounts of polysaccharide when grown on 1% to 5% sucrose agar.

Other members of *Neisseria* considered to be predominantly normal flora include *N. flavescens*; *N. sicca*; *N. lactamica*; *N. subflava* biovars *subflava*, *flavis*, and *perflava*; *N. lactamica*, a rare cause of bacteremia and meningitis, may grow on selective media for *Neisseria*. Thus, it must be differentiated from *N. gonorrhoeae* and *N. meningitidis*. *N. lactamica* produces the enzyme β-galactosidase and can produce acid from glucose, maltose, and lactose.

TABLES 9-1 and **9-2** summarize the growth and biochemical characteristics of the *Neisseria*. Generally, the saprophytic *Neisseria* are not identified unless their identification is determined to be clinically significant.

Laboratory Procedures

Procedure

Cytochrome oxidase

Purpose

Cytochromes are iron-containing heme proteins that transfer electrons to oxygen in the last reaction of aerobic respiration. The cytochrome system is found in the following genera: *Neisseria, Aeromonas, Pseudomonas, Campylobacter,* and *Pasteurella*, but not in any of the Enterobacteriaceae.

TABLE 9-1 Growth Characteristics of *Neisseria* Species and *Moraxella catarrhalis*

Species	Colonial morphology	MTM, ML, or NYC*	Chocolate or blood agar at 22°C	Nutrient at 35°C
N. gonorrhoeae	Gray to white, smooth, five colony types on subculture	Growth	NG	NG
N. meningitidis	Nonpigmented or gray to white, some yellowish. Smooth, transparent encapsulated strains are mucoid.	Growth	NG	NG
N. lactamica	Nonpigmented or yellowish, smooth, transparent	Growth	V	Growth
N. cinerea	Grayish white, slightly granular	V	V	Negative
N. sicca	Nonpigmented, wrinkled, coarse dry, adherent	NG	V	Growth
N. subflava	Greenish yellow, smooth, adherent	NG	Growth	Growth
N. mucosa	Sometimes yellowish, mucoid appearance from capsule production	NG	Growth	Growth
N. flavescens	Yellow, opaque, smooth	NG	Growth	Growth
N. elongata	Gray-white, slight yellow tinge, flat, glistening, dry claylike consistency	NG	Growth	Growth
M. catarrhalis	Nonpigmented or gray, opaque, smooth	V	Growth	Growth

Growth, most strains will grow; NG, most strains will not grow; V, variable growth is positive
*MTM, modified Thayer-Martin agar; ML, Martin-Lewis agar; NYC, New York City medium

TABLE 9-2 Biochemical Reactions of *Neisseria* Species and *Moraxella catarrhalis*

	Acid produced from						Reduction of		Polysaccharide from sucrose
Species	Glucose	Maltose	Lactose	Sucrose	Fructose	DNase	NO_3	NO_2	
N. gonorrhoeae	+	–	–	–	–	–	–	–	–
N. meningitidis	+	+	–	–	–	–	–	V	–
N. lactamica	+	+	+	–	–	–	–	V	–
N. cinerea	–	–	–	–	–	–	–	+	+
N. flavescens	–	–	–	–	–	–	–	+	+
N. sicca	+	+	–	+	+	–	–	+	+
N. subflava	+	+	–	V	V	–	–	+	–
M. mucosa	+	+	–	+	+	–	+	+	+
N. elongata	–	–	–	–	–	–	–	+	–
N. polysaccharea	V	+	+	–	–	–	–	V	+
M. catarrhalis	–	–	–	–	–	+	+	+	–

+, most strains are positive; –, most strains are negative; V, variable reactivity

Principle

Cytochrome oxidase in the presence of atmospheric oxygen oxidizes tetramethyl-*para*-phenylenediamine dihydrochloride (oxidase reagent) to form a colored compound, indophenol.

Reagents and Media

Oxidase reagent: 1% N,N,N9,N9-tetramethyl-*para*-phenylenediamine dihydrochloride (freshly prepared)

Whatman no. 1 filter paper

Sterile petri plate

Procedure

1. Place a piece of filter paper into a sterile petri plate.
2. Invert and add one drop of oxidase reagent to the filter paper.
3. With a sterile disposable needle or loop, pick one 18- to 24-hour-old colony and streak to saturated filter paper.

Interpretation

Positive reaction is indicated by the formation of a maroon-violet color immediately or within 10 to 30 seconds. Negative results remain colorless.

Quality Control

Positive control: *Neisseria gonorrhoeae* or *Moraxella catarrhalis*

Negative control: *Escherichia coli*

Notes

1. Alternatively, the test can be performed by touching the top of a well-isolated colony with a sterile swab that has been saturated with reagent.
2. Iron-containing wire can cause false-positive reactions.
3. Excess reagent may cause a fading of oxidase-positive organisms.
4. Colorless colonies growing on selective media or media containing glucose may result in false-positive reactions because fermentation may inhibit the oxidase activity.
5. Reactions from weakly oxidase-positive organisms, such as *Pasteurella*, may not be accurate.
6. Do not use nutrient or Mueller-Hinton medium because it may lead to inconsistent results.

Procedure

Cystine trypticase agar (CTA) sugars

Purpose

Differentiation of *Neisseria* species can be accomplished through observing acid production from carbohydrates in cystine trypticase agar.

Principle

CTA is an excellent all-purpose medium because it supports the growth of many organisms, including the fastidious *Neisseria*. Various carbohydrates, such as glucose, maltose, sucrose, fructose, and lactose, are added to give a final concentration of 1% in the CTA medium. The test for breakdown of o-nitrophenyl-β-D-galactopyranoside (ONPG) can be replaced for lactose. In a positive reaction the carbohydrate is oxidized to an organic acid that produces a yellow color in the upper layer of the medium as the result of a shift in the phenol red indicator to its acidic color at pH less than 6.8.

To ensure correct results, it is essential to use a heavy inoculum and to test only pure cultures. Both can be obtained by not inoculating the carbohydrates directly from a selective plate; instead, first subculture pure colonies of the isolate to two plates of chocolate agar. Incubate the chocolate plates for 18 hours in increased CO_2, and examine for pure colonies. Perform the oxidase test and Gram stain on the growth to ensure the presence of pure gram-negative diplococci. The CTA medium can then be inoculated as described next. Reagent-grade carbohydrates must be used to provide accurate results.

Reagents and Media

CTA agar deeps or agar slants containing reagent-grade glucose, maltose, sucrose, fructose, and lactose (or ONPG) to a final concentration of 1%

Procedure

1. Subculture suspected *Neisseria* colonies to two plates of chocolate agar. Incubate for 18 hours under increased CO_2.
2. Examine chocolate agar plates for purity by using a hand lens. Perform oxidase test on colonies, and perform a Gram stain to confirm the presence of gram-negative diplococci.
3. CTA medium may be inoculated by either of the following methods:
   a. Prepare a heavy bacterial suspension from the subcultured chocolate agar plate. This is prepared by harvesting the entire growth in 0.5 ml of sterile saline or trypticase soy broth. With a sterile pipette, deposit a few drops of the suspension on the agar surface. Next, stab the inoculum into the upper third of the agar surface.
   b. For each tube, scrape a full 3 mm of growth from the subcultured chocolate agar, and deposit a few millimeters below the surface of the medium.
4. Tighten the caps (or parafilm) and incubate at 35°C to 37°C in a non-CO_2 incubator for 24 hours. If CO_2 enters the tubes, carbonic acid forms, which may be sufficient to drop the pH below 6.8, causing false-positive results.

Interpretation

1. Examine tubes for production of acid (yellow) in the upper portion of the medium periodically for 24 hours. Positive results are indicated by a yellow color caused by a change in the color of the phenol red indicator. Positive reactions should occur within this period.
2. Perform a Gram stain for all positive tubes to check for purity. A bright-yellow color in any tube may signify contamination and should be stained for purity.

Quality Control
Neisseria gonorrhoeae: Glucose positive (yellow)
All others: Negative (red)
Moraxella catarrhalis: All tubes negative (red)

Note
CTA agar slants prepared with CTA (1.5%) and 2% carbohydrates, which are inoculated with a full loopful of growth deposited on the surface of the agar slant, will provide a larger aerobic surface for *Neisseria*. A positive reaction is first detected in the area of the slant under the inoculum within 1 to 4 hours.

There are several commercially available methods that utilize the detection of acid from carbohydrate utilization. These methods are less likely to be contaminated and can be read in 2 to 4 hours.

Laboratory Exercises

1. Compare the growth of the following *Neisseria* species on the media (MTM, modified Thayer-Martin; ML, Martin-Lewis) and at the temperature listed.

Colonial Morphology	MTM (ML)	Chocolate	Nutrient
	35°C	22°C	35°C
Neisseria gonorrhoeae			
Neisseria lactamica			
Neisseria sicca			
Moraxella catarrhalis			
Neisseria flavescens			

2. Perform the cytochrome oxidase test on the following bacteria and record your results. Explain why the oxidase test is useful in preliminary identification of bacteria.
   N. gonorrhoeae
   Proteus vulgaris
   N. lactamica
   M. catarrhalis
3. Perform the cystine trypticase agar (CTA) reactions on the bacteria listed and record your results. Why is it important to ensure a CO_2-free incubation environment?

	Glucose	Maltose	Lactose	Sucrose	Fructose
N. gonorrhoeae					
N. lactamica					
M. catarrhalis					
N. sicca					
N. flavescens					

4. Which species of *Neisseria* is typically DNase positive? What specie(s) (one or more) should be tested for β-lactamase activity?

____

____

Review Questions

Multiple Choice

1. Pili antigens are associated with:
   a. *Staphylococcus aureus*
   b. *Streptococcus pyogenes*
   c. *Streptococcus pneumoniae*
   d. *Neisseria gonorrhoeae*
2. A gram-negative diplococcus isolated from a middle ear aspirate grew on chocolate agar but was inhibited on Martin-Lewis agar. The organism failed to produce acid from glucose, maltose, lactose, and sucrose. It was DNase positive and is most likely:
   a. *Neisseria gonorrhoeae*
   b. *Neisseria meningitidis*
   c. *Neisseria lactamica*
   d. *Moraxella catarrhalis*
3. All *Neisseria* species are positive for the enzyme:
   a. Coagulase
   b. DNase
   c. Oxidase
   d. Penicillinase
4. Cotton swabs are preferred for the culture and transport of specimens to be cultured for *Neisseria gonorrhoeae*.
   a. True
   b. False

5. An isolate recovered from a blood culture specimen was subcultured onto chocolate agar and produced gram-negative diplococci that were oxidase positive and produced acid from glucose and maltose but not from lactose or sucrose. The isolate is most likely:
   a. *Neisseria meningitidis*
   b. *Neisseria gonorrhoeae*
   c. *Moraxella catarrhalis*
   d. *Neisseria lactamica*
   e. *Neisseria sicca*
6. An infant has been diagnosed with bacterial meningitis. Further testing of the spinal fluid would likely indicate:
   a. Increased white blood cells with a predominance of lymphocytes, decreased glucose, and increased protein
   b. Increased white blood cells with a predominance of neutrophils, increased glucose, and decreased protein
   c. Decreased white blood cells, increased protein, and decreased glucose
   d. Increased white blood cells with a predominance of neutrophils, increased protein, and decreased glucose
7. Gram-negative diplococci are observed on a Gram stained smear prepared from a female endocervical genital tract specimen. Which of the following is the *most* appropriate action?
   a. Report "*Neisseria gonorrhoeae* isolated" and perform susceptibility testing.
   b. Report amount of gram-negative diplococci (few, moderate, many) and estimate number of neutrophils present.
   c. Report "normal flora isolated" and discard specimen.
   d. Plate specimen on blood agar.
8. Waterhouse-Friderichsen syndrome is associated with:
   a. Autoimmune response to group A streptococcal infection
   b. Adrenal hemorrhage from *Neisseria meningitidis*
   c. Septicemia from *Neisseria gonorrhoeae*
   d. Hemolytic reaction from *Staphylococcus aureus*
9. Which statement correctly describes the toxins associated with *Neisseria*?
   a. The toxins are released by the living bacterial cell.
   b. The toxins are composed of lipopolysaccharide—components of the cell wall.
   c. The toxins are categorized as exotoxins.
   d. The toxins are similar to the enzymes of *Staphylococcus aureus.*
10. *Neisseria meningitidis* can be carried ______, which serves as a reservoir for infection.
    a. in the nasopharynx
    b. in the blood
    c. in the oral cavity
    d. on the skin
11. There is only one type of capsular antigen for *Neisseria meningitidis*.
    a. True
    b. False
12. Which statement correctly describes the mode of action of the antibiotic listed for modified Thayer-Martin medium?
    a. Vancomycin inhibits gram-negative bacteria.
    b. Colistin inhibits gram-positive bacteria.
    c. Nystatin inhibits fungi and molds.
    d. Trimethoprim lactate inhibits gram-positive bacteria.
13. *Neisseria meningitidis* may be isolated on:
    a. Chocolate agar or sheep blood agar
    b. Colistin-nalidixic acid agar or sheep blood agar
    c. MacConkey or sheep blood agar
    d. Modified Thayer-Martin agar
14. Which of the following organisms is DNase positive?
    a. *Neisseria gonorrhoeae*
    b. *Neisseria meningitidis*
    c. *Moraxella catarrhalis*
    d. *Neisseria lactamica*
    e. *Neisseria sicca*
15. Which of the following *Neisseria* fails to produce acid from glucose, maltose, lactose, and sucrose; produces yellow-pigmented colonies on blood and nutrient agar; and fails to produce DNase?
    a. *Moraxella catarrhalis*
    b. *Neisseria gonorrhoeae*
    c. *Neisseria subflava*
    d. *Neisseria flavescens*
    e. *Neisseria sicca*
16. The Gram stain serves as the definite identification in cases of suspected gonorrhea in female patients.
    a. True
    b. False

Case Studies

I. A Gram stain from the purulent drainage of a synovial fluid reveals numerous gram-negative diplococci. The organism grew on chocolate agar and Martin-Lewis but failed to grow on blood agar, colistin-nalidixic acid, or MacConkey. Further testing revealed the organism to be oxidase positive with positive carbohydrate utilization of glucose. All other carbohydrates were negative. The β-lactamase result was positive.

1. The organism is most likely:
   a. *Streptococcus pneumoniae*
   b. *Neisseria gonorrhoeae*
   c. *Neisseria meningitidis*
   d. *Staphylococcus aureus*
   e. *Moraxella catarrhalis*

2. Based on the information provided, which antibiotic should definitely *not* be used to treat this infection?
   a. Ceftriaxone
   b. Spectinomycin
   c. Penicillin
   d. Tetracycline

II. A gram-negative diplococcus isolated from a nasopharyngeal culture yielded the following results: blood agar—few small, nonhemolytic colonies; chocolate agar—many small, grayish colonies; and oxidase—positive. The organism utilized glucose and maltose in the CTA reactions.

1. Based on the information given, the organism is most likely:
   a. *Streptococcus pneumoniae*
   b. *Neisseria lactamica*
   c. *Neisseria meningitidis*
   d. *Moraxella catarrhalis*
2. Types of infection associated with this organism include:
   a. None; it is generally considered to be nonpathogenic.
   b. Sexually transmitted diseases, such as gonorrhea
   c. Pneumonia and septicemia
   d. Bacteremia and meningitis

Bibliography

Becton, Dickinson and Company. (2003). Environmental Chamber BD Bio-Bag Type C package insert.

Bonin, P., Tanino, T. T., & Handsfield, H. H. (1984). Isolation of *Neisseria gonorrhoeae* on selective and nonselective media in a sexually transmitted disease clinic. *Journal of Clinical Microbiology, 19,* 218.

Boyce, J. M., & Mitchell, E. B., Jr. (1985). Difficulties in differentiating *Neisseria cinerea* from *Neisseria gonorrhoeae* in rapid systems used for identifying pathogenic *Neisseria* species. *Journal of Clinical Microbiology, 22,* 731.

Catlin, B. W. (1990). *Branhamella catarrhalis*: An organism gaining respect as a pathogen. *Clinical Microbiology Reviews, 3,* 293.

Centers for Disease Control and Prevention. (2008, October). Characteristics of *N. gonorrhoeae* and related species of human origin. Retrieved from http://www.cdc.gov/std/Gonorrhea/lab/Ngon.htm

Centers for Disease Control and Prevention. (2008, October). Identification of *N. gonorrhoeae* and related species. Retrieved from http://www.cdc.gov/std/Gonorrhea/lab/ident.htm

Centers for Disease Control and Prevention. (2009, June). Disease information: Causes of bacterial meningitis. Retrieved from http://www.cdc.gov/meningitis/clinical-resources.html

Centers for Disease Control and Prevention. (2009, August). Factsheet: Meningococcal diseases and meningococcal vaccines. Retrieved from http://www.cdc.gov/vaccines/hcp/vis/vis-statements/mening.html#vaccine

Evans, K. D., Peterson, E. M., Curry, J. I., Greenwood, J. R., & de la Maza, L. M. (1986). Effect on holding temperature on isolation of *Neisseria gonorrhoeae. Journal of Clinical Microbiology, 24,* 1109.

Feldman, H. A. (1986). The meningococcus: A twenty-year perspective. *Reviews of Infectious Diseases, 8,* 288.

Forbes, B. A., Sahm, D. F., & Weissfeld, A. S. (2007). *Neisseria* and *Moraxella catarrhalis*. In *Bailey and Scott's diagnostic microbiology* (12th ed.). St. Louis, MO: Mosby Elsevier.

Gen-Probe Incorporated. (2001). AccuProbe packet insert.

Greenwood, J. R., Voss, J., & Smith, R. F. (1986). Comparative evaluation of New York City and modified Thayer Martin media for isolation of *Neisseria gonorrhoeae. Journal of Clinical Microbiology, 24,* 1111.

Hager, H.,Verghese, A., Alvarez, S., & Berk, S. L. (1987). *Branhamella catarrhalis* respiratory infections. *Reviews of Infectious Diseases, 9,* 1140.

Heckels, J. E. (1989). Structure and function of pili of pathogenic *Neisseria* species. *Clinical Microbiology Reviews, 2* (Suppl), S66–S73.

Holt, J. G., King, N. R., & Sneath, P. H. A. (1993). *Bergey's manual of determinative bacteriology* (9th ed.). Baltimore, MD: Lippincott Williams & Wilkins.

Hook, E. W., III, Brady, W. E., Reichart, C. A., Upchurch, D. M., Sherman, L. A., & Wasserheit, J. N. (1989). Determinants of emergence of antibiotic-resistant *Neisseria gonorrhoeae. Journal of Infectious Diseases, 159,* 900.

Janda, W. M., & Gaydos, C. A. (2007). *Neisseria.* In P. R. Murray, E. J. Baron, J. H. Jorgensen, M. L. Landry, & M. A. Pfaller (Eds.), *Manual of clinical microbiology* (9th ed.). Washington, DC: American Society for Microbiology.

Knapp, J. S. (1988). Historical perspectives and identification of *Neisseria* and related species. *Clinical Microbiology Reviews, 1,* 415.

Lossick, J. G., Smeltzer, M. P., & Curan, J. W. (1982). The value of the cervical gram stain in the diagnosis of gonorrhea in women in a sexually transmitted diseases clinic. *Sexually Transmitted Diseases, 9,* 124.

Nassif, X., & So, M. (1995). Interaction of pathogenic *Neisseria* with nonphagocytic cells. *Clinical Microbiology Reviews, 8,* 376–388.

National Foundation for Infectious Diseases. (2012). Facts about meningococcal disease in adults. Bethesda, MD. Retrieved from http://www.adultvaccination.com/vpd/meningitis/facts.html

Oxoid Limited. (2001). CO_2 GenCompact package insert.

Stephens, D. S., Spellman, P. A., & Swartley, J. S. (1993). Effect of the (alpha 2→8)-linked polysialic acid capsule on adherence of *Neisseria meningitidis* to human mucosal cells. *Journal of Infectious Diseases, 167,* 475–479.

NEWS: MENINGOCOCCAL DISEASE AND EPIDEMIOLOGY

Each year, there are 1,000 to 2,000 cases of **invasive** meningococcal disease in the United States. Invasive diseases are those that infiltrate or spread to healthy parts of the body. These may occur as meningitis, meningococcemia, and pneumonia as well as other types of disease. Only a small percentage of these cases (less than 5%) are associated with **outbreaks**, which means that most cases are **sporadic**. Sporadic cases occur singly or occasionally, whereas outbreaks occur in greater numbers within a particular region or area. Worldwide, there is an incidence of 0.5 to 5 cases per 100,000 for **endemic** disease. Endemic indicates that an organism is native to a particular area or population. There are severe **epidemics** throughout parts of Africa, especially in the meningitis belt in sub-Saharan Africa. An epidemic is defined as a disease that affects a large number of people at one time, or a disease that rapidly spreads through a specific demographic part of a population. These epidemics most often are a result of serogroups A and C. Yet serogroup W135 was identified as the cause of a large outbreak in Burkina in West Africa in 2002. Hyperendemics, which are defined as high and sustained amounts of disease in a particular area, have also been associated with meningococcal disease.

Neisseria meningitidis is a leading cause of bacterial meningitis and bacteremia in the United States, with approximately 1,000 cases occurring each year. This is, in part, a result of the successful vaccination of infants against other types of meningitis, such as *Haemophilus influenzae*. Invasive meningococcal disease has a mortality rate of 10% to 14%, and approximately 10% to 20% of survivors have serious health **sequelae**. Sequelae are defined as pathological conditions that result from a disease or injury. Sequelae associated with invasive meningococcal disease include hearing loss, amputations, cognitive impairment, and other neurological disorders.

Risk groups are infants and young children, household contacts of those diagnosed with the disease, college freshmen living in dormitories, and microbiologists who are working with isolates of the organism. Also at risk are military recruits and those who travel to or live in countries where *N. meningitidis* is **epidemic** or **hyperendemic**. Others at risk are those with complement component deficiencies and those who are asplenic.

Infants have the highest rates of meningococcal disease, followed by adolescents who are 18 years of age. College freshmen living in dormitories are at high risk. Approximately 20% of cases occur in young adults aged 14 to 24, while approximately 16% of cases involve infants younger than one year of age. Most cases in infants are a result of serogroup B, and there is currently no vaccine licensed in the United States for serogroup B. The disease is seasonal, with cases peaking in December and January.

The tetravalent meningococcal conjugate vaccination (MCV4) offers protection against serogroups A, C, Y, and W135. The vaccine has been licensed in the United States since 2005 for individuals aged 2 to 55 years. Meningococcal vaccine should be administered to persons in those groups defined as high risk. Use of the vaccine is routine in U.S. vaccination programs and provides an opportunity to control the number of invasive meningococcal disease cases. Currently two doses of the vaccine are recommended for those aged 11 to 18 years of age, with the first dose given at 11 to 12 years of age and the booster given at age 16. A booster is not needed if the first dose is given after the 16th birthday. Vaccination in selected African countries of children and adults may help to control the frequency of outbreaks in endemic areas.

BIBLIOGRAPHY

Centers for Disease Control and Prevention. (2005). Prevention and control of meningococcal disease: Recommendations of the Advisory Committee on Immunization Practice (ACIP). *Morbidity and Mortality Weekly Report, 54* (No. RR-7).

Centers for Disease Control and Prevention. (2011). Recommended adult immunization schedule: United States. *Morbidity and Mortality Weekly Report, 60*(4), 1–4. Meningococcal vaccination.

CHAPTER 10

Enterobacteriaceae

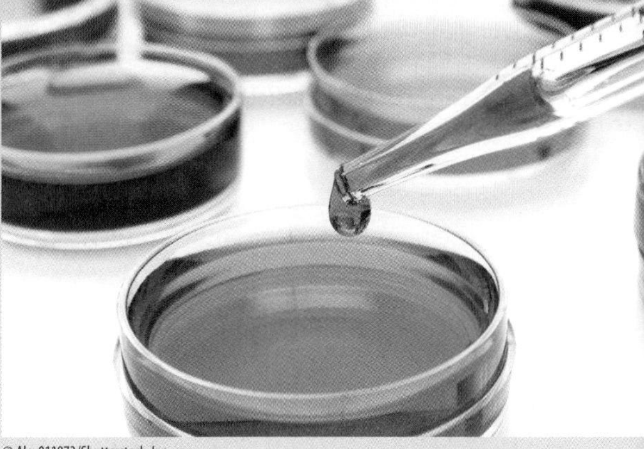

CHAPTER OUTLINE

Characteristics of Enterobacteriaceae
Serological Characteristics
Isolation
Identification
Identification and Significance of Selected Enterobacteriaceae
Antibiotic Susceptibility and Treatment

KEY TERMS

Anaerogenic *E. coli*
Carbohydrate fermentation
Enterohemorrhagic *E. coli*
Enteroinvasive *E. coli*
Enteropathogenic *E. coli*
Enterotoxigenic *E. coli*
Envelope antigen
Flagellar antigen
Kauffman-White classification
Late (slow) lactose fermenters
Outbreak
Pandemic
Serovar
Shiga-producing *E. coli* (STEC)
Shigellosis
Somatic antigen
vero-cytotoxic *E. coli* (VTEC)

LEARNING OBJECTIVES

1. List and describe the serological characteristics of the members of Enterobacteriaceae.
2. Describe the biochemical reactions that are characteristic for the Enterobacteriaceae.
3. State the principle of each of the following biochemical techniques. Perform and interpret each test without error.
   a. Carbohydrate fermentation
   b. Triple sugar iron (TSI)
   c. Indole
   d. Methyl red
   e. Voges-Proskauer
   f. Citrate
   g. Urease
   h. Deaminase (phenylalanine)
   i. ONPG
   j. Hydrogen sulfide (H_2S)
   k. Motility
4. Describe the isolation, identification, and infections of *Escherichia coli*.
5. Discuss the significance of the diarrheagenic *E. coli*.
6. Discuss the identification of the subgroups and species of *Shigella* and the infections associated with *Shigella*.
7. Describe the identification and infections of the *Klebsiella-Enterobacter-Serratia-Hafnia* group. Identify without error members of this group.
8. Describe the currently accepted method for classification of *Salmonella*.
   a. Describe the types of *Salmonella* infections and indicate how each is acquired.
   b. Identify *Salmonella* from a clinical specimen.

9. List the members of the tribe Proteeae (*Proteus* group).
   a. State the important biochemical reactions of the Proteeae group and identify members of this group without error.
   b. Identify significant members of this tribe and state the clinical significance of each.
10. Explain how *Citrobacter* can be differentiated from *Salmonella*. Describe the identification and clinical significance of clinically important members of the genus *Citrobacter*.
11. Describe the identification and clinical significance of the isolation of *Edwardsiella tarda*.
12. List the three species of *Yersinia* and discuss the identification and clinical significance of each.
13. Select and correctly streak the appropriate media for isolation for the following specimen sites when culturing for Enterobacteriaceae:
    a. Urine
    b. Blood
    c. Stool
    d. Wound
14. Identify an unknown from the family Enterobacteriaceae. Select and correctly interpret appropriate media.

The Enterobacteriaceae are a very large and diverse family of bacteria consisting of gram-negative bacilli and coccobacilli. These organisms are frequently encountered in the clinical laboratory and are associated with infections of almost every area of the human body. These bacteria are found in the environment in soil and water and on plants and also are considered to be commensals of the gastrointestinal tract of many animals, including humans. Some of the Enterobacteriaceae are strict pathogens, whereas others are opportunistic pathogens. Still, other Enterobacteriaceae may be isolated from human specimens but are not considered to be clinically significant. Finally, some Enterobacteriaceae are found in animals other than humans and are not considered to play a significant role in human disease.

Humans may develop enteric infections from a variety of situations. Infections may be associated with lapses in personal hygiene through the fecal–oral route, poor sanitation in underdeveloped countries, or colonization of the skin and respiratory tract of hospitalized patients. Humans may acquire these bacteria through ingestion of contaminated food or water, nosocomially through contact with patients or health care personnel or contaminated medical instruments, and endogenously through their own normal flora. Common types of infections attributed to the Enterobacteriaceae include urinary tract, respiratory tract, and wound infections; bacteremia; and gastroenteritis. These bacteria also are known to cause disease in poultry, livestock, fish, and vegetable crops, in addition to being significant human pathogens.

In 1972 Edwards and Ewing described 11 genera and 26 species of the Enterobacteriaceae; in 1985 Farmer noted 22 genera with 69 species. Today, more than 100 species of Enterobacteriaceae exist in over 30 genera. There are various methods of classification, and changes in taxonomy occur frequently, resulting in reclassification as well as the designation of new genera and species. Early classification was based primarily on phenotypical characteristics, such as biochemical reactions and antigenic analysis. Molecular techniques, such as nucleic acid sequencing and hybridization, including deoxyribonucleic acid (DNA) relatedness or homology analysis, have led to reclassification of existing organisms as well as the identification of new species. This chapter focuses on those species that are most frequently found in human infections.

Characteristics of Enterobacteriaceae

All Enterobacteriaceae are glucose fermenters, which means that glucose is utilized anaerobically, with an organic substrate serving as the final hydrogen ion acceptor. In addition, all members of the family are cytochrome oxidase negative, and most species, except for *Erwinia* and *Pantoea agglomerans* (*Enterobacter agglomerans* group), reduce nitrates to nitrites. Most members of this family are motile, with peritrichous flagella, and some species possess pili or fimbriae, which serve as structures for attachment.

The Enterobacteriaceae are facultative anaerobes and grow well in the presence or absence of air. These bacteria also grow very well on blood agar, producing large, dull-gray colonies with variable hemolysis. Isolation is usually accomplished on a differential plate, such as MacConkey medium, with which determination of lactose fermentation can be made.

Serological Characteristics

Members of the Enterobacteriaceae may possess three types of antigenic determinants, which can be used in the serological identification of a particular isolate. These antigens are particularly useful in the characterization of *Escherichia coli*, *Klebsiella*, *Shigella*, and *Salmonella* and are useful for epidemiological purposes.

The **O**, or **somatic, antigen** is found in the outer part of the cell wall and is the heat-stable part of the cell wall. It is known as lipopolysaccharide (LPS) and is released upon cell lysis and as endotoxin. There are over 160 types of O antigen for *E. coli*, and specific types are associated with particular diseases. For example, serotype O111 is known to cause diarrhea in infants, and serotype O157 is associated with verocytotoxin production. Based on the nature of the O antigen, *Shigella* species have been grouped into four serotypes: A, B, C, and D. More than 60 types of O antigen exist for *Salmonella.*

The **K**, or **envelope, antigen** consists of capsular polysaccharide that surrounds the cell wall. It is heat labile and covers the O antigen, thus inhibiting agglutination with type-specific O antisera. After determination of the K antigen, the organism must be boiled for 30 minutes and then retested to detect the O antigen. *Klebsiella*, *Salmonella*, and *E. coli* possess K antigens. The **Vi antigens** of *Salmonella typhi* are categorized as K antigens.

The **H**, or **flagellar, antigen** is found only in motile members of the Enterobacteriaceae. This antigen is found in the flagellum and is protein in nature and heat labile. The H antigen is used to serotype within species of *Salmonella* and other bacteria. *Salmonella* species are known to produce two types of H antigens, which are known as phase 1 and phase 2 antigens.

The **Kauffman-White classification** has been used to classify *Salmonella* species based on their O and H antigens. More than 2,000 serovars (serotypes) of *Salmonella* exist based on typing for the O and H antigens. For epidemiological purposes, *Salmonella* isolates are tested with polyvalent O antisera. If the isolate is positive for the polyvalent antisera, specific monovalent antigen testing is done. Once the serogroup has been determined, the particular serotype should be identified. When agglutination does *not* occur with the polyvalent antisera, a suspension of the organism should be boiled for 15 minutes and then retested. Heating destroys the capsular antigen, which may block the reactivity of the O antigen. Also, *S. typhi* will agglutinate with the Vi antisera before, but not after, boiling. Isolates are usually serotyped in reference laboratories because of the procedure's complexity.

Isolation

The selection of media for the isolation for Enterobacteriaceae depends on the source of the specimen. A combination of MacConkey and blood agars is usually acceptable for specimens other than stool cultures. Eosin-methylene blue (EMB) agar is substituted for MacConkey agar by some laboratories.

Some initial observations on blood agar are helpful in identification of the Enterobacteriaceae. For example, members of the genus *Proteus* produce characteristic swarming motility on blood agar plates, as shown in **FIGURE 10-1** and grow in thin waves over the surface of the agar. *Klebsiella pneumoniae*, which produces a capsule, appears as mucoid colonies, as shown in **FIGURE 10-2**. Organisms that are hydrogen sulfide (H_2S) positive often produce subsurface greening of blood agar. **BOX 10-1** summarizes typical colonial morphology of some common Enterobacteriaceae.

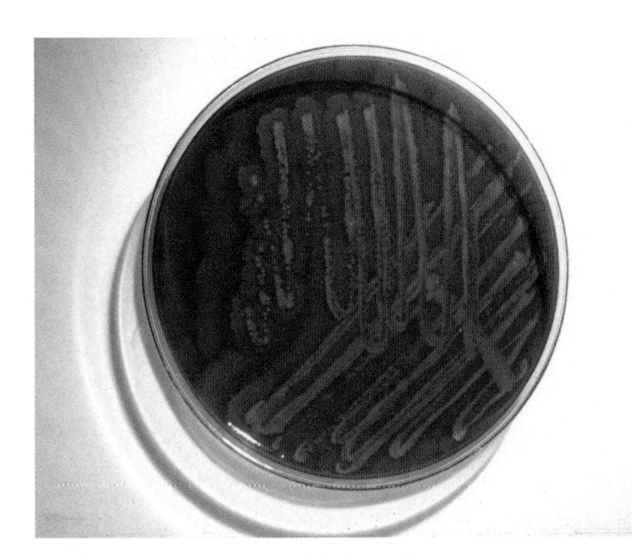

FIGURE 10-1 Swarming motility characteristic of *Proteus* on sheep blood agar.

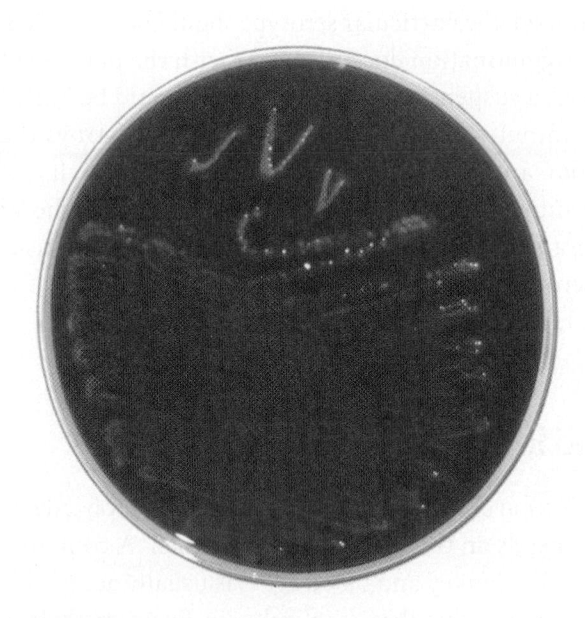

FIGURE 10-2 Mucoid morphology of *Klebsiella pneumoniae* on sheep blood agar.

The members of Enterobacteriaceae most often associated with diarrhea are *Salmonella*, *Shigella*, specific diarrheagenic *E. coli*, and *Yersinia enterolitica*. Stool specimens should be directly plated onto a differential plate (MacConkey or EMB) and onto a selective plate (Hektoen enteric or xylose lysine desoxycholate). In addition, an enrichment broth, such as gram negative, selenite, or tetrathionate, is inoculated. Enrichment broths hold the normal flora coliforms, such as *E. coli*, in a lag period of growth while permitting the pathogenic *Salmonella* and *Shigella* to enter a logarithmic phase of growth. These broths contain a high concentration of bile salts, which inhibit the multiplication of the normal flora coliforms. The selenite broth is subcultured within 8 to 24 hours and gram-negative broth within 4 to 8 hours to a selective plate to ensure proper recovery of pathogens. Enrichment broths can be re-incubated for as long as 24 hours if desired. The normal flora coliforms appear as lactose-positive colonies on differential and selective plates, whereas the pathogenic *Salmonella* and *Shigella* appear as lactose-negative colonies. Sorbitol MacConkey is inoculated in suspected cases of *E. coli* O157:H7 (verocytotoxic *E. coli*); if enterotoxigenic *E. coli* is suspected, a blood agar plate is inoculated. A cefsulodin-irgasan-novobiocin (CIN) plate is inoculated if *Yersinia enterocolitica* is suspected. The CIN agar is incubated at room temperature (22°C to 26°C) for 24 hours to enhance its recovery. A highly selective agar plate, such as brilliant green or bismuth sulfite, can be included for specific *Salmonella*, such as *S. typhi*.

For urine cultures, MacConkey and blood agars are a suitable combination. A colony count should be performed on all urine specimens. If a 1 μl (0.001 ml) calibrated loop is used to inoculate the plate, the number of colonies must be multiplied by 1,000 to gain the colony count per milliliter of urine. For catheterized or suprapubic samples, a 10 μl loop may be used. In this case the number of colonies must be multiplied by 100 to determine the colony count per milliliter of urine. All colony counts for a single organism that are greater than 10^5/ml are considered to be positive for a urinary tract infection.

FIGURES 10-3 and **10-4** illustrate examples of characteristic reactions of the Enterobacteriaceae on MacConkey and Hektoen enteric agars. BOX 10-2 summarizes the media used to isolate Enterobacteriaceae.

BOX 10-1 **Typical Colonial Morphology of Enterobacteriaceae**

Organism on Sheep Blood Agar and MacConkey Agar

E. coli: Smooth, medium 2–3 mm; pink-red, lactose positive

Salmonella: Smooth, medium 2–3 mm; flat, clear, lactose negative

Shigella: Smooth, medium 2–3 mm; flat, clear, lactose negative

Klebsiella pneumonia: Mucoid, large 3–4 mm; pink, mucoid, lactose positive

Enterobacter: Smooth, medium 2–3 mm; pink, lactose positive

Proteus mirabilis and *P. vulgaris*: Swarm in waves from point of inoculation; flat, clear, lactose negative

Morganella, other *Proteus*, *Providentia*: Flat, medium 2–3 mm; clear, lactose negative

Identification

All Enterobacteriaceae grow well on MacConkey medium. After observation of growth on MacConkey, the oxidase test is performed. Any oxidase-negative organism isolated

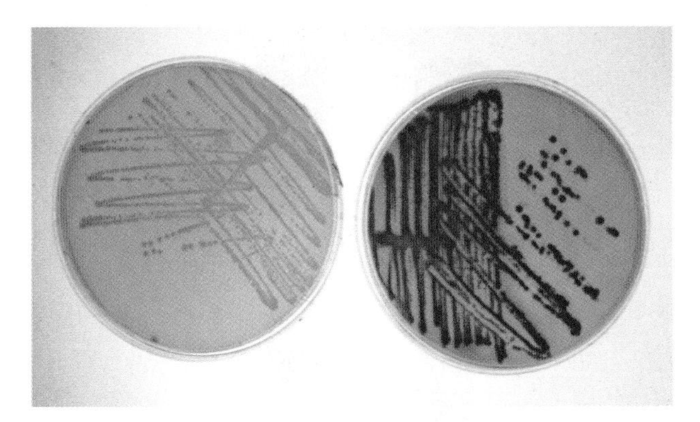

FIGURE 10-3 MacConkey agar showing pink colonies. Plate on left shows colorless colonies which indicate negative lactose fermentation. Plate on right shows pink colonies which indicate positive lactose fermentation.

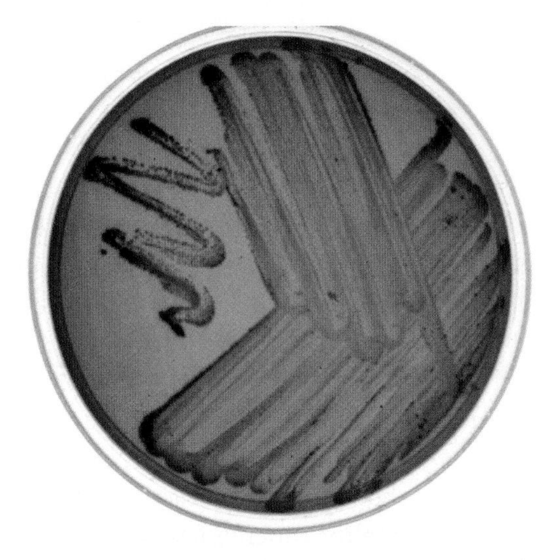

FIGURE 10-4 Hektoen enteric agar showing green growth with black centers. These reactions are typical of organisms that are nonfermenters and are hydrogen sulfide positive.

BOX 10-2 Media Used for Isolation of Enterobacteriaceae

Cefsulodin-irgasan-novobiocin (CIN): Agar selective for *Yersinia* species

Eosin-methylene blue (EMB): Agar used for the isolation and differentiation of lactose fermenters from nonlactose fermenters

Gram-negative (GN) broth: Enrichment broth used to enhance isolation of enteric pathogens

Hektoen enteric (HE): Isolation and differentiation of *Salmonella* and *Shigella*; inhibition of normal flora coliforms

MacConkey: Agar used for the isolation and differentiation of lactose fermenters from nonlactose fermenters

Novobiocin brilliant green (NBG) glucose agar: Isolation and differentiation of *Salmonella*

***Salmonella–Shigella* (SS):** Isolation and differentiation of *Salmonella* and *Shigella*; inhibition of normal flora coliforms

Selenite broth: Enrichment broth used to enhance recovery of *Salmonella* and *Shigella*

Tetrathionate broth: Enrichment broth used to enhance recovery of *Salmonella* and *Shigella*

Xylose lysine desoxycholate (XLD): Agar used to isolate and differentiate *Salmonella* and *Shigella* from other Enterobacteriaceae

from MacConkey agar can be suspected of being a member of the Enterobacteriaceae family. Identification is based on a series of biochemical reactions that historically have been performed in media prepared in test tubes. Today, these reactions are available as packaged test systems using small, concentrated reagent wells, coding indices, and automated instrumentation for identification. The biochemical principles of the reactions for manual, tubed media and the packaged and automated systems are generally the same. A brief summary of the significant biochemical reactions follows, with detailed experimental methods included at the end of this chapter.

The organism's pattern of **carbohydrate fermentation** is an important identifying characteristic for the Enterobacteriaceae. It already has been noted that all members of the Enterobacteriaceae ferment glucose. Through a series of steps, glucose is converted to pyruvic acid and then to lactic acid. The organism's ability to ferment lactose can be determined through observation on MacConkey or EMB agar.

A variety of carbohydrates can be tested for fermentation, and these results are used in the identification of the organism. In addition to lactose, these carbohydrates may include sucrose, mannose, sorbitol, mannitol, xylose, adonitol, cellobiose, dulcitol, and trehalose. In each test, the carbohydrate sugar or sugar alcohol is used to specifically determine the ability of the organism to ferment the compound. Frequently, carbohydrate-like compounds or polyhedral alcohols are used to substitute for the carbohydrate, such as with mannitol, which is actually a sugar alcohol. The system also must contain a pH indicator that changes color as the pH changes from neutral or alkaline to acidic. One such indicator is phenol red, which is orange-red in its original state and becomes yellow in an acidic environment of pH 6.8 or less. The change in indicator color shows that the carbohydrate has been fermented, resulting in the production of acidic end products. A particular pattern of fermentation of the carbohydrates tested assists in the identification of the organism.

Most members of the Enterobacteriaceae produce hydrogen and carbon dioxide (CO_2) gas during fermentation, which can be observed as cracks in the tubed media. Especially large amounts of gas are produced by members of *Klebsiella*, *Enterobacter*, *Hafnia*, and *Serratia*. Of special note is the genus *Shigella*, which cannot produce gas during fermentation of carbohydrates.

The **triple sugar iron (TSI) agar** contains glucose, lactose, and sucrose. The ability of the organism to ferment glucose, lactose, and sucrose, as well as the production of gas from fermentation and H_2S gas production, can be determined using this medium. **FIGURE 10-5** shows typical TSI reactions for selected members of the Enterobacteriaceae.

IMVC is an acronym for the **indole**, **methyl red**, **Voges-Proskauer**, and **citrate** reactions, which have been used in the preliminary identification of the Enterobacteriaceae. The indole reaction uses tryptophan substrate and tests for the presence of the enzyme tryptophanase, which

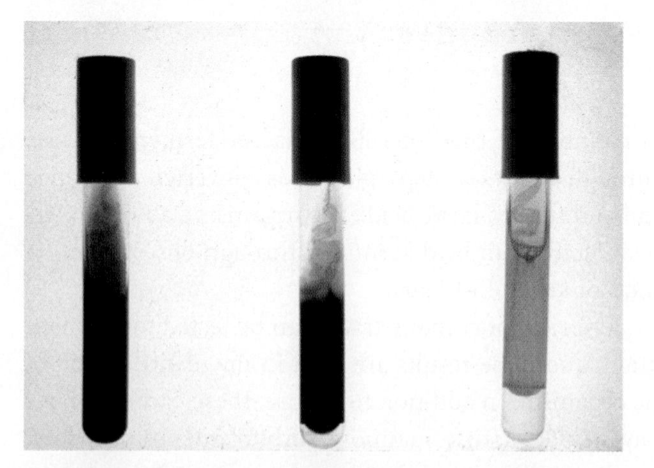

FIGURE 10-5 Triple sugar iron agar showing some characteristic reactions of the Enterobacteriaceae. Tube on left is alkaline over acid with hydrogen sulfide production which is typical of Salmonella. Center tube is acid over acid with hydrogen sulfide production which is seen with Citrobacter fruendii. Tube on right is acid over acid with gas and no hydrogen sulfide production, which is typical of the lactose fermenters such as *E. coli*, *Enterobacter*, and *Klebsiella*.

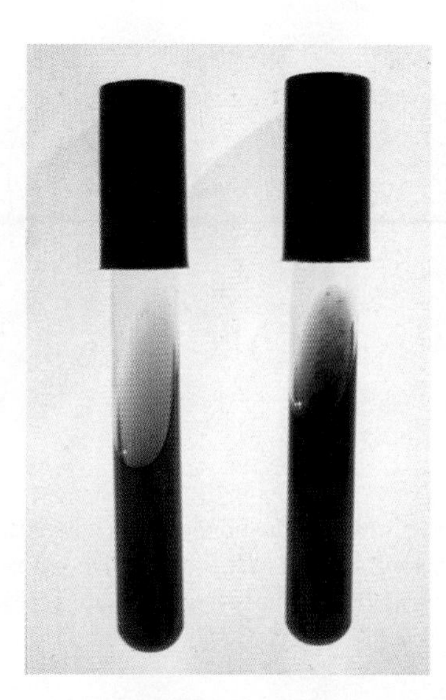

FIGURE 10-6 Citrate reaction. Tube on left shows a negative reaction with no growth. Tube on right shows a positive reaction of growth and a blue color.

converts tryptophan to indole. The methyl red–Voges-Proskauer (MRVP) test identifies the specific pathway for glucose metabolism. In the MR pathway, mixed acids are produced, which results in an acidic pH and a positive methyl red reaction. The VP pathway produces the neutral end product, acetoin, which is detected using potassium hydroxide and α-naphthol. The citrate reaction determines whether an organism can use citrate as its only carbon source. **FIGURE 10-6** shows the citrate reaction. These reactions have been used in the differentiation of the lactose-fermenting Enterobacteriaceae, as indicated in **TABLE 10-1**.

Decarboxylation reactions detect the ability of the organism to enzymatically remove the carboxyl group from a specific amino acid. Generally, the amino acids lysine, ornithine, and arginine are tested. The decarboxylase reactions are useful in the differentiation of *Klebsiella*, *Enterobacter*, and *Pantoea* and also to speciate within the genus *Enterobacter*. **TABLE 10-2** summarizes important decarboxylase reactions, and **FIGURE 10-7** illustrates the

TABLE 10-1 IMVC Reactions for Lactose-Fermenting Enterobacteriaceae

	Indole	MR	VP	Citrate
Escherichia coli	+	+	–	–
Klebsiella	–	–	+	+
Enterobacter	–	–	+	+

MR, methyl red; VP, Voges-Proskauer

TABLE 10-2 Important Decarboxylase Reactions for Enterobacteriaceae

	LDC Lysine	ODC Ornithine	ADH Arginine
Klebsiella pneumoniae	+	–	–
Klebsiella oxytoca	+	–	–
Enterobacter aerogenes	+	+	–
Enterobacter cloacae	–	+	+
Pantoea agglomerans	–	–	–

LDC, lysine decarboxylase; ODC, ornithine decarboxylase; ADH, arginine dihydrolase

ornithine decarboxylase (ODC) and arginine dihydrolase (ADH) reactions.

Deaminase reactions use the amino acid lysine, tryptophan, or phenylalanine as a substrate to detect the removal of the amino group from each amino acid. The reactions are helpful in the identification of *Proteus, Providencia*, and *Morganella*, which are the only deaminase-positive members of Enterobacteriaceae.

Lysine iron agar (LIA) allows for the determination of both deamination and decarboxylation of lysine. Hydrogen sulfide production also can be detected using LIA agar. **FIGURE 10-8** shows characteristic reactions that can be observed in LIA.

Late or slow lactose fermenters are identified in the **ortho-nitrophenyl-β-D-galactopyranoside (ONPG) reaction**. The ONPG reaction is valuable in the differentiation of *Citrobacter* species, which are ONPG positive, from most *Salmonella* species, which are ONPG negative. *Salmonella arizonae* is the only ONPG-positive *Salmonella* serotype.

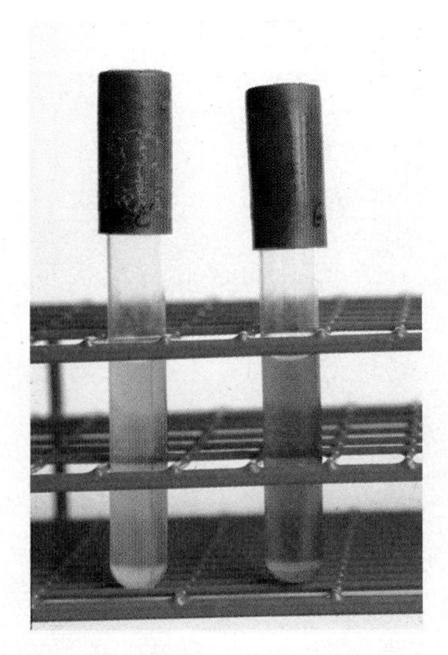

FIGURE 10-7 Ornithine decarboxylase and arginine dihydrolase reactions. Tube on left shows negative decarboxylation (ODC negative) as evidenced by yellow color; tube on right shows positive decarboxylation (ADH positive) as indicated by purple color.

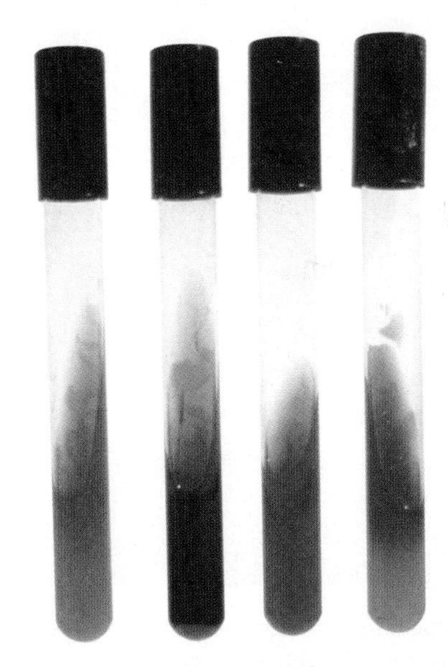

FIGURE 10-8 Lysine iron agar showing typical reactions of Enterobacteriaceae. Left is purple over yellow which indicated negative decarboxylation. Second tube from bottom is purple over purple with blackening which indicates positive lysine decarboxylation and production of hydrogen sulfide. Third tube from left show purple over purple which indicates positive lysine decarboxylase and negative hydrogen sulfide production. Tube on right is red over yellow which indicates positive lysine deaminase production.

The production of **hydrogen sulfide (H_2S) gas** is detected in many media, including TSI, LIA, sulfur indole motility (SIM) medium, and Hektoen enteric agar. For H_2S production to be detected, the system requires a source of sulfur, such as sodium thiosulfate, cysteine, or methionine, and an H_2S indicator, which is usually an iron salt, such as ferrous sulfate, ferrous citrate, or ferric ammonium citrate. Organisms that possess H_2S-producing enzymes liberate sulfur from the sulfur-containing compound to form the colorless gas H_2S. The H_2S then reacts with the iron salt to form the black precipitate of ferrous sulfide (FeS). Media differ in their sensitivity in the detection of H_2S; for example, SIM medium is considered to be very sensitive for H_2S detection.

H_2S production is helpful in differentiating *Salmonella* species, which are positive, from *Shigella* species, which are negative. For example, stool specimens are plated onto Hektoen enteric agar in cases of suspected gastroenteritis caused by *Salmonella* or *Shigella*. Although both are negative for lactose fermentation, *Salmonella* produces colonies

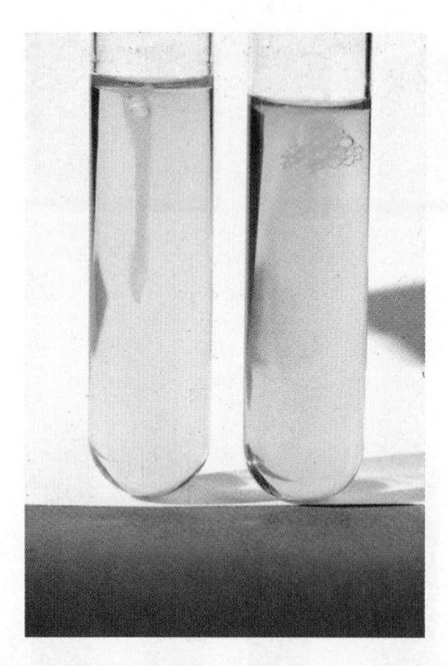

FIGURE 10-9 Semisolid motility media. Tube on the left shows a nonmotile organism as growth is only present along the stab line; tube on the right shows a motile organism with growth present throughout the medium.

with black centers, indicating H_2S production, whereas *Shigella* produces clear colonies, which are H_2S negative.

Most tests for **motility** involve the use of semisolid media, which typically contain 0.4% agar. A motility medium is often incorporated into a test battery, as with SIM medium and motility indole ornithine (MIO) medium. **FIGURE 10-9** shows semisolid motility media with motile and nonmotile bacteria. Motility reactions are very useful in the identification of *Shigella* and *Klebsiella*, the only nonmotile members of Enterobacteriaceae. The reaction also is useful in the identification of *Yersinia* species, which are nonmotile at 37°C but are motile when incubated at 22°C. The **urease reaction** is particularly useful in the identification of the genera *Proteus* and *Morganella*, which are rapid urease producers, as well as in the identification of slower urease producers, such as *Klebsiella* and some members of the genus *Enterobacter.* Urease degrades the substrate urea into alkaline end products, which are detected using a pH indicator.

The identification of the Enterobacteriaceae has been enhanced greatly through the use of packaged microsystems, which are composed of a battery of biochemical tests. The concentrated reagents are inoculated with a suspension of the organism and incubated. Reactions are read, and a profile number is determined that can be matched with its species in a code book, which contains the database. One such example is the API-20E, which contains a series of biochemical tests and is available from bioMérieux. Most principles that are used in the manual tubed media are the same as those for packaged microsystems.

Identification and Significance of Selected Enterobacteriaceae

This section discusses the identification and clinical significance of those members of Enterobacteriaceae most frequently associated with human infection.

ESCHERICHIA COLI

There are six species of *Escherichia* of which *E. coli* is the most common clinical isolate. *E. coli* is normal flora of the human lower gastrointestinal tract and is therefore found in the normal stool. It is the most common clinical isolate in the family Enterobacteriaceae. *E. coli* is closely related through DNA homology to *Shigella*; however, they are easily differentiated because *E. coli* is lactose positive, whereas *Shigella* species are lactose negative.

E. coli is identified by the presence of pink-red colonies on MacConkey agar or by its characteristic green metallic sheen on EMB (**FIGURE 10-10**) and a positive indole reaction. It can be presumptively identified if lactose-positive, oxidase-negative, and indole-positive gram-negative bacilli are isolated. A complete identification requires additional biochemical testing, which may include the following reactions, as shown in **TABLE 10-3**.

E. coli is the cause of many types of infections. Urinary tract infections are frequently attributed to *E. coli*

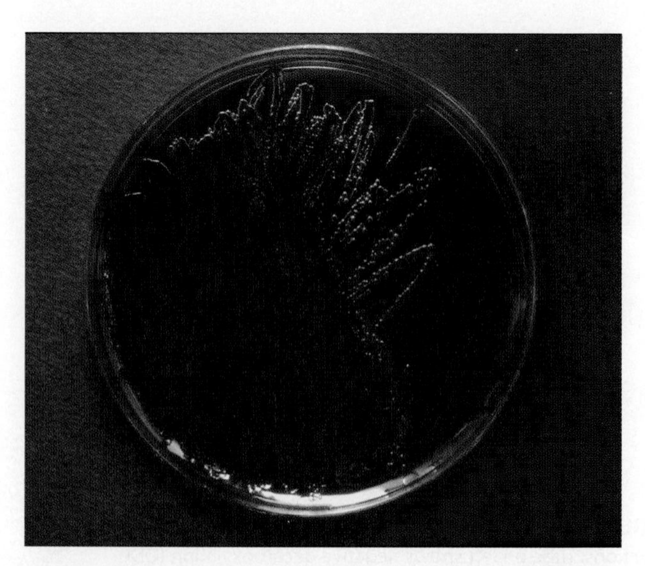

FIGURE 10-10 Eosin-methylene blue medium with *Escherichia coli* with its typical green metallic sheen.

TABLE 10-3 Identifying Characteristics of *E. coli*

TSI: Acid slant over acid deep (A/Ⓐ)
H_2S: Negative
MacConkey: Pink-red colonies
EMB: Green metallic sheen
Indole: Positive
Methyl red (MR): Positive
Voges-Proskauer (VP): Negative
Citrate: Negative
Motility: Positive (most)
Deaminase (phenylalanine): Negative
Urease: Negative
LDC: Positive
ODC: Most strains positive
ADH: Most strains negative
ONPG: Positive
Fermentation of:
Adonitol: Negative
L-arabinose: Positive
Cellobiose: Negative
Dulcitol: Variable
Maltose: Positive
D-mannitol: Positive
D-mannose: Positive
D-sorbitol: Positive
Sucrose: Variable
Trehalose: Positive
D-xylose: Positive

and include cystitis, pyelitis, and pyelonephritis. In fact, it is estimated that approximately 90% of all acute urinary tract infections in nonhospitalized patients are caused by *E. coli*. The source of infection is normal flora *E. coli* from fecal contamination. In addition, approximately 25% of all nosocomial urinary tract infections are attributed to *E. coli*. Other types of infections include appendicitis, peritonitis, gallbladder infections, pneumonia, endocarditis, neonatal meningitis, wound infections, and septicemia. The septicemia may be associated with endotoxic shock from the release of lipopolysaccharide from the gram-negative cell wall.

Specific serotypes of *E. coli* cause diarrhea and gastroenteritis, often with serious consequences. These serotypes differ from those that are found as commensal coliforms and produce virulence factors that contribute to the symptoms of gastroenteritis. Currently, six disease syndromes have been described, which are summarized in BOX 10-3.

TABLE 10-4 *Shigella* Subgroups and Species

Subgroup	Species	Number of serotypes
A	*S. dysenteriae*	15 (type 1: Shiga toxin)
B	*S. flexneri*	8
C	*S. boydii*	19
D	*S. sonnei*	1

Anaerogenic *E. coli*, or ***ªE. coli* inactive**, refers to a particular type of *E. coli* that does not produce gas during fermentation. These bacteria are lactose negative and nonmotile and previously have been known as the alkalescens-dispar group.

SHIGELLA

Shigella organisms resemble *E. coli* but are lactose negative and nonmotile. There are four subgroups and species of *Shigella* and species based respectively on antigenic and biochemical characteristics (TABLE 10-4). Subgroups A, B, and C are biochemically similar. The biochemical reactions to identify the genus *Shigella* are shown in TABLE 10-5.

TABLE 10-5 Biochemical Characteristics of *Shigella*

TSI: Alkaline slant over acid deep (K/A)
H_2S: Negative
Gas in fermentation: Negative
MR: Positive
Motility: Negative
Citrate: Negative
ADH: Negative
LDC: Negative
ODC: Negative
Deaminase (phenylalanine): Negative
Urease: Negative
MacConkey: Clear colonies (lactose negative)
Hektoen enteric: Green colonies (lactose negative)
Fermentation of:
Adonitol: Negative
Dulcitol: Negative
D-mannose: Positive
Sucrose: Negative
Salicin: Negative

BOX 10-3 **Diarrheagenic *E. coli* syndromes**

1. **Enterotoxigenic *E. coli* (ETEC)** grows only on blood agar and produces enterotoxins that result in epidemic diarrhea. It is commonly known as traveler's diarrhea, weanling diarrhea, or Montezuma's revenge or "turista" and is associated with ingestion of contaminated water or food. ETEC is seen more frequently in developing countries. Specific serogroups are associated with severe gastritis. Enterotoxin production occurs in certain serotypes, which include O6, O8, O15, O25, O27, O63, O78, O148, and O159. ETEC may produce a heat-labile toxin (LT) and/or a heat-stable toxin (ST), which leads indirectly to fluid loss. Certain serotypes produce LT and ST, whereas others produce only LT or ST. The intestinal wall is invaded, leading to inflammation and fluid loss. The illness is characterized by nausea, diarrhea without blood, pus or mucus, mild vomiting, chills, and headache. There usually is a low-grade fever or no fever. The incubation period is 1 to 2 days, and the actual illness lasts for 5 to 10 days.
2. **Enteroinvasive *E. coli* (EIEC)** invades the intestinal epithelium, causing a *Shigella*-like infection. The disease is characterized by fever, cramps, and bloody stools that contain red blood cells, neutrophils, and mucus. EIEC may be associated with the following serogroups: O28, O29, O112, O124, O136, O143, O144, O152, and O164. Most strains are nonmotile and late or nonlactose fermenters. EIEC is rare in the United States.
3. **Enteropathogenic *E. coli* (EPEC)** is noninvasive, produces no toxins, and is associated with a limited number of serogroups, which include O55, O86, O111, O114, O127, and O128. This syndrome is usually nosocomial and seen in newborns and infants, causing vomiting, fever, and watery diarrhea with mucus but no blood. EPEC has been the agent of severe outbreaks in newborn nurseries in the United States prior to 1970 but is rarely isolated today in developing countries. It remains an important pathogen in developing countries. EPEC adheres to the intestinal epithelial cells and produces characteristic lesions that attach to and efface the cells. EPEC may be isolated on enteric media.
4. **Enterohemorrhagic *E. coli* (EHEC), Shiga toxin-producing *E. coli* (STEC), or vero-cytotoxic *E. coli* (VTEC)** all refer to serotypes of *E. coli* that cause bloody diarrhea from verotoxin production, which is a cytotoxin resembling that produced by *Shigella*. Hemorrhagic colitis is associated with abdominal cramps, diarrhea that is usually bloody, and lower gastrointestinal hemorrhage. There may be a low-grade fever, or fever may not occur. Infection can range from mild to very severe. Although those of all ages can become infected with STEC, very young children and the elderly are at highest risk to become severely ill and to develop hemolytic uremic syndrome (HUS). While most individuals recover within 5 to 7 days, approximately 5% to 10% of those infected develop HUS. Hemolytic uremic syndrome, the most severe manifestation of EHEC, is a hemorrhagic colitis with bloody diarrhea. STEC is contracted by ingesting the organism in contaminated food products. These organisms may be found in the intestinal tract of many animals, including cattle, sheep, deer, and goats. Consumption of unpasteurized milk, contaminated water, or contaminated food or contact with infected cattle or infected feces are all sources of infection. Implicated foods include undercooked hamburger, unpasteurized apple cider, soft cheeses made from raw milk, and vegetables grown in contaminated soil. Complications of HUS include acute renal failure, thrombocytopenia, and microangiopathic hemolytic anemia. More than 50 serotypes of STEC exist, including O26, O103, O111, O145, and O165, but infection most often is associated with one particular serotype, O157:H7. This particular serotype of *E. coli* is the only strain that is sorbitol negative. It can be isolated on MacConkey agar in which sorbitol has been substituted for lactose (SMAC agar). Outbreaks of EHEC occurred in 1993, when a fast-food chain serving undercooked hamburger was traced as the source of infection. Beef is believed to be contaminated at the slaughterhouse through bovine feces. There have been approximately 200 to 300 cases of HUS reported to the CDC annually since 2005. In 2011, there have been multistate outbreaks of STEC related to Lebanon bologna and hazel nuts. Outbreaks attributed to cheese products, shredded lettuce from one processing facility, and contaminated beef from a single producer/distributer occurred in 2010. Other sources of outbreaks from *E. coli* O157:H7 include prepackaged cookie dough and a variety of beef products. Of special note is the outbreak involving contaminated spinach, which infected 200 individuals from 26 states; several of those infected developed HUS. The organism also can be transmitted via person-to-person contact within families, at petting zoos, and during visits to dairy farms, where unpasteurized milk or apple cider may be consumed.

Sorbitol MacConkey (SMAC) agar is a differential and selective media to detect sorbitol-negative *E. coli*, especially O157:H7. SMAC inhibits gram-positive bacteria with bile salts and the *Enterococcus* with crystal violet. There is no lactose in the medium, but instead D-sorbitol is included. STEC ferment lactose but not D-sorbitol, and thus the medium provides a mechanism to differentiate STEC from other strains of sorbitol-positive *E. coli*. Specimens suspected of harboring STEC are plated directly onto SMAC agar and incubated for 24 hours. Sorbitol-negative colonies are tested with serotype O157 antisera and then confirmed for the H7 flagella antigen. This would confirm the identification of *E. coli* O157:H7.

5. **Enteroaggregative *E. coli* (EAEC)** produces stable and labile toxins and colonization factors that lead to a watery, mucoid diarrhea without red cells or white cells in the stool. EAEC adheres to epithelial cells in a stacking appearance.
6. **Diffusely adherent *E. coli* (DAEC)** adheres to the epithelial cells in a diffuse pattern and also causes a diarrheal syndrome with a watery stool without red cells or white cells present.

Differentiation of *Shigella* subgroups can be based on the biochemical reactions found in **TABLE 10-6**. Because of the biochemical similarities among serogroups A, B, and C, it may be difficult to separate the serogroups based on biochemical reactions. Serogroup D, *S. sonnei*, can be separated from the other serotypes because it is ODC positive and produces β-galactosidase (ONPG positive). Rare strains of *S. sonnei* are slowly lactose and sucrose positive. *S. dysenteriae* is separated from the others by its inability to ferment mannitol.

Shigella is found only in humans and other large primates. Shigellosis, or **bacillary dysentery**, can be caused by all four species of *Shigella*. The disease can occur as sporadic cases or in outbreaks in humans. While most infections are confined to the gastrointestinal tract, *Shigella* infections can be disseminated to other sites in the body. The infection is spread via the fecal–oral route or through contaminated food and water. *Shigella* should be suspected when a nonlactose fermenter, which is nonmotile and H_2S negative, is isolated from the stool.

Shigella infections typically incubate for 1 to 7 days, and shigellosis begins with fever, abdominal cramping and pain, and diarrhea. The first stage of the infection involves a watery diarrhea, which may last up to 3 days. This is followed by less frequent bowel movements and then, the dysenteric phase, characterized by frequent stools with the presence of red and white blood cells and mucus. During the dysenteric phase, the bacteria invade the epithelial lining of the intestine, causing severe inflammation. Fluid and electrolyte loss result from the effects of an enterotoxin, and those with severe illness may require fluid and electrolyte therapy. The severity of the infection depends on the species and the status of the host. More severe infections are seen in infants, children, and the elderly. Because *S. dysenteriae* produces both a neurotoxin and an enterotoxin, infections resulting from this species are the most severe. While the enterotoxin invades the large bowel, the neurotoxin may be associated with paralysis and death. *S. dysenteriae* also produces a Shiga toxin, adding to the severity of infection. The other species produce only an enterotoxin, and thus infections of *S. flexneri*, *S. sonnei*, and *S. boydii* are milder than those caused by *S. dysenteriae*.

S. sonnei is the most prevalent species in the United States and accounts for 65% to 75% of all *Shigella* infections. Many infections occur in the day care setting, where it is most often spread through the fecal–oral route, in children less than 5 years of age. *S. dysenteriae* is the least common species causing infections in the United States, which can be attributed to efficient sanitary disposal systems. Worldwide, the most common species found in infections are *S. flexneri* and *S. dysenteriae*.

The infectious dose for *Shigella* is extremely low, 10 to 200 organisms, which is 100 to 100,000 times smaller

TABLE 10-6 Differentiation of *Shigella* Subgroups

Reaction	*dysenteriae*	*flexneri*	*boydii*	*sonnei*
Fermentation of:				
Lactose	–	–	–	–
Mannitol	–	+	+	+
ODC	–	–	–	+
ONPG	–	–	–	+

than for most other enteric pathogens. Antibiotics are frequently given to lessen the severity of the infection. Currently, the medications of choice are ampicillin and trimethoprim-sulfamethoxazole, although resistance is common. Alternatively, the fluoroquinolones and azithromycin may be given.

KLEBSIELLA-ENTEROBACTER-SERRATIA-HAFNIA GROUP (TRIBE KLEBSIELLEAE)

Prior to molecular diagnostics, the members of the tribe Klebsielleae were grouped together because of their similar biochemical reactions. The tribe includes six genera: *Klebsiella*, *Enterobacter*, *Hafnia*, *Serratia*, *Pantoea*, and *Raoutella*. All members of this tribe are Voges-Proskauer positive and therefore produce acetoin as the end product in glucose metabolism. All members also produce large amounts of gas in the TSI deep portion and grow in potassium cyanide broth; most are also citrate positive.

Klebsiella and *Raoutella*

The nomenclature of the genus *Klebsiella* has been revised based on RNA sequencing, and the genus previously known as *Klebsiella* has been divided into two genera: *Klebsiella* and *Raoutella*. Those organisms that remain in the genus *Klebsiella* are *K. pneumoniae* subspecies *pneumoniae*, *rhinoscleromatis*, and *ozaenae* and *K. oxytoca*. Those organisms placed in the genus *Raoutella* are *R. ornithinolytica*, *R. planticola*, and *R. terrigana*.

Klebsiella and *Raoultella* are found in nature and the gastrointestinal tracts of humans and other animals. These organisms are short, nonmotile bacilli. The most frequently isolated *Klebsiella* species is *K. pneumoniae* subspecies *pneumoniae*. It is carried as normal flora in the upper respiratory and gastrointestinal tracts of approximately 1% to 5% of healthy individuals. This carrier rate is much higher for hospitalized patients, with a prevalence of almost 20%. *K. pneumoniae* subspecies *pneumoniae*, once known as "Friedlander's bacillus," is encapsulated and appears as mucoid colonies that tend to string.

Important reactions to identify *K. pneumoniae* subspecies *pneumoniae* are shown in **TABLE 10-7**. **TABLE 10-8** summarizes the speciation of Klebsiella and the differentiation of *Klebsiella* from *Raoutella*.

TABLE 10-7 Identification of *K. pneumoniae* subspecies *pneumoniae*

MacConkey: Pink, mucoid colonies
TSI: A/Ⓐ H_2S—Negative
Gas: Positive
Indole: Negative
MR: Negative
VP: Positive
Citrate: Positive
Deaminase (phenylalanine): Negative
Motility: Negative
Arginine: Negative
Lysine: Positive
Ornithine: Negative
Urease: Weakly positive
Fermentation of:
Adonitol: Positive
Dulcitol: Variable
D-mannitol: Positive
Salicin: Positive
D-sorbitol: Positive
Sucrose: Positive

TABLE 10-8 Differentiation of *Klebsiella* and *Raoutella*

	K. pneumoniae subsp. *pneumoniae*	*K. pneumoniae* subsp. *ozaenae*	*K. pneumoniae* subsp. *rhinoscleromatis*	*K. oxytoca*	*Raoultella*
Indole	–	–	–	+	+
MR	–	+	+	**V**	+
VP	+	–	–	+	**V**
Urease	+	–	–	+	+
Lysine	+	**V**	–	+	+
Ornithine	–	–	–	–	**V**
Malonate	+	–	+	–	+

V, variable reaction

K. pneumoniae subspecies *pneumoniae* causes primary bacterial pneumonia, which is more frequently found in those individuals with a predisposing lung disease, such as chronic obstructive pulmonary disease, and also in those with other medical conditions, such as diabetes mellitus. The pneumonia is necrotic and hemorrhagic, which leads to the appearance of "currant jelly-like" sputum. There may also be lung abscesses and other complications in the lung. The organism can also cause meningitis, surgical wound infections, urinary tract infections, bacteremia abscesses, neonatal meningitis, infections of the gastrointestinal tract, and other wound infections. Most infections are nosocomial and may occur as a result of colonization from the hands, bowel, and other body sites of hospital personnel and patients. Increases in *Klebsiella* infections are attributed to an increase in the immunosuppressed patient population as well as increased antibiotic resistance. Those at highest risk of *Klebsiella* infections include those on prolonged antibiotic therapy, patients on ventilators, and those with intravenous lines. Many clinical isolates are resistant to ampicillin, carbenicillin, and ticarcillin. Additionally, the production of extended-spectrum β-lactamases (ESBLs) through plasmids have caused increased resistance to many β-lactam antibiotics, including the third-generation cephalosporins.

An additional concern is the organism's capsule, which enables *K. pneumoniae* subspecies *pneumoniae* to resist phagocytosis. A very resilient organism, *K. pneumoniae* subspecies *pneumoniae* also has been isolated from contaminated medications, respiratory care equipment, and intravenous (IV) solutions.

K. pneumoniae subspecies *ozaenae* and *K. pneumoniae* subspecies *rhinoscleromatis* are rarely isolated. *K. ozanenae* causes atrophic rhinitis, a purulent sinus infection, and *K. rhinoscleromatis* causes rhinoscleroma, a granulomatous disease of the nose and oropharynx.

K. oxytoca has been isolated from the stool and the blood. The *Raoultella* bacteria are found in soil and water and also in the respiratory tract and colon. Their role in human infection has not been established, and their presence may indicate colonization. *K. oxytoca* and the *Raoutella* bacteria are indole positive, which differentiates them from the subspecies of *K. pneumoniae*, which is indole negative. *Klebsiella* species can be differentiated from other members of the tribe because they are nonmotile and ODC negative.

Enterobacter

Enterobacter species are motile and ODC positive. Currently 16 species exist, and their habitat includes soil, water, and dairy products. They also are normal flora of the gastrointestinal tract of many animals, including humans.

Important reactions for *Enterobacter* are shown in **TABLE 10-9**.

TABLE 10-9 Biochemical Reactions for *Enterobacter*

TSI: A/Ⓐ
H_2S: Negative
Indole: Negative
MR: Negative
VP: Positive
Citrate: Positive
Motility: Positive
Ornithine: Positive
Deaminase (phenylalanine): Negative
Fermentation of:
L-arabinose: Positive
D-mannitol: Positive
D-mannose: Positive
Rhamnose: Positive
Trehalose: Positive
D-xylose: Positive

The significant *Enterobacter* species can be biochemically distinguished by using the reactions found in **TABLE 10-10**.

Most *Enterobacter* infections are opportunistic and include urinary and respiratory tract and wound infections. *E. cloacae* and *E. aerogenes* are the most frequent clinical isolates. *E. cloacae* is associated with urinary and respiratory tract and wound infections as well as infections of the blood. *E. cloacae* has been isolated from contaminated intravenous fluids and other medical instrumentation. *E. cloacae* and *E. aerogenes* also are associated with a variety of other infections, such as endocarditis and meningitis. *E. cancerogenus* (previously *E. taylorae* and CDC enteric group 19) has been isolated from several clinical sources, including bone and wound infections. *E. cancerogenus* is unique in the genus *Enterobacter* because it is lactose negative but ONPG positive. *E. sakazakii* biochemically resembles *E. cloacae* but can be differentiated by its yellow pigment, which intensifies at 25°C. *E. sakazakii* has been associated with neonatal sepsis and meningitis. *E. gergoviae* resembles *E. aerogenes* but can be differentiated by its strong urease activity and inability to ferment adonitol and sorbitol. *E. gergoviae* has been isolated as the agent in infections of the urinary and respiratory tracts

TABLE 10-10 Characteristics of *Enterobacter*

Reaction	*E. aerogenes*	*E. cloacae*	*E. gergoviae*	*E. sakazakii*	*E. cancerogenus taylorae*	*E. hormaechei*
Lysine	+	–	+	–	–	–
Arginine	–	+	–	+	+	**V**
Ornithine	+	+	+	+	+	+
VP	+	+	+	+	+	+
Fermentation of:						
Adonitol	+	**V**	–	–	–	–
D-arabitol	+	–	+	+	–	–
Lactose	+	+	**V**	+	–	–
Melibiose	+	+	+	+	–	–
Raffnose	+	+	+	+	–	–
Sucrose	+	+	+	+	–	+
Salicin	+	+	+	+	+	**V**
Sorbitol	+	+	–	–	–	–
Urease	–	**V**	+	–	–	+
Yellow pigment	–	–	–	+	–	–

V, reactions are variable

and blood. *E. hormaechei* (formerly enteric group 75) is both urease and sucrose positive and has been found to cause a variety of infections, including septicemia.

Serratia

Serratia organisms are opportunistic pathogens that are unique in their ability to produce the enzymes deoxyribonuclease (DNase), lipase, and gelatinase. Significant reactions of this genus are shown in **TABLE 10-11**.

There are seven species of *Serratia* found in humans. The most significant species is *S. marcescens*, which is associated with pneumonia and septicemia in immunosuppressed patients, including those undergoing chemotherapy. The organism is found in the environment and also as a commensal and may colonize the hands of health care personnel. Thus, nosocomial infections in patients undergoing catheterization and other types of medical instrumentation also may result from *S. marcescens*. The organism also has been isolated as a neonatal pathogen, causing septicemia. Because of its production of proteolytic enzymes and its ability to resist the actions of antibiotics, including cephalothin and colistin, *S. marcescens* is particularly invasive and destructive. Although almost half of all *S. marcescens* isolates produce a red pigment when incubated at room temperature, less than 5% produce this pigment when incubated at 37°C.

TABLE 10-11 Biochemical Reactions for *Serratia*

TSI: K/A H_2S—Negative
VP: Positive
ADH: Negative
LDC: Positive
Urease: Negative
Deaminase (phenylalanine): Negative
Lipase: Positive
Gelatinase: Positive
DNase: Positive
MacConkey: Clear colonies (lactose negative)

S. liquefaciens is differentiated from *S. marcescens* by its ability to ferment arabinose. *S. rubidaea* produces a red pigment, whereas *S. oderifera* produces a rancid, potato-like odor. *S. rubidaea* and *S. oderifera* are rare causes of human infections.

Hafnia

Hafnia alvei (formerly *Enterobacter alvei*) resembles the genus *Enterobacter* but can be distinguished by its inability to ferment lactose, sucrose, sorbitol, and raffinose.

H. alvei also is citrate negative. *H. alvei* is differentiated from *Serratia* because it is DNase negative and lipase negative. Although it has been recovered from a number of human sources, including stools and wounds, the clinical significance of *H. alvei* is still questionable. The organism is found in the gastrointestinal tract of many mammals and also in a variety of foods, including minced pork and beef products. *Hafnia* is an infrequent human pathogen but has been isolated in cases of bacteremia, respiratory tract infections, and gastroenteritis.

Pantoea

Pantoea agglomerans (formerly *Enterobacter agglomerans* group) has been isolated from several sources in nature and in the environment, including animal sources. Of particular note is the organism's isolation from contaminated intravenous fluids in a large outbreak of septicemia in the 1970s. In addition to having a yellow pigment, *P. agglomerans* can be identified by negative reactions for arginine, lysine, and ornithine, which is referred to as triple decarboxylase negative.

TABLE 10-12 summarizes reactions of *Pantoea*, *Hafnia*, and *Serratia*.

Salmonella

Salmonella is a very complex genus and the only genus in the tribe Salmonelleae. There are more than 2,400 serotypes with the Kauffman-White classification based on somatic (O) and flagellar (H) antigens. *Salmonella typhi* also has a capsular, or virulence (Vi), antigen. The *Salmonella* species are grouped according to the somatic, or O, antigen (A, B, C, etc.) and subdivided into serotypes (1, 2, 3, etc.) on the basis of the flagellar (H) antigen. The serogroups are designated as A_1, A_2, B, B_2, etc.). Before 1983 three species of *Salmonella* existed: *S. typhi*, *S. choleraesuis*, and *S. enteritidis*. Unique serotypes are given names that describe the disease or animal from which the organism was isolated. Also, serotypes are named for the specific geographic location where the organism was isolated. In 1983 it was determined through DNA hybridization that only one species of *Salmonella* existed, *S. choleraesuis*. *S. choleraesuis* was subsequently divided into seven subspecies. *Arizonae*, once considered a separate genus (*Arizona*), was then classified as a *Salmonella* subspecies. Later, *S. bongori* was determined to be significantly different from the other *Salmonella* and was classified in a separate species. Later, a determination was made that *S. enterica* was a more appropriate species name for the other *Salmonella*. Current classification names for *S. enterica*, which has six subspecies, and *S. bongori* are shown in BOX 10-4.

Subgroup I is usually isolated from humans and other warm-blooded animals. It is highly pathogenic for humans and is usually not found in environmental sources or in cold-blooded animals. The other subgroups (II, IIIa, IIIb, IV, and VI) and *Salmonella bongori* (formerly subgroup V) are usually isolated from cold-blooded animals and the environment but not from humans or other warm-blooded animals. Almost all pathogenic clinical isolates of *Salmonella* are from subgroup I. This subgroup includes *Salmonella enterica* serotype Typhi, *Salmonella enterica* serotype Paratyphi, *Salmonella enterica* serotype Choleraesuis, *Salmonella enterica* serotype Gallinarum, and

TABLE 10-12 Summary of Reactions of *Pantoea*, *Hafnia*, and *Serratia*

Reaction	*Pantoea*	*H. alvei*	*S. marcescens*	*S. liquefaciens*
LDC	–	+	+	+
ADH	–		–	–
ODC	–	+	+	+
DNase (25°C)	–	–	+	+
Gelatinase (22°C)	–		+	+
Fermentation of:				
L-arabinose	+	+		+
Adonitol	–	–	**V**	–
myo-Inositol		–	+	+
Sucrose	**V**	–	+	+

V, reactions are variable

BOX 10-4 ***Salmonella* Nomenclature**

Salmonella subgroup	Former genus	Subspecies	Serotypes within subspecies
I	*Salmonella*	*enterica subsp. enterica*	1,454
II	*Salmonella*	*enterica subsp. salamae*	489
IIIa	*Arizona*	*enterica subsp. arizonae*	94
IIIb	*Arizona*	*enterica subsp. diarizonae*	324
IV	*Salmonella*	*enterica subsp. houtenae*	70
VI	*Salmonella*	*enterica subsp. indica*	12
	Salmonella	*bongori [formerly subsp. V]*	20
		Total serotypes	2,463

Subgroup I habitat is warm-blood animals; all other subgroups and S. bongori are found in the environment and in cold-blooded animals.

Salmonella enterica serotype Pullorum. *Salmonella* nomenclature is found in BOX 10-4

Salmonella should be suspected when lactose-negative, H_2S-positive colonies are isolated from a stool culture. Important reactions for the genus *Salmonella* are shown in **TABLE 10-13**.

S. typhi should be suspected if a lactose-negative organism produces a small amount of H_2S in the TSI agar at the point of inoculation, appearing as a curved wedge. The organism is citrate negative, ornithine negative, fails to produce gas in the TSI medium, and is generally less biochemically active when compared to other *Salmonella*.

TABLE 10-13 Biochemical Reactions of *Salmonella*

TSI: K/ⒶH_2S—Positive
Motility: Positive
MR: Positive
VP: Negative
Indole: Negative
Lysine: Positive
Urease: Negative
Deaminase (phenylalanine): Negative
Fermentation of:
D-mannitol: Positive
***myo*-Inositol:** Negative
Sucrose: Negative
MacConkey: Clear (lactose negative)
Hektoen enteric: Green with black centers (lactose negative, H_2S positive)

Salmonella subgroups can be differentiated through the reactions found in **TABLE 10-14.**

There are over 1 million cases of *Salmonella* in the United States each year, which result in over 500 deaths annually. Types of *Salmonella* infections include the **enteric fevers**, which result from infection by *Salmonella enterica* serotype Typhi. Humans are the only source for this infection, which is acquired through ingestion of fecally contaminated food or water. The incidence of typhoid fever is high in developing countries, and there are approximately 400 cases each year in the United States. Many of these infections are acquired during foreign travel. The incubation period is approximately 1 to 2 weeks. Fever, headache, and vomiting occur, and the patient appears ill in 2 to 3 weeks. The fever eventually declines, and the patient usually recovers in the fourth week with appropriate therapy. *S. typhi* attacks the lymphoid tissue and the reticuloendothelial system and is able to grow intracellularly within monocytes. The organism can be isolated from blood cultures early in the illness (weeks 1 and 2), from the urine later in the illness (weeks 3 and 4), and indefinitely from the stool. Bismuth sulfite and brilliant green agar are suitable for the isolation of *Salmonella* serotype Typhi. The organism produces characteristic metallic colonies, with a black ring, on bismuth sulfite agar. Most other Enterobacteriaceae cannot grow on these highly selective media. The Widal test, which is usually performed in reference laboratories, detects an individual's antibody to the specific O and H antigens of *S. typhi*.

The most common *Salmonella* infection is gastroenteritis, which can be spread through asymptomatic human

TABLE 10-14 Differentiation of *Salmonella* Subgroups

Reaction	I	II	IIIa	IIIb	IV	VI	*S. bongori*
ONPG	–	–	+	+	–	**V**	+
Potassium cyanide (KCN) growth	–	–	–	–	+	–	+
Dulcitol fermentation	+	+	–	–	–	**V**	+
Gelatinase (37°C)	–	+	+	+	+	+	–
Lactose fermentation	–	–	–	+	–	–	–
Malonate utilization	–	+	+	+	–	–	–
Salicin	–	–	–	–	+	–	–

V, reactions are variable

carriers, the fecal–oral route, contaminated water or food products, and direct contact with infected pets or animals. Contamination rates from *Salmonella* are high in slaughterhouses, where the organism can be spread easily from animal to animal. *Salmonella* organisms are primarily pathogenic for humans and animals; many animal sources, including poultry (chicken, ducks, turkeys), pets (dogs, cats, hamsters, turtles), and numerous other animals (pigs, sheep, cows, donkeys, snakes, parrots) are known to harbor nontyphoid *Salmonella*. Human infection is acquired by ingestion of contaminated food or food products and water or milk contaminated by human or animal feces or through contaminated hands. Approximately half of all *Salmonella* infections are relegated to contaminated poultry or poultry products. The organism can enter hen eggs through small cracks in the shell and then contaminate the egg. The Egg Products Inspection Act of 1970 requires pasteurization of all egg products and has reduced the amount of contamination of egg products in the United States.

The most frequently isolated serotypes of *Salmonella* in the United States are *S.* Typhimurium (~20%), *S.* Enteritidis (~18%), and *S.* Newport (~10%). There are several historic *Salmonella* **outbreaks** that are worthy of discussion. In 1985, the Illinois water supply was contaminated by a faulty valve in a large commercial milk supply. There were 16,000 culture-confirmed cases and 150,000 to 200,000 individuals believed to be actually infected. In 1990, *Salmonella*-contaminated eggs were reported to be used in foods prepared using raw or undercooked eggs, including homemade eggnog and homemade mayonnaise, which served as vehicles for the infection. Also in 1990, *Salmonella* serotype Enteritidis was implicated in an outbreak with a nationally distributed ice cream brand that involved 41 states and over 200,000 people infected. Investigations determined that contaminated eggs in a truck that transported ice cream were the source of infection.

Reptiles are commonly colonized with *Salmonella* and shed the organism in their feces. There have been incidences of infection related to children playing with reptiles; one such incident occurred in the 1970s when there were many cases of salmonellosis related to small pet turtles. The Food and Drug Administration banned the sale of pet turtles to prevent infection. Since 1986, the frequency of iguanas and other reptiles as pets has increased, leading to increased salmonella infections. Reptile-associated *Salmonella* infections account for approximately 70,000 cases in the United States each year, or over 5% of all occurrences. Young children and the immunocompromised are at high risk for reptile- and amphibian-associated salmonellosis with complications such as bacteremia.

More recent outbreaks of *Salmonella* are summarized in BOX 10-5. This box illustrates the wide range of infection sources and serotypes isolated in recent outbreaks. Public health investigators use DNA "fingerprints" of the bacteria collected during the outbreaks and pulsed-field gel electrophoresis (PFGE) to identify cases of illness that may be included in a particular outbreak. PulseNet, a national subtyping network made up of state and local public health laboratories and federal food regulatory laboratories, performs molecular surveillance of food-borne infection in the investigation of these outbreaks.

Salmonella Enteritidis can be mild or severe and is characterized by a low fever, nausea, vomiting, and diarrhea. The signs typically occur within 1 day after ingestion of the organism. However, *Salmonella* infections also can present as bacteremia or septicemia. In addition to gastrointestinal signs, the patient may have a high, spiking fever. Blood cultures usually are positive. *Salmonella* also

BOX 10-5 ***Salmonella* Outbreaks**

Year	Source of infection	Serotype	Description
2006	Tomatoes	*Salmonella* Typhimurium	183 cases in 21 states; tomatoes eaten in restaurants
2007	Pot pies	*Salmonella* I 4,[5],12:i:–	272 cases in 35 states associated with specific brand of pot pies
	Pet food	*Salmonella* Schwarzengrund	65 cases in 20 states who had eaten specific brands of pet food
	Peanut butter	*Salmonella* Tennessee	425 cases in 44 states; linked to specific peanut butter brands
2008	Raw produce	*Salmonella* Saintpaul	1,442 cases in 42 states; jalapeño and serrano peppers and a contaminated water source
	Rice/wheat cereals	*Salmonella* Agona	
	Cantaloupes	*Salmonella* Litchfield	51 cases in 16 states linked to one supplier
2009	Alfalfa sprouts	*Salmonella* Saintpaul	235 cases in 14 states; contaminated alfalfa seeds
	Peanut butter	*Salmonella* Typhimurium	714 cases in 44 states; specific brands of peanut butter
2010	Alfalfa sprouts	*Salmonella* I 4,[5],12:i:–	140 cases from 26 states; related to a restaurant chain
	Shell eggs	*Salmonella* Enteritidis	1,939 cases from specific egg suppliers; ingestion of raw or undercooked eggs
	Frozen fruit pulp	*Salmonella* Typhi (typhoid fever)	9 cases in one state through ingestion of bacteria in smoothie-type drink; this is the agent of typhoid fever
	Restaurant chain	*Salmonella* Hartford and *Salmonella* Baildon	155 cases in 21 states; no specific food item could be identified
	Frozen rodents	*Salmonella* I 4,[5],12:i:–	34 cases in 17 states; frozen food for pet reptiles
	Alfalfa sprouts	*Salmonella* Newport	44 cases in 11 states; wholesale distributors and restaurants
	Red and black pepper/ luncheon meats	*Salmonella* Montevideo	272 cases in 44 states; pepper used in salami meats
	Water frogs	*Salmonella* Typhimurium	85 cases in 31 states; majority were children handling pet frogs that carried the organisms
2011	Clinical and teaching microbiology laboratories	*Salmonella* Typhimurium	
	African dwarf frogs	*Salmonella* Typhimurium	Over 200 cases in 41 states; water frogs that carried the organism
	Turkey burgers	*Salmonella* Hadar	12 cases in 10 states; raw turkey meat produced by one company
	Cantaloupe	*Salmonella* Panama	11 cases in 5 states; cantaloupe sold in national warehouse-type store
2012	Chicken	*Salmonella* Heidelberg	128 persons infected from 13 states
	Peanut butter	*Salmonella* Bredeney	42 individuals from 20 states from peanut butter produced in one warehouse
	Live poultry	*Salmonella* Hadar	46 persons from 11 states; infections were linked to chicks, ducklings, and other live poultry from a single hatchery
	Frozen raw yellow fin tuna	*Salmonella* Bareilly and *Salmonella* Nchanga	425 persons from 28 states were infected with frozen raw yellow fin tuna product, known as Nakaochi Scrape
2013	Hedgehogs	*Salmonella* Typhimurium	20 persons from 8 states through contact with hedgehogs, including African pygmy hedgehogs, or their environments
	Ground meat	*Salmonella* Typhimurium	22 persons from 6 states from a single source of ground meat
	Turtles	*Salmonella* Sandiego, strains A and C; *Salmonella* Newport, strain A; *Salmonella* Pomona, strain A; *Salmonella* Poona, strain A	371 persons from 40 states from contact with small turtles
	Chicken	*Salmonella* Heidelberg	28 individuals from 13 states from consumption of contaminated chicken

Data from Centers for Disease Control, http://www.cdc.gov/salmonella/outbreaks.html

may be carried by those who have had a prior infection. The organism is shed in the stool for up to 1 year after the active infection, which may serve as a reservoir for infection. Infections are most serious in the very young and very old, as well as in those who are immunocompromised.

Salmonella enterica subspecies *arizonae*, formerly *Arizonae hinshawii*, is identified through positive malonate and negative dulcitol fermentation. It is ONPG positive, whereas all other *Salmonella* are negative. It is primarily found in reptiles and may cause a range of infections, from mild gastroenteritis to enteric fever and septicemia.

Full serotyping of *Salmonella* is important for public health and is generally performed in reference or public health laboratories. Serotyping is needed to confirm the specific serotype.

PROTEEAE

The tribe Proteeae includes the genera *Proteus*, *Providencia*, and *Morganella*. Important characteristics of the Proteeae are shown in **TABLE 10-15**.

Proteus

Proteus organisms are found in the environment in soil and water and are normal flora of the human gastrointestinal tract. The genus is characterized by its rapid urease activity and its typical swarming motility on blood agar. There are five recognized species: *P. mirabilis*, *P. penneri*, *P. vulgaris*, *P. myxofaciens*, and *P. hauseri*. Important biochemical reactions and characteristics for the genus *Proteus* are shown in **TABLE 10-16**.

P. mirabilis is the most frequently isolated species of *Proteus* in human infection. It is an important cause of urinary tract infections, such as cystitis and pyelonephritis and also has been shown to be a cause of pneumonia and septicemia. *P. mirabilis* is indole negative and susceptible to both ampicillin and the cephalosporins. Another human pathogen, *P. vulgaris*, is associated with similar infections, causing urinary tract infections that may be nosocomial and affect immunosuppressed patients and those receiving prolonged antibiotic therapy. *P. vulgaris* is indole positive.

TABLE 10-15 Biochemical Reactions of Tribe Proteeae

Lactose fermentation: Negative
Deaminase (phenylalanine): Positive
Arginine: Positive
Malonate: Negative
Motility: Positive

TABLE 10-16 Biochemical Reactions and Characteristics of *Proteus*

TSI: K/ⒶH_2S—Positive
Swarming motility on sheep blood agar:
Urease: Rapidly positive (within 4 hours)
Blood agar: Growth in waves or swarms
KCN growth: Positive
MR: Positive
Lysine: Negative
Arginine: Negative
ONPG: Negative
Acid production from:
D-adonitol: Negative
L-arabinose: Negative
Cellobiose: Negative
Glucose: Positive
Lactose: Negative
D-mannitol: Negative
MacConkey: Clear colonies (lactose negative)

P. penneri resembles *P. vulgaris*, but it is H_2S, salicin, and indole negative. *P. penneri* has been associated with urinary tract and wound infections. *P. myxofaciens*, a rare human isolate, also is indole negative. In general, the indole-negative *P. mirabilis* is more susceptible to antibiotics when compared to *P. vulgaris* and *P. penneri*. *P. mirabilis* has intrinsic resistance to tetracycline and nitrofurantoin but is usually susceptible to ampicillin, amoxicillin, the cephalosporins, and other antibiotics. *Proteus* can be presumptively identified if colonies on sheep blood agar are swarming and oxidase negative. Indole-positive colonies that give a positive ODC reaction are most likely *P. mirabilis*, whereas colonies that are both indole and ODC negative are most likely *P. penneri*. If the colonies are indole positive, the organism is most likely *P. vulgaris*. *Proteus* species can be differentiated using the reactions found in **TABLE 10-17**.

Providencia

Providencia organisms are lactose-negative, deaminase-positive, H_2S-negative, motile members of Proteeae. The organisms ferment mannose and do not swarm on blood agar, and most species are citrate positive. There are currently five species of *Providentia*: *P. alcalifaciens*,

TABLE 10-17 Differentiation of *Proteus*

Reaction	*P. mirabilis*	*P. vulgaris*	*P. penneri*	*P. myxofaciens*
Indole	–	+	–	–
ODC	+	–	–	–
Fermentation of:				
Maltose	–	+	+	+
D-xylose	+	+	+	–
Salicin	–	+	–	–
Sucrose	–	+	+	+
Esculin hydrolysis	–	+	+	+
Chloramphenicol	S	R	R	S

R = organism is resistant
S = organism is susceptible

TABLE 10-18 Important Biochemical Reactions for *Providentia*

Deaminase (phenylalanine): Positive
Arginine: Negative
Lysine: Negative
Ornithine: Negative
VP: Negative
H_2S: Negative
Citrate: Positive
ONPG: Negative
Esculin hydrolysis: Negative
Acid production from:
D-arabinose: Negative
D-mannose: Positive
Maltose: Negative
D-sorbitol: Negative

P. heimbachae, *P. rettgeri*, *P. rustigianni*, and *P. stuartii*. Their biochemical reactions are summarized in **TABLE 10-18**.

Providentia species have been found in specimens from the urine, throat, stool, and blood and from wounds. *P. rettgeri* and *P. stuartii* have been associated with human infections. *P. rettgeri* is the only urease-positive *Providencia* species and is associated with nosocomial infections of the urinary tract and skin. The urinary tract infections may involve patients with predisposing urological problems, whereas the skin infections are often found in burn patients.

P. stuartii also has been associated with urinary tract infections in those with indwelling urinary catheters.

TABLE 10-19 Differentiation of *Providencia* Species

Reaction	*P. rettgeri*	*P. stuartii*	*P. alcalifaciens*
Urease	+	*	–
Fermentation of:			
D-adonitol	+	–	+
D-arabitol	+	–	–
D-mannitol	+	–	–
L-rhammose	+	+	–
Trehalose	–	+	–

*Most strains are negative.

P. rettgeri has been found occasionally in nosocomial urinary tract and wound infections, especially in those with burn wounds. *P. rettgeri* and *P. stuartii* usually are susceptible to amikacin but resistant to gentamycin and tobramycin; urinary tract infections can be treated with extended spectrum cephalosporins and other antibiotics. The *Providentia* species can be differentiated, as shown in **TABLE 10-19**.

Morganella

M. morganii is the only species within the genus *Morganella*. *Morganella* organisms give negative reactions for lactose, citrate, H_2S, and LDC. The genus is urease and deaminase positive. *Morganella* is an opportunistic pathogen, and infections include gastrointestinal disease and urinary tract and wound infections. Infections are most frequently seen in immunosuppressed patients and those undergoing prolonged antibiotic therapy. More serious infections include septicemia and abscesses.

Important biochemical reactions of *Morganella morganii* are found in **TABLE 10-20**.

TABLE 10-21 summarizes the important reactions to differentiate members within the tribe Proteeae.

Citrobacter

Citrobacter organisms resemble *Salmonella* but are ONPG positive and LDC negative. There are 11 species of *Citrobacter*; the *Citrobacter freundii* complex includes the species *C. freundii*, as well as other species. The important human pathogens are *C. freundii* and *C. diversus*, which are associated with urinary and respiratory tract infections. Many of the infections are nosocomial or community acquired. *C. freundii* also is associated with septicemia, wound infections, and gastroenteritis. *C. diversus* has been found to cause meningitis.

TABLE 10-20 Biochemical Reactions of *Morganella morganii*

Indole: Positive
Methyl red: Positive
VP: Negative
H_2S: Negative
Citrate: Negative
Urease: Positive
Deaminase (phenylalanine): Positive
Arginine: Negative
Growth in KCN: Positive
Esculin hydrolysis: Negative
Acid production from:
D-arabinose: Negative
D-mannose: Positive
Maltose: Negative
D-sorbitol: Negative

TABLE 10-22 lists important biochemical reactions in the identification of *Citrobacter* species.

TABLE 10-23 describes how to differentiate *Salmonella* from *Citrobacter.*

TABLE 10-22 Differentiation of *Citrobacter* Species

Reaction	*C. freundii*	*C. diversus*
TSI	A/Ⓐ* or K/A	K/A
Gas	+	+
H_2S	+	–
MR	+	+
VP	–	–
Indole	–	+
Citrate	+	+
Deaminase (phenylalanine)	–	–
Urease	**V**	**V**
Motility	+	+
LDC	–	–
ADH	**V**	**V**
ODC	**V**	+
ONPG	+	+
MacConkey	Pink or clear	Clear
KCN (growth)	+	–

A/Ⓐ acid slant over acid deep; K/A, alkaline slant over acid deep; **V**, variable

Certain strains of *C. freundii* produce a unique TSI of A/A, H_2S positive.

Edwardsiella

Edwardsiella has been isolated from the environment and many cold-blooded and warm-blooded animals, including reptiles, freshwater and aquarium fish, frogs, and turtles. The most important species for human infections is *E. tarda*, which has been identified as the source of gastrointestinal infection, mainly in the tropics and subtropics.

TABLE 10-21 Differentiation of Clinically Important Members of the Tribe Proteeae

Reaction	*P. vulgaris*	*P. mirabilis*	*M. morganii*	*Providentia rettgeri*	*Providentia stuartii*
TSI	K/Ⓐ	K/Ⓐ	K/A	K/A	K/A
H_2S	+	+	–	–	–
Gas	+	+	+	–	–
MR	+	+	+	+	+
VP	–	**V**	–	–	–
Indole	+	–	+	+	+
Citrate	–	**V**	–	+	+
Deaminase (phenylalanine)	+	+	+	+	+
Urease	+	+	+	+	*
Motility	**S**/+	**S**/+	+	+	+
LDC	–	–	–	–	–
ADH	–	–	–	–	–
ODC	–	+	+	–	–

K/A, alkaline slant over acid deep; **V**, variable; **S**, swarms

*Most strains are negative.

TABLE 10-23 Differentiation of *Salmonella* from *Citrobacter*

Reaction	*Salmonella*	*Citrobacter*
Potassium cyanide (KCN) growth	−	+
Lysine	+	−
ONPG	−	+

It is the agent of wound infections, abscesses, and systemic infections in those with existing liver disease. Infections may occur following trauma or accidents involving the aquatic environment. *Edwardsiella* is identified by the abundance of H_2S in the TSI agar. It biochemically resembles *E. coli*, except *Edwardsiella* is H_2S positive and lactose negative. Important reactions for *Edwardsiella* are as follows in **TABLE 10-24**.

Yersinia

Yersinia organisms are small coccobacilli that exhibit bipolar staining. They are classified in the tribe Yersinieae and were originally named *Pasturella* but later were named for the French bacteriologist Yersin in 1894. *Yersinia* produce small, pinpoint colonies on MacConkey agar; optimal growth is observed at 25°C to 30°C, and growth is enhanced by continued incubation at room temperature. *Yersinia* are facultative anaerobes and catalase positive and oxidase negative. *Yersinia* should be suspected if

TABLE 10-24 Biochemical Reactions of *Edwardsiella*

TSI: K/A H_2S—Positive
Lactose: Negative
Indole: Positive
MR: Positive
VP: Negative
Citrate: Negative
Motility: Positive
Urease: Negative
Deaminase (phenylalanine): Negative
ONPG: Negative
Lysine: Positive
Arginine: Negative
Ornithine: Positive
Fermentation of:
Maltose: Positive
Mannitol: Negative
Sucrose: Negative

TABLE 10-25 Biochemical Reactions of *Yersinia*

TSI: Alk/A or A/Alk (*Y. pestis*)
H_2S: Negative
Deaminase: Negative
Motile at 22°C and nonmotile at 37°C

the TSI is yellow over orange at 24 hours. This reaction occurs because of weak acid production in the slant with no change in the deep. *Yersinia* species are also nonmotile at 37°C, and all except *Y. pestis* are motile at room temperature (25°C to 30°C).

There are three important human pathogens: *Y. pestis*, the agent of plague; *Y. enterocolitica*, and *Y. pseudotuberculosis*. Important reactions for *Yersinia* are shown in **TABLE 10-25**, and speciation of *Yersinia* is shown in **TABLE 10-26**.

Y. pestis is the agent of **plague**, which is a zoonosis and transmitted via the flea–rodent life cycle. Plague is an ancient disease; however, it persists even today. Three types of plague exist: bubonic, septicemic, and pneumonic, of which bubonic plague is the most common. Bubonic plague is a highly fatal zoonosis and has been associated with three **pandemics**. The Justinian Plague, or 1st Pandemic of Plague, occurred from 541–544 CE and was found in the areas of Egypt to the Middle East and Mediterranean Europe. The second pandemic, known as the Black Death, occurred from 1347–1351 CE and involved areas of the Black Sea to Sicily and all of Europe. It is estimated that 17 to 28 million Europeans, or 30% to 40% of the entire population of Europe, was affected. Pandemics continued to occur in 2- to 5-year cycles and then occurred less frequently into the 17th century. The third pandemic, or the Modern Pandemic, began in 1855 in China and then

TABLE 10-26 Speciation of *Yersinia*

Reaction	*Y. pestis*	*Y. pseudotuberculosis*	*Y. enterocolitica*
Motility (25°C)	−	+	+
Ornithine	−	−	+
Urease	−	+	+
Fermentation of:			
Sucrose	−	−	+
Rhamnose	−	+	−
Sorbitol	−	−	+

spread to Hong Kong and Bombay in 1896. It continued to spread to Egypt, Portugal, Japan, Paraguay, and Eastern Africa and to Manila by 1899. The disease reached San Francisco by boat in 1900 and also appeared in New York, New Orleans, and Brazil. Local epidemics continued over the world until the 1950s when the pandemic ended. There have been 400 cases of plague reported in the United States between 1947 and 1996, with 60 deaths. Bubonic plague accounts for over 80% of the cases.

The route of infection is either rodent to rodent or rodent to flea to human. Thus, humans acquire the infection by an infected flea bite or by handling infected animal hides or products. The organism is endemic in the southwestern and Pacific areas of the United States and is concentrated in the four corners region of Utah, Colorado, Arizona, and New Mexico. The organism is harbored in rats, squirrels, rabbits, chipmunks, and prairie dogs. Sylvatic plague is concentrated in the four corners region, while urban plague is associated with the urban rat population throughout the country. Peridomestic exposure occurs when domestic animals, such as cats or rodents, carry fleas into the house. Individuals may acquire *Y. pestis* infection if bit by an infected flea.

The bacteria either invade the skin through the flea bite or are inhaled and then enter the macrophage and polymorphonuclear neutrophils. *Y. pestis* multiplies within the white blood cells, producing a protein and lipoprotein antigen. It then lyses the cell and escapes. *Y. pestis* is resistant to phagocytosis because of a protective antigen that enters the host's white blood cells. Clinical symptoms include swelling of the cervical, axillary, and inguinal lymph nodes, and it may be hematogenously spread to organs and tissues. Additional effects include disseminated intravascular coagulation, endotoxic shock, and dark discoloration of extremities.

Plague is diagnosed through blood cultures and Gram stains of lymph nodes (buboes), as well as through Wright stained blood smears. The organism stains as a small, gram-negative coccobacillus. On blood smears, it may be intracellular to macrophage and exhibit a bipolar or "safety pin" appearance. It is slow growing on ordinary media and has the appearance of beaten copper under a stereoscope, and the TSI shows weak acid in slant with little or no change in deep (yellow/red).

Y. enterocolitica is the most common *Yersinia* species isolated from humans. It is the agent of **enterocolitis**, and occurs most frequently in infants and children. In adults the bacterium is also an agent for enterocolitis, ileitis, and septicemia. Animals serve as the major route of infection, and humans may acquire the infection through ingestion of contaminated water, pork, beef, or milk products. Fecal–oral transmission also has been implicated as a route of infection.

Because *Y. enterocolitica* produces small colonies on selective media, it may be overgrown by other Enterobacteriaceae. Also, because it ferments sucrose, *Y. enterocolitica* may be mistaken as normal flora coliform on EMB and Hektoen enteric agars. For these reasons, it is recommended that cefsulodin-irgasan-novobiocin (CIN) medium be used to enhance the isolation of *Y. enterocolitica*. CIN medium contains mannitol, peptones, yeast, neutral red indicator, and the inhibitory agents crystal violet, novobiocin, irgasan, and cefsulodin. The crystal violet is inhibitory for gram-negative bacteria. Novobiocin inhibits gram-positive cocci, and cefsulodin is a cephalosporin that inhibits gram-positive bacteria (except the *Enterococcus*) and most gram-negative bacilli. CIN is selective for *Y. enterocolitica*, *Aeromonas* species, and *Plesiomonas shigelloides*. *Y. enterocolitica* ferments mannitol and appears as red "bull's-eye" colonies surrounded by a colorless halo. The species is ODC positive and ferments both sucrose and sorbitol.

Y. pseudotuberculosis is endemic in many wild animals and game fowl and is a rare cause of lymphadenitis in children. The species is ODC negative and fails to ferment both sucrose and sorbitol. Table 10-25 summarizes the important reactions for *Yersinia* species.

Miscellaneous Members of Enterobacteriaceae

There are many new members of Enterobacteriaceae that are less frequently associated with human infection than those that have been discussed in this chapter. These include *Arsenophonus*, *Buttiauxella*, *Cedecea*, *Erwinia*, *Ewingella*, *Kluyvera*, *Leminorella*, *Moellerella*, *Plesiomonas*, *Photorhabdus*, *Tatumella*, and *Xenorhabdus*.

Antibiotic Susceptibility and Treatment

Many members of Enterobacteriaceae produce extended spectrum β-lactamases and other β-lactamases that produce resistance against many β-lactam drugs. Thus, all clinical isolates must be tested using appropriate antibiotic susceptibility procedures. Aminoglycosides, β-lactams, and quinolones may be used to treat most infections from *E. coli*, *Enterobacter*, *Proteus*, *Providentia*, *Citrobacter*, and *Serratia* infections. Gastrointestinal infections require rehydration therapy, in addition to antibiotics when appropriate.

Laboratory Procedures

Procedure
MacConkey agar

Purpose
MacConkey agar is a selective differential media that isolates gram-negative bacteria and also differentiates lactose fermenters from nonlactose fermenters.

Principle
The medium contains bile salts, neutral red, crystal violet, and lactose. Bile salts inhibit gram-positive bacteria, which allows for the isolation of gram-negative bacteria. Neutral red and crystal violet further inhibit the gram-positive bacteria. Neutral red indicator is brown in pH 6.8 to 8.0 and pink-red at pH less than 6.8. Lactose is the only carbohydrate source, and those gram-negative bacteria that ferment lactose appear pink to red, whereas those that cannot ferment lactose are colorless.

Procedure

1. Streak agar for isolation.
2. Incubate at 35°C to 37°C for 18 to 24 hours and observe for growth and color.

Interpretation
If lactose is fermented, the medium is acidified, and bile salts are precipitated. The precipitated dye is absorbed, resulting in a pink-to-red complex.

Quality Control
Enterococcus faecalis: Partial to complete inhibition
Escherichia coli: Growth and lactose fermentation—pink-to-red colonies
Proteus mirabilis: Growth—colorless colonies

Procedure
Eosin-methylene blue (EMB) agar

Purpose
EMB agar is a selective differential medium that isolates for gram-negative enteric bacteria and also differentiates lactose fermenters (purple color to green metallic sheen) from nonlactose fermenters (colorless).

Principle
Eosin and methylene blue are dyes that inhibit the gram-positive bacteria and also indicate lactose fermentation. Lactose is the only carbohydrate source in most formulations, and its utilization results in an acidic pH. The eosin-methylene blue dye complex is taken up by lactose fermenters, which produce purple colonies. Those gram-negative enterics that cannot ferment lactose produce colorless, clear colonies

Procedure

1. Streak agar for isolation.
2. Incubate at 35°C to 37°C for 18 to 24 hours and observe for growth and color.

Interpretation
If lactose is fermented, precipitated eosin and methylene blue are absorbed, resulting in a purple color in the medium. A classic green metallic sheen is produced by *Escherichia coli*, which is a rapid lactose fermenter. Nonlactose fermenters produce colorless colonies on EMB.

Quality Control
Enterococcus faecalis: Partial to complete inhibition
Escherichia coli: Good growth with large colonies and a green metallic sheen
Proteus mirabilis: Good growth with large clear colonies

Notes
Some gram-positive bacteria, such as *Enterococcus* and staphylococci and yeast, may grow on EMB.

Procedure
Hektoen enteric agar

Purpose
Hektoen enteric medium is a moderately selective agar to isolate stool pathogens by inhibiting the normal flora coliforms of the lower gastrointestinal tract.

Principle
A high concentration of bile salts inhibits gram-positive bacteria and gram-negative coliforms. Lactose, sucrose, and salicin are the carbohydrate sources. Bromthymol blue is the pH indicator, which has a blue color for pH greater than 7.6, a green color for pH of 6.0 to 7.6, and a yellow color for pH less than 6.0. Sodium thiosulfate is the sulfur source for H_2S detection. H_2S combines with ferric ammonium citrate to form ferric sulfide (FeS), which is represented by

black-centered colonies. If one, two, or three of the carbohydrates are fermented, the colonies are orange in color. Nonfermenters produce greenish blue colonies.

Procedure

1. Streak agar for isolation.
2. Incubate at 35°C to 37°C for 18 to 24 hours and observe for growth and color. Observe color of colonies and color of medium surrounding colonies.

Interpretation

Pathogens appear as green colonies or green colonies with black centers. Yellow or orange colonies are considered normal flora except for *Yersinia enterocolitica,* which produces yellow colonies because of its fermentation of sucrose. Yellow, orange, or salmon-colored colonies indicate fermentation of one, two, or all of the carbohydrates. A black precipitate indicates production of hydrogen sulfide gas.

Quality Control

Escherichia coli: Partial inhibition—salmon-to-orange-colored growth
Salmonella enterica subspecies *enterica* serotype Typhimurium: Good growth—greenish blue with black centers
Shigella flexneri: Good growth—greenish blue

Procedure

Xylose lysine desoxycholate (XLD) agar

Purpose

XLD medium is a selective differential medium used for the isolation and differentiation of enteric pathogens.

Principle

The medium contains sodium desoxycholate, lysine, xylose, lactose, sucrose, phenol red, sodium thiosulfate, and ferric ammonium citrate. Sodium desoxycholate inhibits gram-positive bacteria, partially inhibits the growth of *Escherichia coli*, and inhibits the swarming of *Proteus.*

Phenol red indicator becomes yellow in acidic environments. Fermentation of xylose results in yellow colonies. Most members of Enterobacteriaceae are xylose positive, except for *Shigella*. Most strains of *Shigella* cannot ferment lactose and thus produce red colonies. Lysine permits the differentiation of *Salmonella*. Lysine-positive bacteria first produce yellow colonies as xylose is fermented, followed by red colonies, indicating lysine decarboxylation. Sodium thiosulfate provides a sulfur source, and H_2S-positive bacteria produce black centers from the reaction of H_2S with ferric ammonium citrate.

Procedure

1. Streak agar for isolation.
2. Incubate at 35°C to 37°C for 18 to 24 hours and observe for growth and color.

Interpretation

Salmonella typically produces red colonies with black centers, whereas *Citrobacter* and *Proteus* produce yellow colonies with black centers.

Quality Control

Escherichia coli: Good growth—yellow colonies
Salmonella enterica subspecies *enterica* serotype Typhimurium: Good growth—red colonies with black centers
Shigella flexneri: Good growth—red colonies

Notes

Salmonella will use all of the available xylose and then will decarboxylate lysine, which causes the pH to revert back to its alkaline color. Utilization of xylose, lactose, or sucrose causes the pH to become acidic, resulting in a yellow color.

Procedure

Salmonella–Shigella agar

Purpose

Salmonella–Shigella medium is a moderately selective and differential agar that provides for isolation and differentiation of enteric pathogens.

Principle

The medium contains bile salts, lactose, brilliant green agar, and neutral red indicator. Bile salts inhibit gram-positive bacteria, and brilliant green agar and bile salts inhibit the gram-negative coliforms. Lactose is the sole carbohydrate source. Neutral red indicator is red in acidic conditions. Lactose fermenters appear pink-red, whereas nonlactose fermenters appear clear. To detect H_2S production, sodium thiosulfate serves as a sulfur source. When H_2S is formed, it combines with ferric ammonium citrate to form ferric sulfide (FeS), which is represented by black-centered colonies.

Procedure

1. Streak agar for isolation.
2. Incubate at 35°C to 37°C for 18 to 24 hours and observe for growth and color.

Interpretation

Normal flora coliforms appear as pink-to-red colonies. *Shigella* appears as colorless colonies without black centers. *Salmonella* appears as colorless colonies with black centers.

Quality Control
Enterococcus faecalis: Partial to complete inhibition
Escherichia coli: Partial inhibition—pink-to-red colonies
Salmonella enterica subspecies *enterica* serotype Typhimurium: Good growth—colorless colonies with black centers
Shigella flexneri: Good growth—colorless colonies

Procedure
Triple sugar iron (TSI) agar

Purpose
TSI agar can be considered an initial step in the identification of the Enterobacteriaceae based on carbohydrate fermentation and hydrogen sulfide production.

Principle
TSI agar contains protein sources (beef extract, peptone, yeast extract, proteose peptone), which permit the growth of most bacterial strains. Three carbohydrates, lactose, sucrose, and glucose, are present. Glucose is in a concentration one-tenth that of the other carbohydrates. Ferrous sulfate is present as an indicator of hydrogen sulfide (H_2S) production. The indicator is phenol red, which is yellow in an acidic environment and red in an alkaline environment.

The TSI is a two-reaction chamber, with an aerobic slant portion and an anaerobic deep portion. The slant portion of the tube is exposed to atmospheric oxygen and will become alkaline as a result of oxidative decarboxylation of peptides and amino acids. The slant tends to become and remain alkaline (red). Amino acid degradation is minimal in the deep (anaerobic) portion, and thus a small quantity of acid produced can be detected because few amines are being formed from amino acids.

Bacteria that ferment glucose, but not lactose or sucrose, produce only small quantities of acid and cannot counteract the degradation of amino acids at the slant, which results in an alkaline pH resulting from oxidative decarboxylation. Such organisms characteristically produce an alkaline slant over an acid deep (K/A).

Organisms that ferment both glucose and lactose and/or sucrose produce large quantities of acid, which overcome the alkaline reaction of the slant, yielding an acid slant over an acid deep (A/A).

An organism incapable of fermenting glucose produces no change in the indicator and is characterized by an alkaline slant over an alkaline deep (K/K).

A sulfur source, sodium thiosulfate, provides sulfur atoms to detect the production of H_2S gas. H_2S reacts with iron salts (ferrous sulfate or ferric ammonium citrate) to produce the black precipitate of ferrous sulfide.

The production of gas during fermentation is indicated by the presence of cracks in the medium or the pulling away of the medium from the walls of the test tube. See Figure 10-5 for typical TSI reactions.

Materials
Selected members of Enterobacteriaceae nonfermentative gram-negative bacilli TSI slants

Procedure

1. Use a single, isolated 18- to 24-hour colony.
2. Select colony with sterile needle and stab within 0.5 inch of the bottom of the agar.
3. Streak colony up slant.
4. Leave cap on loosely and incubate at 35°C to 37°C for 18 to 24 hours.
5. Read and interpret results.

Interpretation
Yellow deep indicates fermentation of glucose only.
Yellow slant and yellow deep indicates fermentation of glucose and lactose and/or sucrose.
Red slant and red deep indicates a nonfermentative organism.
Black precipitate in deep indicates production of hydrogen sulfide.
Splitting or cracking of medium indicates gas production during fermentation process.

Quality control:
Escherichia coli: A/Ⓐ H_2S negative
Salmonella enterica subspecies *enterica* serotype Typhimurium: K/Ⓐ H_2S positive
Shigella flexneri: K/A H_2S negative

Notes

1. When all of the glucose has been used, organisms will use lactose and sucrose if they are able. The low oxygen concentration in the deep helps maintain an acidic pH once glucose has been fermented.
2. Incubating over 24 hours may cause acidic reactions in the slant to revert to alkaline.
3. If the caps are tightly closed, a false acidic reaction may occur in the slant. Loosened caps enhance alkaline conditions on the slant and allow the required free exchange of air.

4. Do not use an inoculating loop to stab the deep because it may split the medium and cause a false-positive gas production.
   A summary of TSI reactions follows:

Reaction	Carbohydrate fermented	Typical organisms
A/ⒶH_2S–	Glucose with acid and gas Lactose and/or sucrose with acid and gas	*Escherichia, Klebsiella, Enterobacter*
K/ⒶH_2S+	Glucose with acid and gas Lactose or sucrose not fermented	*Salmonella, Proteus, Citrobacter*
K/A H_2S–	Glucose with acid; no gas Lactose or sucrose not fermented	*Shigella, Providencia, Serratia, anaerogenic Escherichia coli*
A/ⒶH_2S+	Glucose fermented with gas Lactose or sucrose fermented	*Citrobacter freundii*
K/K H_2S–	Glucose not fermented Lactose or sucrose not fermented	*Pseudomonas, Alcaligenes*

Those species of *Proteus* that ferment sucrose may produce an acidic slant.

A, acid; Ⓐ, acid and gas; K, alkaline (no change)

Procedure

Indole broth

Purpose

Indole (tryptophan) broth is used for distinguishing Enterobacteriaceae based on the ability to produce indole from tryptophan. The test is particularly useful for the identification of lactose-fermenting members of Enterobacteriaceae. *Escherichia coli* is indole positive, whereas most *Enterobacter* and *Klebsiella* are indole negative. Indole also is useful in the speciation of *Proteus: P. mirabilis* is indole negative, whereas *P. vulgaris* is positive.

Principle

Tryptophan present in peptone is oxidized by certain bacteria to indole, skatole, and indoleacetic acid by the enzyme tryptophanase. Indole is detected in broth cultures of bacteria with an alcoholic *p*-dimethylaminobenzaldehyde reagent. Indole reacts with the aldehyde to form a red product. Either Kovach's or Erlich's reagent is used to detect indole. The reaction is summarized as follows:

Tryptophan → Indole + Pyruvic acid + Ammonia
tryptophanase

Indole + *p*-Dimethylaminobenzaldehyde → Red

Reagents and Media

Tryptophan (1%) broth
Kovac's or Ehrlich's reagent
Xylene or chloroform for extraction if using Ehrlich's reagent

Procedure

1. Inoculate indole broth with pure isolates of organisms.
2. Replace cap loosely and incubate at 35°C for 18 to 24 hours.
3. Add five drops of Kovac's reagent directly to the broth culture. Observe for a red color in the upper alcohol layer.
4. If using Ehrlich's reagent, first add 1 ml xylene or chloroform to the broth culture. Shake gently and then add five drops of reagent.

Interpretation

Negative reaction: No color development
Positive reaction: Red ring at the interface of reagent and broth (or reagent and xylene or chloroform)
Variable reaction: Orange color, indicates production of skatole, a methylated intermediate that may be a precursor to indole production

Quality Control

E. coli: Positive control—red ring
Enterobacter cloacae: Negative control—no color development

Note

Erlich's reagent is believed to be more sensitive than Kovac's and is recommended for indole detection in anaerobes and nonfermentative bacteria. Kovac's reagent was initially used to classify members of the Enterobacteriaceae and should be used with these organisms.

Procedure

Methyl red–Voges-Proskauer (MR-VP) tests

Purpose

MR-VP broth is a dextrose broth medium that is buffered with peptone and used to differentiate gram-negative bacteria. The tests are particularly useful for the lactose-fermenting Enterobacteriaceae. *Escherichia coli* is MR positive and VP negative, whereas most members of the *Klebsiella-Enterobacter-Serratia-Hafnia* group are VP positive.

Principle

MR-positive bacteria produce large amounts of mixed acid products (lactic, acetic, formic, and succinic) from the fermentation of glucose, leading to a decrease in the pH of the medium and a positive MR test. The pH must drop to 4.4 or less for the MR indicator to take on its acidic color of red.

VP-positive bacteria produce acetylmethyl carbinol (acetoin) as an intermediate product to butylene glycol during the fermentation of glucose. Acetoin is the neutral product detected in the VP reaction. In the presence of oxygen and 40% potassium hydroxide (KOH), acetoin is converted to the diacetyl form, which results in a red color in the presence of α-naphthol.

Media and Reagents

MR-VP broth: Glucose base
MR pH indicator
5% α-naphthol in absolute methyl alcohol
40% KOH containing 0.3% creatine

Procedure

1. Inoculate medium with a light inoculum of an 18- to 24-hour culture.
2. Incubate for at least 48 hours or until sufficient growth occurs in broth.
3. Pipette 1 ml of the broth to a clean test tube for the VP test.
4. Perform the MR test on a portion of the remaining aliquot:
   a. Add five drops of MR indicator to the aliquot with a Pasteur pipette.
   b. Interpret color result immediately.
5. Perform the VP test on the 1 ml aliquot:
   a. Add 1.5 ml (15 drops) of α-naphthol reagent to the VP aliquot and shake well.
   b. Add 0.5 ml (five drops) of 40% KOH reagent to aliquot.
   c. Gently shake the tubes for 30 seconds to 1 minute to expose reaction to atmospheric oxygen. This oxidizes acetoin to obtain a color reaction.
   d. Allow tubes to stand at least 10 to 15 minutes before attempting to interpret color results, although the reaction is often immediate.

Interpretation

Positive MR: Distinct red color at surface of the medium
Negative MR: Yellow color at surface of the medium
Delayed reaction: Orange color. Continue incubation and repeat test in 4 days.
Positive VP: Pink-red color at surface of the medium
Negative VP: Yellow color at the surface of the medium
A copper-like color is interpreted as negative because this is caused by the action of the reagents when mixed.

Quality Control

E. coli: MR positive—red; VP negative—no pink-red color
Enterobacter cloacae: MR negative—no red color; VP positive—pink-red color

Notes

1. Most Enterobacteriaceae give either a positive MR or a positive VP. However, some bacteria, such as *Hafnia alvei* and *Proteus mirabilis* may give a positive for both the MR and the VP.
2. VP reagents must be added in the correct order and correct amounts, or a false-negative result may occur.
3. The MR incubation should not be decreased by increasing the glucose concentration or by using a heavy inoculum.
4. Re-incubate MR reactions that are negative at 48 hours and retest.
5. Read the VP at 48 hours. Increasing the incubation time can lead to false-negatives resulting from the production of acid.

Procedure

Simmons citrate reaction

Purpose

The citrate reaction is used to differentiate members of the Enterobacteriaceae based on citrate utilization. The reaction is useful in identification of the lactose-fermenting Enterobacteriaceae. *Escherichia coli* is citrate negative, whereas *Enterobacter* and *Klebsiella* are positive.

Principle

Simmons citrate agar contains sodium citrate, which is the only carbon source in the medium. If an organism can utilize citrate, sodium citrate is converted to ammonia, which is then converted to ammonium hydroxide. The alkalinity of the compound formed raises the pH of the medium, and bromthymol blue indicator takes on its alkaline color, which is blue. See Figure 10-6 for the citrate reaction.

Media and Reagents

Simmons citrate agar

Procedure

Use a single, well-isolated 18- to 24-hour colony.
Select colony with sterile needle and streak citrate slant lightly.
Leave cap on loosely and incubate at 35°C ± 2°C for 18 to 24 hours.

Interpretation
A positive test is indicated by growth with an intense blue color on the slant or solely the presence of growth. Compare to an uninoculated tube for correct interpretation. A negative test is indicated by the absence of growth and no color change in the medium (remains green). False-positive results may occur with an inoculum that is too heavy.

Quality Control
Klebsiella pneumoniae: Positive—blue (alkaline) with good growth
E. coli: Negative—no growth with no color change

Procedure
Motility test medium

Purpose
This procedure determines the motility of bacteria through semisolid media. *Shigella* and *Klebsiella* are nonmotile members of Enterobacteriaceae. *Yersinia enterocolitica* is nonmotile at 37°C but motile at 22°C.

Principle
The semisolid medium contains a small amount of agar, which allows motile bacteria to move out from the line of inoculation. Nonmotile organisms grow only along the line of inoculation. Highly motile bacteria show growth throughout the medium.

To aid visualization of the reaction, 1% triphenyltetrazolium chloride may be added to the medium. Bacteria incorporate this colorless dye and reduce it to a red pigment. Thus, reddening of the medium can be used as an indication for the extent of bacterial growth. See Figure 10-9 for the motility test.

Procedure
1. With a sterile inoculating needle, select one colony and stab the center of the medium. Stab to a depth greater than half of the tube's depth, near the bottom of the agar.
2. Incubate at 35°C ± 2°C for 24 to 48 hours, and examine for growth around the line of inoculation.

Interpretation
Motile: Diffuse growth extending laterally from line of inoculation or growth present throughout the medium
Nonmotile: Growth only along line of inoculation

Quality Control
Proteus mirabilis: Motile—growth extending laterally from line of inoculation
Klebsiella pneumoniae: Nonmotile—growth only along line of inoculation

Procedure
Decarboxylase reactions

Purpose
Moeller decarboxylase medium is used for determining the production of decarboxylase enzymes by the enteric bacteria. Specific enzymes are detected by incorporating lysine, ornithine, and arginine into a media base. The reactions are useful in differentiating *Klebsiella*, which is nonmotile, from *Enterobacter*. All *Klebsiella*, except *K. ornitholytica*, are ornithine decarboxylase (ODC) negative. All *Enterobacter* are ODC negative; *Pantoea agglomerans* is negative for all three decarboxylase enzymes. Lysine decarboxylase (LDC) is useful in differentiating *Salmonella*, for which most serotypes are LDC positive, from *Citrobacter*, which is LDC negative.

Principle
The decarboxylases are enzymes that attack the carboxyl group of specific amino acids, forming amines and carbon dioxide. The amines formed are alkaline and alter the color of the pH indicator. The basal medium contains peptones, beef or yeast extract, and other nutrients for bacterial growth. Glucose is present as a fermentable carbohydrate. Bromcresol purple and cresol red are the pH indicators, which are purple in alkaline conditions and yellow in acid.

The amino acid to be tested is added to the Moeller base medium in a 1% concentration. Each decarboxylase reaction is specific for a particular amino acid. Tests for **lysine decarboxylase** (LDC), **ornithine decarboxylase** (ODC), and **arginine dihydrolase** (ADH) are used. **Lysine** is decarboxylated to **cadaverine**, **ornithine** is decarboxylated to **putrescine**, and **arginine** undergoes a dihydrolase reaction to form **citrulline,** which is then converted to **ornithine** in a decarboxylation.

A control tube of Moeller decarboxylase medium, which contains glucose but no amino acid, is inoculated with each set of reactions. Conversion of the control tube to yellow indicates the organism is viable and has fermented glucose. During the early part of a decarboxylation reaction, glucose is fermented, leading to a yellow color. As the pH decreases, an optimal environment for decarboxylation occurs, and the amino acid is decarboxylated. This leads to the formation of alkaline amines, which increase the pH, giving a red-purple color. In the absence of decarboxylation, the medium remains yellow or acidic.

All tubes are overlaid with mineral oil to protect the reaction from air, which may cause alkalinization and false-positive decarboxylase reactions.

Media and Reagents

Moeller decarboxylase broths containing:
1% Lysine
1% Ornithine
1% Arginine
Control tube with only glucose
Sterile mineral oil

Procedure

1. Inoculate test cultures into the tubes of decarboxylase media for each amino acid to be tested. Include a control tube for each organism.
2. Overlay all tubes with 5 mm to 10 mm (or 1 ml) of sterile mineral oil. Replace cap.
3. Incubate at 35°C ± 2°C for 24 hours.

Interpretation

Glucose fermentation indicates the organism is viable and the medium turns yellow.
Positive decarboxylation is indicated by a red-purple color in the medium.
Incubate all tubes negative for decarboxylation for another 24 hours and read again.

Quality Control

All tubes should be read at 24 hours.

Arginine:
Enterobacter cloacae: Positive (purple), alkaline
Klebsiella pneumoniae: Negative (yellow), acidic

Lysine:
Klebsiella pneumoniae: Positive (purple), alkaline
Enterobacter cloacae: Negative (yellow), acidic

Ornithine:
Enterobacter cloacae: Positive (purple), alkaline
Klebsiella pneumoniae: Negative (yellow), acidic

Control: Inoculate the control with the same organisms that are tested in the amino acid tubes. All reactions for the control should be negative (yellow), acidic.

Notes

1. If control tube shows an alkaline reaction, the test is invalid.
2. Organisms should be subcultured to nutrient or sheep blood agar before inoculating decarboxylase media.
3. If layers of yellow or purple are observed after incubation, gently shake tubes and then interpret reactions.
4. If reactions are difficult to interpret, compare tubes to an uninoculated control tube. Any trace of purple after 24 hours is positive.
5. A gray color may be observed when the indictor has been reduced. Add additional indicator before interpreting the reaction.

Procedure

Phenylalanine agar (deaminase reaction)

Purpose

Deaminase activity is determined using the amino acid phenylalanine. Only *Proteus, Providencia*, and *Morganella* species possess the deaminase enzyme. The amino acid tryptophan may be substituted.

Principle

Deamination of the amino acid results in a colored compound with the addition of 10% ferric chloride ($FeCI_3$)
Phenylalanine $\rightarrow$ Phenylpyruvic acid + 10% $FeCl_3$ $\rightarrow$ Green
Phenylalanine deaminase (PDA)
Tryptophan $\rightarrow$ Indole pyruvic acid + 10% $FeCl_3$ $\rightarrow$ Brown
Tryptophan deaminase (TDA)
Alternatively, deaminase activity can be determined using lysine iron agar (LIA) to detect the enzyme lysine deaminase.

Media and Reagents

Phenylalanine or tryptophan agar
10% $FeCI_3$

Procedure

1. Streak the agar slant with a heavy inoculum of pure isolates of the bacteria and replace cap.
2. Incubate 24 hours at 35°C ± 2°C.
3. Add four or five drops of 10% $FeCI_3$ to the slant. Rotate the tube and mix gently to loosen the growth and to provide proper contact for reagent and medium. Observe for color formation within 1 to 5 minutes.

Interpretation

Appearance of an intense green color indicates a positive deamination for phenylalanine.
Appearance of a brown color indicates a positive deamination for tryptophan.

Quality Control

Proteus vulgaris: Positive—green for PDA or brown color for TDA with $FeCl_3$
Escherichia coli: Negative—no color development with $FeCl_3$

Procedure
Lysine iron agar (LIA)

Purpose
LIA can be used in the differentiation of enteric bacteria based on its ability to deaminate or decarboxylate lysine and to produce hydrogen sulfide. It is useful in the identification of *Salmonella, Proteus, Providencia,* and *Morganella.* Members of the *Proteus* group (*Proteus, Providencia,* and *Morganella)* are the only members of the Enterobacteriaceae that are deaminase positive.

Principle
LIA contains a small amount of protein, glucose, lysine, sodium thiosulfate, ferric ammonium citrate, and the pH indicator bromcresol purple. Lysine is the enzyme substrate, and glucose is the fermentable carbohydrate. Sodium thiosulfate is the sulfur source to detect hydrogen sulfide, which reacts with ferric ammonium citrate.

As glucose fermentation occurs, the deep of the tube turns yellow. Lysine decarboxylation produces alkaline cadaverine and leads to reversion of the deep from yellow to purple.

Lysine deamination occurs in the presence of oxygen (on the slant) and results in production of a red color. Bromcresol purple indicator is purple (alkaline) at pH of 6.8 or greater and yellow (acidic) at pH of 5.2 or lower. H_2S production is noted by a black precipitate in the deep as H_2S gas reacts with ferric ammonium citrate. See Figure 10-8 for LIA reaction.

Media and Reagents
LIA slants

Procedure
1. Inoculate LIA by using a straight wire to stab the deep and streak the slant.
2. Incubate at 35°C ± 2°C for 18 to 24 hours. If necessary, incubate for 48 hours.

Interpretation
Lysine decarboxylase positive: Purple deep (alkaline)
Lysine decarboxylase negative: Yellow deep (acidic); glucose fermented
Deaminase positive: Red slant
H_2S positive: Black precipitate

Quality Control
Salmonella Typhimurium: LDC positive (alkaline)—purple deep and H_2S positive
Shigella flexneri: LDC negative (acidic)—yellow deep and H_2S negative
Proteus vulgaris: LDA positive—red slant and yellow deep

Notes
1. H_2S-producing strains of *Proteus* may not blacken this medium.
2. *Morganella morganii* does not consistently produce a red color after 24 hours of incubation.

Procedure
ONPG reaction

Purpose
The o-nitrophenyl-β-D-galactopyranoside (ONPG) reaction identifies the presence of late or slow lactose-fermenting strains. The test is useful in detecting late lactose-fermenting strains of *Escherichia coli* and distinguishing some *Citrobacter* species and *Salmonella arizonae* subspecies, which are ONPG positive, from similar *Salmonella* subspecies, which are ONPG negative. It also is useful in speciation of *Shigella. S. sonnei* is the only ONPG-positive *Shigella* species.

Principle
Lactose fermentation requires two enzymes: **lactose permease**, which actively transfers lactose into the bacterial cell, and **β-galactosidase**, which degrades lactose into glucose and galactose. Nonlactose fermenters lack both enzymes, and those bacteria that are slow or late lactose fermenters possess the β-galactosidase but lack the permease. Lactose fermenters possess both enzymes.

The substrate ONPG is useful in detecting late lactose fermenters because the ONPG molecule is structurally similar to that of lactose. ONPG can enter the bacterial cell without a permease. In the presence of β-galactosidase, ONPG (colorless) is converted into galactose and o-nitrophenyl, which is yellow chromogen and the alkaline end product.

Media and Reagents
ONPG tablets or disks
Sterile distilled water
Sterile 1.0 ml pipettes
Sterile test tubes

Procedure
1. If using ONPG tablets, dissolve one tablet in 1.0 ml of sterile distilled water. ONPG disks are dissolved in 0.5 ml sterile distilled water.
2. Mix and allow tablet to dissolve (5 to 10 minutes).

3. Inoculate with four or five colonies of an 18- to 24-hour culture. Use sterile needle to select colonies and mix well.
4. Cover each tube with parafilm and incubate at 35°C ± 2°C for 4 to 6 hours. Re-incubate all negative tubes for up to 24 hours.

Interpretation

Positive reaction: Yellow color within 20 minutes to 24 hours
Negative reaction: Colorless after 24 hours

Quality Control

E. coli: Positive—yellow
Salmonella Typhimurium: Negative—no color change

Procedure

Urease reaction

Purpose

Urease is an enzyme that splits urea into alkaline end products. The reaction is useful in the identification of rapid urease producers, such as *Proteus* and *Morganella*, as well as weak urease producers, such as *Klebsiella pneumoniae* and some species of *Enterobacter* and *Citrobacter*.

Principle

Urease splits the urea molecule into ammonia (NH_3), carbon dioxide (CO_2), and water (H_2O). Ammonia reacts in solution to form an alkaline compound, ammonium carbonate, which results in an increased pH of the medium and a color change in the indicator to pink-red.

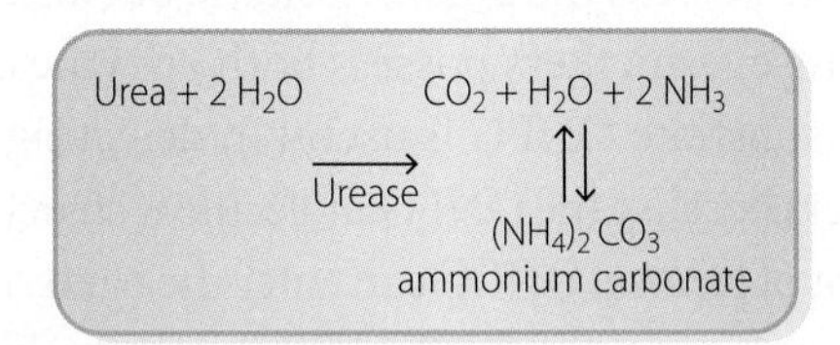

Media and Reagents

Christensen's (urea) agar tubes or Stuart (urea) broth

Procedure

1. Use an 18- to 24-hour culture to inoculate medium. If using urea broth, use a heavy inoculum (approximately 2 loopfuls). Gently shake tubes to suspend the bacteria. If using urea agar, streak slant over entire agar surface with a heavy inoculum. Do not stab the deep, because this will be the negative control.
2. Replace cap loosely.
3. Incubate at 35°C ± 2°C for 18 to 24 hours.

Interpretation

Broth

Positive: Red color in medium
Negative: No color change. Broth remains buff to pale yellow. Strong positive reactions are seen only with *Proteus* species (*Proteus* and *Morganella*) and may be interpreted as early as after 4 hours of incubation. Weakly positive reactions (pink to orange) may be seen with *K. pneumoniae* and other slow urease producers.

Agar

Positive (rapid urease activity): Red throughout medium (seen only with *Proteus* and *Morganella*)
Positive (slow urease activity): Red in slant (*K. pneumoniae*)
Negative (no urease activity): Medium remains yellow

Quality Control

Proteus vulgaris: Positive—rapid urease producer
K. pneumoniae: Positive—slow urease producer
Escherichia coli: Negative—no urease production

Notes

1. When using urea agar, a false-positive may occur from utilization of peptones or other proteins, which increase the pH.
2. Compare the broth with an uninoculated tube to assist in determining results. The high buffering capacity may obscure urease action in slow urease producers.
3. The extent of the color formation is related to the rate of urease action.

Laboratory Exercises

1. Streak the organisms on the plates listed and incubate for 18 to 24 hours at 35°C ± 2°C. Describe the appearance of each of the following on the media listed. Interpret the reactions that have occurred. Contrast the growth on Hektoen enteric (HE) with that on MacConkey and EMB.

	MacConkey	Eosin-methylene blue	Hektoen enteric	Sheep blood agar
Escherichia coli				
Klebsiella pneumoniae				
Proteus mirabilis				
Salmonella enteritidis				

How does the growth of *E. coli* on MacConkey compare to its growth on HE? Explain why.

____

What is unique about the appearance of *Proteus* on sheep blood agar? ______________

What is unique about the appearance of *E. coli* on EMB? ______________

What accounts for the mucoid appearance of *Klebsiella* on sheep blood agar? ______________

2. Perform the cytochome oxidase test on the following bacteria. Why is this an important biochemical test in the initial workup of gram-negative bacilli?

Escherichia coli
Observations: __________ Interpretation: __________
Klebsiella pneumoniae
Observations: __________ Interpretation: __________
Proteus vulgaris
Observations: __________ Interpretation: __________
Enterobacter cloacae
Observations: __________ Interpretation: __________

3. Perform a TSI on the following bacteria. Record your observations and interpret your results:

Escherichia coli
Observations: __________ Interpretation: __________
Klebsiella pneumoniae
Observations: __________ Interpretation: __________
Salmonella enteritidis
Observations: __________ Interpretation: __________
Proteus mirabilis
Observations: __________ Interpretation: __________
Citrobacter freundii
Observations: __________ Interpretation: __________
Shigella sonnei
Observations: __________ Interpretation: __________

Describe how each of the following is observed in the TSI:

Glucose fermentation: ______________
Gas production: ______________
Lactose/sucrose fermentation: ______________
Hydrogen sulfide production: ______________

How are results affected if the caps are tightened too tightly on the TSI medium? ______________

____

4. Describe the appearance of a positive MR: ______________

____

Describe the appearance of a positive VP: ______________

What end products are detected in the MR? ______________ in the VP? ______________

Perform the MR-VP on the following bacteria. Record your observations and interpret your results.

Escherichia coli
MR: Observations: __________ Interpretation: __________
VP: Observations: __________ Interpretation: __________
Klebsiella pneumoniae
MR: Observations: __________ Interpretation: __________
VP: Observations: __________ Interpretation: __________
Proteus mirabilis
MR: Observations: __________ Interpretation: __________
VP: Observations: __________ Interpretation: __________
Enterobacter cloacae
MR: Observations: __________ Interpretation: __________
VP: Observations: __________ Interpretation: __________

5. Perform the indole reaction on the following bacteria. Record your observations and interpret your results. Give the principle of this reaction: ______________

____

Escherichia coli
Observations: __________ Interpretation: __________
Klebsiella pneumoniae
Observations: __________ Interpretation: __________
Proteus mirabilis
Observations: __________ Interpretation: __________
Proteus vulgaris
Observations: __________ Interpretation: __________
Enterobacter cloacae
Observations: __________ Interpretation: __________

6. Describe the appearance of a positive citrate reaction. Perform the citrate test on the following bacteria. Record your observations and interpret your results.

Escherichia coli
Observations: __________ Interpretation: __________
Klebsiella pneumoniae
Observations: __________ Interpretation: __________
Enterobacter cloacae
Observations: __________ Interpretation: __________
Citrobacter freundii
Observations: __________ Interpretation: __________

7. What does a yellow color in a decarboxylase tube indicate? ______________

Describe the appearance of a positive decarboxylase reaction: ______

What is the purpose of overlaying the medium with mineral oil? ______

______

Perform and interpret the following decarboxylase reactions. Record your observations and interpret your results.

Escherichia coli

ADH: Observations: ______ Interpretation: ______

ODC: Observations: ______ Interpretation: ______

LDC: Observations: ______ Interpretation: ______

Klebsiella pneumoniae

ADH: Observations: ______ Interpretation: ______

ODC: Observations: ______ Interpretation: ______

LDC: Observations: ______ Interpretation: ______

Enterobacter cloacae

ADH: Observations: ______ Interpretation: ______

ODC: Observations: ______ Interpretation: ______

LDC: Observations: ______ Interpretation: ______

Enterobacter aerogenes

ADH: Observations: ______ Interpretation: ______

ODC: Observations: ______ Interpretation: ______

LDC: Observations: ______ Interpretation: ______

Salmonella enteritidis

ADH: Observations: ______ Interpretation: ______

ODC: Observations: ______ Interpretation: ______

LDC: Observations: ______ Interpretation: ______

8. Perform the motility test on the following bacteria. What members of Enterobacteriaceae are nonmotile?

______

Escherichia coli

Observation: ______ Interpretation: ______

Klebsiella pneumoniae

Observation: ______ Interpretation: ______

Proteus mirabilis

Observation: ______ Interpretation: ______

Shigella sonnei

Observation: ______ Interpretation: ______

9. Which bacteria are deaminase positive? ______

How is deaminase activity determined? ______

Perform the deaminase test on the bacteria listed. Record your observations and interpret the results.

Escherichia coli

Observation: ______ Interpretation: ______

Klebsiella pneumoniae

Observation: ______ Interpretation: ______

Proteus mirabilis

Observation: ______ Interpretation: ______

Providentia stuartii

Observation: ______ Interpretation: ______

10. Which bacteria are strong urease producers? ______

______

Which bacteria are weak urease producers? ______

______

Perform and interpret the urease reaction on the following bacteria.

Escherichia coli

Observations: ______ Interpretation: ______

Klebsiella pneumoniae

Observations: ______ Interpretation: ______

Proteus vulgaris

Observations: ______ Interpretation: ______

Proteus mirabilis

Observations: ______ Interpretation: ______

Providentia stuartii

Observations: ______ Interpretation: ______

11. What is determined in the ONPG reaction? ______

Perform and interpret the ONPG reaction on the following bacteria:

Escherichia coli

Observations: ______ Interpretation: ______

Salmonella enteritidis

Observations: ______ Interpretation: ______

Citrobacter freundii

Observations: ______ Interpretation: ______

Shigella sonnei

Observations: ______ Interpretation: ______

12. Describe how you would differentiate the following paired bacteria. Give a biochemical reaction and the expected result.

Escherichia coli from *Enterobacter cloacae:* ____________

____

Proteus mirabilis from *Proteus vulgaris:* ____________

____

Klebsiella pneumoniae from *Enterobacter aerogenes:*

____

Shigella sonnei from *Salmonella enteritidis:* ____________

____

Proteus mirabilis from *Salmonella enteritidis:* ________

____

Citrobacter freundii from *Salmonella enteritidis:* _____

____

Proteus mirabilis from *Providencia stuartii:* ____________

____

13. Identify an unknown member of the family Enterobacteriaceae. Include a log of all media inoculated and tests performed, with observations and results. Interpret your reactions and justify your identification.
Unknown number: ______________________________

Media inoculated	Observation	Result
Procedures performed	**Observation**	**Result**
Identification and explanation		

Review Questions

Matching

Match the species of Enterobacteriaceae with its unique characteristic:

1. Mucoid colonies
2. Swarming motility
3. Production of DNase, lipase, and gelatinase
4. Possesses Vi antigen
5. Green metallic sheen on EMB
   a. *Salmonella enterica* serotype Typhi
   b. *Escherichia coli*
   c. *Serratia marcescens*
   d. *Proteus mirabilis*
   e. *Klebsiella pneumoniae*

Match the description given for the following gram-negative bacilli with the correct name for each:

	6.	7.	8.	9.	10.
TSI	K/ⒶH_2S+	A/ⒶH_2S–	A/ⒶH_2S+	A/ⒶH_2S–	K/A H_2S+
MacConkey	Lactose–	Lactose+	Lactose+	Lactose+	Lactose–
Methyl red	+	+	+	–	+
Indole	–	+	–	–	–
Urease	+	–	–	weak+	–
ONPG	–	+	+	+	–
Deaminase	+	–	–	–	–
Motility	+	+	+	–	+
ADH	–	–	–	–	+
ODC	+	+	+	–	+
LDC	–	+	–	+	+

a. *Citrobacter freundii*
b. *Proteus mirabilis*
c. *Salmonella enterica* serogroup I
d. *Escherichia coli*
e. *Klebsiella pneumoniae*

Multiple Choice

11. All members of the family Enterobacteriaceae:
    a. Oxidize glucose
    b. Ferment glucose
    c. Ferment lactose
    d. Ferment sucrose
12. In the grouping of *Shigella* organisms, agglutination by group C antisera indicates that the species is:
    a. *S. dysenteriae*
    b. *S. boydii*
    c. *S. flexneri*
    d. *S. sonnei*
13. Enteric pathogens, such as *Shigella* and *Salmonella,* are most easily differentiated from normal intestinal gram-negative bacilli by their failure to:
    a. Ferment glucose
    b. Produce H_2S gas
    c. Ferment lactose
    d. Produce urease
14. Select the most appropriate combination for plating a urine culture:
    a. EMB and MacConkey
    b. MacConkey and blood
    c. Hektoen enteric and EMB
    d. Chocolate and CNA
15. Which of the following reactions is *incorrect* for *Salmonella enterica* subgroup I?
    a. H_2S positive
    b. Motile
    c. ONPG positive
    d. ODC positive
    e. Lactose negative
16. An organism that is a late or slow lactose fermenter possesses:
    a. β-galactosidase and lactose permease
    b. Only β-galactosidase
    c. Only lactose permease
    d. Neither β-galactosidase nor lactose permease
    e. Cytochrome oxidase
17. A burn patient develops a wound infection, which is cultured and sent to the laboratory for identification. Pink colonies are found on MacConkey medium, and abundant gray colonies are observed on blood agar. The following results are obtained:
    TSI: A/(A) H_2S negative
    IMVC: – – + +
    Ornithine: Positive
    Lysine: Negative
    Arginine: Positive
    Urease: Negative
    Motility: Positive
    Identify the isolate:
    a. *Escherichia coli*
    b. *Klebsiella pneumoniae*
    c. *Enterobacter cloacae*
    d. *Enterobacter aerogenes*
    e. *Citrobacter freundii*
18. A catheterized urine specimen collected from a female patient who is residing in a nursing home reveals the following:
    TSI: K/A H_2S negative
    MacConkey: Clear colonies
    Indole: Positive
    Citrate: Positive
    Motility: Positive
    Urease: Negative
    Deaminase: Positive
    Identify the isolate:
    a. *Escherichia coli*
    b. *Proteus mirabilis*
    c. *Klebsiella pneumoniae*
    d. *Providencia stuartii*
    e. *Serratia marcescens*
19. *Salmonella* has been isolated as the source of contamination in an outbreak of gastroenteritis associated with eggs. Which of the following reactions is correct for this genus?

	H_2S	Urease	Motility	ONPG	LDC	Potassium cyanide
a.	+	–	–	+	–	+
b.	+	–	+	–	+	–
c.	–	+	+	+	+	–
d.	+	–	–	–	–	+

20. Which statement correctly describes the antigens of Enterobacteriaceae?
    a. The O antigen is heat labile.
    b. The O antigen is located on the cell wall.
    c. The Vi antigen is an example of a flagellar antigen.
    d. The K antigen is also known as the somatic antigen.

Bibliography

Brenner, F. W., Villar, R. G., Tauxe, A. R., & Swaminathan B. (2000). *Salmonella* nomenclature: Guest commentary. *Journal of Clinical Microbiology, 38,* 2465–2467.

Centers for Disease Control and Prevention. (1985). Update: Milk-borne salmonellosis—Illinois. *Morbidity and Mortality Weekly Report, 34,* 200. Retrieved from http://www.cdc.gov/mmwr/preview/mmwrhtml/00000520.htm

Centers for Disease Control and Prevention. (1990). Update: *Salmonella enteritidis* infections and shell eggs—United States, 1990. *Morbidity and Mortality Weekly Report, 39,* 909. Retrieved from http://www.cdc.gov/mmwr/preview/mmwrhtml/00001862.htm

Centers for Disease Control and Prevention. (2010). *Escherichia coli* O157:H7. Retrieved from http://www.cdc.gov/ecoli/index.html

Centers for Disease Control and Prevention. (2011). *Salmonella* outbreaks. Retrieved from http://www.cdc.gov/salmonella/outbreaks.html

Clark, S. C., Haigh, R. D., Freestone, P. P. E., & Williams, P. H. (2003). Virulence of enteropathogenic *Escherichia coli,* a global pathogen. *Journal of Clinical Microbiology, 16,* 365–378.

Endimiani, A., Luzzaro, F., Brigante, G., Perilli, M., Lombardi, G., Amicosante, G., . . . & Toniolo, A. (2005). *Proteus mirabilis* bloodstream infections: Risk factors and treatment outcome related to the expression of extended spectrum beta-lactamases. *Journal of Clinical Microbiology, 49,* 2598–2605.

Farmer, J. J., III, Boatwright, K. D., & Janda, J. M. (2007). Enterobacteriaceae: Introduction and identification. In P. R. Murray, E. J. Baron, J. H. Jorgensen, M. L. Landry, & M. A. Pfaller (Eds.), *Manual of clinical microbiology,* 9th ed. Washington, DC: American Society for Microbiology.

Janda, J. M., & Abbott, S. L. (2006). The genus *Hafnia*: From soup to nuts. *Journal of Clinical Microbiology, 19,* 12–18.

O'Hare, C. M. (2005). Manual and automated instrumentation for identification of Enterobacteriaceae and other aerobic gram-negative bacilli. *Clinical Microbiology Reviews, 18,* 147–162.

O'Hare, C. M., Brenner, F. W., Miller, J. M. (2000). Classification, identification, and clinical significance of *Proteus, Providentia* and *Morganella. Clinical Microbiology Reviews, 13,* 534–546.

Pignata, S., Giammanco, G. M., Grimont, F., Grimont, P. A., & Giammanco, G. (1999). Molecular characterization of the genera *Proteus, Morganella,* and *Providentia* by ribotyping. *Journal of Clinical Microbiology, 37,* 2840–2847.

Podschun, R., & Ullman, U. (1998). *Klebsiella* species as nosocomial pathogens: Epidemiology, taxonomy, typing methods and pathogenicity factors. *Clinical Microbiology Reviews, 11,* 589–603.

Qadri, F., Svennerholm, A. M., & Farugue, A. S. G. (2005). Enterotoxigenic *Escherichia coli* in developing countries: Epidemiology, microbiology, clinical features, treatment, and prevention. *Journal of Clinical Microbiology, 18,* 465–483.

Wagner, A. *Yersinia.* In P. R. Murray, E. J. Baron, J. H. Jorgensen, M. L. Landry, & M. A. Pfaller (Eds.), *Manual of clinical microbiology,* 9th ed. Washington, DC: American Society for Microbiology.

Winn, Jr., W., Allen, S., Janda, W., Konemen, E., Procop, G., Schreckenberger, P., & Woods, G. (Eds.). (2005). Enterobacteriaceae. In *Koneman's color atlas and textbook of diagnostic microbiology* (6th ed.). Philadelphia, PA: Lippincott Williams & Wilkins.

Zimbro, M. J., Power, D. A., Miller, S. M., Wilson, G. E., & Johnson, J. A. (Eds.). (2009). *Difco and BBL manual: Manual of microbiological culture media* (2nd ed.). Sparks, MD: BD Diagnostics–Diagnostic Systems.

NEWS: NOMENCLATURE AND SEROVARS OF *SALMONELLA*

Salmonella nomenclature is complex and can be confusing. Names are based on different systems, which may be communicated in a variety of ways by scientists, health officials, media, and authors. Nomenclature systems that have evolved include division of the genus *Salmonella* into species; subspecies; subgenera; groups; subgroups; and serotypes, or serovars.

When a **serovar** designation is used, it is indicated by using a "var" suffix. The serotype, or serovar, is a serological variant and represents the testable antigenic composition of the organism based on the somatic, or O, and flagellar, or H, antigens. Thus, each identified strain has an antigenic formula, with specific numbers and letters that refer to those antigens. Using the current nomenclature system, the serovar is capitalized and written after the genus, species, or subspecies name.

Currently, there are over 2,400 serotypes of *Salmonella* based on the Kauffman-White serologic identification of O and H antigens. When species were initially named, each serotype was considered to be a separate species, which today, would result in over 2,400 species! Other methods of nomenclature included naming the species for the nature of the clinical disease. Examples include *S. typhi*, the agent of typhoid fever, and *S. enteritidis*, the agent of gastroenteritis. Geographic location and animal species of the original isolate were also used in the nomenclature process.

The Subcommittee of Enterobacteriaceae of the International Committee on Systematic Bacteriology investigates classification and nomenclature revisions for *Salmonella*. In 1973, DNA–DNA hybridization determined that all serotypes and subgenera I, II, and IV of *Salmonella* and all serotypes of Arizona were related at the species level and therefore belonged in a single species. Subspecies V, *S. bongori*, was not related to the others at the species level and thus is classified in its own species. During this time, *S. choleraesuis* was designated the type species for *Salmonella*. Later, this committee determined that *S. choleraesuis* did not represent all of the genotypes because of the biochemical reactions as well as the confusion, because it is a species and a serotype name. Thus, in 1986, the type species was changed to *S. enterica*. Challenges to this also have occurred.

Today, the current system used by the Centers for Disease Prevention and Control (CDC) is based on recommendations of the World Health Organization. See Box 10-4 in the text. These recommendations are that the genus *Salmonella* contains two species, and each contains many serotypes. The species are *S. enterica* (which is the type species) and *S. bongori*, which was formerly subspecies V. There are six subspecies in the species *S. enterica*, which are designated by a Roman numeral and a name. The subspecies are differentiated on the basis of biochemical reactions and genomic relatedness.

Serotypes in subspecies I, which contains the majority of *Salmonella* involved in human infection, also have a name. The name is generally related to the geographic location where the serotype was first isolated. The serotype name is not italicized, and the first letter is capitalized. Unnamed serotypes in subspecies II, IV, VI, and *S. bongori* have antigenic formulas. When the serotype is first mentioned within a text or article, the genus name is given, followed by either the word "serotype" or "ser.," and then the serotype name is written. When cited again, the name is written with the genus, followed directly by the serotype name.

The code to the antigenic formula is as follows:

Antigenic formula

Subspecies designation (I though VI)

O antigens, followed by a colon

H antigens (phase 1), followed by a colon

H antigens (phase 2, when present)

For example:

Complete name	CDC name	Also known as . . .
S. enterica subsp. *enterica* ser. Typhi	*Salmonella* ser. Typhi	*Salmonella typhi*
S. enterica subsp. *salamae* ser. Greenside	*Salmonella* ser. Greenside	S. II 50:z:e,n,x, and *S. greenside*
S. enterica subsp. *arizonae* ser. 18:z_4z_{23}:–	*Salmonella* IIIa: 18:z_4z_{23}:–	"*Arizona hinshawii*" ser. 7a,7b:1,2,5:–

Prior to 1966, all serotypes in all subspecies were given names, except in serotypes IIIa and IIIb. Beginning in1966, names were given only for subspecies I, and all existing serotype names in subspecies II, IV, VI, and *S. bongori* from the Kaufmann-White scheme were no longer used.

Within *S. enterica*, the most common O antigens are serogroups A, B, C1, C2, D, and E, which together cause almost 99% of all infections in humans and warm-blooded animals. Serotyping is a useful tool for epidemiology and to confirm the identification of the genus. However, it does not enable one to determine whether the organism can cause enteric fever because of cross-reacting antigens within the serogroups. For example, serogroup C1 includes both serotypes Infantis and Choleraesuis. Serotype Infantis generally causes gastroenteritis, whereas serotype Choleraesuis is an important cause of invasive, systemic infections, such as septicemia, without gastroenteritis. In the United States, the most frequently isolated *Salmonella* serotypes are Typhimurium, Enteritidis, and Newport. However, serotype Choleraesuis is one of the most frequent *Salmonella* serotypes isolated from humans in Asian countries.

BIBLIOGRAPHY

Brenner, F. W., Villar, R. G., Tauxe, A. R., & Swaminathan, B. (2000). *Salmonella* nomenclature: Guest commentary. *Journal of Clinical Microbiology, 3,* 2465–2467.

Chiu, C.-H., Su, L.-H., & Chu, C. (2004). *Salmonella enterica* serotype Choleraesuis: Epidemiology, pathogenesis, clinical disease and treatment. *Journal of Clinical Microbiology, 17,* 311–322.

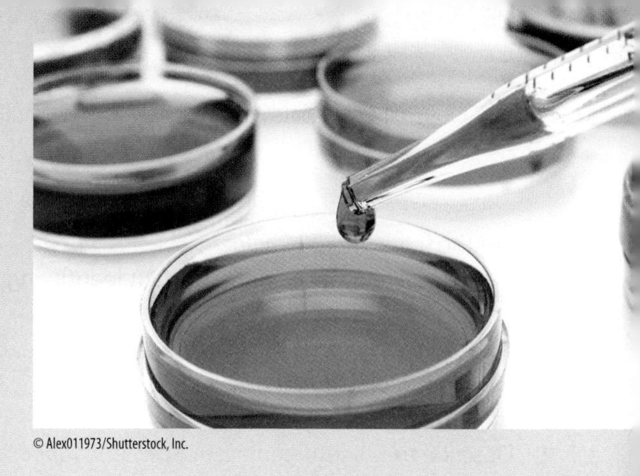
© Alex011973/Shutterstock, Inc.

CHAPTER 11

Nonfermentative Gram-Negative Bacilli

CHAPTER OUTLINE

Characteristics of Nonfermenters
Family Pseudomonadaceae
Burkholderia
Ralstonia
Acinetobacter
Stenotrophomonas
Alcaligenes
Achromobacter
Moraxella
Oligella
Chryseobacterium
Kingella

KEY TERMS

Alginate
Exotoxin A
Fermentative
Glanders
Melioidosis
Nonsaccharolytic
Oxidative
Oxidative-fermentative (OF) medium
Pyocyanin
Pyoverdin

LEARNING OBJECTIVES

1. Describe environmental sources and types of infections attributed to the nonfermentative gram-negative bacilli.
2. Contrast the peptone-to-carbohydrate ratio in fermentative and oxidative-fermentative media, and explain why this concentration is well suited for nonfermenters.
3. State the principle and use of and interpret oxidative-fermentative medium. Differentiate nonfermenters, fermenters, and nonsaccharolytic organisms.
4. Discuss the classification and characteristics of the Pseudomonadaceae.
    a. List the significant groups, the unique characteristics of each, and the representative organism.
5. Explain how *Pseudomonas aeruginosa* is identified and describe its unique characteristics.
    a. Identify *P. aeruginosa* as an unknown without error.
6. Describe the types of infections for *P. aeruginosa* and state which populations are most susceptible to infection.
7. List and describe the virulence factors produced by *P. aeruginosa* that are associated with its pathogenicity and the role of each.
8. Briefly discuss the identification and clinical significance of the following *Pseudomonas* species:
    a. *P. fluorescens*
    b. *P. putida*
    c. *P. stutzeri*
    d. *P. mendocino*

9. For the following *Burkholderia* species, discuss the clinical relevance and important identifying characteristics:
   a. *B. mallei*
   b. *B. pseudomallei*
   c. *B. cepacia*
10. Describe the clinical significance of *Stenotrophomonas maltophilia* and explain how it is identified.
11. State the clinical significance and characteristics of *Acinetobacter.*
    a. Differentiate *A. baumannii* from *A. lwoffii.*
    b. Differentiate *Acinetobacter* from *Neisseria.*
12. Describe the clinically significant *Alcaligenes* and state the important morphological and biochemical characteristics.
13. Describe the clinically significant *Achromobacter* and state the important morphological and biochemical characteristics.
14. Describe the clinically significant *Moraxella* and *Oligella* and explain how each is identified in the laboratory.
15. State a unique characteristic of *Chryseobacterium* and describe infections associated with *C. indologenes* and *C. meningosepticum*.
16. Identify an unknown gram-negative nonfermenter through biochemical reactions and morphological characteristics.

Characteristics of Nonfermenters

The nonfermentative, or **oxidative**, gram-negative bacilli metabolize carbohydrates oxidatively and require molecular oxygen as the final hydrogen ion acceptor. These organisms are unable to ferment glucose or other carbohydrates in the absence of oxygen. This oxidative process results in the formation of very weak acids as metabolic end products. Other gram-negative bacilli discussed in this chapter are termed **nonsaccharolytic**, or **nonoxidizers**. These bacteria cannot utilize carbohydrates either in the absence or presence of oxygen and must rely on compounds other than carbohydrates for sources of energy.

The nonfermentative gram-negative bacilli (**FIGURE 11-1**) are nonspore formers and obligate aerobes.

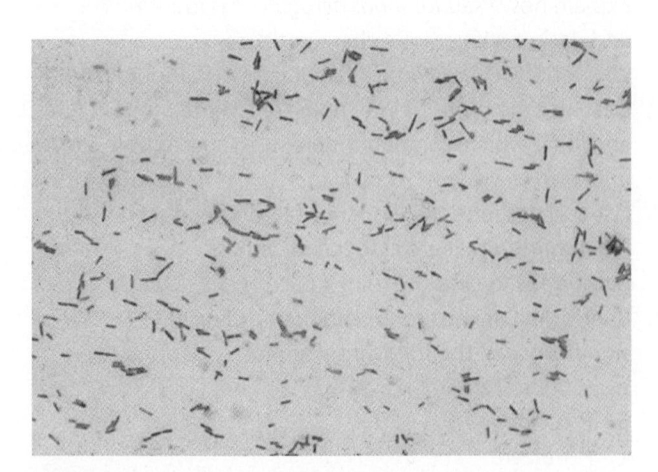

FIGURE 11-1 Photomicrograph of *Pseudomonas aeruginosa* illustrating long, narrow, gram negative bacilli.

Typically, the triple sugar iron (TSI) agar shows no reaction or a K/K H_2S negative reaction. Some of the bacteria can grow on the TSI slant, where oxygen is present (**FIGURE 11-2**).

The nonfermentative gram-negative bacilli bacteria are usually found in natural water sources as well as in contaminants in medical devices, respiratory care equipment, water baths, and sinks. In addition, some nonfermenters

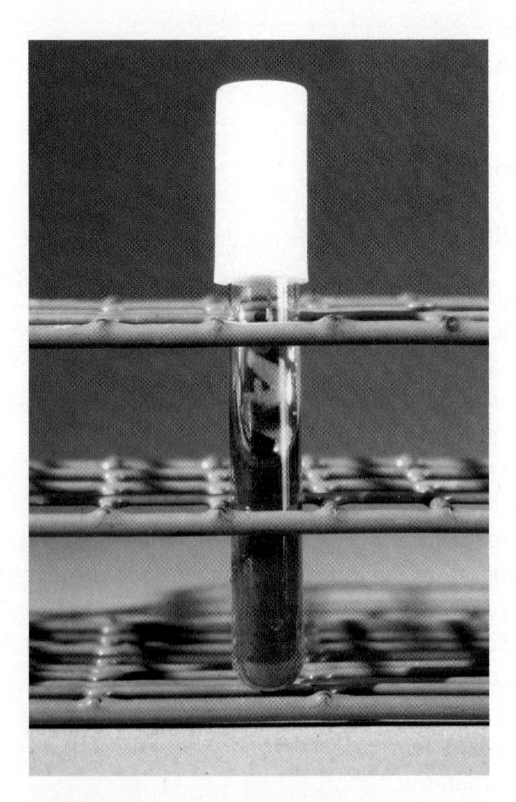

FIGURE 11-2 TSI of K/K typical of nonfermenters.

can colonize the mucous membranes and skin of humans, especially when present in the hospital environment. Some nonfermenters have been implicated as contaminants in pharmaceutical compounds and intravenous solutions. These organisms are associated also with nosocomial or hospital-acquired infections (HAI).

The nonfermenters are opportunistic pathogens and can colonize and cause infections in debilitated and immunosuppressed hosts. Those at increased risk include patients receiving prolonged antibiotic therapy, burn patients, and those receiving immunosuppressive therapy or chemotherapy as well as individuals receiving prolonged or invasive medical instrumentation, such as intravenous catheters. The bacteria have an opportunity to gain access to normally sterile sites through trauma, burns, or wounds. The source may be endogenous—from the site of the individuals' own colonized site—or exogenous—from an environmental source.

There have been many changes in the nomenclature and classification of the nonfermentative gram-negative bacilli based on nucleic acid sequencing and molecular technology. New genera have been established, and existing species have been renamed and reclassified. There are ever increasing species identified, which may or may not be considered to be clinically significant. This chapter will focus on those nonfermenters that are most clinically relevant.

IDENTIFICATION OF NONFERMENTERS

A nonfermenter is suspected if an oxidase-positive, gram-negative bacillus is found growing better on sheep blood agar than on MacConkey agar. A TSI showing K/K also indicates the presence of a nonfermenter. Differential reactions used to identify nonfermenters are summarized in BOX 11-1.

BOX 11-1 Differential Methods to Identify Nonfermentative Gram-Negative Bacilli

Cellular morphology of the flagellum: Type, number, and arrangement
Modified indole test
Growth on MacConkey agar (positive or negative)
Motility
Oxidative-fermentative carbohydrate utilization patterns
Decarboxylation reactions
Nitrate reduction
Acetamide
Urease

Many of these methods have been described previously in Chapter 10 but must be modified when identifying the nonfermenters. For example, because nonfermenters produce only small amounts of indole, the method must be adapted for nonfermenters. Indole must be extracted to be detected. In the modified indole test, indole produced from the breakdown of tryptophan by tryptophanase is extracted with xylene before detection. Tryptone both is inoculated with the organism and incubated for 48 hours at 25°C to 37°C. Then, 1.0 ml of xylene is added to the tube, which is then shaken and left undisturbed until the solvent rises to the top. Next, 0.5 ml of Ehrlich's reagent is added gently down the sides of the tube, forming a ring between the test medium and solvent. In a positive reaction, a bright red ring forms just below the solvent layer after addition of Ehrlich's reagent. This modified indole procedure is the recommended method to determine indole production by nonfermenters.

Triple sugar iron (TSI) agar is not suitable to study carbohydrate use by the nonfermenters because the bacteria are slow growing and produce only minimal amounts of acidic end products. A special medium for this purpose, the **oxidative-fermentative (OF) medium of Hugh and Leifson**, has been formulated to study carbohydrate utilization by the nonfermenters. OF media has a high concentration of carbohydrate (1.0%) and a low concentration of peptone or protein (0.2%). This high carbohydrate concentration enhances the production of acidic end products, which can be detected. The low concentration of peptone decreases the formation of oxidative products and amino acids. These end products can neutralize the pH and obscure a positive reaction. The concentration of peptone to carbohydrate is 1:5 in OF medium, whereas a concentration of 2:1 is used in media used for Enterobacteriaceae.

In the OF determination, many carbohydrates can be tested; these include glucose, maltose, lactose, mannitol, and xylose. The medium also contains bromthymol blue indicator, which is yellow in an acidic pH, indicating a positive reaction, and green to blue in an alkaline pH, indicating a negative reaction.

BOX 11-2 Summary of Oxidative-Fermentative Reactions

Oxidative: Positive (yellow) in the open tube and negative (green or blue-green) in the closed tube. The organism can use the carbohydrate only when oxygen is present (**FIGURE 11-3**).

Fermentative: Positive (yellow) in both the open and the closed tubes. Acid is produced in both tubes; this is typical of the Enterobacteriaceae, which indicates the activity of facultative anaerobes (**FIGURE 11-4**)

Nonsaccharolytic (nonoxidative): No change or an alkaline (blue-green) reaction in both tubes. The organism cannot use the carbohydrate and must seek other sources of energy (**FIGURE 11-5**).

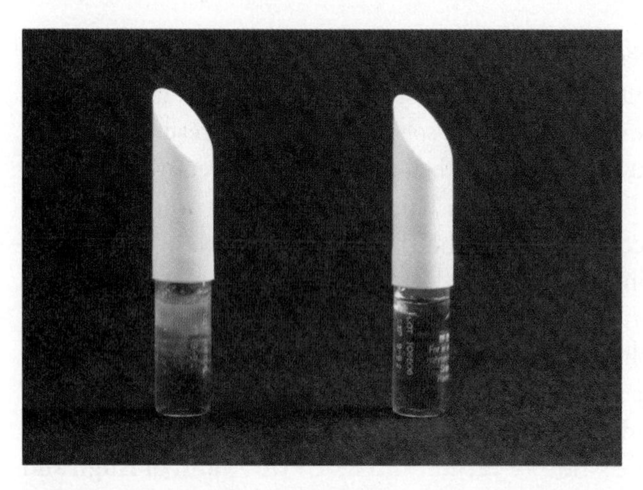

FIGURE 11-3 OF media-positive in open tube which indicates an oxidative organism.

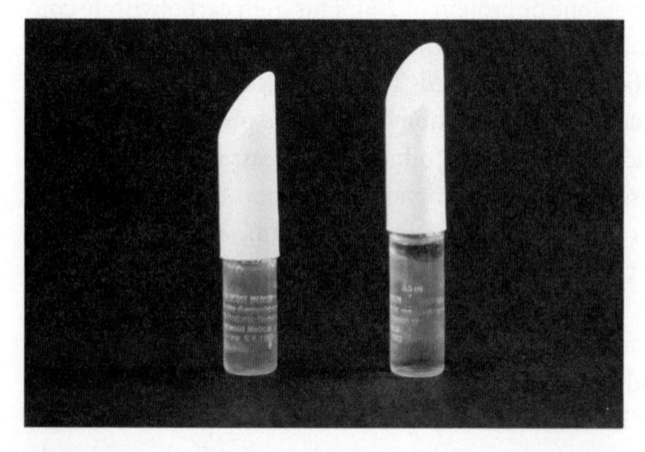

FIGURE 11-4 OF media-positive in both open and closed tubes which indicates a fermentative organism.

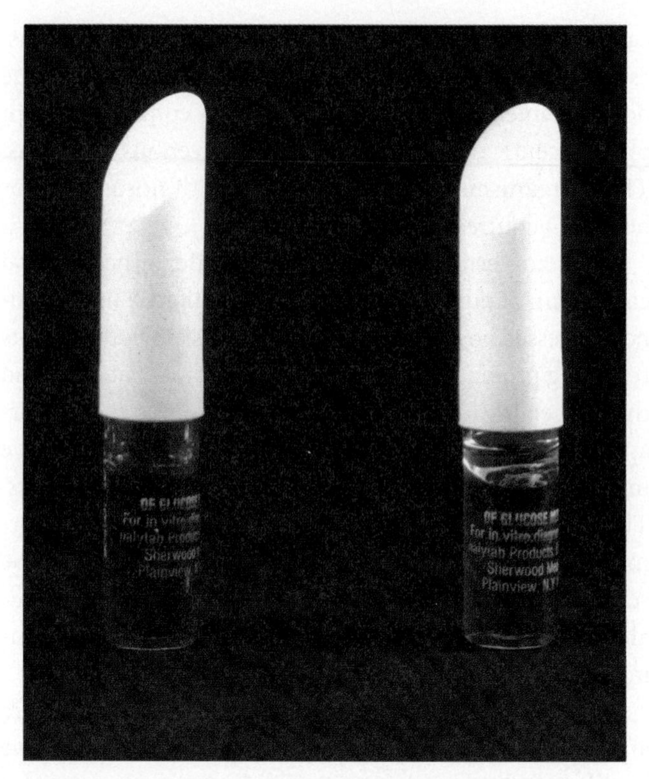

FIGURE 11-5 OF media-both open and closed tubes are negative which indicates a nonsaccharolytic organism.

For each organism and carbohydrate to be tested, two tubes of that specific medium are needed. One tube is exposed to the air, providing an oxidative environment, and is known as the open tube; the second tube is overlaid with mineral oil, providing a fermentative environment, and is known as the closed tube. After inoculation and incubation, an organism can be classified into one of three categories, as shown in BOX 11-2.

The reduction of nitrates (NO_3) to nitrites (NO_2) is another useful reaction for the identification of nonfermenters. Although some bacteria convert NO_3 to NO_2, others convert nitrates completely to nitrogen gas (N_2). N_2 can be detected by adding zinc to the final reaction. A red color with zinc indicates the presence of NO_3 and therefore a negative reaction for nitrogen reduction. No change with the addition of zinc indicates that nitrates have been reduced completely to N_2, which indicates a positive reaction.

The nonfermenters also can be identified by semiautomated and automated identification systems. There are many nonfermentative gram-negative bacilli and various classification methods. This chapter will focus on those most commonly encountered in the clinical microbiology laboratory.

Family Pseudomonadaceae

The classification of *Pseudomonas* bacteria has continued to evolve from when *Pseudomonas aeruginosa* was first isolated in 1882 from soldiers' wounds, which oozed a green and blue exudate. The genus name was first applied to all gram-negative aerobic bacilli with polar flagella, resulting in over 100 species of *Pseudomonas* by the 1980s. With the advent of molecular technology based on 16S ribosomal RNA sequencing, many of the pseudomonads have been reclassified into different genera. Hybridization studies divided the genus into five rRNA groups (I through V). Later, groups II, III, IV, and V were classified into different genera, which are *Burkholderia* and *Ralstonia*. Today, rRNA group I remains and includes the following *Pseudomonas* species: *P. aeruginosa* (including *P. mendocina*), *P. fluorescens*, *P. putido*, and *P. stutzeri*.

The family Pseudomonadaceae includes nonfermentative gram-negative bacilli that are motile with polar flagella. *Pseudomonas* can utilize many nutrients, both in the environment and in many types of media. These organisms oxidize glucose and other carbohydrates and are strict aerobes and usually are cytochrome oxidase positive. Infections most commonly are seen in neutropenic patients, burn patients, and those with other underlying medical disorders. The most clinically relevant species will be discussed in this chapter. BOX 11-3 summarizes the relevant groups and species of current and former Pseudomonadaceae groups.

PSEUDOMONAS AERUGINOSA

The most frequently isolated nonfermenter is *Pseudomonas aeruginosa*, an important opportunistic pathogen. In fact, this organism accounts for approximately 75% to 80% of all nonfermenters isolated from clinical specimens. It is classified as a fluorescent pseudomonad and is a strict aerobe. Identification of the organism is usually aided by characteristic pigments, which are **pyocyanin**, a water-soluble blue pigment, and **fluorescein**, or **pyoverdin**, a yellow fluorescing pigment. Together, the pigments produce the notable blue-green color of *P. aeruginosa* (**FIGURE 11-6**). Pyocyanin

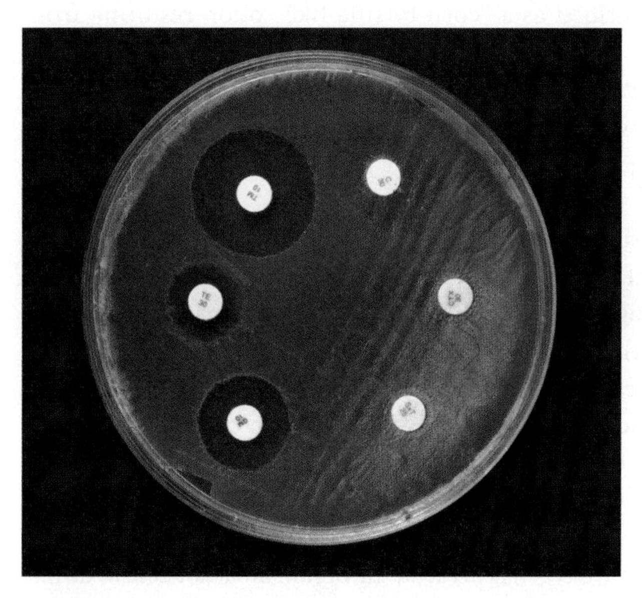

FIGURE 11-6 *P. aeruginosa* on Mueller-Hinton agar illustrating its characteristic blue-green pigment.

BOX 11-3 Pseudomonadaceae Characteristics and Species

Group	Characteristics	Species
Fluorescent Group	Produce pyoverdin, yellow	*P. aeruginosa*
	fluorescent pigment	*P. fluorescens*
		P. putida
Stutzeri Group	Soil denitrifiers	*P. stutzeri*
		P. mendocina
Pseudomallei Group	Resistant to polymyxin B and colistin	*Burkholderia mallei*
		B. pseudomallei
		B. cepacia
		Stenotrophomonas maltophilia

is produced only by *P. aeruginosa* and can be extracted with chloroform. This pigment is responsible for the blue exudate that may be seen with *P. aeruginosa* wound infections. Fluorescein must be visualized using an ultraviolet light. These pigments are visible on most clear agars, and their colors can be enhanced through use of Flo Agar, or Pseudomonas F Agar, and Tech Agar, or Pseudomonas P Agar (Becton Dickinson Microbiology Systems). Other strains of *P. aeruginosa* also may produce pyorubin pigment (red color) or pyomelanin pigment (brown color).

Another significant characteristic of *P. aeruginosa* is its fruity odor of overripened grapes, which also has been described as a "corn tortilla-like" odor, resulting from the production of 2-aminoacetophenone. Other important factors include the organism's ability to grow at 42°C, as well as at room temperature and at 35°C to 37°C. The organism is motile with a single, polar flagellum.

P. aeruginosa grows well on MacConkey agar and eosin-methylene blue (EMB) as a lactose-negative organism. On blood agar the bacterium typically produces large, rough, dull grayish, spreading colonies that are opalescent with the appearance of ground lead. The colonies have a feathery edge and are β-hemolytic (**FIGURE 11-7**). The mucoid strain, isolated in those with cystic fibrosis, produces large amounts of capsular alginate, which can give the colonies a mucoid appearance.

Although *P. aeruginosa* will grow on the TSI slant, where oxygen is present, the organism is not able to utilize carbohydrates in the TSI, so a reaction of K/K is observed. *P. aeruginosa* is oxidase positive and oxidizes glucose but not maltose in the OF medium. It is an obligate aerobe but also can use nitrate and arginine as a final electron acceptor when oxygen is not present. **TABLE 11-1** lists important reactions to identify *P. aeruginosa*.

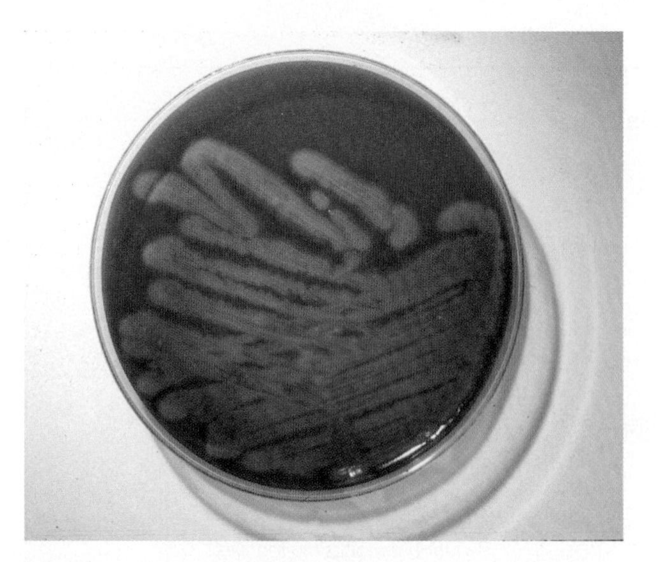

FIGURE 11-7 *P. aeruginosa* on sheep blood agar showing opalescent colonies with a feathered edge and beta hemolysis.

TABLE 11-1 Identification of *Pseudomonas aeruginosa*

Oxidase: Positive
Pyocyanin: Positive
Fluorescein (pyoverdin): Positive
Oxidizes glucose, fructose, and xylose in oxidative-fermentative (OF) medium
Cannot utilize maltose, sucrose, or lactose in OF medium
Grows well on MacConkey agar as lactose-negative colonies
Arginine: Positive
Lysine: Negative
Ornithine: Negative
Acetamide: Positive
Nitrates denitrified to nitrites (NO_3 to NO_2)
Citrate: Positive
Urease: Variable
Indole: Negative
Growth at 42°C: Positive
Motile by one or two polar flagella
Resistant to kanamycin
Susceptible to carbenicillin

P. aeruginosa is an important pathogen, especially in the immunocompromised host; it is the agent of both acute and chronic lung infections, urinary tract infections, and sepsis. Infections typically occur at sites where water or moisture accumulate, such as in the ears, eyes, and indwelling catheters and most often at sites of burns and wounds. The organism is found throughout the environment and nature and is known to cause infections in mammals, insects, birds, fish, and plants. *P. aeruginosa* also has been isolated from contact lens solutions, cosmetics, hot tubs, and fruits and vegetables. It is able to survive the harsh environment of soap solutions, water faucets, disinfectants, and whirlpools and has been isolated even on flowers and plants in patients' rooms. Thus, the organism is often associated with nosocomial infections, such as whirlpool-associated dermatitis, wound infections, urinary tract infections, and lower respiratory tract infections following respiratory ventilation in patients with preexisting lung disorders. It is not considered to be a major normal flora of humans but can be found in the

BOX 11-4 Infections Associated with *P. aeruginosa*

Nosocomial, or HAI:

Severe wound infections in burn patients

Urinary tract infections

Pneumonia

Septicemia

Chronic lung infections in cystic fibrosis patients

Meningitis

Community acquired:

Destructive eye infections, such as keratitis or corneal ulcers in contact lens wearers

Otitis externa, or swimmer's ear

Otitis media

Folliculitis ("hot tub folliculitis")

gastrointestinal tract and can colonize moist skin areas and the throat and nose.

The incidence of hospitalized-acquired infections (HAI), or nosocomial infections, caused by *P. aeruginosa* has increased in recent years (BOX 11-4). There is an exogenous acquisition through the environment and also an endogenous route from the site of colonization. Ventilator-associated pneumonia and bacteremia are also associated with *P. aeruginosa*.

A mucoid strain of *P. aeruginosa* occurs in those with cystic fibrosis, causing a severe and chronic lung disease. Individuals with cystic fibrosis activate the alginate gene, resulting in the production of alginate, which surrounds the bacterial cell wall and protects it from phagocytosis.

P. aeruginosa has several virulence factors that contribute to its pathogenesis, including fimbriae, which enable it to attach to respiratory epithelial cells. **Flagella** also enable the organism to adhere to host cells, and **alginate** is associated with inhibition of **chemotaxis** and **phagocytosis**. **Elastase**, which digests elastin of the arterial walls; **collagenase**, which breaks down collagen; and **protease**, which degrades protein, are all important enzymes produced by the organism that destroys tissues. The pigment pyocyanin is known to inhibit lymphocytes and cilia, and **exotoxin A** inhibits protein synthesis, which leads to tissue destruction and an aggravated host immune response. *P. aeruginosa* also produces hemolysins, which destroy red cells, and

BOX 11-5 Virulence Factors of *Pseudomonas aeruginosa*

Attachment

Fimbriae attach to host cells; activate proinflammatory genes

Polar flagella attach to host cells; motility, and inactivate interleukin 8

Tissue invasion and immune inhibition

Pyoverdin: Binds iron

Elastase tissue invasion: Digests elastin

Protease tissue invasion: Protein degradation

Collagenase tissue invasion: Collagen destruction

Hemolysin tissue invasion: Lyse red blood cells

Leukocidan tissue invasion: Lyse white blood cells

Lipopolysaccharide endotoxin effects

Alginate capsule: Inhibits phagocytosis and chemotaxis of neutrophils, and activation of complement

Exotoxin A: Inhibits protein synthesis and facilitates infection

Type III secretion system: Injects toxins into host cells (ExoS, ExoT, ExoU, ExoY)

ExoS, ExoT, ExoU, ExoY: Toxins that have cytotoxic and other effects

lipopolysaccharide, which functions as endotoxin. These are summarized in BOX 11-5.

Another significant characteristic is the organism's resistance to many antibiotics used to treat gram-negative infections. *P. aeruginosa* has exhibited both intrinsic and extrinsic resistance to several antibiotics. Infections may be treated with the aminoglycosides, such as tobramycin, gentamycin, or amikacin; β-lactams, such as third- and fourth-generation cephalosporins, ticarcillin, and piperacillin; the carbapenems, such as imipenem; or the fluoroquinolones, such as ciprofloxacin, levofloxacin, and ofloxacin. Antibiotic susceptibility testing is performed to determine suitable antibiotic choices.

PSEUDOMONAS FLUORESCENS AND *P. PUTIDA*

P. fluorescens and *P. putida* are grouped as fluorescent pseudomonads because they produce pyoverdin, a yellow

BOX 11-6 Summary of Characteristics for *Pseudomonas fluorescens* and *Pseudomonas putida*

Motile by a polar tuft of flagella
Growth at 42°C: Positive
Oxidase: Positive
Oxidize glucose in OF medium
Pyocyanin: Negative
Pyoverdin: Positive
Acetamide: Negative
Arginine: Positive
Resistant to carbenicillin
Susceptible to kanamycin

fluorescent pigment. Both of these organisms are found in environmental sources and are associated with nosocomial infections. They are not considered to be part of the human normal flora and rarely are associated with opportunistic infections. *P. fluorescens* is found in the soil and water as an environmental contaminant and is associated with food spoilage and plant infections. It also is a rare cause of urinary tract and wound infections in humans. *P. putida* has been the cause of isolated cases of septicemia, urinary tract infections, and pneumonia. The organisms also have been isolated from hospital environmental sources, including sinks. BOX 11-6 lists important characteristics of *P. fluorescens* and *P. putida*.

To differentiate *P. fluorescens* from *P. putida*, *P. fluorescens* is proteolytic and can hydrolyze gelatin, whereas *P. putida* is nonproteolytic and cannot hydrolyze gelatin.

P. STUTZERI AND *P. MENDOCINA*

P. stutzeri and *P. mendocina* are categorized as "soil denitrifiers" because these bacteria use ammonium (NH_4) as the sole nitrogen source and acetate as the sole carbon source, grow anaerobically, and produce nitrogen gas. They have been isolated from straw and manure and also from contaminated cosmetics and baby formula. These organisms have been cited as rare causes of otitis media, eye infections, and pneumonia. *P. stutzeri* is found in soil, marine water, and stagnant water, as well as in medical devices. Colonies are dry and wrinkled with a buff or light-brown color. The colonies are often tough and adherent. The organism is arginine dehydrolase (ADH) negative and positive for starch hydrolysis. *P. mendocina* appears as smooth, buttery, flat, unwrinkled colonies on blood agar. It is motile by polar monotrichous flagella, grows at 42°C, and is ADH positive and negative for starch hydrolysis.

Burkholderia

Burkholderia mallei is the cause of **glanders**, primarily an infectious disease of horses, goats, sheep, and donkeys. Although extremely rare, humans can acquire the infection through direct contact with the body fluids or tissues of infected animals through skin abrasions. It also can be acquired through inhalation of contaminated aerosols or through the mucous membranes of the eyes or nose. The infection is most commonly seen in domestic animals in Asia, Africa, and the Middle East; there have been no naturally acquired cases of glanders in the United States for over 60 years. However, there have been laboratory-acquired infections and rare sporadic cases in veterinarians and animal handlers. Human-to-human infection has not been reported in the United States.

Types of glanders infections depend on the route of infection and include acute and chronic cutaneous infections, lung infections, bacteremia, and chronic infections.

B. mallei is the only nonmotile pseudomonad and is resistant to polymyxin B. Colonies are smooth and cream to white in color on blood agar. The organism is weakly oxidase positive and fails to grow at 42°C.

Burkholderia pseudomallei is the agent of **Melioidosis**, a glanders-like disease found in humans and other animals in Southeast Asia and Australia. Melioidosis is believed to be a relatively common disease in the tropics in areas where it is endemic in the environment. *B. pseudomallei* is found in contaminated water, soil, and vegetation in endemic areas. It is endemic in Southeast Asia and was the source of infections in American soldiers during the Vietnam conflict. Melioidosis, also known as Whitmore's disease, is a seasonal disease and is more prevalent during the monsoon rain season. It is rarely found in the United States or other western parts of the world; there are approximately five cases reported each year in the United States. Travelers may acquire the disease during travel to endemic areas and may bring the disease to the United States.

The infection most often is characterized by an acute and severe pneumonia that can lead to septicemia. It also can cause acute and chronic skin infections and abscesses through skin inoculation. This bacterium is easily aerosolized, and infections in the United States may be laboratory acquired through inhalation in aerosols.

B. pseudomallei grows on sheep blood agar as wrinkled cream-to-tan colonies. The organism is oxidase positive and motile via a polar tuft of multitrichous flagella and is arginine positive. It is highly oxidative and can oxidize glucose, maltose, lactose, mannitol, and cellobiose. The wrinkled colonies may be confused with *P. stutzeri*, which is arginine negative.

In recent years, both *B. mallei* and *B. pseudomallei* have been cited as possible agents of bioterrorism.

B. cepacia, the cause of onion bulb rot in plants and foot rot in humans, is found in soil, water, and plants and also survives well in the hospital environment. It has been isolated from environmental sources of water and in intravenous fluids, detergents, and disinfectants, including chlorohexidine. It is being found with increasing frequency as an opportunistic and nosocomial pathogen, causing pneumonia, urinary tract infections, septicemia, and endocarditis in patients with contaminated heart valves.

B. cepacia is not normal flora of humans and is not pathogenic in a healthy host. The organism colonizes the skin and respiratory tract of hospitalized patients. It is an opportunistic pathogen and causes infections of the respiratory and urinary tracts, as well as wound infections. It also is associated with a pneumonia in individuals with cystic fibrosis and chronic granulomatous disease. The organism is intrinsically resistant to the aminoglycosides and must be treated with sulfamethoxazole, chloroamphenicol, or the third-generation cephalosporins.

B. cepacia produces yellow, serrated colonies that are weakly oxidase positive. This bacterium acidifies the open glucose, maltose, lactose, and mannitol tubes and is arginine negative and lysine positive.

Ralstonia

Ralstonia pickettii and *R. radiobacter* are slow-growing nonfermenters that are rare opportunistic pathogens. *R. pickettii* is nonpathogenic in the healthy host and is not normal flora in humans. It has been isolated from environmental sources, including contaminated medical instruments, intravenous fluids, and medications. The organism has been isolated from a variety of clinical sources, including blood, urine, and sputum.

TABLE 11-2 summarizes the biochemical reactions used to identify *Pseudomonas* and *Burkholderia* species.

TABLE 11-2 Identification of Important *Pseudomonas*, *Burkholderia*, and *Stenotrophomonas* Species

	P. aeruginosa	*P. fluorescens*	*P. mendocina*	*P. putida*	*P. stutzeri*	*B. cepacia*	*B. pseudomallei*	*Stenotrophomonas maltophilia*
Oxidase	+	+	+	+	+	Weak +	+	–
Motility	+	+	+	+	+	+	+	+
Pyoverdin	+	+	–	+	–	–	–	–
Oxidation of:								
Glucose	+	+	+	+	+	+	+	Weak+
Maltose	–	V	–	V	+	+	+	Strong+
Lactose	–	–	–	–	–	+	+	+
Mannitol	+	+	–	–	V	+	+	–
Arginine	+	+	+	+	–	+	+	–
Lysine	–	–	–	–	–	+	–	Slow+
Nitrate to nitrite	+	V	+	–	+	V	+	V
Nitrate to nitrogen gas	V	–	+	–	+	–	+	–
DNase	–	–	–	–	–	–	–	+
Polymyxin susceptibility	S	S	S	S	S	R	R	R

+, most strains positive; –, most strains negative; V, variable reaction; S, susceptible; R, resistant

Acinetobacter

Acinetobacter species are oxidase-negative, catalase-positive, nonmotile coccobacilli appearing as plump, paired rods or diplococci in direct smears (**FIGURE 11-8**). The organisms grow well on MacConkey and sheep blood agars, with a translucent appearance. There are currently over 20 genospecies of *Acinetobacter* based on deoxyribonucleic acid (DNA) hybridization. The most prevalent human pathogen is *A. baumannii*, previously known as *Acinetobacter calcoaceticus* var. *anitratus*. Key reactions are as follows in BOX 11-7.

A. baumannii produces large, gummy, translucent, gray-to-white, convex, entire colonies on sheep blood agar. A bluish or peach-to-pink tint may be observed on MacConkey agar, and a cornflower blue color is produced on EMB. Growth on MacConkey agar and the negative oxidase test may lead one to identify the organism mistakenly as a member of the Enterobacteriaceae.

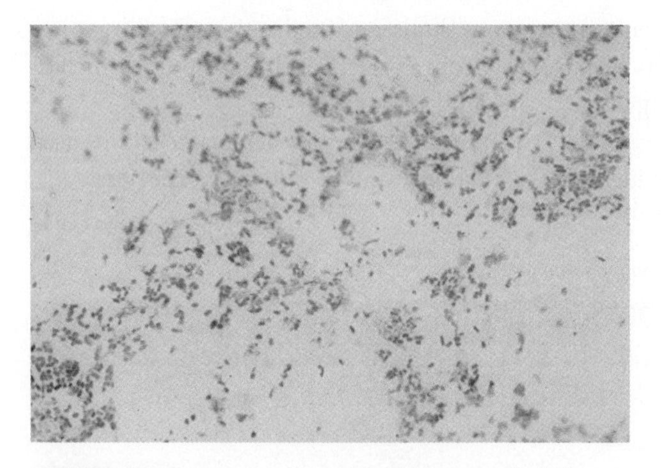

FIGURE 11-8 Gram stained *Acinetobacter baumannii* which shows plump coccobacilli arranged in pairs.

BOX 11-7 Characteristics of *Acinetobacter*

- Obligate aerobe
- Nonmotile
- Oxidase negative
- Nonhemolytic
- Grows well on MacConkey agar
- Resistant to penicillin

TABLE 11-3 Differentiation of *Acinetobacter* Species

	A. baumannii	*A. lwoffii*
Oxidase	Negative	Negative
Growth at 42°C	Positive	Negative
Lysine	Negative	Negative
Carbohydrate utilization	Saccharolytic	Asaccharolytic
Glucose	Ferments rapidly	Asaccharolytic
Lactose assimilation	Rapid assimilation	Negative

Acinetobacter lwoffii (formerly known as *Acinetobacter calcoaceticus* var. *lwoffii*), the second most common *Acinetobacter* isolate, is also oxidase negative and nonmotile. However, in contrast to *A. baumannii*, this bacterium is asaccharolytic. It grows on MacConkey agar, producing an ammonia-like odor, and is resistant to penicillin. **TABLE 11-3** summarizes the differentiation of *A. baumannii* from *A. lwoffii*.

Acinetobacter is associated with nosocomial and opportunistic infections. The bacteria colonize moist areas of human skin and are normally found in the oropharynx and vaginal and gastrointestinal tracts. The organisms also are found in the hospital environment, soil, and water. Infections include urinary and respiratory tract infections, wound infections associated with soil and water contamination, bacteremia, and meningitis. Hospital equipment that has been contaminated by *Acinetobacter* species includes endotracheal tubes, respiratory care and dialysis equipment, and venous catheters.

In the past, *Acinetobacter* was known as "*Mima*" because it was said to mimic the appearance of *Neisseria* in the Gram stain in female genital tract specimens. Thus, *Acinetobacter* must be differentiated from *Neisseria*. Using, the oxidase reaction, *Neisseria* is oxidase positive, whereas *Acinetobacter* is oxidase negative.

Stenotrophomonas

Stenotrophomonas maltophilia is present in food and water sources, soil, animals, and plants. It also has been isolated from a variety of clinical sites and is considered to be a contaminant or commensal on humans. It is a part of the transient flora that a patient acquires while in the hospital and may colonize the respiratory, urinary, and genitourinary tracts. Most infections are nosocomial, such

BOX 11-8 Identification of *Stenotrophomonas maltophilia*

Yellow-to-tan pigment on trypticase soy agar

Lavender-green to pale lavender pigment on sheep blood agar

Growth at 42°C: Positive

Oxidase: Negative

Oxidizes glucose in OF medium: Weakly positive

Oxidizes maltose in OF medium: Strongly positive

Pyoverdin: Negative

ONPG: Positive

DNase: Positive

Nitrates are not reduced to nitrogen gas

Lysine: Slowly positive

Arginine: Negative

Ornithine: Negative

as pneumonia, including ventilator-associated pneumonia; septicemia; urinary tract infections; and meningitis. It also has been the agent of wound infections from contact with contaminated farming equipment. The organism is resistant to many antibiotics, including the aminoglycosides and β-lactams and is susceptible to trimethoprim-sulfamethoxazole.

S. maltophilia produces large, smooth, glistening colonies with a yellow to tan pigment on trypticase soy agar (TSA) and a lavender-green to light purple pigment on sheep blood agar. It will grow at 42°C and is unique for *Pseudomonas* in being oxidase negative. The organism produces a weakly positive reaction for glucose in the open tube and a strongly positive reaction in the open maltose tube. An ammonia-like odor is sometimes produced by the *S. maltophilia*. BOX 11-8 lists important reactions of *S. maltophilia*.

Alcaligenes

Alcaligenes organisms are tiny gram-negative bacilli that are motile by peritrichous flagella. All species are oxidase and catalase positive and grow on MacConkey agar.

Alcaligenes faecalis is the species most often associated with human infections; this species includes the strain formerly known as *A. odorans*. *A. faecalis* is associated with opportunistic infections of the blood, cerebrospinal fluid, urinary tract, and pleural cavity; wound infections; and abscesses. It is found in soil and water sources and grows as flat, dull colonies with an irregular edge on sheep blood agar. The organism produces strong alkaline reactions in oxidative-fermentative medium. It is unable to reduce nitrates to nitrites or nitrates to nitrogen gas but is able to reduce nitrites to nitrogen gas. *A. faecalis* can grow in 6.5% sodium chloride (NaCl). The strain formerly known as *A. odorans* has a fruity odor of apples or pears.

A. piechaudii is rarely clinically significant and reduces nitrates to nitrites, grows in 6.5% NaCl, and produces alkaline reactions in OF glucose and xylose tubes.

Achromobacter

Achromobacter denitrificans and *A. xylosoxidans* were previously classified in the genus *Alcaligenes*. *A. xylosoxidans* is a rare opportunistic pathogen, which has been isolated from various clinical sites. An important reaction is its ability to oxidize both glucose and xylose in oxidative fermentative media. *A. xylosoxidans* cannot grow in 6.5% NaCl broth; it is able to reduce nitrates to nitrites but cannot reduce nitrites to nitrogen gas. TABLE 11-4 differentiates *Achromobacter xylosoxidans* from *Alcaligenes faecalis*.

TABLE 11-4 Differentiation of *Alcaligenes* and *Achromobacter* Species

	Alcaligenes faecalis	*Achromobacter xylosoxidans*
Oxidase	Positive	Positive
Motility	+ with peritrichous flagella	+ with peritrichous flagella
MacConkey agar	Growth	Growth
Oxidation of:		
Glucose	Negative (alkaline)	Positive (acidic)
Xylose	Negative (alkaline)	Positive (acidic)
Nitrate to nitrite	Negative	Positive
Nitrate to nitrogen gas	Negative	Variable
Nitrite to nitrogen gas	Positive	Negative
Growth in 6.5% NaCl	Positive	Negative

A. denitrificans is a rare clinical isolate that reduces nitrates to nitrites and nitrogen gas and nitrites to nitrogen gas. Alkaline reactions are observed in the OF glucose and xylose tubes.

Moraxella

Moraxella organisms are nonmotile, tiny gram-negative diplococci or diplobacilli. The organisms are free living in soil and water and are found as normal flora on the mucous membranes and skin of humans. Small, pinpoint, nonpigmented colonies are observed on sheep blood agar after 24 hours of incubation. The organism grows poorly or not at all on MacConkey agar. *Moraxella* is oxidase and catalase positive and nonsaccharolytic. In fact, most *Moraxella* species are considered to be biologically inactive, producing very few positive biochemical reactions. *Moraxella* species are very susceptible to low levels of penicillin.

To differentiate *Moraxella* from *Acinetobacter*, the oxidase test is used. *Moraxella* is oxidase positive, whereas *Acinetobacter* is oxidase negative. Because *Moraxella* may be confused with *Neisseria* in a Gram stain smear, it must be differentiated from *Neisseria*. Using the cysteine trypticase agar (CTA) reactions, *Moraxella* does not utilize any carbohydrates because it is nonsaccharolytic, whereas *N. gonorrhoeae* will use glucose only. Furthermore, some *Moraxella* will grow on sheep blood agar, and *N. gonorrhoeae* cannot grow on sheep blood agar. In addition, a Gram-stained smear prepared from the outer zone of inhibition around a penicillin susceptibility disk will produce elongated forms for *Moraxella*, whereas *Neisseria* will remain as cocci.

Clinically important *Moraxella* include *M. catarrhalis* (discussed in Chapter 9), *M. lacunata*, *M. nonliquefaciens*, and *M. osloensis*. *M. lacunata* may cause conjunctivitis and needs enriched media, such as rabbit serum, to grow. *M. nonliquefaciens* has been found to cause infections of the eye and respiratory and genital tracts. *Moraxella* is normal flora on the mucous membranes of the respiratory tract.

Oligella

Oligella organisms are nonsaccharolytic, oxidase-positive, catalase-positive, nonmotile coccobacilli. The significant human species are *O. urethralis* (formerly *Moraxella urethralis*) and *O. ureolytica*. *O. urethralis* is typically found in urethral specimens and is commensal in the genitourinary tract. It is unable to utilize carbohydrates and is phenylalanine deaminase positive. *O. ureolytica* is motile by peritrichous flagella and produces a rapid urease reaction. It has been isolated in clinical cultures, mainly as a cause of urinary tract infections.

Chryseobacterium

Chryseobacterium is a member of the family Flavobacteriaceae. Other genera in this family include *Flavobacterium* and *Caponocytophagia*. Important members of *Chryseobacterium* include *C. indologenes* and *C. meningosepticum*, which were previously classified in the genus *Flavobacterium*. All members of this family generally fail to grow or grow poorly on MacConkey agar, are oxidase positive and nonmotile, and fail to reduce nitrates. Most species produce yellow-colored colonies on nutrient and sheep blood agar, which intensifies with prolonged incubation at room temperature. (**FIGURE 11-9**)

Chryseobacterium organisms are widely distributed in the environment in soil and water and on plants. They also are found in water sources within the hospital environment. Key reactions for this genus include resistance to penicillin and polymyxin B. They may produce a lavender-green color on sheep blood agar because of the proteolytic enzyme gelatinase. *C. indologenes* is the most

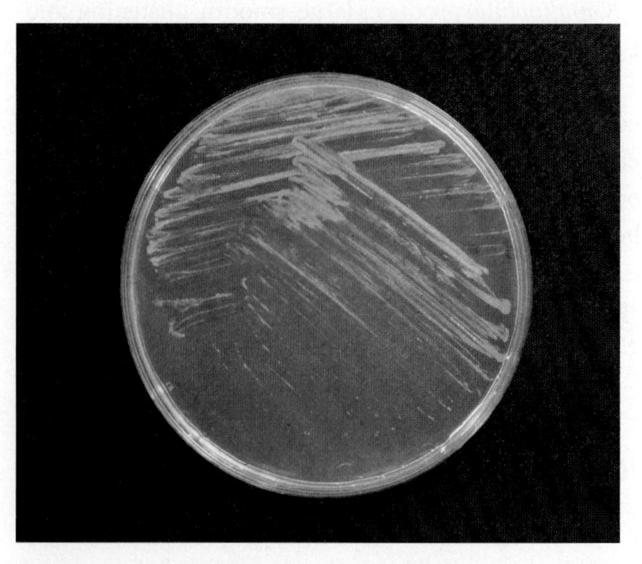

FIGURE 11-9 *Chryseobacterium meningosepticum* on nutrient agar which shows its characteristic yellow pigment.

frequent human isolate, although it is usually not clinically significant. It is an occasional cause of bacteremia in the immunosuppressed individual. *C. indologenes* produces dark-yellow colonies on blood agar and is indole positive when using the modified indole method, which uses xylene extraction. The organism oxidizes glucose, but not mannitol, in the OF media.

C. meningosepticum is the species most often found causing significant infections in humans. It has been isolated from several water sources, including ice machines, water fountains, sinks, incubators, and water baths. The organism is nosocomial and extremely opportunistic, causing meningitis in newborns and pneumonia, endocarditis, bacteremia, and wound infections in immunosuppressed adults. Newborn infections have a high mortality rate and epidemics have occurred. *C. meningosepticum* produces delayed positive reactions in the open OF glucose and mannitol tubes, is indole positive (with the modified method), and is positive for esculin hydrolysis, ONPG, and deoxyribonuclease. It is urease negative. Colonies are pinpoint and glistening, and a pale-yellow pigment is observed that is enhanced with additional incubation at room temperature. The organism is resistant to penicillin and to the aminoglycosides.

Kingella

Kingella organisms are oxidase-positive, catalase-negative bacteria that are indole positive and ferment glucose. *Kingella* species require blood for growth and may "pit" the agar surface. *Kingella denitrificans* and *Kingella kingae* are rare pathogens.

The nonfermenters are being isolated as increasing causes of human infection. Identification is facilitated by the use of several packaged identification systems, including the Crystal™ Enteric/Nonfermenter ID Kit (Beckton Dickinson Microbiological Systems), RapID NF Plus (Remel Laboratories), and the API® 20E (bioMérieux). BOX 11-9 categorizes the significant nonfermentative gram-negative bacilli.

BOX 11-9 **Significant Nonfermentative Gram-Negative Bacilli**

Motile with polar flagella

Pseudomonas

Burkholderia

Ralstonia

Stenotrophomonas

Motile with peritrichous flagella

Alcaligenes

Achromobacter

Oligella

Nonmotile and oxidase positive

Chryseobacterium

Flavobacterium

Moraxella

Nonmotile and oxidase negative

Acinetobacter

Laboratory Procedures

Procedure

Oxidative-fermentative (OF) medium

Purpose

OF medium is used to determine whether an organism can utilize carbohydrates in an oxidative or a fermentative manner. Those bacteria that are nonsaccharolytic, or unable to break down carbohydrates, are also identified. OF medium can be used as a single test for glucose or as a set of OF carbohydrates. Lactose, maltose, sucrose, xylose, and fructose are usually tested.

Principle

OF medium contains a high concentration of carbohydrate (1%) and a small concentration of peptone (0.2%), which facilitates the oxidative use of carbohydrates by nonfermenting gram-negative bacilli.

Medium used to identify Enterobacteriaceae is not suitable for the nonfermenters for two reasons. First, the amount of acid produced during the oxidative process is not sufficient for the indicator to take on its acidic color. Second, the alkaline end products produced during the reaction neutralize the acid produced.

In OF medium, positive reactions are indicated by a yellow color, as the bromthymol blue indicator becomes yellow in an acidic environment. Green or blue-green is interpreted as negative.

Reagents and Media

OF basal medium containing glucose in a final concentration of 1% OF basal medium containing other desired carbohydrates (lactose, maltose, sucrose, xylose, fructose) in a final concentration of 1%

Procedure

1. Inoculate the top portion of the medium of two OF tubes (for each carbohydrate tested) with growth taken from colonies with a needle.
2. Overlay the surface of one tube with 0.25 inch of sterile mineral oil.
3. Replace caps of both tubes.
4. Incubate at 35°C for 18 to 24 hours. Interpret reactions at 24 hours. If no change has occurred, re-incubate for an additional 18 to 24 hours.

Interpretation

Oxidative: Open tube (without oil) turns yellow; closed tube (with oil) remains green or blue-green.
Fermentative: Both open and closed tubes turn yellow.
Nonsaccharolytic: Both open and closed tubes remain green or become blue-green.

Quality Control

Glucose fermented: *Escherichia coli*
Glucose oxidized: *Pseudomonas aeruginosa*
Glucose neither oxidized nor fermented: *Alcaligenes faecalis*
Oxidation of:
Maltose: Positive—*Burkholderia cepacia*; negative—*Alcaligenes faecalis*
Lactose: Positive—*B. cepacia*; negative—*A. faecalis*
Mannitol: Positive—*B. cepacia*; negative—*A. faecalis*
Fructose: Positive—*P. aeruginosa*; negative—*A. faecalis*
Sucrose: Positive—*B. cepacia*; negative—*A. faecalis*
Xylose: Positive—*P. aeruginosa*; negative—*A. faecalis*

Notes

1. Some microbiologists state that only one type of OF medium needs to be inoculated. The rationale is that oxidizers will acidify only the top portion of the agar, while fermenters will acidify the entire tube.
2. Enteric media, such as the triple sugar iron (TSI) agar, also will determine whether the organism is a fermenter.

Procedure

Nitrate reaction

Purpose

The nitrate reaction is used to determine whether aerobes and facultative anaerobes can reduce nitrates.

Principle

Nitrate broth contains potassium nitrate. After inoculation and incubation, the medium is evaluated for reduction of nitrates. An inverted Durham fermentation tube is used to detect production of nitrogen gas. If gas is present and the organism is a nonfermenter, the test is positive for denitrification, and nitrate has been reduced to nitrogen gas. If a red color develops after addition of 0.8% sulfanilic acid in 5N acetic acid, followed by 0.6% N,N-dimethyl-α-naphthylamine in 5N acetic acid, nitrates have been reduced to nitrites. Zinc dust is added to negative reactions to detect unreduced nitrate. If there is no color development after the addition of zinc, nitrate was reduced beyond nitrite, and the test is positive. If a red color develops after the addition of zinc, unreduced nitrates are present, indicating a negative test.

Reagents and Media

Nitrate broth
Reagent A: 0.8% sulfanilic acid in 5N acetic acid
Reagent B: 0.6% N,N-dimethyl-α-naphthylamine in 5N acetic acid
Zinc dust

Procedure

1. From a pure culture, use a sterile inoculating loop to remove several colonies and inoculate nitrate broth.
2. Replace cap loosely and incubate at 35°C to 37°C.
3. Examine tubes at 18 to 24 hours and at 42 to 48 hours for growth and presence of gas in the Durham tube.
4. If gas is present and the organism is a nonfermenter, the test is positive for denitrification, indicating that nitrate has been reduced to nitrogen gas. If the organism is a ferment, gas may or may not be present.
5. Add 10 drops of reagent A (0.8% sulfanilic acid in 5N acetic acid) and 10 drops of reagent B (0.6% N,N-dimethyl-α-naphthylamine in 5N acetic acid) to the tube. Development of a red color within 2 minutes indicates a positive test for the reduction of nitrate to nitrite.
6. If there is no color development, add a small amount of zinc dust to the tube. If no color develops within 5 to 10 minutes, nitrate was reduced beyond nitrite, and the test is positive. The development of a red color indicates the presence of unreduced nitrate and a negative test.

Quality Control
Acinetobacter calcoaceticus: Negative
Escherichia coli: Positive
Pseudomonas aeruginosa: Positive

Interpretation
Gas in Durham tube: Positive for nonfermenters
Red after addition of reagent A and reagent B: Positive reduction of nitrates to nitrite
Red after addition of zinc dust: Negative for nitrate reduction
No color development after addition of zinc dust: Positive reduction of nitrates to nitrite

Notes

1. Because the test is very sensitive, an uninoculated control should be tested with reagents to ensure that the medium is nitrate free and that the glassware and reagents have not been contaminated with nitrous oxide.
2. Adding too much zinc may result in a false-negative reaction or a brief reaction that could be interpreted incorrectly as negative.

Laboratory Exercises

1. Streak the following nonfermenters on blood, chocolate, and MacConkey agars. Incubate at 35°C, and record your observations at 24 and 48 hours.

	Blood	Chocolate	MacConkey
Pseudomonas aeruginosa			
Acinetobacter baumannii			
Alcaligenes faecalis			
Chryseobacterium meningosepticum			
Stenotrophomonas maltophilia			
Burkholderia cepacia			

2. Perform the cytochrome oxidase technique on each of the organisms from Exercise 1. List which organisms gave a positive or a negative result.

Oxidase result	Organisms
Positive	
Negative	

3. Explain why both an open and a closed tube are needed in the oxidative-fermentative (OF) medium. __________

   Perform the following OF reactions and interpret your results.

	Glucose	Lactose	Maltose	Fructose
	Open Closed	Open Closed	Open Closed	Open Closed
P. aeruginosa				
A. baumannii				
A. faecalis				
C. meningosepticum				
B. cepacia				
S. maltophilia				

4. Perform the nitrate reduction technique on the following organisms. Record your observations and interpretations. What is the purpose of the the inverted Durham tube? __________

   When is it necessary to add zinc dust? __________
   Why? __________

	Observations after reagents A and B	Observations after zinc (if needed)	Interpretation
P. aeruginosa			
A. baumannii			
A. faecalis			
C. meningosepticum			
B. cepacia			
S. maltophilia			

5. Identify an unknown in pure culture prepared by your instructor. Include a log of media and procedures performed, with results. Inoculate appropriate media and perform necessary tests. Record your observations and results, and identify the unknown.
   Unknown number: __________

Media inoculated	Observation	Result
Procedures performed	**Observation**	**Result**
Identification and explanation		

Review Questions

Multiple Choice

1. Infection associated with the nonfermentative gram-negative bacilli:
   a. Can be classified as true pathogens and are generally community acquired
   b. Are opportunistic and often nosocomial
   c. Are the most common clinical infections
   d. Are declining in number
2. Oxidative-fermentative (OF) medium of Hugh and Leifson is well suited for nonfermenters because of a:
   a. High concentration of peptone and low concentration of carbohydrate
   b. High concentration of both peptone and carbohydrate
   c. High concentration of carbohydrate and low concentration of peptone
   d. Low concentration of both peptone and carbohydrate
3. An organism producing a yellow color in the open tube and a blue-green color in the closed tube of an OF glucose determination is said to:
   a. Ferment glucose
   b. Oxidize glucose
   c. Be unable to utilize carbohydrate
   d. Give a TSI of A/A
4. Which reaction is incorrect for *Pseudomonas aeruginosa*?
   a. Produces pyocyanin pigment
   b. Produces pyoverdin pigment
   c. Positively alkalizes acidamide
   d. Fails to grow at 42°C
5. Which statement most correctly describes infections attributed to *Pseudomonas aeruginosa*?
   a. Common cause of wound infections in burn patients
   b. Resistant to many antibiotics typically used to treat gram-negative infections
   c. Cause of pneumonia in patients with cystic fibrosis
   d. Both a and b are correct.
   e. All are correct.
6. Which of the following does not produce pyoverdin pigment?
   a. *Pseudomonas aeruginosa*
   b. *Burkholderia cepacia*
   c. *Pseudomonas fluorescens*
   d. *Pseudomonas putida*
7. *Burkholderia mallei* is the causative agent in:
   a. Glanders
   b. Melioidosis
   c. Neonatal sepsis
   d. Onion bulb rot
8. Which of the following correctly lists the characteristics of *Stenotrophomonas maltophilia*?
   a. Blue-green pigment, oxidase positive, oxidizes glucose
   b. Yellow pigment, oxidase positive, oxidizes maltose
   c. Nonpigmented, oxidase negative, deoxyribonuclease positive
   d. Yellow pigment, oxidase negative, oxidizes maltose
9. *Acinetobacter baumannii* is:
   a. Oxidase positive
   b. Nonsaccharolytic
   c. Resistant to penicillin
   d. Motile
10. *Acinetobacter* can be differentiated from *Neisseria* by:
    a. A positive oxidase reaction for *Neisseria*
    b. Gram stain
    c. Carbohydrate utilization patterns
    d. Pigment production
11. A yellow-pigmented gram-negative bacillus, isolated from a sink in a neonatal nursery where an outbreak of meningitis occurred, oxidized glucose but failed to oxidize mannitol in the OF reactions. It produced tiny pinpoint colonies on MacConkey agar. The organism is most likely:
    a. *Stenotrophomonas maltophilia*
    b. *Pseudomonas aeruginosa*
    c. *Chryseobacterium meningosepticum*
    d. *Alcaligenes faecalis*

Bibliography

Athan, E., Allworth, A. M., Engler, C., Bastian, I., & Cheng, A. C. (2005). Melioidosis in tsunami survivors. *Emerging Infectious Diseases, 11,* 1638–1639.

Blondel-Hill, E., Henry, D. A., & Speert, D. P. (2007). *Pseudomonas.* In P. R. Murray, E. J. Baron, J. H. Jorgensen, M. L. Landry, & M. A. Pfaller (Eds.), *Manual of clinical microbiology* (9th ed.). Washington, DC: American Society for Microbiology.

Camp, C., & Tatum, O. (2010). A review of *Acinetobacter baumannii* as a highly successful pathogen in times of war. *Laboratory Medicine, 41,* 649–657.

Centers for Disease Control and Prevention. (2000). Laboratory-acquired human glanders—Maryland, May 2000. *Morbidity and Mortality Weekly Report, 49,* 532–535. Retrieved from http://www.cdc.gov/mmwr/preview/mmwrhtml/mm4924a3.htm

Centers for Disease Control and Prevention. (2004). *Acinetobacter baumannii* infections among patients at military medical facilities treating injured U.S. service members, 2002–2004. *Morbidity and Mortality Weekly Report, 53,* 1063–1066. Retrieved from http://www.cdc.gov/mmwr/preview/mmwrhtml/mm5345a1.htm

Centers for Disease Control and Prevention. (2004). Laboratory exposure to *Burkholderia pseudomallei*—Los Angeles, California, 2003. *Morbidity and Mortality Weekly Report, 53,* 988–990. Retrieved from http://www.cdc.gov/mmwr/preview/mmwrhtml/mm5342a3.htm

Centers for Disease Control and Prevention. (2012). Glanders. Retrieved from http://www.cdc.gov/glanders

Centers for Disease Control and Prevention. (2012). Melioidosis. Retrieved from http://www.cdc.gov/meliodosis

Moore, N. M., & Flaws, M. L. (2011). Epidemiology and pathogenesis of *Pseudomonas aeruginosa* infections. *Clinical Laboratory Science, 24,* 43–46.

Moore, N. M., & Flaws, M. L. (2011). Treatment strategies and recommendations for *Pseudomonas aeruginosa infections. Clinical Laboratory Science, 24,* 52–56.

Pickett, M. J., Hollis, D. G., & Bottone, E. J. (1991). Miscellaneous gram negative bacteria. In A. Balows (Ed.), *Manual of clinical microbiology* (5th ed.). Washington, DC: American Society for Microbiology.

Schreckenberger, P. C. (1992). Classification of nonfermenting gram-negative bacilli. *Clinical Microbiology Update.* Western Pennsylvania Society for Clinical Microbiology.

Schreckenberger, P. C., Daneshvar, M. I., & Hollis, D. A. (2007). Nonfermentative gram-negative rods. In P. R. Murray, E. J. Baron, J. H. Jorgensen, M. L. Landry, & M. A. Pfaller (Eds.), *Manual of clinical microbiology* (9th ed.). Washington, DC: American Society for Microbiology.

Winn, Jr., W., Allen, S., Janda, W., Koneman, E., Procop, G., Schreckenberger, P., & Woods, G. (2006). The nonfermentative gram-negative bacilli. In *Koneman's color atlas and textbook of diagnostic microbiology* (pp. 309–391). Philadelphia, PA: Lippincott Williams & Wilkins.

NEWS: BIOLOGICAL WARFARE AND GLANDERS

Glanders, an ancient and infectious disease of equines, is caused by *Burkholderia mallei*. Aristotle first described the disease in horses in 330 BCE and named it "malleus," which means hammer or mallet. Glanders was first studied in the 19th century, and in 1892, *B. mallei* was identified as its causative agent. The first recorded infected humans were documented in 1821. History speaks to its use as an agent of biological warfare, and today it is considered to be one of several possible agents of bioterrorism.

Glanders is a highly contagious zoonosis with a high mortality rate that infects horses, mules, and donkeys. There are ulcerating skin lesions, and the disease may progress through the lymph nodes into the blood. Naturally occurring glanders has been eradicated in most parts of the world; it was eliminated from U.S. animals in the 1940s. However, glanders is still found in the Middle East, South America, Eastern Europe, and Africa. It is rare in humans, and no epidemics have been reported. The mortality rate for the pulmonary form is 90% to 95% if untreated and 40% if treated.

B. mallei was one of the first biological warfare agents. It was used in sabotage campaigns during World War I in many countries, including the United States, Russia, France, Mesopotamia, and Romania. In 1914, an American educated physician who was a member of the German army returned to live in the United States after an illness. He grew both *B. mallei* and *Bacillus anthracis* (the agent of anthrax) in a home laboratory. Through another contact, horses were inoculated with the bacteria, which were then shipped to the Allies in Europe, thus infecting substantial livestock. Other German agents infected mules in Mesopotamia and mules and horses on the Russian front. These acts harmed artillery movement as well as the convoys of troops and materials.

It also is reported that between 1932 and 1945, Japan used *B. mallei* to infect horses, civilians, and prisoners of war. In China during World War II, it is estimated that 30% of horses tested were infected with glanders. The United States began to develop biological warfare agents in 1942 at Camp Detrick (Fort Detrick) in Maryland. Glanders was studied for possible use but was never weaponized. There were seven laboratory-acquired cases of glanders from 1944 to 1953 at Camp Detrick. In 1972, the United States signed the Prohibition of the Development, Production and Stockpiling of Bacteriological (Biological) and Toxin Weapons and on their Destruction. While most of the biological warfare research had been completed at Fort Detrick, all remaining biological weapons were destroyed by 1973.

The former Soviet Union was suspected of using *B. mallei* as an agent of biological warfare in Afghanistan between 1982 and 1984. There was one laboratory-acquired case in March 2000 during defensive research on *B. mallei*. This was the first human case of glanders in the United States since 1945. Research regarding biodefense of *B. mallei* continues; however, no known current attempts by terrorists have been noted.

Glanders is a category B disease of concern for bioterrorism by the CDC. In the aerosolized form, *B. mallei* is highly infectious when inhaled. The organism is relatively easy to grow in the laboratory and resistant to many commonly used antibiotics.

BIBLIOGRAPHY

Centers for Disease Control and Prevention. (2000). Laboratory-acquired human glanders—Maryland, May 2000. *Morbidity and Mortality Weekly Report, 49,* 532–535. Retrieved from http://www.cdc.gov/mmwr/preview/mmwrhtml/mm4924a3.htm

Gregory, B.C., & Waag, D. M. (2007). Glanders. In Z. F. Dembek (Ed.), *Medical aspects of biological warfare* (pp. 121–146). Washington, DC: U.S. Army Medical Department.

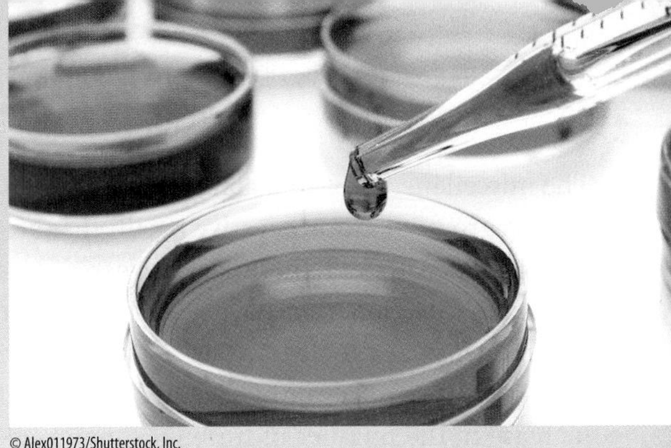

CHAPTER 12

Miscellaneous Gram-Negative Bacilli: Part 1

CHAPTER OUTLINE

Vibrio
Campylobacter
Helicobacter
Aeromonas
Plesiomonas

KEY TERMS

Capnophilic
Choleragen
Halophilic
Microaerophilic

LEARNING OBJECTIVES

1. Explain why the number of miscellaneous gram-negative bacilli associated with human infections has increased.
2. Define and differentiate the following terms:
   a. Halophilic
   b. Capnophilic
   c. Microaerophilic
3. Discuss the clinical relevance of *V. cholerae* O1.
   a. Differentiate classic cholera from El Tor cholera.
   b. Explain how cholera is transmitted.
   c. Describe how *V. cholerae* is identified.
4. Discuss the clinical significance and identification of other *Vibrio*, including *V. parahemolyticus*, *V. vulnificus*, and *V. mimicus*.
   a. Describe how TCBS medium is used to isolate and differentiate *Vibrio*.
5. Describe the unique characteristics of the genus *Campylobacter*.
   a. Explain how *Campylobacter* infections are transmitted.
   b. Differentiate *C. jejuni* subspecies *jejuni* from *C. coli*.
6. Explain the clinical significance of *Helicobacter pylori* and state its unique characteristics.
7. Describe the clinical significance of *Aeromonas* and *Plesiomonas* and describe how each is identified.
   a. Differentiate *Aeromonas* from *Plesiomonas*.

The miscellaneous or unusual gram-negative bacilli are a diverse group of gram-negative bacilli that are not easily categorized. Although these bacteria were once rare causes of human infection, they have been isolated with increasing frequency as agents in a variety of human infections. This increase is a result of several factors, including the increase in the number of immunosuppressed hosts and increased medical instrumentation. In addition, methods of detection, including the use of highly selective media and immunological techniques, have been developed that facilitate the detection and identification of these bacteria. Finally, changes in social factors, such as eating habits and international travel, also may have contributed to the increased incidence of the unusual gram-negative bacilli.

Some of these organisms are associated with **zoonoses**, infections in which the bacteria are transmitted from animals to humans. Transmission also may follow a direct route through direct contact with an infected animal, ingestion of contaminated animal products, or an indirect route through tick or flea vectors.

Common characteristics of some of these bacteria include slow or poor growth on blood, chocolate, and MacConkey agar. Growth is usually enhanced with increased carbon dioxide (CO_2) and humidity.

This chapter focuses on those unusual gram-negative bacilli that are fermentative and cytochrome oxidase positive. Most of these bacteria are curved bacilli.

Vibrio

Vibrio organisms are natural habitants of sea water, and all species except *V. cholerae* and *V. mimicus* require increased sodium chloride (NaCl) for growth. All species of *Vibrio* can grow in the presence of increased sodium chloride. In fact, many require salt to grow. This preference for increased salt is known as **halophilic** and is attributed to the organism's need for increased sodium ions. To determine whether the organism is halophilic, it is grown in medium without salt and also in medium with 1% NaCl. The amount of growth is compared, and if there is increased growth in the medium containing NaCl, the organism is determined to be halophilic.

Most species of *Vibrio* are associated with infections caused by contaminated water or seafood. *Vibrio* species have been isolated from the gastrointestinal tract as causes of gastritis and also have been found in blood and wound infections.

Vibrio organisms grow on blood agar, and selective media also are used in their isolation and identification. The organisms grow on some differential media, including MacConkey agar, but may be overgrown by the normal flora coliforms. Thiosulfate citrate bile salts sucrose (TCBS) agar can be used to isolate most *Vibrio* species. TCBS agar contains sucrose, oxgall, sodium cholate, and bromthymol blue and thymol blue indicators. The medium is alkaline (pH of 8.6), which enhances the growth of *Vibrio*. The high pH of TCBS, oxgall, and cholate inhibit gram-positive bacteria and some lactose-fermenting gram-negative bacilli. A yellow to orange color indicates sucrose fermentation on TCBS, which can be used in the speciation of *Vibrio*. Sucrose fermentation is positive for *V. cholerae* but negative for *V. parahaemolyticus*.

Vibrio organisms are gram-negative straight, comma-shaped, or curved rods (**FIGURE 12-1**) and are motile with a single polar flagellum. They are facultative anaerobes or aerobic, and some prefer increased CO_2. *Vibrio* species are oxidase positive and fermentative in their metabolism of carbohydrates. There are more than 20 species, with 12 known to cause human infection. These 12 clinically significant *Vibrio* species are divided into six groups, using differential biochemical tests.

Vibrio infections have a low incidence in the United States and should be suspected if one has traveled to a foreign country, ingested shellfish, or had contact with seawater. Certain species are seen more frequently near the Chesapeake Bay area.

VIBRIO CHOLERAE

Vibrio cholerae is the cause of cholera. There are over 130 serogroups of the organism based on typing for the

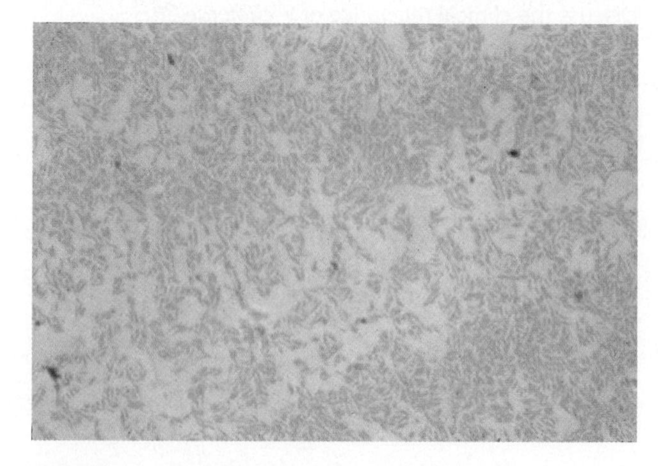

FIGURE 12-1 *Vibrio parahaemolyticus* illustrating its morphology of curved gram negative bacilli.

O antigen, although all share a common H antigen. The cholera-producing strains belong to the O1 type, which means that the organisms agglutinate with a single antisera against serotype O, subgroup 1. The O1 strains are associated with pandemics and epidemics, while the other strains (non-O1) are not. *V. cholerae* O1 is serotyped into three serogroups: Ogawa, Inaba, and Hikojima. These serogroups are used to follow pandemics or epidemics. Epidemic strains also are categorized into two biotypes, classic and El Tor.

The classic strain, responsible for pandemics in the past, is nonhemolytic on sheep blood agar, Voges-Proskauer (VP) negative, and susceptible to polymyxin B and fails to agglutinate chicken red blood cells. The El Tor strain, which has been associated with more recent pandemics, is β-hemolytic, more resistant to environmental changes, VP positive, and resistant to polymyxin B and agglutinates chicken red blood cells.

There have been seven pandemics of cholera occurring in 1816–1817, 1829, 1852, 1863, 1881, and 1889 and the currently occurring pandemic, which began in 1961. The current pandemic began in Indonesia and spread to Asia, Europe, and Africa and then to South and Central America in 1991. There were 13 cases of *Vibrio cholerae* O1 isolated in 1978 in Louisiana and 18 in Texas, which were attributed to contaminated seafood that had been harvested along the Gulf of Mexico.

Toxigenic cholera infections are infrequent in the United States. According to the CDC, there were 12 total cases in 2010.

Most cholera infections are acquired through the ingestion of contaminated seafood, especially undercooked shellfish, or by drinking contaminated water. The infection ranges from a mild infection to a very severe form with a high mortality rate. The severe diarrheal disease is a result of the production of the potent cholera enterotoxin, known as **choleragen**, which attacks the bowel mucosa. This leads to a tremendous outpouring of water and electrolytes and the production of the characteristic "rice-water stool," which is watery and gray with mucin. There is severe dehydration, fluid and electrolyte loss and imbalance, severe muscle cramping, and anuria. Death may result from hypovolemic shock and circulatory collapse. Other individuals may have asymptomatic infections or self-limiting diarrhea. Mildly infected or asymptomatic individuals may excrete the organism and serve as a source of transmission.

Cholera is treated with an aggressive replacement of fluids and electrolytes. There are two oral vaccines currently available; however, neither is licensed, available, or recommended in the United States. The vaccines offer incomplete protection for a short time period. Cholera is prevented through proper sanitation methods, appropriate water treatment, and good personal hygiene. Seafood can be contaminated, and the ingestion of undercooked, contaminated seafood should be avoided.

V. cholerae non-O1 is isolated in cases of diarrheal disease. The non-O1 strains produce an enterotoxin but not choleragen. These strains also may cause wound infections.

V. cholerae O139 was first identified as the cause of epidemic cholera in India and Bangladesh in 1992 and quickly spread through Asia. It is closely related to *V. cholerae* O1 El Tor stains. It produces an enterotoxin and other virulence factors and has been postulated as the possible agent of an eventual eighth pandemic.

Identification

V. cholerae produces smooth, yellow colonies on TCBS agar because it is a sucrose fermenter. The organism produces a positive string test. In this procedure, 0.5% sodium desoxycholate is mixed with the suspected colony on a glass slide and mixed with an inoculating loop. Viscous stringing resulting in the production of a long, tenacious string occurs in a positive test. The stringing must be evident after sixty seconds to be interpreted as a positive string test.

OTHER *VIBRIO*

Vibrio parahaemolyticus is a cause of wound and diarrheal infections. It is seen more frequently in the Far East and has been implicated as the cause of almost half of all cases of food-borne disease in Japan. Infection follows ingestion of contaminated, undercooked or raw fish or shellfish or by direct skin contact with contaminated water. It also is found in specific coastal areas of the United States, such as in the Chesapeake Bay area, where it is associated with contaminated crab. *V. parahaemolyticus* does not ferment sucrose and produces green colonies on TCBS. It is halophilic and nonhemolytic on sheep blood agar.

Vibrio vulnificus has been isolated from marine sources and primarily causes wound infections and septicemia. In many cases, raw, contaminated oysters are the source of infection. Infections are most often seen in those handling seafood or working in the marine environment who have

TABLE 12-1 Clinically Significant *Vibrio* Species: Summary of Characteristics

***Vibrio cholerae* (serogroup O1)**

Nonhalophilic

Sucrose fermented

	Classic	El Tor
Red blood cell hemolysis	Negative	Positive
Voges-Proskauer	Negative	Positive
Polymyxin B (50 U)	Susceptible	Resistant
Agglutination of chicken RBCs	Negative	Positive
Clinical significance	Cholera First six pandemics	Cholera Seventh pandemic

Vibrio parahaemolyticus

Halophilic

Lysine decarboxylase (LDC): Positive

Arginine dehydrolase (ADH): Negative

Fermentation of:

Sucrose: Negative

Salicin: Negative

Celloblose: Negative

Clinical significance: Gastroenteritis, usually from ingestion of contaminated seafood

Vibrio vulnificus

Halophilic

LDC: Positive

ADH: Negative

Fermentation of:

Sucrose: Negative

Salicin: Positive

Cellobiose: Positive

Clinical significance: Septicemia and wound infections involving marine environment

Vibrio mimicus

Nonhalophilic

Sucrose fermentation: Negative

Voges-Proskauer: Negative

Clinical significance: Gastroenteritis and ear infections involving marine environment

Vibrio anginolyticus

Halophilic

LDC: Positive

ADH: Negative

Voges-Proskauer: Positive

Fermentation of:

Sucrose: Positive

Arabinose: Negative

Salicin: Negative

Cellobiose: Negative

Clinical significance: Wound and ear infections associated with marine environment

Vibrio fluvialis* and *Vibrio furnissii

Halophilic

ADH: Positive

Voges-Proskauer: Negative

Citrate: Positive

Fermentation of sucrose: Positive

Clinical significance: Gastroenteritis and diarrhea involving marine environment

a predisposing medical condition, such as liver disease or immunosuppression. *V. vulnificus* produces a cytolysin, which contributes to its virulence and high mortality rate from septicemia. Most strains produce green colonies on TCBS; the organism is a lactose fermenter and is positive for ONPG (o-nitrophenyl-β-D-galactopyranoside).

V. mimicus, *V. fluvialis*, and *V. furnissii* are agents of gastroenteritis, and *V. alginolyticus* causes ear, eye, and blood infections. **TABLE 12-1** summarizes the clinically relevant *Vibrio*.

Campylobacter

Campylobacter species are curved, gram-negative bacilli that are motile with one polar flagellum. These organisms are both **microaerophilic**, preferring decreased amounts of oxygen, and **capnophilic**, preferring increased levels of carbon dioxide. The organisms are oxidase positive and unable to ferment carbohydrates and thus must obtain their energy from other sources, such as amino acids.

Campylobacter has a diverse reservoir in many animals; it is notably the agent of abortion and sterility in cattle. *Campylobacter* is an agent of gastroenteritis and diarrhea in humans. In fact, *Campylobacter* is the most common bacterial cause of diarrheal disease in the United States even surpassing Salmonella, with an incidence of 13 cases per 100,000 according to the Centers for Disease Control (CDC). There are over two million individuals affected annually. Humans become infected by ingestion of contaminated animal products, direct contact with contaminated animal feces, or though contact with another infected human. Animals known to harbor *Campylobacter* include farm animals, birds, cows, poultry, domestic pets, and water fowl. Chicken flocks are infected with the organism because it is spread between birds through infected feces or through a common contaminated water source. When infected poultry are slaughtered, the organism can be transferred from their intestines to the poultry product. It is estimated that almost 50% of poultry contains *Campylobacter* in the United States. Humans acquire the infection by ingesting contaminated raw milk, undercooked poultry, or contaminated water. The organism also has been isolated from environmental sources, such as soil and water. Individuals also may acquire *Campylobacter* by direct contact with infected domestic pets, which is a concern for children and other household contacts.

The clinical signs of *Campylobacter* infection include fever, abdominal pain, cramping, and bloody diarrhea. The stool characteristically contains segmented neutrophils and red blood cells. In its severe form the gastroenteritis may lead to intestinal bleeding that may mimic inflammatory bowel disease. The organism may invade the bloodstream and also cause endocarditis, septic arthritis, or meningitis. There are approximately 124 fatal cases of *Campylobacter* each year in the United States. Approximately one in 1,000 diagnosed cases lead to Guillain-Barre syndrome, a paralytic disease that can last for weeks and requires intensive medical care. Some individuals are asymptomatic carriers and serve as a source of *Campylobacter* infection.

Virulence factors for *Campylobacter* include the production of cytotoxin, cytotonic factor, and an enterotoxin.

There are currently 19 species of *Campylobacter*, and the most frequently isolated species in humans is *Campylobacter jejuni* subspecies *jejuni*, followed by *C. coli*. *Campylobacter* species require selective media, such as *Campylobacter* blood agar (Becton-Dickinson), which contains a blood agar base with the antibiotics vancomycin, polymyxin, cephalothin, trimethoprim, and amphotericin B added. *Campylobacter* agar skirrow is a blood agar base with the antibiotics vancomycin, trimethoprim, and polymyxin B added. Several other media selective for *Campylobacter* are available commercially.

The enteric *Campylobacter* grow optimally at 42°C to 43°C in a microaerophilic, capnophilic environment of 85% nitrogen, 5% oxygen, and 10% CO_2. However, *Campylobacter* also grow at 37°C. Disposable plastic bags with generators providing this environment can be commercially purchased. An example is the Bio-Bag Type Cf, available from Becton-Dickinson, which generates an environment of 5% to 10% oxygen and 8% to 10% CO_2. This disposable, individual chamber uses a gas generator of potassium borohydride-sodium bicarbonate and an ampule of hydrochloric acid to produce a microaerophilic environment. Candle jars or standard CO_2 incubators should not be used for *Campylobacter* because the oxygen concentration is too high.

Growth is generally present within 48 hours, and *Campylobacter* produces colonies that are gray to pink or yellow to gray in color. Their appearance varies from dry to moist and convex to flat, with an irregular margin. Colonies are nonhemolytic and slightly mucoid.

A wet preparation should be prepared from any organism growing on *Campylobacter*-selective media at 42°C to 43°C. Characteristic darting motility is observed in the wet preparation, as well as in a darkfield examination. Gram stains of *Campylobacter* are improved by substituting carbolfuchsin for safranin O in the final step. The organism appears as gram-negative S-shaped or spiral forms and frequently is said to resemble the wings of sea gulls (**FIGURE 12-2**).

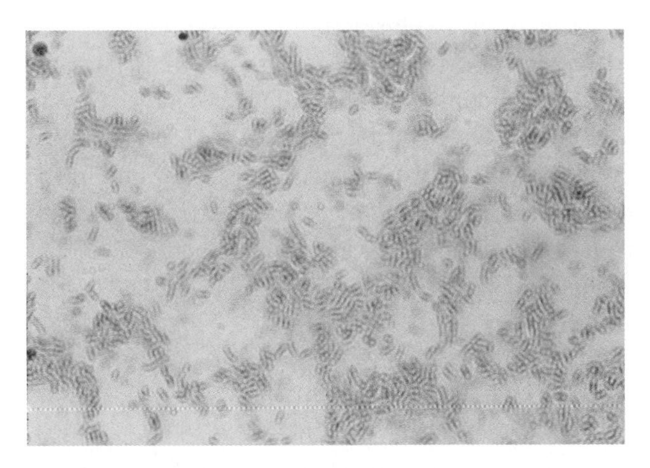

FIGURE 12-2 *Camplyobacter* in a Gram stained smear showing curved gram negative bacilli that may join to form "gull wings."

TABLE 12-2 Differentiation of *Campylobacter* and *Helicobacter* Species

	C. jejuni subsp. *jejuni*	*C. coli*	*C. fetus* subsp. *fetus*	*Helicobacter pylori*
Catalase	+	+	+	+
Nitrate	+	+	+	–
Urease	–	–	–	++
Hippurate hydrolysis	+	–	–	–
Growth at 25°C	–	–	+	V
Growth at 37°C	+	+	+	+
Growth at 42°C	+	+	–	V
Susceptible to:				
Nalidixic acid	S	S	V	R
Cephalothin	R	R	S	S

+, most isolates give positive reaction; –, most isolates give negative reaction; V, variable reaction; S, susceptible; R, resistant

Another species of *Campylobacter* is *C. coli*, which causes food-borne illness in humans, accounting for approximately 5% to 10% of the reported *Campylobacter* cases in the United States. This species also grows at 42°C and is resistant to cephalothin but is susceptible to nalidixic acid. *C.coli* is negative for hippurate hydrolysis, which differentiates it from *C. jejuni* subspecies *jejuni*. *C. fetus* subspecies *fetus* is the cause of infective abortion in cattle and sheep. It is a rare human pathogen and may infect immunocompromised hosts and those with underlying medical disorders. This species does not grow at 42°C.

Campylobacter species can be differentiated by the reactions shown in **TABLE 12-2**.

Helicobacter

Helicobacter pylori was formerly known as *Campylobacter pylori*. The organism is differentiated from *Campylobacter* by the presence of four to six polar flagella and its very strong urease activity. The natural habitat for *H. pylori* is only in the human stomach, where the organism is found in the mucous-secreting cells. *H. pylori* is a factor in the development of chronic antral gastritis and in peptic ulcer disease. It also may play a role in duodenal ulcers and gastric adenocarcinoma.

H. pylori is microaerophilic, preferring 85% nitrogen, 10% CO_2, and 5% oxygen. It grows optimally at 35°C to 37°C and prefers increased humidity. The organism appears as a small, curved bacillus in Gram-stained smears and may show "U" forms and the appearance of gull wings. It is positive for catalase and oxidase. Its rapid production of urease is a significant characteristic used to identify *H. pylori*. The gold standard to identify *H. pylori* is through histological staining and culture of biopsies obtained from the stomach or duodenum. The tissue is ground and plated onto nonselective agar, such as 5% sheep blood agar, and incubated at 37°C in a microaerophilic environment and increased humidity. Typical growth shows small gray, translucent colonies that are slightly β-hemolytic. Identification is confirmed through biochemical reactions, especially strong urease production. There are other non-invasive methods to identify *Helicobacter*. These include the urease breath test, which detects urease in the individual's breath. There are also enzyme linked immunosorbent assays to detect *Helicobacter* antigen in the stool and serological methods to detect IgG antibody in the serum.

Aeromonas

Aeromonas organisms are oxidase-positive, fermentative, gram-negative bacilli that are generally motile with polar monotrichous flagella. *Aeromonas* is naturally found in freshwater and seawater and is known to cause disease in cold-blooded animals. The organism is also found in drains, sink traps, distilled water, and tap water. The most common types of human infections include cellulitis and wound infections, acquired through contact with contaminated water or soil, as well as gastrointestinal disease.

Miscellaneous types of infections associated with *Aeromonas* include septicemia, urinary tract infections, and ear infections.

Aeromonas organisms grow on MacConkey agar, eosin-methylene blue (EMB) agar, and *Salmonella–Shigella* (SS) agar but can be differentiated from Enterobacteriaceae by a positive oxidase reaction. *Aeromonas* also grows on cefsulodin-irgasan-novobiocin (CIN) medium, which is used to isolate *Yersinia* species. It can be differentiated from *Pseudomonas aeruginosa* by its ability to ferment glucose and produce indole. *P. aeruginosa* oxidizes glucose and is indole negative.

The most common human isolate is *A. hydrophilia*, which means "water loving" and is the species that most often causes gastrointestinal disease. The organism produces a heat-labile enterotoxin and a heat-stable cytotoxic enterotoxin. *A. hydrophilia* also produces protease, lipase, and nuclease.

Plesiomonas

Plesiomonas is a straight, round, gram-negative bacillus, which is motile with polar lophotrichous flagella. *P. shigelloides* is an important infectious agent in Japan and in the tropics and subtropics as a cause of gastroenteritis. The infection is generally mild with no blood or mucus in the stool. The organism is carried on various cold-blooded animals and is found in the water and soil. Infection is acquired through the ingestion of contaminated or unwashed foods. *P. shigelloides* grows on blood agar and as a nonlactose fermenter on MacConkey agar, and eosin-methylene blue. It can be differentiated from Enterobacteriaceae by a positive oxidase reaction.

TABLE 12-3 cites important biochemical reactions that can differentiate *A. hydrophila* from *P. shigelloides.*

TABLE 12-3 Differentiation of *Aeromonas hydrophila* from *Plesiomonas Shigelloides*

Reaction	*A. hydrophilia*	*P. shigelloides*
Hemolysis of blood agar	–	–
Oxidase	+	+
Indole	+	+
Glucose fermented	+	+
Gas from glucose	+	–
Motility	+	+
Deoxyribonuclease (DNase)	+	–
Esculin hydrolyzed	+	–
ADH	+	+
ODC	–	+
LDC	+	+

Laboratory Procedures

Procedure
Thiosulfate citrate bile salts sucrose (TCBS) agar

Purpose
TCBS medium selectively isolates *Vibrio* in specimens, such as stools, that contain mixed flora.

Principle
The medium contains sucrose, bile in the forms of oxgall and sodium cholate, sodium citrate, proteins, yeast, and pH indicators. *Vibrio* species prefer a high salt concentration and a high pH and thus grow well on TCBS, whereas other flora, such as *Proteus* and other members of the Enterobacteriaceae, are inhibited.

Fermentation of sucrose is indicated by a yellow color and is characteristic of certain *Vibrio* species, such as *V. cholerae* and *V. alginolyticus. V. parahaemolyticus* and *V. vulnificus* cannot ferment sucrose and appear as blue-green colonies.

Method

1. Inoculate plate and streak for isolation using stool culture suspected of containing *Vibrio.*
2. Incubate at 35°C to 37°C for 24 to 48 hours.

Interpretation
Growth usually indicates a *Vibrio* species. Occasionally, *Aeromonas* or *Pseudomonas* may grow on the medium.
Yellow colonies indicate a sucrose-fermenting *Vibrio.*
Blue-green colonies usually indicate a non–sucrose-fermenting *Vibrio.*

Quality Control
Growth and fermentation of sucrose: *V. alginolyticus*—yellow colonies
Growth and lack of fermentation of sucrose: *Vibrio parahaemolyticus*—blue-green colonies

Review Questions

1. Thiosulfate citrate bile salt sucrose agar is used to isolate and differentiate:
   a. *Campylobacter*
   b. *Vibrio*
   c. *Aeromonas*
   d. *Plesiomonas*
2. Halophilic means that the organism requires:
   a. Increased oxygen
   b. Increased carbon dioxide
   c. Decreased oxygen
   d. Increased sodium chloride
3. Which is *not* a characteristic of *Vibrio cholerae*?
   a. Motile with single polar flagellum
   b. Oxidase negative
   c. Ferments glucose and sucrose
   d. Positive string test
4. *Vibrio cholera* O1 El Tor strain:
   a. Is nonhemolytic on sheep blood agar
   b. Is associated with the first six pandemics
   c. Agglutinates chicken red blood cells
   d. Is halophilic
5. Which description is correct for *Campylobacter jejuni* subspecies *jejuni*?
   a. Motile curved rod, halophilic, catalase negative
   b. Nonmotile curved rod, grows at 42°C, catalase negative
   c. Motile curved rod, grows at 42°C, catalase positive
   d. Motile curved rod, cannot grow at 42°C, capnophilic
6. A *Vibrio* yielded the following biochemical reactions:
   Growth in nutrient broth: Negative
   Growth in nutrient broth with 1% NaCL: Positive
   Oxidase: Positive
   Nitrates reduced to nitrites
   ADH: Negative
   LDC: Positive
   Fermentation of:
   Sucrose: Negative
   Salicin: Negative
   Cellobiose: Negative
   This *Vibrio* species most likely can be identified as:
   a. *V. cholerae*
   b. *V. mimicus*
   c. *V. parahaemolyticus*
   d. *V. fluvialis*
7. Characteristics of *Aeromonas* include each of following *except*:
   a. Motile
   b. Ferments glucose
   c. Esculin hydrolysis negative
   d. Cytochrome oxidase positive
8. *Plesiomonas* infections are:
   a. Found worldwide and associated with the ingestion of contaminated meat products
   b. Found in Japan and South and Central America and associated with ingestion of contaminated food or drinking water
   c. The most prevalent type of food- and water-borne disease in the United States.
   d. None of the above

Bibliography

Abbott, S. L., Janda, J. M., Johnson, J. A., & Farmer III, J. J. (2007). *Vibrio* and related organisms. In P. R. Murray, E. J. Baron, J. H. Jorgensen, M. L. Landry, & M. A. Pfaller (Eds.), *Manual of clinical microbiology* (9th ed.). Washington, DC: American Society for Microbiology.

Alam, M., Nusrin, S., Islam, A., Bhuiyan, N. A., Rahim, N., Delgado, G., . . . Cravioto, A. (2010). Cholera between 1991 and 1997 in Mexico was associated with infection by classical, El Tor, and El Tor variants of *Vibrio cholerae*. *Journal of Clinical Microbiology, 48,* 3666–3674.

Bannerman T. L., & Peacock, S. J. (2007). *Staphylococcus, Micrococcus,* and other catalase positive cocci. In P. R. Murray, E. J. Baron, J. H. Jorgensen, M. L. Landry, & M. A. Pfaller (Eds.), *Manual of clinical microbiology* (9th ed.). Washington, DC: American Society for Microbiology.

Blaser, M. J., Berkowitz, I. D., LaForce, F. M., Cravens, J., Reller, L. B., & Wang, W. L. (1979). *Campylobacter enteritis:* Clinical and epidemiologic features. *Annals of Internal Medicine, 91,* 179–185.

Centers for Disease Control and Prevention. (1986). Cholera in Louisiana: Update. *Morbidity and Mortality Weekly Report, 35,* 687–688.

Centers for Disease Control and Prevention. (1995). Update: *Vibrio cholera* O1—Western Hemisphere, 1991–1994, and *V. cholerae* O139—Asia, 1994. *Morbidity and Mortality Weekly Report, 44,* 215–219.

Centers for Disease Control and Prevention. (2010). Cholera. Retrieved from http://www.cdc.gov/cholera/general

Centers for Disease Prevention and Control. (2010). *Campylobacter.* Retrieved from http://www.cdc.gov/nczved/divisions/dfbmd/diseases/campylobacter/technical.html

Centers for Disease Control and Prevention. (2009). *Camplylobacter jejuni* infection associated with unpasteurized milk and cheese—Kansas, 2007. *Morbidity and Mortality Weekly Report, 57,* 1377–1399.

Centers for Disease Control and Prevention. (1991). Cholera—Peru, 1991. *Morbidity and Mortality Weekly Report, 40,* 108.

Fitzgerald, C., & Nachamkin, I. *Camplyobacter* and *Arcobacter.* In P. R. Murray, E. J. Baron, J. H. Jorgensen, M. L. Landry, & M. A. Pfaller (Eds.), *Manual of clinical microbiology* (9th ed.). Washington, DC: American Society for Microbiology.

Janda, J. M., & Abbott, S. L. (2010). The genus *Aeromonas*: Taxonomy, pathogenicity, and infection. *Clinical Microbiology Reviews, 23,* 35–73.

Janssen, R., Krogfelt, K. A., Cawthraw, S. A., van Pelt, W., Wagenaar, J. A., & Owen, R. J. 2008. Host-pathogen interactions in *Campylobacter* infections: The host perspective. *Clinical Microbiology Reviews, 20,* 505–518.

World Health Organization. (2011). Cholera. Retrieved from http://www.who.int/topics/cholera/en/

NEWS: CHOLERA: A PAST AND CURRENT CONCERN

There have been seven cholera pandemics, with the first pandemic documented in 1817. The first pandemic began in Southeast Asia and spread to other parts of the world. The first six pandemics were caused by the classic biotype of *V. cholerae* serogroup O1, and all of them spread from India to most of the world, killing millions of people. The current, or seventh, cholera pandemic began in 1961 and was caused by the El Tor biotype of *V. cholerae* serogroup O1. This pandemic began in Indonesia and reached Africa by 1971; spread quickly to other countries in Asia, Europe, and Africa; and in 1991 reached Latin America. Until that time, there had been no cholera in Latin America for over 100 years. Cholera is now endemic in many countries. Many countries in the Western hemisphere were previously not exposed to cholera, and the populations, therefore, lacked immunity. From 1997 to 1998, the number of cases in the Western hemisphere increased from 17,760 to 57,106, with the increase predominantly in Peru but also affecting Ecuador, Guatemala, and Nicaragua. The effects of major disasters, including El Nino and hurricanes, may be related to this increase.

Cholera remains a major public health concern. The World Health Organization (WHO) estimates that there are three to five million cases in the world and 100,000 to 120,000 deaths from cholera. There is an incubation period of two hours to five days, which enhances the potential for outbreaks. From 2004 to 2008, there was a 24% increase in cholera cases compared to the time period of 2000 to 2004. In 2008, cholera was found in 56 countries. It is believed to be underestimated because of limitations in surveillance and other factors. In 2009, the number of cases of cholera reported to WHO increased by 16% when compared with 2008. There were 221,226 cases reported and almost 5,000 deaths. Cholera was reported from 45 countries. Africa accounted for 217,333, or 98%, of the cases globally. There were 10 cholera cases in the United States in 2009, of which eight were imported.

Following the earthquake in Haiti in 2010, cholera was confirmed in October 21, 2010. This was somewhat surprising because cholera had not been documented in Haiti for several decades. For this to happen, *Vibrio* cholera had to be present in the environment, and there also had to be a breakdown in the water and sanitation systems in Haiti. The first isolate in the outbreak was identified as *V. cholerae* O1 serotype Ogawa, biotype El Tor. Within one week, there were almost 5,000 cholera cases and over 300 deaths reported.

Approximately 75% of those infected with cholera do not have symptoms and can carry the organism. *Vibrio* can shed it in the stool for up to two weeks after infection, which serves as a source of infection from individuals who may not know that they carry the organism. Of the 25% who develop symptoms, 80% have mild or moderate symptoms. The other 20% develop acute watery diarrhea and severe electrolyte imbalance and dehydration.

Cholera is transmitted through fecally contaminated food or water. Because epidemic cholera was never reported from Haiti, the population was immunologically naive and very susceptible to infection. The infection spread from two regions of Haiti to seven within one month. During this time over 16,000 were hospitalized with acute symptoms, and there were almost 1,000 deaths. Disruption of water and sanitation systems and displacement of people to overcrowded shelters increased the rate of transmission. Cholera is prevented by maintaining adequate water and sanitation systems. It is treated by rehydration and electrolyte therapy, including intravenous fluids.

By December 3, 2010, there were almost 92,000 cases of cholera, and all regions of Haiti were affected. There were over 2,000 deaths. By December 17, there were 121,518 cases reported in Haiti. Additionally there were confirmed cases in the Dominican Republic and Florida. While a few of the cases in the Dominican Republic were imported by travelers from Haiti, most of the cases were attributed to local transmission through household contacts and contaminated canal and untreated river water. There were five cases in the United States, all of which have been imported from individuals who had traveled from Haiti.

Cholera continues to be a major public health issue worldwide.

BIBLIOGRAPHY

Centers for Disease Control and Prevention. (2010). Cholera confirmed in Haiti. Retrieved from http://www.cdc.gov/haiticholera/situation

Centers for Disease Control and Prevention. (2010). Haiti cholera outbreak. Retrieved from http://www.cdc.gov/haiticholera

World Health Organization. (2010). Cholera. *Weekly Epidemiological Record, 85,* 293–308. Retrieved from http://www.who.int/wer/2010/wer8531/en/index.html

World Health Organization. (2010). Cholera fact sheet. Retrieved from http://www.who.int/mediacentre/factsheets/fs107/en/index.html

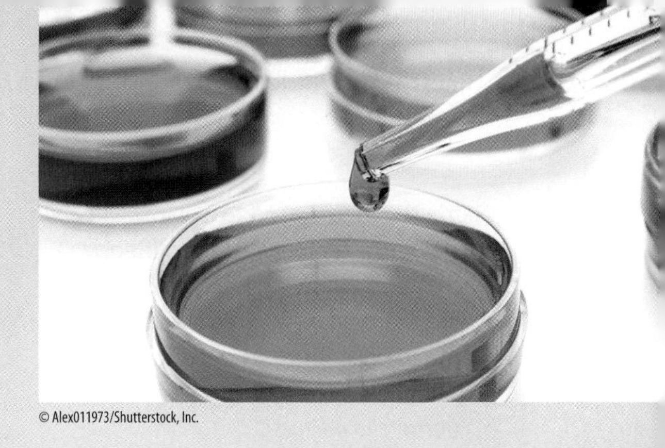
© Alex011973/Shutterstock, Inc.

CHAPTER 13
Miscellaneous Gram-Negative Bacilli: Part 2

CHAPTER OUTLINE

Haemophilus
Legionella
Bordetella
Brucella
Pasteurella
Francisella
Streptobacillus
HACEK Group
Chromobacterium

KEY TERMS

δ-aminolevulinic acid
Chancroid
Fastidious
HACEK
Haemophilus influenzae serotype b
Hematin
Legionellosis
Legionnaires' disease
Nicotinamide-adenine dinucleotide (NAD)
Pasteurellosis
Pertussis
Pleomorphic
Satellitism
Tularemia
Undulant fever
Zoonoses

LEARNING OBJECTIVES

1. Describe the general morphological and biochemical characteristics of *Haemophilus*.
2. Describe X and V factors and indicate a source for each. Perform and interpret the test for X and V factors.
3. List the media used to isolate *Haemophilus* and indicate why sheep blood agar is usually not acceptable.
4. State the principle and purpose of satellitism and the δ-aminolevulinic acid (ALA) test.
5. Explain how *H. influenzae* is identified from a clinical specimen and list important biochemical characteristics of this organism.
   a. Identify *H. influenzae* in a clinical sample or stock culture.
6. List the serotypes of *H. influenzae* and indicate which is found most frequently in human infection.
7. List the infections associated with *H. influenzae* and indicate which population is most affected.
8. Briefly describe the identification and clinical relevance of:
   a. *H. ducreyi*
   b. *H. aegyptius*
   c. *H. parainfluenzae*
   d. *H. haemolyticus*
9. Discuss the important characteristics and clinical relevance of the *Aggregatibacter* species.
10. Name the etiologic agent of Legionnaires' disease.
    a. Describe and compare the types of legionellosis.

b. Name the media used to isolate *Legionella*.
c. Explain how *Legionella* is identified.

11. For each of the following bacteria:
    a. Name the media required for isolation.
    b. Name or describe the infectious process.
    c. Explain how the organism is identified.
       (1) *Bordetella pertussis*
       (2) *Brucella*
       (3) *Pasteurella*
       (4) *Francisella*
12. Name four species of *Brucella* and list the animal source of each. Differentiate the species based on biochemical reactions and growth characteristics.
13. Name and describe the gram-negative bacillus associated with rat-bite fever.
14. Explain what the acronym HACEK represents, list the bacteria included in this designation, and briefly describe the clinical significance.

This chapter discusses additional miscellaneous gram-negative bacilli. These organisms are associated with a variety of infections, and most require specialized media or techniques for identification. Most of the bacteria in this group grow slowly on blood and chocolate agar and do not grow on MacConkey agar. Growth is usually enhanced with increased carbon dioxide (CO_2) and humidity. Others, such as *Bordetella*, *Legionella*, and *Brucella*, need unique media with specific supplements. Some, such as *Haemophilus influenzae*, are transmitted in specific populations. Others require a particular environment to grow as is seen with *Legionella*. Still others are associated with **zoonoses**, such as *Brucella*, *Pasturella*, and *Francisella*.

Haemophilus

The genus *Haemophilus* consists of tiny gram-negative coccobacilli that are nonmotile. In clinical cultures the organisms may form long, threadlike or filamentous strands. The organisms are facultative anaerobes, reduce nitrates, and utilize carbohydrates either fermentatively or by using oxygen as the final hydrogen ion acceptor. Most species are oxidase and catalase positive and prefer incubation temperatures of 35°C to 37°C with 5% to 10% CO_2. *Haemophilus* species are very sensitive to drying and chilling; thus abrupt fluctuations in temperature must be avoided.

Many species of *Haemophilus* are nonpathogenic, or opportunistic, pathogens except for *H. influenzae* and *H. ducreyi*. Several species are considered to be indigenous flora of the mucous membranes of the upper respiratory tract and oral cavity of humans.

Haemophilus, which means "blood loving," has special growth requirements, which include a group of iron-containing compounds known as **hemin**, **hematin**, or protoporphyrin X. These compounds, commonly known as X factor, are heat-stable products that are released upon the breakdown of hemoglobin. Most *Haemophilus* species also require **nicotinamide-adenine dinucleotide (NAD)** or coenzyme I, also known as V factor. NAD is a heat-labile compound produced by certain bacteria and yeast. It also can be obtained through exogenous sources, such as potato or yeast extracts.

ISOLATION

The *Haemophilus* species that require NAD cannot grow on sheep blood agar. Sheep red blood cells release NADase, which inactivates the NAD present in the medium. However, horse or rabbit blood agar can be used to isolate *Haemophilus* because these types of blood agar do not contain NADase. Because these media are not routinely used in the microbiology laboratory, *Haemophilus* is most often isolated on chocolate agar. Chocolate agar is prepared by either heating sheep red blood cells to at least 80°C or using enzyme treatment. Either method will release hematin (X factor) and inactivate NADase. Additional cofactors and supplements are added to the medium. Chocolate agar is commercially available; there also is synthetic chocolate agar, which contains NAD, iron, vitamin B_{12}, thiamin, iron, magnesium, glucose, cysteine, and glutamine. It is important to note that hemolysis cannot be interpreted using chocolate agar. β-hemolysis is an important criterion in differentiating certain species of *Haemophilus*.

The ***Staphylococcus* streak** also can be used for primary isolation. In this technique the specimen or culture is heavily streaked onto a sheep blood agar plate. Next, a single inoculation of β-hemolytic *Staphylococcus aureus* is streaked through the inoculum. Because many

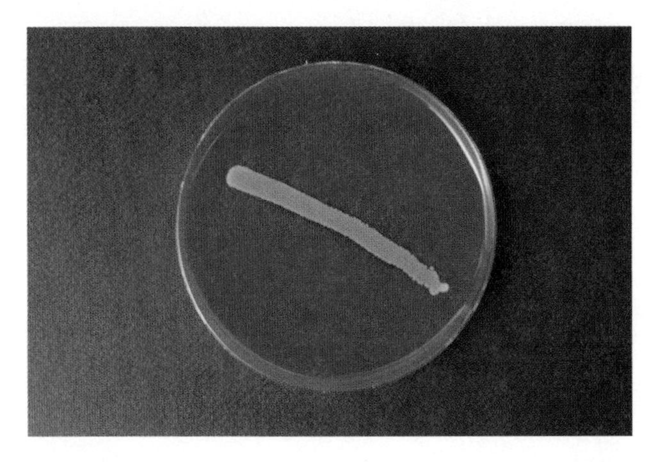

FIGURE 13-1 Satellitism showing Haemophilus species growing in beta hemolytic zones that surround S. aureus.

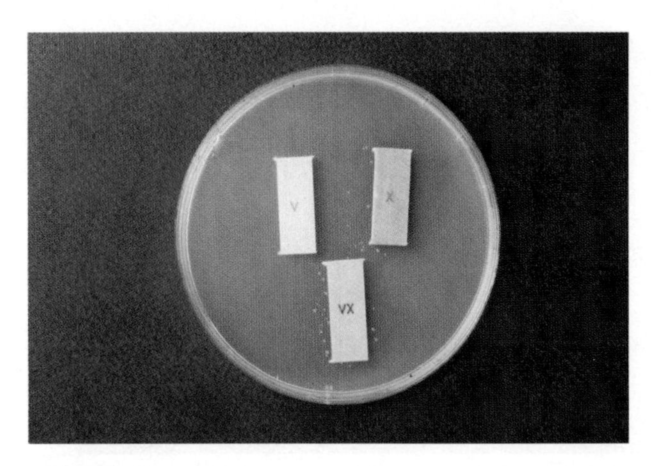

FIGURE 13-2 *H. influenzae*: X and V strips illustrating the requirement for both X and V factors.

bacteria, including *S. aureus*, synthesize NAD (V factor) and because hematin is released upon β-hemolysis, both growth requirements are met for *Haemophilus* species. *Haemophilus* species that require both X and V factors appear as tiny satellite colonies around the *S. aureus* after incubation. Other organisms also produce NAD and allow satelliting. **Satellitism** is illustrated in **FIGURE 13-1**.

Haemophilus isolation media such as horse blood–bacitracin agar also can be used. This medium contains beef heart infusion, peptone, yeast, 5% defibrinated horse blood (which provides X and V factors), and 300 mg/l of bacitracin. The bacitracin inhibits normal flora, which enhances the recovery of *Haemophilus* species. Hemolysis also can be detected using blood–bacitracin agar. Levinthal agar is a clear medium containing hemin, NAD, and other growth factors, which also can be used to isolate *Haemophilus*. Encapsulated colonies of *H. influenzae* appear iridescent when viewed with an oblique light, whereas nonencapsulated strains appear transparent, bluish, and noniridescent.

IDENTIFICATION

Most species of *Haemophilus* are catalase and oxidase positive. *Haemophilus* species are identified through hemolytic reactions on horse blood agar and through growth requirements for hemin and NAD. One method to determine the organism's growth requirements is to use X and V filter paper strips. In this method, the isolated organism is inoculated onto a medium deficient in hemin and NAD, such as Mueller-Hinton or trypticase soy agar. The strips are then applied, and the plate is incubated under increased CO_2 at 35°C for 24 hours, at which time the plate is examined for growth. If growth occurs around only the X strip, the organism requires only X factor for growth. If growth occurs around only the V strip, the organism requires only V factor for growth. If growth occurs between only the X and V strips, the organism requires both X and V factors. In performing the test for X and V factors, it is essential not to transfer any chocolate- or blood-containing medium to prevent carryover of the factors, which could lead to false results. X and V factor strips for *H. influenzae* are illustrated in **FIGURE 13-2**.

The **δ-aminolevulinic acid** test (ALA porphyrin test) also can be used to assess the requirement for hemin. The ALA porphyrin test is not affected by carryover, which might occur in X factor testing. In this procedure the synthesis of protoporphyrin from the substrate ALA is determined. Species, such as *H. parainfluenzae*, that do not require exogenous X factor, are ALA positive because they possess the necessary enzymes to convert ALA to porphobilinogen and porphyrin to hemin. Species that require exogenous X factor for growth and do not have the needed enzymes, such as *H. influenzae*, are ALA negative.

Haemophilus identification plates are available commercially from several manufacturers as tri-plates and quad-plates. Quad-plates have one quadrant each for horse blood to determine growth and hemolysis, X factor–enriched medium, V factor–enriched medium, and both X and V factor–enriched medium. The plate can be used instead of the technique for X and V factors. Reactions for *H. influenzae* and *H. parainfluenzae* on *Haemophilus* identification plates are illustrated in **FIGURES 13-3** and **13-4**.

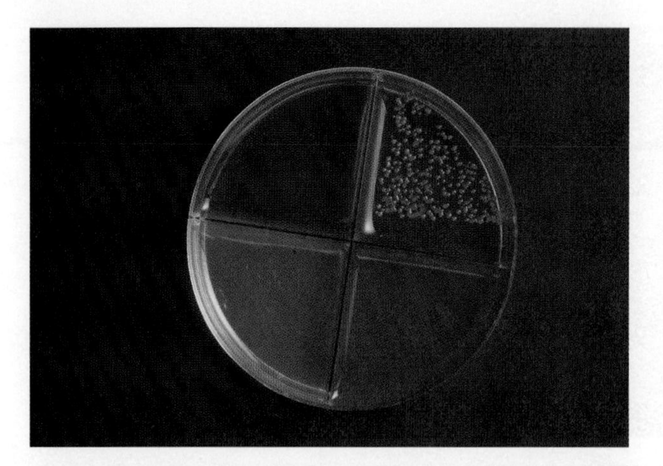

FIGURE 13-3 *Haemophilus* quad-plate with *H. influenzae* showing growth only in the quadrant that contains both X and V factors.

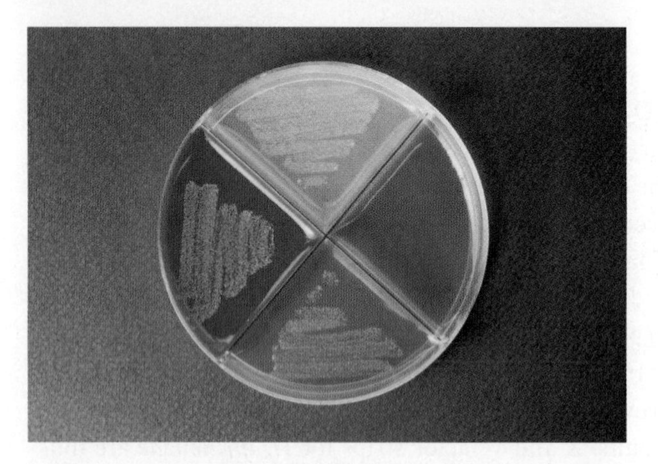

FIGURE 13-4 *Haemophilus* quad-plate with *H. parainfluenzae* showing growth in those quadrants that contain V factor and the lack of hemolysis on quadrant with horse red blood cells.

Carbohydrate fermentation reactions also can be used to speciate *Haemophilus*. **TABLE 13-1** summarizes the biochemical reactions of the clinically important *Haemophilus*.

HAEMOPHILUS INFLUENZAE

The most frequent clinically isolated *Haemophilus* is *H. influenzae*, formerly known as "Pfeiffer's bacillus." There are six serotypes of *H. influenzae* designated as a, b, c, d, e, and f, which are serotyped based on the characteristics of the capsule. The serotype can be determined through identification of the distinct capsular antigen through latex agglutination, capsular swelling, or immunofluorescence with type-specific antisera. **Haemophilus influenzae serotype b** is encountered most frequently in infections.

There are also currently eight identified biotypes of *H. influenzae*: I, II, III, IV, V, VI, VII, and VIII. Biotypes are based on biochemical reactions, including carbohydrate fermentation, indole, urease, and ornithine decarboxylase (ODC). Table 13-1 above lists biochemical reactions used to identify the biotypes of *H. influenzae*.

TABLE 13-1 Identification of *Haemophilus influenzae* Biotypes

Haemophilus influenzae biotype	Indole	Urease	ODC
I	+	+	+
II	+	+	–
III	–	+	–
IV	–	+	+
V	+	–	+
VI	–	–	+
VII	+	–	–
VIII	–	–	–

Note: Biotypes are based on the biochemical reactions with indole, urease, and ornithine decarboxylase (ODC). Certain biotypes more frequently cause certain diseases. For example, biotype I is found most often in human infections and is associated with meningitis and septicemia. Biotypes II and III have been found in the eye and respiratory tract, and biotypes IV and V have been found in the ear and respiratory tract.

H. influenzae may be carried as normal flora of the upper respiratory tract. The nonencapsulated strain, which is generally not virulent, is estimated to be carried asymptomatically by more than 50% of the general population. Encapsulated strains are able to reduce phagocytosis and are very pathogenic, producing rapid, devastating disease in nonvaccinated children and other susceptible individuals.

Before the first immunizations were available, *H. influenzae* was the major cause of meningitis in children less than five years of age. The first conjugate vaccine was licensed in the United States for children in 1987 and for infants in 1990. Rates of disease in infants and young children have decreased by 99% to fewer than one case per 100,000 children under five years of age, according to the CDC. Today, in the United States, *H. influenzae* b disease is found most often in infants too young to have completed the immunization series and in underimmunized children. The infection is spread through direct contact with respiratory droplets from a carrier or another infected individual. Thus, household contacts, day care classmates and infants, and young children are at risk for infection. The organism spreads from the nasopharynx to the regional lymph nodes, to the blood, and finally to the meninges. Although some children may become asymptomatic carriers, others develop severe infections. Adults who develop *H. influenzae* meningitis may have a predisposing condition, such as chronic sinus infection, alcoholism, head trauma, diabetes, ear infections, or heart valve disease. More than 90% of the cases of meningitis are caused by serotype b.

Symptoms *of H. influenzae* infection resemble those of an upper respiratory tract infection, which may develop either slowly or rapidly. Invasive diseases include pneumonia, bacteremia, meningitis, epiglottitis, septic arthritis, pericarditis, and otitis media. Epiglottitis is most often seen in young children and is characterized by a red, swollen epiglottis, which may lead to respiratory distress. Other respiratory infections attributed to *H. influenzae* include acute sinusitis and chronic bronchitis.

Systemic infections, including meningitis, bacteremia, septicemia, and endocarditis, are also seen in immunosuppressed adults. Nonencapsulated strains of *H. influenzae* are associated with upper respiratory tract infections and bronchitis in immunosuppressed adults.

Because *H. influenzae* is very **fastidious** and adversely affected by changes in temperature and drying, specimens should be held at room temperature and never subjected to cold temperatures. Specimens must be inoculated onto enriched media as soon as possible. Swabs are premoistened, or a transport medium, such as modified Stuart's or Amies charcoal, is used when it is not possible to inoculate the agar in a reasonable time.

Specimen type is dictated by the type of infection. Possible specimen sites include blood, cerebrospinal fluid (CSF), middle ear aspirate, infected joint fluid, nasopharyngeal swabs, and eye swabs.

H. influenzae identification begins with a Gram stain of the infected area. CSF smears are centrifuged, concentrated, and Gram stained. The organism appears in CSF and blood smears as small, pale staining gram-negative coccobacilli, which also may appear **pleomorphic** or tangled. A Gram-stained smear of *H. influenzae* is shown in **FIGURE 13-5**.

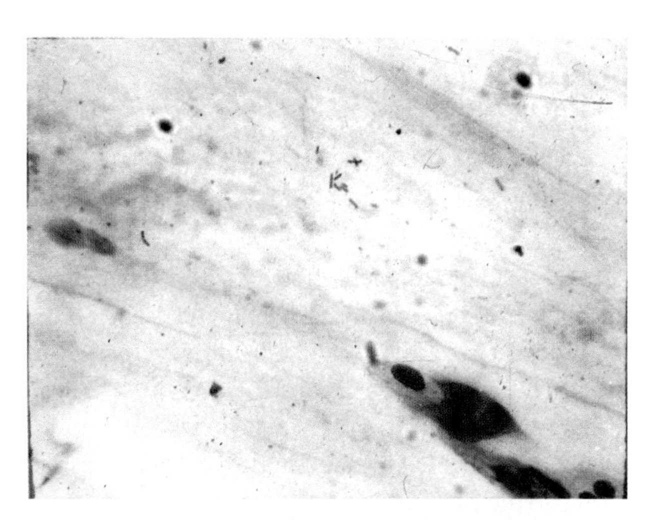

FIGURE 13-5 Gram stain of *H. influenzae* from direct smear showing tiny gram negative bacilli and white blood cells.

Rapid direct identification of the capsular antigen in serum, urine, or cerebrospinal fluid can be accomplished through the Neufeld quellung reaction, or capsular swelling test, in which antisera react with the capsular antigens of the organism, making the capsule more prominent. Other methods for direct antigen detection include staphylococcal coagglutination or latex agglutination. In these methods, the capsular antigen in the body fluid reacts with antisera specific to *H. influenzae* serotype b. Antibodies against *H. influenzae* type b capsular material are fixed to either latex beads or staphylococcal bacteria. The specimen is mixed with the sensitized reagent, and agglutination indicates a positive result. The Directogen Meningitis Combo Test Kit (Becton-Dickinson) uses latex agglutination to demonstrate the type b capsular antigen of *H. influenzae*.

Specimens are plated on chocolate agar, and a staphylococcus streak also may be performed on sheep blood agar. Plates are incubated at 35°C to 37°C under ambient air or 5% to 10% CO_2 with increased humidity. The extremely fastidious *H. ducreyi* and *H. aegyptius* require Mueller-Hinton–based chocolate medium plus 10% IsoVitaleX™ Enrichment (Becton-Dickinson) for enhanced and more rapid growth. This medium also enhances the growth of *H. influenzae*.

Reactions to identify *H. influenzae* can be found in Table 13-1. A summary of important reactions is shown in BOX 13-1.

BOX 13-1 **Key Characteristics of *Haemophilus influenzae***

Fails to grow on sheep blood agar

Nonhemolytic on rabbit or horse blood agar

ALA (porphyrin) negative

Carbohydrate fermentation:

Positive: Glucose, ribose, xylose

Negative: Sucrose, lactose, fructose, mannose

Indole, urease, ODC: Variable based on biotype (see Table 13-1)

All *H. influenzae* isolates should be tested for β-lactamase, an extracellular enzyme produced by certain *H. influenzae*, which hydrolyzes the amide bond in penicillin to penicillic acid and produces resistance to penicillin. Ampicillin remains the drug of choice for those *H. influenzae* isolates that are susceptible to penicillin. In penicillin-resistant cases, chloroamphenicol, amoxicillin-clavulanate, and third-generation cephalosporins may be used.

There are currently four conjugate vaccines used in immunizations against *H. influenzae* type b. These vaccines are produced from purified polyribosyl ribitol phosphate (PRP), which is found in the bacterial capsule. According to the CDC, the current recommended vaccination schedule for *H influenzae* type b is for infants at 2, 4, and 6 months with a booster given at 15 months or older.

MISCELLANEOUS *HAEMOPHILUS* SPECIES

Haemophilus influenzae biogroup *aegyptius*, formerly known as Koch-Weeks bacillus, causes pinkeye, a very contagious conjunctivitis spread through contact with infected secretions of fluids, including the sharing of contaminated handkerchiefs and towels. The infection occurs in seasonal epidemics, especially in the warmer climates. This biogroup also has been isolated as the cause of Brazilian purpuric fever, which was first found in children in rural Brazil in the 1980s. Symptoms of this disease include fever, abdominal pain, a petechial rash, shock, and vascular collapse.

Haemophilus ducreyi is the infective agent of **chancroid**, a soft chancre venereal disease characterized by the appearance of a ragged, painful ulcer on the genitalia. Chancroid is found more frequently in Africa, Asia, and the tropics and less frequently in Europe and North America. The organism appears as tiny gram-negative bacilli, which are intracellular to polymorphonuclear neutrophils on direct examination of the genital ulcer, and is said to resemble "schools of fish." The organism is extremely fastidious, requiring freshly clotted rabbit, sheep, or human blood to grow. It also can be cultured on chocolate agar supplemented with 1% IsoVitaleX™ or gonococcus agar with 1% to 2% hemoglobin, 5% bovine fetal serum, and 3 μg/ml vancomycin. *H. ducreyi* requires X but not V factor.

Haemophilus haemolyticus is occasional normal flora of the upper respiratory cavity. It requires both X and V factors and shows a wide zone of β-hemolysis on horse blood agar. It may be mistaken for group A *Streptococcus* on the blood agar plate; the differentiation can be made through the Gram stain. ***Haemophilus parainfluenzae*** is normal flora of the upper respiratory tract. It is rarely infectious and requires only the V factor.

Species of *Haemophilus* that are now classified in the genus *Aggregatibacter* include *H. aphrophilus* and *H. paraphrophilus*. *Aggregatibacter* organisms are small, fastidious, nonmotile, slow-growing capnophilic gram-negative coccobacilli. Their name is derived from their tendency to grow in broth cultures as small granules that adhere to the walls of the test tube. *H. aphrophilus* and *H. paraphrophilus* are now classified within the single species *Aggregatibacter aphrophilus*. They are a normal component of the oral cavity and have been found in the gums and dental plaque of healthy adults. While considered to be of low pathogenicity, *A. aphrophilus* is a rare cause of several infections, including endocarditis, bone and joint infections, meningitis, brain abscess, bacteremia, and skin and soft tissue infections.

Some of the *Haemophilus* species are included in the HACEK group, discussed later in this chapter.

The identification of these miscellaneous *Haemophilus* species is summarized in **TABLE 13-2**.

Legionella

Legionella organisms are fastidious, narrow, gram-negative, non–spore-forming bacilli that are motile by one or more polar or subpolar flagella. The family Legionellae contains a single genus, *Legionella*, which includes the species *L. pneumophila*, the etiologic agent in **Legionnaires' disease**. This was first documented in July 1976 as a pneumonia outbreak in Philadelphia at the American Legion Convention. The infectious agent was previously unknown. Legionellae is also associated with Pontiac fever, a milder form of Legionnaires' disease.

In 1977, Dr. Joseph McDade of the Centers for Disease Control isolated the agent of Legionnaires' disease. Two years later, the name *Legionella pneumophila* was proposed for this bacterium. Today, there are 15 serogroups of *L. pneumophila* and 48 species of *Legionella*. Many of the species are considered to be potentially pathogenic for humans, and most have been isolated from environmental

TABLE 13-2 Identification of *Haemophilus* Species

Species	Requirement for		β-hemolysis	ALA	Fermentation of:			
	X factor	V factor			Glucose	Sucrose	Lactose	Fructose
H. influenzae	+	+	–	–	+	–	–	–
H. influenzae biogroup *aegyptius*	+	+	–	–	+	–	–	–
H. parainfluenzae	–	+	–	+	+	+	–	+
H. haemolyticus	+	+	+	–	+	–	–	wk+
H. parahaemolyticus	–	+	+	+	+	+	–	+
H. aphrophilus	–	–	–	+	+	+	+	+
H. paraphrophilus	–	+	–	+	+	+	+	+
H. ducreyi	+	–	wk+	–	–	–	–	–

ALA, δ-aminolevulinic acid; +, positive reaction; –, negative reaction; wk+, weakly positive

sources. The most common type of infection involves sporadic cases or clusters of pneumonia.

Legionella organisms are naturally found in both natural and artificial water sources. The bacteria have been found in ponds, creeks, streams, and wet soil. Potable water systems, whirlpool spas, cooling towers for air-conditioning and heating systems, showerheads, and plumbing systems are sources of infection. It is believed that susceptible individuals inhale the organism from aerosols produced through these water sources. There also are nosocomial cases caused by patients inhaling aerosols from contaminated water in showers, baths, and humidifiers. There also are several cases associated with building construction, which have been attributed to descalement of plumbing systems from pressure changes during construction. *Legionella* multiplies between temperatures of 25°C and 42°C and optimally grows at 35°C. *Legionella* infections are most often attributed to temperature alterations in water systems, which promotes the rapid multiplication of the organism. Freshwater sources of *Legionella* are generally not associated with infection; by contrast, altering the environment seems to promote its survival and transmission to humans. *Legionella* cannot survive in dry environments. It is important to note that person-to-person transmission does not seem to occur.

There are approximately 8,000 to 18,000 cases of Legionnaires' disease that require hospitalization each year in the United States. It is believed that the disease is underreported. Legionnaires' disease is an important cause of severe pneumonia, with the majority of cases being sporadic. However, there also are community, nosocomial, occupational, and travel-associated cases.

L. pneumophila accounts for approximately 90% of all cases of legionellosis in the United States, and most confirmed cases are caused by *L. pneumophila* serogroup 1.

Legionellosis includes both Legionnaires' disease, an acute pneumonia, and Pontiac fever, a nonpneumonia illness. Risk factors for Legionnaires' disease include age, smoking, male sex, chronic lung disease, lung cancer, diabetes, hematologic malignancies, and renal disease. Symptoms of Legionnaires' disease include fever, a nonproductive or dry cough, fatigue, myalgia, arthralgia, headache, difficulty breathing, and diarrhea. These symptoms are followed by pneumonia and pleural effusions. Bacteremia and dissemination to other organs, resulting in a multisystemic disease, also may occur. Outbreaks of legionellosis have also occurred in potable water sources found in hotels, cruise ships, at excavation sites, and in industrial plants.

The milder manifestation, Pontiac fever, is associated with mild flu-like symptoms, such as low-grade fever and chills; it is generally self-limiting. There may be a cough, headache, fever, and myalgia, but there is no pleural effusion or pneumonia. Patients usually recover uneventfully.

Although most cases of legionellosis are attributed to *L. pneumophila*, other species have also been implicated in pneumonia. These species include *L. micdadei*, also known as Pittsburgh pneumonia agent, which has been isolated from respiratory care equipment and cooling towers. It also is the cause of severe pulmonary infections in patients with leukemia, those undergoing corticosteroid therapy, and those who have had renal transplants. *L. bozemanii* also has been isolated as an agent of pneumonia.

Legionella species do not grow on ordinary laboratory media and require L-cysteine and a soluble form of iron to grow. They are isolated on an enriched media of buffered charcoal yeast extract (BCYE) agar. BCYE contains L-cysteine, activated charcoal, α-ketoglutarate, and other growth factors. Colonies of *Legionella* on BCYE are circular, glistening, and convex with an entire margin and may require up to four days to grow. Subcultures of suspected *Legionella* species growing on BCYE medium onto blood agar can be a useful tool to identify *Legionella* because *Legionella* will not grow on blood agar. Biochemical reactions for *Legionella* include a weakly positive catalase reaction, positive gelatinase, and positive motility. Reactions for urease, carbohydrate use, and nitrate reduction are all negative. The organism Gram stains poorly, and Giemsa or basic fuchsin should be substituted for safranin O to improve the quality of the stain.

Legionella can be isolated from many specimens, including blood; lung tissue; respiratory secretions, such as sputum or bronchial aspirates; and stool. However, respiratory specimens are preferred.

Culture diagnosis remains the gold standard for identification of *Legionella*, but other diagnostic tools also are very helpful. A direct fluorescent antibody (DFA) can be used to detect *Legionella* antigen in lung tissue and respiratory secretions. The specimen is fixed on a microscope slide and overlaid with *Legionella*-specific antisera labeled with conjugated fluorescein isothiocyanate. The antigen, if present, binds to the globulin in the labeled antibody, forming an antigen–antibody complex that fluoresces as short rods under ultraviolet light. This method provides a rapid identification and also can be used to identify *Legionella* antigen from isolates on BCYE agar. Serological diagnosis by indirect immunofluorescence, enzyme immunoassay, and microhemagglutination can be used to detect antibodies to *Legionella*. Urine antigen testing detects primarily *L. pneumophila* serogroup 1. This method provides an early diagnosis and is useful in screening large groups but is limited because the method detects only the serogroup 1 antigen. Polymerase chain reaction continues to be developed to enhance detection of *Legionella*.

Legionella infections are treated with erythromycin. The infection can be prevented by appropriate treatment and maintenance of water sources. Nosocomial infection remains a concern because this setting provides a combination of an at-risk population with plumbing systems that are often aging, which promotes the growth of *Legionella*.

Bordetella

Bordetella organisms are aerobic, oxidative obligate parasites in animals and humans. The organisms bind to the ciliated epithelial cells in the mucous membranes of the respiratory tract. There are currently seven species: *B. pertussis*, *B. parapertussis*, *B. bronchiseptica*, *B. avium*, *B. hinzii*, *B. holmesii*, and *B. trematum*. All of these species are capable of infecting humans except *B. avium*. *B. bronchiseptica* is found in many animals, including dogs, cats, rabbits, and horses, and rarely in humans. Human infection with *B. bronchiseptica* usually involves transmission from animals.

B. avium and *B. hinzii* are found in birds and turkeys. *B. trematum* has been found in human wounds and ear infections, and *B. holmesii* has been isolated from a variety of clinical infections.

The most important human species, *B. pertussis*, the agent of **pertussis**, is found only in humans. Pertussis is very contagious, with an attack rate of over 90% in those who are not immunized. The first recognized case of pertussis occurred in 1640, and it continued as a major cause of childhood illness and death until the introduction of the first whole-cell vaccine in the 1940s. Since that time, the disease steadily declined in the United States until the 1980s, when there was an increase in the number of cases in teenagers and babies younger than 6 months of age. This increase is attributed to declining vaccination because of fears of side effects from the cellular vaccine. Acellular vaccines were introduced in 1999, and compliance improved. The incidence of pertussis is cyclical, with peaks observed every 3 to 5 years in the United States. In 2009, there were almost 17,000 reported cases of pertussis and 14 deaths, whereas in 2010, there were over 11,000 cases reported. There have been outbreaks in California in 2010, when there were over 9,000 cases reported, which was the most cases reported since 1945, when there were over 13,000 cases. There also have been outbreaks in Michigan in 2008 and in Ohio in 2010, as well as in other states.

The recommended vaccination for infants and children is known as the DTaP, which consists of vaccines for diptheria, tetanus, and pertussis. There are a series of five immunizations given at 2, 4, and 6 months, between

15 and 18 months, and when the child begins school at age 5 to 7 years. A booster vaccination also is given at age 11 to 12 years; adults who did not receive DTaP should also receive the vaccination.

B. pertussis has several virulence factors, including a capsule, pertussis toxin, hemolysins, lipopolysaccharide or endotoxin, tracheal cytotoxin, and agglutinogens. Agglutinogens, or fimbriae, are involved in the initial attachment and colonization in pertussis. Pertussis toxin elicits several effects, such as clinical symptoms, lymphocytosis, and impairment of neutrophil chemotaxis and phagocytosis. This absolute and relative lymphocytosis is a unique response to a bacterial infection. Filamentous hemagglutinin is believed to enable the organism to attach to mucosal cells, thus allowing the atracheal cytotoxin to damage the ciliated respiratory epithelial cells after the organism attaches. In addition, endotoxin is released upon cell lysis, which induces systemic effects, such as fever and toxicity. Heat-labile toxin or dermonecrotic toxin causes inflammation and necrosis of the skin.

Pertussis infection is acquired through exposure to infectious respiratory droplets. There are three stages to pertussis: catarrhal, paroxysmal, and convalescent. The incubation period ranges from 7 to 20 days. During the catarrhal stage, the individual may have flu-like symptoms, as seen in a mild common cold, such as rhinorrhea, a mild cough, and a low-grade fever. During the catarrhal stage, bacteria multiply, spread to contiguous areas, and become concentrated in the ciliated epithelial cells and mucous membranes in the respiratory tract. Recovery of the organism from the nasopharynx is highest during this stage of the illness.

As the catarrhal stage progresses, the coughing becomes more severe after several weeks, and then the paroxysmal coughing phase occurs. The coughing continues to become more violent and severe, with several paroxysms occurring each day. The coughing clears the airways that have become clogged with mucus, and air is rapidly inspired over the glottis. This may produce a characteristic "whoop," which occurs as the patient inhales after a coughing spell. Whooping cough has been used in the past as a synonym for pertussis. There are many complications during the catarrhal stage, which include vomiting and extreme exhaustion. More-serious complications include hernia, pneumothorax, pulmonary complications, seizures, and encephalopathy. There also may be secondary bacterial infections and death. The paroxysmal stage may last for 1 to 4 weeks, and symptoms slowly subside.

The convalescent phase, which lasts for 4 to 8 weeks in some cases, but as long as 6 months in other cases, may be accompanied by coughing. The cough eventually subsides, but secondary bacterial infections may occur.

Bordetella organisms appear as tiny, gram-negative coccobacilli on primary isolation. The organisms are often pleomorphic on subculture. The bacteria are obligate aerobes and are not very active metabolically. All species except *B. bronchiseptica* are nonmotile.

Primary isolation of *B. pertussis* requires a special medium known as Bordet-Gengou (B-G) agar, which contains potato, glycerol, and blood. In the past, patients suspected of pertussis simply coughed onto a B-G plate. This technique was referred to as a "cough plate." Today the specimen of choice is a nasopharyngeal swab or washings, which are plated onto B-G agar or Regan-Lowe medium. B-G medium with methicillin or cephalexin, which inhibits normal flora, is preferable to the original B-G agar. Regan-Lowe medium contains horse blood, charcoal agar, cephalexin, and amphotericin B and is preferred by many microbiologists. Ideally, two specimens are collected from the nasopharynx to increase the chances of isolation; Dacron swabs are recommended.

B. pertussis produces small, smooth colonies in 7 days on B-G or Regan-Lowe medium in ambient air or increased CO_2 at 35°C to 37°C in 7 to 10 days. The colonies are shiny and said to resemble mercury droplets or pearls. Colonies are slightly β-hemolytic. The organism appears as a tiny, gram-negative coccobacillus on the Gram stain. Once isolated, identification can be confirmed by testing for the presence of *B. pertussis* antigen through use of a fluorescent assay. Important biochemical reactions for *B. pertussis* are shown in BOX 13-2.

BOX 13-2 **Key Reactions for *Bordetella pertussis***

Nonmotile

Sheep blood agar: No growth

MacConkey agar: No growth

Bordet-Gengou agar: Convex, shiny, silver, mercury-like droplets in 7 days with slight hemolysis

Catalase: Positive

Citrate: Negative

Indole: Negative

TABLE 13-3 Differentiation of *Bordetella* Species

	Urease	Nitrate	Motility	Oxidase
B. pertussis	–	–	–	+
B. parapertussis	+ (18 hours)	–	–	–
B. bronchiseptica	Strong + (4 hours)	+	+	+

B. pertussis can be directly identified from nasopharyngeal specimens by using the direct fluorescent antibody test (DFA). In this technique, a smear is made from a nasopharyngeal specimen and conjugated fluorescein isothiocyanate *B. pertussis* antibodies are added. After incubation, the slide is washed and examined under the fluorescent microscope. In a positive test for *B. pertussis*, short rods with a rim of bright-green fluorescence are observed. DFA testing can be performed using polyclonal or monoclonal antibodies.

Newer technologies developed to detect *B. pertussis* include the use of monoclonal antibodies to directly detect lipopolysaccharide and filamentous hemagglutinin. Polymerase chain reaction methods that directly detect the organism in nasopharyngeal specimens or from culture are also available.

B. parapertussis produces a brown pigment on Bordet-Gengou agar. It is nonmotile and has been associated with a pertussis-like syndrome, which is a milder infection than seen with *B. pertussis*.

B. bronchiseptica is motile with peritrichous flagella and has been found to be a cause of a variety of infections, including septicemia and meningitis, in immunosuppressed hosts. It is a rapid urease producer.

Some general biochemical reactions used to speciate *Bordetella* are found in **TABLE 13-3**.

Brucella

Brucella organisms are catalase-positive, oxidase-positive, nonsaccharolytic, strictly aerobic gram-negative bacilli. The organisms are normal flora of the urinary and gastrointestinal tracts of goats, pigs, cows, and dogs and are agents of brucellosis in animals and humans. Brucellosis is a zoonosis and may be the cause of outbreaks in animals, which may lead to severe economic loss from damage to livestock. It occurs throughout the world and is most prevalent in the countries around the Mediterranean Gulf and Persian Gulf, Central and South America, Mexico, and India.

Humans acquire *Brucella* infections through the ingestion of contaminated animal products, including meats and milk; through inhalation of aerosolized particles; or through direct contact through skin abrasions from handling infected animals. *Brucella* species and their primary animal reservoirs include *B. abortus* (cattle), *B. melitensis* and *B. ovis* (sheep and goats), *B. suis* (pigs), and *B. canis* (dogs). Humans can acquire the infection from any of these animal sources. There are approximately 100 cases of human *Brucella* infections each year in the United States. Those at increased risk include handlers of livestock, slaughterhouse workers, farmers, veterinarians, and laboratory personnel.

Brucella species are obligate parasites and can survive intracellularly in the reticuloendothelial system, bone, liver, and central nervous system of humans. The organism causes **undulant fever** (brucellosis), which is a chronic and recurring fever that causes rising and falling fevers, following a pattern that is described as a wave. The acute form of the disease shows flu-like symptoms, including fever, malaise, anorexia, weight loss, and muscle and back pain. The undulant form occurs within one year of the initial symptoms and includes undulant fevers, arthritis, and possibly arthritis and chronic fatigue. Granulomatous infections occur in the reticuloendothelial system and in the bones; lymphoadenopathy and splenomegaly also may occur. The infections become chronic because the organism resides intracellularly, protected from cell-mediated immunity.

Brucella can be isolated from bone marrow, cerebrospinal fluid, and wounds; however, it is most frequently isolated from the blood. The blood culture system recommended is the biphasic Castaneda method, which uses both solid and liquid media in the same container. Blood cultures are more likely to be positive between the first and third weeks of febrile illness. Blood cultures generally become negative following the fourth week, after the acute symptoms subside, because antibody production has begun. Although *Brucella* grows on blood and chocolate agar, *Brucella* agar plus 5% horse or rabbit serum is recommended for isolation. *Brucella* agar contains a pancreatic digest of casein, a peptic digest of animal tissue, yeast, and sodium bisulfite. Plates are incubated in 5% to 10% CO_2 and are held for 3 weeks.

In direct Gram-stained smears, *Brucella* organisms are tiny, gram-negative coccobacilli, which may appear intracellular in tissue specimens. Carbolfuchsin should be substituted for safranin O to improve the quality of the Gram stain. The Gram stain morphology is not specific for *Brucella*.

Because of the difficulty in culturing *Brucella*, the **serum agglutination test** (SAT), which is a serological test for antibodies in the patient's serum, may be used to confirm the infection. Antibodies that react with the major antigens of *Brucella*, which include the smooth (S) and the lipopolysaccharide (LPS) of the outer cell membrane and the internal cytosolic proteins, are detected using ELISA or immunofluorescence. The immune response to *Brucella* begins with production of IgM isotype antibodies, followed after a long period by production of IgG isotype antibodies. A fourfold increase between the acute and convalescent titer or a titer of at least 1:160 is considered significant. SAT detects antibodies to *B. abortus*, *B. suis*, and *B. melitensis*, but not to *B. canis*.

Brucella is a Biosafety Level 3 biohazard, which includes common and unusual pathogens; the World Health Organization (WHO) identifies *Brucella* as a pathogen that presents a high risk to laboratory workers. Laboratory-acquired infections occurred in 2006 in Indiana and Minnesota, where two microbiologists acquired brucellosis through cultures that contained *B. melitensis*. In 2007, New York state laboratory workers were exposed to *B. abortus* through an isolate used in a laboratory preparedness survey as part of a proficiency testing program. To prevent laboratory-acquired infections, a biological class II or higher safety cabinet must be used to minimize the generation of aerosols and protect against splashing. Also, specific primary barriers, including safety centrifuge cups and personnel protective equipment, must be in place. Secondary barriers, including restricted access to the laboratory and appropriate maintenance of the laboratory air-handling system, are also required. All positive results are sent to the state or another reference laboratory for confirmation and then reported to the CDC.

The species of *Brucella* can be identified using the biochemical reactions as shown in **TABLE 13-4**.

Pasteurella

Pasteurella is a nonmotile, oxidase-positive, fermentative, facultative anaerobic gram-negative bacillus. There are several species, including *P. multocida*, which is the etiologic agent of **pasteurellosis**. *Pasteurella* is encapsulated, which enables it to resist phagocytosis. The organism is carried in the oral cavity and respiratory and gastrointestinal tracts of healthy domestic cats and dogs and also is normally found in many wild animals, including rodents, rabbits, and birds. It is the agent of "shipping fever" in cattle, which is a hemorrhagic septicemia.

Humans may acquire the infection following contact with domestic animals that harbor the bacterium. Most frequently the route of infection is from the bite or scratch of an infected animal, usually a cat. Local wound infections are the most common type of pasteurellosis, which is characterized by pain, redness, swelling, cellulitis, and a purulent discharge. There is a rapid onset of inflammation, with a fever developing 3 to 5 days after the infection has been acquired. Complications of pasteurellosis include osteomyelitis, meningitis, and joint infections. Bacteremia also can result from the primary bite infection. A second route of infection is inhalation of the bacterium, which can lead to pneumonia, bronchitis, or sinusitis. Those at occupational risk for acquiring pasteurellosis via the respiratory route include those who handle or raise animals and those with an existing respiratory disorder. Other types of

TABLE 13-4 Speciation of *Brucella*

	B. abortus	*B. melitensis*	*B. suis*	*B. canis*
Animal source	**Cattle**	**Sheep and goats**	**Pigs**	**Dogs**
Urease (positive in)	1–2 hr	1–2 hr	0–30 min	0–30 min
Hydrogen sulfide (H_2S)	+	–	–	–
Growth on media containing:				
Thionin (20 µg)	–	+	+	+
Basic fuchsin (20 µg)	+	+	–	–
Thionin blue (2 mg/ml)	+	+	–	–

BOX 13-3 **Key Reactions for *Pasturella multocida***

Oxidase: Positive

Catalase: Positive

Nitrate: Positive

Indole: Positive

Urease: Negative

Acid but no gas produced from glucose, sucrose, and mannose

Acid not produced from maltose and lactose

Starch hydrolysis: Negative

infections attributed to *Pasteurella* include endocarditis, peritonitis, and postoperative wound infections.

To identify *P. multocida*, the Gram stain reveals a small, gram-negative rod with bipolar staining. The bacterium grows well on both blood agar and chocolate agar, but growth is not enhanced under increased CO_2. On sheep blood agar the colonies are small, smooth, gray or translucent, and nonhemolytic. Colonies may be either rough or mucoid depending on the strain. The organism cannot grow on MacConkey agar. *P. multocida* produces a musty or mushroom-like odor. Important biochemical reactions to *P. multocida* are shown in BOX 13-3.

Francisella

Francisella tularensis, a small, nonmotile, pleomorphic gram-negative bacillus, is the agent of **tularemia**, a disease of rodents, primarily rabbits. In 1911, plague-like disease in rodents in Tulare City, California, marked the first isolation of *Bacterium tulareri*, which is now known as *Francisella tularensis*. The organism is carried on many wild animals, including rodents, rabbits, lemmings, squirrels, muskrats, birds, fish, beavers, and other mammals. Tularemia is also known as rabbit fever, hare fever, and lemming fever. Individuals at increased risk include farmers, hunters, forest workers, and others who have contact with infected animals. This zoonosis is acquired through direct contact with blood or through an animal bite or scratch. The bacterium also can be acquired indirectly through insect vectors, primarily biting flies and ticks, which harbor *F. tularensis*. Infection also may result from the ingestion of contaminated water or food or inhalation of contaminated aerosols. It is highly infective when grown in culture, and extreme caution must be used in the clinical laboratory to avoid laboratory-acquired infections.

There are several forms of tularemia, which may range from severely debilitating to less virulent forms of illness. There is a 2-day to 3-week incubation period after exposure, followed by fever, chills, sore throat, and headache. There is also weight loss and lymphoadenopathy. The ulceroglandular form of the disease results from the bite of an infected arthropod vector or from handling contaminated animal products. An ulcer forms at the site of infection and may persist for months. *F. tularensis* possesses a capsule that enables it to resist phagocytosis and also has invasive properties that allow the bacterium to penetrate intact skin. Once skin entry has occurred, the organism can disseminate through the lymphatic system to the lymph nodes, where regional lymphoadenopathy occurs. The organism can cause bacteremia, living as an intracellular parasite within the reticuloendothelial system and lymph nodes of the host. When acquired through inhalation, the most common type of infection is pneumonia. Another type of tularemia is oculoglandular disease, which affects the conjunctiva of the eye and is acquired through splashing or infecting the eye with contaminated hands. Oropharyngeal tularemia results from ingesting contaminated food or water, and the primary lesion is found in the pharynx. Pneumonic tularemia results from inhalation of the organism or also may occur as a complication of the other forms.

F. tularensis requires a special medium, blood-cysteine-glucose agar with thiamine, to grow. It takes 2 to 4 days to grow and is a strict aerobe. Colonies are smooth, bluish gray, and slightly mucoid with a narrow α-hemolytic zone. It also grows on modified charcoal-yeast agar and chocolate agar with IsoVitaleX™. Biochemical reactions used to identify *Francisella* include catalase-positive, oxidase-negative, and positive fermentation of glucose, maltose, and mannose.

Serological techniques are the recommended method for identification. The DFA stain is used to detect antibodies to *F. tularensis* in the patient's serum. Enzyme linked immunoassay techniques also are available.

Extreme caution should be exhibited when *F. tularensis* is suspected because it readily can penetrate through small breaks in the skin. It is a Biosafety Level 2 pathogen, which requires that laboratory workers wear gloves and work in a biological safety cabinet.

Cases of tularemia have declined in the United States from several thousands in the 1930s to several hundred in the 1980s. During 1990 to 2000, a total of 1,368 cases of tularemia were reported to the CDC from 44 states. Most cases are acquired through arthropod vectors. *Francisella tularensis* has been identified as a possible agent of bioterrorism. Its extremely low infectious dose of 10 to 50 organisms further contributes to its virulence.

Streptobacillus

Streptobacillus moniliformis is a fastidious, gram-negative, very pleomorphic, filamentous bacillus normally found in the oropharynx of rodents, primarily wild and laboratory rats. Humans most frequently acquire the infection, **rat-bite fever**, through the bite of an infected animal. Other routes of infection include scratches or direct contact with rodents. Rat-bite fever begins with fever, chills, and muscle aches. There also may be symptoms resembling an upper respiratory tract infection, headache, nausea, and vomiting. As the disease continues, there is joint pain in the extremities and development of a skin rash on the palms of the hands and on the soles of the feet. Although the bite heals, complications include lymphadenitis, hepatic and splenic disorders, endocarditis, and meningitis. The disease often is difficult to diagnose because it resembles several other infections. *Spirillum minus*, a helical gram-negative bacterium, also causes rat bite fever. Another type of *Streptobacillus* infection, known as Haverhill fever, is acquired by ingesting milk contaminated with *S. moniliformis*. It resembles rat-bite fever, but gastrointestinal signs are more pronounced. The infection is named for an outbreak that occurred in Haverhill, Massachusetts, in 1926.

There are over two million animal bites reported each year in the United States, and rats are responsible for 1% of the cases. The typical victim is a child less than 5 years of age living in poverty where there is an infected rat population. With the increased popularity of rodents, including rats as pets, and their use in scientific studies, the affected population has widened to include other children, laboratory technicians, and pet store employees.

Streptobacillus is treated with penicillin, in combination with streptomycin or gentamycin for more serious infections.

The organism is difficult to identify and is rarely isolated from culture. It is extremely fastidious and requires media enriched with whole blood, serum, or ascitic fluid for growth. Growth occurs slowly and may be apparent in as early as 2 to 3 days but may take as long as 7 days. Colonies have a "cotton ball" or "bread crumb" appearance in the bottom of liquid media and appear as circular, convex, gray, smooth, glistening colonies on agar. A "fried egg" appearance may be present after 5 days of growth. *Streptobacillus* is biochemically inactive, and most reactions, including indole, catalase, oxidase, urease, and nitrates, are negative. Serological identification for serum agglutinins against *S. moniliformis*, in which a fourfold increase between the acute and convalescent titers occur, is an important tool for diagnosis.

HACEK Group

The **HACEK** group colonizes the oropharynx; these are a group of slow-growing gram-negative bacilli whose growth is enhanced under increased CO_2. The HACEK bacteria are rare causes of bacterial endocarditis and peritonitis. Generally, infection occurs after the bacteria enter a normally sterile site. These infections are usually treated with β-lactam antibiotics with an aminoglycoside. The acronym HACEK refers to the first letter of the genera of bacteria that fit the above description and include *Haemophilus* (H), *Aggregatibacter* (A), *Cardiobacterium* and *Capnocytophaga* (C), *Eikenella* (E), and *Kingella* (K).

Haemophilus influenzae, *H. parainfluenzae*, and *Aggregatibacter aphrophilus* are included in the HACEK group and were discussed earlier in this chapter.

Aggregatibacter actinomycetemcomitans was previously classified in the genus *Actinobacillus* and has been transferred to the *Aggregatibacter* genus, along with *A. aphrophilus*, based on DNA homology and 16S rRNA sequencing. *A. actinomycetemcomitans* is a small, gram-negative bacillus that is nonmotile and resembles *Pasteurella*; in fact the *Aggregatibacter* genus is classified within the family Pasteurellaceae. It is normal flora of the human oral cavity and a rare agent of endocarditis. The infection follows an endogenous route whereby the bacterium invades deeper tissues following dental procedures. Other infections include perodontitis, soft tissue infections, septic arthritis, abscesses, septicemia, and human bite infections. *A. actinomycetemcomitans* is also found with *Actinomyces* in cases of actinomycoses.

A. actinomycetemcomitans grows on sheep blood agar with enhanced growth in humid conditions under increased CO_2. Colonies are pinpoint and rough and sticky at 24 hours of incubation. On clear media, such as brain-heart infusion, there may be a star-shaped configuration in the middle of the mature colony. *A. actinomycetemcomitans* does not grow on MacConkey agar. It is catalase positive and reduces nitrates and is negative for indole, urease, and esculin hydrolysis.

Cardiobacterium hominis is normally found in the upper respiratory tract and is isolated as a rare cause of endocarditis, especially in those with an existing heart defect. *C. hominis* grows on blood agar, producing small, opaque, glistening colonies that are α-hemolytic. Growth is enhanced at increased CO_2. It is nonmotile, oxidase positive, catalase negative, and indole positive when using the modified method with xylene extraction. The organism ferments mannitol and sorbitol.

Capnocytophaga species include *C. gingivalis*, *C. sputigena*, *C. hominis*, and *C. canimorsus*. *C. canimorsus* is found as normal flora of dogs and causes human infections following dog bites, which can range from a mild local infection to bacteremia. *C. gingivalis*, *C. sputigena*, and *C. hominis* are a part of the normal flora of the human oral cavity and may serve as endogenous causes of periodontitis and bacteremia in immunosuppressed patients. *Capnocytophaga* grow on sheep blood agar and at 48 to 72 hours appear as small, opaque, yellow-pigmented, shiny colonies, which are nonhemolytic. A gliding motility that appears as a film on the agar's surface may be observed. *Capnocytophaga* appear as thin, gram-negative bacilli with tapered ends.

Eikenella corrodens, or "corroding bacterium," pits or corrodes the surface of agar. It is normal flora of the human mouth and upper respiratory tract and is an agent of human bite wounds, meningitis, endocarditis, brain and intra-abdominal abscesses, and peritonitis. Infections are usually polymicrobic in nature. It most frequently is isolated from blood cultures after tooth extractions in patients who subsequently develop facial and neck abscesses, cellulitis, and septicemia.

The organism is a facultative aerobe and requires hemin for growth, preferring chocolate agar. Colonies on blood agar are minute and often require several days to grow. The organism has a characteristic bleach-like odor. *E. corrodens* is nonsaccharolytic, oxidase positive, catalase negative, and nonmotile.

Kingella organisms are oxidase positive and ferment glucose. *Kingella* gives negative reactions for catalase, indole, urea, and esculin hydrolysis. *Kingella* is a short coccobacillus with rounded ends, which may arrange in chains. As with *Eikenella*, *Kingella* species require blood for growth and may "pit" the agar surface. *Kingella denitrificans* and *Kingella kingae* are rare pathogens, which are normal flora of the upper respiratory tract and genitourinary tract. They may cause endocarditis and other infections in immunocompromised hosts. *K. kingae* also causes bone, blood, and joint infections in children. *K. denitrificans* is nonhemolytic, whereas *K. kingae* shows a narrow zone of β-hemolysis on sheep blood agar. *Kingella* grows on selective agar for *Neisseria*, such as Thayer Martin, and must be differentiated from *Neisseria*. A negative catalase reaction is important to differentiate *Kingella* from catalase-positive *Neisseria*. Also, nitrate reduction is positive for *K. denitrificans* and negative for *Neisseria*.

Chromobacterium

Chromobacterium violaceum, a motile, oxidase-positive facultative anaerobe, is a rare cause of human infection. It is found in soil and water in the tropics and subtropics. It is not part of the normal flora, and infection occurs following contact of wounds with contaminated soil or water. The infection begins as cellulitis or lymphadenitis and may extend to systemic infections, such as abscesses and septicemia. *Chromobacterium* grows on sheep blood agar and MacConkey's agar as a nonlactose fermenter. It produces round, smooth colonies with a unique purple to dark purple pigment because of the production of violaceum.

Laboratory Procedures

Procedure
Staphylococcus streak

Purpose
Haemophilus can be isolated on blood agar by streaking the culture with β-hemolytic *Staphylococcus aureus* and observing for satellitism.

Principle
Many microorganisms, including *S. aureus*, *Neisseria*, and certain yeasts, are capable of synthesizing NAD (V factor).

When these organisms appear in mixed culture, those species of *Haemophilus* that require V factor appear as small "dewdrop" colonies around those bacterial colonies producing NAD. This phenomenon is known as satellitism. When grown on sheep blood agar, β-hemolytic strains of *S. aureus* release X factor (hemin) as the red cells are hemolyzed.

Materials and Media

Sheep blood agar plate *S. aureus* (β-hemolytic strain)
Species of culture suspected of containing *Haemophilus*

Procedure

1. Streak the *Haemophilus* culture heavily on the sheep blood agar plate. Use a swab if necessary.
2. Make a single, narrow streak of *S. aureus* through the area where the *Haemophilus* was streaked.
3. Incubate at 35°C to 37°C under 3% to 10% CO_2 for 18 to 24 hours.

Interpretation

Observe the plate for satellitism. *Haemophilus* colonies appear as moist, small, dewdrop colonies adjacent to the *S. aureus* colonies. The plate also can be observed for hemolysis and growth in the hemolyzed areas, indicating that the species requires factor X.

Quality Control

Haemophilus influenzae: Growth in β-hemolytic zone surrounding *S. aureus*

Procedure

X and V factors

Purpose

Haemophilus organisms can be identified based on their specific growth requirements for X and V factors.

Principle

X factor (hemin or hematin) is derived from the digestion or degradation of blood. V factor (coenzyme I or NAD) is obtained from yeast or potato extract and also is produced by some bacteria, such as *Staphylococcus aureus*. These factors are required either singly or in combination by various *Haemophilus* species and are thus used as a method of species differentiation. The growth requirements are tested through use of filter paper strips impregnated with X factor and V factor and both X and V factors. A nutrient-poor medium, such as Mueller-Hinton agar, is used.

Materials and Media

Mueller-Hinton agar
Brain-heart infusion broth or trypticase soy broth
X factor, V factor, and XV factor filter paper disks

Procedure

1. From a pure *Haemophilus* isolate, prepare a light suspension in brain-heart infusion broth or trypticase soy broth. It is important not to carry any chocolate agar over into the broth because this may lead to inaccurate results.
2. Inoculate the Mueller-Hinton plate with a sterile swab. Streak the plate for maximum growth in three directions to obtain a lawn of growth.
3. Using sterile forceps, place the filter paper disks on the agar surface approximately 20 mm apart. Gently tap into place.
4. Incubate 18 to 24 hours under 3% to 10% CO_2 at 35°C to 37°C.
5. Observe the plates for visible growth about each filter paper disk.

Interpretation

Growth about X factor and XV: X factor is required
Growth about V factor and XV: V factor is required
Growth about XV: both X and V factors are required

Expected Results

Haemophilus species	Growth around XV	Growth around X	Growth around V	Needs
H. influenzae	+	−	−	X and V
H. parainfluenzae	+	−	+	V
H. haemolyticus	+	−	+	X and V
H. parahaemolyticus	+	−	+	V

Quality Control

H. influenzae: Growth about XV strip
H. parainfluenzae: Growth around V and XV strips

Procedure

Haemophilus identification quad-plate

Purpose

The *Haemophilus* identification plate is used to determine the hemolytic properties and requirements for X and V factors for particular *Haemophilus* species.

Principle

The plate consists of four quadrants: quadrant I—hemin (X), quadrant II—NAD (V), quadrant III—NAD (V) and hemin (X), and quadrant IV—5% defibrinated horse sheep blood agar. Presence or absence of growth in each quadrant and hemolysis on horse blood agar are used for the identification of *Haemophilus* species.

Reagents and Media

Haemophilus identification plate (Hemo ID QUAD, available through Becton-Dickinson)
Trypticase soy broth

Procedure

1. Pick several colonies of suspected organisms with a sterile inoculating needle or sterile cotton swab.
2. Suspend organism in trypticase soy broth until a turbidity of 0.5 McFarland is obtained.
3. Streak one loopful of this suspension on each quadrant of the plate. Streak the entire quadrant. Stab blood agar quadrant. Sterilize loop between quadrants, or use a new disposable loop for each quadrant.
4. Incubate plate in 3% to 10% CO_2 at 35°C for 24 to 48 hours.

Interpretation

1. Interpret plate for visible growth and hemolysis. The organism should grow in quadrants III and IV. Read quadrant IV for hemolysis. Growth in quadrants II, III, and IV indicates requirement for X factor. Growth in quadrants I, III, and IV indicates requirement for X factor. Growth in only quadrants III and IV indicates requirement for both X and V factors.
2. Perform a Gram stain to obtain expected results to ensure purity and to obtain morphological characteristics of *Haemophilus.*

Expected Results

Haemophilus species	Growth in quadrants			
	I (X)	II (V)	III (XV)	IV (HEMOLYSIS)
H. influenzae	–	–	+	–
H. parainfluenzae	–	+	+	–
H. haemolyticus	–	–	+	+
H. parahaemolyticus	–	+	+	+

Quality Control

H. influenzae: Nonhemolytic; growth in quadrants III and IV
H. parainfluenzae: Nonhemolytic; growth in quadrants II, III, and IV
(Source: Package insert, Hemo ID QUAD, Becton-Dickinson)

Laboratory Exercises

1. Perform the tests for X and V factors for *Haemophilus influenzae* and *Haemophilus parainfluenzae.* Record your results.

Haemophilus species	X factor	V factor	XV factor	Observations	Interpretation
H. influenzae					
H. parainfluenzae					

2. Perform the staph streak on *H. influenzae* and *H. parainfluenzae.* Describe your results.

Haemophilus species	Observations	Interpretation
H. influenzae		
H. parainfluenzae		

How does β-hemolytic *Staphylococcus aureus* supply the growth requirements for *Haemophilus*?

____

____

3. Streak one *Haemophilus* identification plate each for *H. influenzae, H. parainfluenzae,* and an unknown *Haemophilus.* Incubate, record observations, and interpret results.

Organism	X quadrant	V quadrant	XV quadrant	Horse blood (hemolysis)	Interpretation
H. influenzae					
H. parainfluenzae					
Unknown ________					

Review Questions

Matching

Identify the *Haemophilus* species by matching each with its correct biochemical reactions.

	Requirement for					Fermentation of		
	X factor	V factor	Hemolysis	ALA	Glucose	Sucrose	Lactose	Fructose
1.	–	+	–	+	+	+	–	+
2.	+	+	–	–	+	–	–	–
3.	+	–	–	–	–	–	–	–

a. *H. influenzae*
b. *H. parainfluenzae*
c. *H. haemolyticus*
d. *H. parahaemolyticus*
e. *H. ducreyi*

Multiple Choice

4. Which statement correctly describes X factor?
   a. Heat labile
   b. Known as hemin or hematin
   c. Derived from yeast and potato extract
   d. Produced by *Staphylococcus aureus*
5. *Haemophilus influenzae* is most frequently isolated on:
   a. Sheep blood agar
   b. Rabbit blood agar
   c. Chocolate agar
   d. CNA

   Use the following information for questions 6 and 7: In a determination of requirements for X and V factors, a suspected *Haemophilus* species grew only between the X and V strips.
6. This *Haemophilus* species requires:
   a. Only V factor
   b. Only X factor
   c. Both X and V factors
   d. Neither X nor V factor
7. Which of the following is *not* a possible species for these results?
   a. *H. influenzae*
   b. *H. aegyptius*
   c. *H. parainfluenzae*
   d. *H. hemolyticus*
8. Those *Haemophilus* species that are porphyrin positive:
   a. Require exogenous NAD
   b. Do not require exogenous NAD
   c. Require exogenous hemin
   d. Do not require exogenous hemin
9. The serotype of *H. influenzae* found most frequently in infections is:
   a. a
   b. b
   c. c
   d. d
   e. e
10. The population most frequently infected by *H. influenzae* is:
   a. Newborns
   b. Nonimmunized infants and children less than 3 years of age
   c. Nonimmunized preschool-age children, ages 3 to 5 years
   d. School-age children, ages 6 to 10 years
   e. Immunosuppressed adults
11. The infectious agent of chancroid is:
   a. *H. aegyptius*
   b. *H. haemolyticus*
   c. *H. ducreyi*
   d. *H. influenzae* biotype V

For questions 12 to 15, match the isolation medium with the bacterium that the agar primarily is used to isolate:

12. Whole blood or serum-enriched media
13. Bordet-Gengou agar
14. Buffered charcoal-yeast extract
15. Blood-cysteine-glucose agar
   a. *Bordetella pertussis*
   b. *Francisella tularensis*
   c. *Pasteurella multocida*
   d. *Legionella pneumophila*
   e. *Streptobacillus moniliformis*

For questions 16 to 19, match the organism with its associated infection:

16. Pertussis
17. Undulant fever
18. Pontiac fever
19. Rat-bite fever
20. Tularemia
   a. *Pasteurella*
   b. *Streptobacillus*
   c. *Bordetella*
   d. *Legionella*
   e. *Brucella*
   f. *Francisella*
21. The population with increased susceptibility to *Legionella* infection is:
   a. Newborns
   b. Middle-aged females with autoimmune illness
   c. Infants between ages 6 months and 4 years
   d. Middle-aged males with an underlying medical problem

22. Legionnaires' disease is spread through:
    a. Inhalation of aerosols from contaminated water
    b. Ingestion of contaminated water
    c. Direct contact with respiratory secretions of an infected individual
    d. Direct contact with an infected animal or animal products
23. On Bordet-Gengou medium, *B. pertussis* appears:
    a. Dry, heaped, serrated
    b. Iridescent brown
    c. Smooth and shiny, resembling mercury droplets
    d. White, raised, rough
24. A *Brucella* species gave the following reactions:
    Urease positive in 1.5 hours
    H_2S negative
    Growth in presence of:
    20 μg thionin: Positive
    2 μg thionin blue: Positive
    20 μg basic fuchsin: Positive

    This *Brucella* species is most likely:
    a. *B. abortus*
    b. *B. melitensis*
    c. *B. suis*
    d. *B. canis*
25. Which set of reactions is correct for *Pasteurella multocida?*

	Oxidase	Catalase	Growth on blood agar	Glucose fermented	Acid from glucose
a.	+	+	–	–	–
b.	–	+	+	+	–
c.	–	–	+	+	+
d.	+	+	+	+	–

26. The HACEK bacteria:
    a. Are fastidious gram-negative bacilli, which are normal flora of the oral cavity
    b. Are associated with endogenous endocarditis
    c. Are treated with β-lactam antibiotics with an aminoglycoside
    d. All of the above

Bibliography

Brouqui, P., & Raoult, D. (2001). Endocarditis due to rare and fastidious bacteria. *Clinical Microbiology Review, 14,* 177–207.

Centers for Disease Control and Prevention. (2008). *Haemophilus influenzae* disease (including Hib). Retrieved from http://www.cdc.gov/hi-disease/clinicians.html

Centers for Disease Control and Prevention. (2011). Top 10 things every clinician needs to know about legionellosis. Retrieved from http://www.cdc.gov/legionella/clinicians.html

Centers for Disease Control and Prevention. (2010). *Brucellosis.* Retrieved from http://www.cdc.gov/brucellosis/

Centers for Disease Control and Prevention. (2005). Legionnaires' disease associated with potable water in a hotel—Ocean City, Maryland, October 2003–February 2004. *Morbidity and Mortality Weekly Reports, 54,* 165–168. Retrieved from http://www.cdc.gov/mmwr/preview/mmwrhtml/mm5407a1.htm

Centers for Disease Control and Prevention. (2005). Cruise-ship-associated Legionnaires' disease, November 2003–May 2004. *Morbidity and Mortality Weekly Reports, 54,* 1153–1155. Retrieved from http://www.cdc.gov/mmwr/preview/mmwrhtml/mm5445a2.htm

Centers for Disease Control and Prevention. (2001). Outbreak of Legionnaires' disease among automotive plant workers—Ohio, 2001. *Morbidity and Mortality Weekly Report, 50,* 357–359. Retrieved from http://www.cdc.gov/mmwr/preview/mmwrhtml/mm5018a1.htm

Centers for Disease Control and Prevention. (2009). *Brucella suis* infection associated with feral swine hunting—Three states, 2007–2008. *Morbidity and Mortality Weekly Report, 58,* 618–621. Retrieved from http://www.cdc.gov/mmwr/preview/mmwrhtml/mm5822a3.htm

Centers for Disease Control and Prevention. (2008). Laboratory-acquired *Brucellosis*—Indiana and Minnesota, 2006. *Morbidity and Mortality Weekly Report, 57,* 39–42. Retrieved from http://www.cdc.gov/mmwr/preview/mmwrhtml/mm5702a3.htm

Centers for Disease Control and Prevention. (2002). Tularemia—United States 1990–2000, *Morbidity and Mortality Weekly Report, 61,* 182–184. Retrieved from http://www.cdc.gov/mmwr/preview/mmwrhtml/mm5109a1.htm

Elliott, S. P. (2007). Rat bite fever and *Streptobacillus moniliformis. Clinical Microbiology Reviews, 20,* 13–22.

Ellis, J., Oyston, P. C., Green, M., & Titball, R. W. (2002). Tularemia. *Clinical Microbiology Reviews, 15,* 631–646.

Fields, B. S., Benson, R. F., & Besser, R. E. (2002). *Legionella* and Legionnaires' disease: 25 years of investigation. *Clinical Microbiology Reviews, 15,* 506–526.

Friedman, R. L. (1988). Pertussis: The disease and new diagnostic methods. *Clinical Microbiology Reviews, 1,* 365–376.

Mattoo, S., & Cherry, J. D. (2005). Molecular pathogenesis, epidemiology and clinical manifestations of respiratory infections due to *Bordetella pertussis* and other *Bordetella* subspecies. *Clinical Microbiology Reviews, 18,* 326–382.

Pasculli, A. W., & Rogers, F. G. (1991). *Legionella.* In A. Balows (Ed.), *Manual of clinical microbiology* (5th ed.) (pp. 442–453). Washington, DC: American Society for Microbiology.

Taylor, S. L., & Lang, S. D. R. (2012). *Aggregatibacter actinomycetemcomitans* (*Actinobacillus actinomycetemcomitans*). Retrieved from http://www.antimicrobe.org/new/b72.asp

Winn, Jr., W. C. (1988). Legionnaires' disease: Historical perspective. *Clinical Microbiology Reviews, 1,* 60–81.

Winn, Jr., W., Allen, S., Janda, W., Konemen, E., Procop, G., Schreckenberger, P., & Woods, G. (Eds.). (2005). Miscellaneous fastidious gram-negative bacilli. In *Koneman's color atlas and textbook of diagnostic microbiology* (6th ed.). Philadelphia, PA: Lippincott Williams & Wilkins.

Wright, P., Keane, C., Ricketts, H. C., & McKay, A. (2012). *Aggregatibacter aphrophilus* endocarditis: A case report. *Scottish Medical Journal, 57,* 247–251.

NEW: THE MICROBIAL ECOLOGY OF *LEGIONELLA*

Legionella has been detected in up to 40% of freshwater environments by culture and almost 80% of freshwater sites by polymerase chain reaction. Most cases of legionellosis are related to human-made aquatic environments in which the water temperature is higher than that of the natural environment. This temperature adjustment alters the balance between protozoa and bacteria, promoting the rapid multiplication of *Legionella*.

Legionella has unique nutritional needs, including iron and sulfur. These compounds are rarely found in freshwater sources. How does *Legionella* survive in freshwater that does not meet its nutrient needs? *Legionella* survives by growing as an intracellular parasite of free-living protozoans. There are 14 species of amoeba, two species of ciliated protozoa, and one species of slime mold, all of which support the amplification of *Legionella* bacteria. These include *Naegleria* species and *Acanthamoeba* species, which are ubiquitous in water. Thus, protozoans serve as the natural host for *Legionella,* whereas human host cells serve as an opportunistic host. Warming the water temperature enhances the multiplication of *Legionella,* which grows optimally at 35°C.

Also, *Legionella* survives within biofilms in building water systems. Biofilms are complex aggregates of microorganisms on a solid substrate, which is generally in an aquatic environment. Biofilms begin with the attachment of bacteria to a surface, anchoring the microbial cells to the surface, followed by the attachment of additional bacterial cells. Bacteria in a biofilm may have different characteristics from those that are free floating and not attached. The biofilm environment provides protection against antibiotics and disinfectants because of its dense extracelluar matrix. The biofilm also serves as a nutrient source for the bacteria. Biofilms are very common in water systems.

Legionella organisms multiply intracellularly within human macrophages, including alveolar macrophages in the lungs. They multiply in a membrane-bound vacuole that cannot be destroyed by the usual phagocytosis mechanisms. This arrangement also serves to protect the organism from the effects of antibiotics. Cell-mediated immunity plays the most important role in combating *Legionella* infections.

It is not surprising that the major source of *Legionella* infections involves human-made water sources, which include air-conditioning ducts and cooling towers, warm-water plumbing systems, humidifiers, whirlpool spas, and medical equipment. With diminished immunity in a susceptible host, *Legionella* is able to multiply and establish infection. The organism also secretes proteins that permit it to use host cell functions to produce proteins that enable it to survive. Other cellular products produced by *Legionella* include an extracellular cytotoxin and enzymes associated with virulence.

BIBLIOGRAPHY

Fields, B. S., Benson, R. F., & Besser, R. E. (2002). *Legionella* and Legionnaires' disease: 25 years of investigation. *Clinical Microbiology Reviews, 15,* 506–526.

Winn, Jr., W. C. (1988). Legionnaires' disease: Historical perspective. *Clinical Microbiology Reviews,* 1, 60–81.

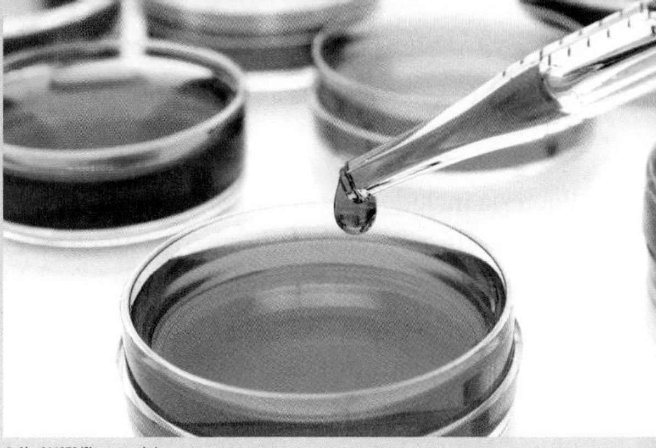

CHAPTER 14
Gram-Positive Bacilli

CHAPTER OUTLINE

Spore Formers

Nonspore Formers

KEY TERMS

Anthrax
Diphtheroid
Listeriosis
Metachromatic granules
Mycetoma
Partially acid fast

LEARNING OBJECTIVES

1. Describe the significant morphological and microscopic characteristics of the genus *Bacillus*.
2. List and describe the types of anthrax.
3. Compare and contrast *Bacillus anthracis* and *Bacillus cereus*, including biochemical reactions, morphological characteristics, and diseases.
4. List those gram-positive bacilli that are catalase positive and nonbranching.
5. Describe and recognize the following:
   a. Diphtheroid
   b. Metachromatic granules
   c. Pleomorphic
6. State the purpose of the following media:
   a. Tellurite medium
   b. Loeffler serum medium
7. Discuss the identification and infectious process of *Corynebacterium diphtheriae*. Describe the significance and technique used to identify diptheria exotoxin.
8. Describe the identification and clinical significance of *C. jeikeium*.
9. Discuss the relevance of isolating:
   a. *Corynebacterium ulcerans*
   b. *Corynebacterium pseudodiphtheriticum*
10. Describe the identification and clinical significance of *Listeria monocytogenes*.
    a. List the outstanding characteristics of this organism.
    b. Describe the transmission and types of listeriosis.
11. Discuss the clinical relevance and identification of:
    a. *Lactobacillus*
    b. *Erysipelothrix rhusiopathiae*
12. Based on colonial morphology and biochemical reactions, differentiate *Lactobacillus*, *Erysipelothrix*, and *Listeria*.
13. Discuss the clinical significance and important characteristics of the aerotolerant actinomyces and aerobic actinomycetes.
    a. Relate epidemiological, clinical, and pathological aspects of *Nocardia*.
    b. Differentiate *Nocardia* from other aerobic actinomycetes.
14. Describe the characteristics of *Gardnerella* and relevance of its isolation.

Bacteria included in this chapter are the aerobic and facultative gram-positive bacilli. There is much diversity within this group relating to morphological and biochemical characteristics as well as types and severity of infectious diseases. The gram-positive bacilli can be categorized as spore formers or nonspore formers, whether the morphology is pleomorphic or straight or branching and whether the organism is partially acid fast.

Spore Formers

BACILLUS

Bacillus organisms are large gram-positive aerobic or facultative anaerobic bacilli. The spores may be either small and contained within the cell or large and swollen beyond the width of the cell. Although more than 50 species of *Bacillus* are known, most are saprophytic, contaminants, and nonpathogenic or low virulence to humans. *Bacillus* species are found in the environment, in soil and water, and in a variety of climates and temperatures. In fact, *Bacillus* species can survive in temperatures ranging from −5°C to thermophilic species, which can be found at temperatures as high as 75°C! The endospores, which remain dormant in the environment, germinate in favorable conditions. Many species are normal flora of the gastrointestinal tract of animals. While most species of *Bacillus* are not pigmented, others may form pigments that are pink to blue to black in color. Although other *Bacillus* species have been found increasingly in human infection, the important pathogenic human species are *B. anthracis*, the agent of anthrax, and *B. cereus*, a cause of food-borne disease. **FIGURE 14-1** illustrates a photomicrograph of *Bacillus subtilis*, which is considered to be a nonpathogen.

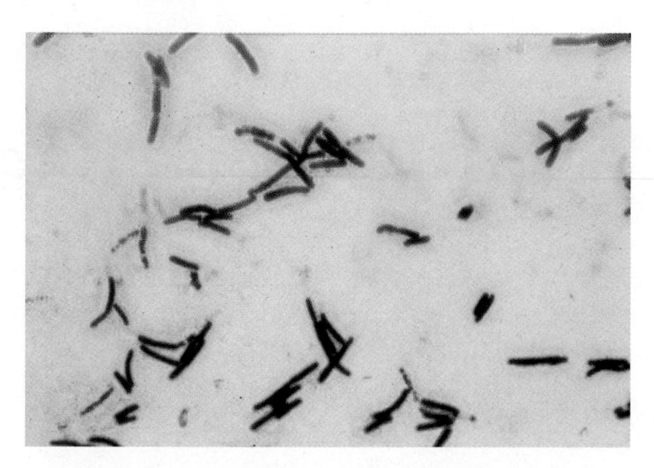

FIGURE 14-1 *Bacillus* Gram stain showing typical large Gram positive bacilli.

Bacillus species are catalase positive and form spores aerobically. These are important characteristics in differentiating *Bacillus* from *Clostridium*, which is an anaerobic, spore-forming, gram-positive bacilli. *Clostridium* species are usually catalase negative. Most species of *Bacillus* are motile with peritrichous flagella, except for *Bacillus anthracis*.

B. anthracis

B. anthracis is the agent of **anthrax** and also is a possible agent in bioterrorism. Anthrax is associated with cattle hides, goat hairs, and other herbivorous animals. Humans acquire the infection through direct contact with infected animal products, wool, or hair. Anthrax is an occupational hazard for those who handle livestock. Although rarely found in the United States in Texas, Louisiana, and Nebraska, the infection has a worldwide distribution and occurs in Europe, Asia, and Africa. The decline in animal cases in the United States is attributed to vaccines and the use of synthetic fibers instead of animal hides and hairs, as well as safety improvements in the processing and manufacture of animal products.

Once the disease is established in an area, bacterial spores from dead infected animals can contaminate the soil. The resistant spore form can remain dormant indefinitely in the soil, and the area can remain infected for years.

There are four types of anthrax. **Cutaneous anthrax** is the most common, comprising 95% of the cases, but least severe form of the disease. Infection occurs through direct mucosal contact with infected animals, their hide or hairs, or contact with soil contaminated with the organism or its spores. A lesion occurs at the site of contact, usually on the hands, arms, or face. The lesion is typically red and fluid filled but eventually becomes black and necrotic from bleeding. There are localized signs of infection and general lymphadenopathy and possible bacteremia. **Woolsorters' disease**, or **pulmonary (inhalation) anthrax**, results from the inhalation of spores during shearing or sorting of animal hair or hides. Although this form occurs less frequently than cutaneous anthrax, the mortality rate is 80% to 90% without treatment. There is an incubation period of 1 to 3 days. The spores attach to the lymph nodes in the lungs and germinate into bacterial cells within the macrophage. There are pleural effusions, the macrophages rupture, and the bacteria are released into the blood. The organism spreads through the blood to various sites, including the gastrointestinal tract and central nervous system. Symptoms include fever, chills, a dry cough, chest pain, nausea, and vomiting. Death occurs from septic shock. **Gastrointestinal anthrax** and **oropharyngeal anthrax** result from ingestion of the bacilli or spores in contaminated food. Oropharyngeal anthrax is characterized by mouth or neck pain with edema, lesions in the throat, and throat pain. Gastrointestinal anthrax and oropharyngeal anthrax may become systemic, resulting in septic shock and death.

Extreme safety precautions are required when working with a suspected case of anthrax. Biosafety Level 3 precautions, with the avoidance of aerosols; a biosafety hood; and protective laboratory gowns, gloves, and masks are all necessary.

B. anthracis is a large gram-positive bacillus. The cells typically occur in long chains, which give the organism a "bamboo rod" appearance. Virulent strains may be encapsulated. The spores are oval, located centrally to subterminally, and usually not swollen.

The specimen collected for diagnosis depends on the type of anthrax suspected. Thus, specimens may include skin swabs, lesion drainage, gastric aspirates, and blood cultures. The organism grows well on sheep blood agar but is somewhat inhibited on colistin-nalidixic acid (CNA) by nalidixic acid. Colonies are medium to large in size, with a diameter of 4 mm to 6 mm, and gray-white in color. Colonies are raised with an irregular curled margin and whirling projections. This has been described as a "Medusa head" appearance when seen under the dissecting microscope. When the colony is lifted with an inoculating loop, it has the consistency of a beaten egg white. *B. anthracis* is nonhemolytic on blood agar, an important reaction in differentiating it from other *Bacillus* species. Special media to isolate *B. anthracis* include polymyxin, lysozyme, EDTA, thallous acetate (PLET) media, and bicarbonate media.

Important biochemical reactions to identify *B. anthracis* are shown in BOX 14-1.

B. anthracis also produces a "string of pearls" when it is streaked on Mueller-Hinton agar and a 10 U penicillin disk is added and a cover slip applied. The plate is incubated 3 to 6 hours at 37°C, and the growth beneath the cover slip is viewed microscopically. Serodiagnostic methods, such as ELISA, are also available.

BOX 14-1 **Important Biochemical Characteristics of *Bacillus anthracis***

Nonmotile

Produces acid from glucose, sucrose, and maltose

Fails to produce acid from xylose, mannitol, lactose, or salicin

Lecithinase: Most strains positive

Starch hydrolysis: Positive

Casein hydrolysis: Positive

B. anthracis has become a concern as a possible agent of bioterrorism by many countries, including Japan, the former Soviet Union, and Iraq. In 2001, anthrax spores were mailed in envelopes in the United States, resulting in several cases of inhalation and cutaneous anthrax. The Bioterrorism Preparedness Initiative has been developed to respond to bioterrorism threats from anthrax and other potential agents of bioterrorism.

B. anthracis produces several virulence factors, which include a protective capsular antigen, edema factor, and lethal factor. These toxins are associated with a variety of biological effects that include resisting phagocytosis by macrophages and neutrophils.

Bacillus cereus

Bacillus cereus is associated with food poisoning isolated from several sources. The organism is found in the environment in soil and water and on vegetation. Foods implicated in *B. cereus* food poisoning include rice and other cereal grains, vegetables, meats, seafood, chicken, pasta, and milk. The spores may resist pasteurization, and the organism can grow at lower temperatures and even in refrigerated food products. *B. cereus* produces hemolysins, enterotoxins, and phosopholipase enzymes, which contribute to its virulence.

There two types of food-borne illness associated with *B. cereus*: a short incubation form and a longer incubation form. The short incubation form is associated with vomiting, which results from the production of an emetic toxic. This toxin is heat stable, with vomiting occurring within 1 to 6 hours after ingestion of the contaminated food. Most patients recover without medical intervention. The emetic toxin has been isolated primarily from boiled

BOX 14-2 Important Biochemical Characteristics of *Bacillus cereus*

Motility: Positive

Hemolysis: Wide-zone β

Produces acid from glucose, maltose, and salicin

Fails to produce acid from xylose, mannitol, or lactose

Lecithinase: Positive

Starch hydrolysis: Positive

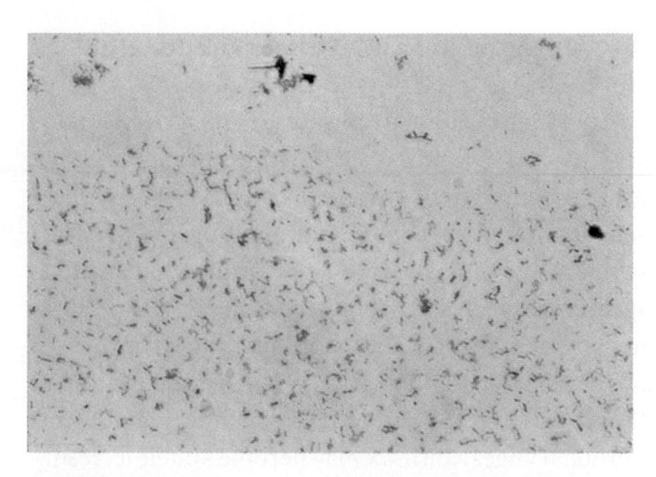

FIGURE 14-2 Gram stain showing diphtheroid morphology.

rice allowed to remain at room temperature or held warm. The spores are not killed during cooking and germinate when left unrefrigerated. Symptoms of long-term incubation infection occur 8 to 16 hours after ingestion of the contaminated food. These include a diarrheal syndrome that results from the release of a heat-labile enterotoxin. Foods associated with long-term incubation include meat, poultry, dairy products, and desserts; the toxin is produced while the foods are left at room temperature. Proper cooking and refrigeration of foods decreases the likelihood of toxin production.

In addition to food poisoning, *B. cereus* also has been isolated from a variety of opportunistic infections, including septicemia, pneumonia, meningitis, and peritonitis.

B. cereus produces various colonial types on blood agar, ranging from small, shiny colonies to large, spreading ones. The organism may produce a grayish to lavender color on sheep blood agar and produces a wide zone of β-hemolysis. Important biochemical reactions for *B. cereus* are shown in BOX 14-2.

Nonspore Formers

The gram-positive, nonspore-forming bacilli that are clinically important include *Listeria* and *Corynebacterium*. Many of the bacteria in this section have a **diphtheroid** microscopic appearance. Diphtheroid cells have variable shapes and sizes and have been described as Chinese letters or picket fences (**FIGURE 14-2**). This pleomorphic appearance is believed to result from irregular snapping during cell division. Bacteria in the genus *Corynebacterium* exhibit a diphtheroid appearance. In addition, *Lactobacillus*, *Listeria*, *Erysipelothrix*, *Rothia*, and *Nocardia* may also appear as diphtheroids.

CATALASE POSITIVE AND NONBRANCHING

Corynebacterium

Corynebacterium organisms are slender, pleomorphic, club-shaped, nonbranching gram-positive bacilli, which are aerobes or facultative anaerobes. Klebs first isolated the *Corynebacterium* in 1883, and the discovery of diphtheria is attributed to Loeffler. Thus a common name for *Corynebacterium diphtheriae*, the agent of diphtheria, has been Klebs-Loeffler bacillus. *Corynebacterium* bacteria are nonspore formers, nonmotile, and positive for both catalase and oxidase reactions. The diphtheroid appearance in Gram-stained and methylene blue smears is evident. There are many species of *Corynebacterium*, including the very virulent *C. diphtheriae*, as well as several species that are normal flora of the upper respiratory tract and skin.

The *Corynebacterium* can be divided into three groups: Group I—human and animal pathogens, Group II—plant pathogens, and Group III—nonpathogenic. The bacteria are widely distributed in nature and can be found in soil and water. Some species are found as normal flora of the mucous membranes of humans and other animals. Unless isolated from the blood or spinal fluid, species other than *C. diphtheriae* are generally considered to be commensal. However, they are found with increasing frequency in causing infection in immunocompromised hosts.

CORYNEBACTERIUM DIPHTHERIAE

The most virulent species is *Corynebacterium diphtheriae*, the etiologic agent of **diphtheria**, a severe and acute infection. Infection is transmitted through direct contact with contaminated respiratory droplets, such as through coughing or sneezing. Its virulence is related to the production of a very powerful diphtheria exotoxin, which first attacks the mucous membranes of the respiratory tract. This results in severe inflammation and the formation of a diphtheritic pseudomembrane formation of the oropharynx. The pseudomembrane contains bacteria, inflammatory cells, and necrotic tissue. As the bacteria grow, more exotoxin is produced, leading to more inflammation and necrosis. This may eventually result in respiratory obstruction. The pseudomembrane also may spread to the nasopharynx, middle ear, face, or eye. The exotoxin may be absorbed, resulting in damage to the heart, liver, kidney, and central and peripheral nerves. *C. diphtheriae* can be carried in the nasopharynx of infected individuals or healthy carriers, which leads to the spread of the infection. As a result of childhood immunizations through the DPT (diphtheria-pertussis-tetanus), the incidence of diphtheria is very low in the United States. The current recommended vaccination schedule includes a series of three intramuscular injections at 2 and 4 months, followed by another injection at 1 year of age. Toxigenic strains from unvaccinated individuals in developing countries continue to contribute to a worldwide public health concern. A cutaneous form of diphtheria characterized by ulcerative, necrotic lesions on the extremities occurs in the tropics and subtropics.

Nasopharyngeal swabs of the inflamed areas or a vigorously swabbed culture of the pseudomembrane is collected to diagnose diphtheria. Swabs of skin lesions can be used to diagnose cutaneous diphtheria. Dacron swabs should be used for specimen collection. A direct smear using both Gram stain and Loeffler methylene blue should be performed. The Chinese letters, typical of *Corynebacterium*, are better visualized with the methylene blue smear, as are **metachromatic granules** (or **Babes-Ernst bodies**). Metachromatic granules are irregularly staining granules, which appear as beads. It is believed that these areas serve as storage depots for materials needed by the bacterial cell. These staining characteristics are typical for most *Corynebacterium*, including those species that are normal flora of the throat. Thus, a diagnosis of diphtheria cannot be made from the smear alone.

The specimen is transported in semisolid transport medium and plated onto sheep blood agar, CNA, cysteine or potassium tellurite media, and Loeffler serum medium. The organism generally produces a narrow zone of β-hemolysis on sheep blood agar; however, colonies of *C. diphtheriae* also may be nonhemolytic. Loeffler medium enhances metachromatic granule formation. *C. diphtheriae* produces gray to black colonies on potassium tellurite medium. This is an important medium for primary isolation because it inhibits most of the normal flora of the upper respiratory tract. Isolates from Loeffler medium should be subcultured onto modified Tinsdale medium, which also contains tellurite. *C. diphtheriae* produces black colonies with a brown halo, which are distinct from the normal flora species of *Corynebacterium*.

There are four colonial types, or biotypes, of *C. diphtheriae*, gravis, mitis, belfanti, and intermedius. These biotypes differ slightly in their colonial morphology and biochemical reactions. The intermedius type can be identified on its colonial morphology of small, gray or lipophilic colonies. Intermedius type colonies are small with a diameter of 0.5 mm on blood agar. The other biotypes produce larger, white or opaque colonies. For example, the gravis type produces the largest colonies with convex colonies and a diameter of 1 mm to 2 mm on sheep blood agar. The mitis type shows colonies with a "fried egg" appearance, which are clear with white centers, on blood agar. Mitus colonies may produce a bleach-like odor on tellurite medium. The belfanti biotype resembles the mitus biotype, and rarely carries the diphtheria toxin gene.

Because nontoxigenic strains of *C. diphtheriae* may exist, it is necessary to demonstrate the exotoxin. In vivo toxigenicity tests include direct animal inoculation into guinea pigs. However, in vitro toxigenicity tests are more likely performed. One example is the modified Elek test. In this procedure a filter paper strip impregnated with diphtheria antitoxin is placed in a medium containing rabbit serum, potassium tellurite, and prepared agar. The medium is allowed to solidify, and the antitoxin diffuses through the medium. The plate is inoculated with a toxigenic strain of *C. diphtheriae*, which is made at a right angle to the strip of antitoxin. A negative (nontoxigenic) control is streaked in the same manner. The unknown culture is streaked parallel to the positive and negative controls. After incubation at 35°C for 24 to 48 hours, the plate is observed for precipitin lines. If the diphtheria toxin is present, precipitin lines form at a 45° angle between the inoculum and the antitoxin strip.

C. diphtheria infection is treated by giving equine antitoxin, which will neutralize any unbound diphtheria toxin. Penicillin or erythromycin is given as supportive respiratory and cardiac care.

Corynebacterium jeikeium

Corynebacterium jeikeium (formerly **group JK**) was first recognized in 1976 when the Centers for Disease Control characterized 95 diphtheroid bacilli. The bacteria were isolated from a number of nosocomial infections, including blood, spinal fluid, and wounds. All held one unique characteristic: They were resistant to a number of antibiotics. Today it is known that the *C. jeikeium* is associated with both nosocomial and community-acquired infections, including bacteremia, endocarditis, meningitis, pneumonia, and peritonitis. These bacteria colonize the skin of hospitalized individuals and are lipophilic, with enhanced growth in the presence of lipid. Infections may be seen in those persons on broad-spectrum antibiotic therapy or those who have indwelling central venous catheters. This bacterial group consists of pleomorphic, nonsporeforming, gram-positive bacilli, which produce pinpoint white colonies on sheep blood agar after incubation at increased carbon dioxide (CO_2) at 30°C for 24 hours. They are generally resistant to many antibiotics.

Other Corynebacterium

Corynebacterium amycolatum is resistant to many antibiotics and has been isolated in cases of sepsis, endocarditis, and surgical wound infections. ***Corynebacterium striatum*** is found in cattle and as normal flora in the human nasal cavity. It is an emerging pathogen and is found causing infections in the immunocompromised host. ***Corynebacterium ulcerans*** produces a diphtheria-like toxin and causes a diphtheria-like infection in humans and mastitis in cattle. Infections in humans frequently follow exposure to cattle or ingestion of contaminated milk. ***Corynebacterium pseudotuberculosis***, formerly known as *C. ovix*, is a rare cause of lymphadenitis in humans, frequently following contact with infected livestock through direct contact or ingestion of contaminated or raw goat or cow milk. ***Corynebacterium xerosis*** is part of the normal flora of human skin, the nasopharynx, and the conjunctival sac and is a rare cause of endocarditis. ***Corynebacterium pseudodiphtheriticum*** is found in the normal flora of the human oropharynx and is a rare cause of endocarditis and respiratory tract infections. ***Corynebacterium urealyticum*** is associated with chronic urinary tract infections, bacteremia, and wound infections in the immunocompromised host. It is unique in its ability to hydrolyze urea.

Biochemical reactions for *Corynebacterium* species are summarized in **TABLE 14-1**.

Listeria

Listeria is found in the environment in soil, water, sewage, and decaying vegetation and in the feces of humans, swine, and poultry. Animals, soils, and plants can become contaminated through contact with animal products. Although primarily an animal pathogen, human infections may be initiated through contact with infected animals or animal products. There are currently seven species of *Listeria*, and ***Listeria monocytogenes*** is the most significant human isolate. The major source of infection is contaminated food, and those at highest risk include pregnant females and their fetuses, newborns, the elderly, and the immunosuppressed. Foods contaminated with *Listeria* include cabbage, raw fruit and vegetables, fish, poultry, fresh and processed meats, and pasteurized and unpasteurized dairy products. *Listeria* can grow on biofilms and

TABLE 14-1 Biochemical Reactions of *Corynebacterium* Species

Species	Lipophilic	Hemolysis on SBA	PYZ	Alk phos	Urease	Esculin hydrolysis	Fermentation of		
							Glucose	Maltose	Sucrose
C. amycolatum	–	–	+	+	–	–	+	+	+
C. diphtheriae	–	Narrow β +/–	–	–	–	–	+	+	–
C. jeikeium	+	–	+	+	–	–	+	V	–
C. pseudodiphthericum	–	–	+	V	+	–	–	–	–
C. pseudotuberculosis	–	β	–	V	+	–	+	+	–
C. striatum	–	–	+	+	–	–	+	–	+
C. urealyticum	+	–	+	V	Rapid +	–	–	–	–
C. xerosis	–	–	+	+	–	–	+	+	+

+, most are positive; –, most are negative; +/–, more likely to be positive to negative; V, variable reaction; PYZ, pyrazinamidase; Alk phos, alkaline phosphatase food surfaces and may even show enhanced growth at 4°C. Thus, it is found on many food products. *Listeria* also is found as transient normal flora in the feces in 1% to 10% of the population.

In the fetus and newborn, the most common manifestation of **listeriosis** is meningitis. In early onset listeriosis the fetus becomes infected either in utero or during the first days following birth. These affected newborns have septicemia, pneumonia, brain abscess, or meningoencephalitis. They also may have lesions in the liver, spleen, or other organs. In severe cases, the infection may result in spontaneous abortion or stillbirth. In late-onset listeriosis, the infant encounters *Listeria* from the normal flora of the mother during birth; the infection occurs 1 to 2 weeks after birth. Meningitis is typically associated with late-onset listeriosis, as is conjunctivitis and septicemia. In immunosuppressed adults, particularly those who have undergone transplants or treatment for malignancies, *Listeria* may cause meningitis, endocarditis, septicemia, conjunctivitis, and urethritis.

L. monocytogenes is a classical intracellular parasite that can resist phagocytosis. It is taken up by the cells of the host's reticuloendothelial system. There is a high mortality rate for newborns infected with *Listeria*. Antibiotic treatments include penicillin, ampicillin, aminoglycosides, erythromycin, and tetracycline.

Listeriosis can be prevented through cooking raw foods from animal sources and avoiding raw and unpasteurized milk or dairy products. *Listeria* can enter the food product at the food processing plant, where the organism can be viable for years. It also is found in many raw foods, such as uncooked meats and vegetables. Foods that become contaminated after processing, such as hot dogs, delicatessen meats, smoked seafood, and soft cheeses, also have been implicated in listeriosis. Unpasteurized or raw milk and cheeses made from unpasteurized milk also may contain *Listeria*. An additional route of contamination is seen in ready to eat foods, where contamination may occur after factory cooking but prior to packaging. Other foods to avoid at high risk for listeriosis include soft cheeses, such as feta, brie, and Mexican-style cheeses. Hotdogs should be heated to boiling and never consumed raw.

There are approximately 1,500 reported cases of *Listeria* each year in the United States, with a mortality of approximately 250 annually. There have been a number of cases of listeriosis attributed to a variety of contaminated food products. These include cases associated with contaminated soft Mexican-style cheese (1985, 2000), shrimp (1994), turkey delicatessen meat (2002), dairy milk (2007), and hog head cheese (2010).

L. monocytogenes is a tiny, gram-positive, motile diphtheroid and a facultative anaerobe. The organism is most frequently isolated from blood cultures or cerebrospinal fluid. It grows on blood agar, producing smooth, clear to gray colonies, 1 mm to 2 mm in diameter, with a narrow band of β-hemolysis. The organism grows best at 25°C to 35°C, slowly at 4°C, and poorly at 42°C.

The organism possesses unique motility characteristics. First, *L. monocytogenes* produces a characteristic tumbling motility when observed in a wet mount or through a hanging-drop technique. The bacillus flips end over end. Also, when a semisolid agar is used to demonstrate motility, the organisms produce an umbrella-like growth 2 mm to 5 mm below the agar surface. Others have described this pattern as an inverted Christmas tree. The organism has optimal motility at 25°C, and these unique characteristics are best observed at this temperature when compared with those observed at 35°C. Molecular diagnostic tests, including DNA probes, are available to identify *L. monocytogenes*.

Important reactions to identify *L. monocytogenes* are shown in BOX 14-3.

CATALASE NEGATIVE AND SIMPLE BRANCHING

Erysipelothrix rhusiopathiae

Erysipelothrix (red skin, thread) *rhusiopathiae* (red disease) is a veterinary infection and an occupational hazard for those handling meat, poultry, fish, and rabbits. The

BOX 14-3 Important Biochemical Reactions of *L. monocytogenes*

Catalase: Positive

Oxidase: Negative

Indole: Negative

Hydrogen sulfide (H_2S): Negative

CAMP reaction: Positive rectangle observed with β-hemolytic *Staphylococcus aureus*

Bile-esculin hydrolysis: Positive

VP: Positive

Ferments glucose, trehalose, and salicin

organism is carried asymptomatically or causes infection in fish, cattle, horses, turkeys, and pigs. Erysipelas infection may occur in swine and cattle. Human infections, or erysipeloid, can develop from direct contact or ingestion of contaminated water or animal products. Human infections most frequently occur as a cutaneous red inflammation, spreading on the hands or fingers. Most infections remain localized, but rarely they may disseminate to the lymph nodes and blood and may result in bacteremia and arthritis. Virulence factors include a capsule, neuraminidase, and hyaluronidase. Infections are treated with penicillin, cefotaxime, or piperacillen.

The organism is a thin gram-positive bacillus, which may appear as chains of nonbranching bacilli that decolorize easily. It is nonmotile and grows as α-hemolytic or nonhemolytic colonies on sheep blood agar. Specimens collected for diagnosis include skin biopsies, tissue aspirates, and blood cultures. Important biochemical reactions for *E. rhusiopathiae* are shown in BOX 14-4.

Lactobacillus

Lactobacillus is found in the environment in water and sewage and as the normal flora of many animals. It is found also in the human oropharynx, gastrointestinal tract, and vaginal canal. *Lactobacillus* is found also in foods, meats, dairy products, and yogurt and as probiotics in many foods. It is usually nonpathogenic and has little clinical significance. The organism is a rare opportunistic pathogen and the cause of bacteremia, endocarditis, and pneumonia.

The organism helps to maintain the normal homeostatic environment by producing large quantities of lactic acid. This acidic environment is intolerable to many pathogenic bacteria and candida and thus inhibits their growth. *Lactobacillus* tolerates this highly acidic environment and can grow at a pH of 3 to 4.

Lactobacillus is a gram-positive, catalase-negative, pleomorphic bacillus, which may show a long and thin morphology or a more rounded or diphtheroid appearance. It is nonmotile and unable to produce H_2S or hydrolyze esculin. Important biochemical reactions for *Lactobacillus* are shown in BOX 14-5.

TABLE 14-2 summarizes important characteristics of the gram-positive, nonspore-forming bacilli.

BOX 14-4 Biochemical Reactions of *Erysipelothrix rhusiopathiae*

Catalase: Negative

Indole: Negative

VP: Negative

Nitrate: Negative

H_2S: Positive

Weakly ferments glucose, galactose, fructose, and lactose

BRANCHING OR PARTIALLY ACID FAST GRAM-POSITIVE BACILLI

Aerotolerant *Actinomyces*

Actinomyces are gram-positive facultative anaerobes or microaerophiles. They show a diphtheroid appearance and rudimentary branching and are nonmotile. They are non-acid fast, an important characteristic in differentiating them from *Nocardia*, which is partially acid fast. Most *Actinomyces* grow better anaerobically; however, they also will grow aerobically under increased CO_2. *Actinomyces* may be a part of the normal flora of the oral cavity and causes periodontitis, gingivitis, wound infections, abscesses, genital tract infections, and actinomycoses. Actinomycoses are draining abscesses, which contain small, hard granules of the organism. *Actinomyces* is most often found in the head, neck, or jaw area but may also involve the thoracic area and chest, abdomen, pelvic area, and central nervous system. There are many species of *Actinomyces*, including *A. bovis, A. israelii, A. oricola,* and *A. georgiae. A. israelii* is the species most often isolated in actinomycoses.

Actinomyces forms small colonies, with a granular center and branches, and may be described as resembling a spider. Typically colonies take 1 to 2 weeks to grow.

BOX 14-5 Biochemical Reactions of *Lactobacillus*

Catalase: Negative

Oxidase: Negative

Indole: Negative

Nitrate: Negative

H_2S: Negative

TABLE 14-2 Biochemical Reactions to Differentiate Gram-Positive Nonspore-Forming Bacilli

	Listeria monocytogenes	*Erysipelothrix rhusiopathiae*	*Lactobacillus* species	Corynebacterium diphtheriae	Corynebacterium jeikeium
β-hemolysis	+	–	–	V	–
Catalase	+	–	–	+	+
Motility	+*	–	–	–	–
H_2S	–	+	–	–	–
Esculin hydrolysis	+	–	–	–	–
Fermentation of:					
Glucose	+	+	+	+	+
Mannitol	–	–	V	+	–
Salicin	+	–	V	–	–

+, most isolates give a positive reaction; –, most isolates give a negative reaction; V, variable reaction.
*Umbrella growth in semisolid media. Motile at 25°C.

Generally, growth is enhanced anaerobically, and some species are categorized as anaerobes.

Aerobic Actinomycetes

Members of the aerobic actinomycetes include *Nocardia*, *Nocardiopsis*, *Streptomyces*, *Actinomadura*, *Rhodococcus*, *Gordonia*, and *Dermatophilus*. The aerobic actinomycetes are gram-positive bacilli that develop thin, branching filaments, which may show beading. Some species form aerial mycelium, which extend into the air, and vegetative mycelium, which extend into the substrate. Some actinomyctes are partially acid fast. The colonies require at least 48 to 72 hours to grow and may not show growth for 14 days.

Nocardia is the most frequent isolate in human infection. It is found in soil and water, and humans can become infected through inhalation of the organism. The species most frequently found in human infections is *Nocardia asteroides*. Other species include *N. brasiliensis* and *N. caviae*. Infections are usually chronic in nature and most frequently involve the respiratory tract and central nervous system. The organism typically infects immunosuppressed hosts, and the infection is characterized by necrosis and abscesses. *Nocardia* also can cause skin infections. Because the organism can resist phagocytosis, it can remain within the host indefinitely.

Nocardia species are unique in their ability to retain carbolfuchsin after decolorization with mild acid. They are thus termed "**partially acid fast**." A specimen of a lesion of sputum will yield long, thin, branching gram-positive bacilli. The organism grows well on Sabouraud dextrose agar but is inhibited by chloroamphenicol. Growth is enhanced in 10% CO_2 and appears in 3 days to 4 weeks as waxy, bumpy, velvety, yellow-orange colonies. This growth may resemble that of the mycobacteria, which are acid fast.

Actinomadura, *Dermatophilus*, *Nocardiopsis*, and *Streptomyces* are associated with chronic granulomas of the skin and subcutaneous tissue. **Mycetoma**, a swelling, draining lesion of the extremities, neck, or head can be caused by fungi as well as by the aerobic actinomycetes. The infection, termed actinomycetoma, is acquired through penetrating wounds, such as inoculation through a thorn, or abrasions from contact with the organism on vegetation or in the soil. Mycetoma is usually an opportunistic infection.

MISCELLANEOUS GRAM-POSITIVE BACILLI

Gardnerella

Gardnerella vaginalis is a pleomorphic, gram-variable to gram-positive, nonmotile bacillus. It has an unusual cell wall composition and was previously known as *Corynebacterium vaginalis* and *Haemophilus vaginalis*. The organism is associated with **bacterial vaginosis**, which is characterized by a malodorous, grayish vaginal discharge. Characteristics of bacterial vaginosis include an excessive vaginal discharge, the presence of clue cells, and a vaginal pH greater than 4.5. Although *G. vaginalis* is normally found in many healthy females, it is found in higher numbers in those with bacterial vaginosis. In addition, the normal vaginal flora, including *Lactobacillus*, may be decreased.

Thus the isolation of *Gardnerella* is not always diagnostic for bacterial vaginosis.

Direct examination of vaginal secretions is an important diagnostic tool for bacterial vaginosis. The clue cell is a vaginal epithelial cell to which organisms are attached, obscuring the border of the epithelial cell. In addition, the vaginal secretions reveal a mixed flora with many small gram-negative and gram-variable rods. There are few or no lactobacilli, which are large gram-positive bacilli that constitute a part of the normal flora of the vaginal tract.

G. vaginalis is fastidious but will grow as small, pinpoint nonhemolytic colonies on sheep blood agar. It can be isolated on chocolate agar, CNA, and Columbia agar, which contains biotin, folic acid, niacin, and thiamine. The best medium for isolation is human blood bilayer Tween (HBT) agar, on which the organism grows as small, opaque, β-hemolytic colonies. Plates should be incubated under increased CO_2. Significant characteristics of *Gardnerella* are shown in BOX 14-6.

BOX 14-6 Characteristics of *Gardnerella*

HBT agar: Small colonies with β-hemolysis
Oxidase: Negative
Catalase: Negative
Hippurate hydrolysis: Positive
Starch hydrolysis: Positive

Review Questions

Multiple Choice

1. Which of the following is *not* a characteristic of *Corynebacterium diphtheriae*?
   a. Pleomorphic morphology
   b. Gram-positive bacillus
   c. Spore former
   d. Nonmotile
2. To differentiate *Bacillus anthracis* from *Bacillus cereus*:
   a. *B. anthracis* is β-hemolytic on blood agar and nonmotile; *B. cereus* is nonhemolytic and motile.
   b. *B. cereus* is β-hemolytic on blood agar and motile; *B. anthracis* is nonhemolytic on blood agar and nonmotile.
   c. *B. anthracis* produces acid from glucose and maltose; *B. cereus* does not.
   d. *B. anthracis* is lecithinase positive; *B. cereus* is lecithinase negative.
3. *Bacillus cereus* has been implicated in which of the following?
   a. Anthrax
   b. Pseudomembranous colitis
   c. Gastroenteritis
   d. Meningitis
4. On potassium tellurite medium, *Corynebacterium diphtheriae* produces:
   a. β-hemolytic colonies
   b. Enhanced pleomorphic properties
   c. Black colonies
   d. Pink to red colonies
5. Which species of *Corynebacterium* was characterized in 1976 as a multidrug-resistant agent in a variety of clinical infections?
   a. *C. diphtheriae*
   b. *C. ulcerans*
   c. *C. pseudotuberculosis*
   d. *C. jeikeium*
6. Partial acid fastness is a characteristic of:
   a. *Listeria monocytogenes*
   b. *Nocardia*
   c. *Lactobacillus acidophilus*
   d. *Bacillus anthracis*
7. A gram-positive bacillus isolated from the spinal fluid of a 1-month-old infant is catalase positive, β-hemolytic, and bile-esculin positive and exhibits tumbling motility in a wet preparation. This organism is most likely:
   a. *Lactobacillus acidophilus*
   b. *Listeria monocytogenes*
   c. *Erysipelothrix rhusiopathiae*
   d. *Corynebacterium jeikeium*
8. Which statement correctly describes *Lactobacillus*?
   a. Prefers alkaline pH range
   b. Strict pathogen
   c. Produces large quantities of lactic acid
   d. Characteristic tumbling motility
9. *Actinomyces israelii* is associated with:
   a. Abscesses and draining sinuses
   b. Erysipeloid
   c. Meningitis
   d. Anthrax

10. If a branching gram-positive bacillus with a pleomorphic morphology is observed, which of the following can be ruled out?
    a. *Listeria*
    b. *Lactobacillus*
    c. *Nocardia*
    d. *Streptomyces*

11. An organism associated with bacterial vaginosis is:
    a. *Listeria*
    b. *Nocardia*
    c. *Gardnerella*
    d. *Lactobacillus*

Bibliography

Bille, J. (2007). *Listeria* and *Erysipelothrix*. In P. R. Murray, E. J. Baron, J. H. Jorgensen, M. L. Landry, & M. A. Pfaller (Eds.), *Manual of clinical microbiology* (9th ed.). Washington, DC: American Society for Microbiology.

Catlin, B. W. (1992). *Gardnerella vaginalis*: Characteristics, clinical considerations, and controversies. *Clinical Microbiology Reviews, 5,* 1213–237.

Centers for Disease Control and Prevention. (2013). Anthrax: Laboratories. Retrieved from http://emergency.cdc.gov/agent/anthrax/lab-testing/

Centers for Disease Control and Prevention. (2013). *Listeria*: Listeriosis. Retrieved from http://www.cdc.gov/listeria/index.html

Coyle, M. B., & Lipsky, B. A. (1990). Coryneform bacteria in infectious disease: Clinical and laboratory aspects. *Clinical Microbiology Reviews, 3,* 227–246.

Funke, G., von Graevenitz, A., Clarridge, J. E., & Bernard, K. A. (1997). Clinical microbiology of coryneform bacteria. *Clinical Microbiology Reviews, 10,* 125–159.

Gorby, G. L., & Peacock, J. E., Jr. (1988). *Erysipelothrix rhusiopathiae* endocarditis: Microbiologic, epidemiologic, and clinical features of an occupational disease. *Reviews of Infectious Diseases, 10,* 31.

Logan, N. A., Popovic, T., & Hoffmaster, A. (2007). *Bacillus* and other aerobic endospore-forming bacilli. In P. R. Murray, E. J. Baron, J. H. Jorgensen, M. L. Landry, & M. A. Pfaller (Eds.), *Manual of clinical microbiology* (9th ed.) (pp. 455–473). Washington, DC: American Society for Microbiology.

McNeil, M., & Brown, J. M. (1994). The medically important aerobic actinomycetes: Epidemiology and microbiology. *Clinical Microbiology Reviews, 7,* 357–417.

Schuchat, A., Swaminathan, B., & Broome, C. V. (1991). Epidemiology of human listeriosis. *Clinical Microbiology Reviews, 4,* 169–183.

Tiwari, T. S. P. (2013). Infectious diseases related to travel: Diphtheria. Retrieved from http://wwwnc.cdc.gov/travel/yellowbook/2012/chapter-3-infectious-diseases-related-to-travel/diphtheria.htm

NEWS: LISTERIOSIS—VETERINARY TO HUMAN PATHOGEN

The first cases of listeriosis were veterinary diseases, with a disease in rabbits first described in 1926. Listeria also causes abortions and "circling disease," or meningoencephalitis, in herds of cattle and sheep. Epizootics of listeriosis were observed in animals prior to their association with human infection. An **epizootic** refers to an outbreak of disease in an animal herd or population, which may affect many animals of one kind at the same time. Often, the infection has the risk of spreading to humans, which was the case for *Listeria*.

Listeria has been isolated from many animals, including cattle, sheep, pigs, ducks, turkeys, and chickens. Listeriosis was first considered to be a zoonosis, with human disease occurring only after direct contact with an animal host that was the primary reservoir. For example, conjunctivitis was noted in poultry workers who handled infected chickens. Skin infections were found in veterinarians and ranchers who had direct contact with infected cattle. However, most cases of reported listeriosis did not indicate a history of direct contact with animals; in fact, most cases were reported in urban and not rural areas. Thus, evidence began to support the notion that *Listeria* could be spread through the indirect route of ingestion of contaminated animal products.

Human listeriosis may range from mild, noninvasive gastroenteritis to severe, invasive disease that can result in meningitis, sepsis, and stillbirth.

Listeria is found throughout the environment in soil, water, plants, and decaying vegetation. Because of its wide distribution, both in animals and in nature, and its ability to survive at 4°C, *Listeria* easily can enter the food production environment. It has been implicated in both sporadic and epidemic cases of food-borne infection. Depending on the handling, processing and shelf life of the food product, a low initial inoculum of *Listeria* can multiply into a large dose once the product has been consumed.

It is believed that many humans carry *Listeria* but that they don't develop invasive disease. Factors that may determine whether invasive disease occurs include the susceptibility of the host, size of the inoculum, and virulence of the organism.

Once ingested in raw, contaminated food, *Listeria* is able to penetrate the host's epithelial cells. Those with a healthy cell-mediated immunity will eliminate the organism before infection develops. In cases of compromised immunity, *Listeria* multiplies both extracellularly and intracellularly. *Listeria* can multiply within macrophages and parenchymal cells, which have been entered via induced phagocytosis. Virulence factors of *Listeria monocytogenes* include a hemolysin, which is known as **listeriolysin**. This toxin inhibits macrophage presentation of antigen to T cells, which inhibits cell-mediated immunity. *Listeria* is able to escape the phagosome before fusion occurs with the lysosome. Once the phagolysosome forms, *Listeria* can also survive by its ability to produce catalase and superoxide dismutase. Because *Listeria* can multiply intracellularly, the host humoral antibody response and complement-mediated lysis are not very effective. Cell-mediated immunity, including lymphokine production, such as interferon and direct cell lysis, is needed. In the absence of effective cell-mediated immunity, invasive disease may occur.

Those at risk for listeriosis include the elderly and immunosuppressed and those with decreased cell-mediated immunity, including those with lymphomas and transplant patients. Also at risk are pregnant women and their fetuses. *Listeria* also has the unusual ability to penetrate the endothelial layer of the placenta, which poses severe infection risk to the fetus. However, infection also occurs in healthy people with no known risk factors.

It is difficult to determine the actual number of *Listeria* cases each year in the United States because many sporadic cases are not reported. There are approximately 1,500 cases reported to the CDC each year, with approximately 250 deaths.

BIBLIOGRAPHY

Schuchat A., Swaminathan, B., & Broome, C. V. (1991). Epidemiology of human listeriosis. *Clinical Microbiology Reviews, 4,* 169–183.

Todar, K. (2011). *Listeria monocytogenes*. Retrieved from http://www.textbookofbacteriology.net/Listeria.html

CHAPTER 15
Spirochetes

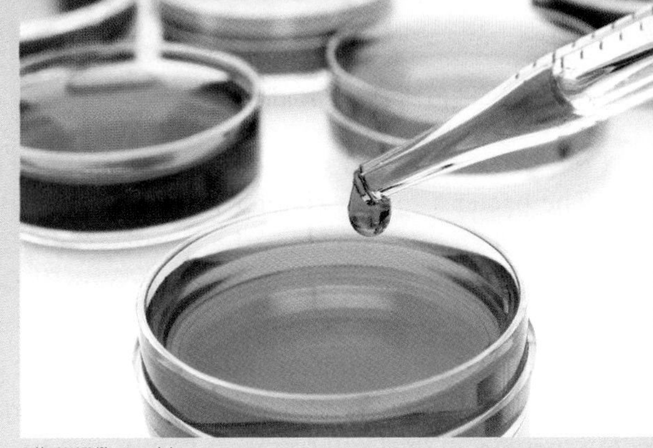

CHAPTER OUTLINE

Borrelia
Treponema
Leptospira

KEY TERMS

Biological false-positives (BFP)
Endemic syphilis
Erythema chronicum migrans
Leptospirosis
Lyme borreliosis
Lyme disease
Nontreponemal tests
Pinta
Relapsing fever
Treponemal tests
Two-tier testing
Venereal syphilis
Yaws

LEARNING OBJECTIVES

1. Name the etiologic agent and tick or louse vectors for the following borreliosis:
   a. Relapsing fever
   b. Lyme disease
2. Explain how Lyme disease is acquired and diagnosed.
   a. List and describe the laboratory methods used to diagnose Lyme disease.
   b. Discuss the stages of Lyme disease.
3. Explain how relapsing fever is acquired and diagnosed.
4. State the etiologic agent for the following diseases:
   a. Syphilis (venereal)
   b. Yaws
   c. Pinta
   d. Endemic syphilis (nonvenereal)
5. List and describe the stages of syphilis. Discuss laboratory methods to identify primary, secondary, and tertiary syphilis.
6. Compare and contrast the treponemal and nontreponemal tests for syphilis.
   a. State the principle for each of the following tests: RPR, VDRL, TPPA, FTA-absorbed, TPI, and MHA.
   b. Discuss biological false-positives (BFPs) and explain how to differentiate a BFP from a true-positive.
7. Name the etiologic agent of leptospirosis and describe its significant characteristics.

The bacteria in this chapter belong to the order Spirochaetales, which includes the families Spirochaetaceae and Leptospiraceae. The pathogenic spirochetes include the following genera: *Borrelia*, *Treponema*, and *Leptospira*. The genera *Treponema* and *Borrelia* are classified in the family Spirochaetaceae, and the genus *Leptospira* is a member of the Leptospiraceae family. These bacteria are helically coiled and motile through periplasmic or endoplasmic flagella. Periplasmic flagella are enclosed within the outer membrane of the bacterial cell. The outer membrane surrounds the protoplasmic cylinder, which contains both cytoplasmic and nuclear regions. One end of each flagellum is inserted near one pole of the protoplasmic cylinder, whereas the other end is not attached. Because of this unique flagellar arrangement, spirochetes can propel through the liquid environment using locomotion, rotation, and flexion. These organisms are motile even in viscous solutions.

Although spirochetes have the characteristics of a gram-negative cell wall, they are neither classified as gram positive nor gram negative. The spirochetes do not Gram stain very well, and thus Gram-staining procedures have limited usefulness.

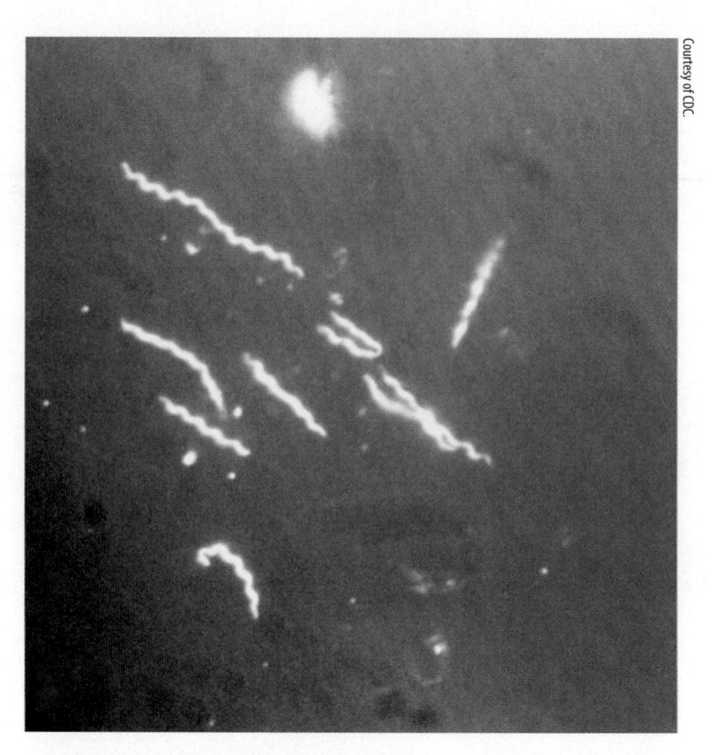
Courtesy of CDC.

FIGURE 15-1 *Borrelia* showing tight coils.

Borrelia

Borrelia organisms are microaerophilic, helically coiled bacteria, which stain well with Giemsa dyes. Typically, *Borrelia* organisms have a length of 8 μm to 30 μm and a width of 0.2 μm to 0.5 μm. These bacteria are very motile via corkscrew or oscillating or swing-like motility. See **FIGURE 15-1**, which shows a darkfield image of *Borrelia*. *Borrelia* infections are transmitted through arthropod vectors, including lice and ticks. *Borrelia* is the cause of various types of relapsing fever and Lyme borreliosis. *Borrelia* bacteria enter the host through the bite of a tick or through lice, which then gain entrance through a damaged skin barrier.

Species of *Borrelia* and their associated vectors, animal reservoirs, and infections are summarized in **TABLE 15-1**.

RELAPSING FEVER

Relapsing fever is transmitted either through soft-bodied ticks of the genus *Ornithodoros* or by the human body louse, *Pediculus humanus humanus*. *Borrelia recurrentis* is the agent of louse-borne epidemic **relapsing fever**, which occurs in South America, Europe, Asia, and Africa. Tick-borne relapsing fever occurs worldwide, and the infection can be attributed to several *Borrelia* species, including *B. hermsii*, *B. duttonii*, *B. hispanica*, *B. persica*, *B. caucasica*, *B. mazzottii*, *B. parkeri*, and *B. venezuelensis*. The vector in relapsing fever is the human body louse, *Pediculus humanus* subspecies *humanus*, and the infection is seen worldwide but most often in developing countries in the Middle East and Asia. Because the body louse feeds on only humans, humans are the only vertebrate reservoir. Ticks of the genus *Ornithodoros*, including *O. hermsii* and *O. parkeri*, are the vectors in tick-borne relapsing fever. These ticks also can feed on rodents, prairie dogs, and squirrels and have been found to inhabit animal dwellings, caves, and decaying vegetation.

Relapsing fever has a dramatic onset with a high fever, muscle and bone pain, and confusion. The organism enters the blood, and multiple lesions may form in the spleen, liver, or kidneys. Hepatosplenomegaly and jaundice also are seen in relapsing fever. The fever persists for 2 to 6 days, and then the patient appears to recover spontaneously, only to relapse days or weeks later. Patients may enter several relapsing phases before recovery. These relapses are attributed to the ability of *Borrelia* to alter its antigenicity and

TABLE 15-1 Summary of *Borrelia* Species and Their Vectors, Reservoirs, and Infections

Relapsing fever *Borrelia*	Arthropod vector	Animal reservoir	Infection
B. recurrentis	*Pediculus humanus humanus* human body louse	Humans	Louse-borne relapsing fever (worldwide)
B. hermsii	*Ornithodoros hermsi*	Rodents	American tick-borne relapsing fever
B. parkeri	*Ornithodoros parkeri*	Rodents	American tick-borne relapsing fever
B. persica	*Ornithodoros tholozani*	Rodents	Asiatic-African tick-borne relapsing fever
B. duttonii	*Ornithodoros moubata*	Humans	African tick-borne endemic relapsing fever
Lyme borreliosis *Borrelia*	**Arthropod vector**	**Animal reservoir**	**Infection**
B. burgdorferi	*Ixodes scapularis*	Rodents	Lyme borreliosis (eastern and midwestern United States)
	Ixodes pacificus	Rodents	Lyme borreliosis (western United States)
	Ixodes ricinus	Rodents	Lyme borreliosis (Europe)
B. garinii	*I. rininus, I. persulcatus*	Rodents	Lyme borreliosis (Europe, Asia)
B. afzelii	*I. ricinus, I. persulcatus*	Rodents	Lyme borreliosis (Europe, Asia)

thus require the host to develop new immunity to each altered strain.

Borrelia is difficult to culture in vitro and requires modified Kelly's medium, also known as Barbour-Stoenner-Kelly medium (BSK-II), to grow. *B. recurrentis* is microaerophilic and will grow on BSK-II in 7 to 14 days when incubated at 30°C to 35°C. However, the preferred diagnostic tool is detection of the organism in peripheral blood smears. Thick blood films are recommended to enhance recovery of *Borrelia* because the number of organisms in blood may be low; the yield also is enhanced in the blood when the specimen is collected during a febrile episode. Giemsa or Wright's aniline dye is used to stain the blood smears, and *Borrelia* stains a blue color using either stain. Although antigen detection and molecular techniques and serological methods are available to diagnose relapsing fever, most of these techniques are performed only in public health or reference laboratories.

BORRELIA BURGDORFERI

Lyme Borreliosis Disease

Borrelia burgdorferi is the agent of **Lyme borreliosis**, or **Lyme disease**. There are 11 *Borrelia* species contained in the *B. burgdorferi* sensu lato complex; three have been found in North America. These are *B. burgdorferi* sensu stricto, *B. andersonii*, and *B. bissetti*. Of these, *B. burgdorferi* sensu stricto is the only human pathogenic species found in North America. Other species are found in Europe and Asia, of which some are human pathogens. *B. burgdorferi* is helically shaped, with three to 10 loose coils and a length of 10 μm to 30 μm. The organism is motile with several endoflagella, which can be visualized using dark-field or phase-contrast microscopy.

Lyme borreliosis was first described in the United States in the late 1970s, although characteristics of the infection had been documented in Europe in previous years. An increased incidence of rheumatoid arthritis in children in Lyme and Old Lyme, Connecticut, was brought to the attention of the state health department. It also was noted that several of the children had developed a unique red skin rash before the arthritis. This rash resembled a rash first described by Arvid Afzelius, of Sweden, in 1909, who noted a red papular rash that spread into a larger lesion. The rash typically appeared after the bite of a tick. He named the rash **erythema chronicum migrans**.

Most of the cases of what is now known as Lyme disease occurred in the summer months. Based on these findings, an arthropod vector was suspected. Because of its minute size, many patients with Lyme disease did not recall a tick bite before the development of the rash. Eventually a tick was isolated from a patient's rash and identified as *Ixodes dammini* (now *Ixodes scapularis*). This particular tick was present in abundant amounts in the wooded areas of Lyme and Old Lyme.

Soon after, Dr. W. Burgdorferi isolated a unicellular, loosely coiled spirochete from the gut of the *Ixodes* tick, and the bacterium was named *Borrelia burgdorferi*. It is now known that *B. burgdorferi* is found in the tissues of several mammals, including field mice and deer.

Several species of the *Ixodes* tick carry *B. burgdorferi*:

- *Ixodes scapularis*, found in the northeastern, eastern, and north-central areas of the United States
- *Ixodes pacificus*, found in the northwestern area of the United States
- *Ixodes ricinus*, found in Europe

Today, Lyme disease is the most common arthropod-borne disease in the United States. The CDC began surveillance for Lyme borreliosis in 1982, and since this time, over 200,000 cases have been reported. Annually, there are approximately 17,000 cases in the United States, with almost 95% of the cases occurring in 12 states in the northeastern, mid-Atlantic, and north-central regions of the country. The disease also has been found in North and South America, Europe, Asia, Africa, and Australia.

The life cycle of the *Ixodes* tick spans 2 years, as shown in BOX 15-1.

Because of its varied presentation, the diagnosis of Lyme disease may be overlooked or confused with other disease syndromes. There are various clinical syndromes that may occur with Lyme disease. Early infection (stage I) follows the tick bite and may consist of a localized lesion, known as the erythema chronicum migrans (EM) rash. The EM rash is a characteristic sign of early Lyme disease infection and begins as a red macule or papule, which enlarges quickly and develops an area of central clearing. Not all individuals with Lyme disease exhibit the EM rash. Some patients may be otherwise asymptomatic, whereas others may exhibit flu-like symptoms of headache, arthralgia, fever, or myalgia.

Within days or weeks of the rash, dissemination (stage II) occurs through the blood to the bones (arthritis), central nervous system (meningitis, facial palsy, and other neurological symptoms, such as dizziness and paralysis), heart (myocarditis, palpitations), skin (multiple EM lesions), or the liver.

Late Lyme borreliosis (stage III), also known as the chronic stage, may develop months or years after the initial infection. The major clinical manifestations are arthritis (most often of the large joints of the knee), skin lesions, peripheral neuropathy, or encephalomyelitis. The symptoms of Lyme disease may vary and can be mistaken for several other diseases, including rheumatoid arthritis, systemic lupus erythematosus, and viral meningitis.

BOX 15-1 Life Cycle of *Ixodes* Tick

First spring: Eggs are deposited and hatch into free-living larvae 1 month later.

First summer: Larvae feed once on a host's blood.

First winter: Larvae enter a resting stage.

Second spring: Larvae molt and enter a second immature stage, known as the nymphal stage; attach to an animal host; and feed. Hosts include many vertebrates, including humans and white-footed mice.

Second summer: Nymphal stage molts into adult stage; ticks are found in brush approximately 1 yard above the ground. Ticks now can attach to larger animals, particularly the white-tailed deer. The adult ticks mate on the host soon after the female attaches and deposit eggs. The life cycle continues.

Diagnosis

There are several laboratory techniques used to identify *B. burgdorferi*, including culture and molecular and serological methods. *B. burgdorferi* can be cultured in modified Kelly's medium or its modifications, such as Barbour-Stoenner-Kelly II medium. Clinical specimens include EM skin lesions, cerebrospinal fluid, blood, and other tissues. Culture is useful for research studies but is not used routinely in the clinical laboratory. Culture is labor intensive and costly and requires incubation for up to 12 weeks. Biopsy of the primary lesion, or the erythema, and subsequent silver impregnation can be used to demonstrate the spirochete in the lesion.

Molecular methods, such as polymerase chain reaction (PCR), may be used either quantitatively or qualitatively to identify *B. burgdorferi* infection. PCR is useful to confirm a diagnosis but may have a low sensitivity and be hampered by possible false-positive reactions. Therefore the patient history and serological methods are most often used to diagnose Lyme disease.

Serological methods that demonstrate the presence of antibody to *B. burgdorferi* are the primary laboratory methods used to diagnosis Lyme borreliosis. These methods include fluorescent immunoassay, indirect immunofluorescence, and enzyme linked immunoassay. A Western blot method offers increased specificity.

In fluorescent immunoassays, *B. burgdorferi* antigen is adsorbed onto an inanimate surface, such as a plastic stick. The antigen is incubated with the patient's serum and fluorescein-labeled antihuman conjugate. If the patient has antibody to *B. burgdorferi*, the antibody will bind to the antigen, which then binds to the fluorescein-labeled antihuman conjugate. The reaction is read for fluorescence using a fluorometer. In enzyme-linked immunoassay methods, *B. burgdorferi* antigen is attached to a solid phase, such as the surface of microtiter wells. When present, the patient's antibody to *B. burgdorferi* will bind to the antigen. Unbound antibodies are washed away, and enzyme-conjugated antihuman immunoglobulin G (IgG) and IgM are added. The enzyme conjugate binds to the antigen–antibody complex. Excess enzyme conjugate is washed away, and then a substrate is added. Bound enzyme conjugate initiates a hydrolytic reaction. The color intensity is read spectrophotometrically, and its intensity is proportional to the amount of *B. burgdorferi* antigen present in the specimen.

The Western blot test may be considered the gold standard in Lyme disease testing because of its high specificity and sensitivity. Some methods detect both IgG and IgM antibodies specific to *B. burgdorferi*. Specific *B. burgdorferi* proteins are separated according to molecular weight by sodium dodecyl sulfate (SDS) polyacrylamide electrophoresis. The separated proteins are transblotted to a microcellulose membrane, which is washed, cut, and packaged. The strip is incubated with the patient's serum, enzyme conjugate (IgG or IgM), and substrate. A hydrolytic reaction enables the visualization of antibodies that specifically bind to various *B. burgdorferi* proteins. The antigen–antibody bands are compared with known positive and negative controls to determine the patient's immune status.

The use of **two-tier testing** for serological diagnosis of Lyme disease is recommended to improve test accuracy. The first test is either an enzyme-linked immunoassay (EIA) or immunofluorescence assay (IFA). If the first test is positive or equivocal and the patient exhibits symptoms of Lyme disease, a Western blot is performed as the second test to confirm the diagnosis. If the symptoms occurred in 30 days or less, an IgG and IgM Western blot is performed; if the symptoms occurred in over 30 days, then an IgG Western blot is performed. For those individuals with a negative first test, a repeat EIA or IFA, collected as a convalescent specimen, is recommended for those individuals who exhibit symptoms of Lyme borreliosis.

Treatment

Patients in the early stages of Lyme disease generally recover. Appropriate antibiotics include doxycycline, amoxicillin, or cefuroxime. Those with neurological or cardiac involvement also may need intravenous ceftriaxone or penicillin. It is estimated that 10% to 20% of those treated for Lyme disease may have persistent symptoms, such as joint pain or fatigue, which may last for over 6 months. This is known as chronic Lyme disease or post-treatment Lyme disease syndrome (PTLDS) and is believed to result from tissue damage.

Prevention

Lyme disease is prevented by avoiding contact with ticks, especially during the summer months, when they are most active. Wooded areas and tick habitats should be avoided. The use of repellants that contain more than 20% DEET (N,N-diethyl-m-toluamide) should be applied to the skin when present in endemic tick areas. Permethrin products can be used on clothing. Individuals should thoroughly examine their bodies for ticks and remove them carefully after activities in endemic areas for ticks or Lyme borreliosis.

Treponema

Treponemes are helically shaped bacteria that either fail to stain or stain very poorly with Gram and Giemsa stains. The organisms characteristically have tight, regular or irregular coils. There are many species of *Treponema*, and most are anaerobic. However, the human pathogenic species are microaerophilic. Some species are human pathogens, whereas others are normally found in the human gingival areas. These organisms have not been cultured in artificial media, although some have been cultivated for one passage in tissue culture. **TABLE 15-2** lists the human treponemal pathogens and their associated diseases. These

TABLE 15-2 Pathogenic Treponemes and Their Associated Infections

Pathogens	Infections
Treponema pallidum subsp. *pallidum*	Venereal syphilis
Treponema pallidum subsp. *pertenue*	Yaws
Treponema pallidum subsp. *endemicum*	Bejel (endemic, nonvenereal syphilis)
Treponema carateum	Pinta

organisms are closely related, both morphologically and serologically.

TREPONEMA PALLIDUM

T. pallidum subspecies *pallidum* (*T. pallidum*) is the etiologic agent of **venereal syphilis**, a chronic disease transmitted through direct, usually sexual, contact with primary or secondary lesions. Infection also may occur through the transplacental route from the infected mother to the fetus. The spirochete enters the body through the mucous membranes or abrasions in the skin. The incubation period varies from 10 to 90 days, with an average of 14 to 21 days.

Syphilis is divided into several stages, summarized as follows:

Primary syphilis. The first stage of the disease is characterized by the appearance of a chancre at the site of inoculation. The chancre develops approximately 3 weeks after exposure and is usually painless, firm, and smooth. Regional lymphadenopathy and early invasions of the blood are other characteristics of this stage. The chancre usually heals spontaneously within 4 to 6 weeks.

Secondary syphilis. The onset of secondary syphilis is 6 weeks to 6 months after the appearance of the chancre, or approximately 3 months after the initial infection. The secondary stage may last for a few days to a few months. It is characterized by a widespread rash of the skin and mucous membranes, typically occurring on the palms of the hands and the soles of the feet. The lesions are filled with treponemes and are considered to be infectious. Systemic signs include lymphadenopathy, fever, and involvement of various organs, including the liver, eyes, bones, and central nervous system. The great variety of symptoms has given secondary syphilis the name "The Great Imitator."

Tertiary (late) syphilis. Tertiary, or late, syphilis can occur 5 to 30 years after primary syphilis and may include central nervous system involvement and neurological disorders, such as paralysis, delusions, blindness, deafness, and the tabes dorsalis gait. There may be cardiovascular abnormalities and granulomatous lesions, known as gummata. Gummata are painless ulcers that enlarge and erupt and contain few, if any, spirochetes. Gummata result from the intense cellular immune response directed against the spirochete that produces the granulomatous inflammation.

Latent syphilis. Latent syphilis is characterized by the absence of clinical symptoms, with positive serological tests for the organism. Relapses are possible during this stage.

Congenital syphilis. Syphilis may be passed from the mother to the fetus during primary, secondary, or latent syphilis. Transplacental transfer usually occurs after the fourth month of pregnancy. This may result in miscarriage, stillbirth, or congenital syphilis upon birth. Newborns with congenital syphilis may be afflicted with bone malformation, a widespread skin rash, meningitis, or hepatosplenomegaly.

Identification and Diagnosis

Because *T. pallidum* cannot be cultured in artificial media, diagnosis is based on clinical symptoms, dark-field examination, and serological detection of antibodies. Dark-field examination and direct immunofluorescence may be used to observe spirochetes in the genital or skin lesions of primary or early secondary syphilis. Spirochetes also are found in cerebrospinal fluid during primary and secondary syphilis.

Serological testing for syphilis is categorized as either nontreponemal or treponemal. **Nontreponemal tests** detect **reagin,** or **Wassermann antibodies**, which are nonspecific antibodies produced in response to *T. pallidum* infection. Such tests use a cardiolipin-lecithin antigen to detect reagin. For example, in the **rapid plasma reagin** (RPR) test, the antigen is coated with carbon to aid detection. Black flocculation against the white background of a reaction card indicates a positive reaction, or a reactive RPR. Negative tests are reported as nonreactive. The **Venereal Disease Research Laboratory** (VDRL) test uses a cardiolipin-lecithin-cholesterol antigen in a flocculation procedure. The VDRL is considered to be more sensitive than the RPR and is recommended for the diagnosis and follow-up of neurosyphilis in cerebrospinal fluid. The VDRL procedure is standardized, and the antigen must be titrated.

The VDRL and RPR are useful for screening because the procedures are relatively inexpensive and simple to perform. These tests have high sensitivity, especially in secondary and latent syphilis. However, these tests are nonspecific because **biological false-positives (BFPs)** may occur in various viral infections; immunological disorders; and autoimmune diseases, such as rheumatoid arthritis and systemic lupus erythematosus. Therefore, any positive nontreponemal test must be confirmed with a treponemal test. Also, nontreponemal tests may yield a false-negative result in some individuals in early primary syphilis. It is important to consider the patient's clinical symptoms and stage of the disease in all serological tests for syphilis.

Treponemal tests use specific treponemal antigens in the reaction system. The hallmark treponemal test was the ***Treponema pallidum* immobilization** (TPI) test, which used live treponemes. In this method, serum is incubated with live treponemes. In a positive test, the spirochetes become immobilized as the specific treponemal antibodies present in the serum bind to the *T. pallidum* antigens. Currently, available treponemal tests include the ***T. pallidum* particle agglutination** (TPPA), enzyme immunoassay, and the **fluorescent treponemal antibody-absorbed** (FTA-absorbed). In the TPPA method, gelatin particles coated with *T. pallidum* subspecies *pallidum* antigens are used. The serum sample is diluted in a microtiter plate, and the sensitized gelatin particles are added. A mat of agglutinated particles indicates a positive reaction. The TPPA method has replaced the **microhemagglutination test for *T. pallidum*** (MHA-TP). In this method, patient serum was mixed with red blood cells that had been sensitized with *T. pallidum* antigens to detect *T. pallidum* antibodies in the patient's serum. The red cells agglutinate in the presence of *T. pallidum* spirochetes.

In enzyme-linked immunoassay, purified *T. pallidum* antigens are used. After incubation with serum and the antigens in a microtiter plate, the plate is washed, and an enzyme-labeled conjugate is added. There is a second incubation and wash, and an enzymatic conjugate is added. If antitreponemal antibodies are present, a color change occurs, which is read spectrophotometrically. In the FTA-absorbed procedure, after mixing patient serum with sorbent, a nonpathogenic treponemal strain, to remove cross-reacting antibodies, the patient's serum is incubated on a slide containing nonviable *T. pallidum*. If the patient's serum contains antibodies to *T. pallidum*, the antibodies will bind to the *T. pallidum* antigen on the slide. Next, fluorescein-labeled antihuman globulin is added to the slide. A positive test is indicated by treponemes staining with the fluorescent dye as the antihuman globulin binds to the antibody–organism complex.

Syphilis remains an important health concern in the United States. The rate of primary and secondary syphilis declined in the 1990s. In fact, in 2000, the rate was the lowest since the CDC began reporting the number of cases in 1941. However, the rate increased from 2001 to 2009, from approximately 32,000 cases in 2001 to over 44,000 cases in 2009. Syphilis is treated with intravenous penicillin.

OTHER TREPONEMES

T. pallidum subspecies *pertenue*, the agent of **yaws**, is similar genetically and morphologically to *T. pallidum* subspecies *pallidum*. Yaws is a chronic, nonvenereal disease of the skin and bones. Transmission occurs through direct contact with the open skin lesions. The disease is found in tropical areas, including Africa, South America, the Caribbean, and Indonesia. The initial lesion appears 3 to 4 weeks after exposure and then heals spontaneously and reappears as a secondary lesion months later. The secondary lesions ulcerate, heal, and then reappear in crops for several years. Tertiary lesions can occur in the skin and bones, which can lead to disfiguration of the face.

T. pallidum subspecies *endemicum* is the agent of bejel, which is nonvenereal **endemic syphilis**. The disease is found in arid climates, including Africa, the Middle East, Asia, and India. Transmission occurs through poor sanitation or personal hygiene, such as through the sharing of eating or drinking utensils. Primary lesions occur in the oral cavity, whereas secondary lesions occur in the oral mucosa. Tertiary lesions are widespread and may occur in the skin, bones, or nasopharynx.

T. carateum, the agent of **pinta**, an ulcerative skin disease, is found in semiarid and warm climates, including South and Central America. The infection is spread through direct contact with infected lesions. The skin lesions are flat and red and become depigmented but do not ulcerate, as is seen in yaws. Unlike the lesions of bejel, those of pinta remain confined to the skin and do not disseminate to the bone.

Antibodies to *T. pallidum* subspecies *pertenue* and *T. carateum* may be indistinguishable and may cross-react with those of *T. pallidum* subspecies *pallidum*. Yaws, pinta, and bejel are treated with penicillin because all currently remain susceptible to penicillin.

MISCELLANEOUS SPIROCHETES

There also are several spirochetes that are found in the gingival plaque in the human oral cavity. These include *Treponema socranskii*, *T. denticola*, *T. pectinovorum*, and others. These bacteria are more likely isolated from individuals with gingivitis or periodontal disease than from those individuals with healthy gums. Treponemes are also found in the colon, rectum, and human feces as well as in the sebaceous glands of the genital tract. These spirochetes are all strict anaerobes and are generally nonpathogenic.

Leptospira

Leptospira organisms are flexible, helical, tightly coiled spirochetes that stain faintly with aniline dyes. One or both ends of the cells are pointed or bent into a hook. The leptospires are obligate aerobes and motile through periplasmic flagella that occur singly at each end of the cell. They are catalase and oxidase positive. *Leptospira biflexa* is nonpathogenic and found in water and soil. *Leptospira interrogans* is the cause of human and animal **leptospirosis**, a zoonosis.

L. interrogans is primarily parasitic on vertebrates other than humans, including rodents, cattle, dogs, cats, raccoons, and bats. Specific serovars of the organism exist, including *icterohaemorrhagiae*, *canicola*, *panama*, *louisiana*, *pomona*, and *autumnalis*.

The leptospires are shed in the urine of these animals, and humans acquire the infection through either direct or indirect contact with the urine of an infected animal. Indirect contact occurs when urine from leptospiruric animals contaminates water or soil. Those individuals at highest risk for acquiring leptospirosis include slaughterhouse workers, farmers, veterinarians, pet owners, sewage workers, campers, and those living in rodent-infested areas. Infection is usually initiated though an abrasion or cut in the skin or through the conjunctiva of the eye. There also may be infection through intact skin after prolonged contact with contaminated water. Waterborne transmission, inhalation of the organism in contaminated aerosols, and animal bites are other routes of infection. Humans may acquire the infection through occupational or recreational exposures.

Leptospirosis shows a wide range of clinical symptoms. Whereas some individuals may have subclinical infections, others suffer from multiple organ failure with a high mortality. Infection typically involves the kidney, liver, or central nervous system. There is a biphasic illness with an acute and septicemia phase, which lasts for about 7 days, followed by an immune phase with antibody product and excretion of the organism in the urine. The infection may be accompanied by muscle pain, nausea, vomiting, fever, headache, and chills in the acute phase. The immune phase follows the acute phase and is associated with antibody production and elimination of the organism. Most patients recover in 2 to 3 weeks.

A rare, severe form of icteric leptospirosis, known as Weil's syndrome, is caused by serovar *icterohaemorrhagiae*. Icteric leptospirosis has a rapid progression, with severe jaundice and hepatic damage, followed by acute renal failure. There also may be cardiac and pulmonary involvement. Approximately 5% to 10% of those with leptospirosis have this severe, icteric form.

In the anicteric form, experienced by 90% to 95% of those with leptospirosis, there is fever, chills, headache, myalgia, abdominal pain, and a transient skin rash. The infection lasts for about 1 week, and the patient usually recovers when antibody production occurs. The fever may be biphasic and recur after 3 to 4 days, accompanied by a severe headache and excruciating muscle pain in the back and legs.

Early in the infection, *L. interrogans* can be detected microscopically using dark-field examination or with immunofluorescence of the blood or spinal fluid. The organism requires rabbit or bovine serum albumin to grow and can grow in either serum or albumin with polysorbate or oleic acid albumin medium. Growth of primary isolates is very slow and may require as long as 13 weeks. Pure subcultures grow within 1 to 2 weeks, with optimal growth occurring at 30°C. Dark-field examination also can be performed on these colonies.

However, most cases are diagnosed serologically; antibodies are found in the blood 5 to 7 days after the onset of symptoms. The microscopic agglutination test (MAT) uses patient sera reacted against live leptospires. After incubation, the serum–antigen mixtures are examined for agglutination microscopically. Paired sera, using acute and convalescent sera, are needed to confirm a diagnosis. A fourfold or greater increase in the antibody titer to *L. interrogans* is needed for diagnosis. Acute infection also can be diagnosed by a single elevated titer in association with an acute febrile illness.

Treatment depends on the severity of the illness and includes supportive care for headache, muscle pain, and hepatic and renal complications. Doxycline is given to reduce the duration and severity of the infection.

Review Questions

Matching

Match the spirochete with its associated disease:

1. *Borrelia recurrentis*
2. *Treponema pallidum* subspecies *pertenue*
3. *Treponema pallidum* subspecies *endemicum*
4. *Treponema pallidum* subspecies *pallidum*
5. *Borrelia burgdorferi*
   a. Syphilis
   b. Lyme disease
   c. Yaws
   d. Relapsing fever
   e. Pinta
   f. Bejel

Multiple Choice

6. Which statement is *incorrect* for the pathogenic spirochetes?
   a. Stain well with Gram stain reagent
   b. Cultured only *in vivo*
   c. Fail to grow on solid culture media
   d. Anaerobic
7. The stage of syphilis characterized by granulomatous lesions in various organs of the body, including cardiovascular and neurological disorders, is:
   a. Primary
   b. Secondary
   c. Tertiary
   d. Latent
   e. Congenital
8. Primary syphilis is best diagnosed by:
   a. Clinical signs and serological testing
   b. Clinical signs and dark-field examination
   c. Dark-field examination and serological examination
   d. Growth on culture media and Gram stain
9. Secondary syphilis is best diagnosed by:
   a. Clinical signs and serological testing
   b. Clinical signs and dark-field examination
   c. Dark-field examination and serological examination
   d. Growth on culture media and Gram stain
10. A patient's serum yields a positive RPR and a negative TPPA. These results most likely indicate:
   a. Reactive for syphilis
   b. False-negative FTA-absorbed from low sensitivity of the test
   c. Biological false-positive RPR from cross-reacting antibodies
   d. Patient in remission for syphilis
11. The most common arthropod-borne disease in the United States is:
   a. Pinta
   b. Relapsing fever
   c. Plague
   d. Lyme disease
12. The diagnosis of Lyme disease can be made by:
   a. Silver impregnation techniques to demonstrate spirochete in tissue
   b. Serological demonstration of antibody in patient's serum using enzyme immunoassay
   c. Growth on blood and chocolate agar
   d. Both a and b
   e. All the above
13. *Ixodes scapularis* is the:
   a. Name of the person who first isolated the agent of Lyme disease
   b. Agent of leptospirosis
   c. Species of one of the tick vectors of Lyme disease
   d. Agent of rat-bite fever
14. All the following are categorized as specific treponemal tests *except*:
   a. RPR
   b. TPI
   c. FTA-absorbed
   d. MHA
   e. TPPA
15. The preferred diagnostic method for relapsing fever is:
   a. Biochemical identification
   b. Giemsa stain of peripheral blood smears
   c. Serological techniques
   d. All the above
16. The characteristic symptom of early Lyme borreliosis is:
   a. The chancre
   b. A mucocutaneous rash
   c. Erythema chronicum migrans
   d. Arthritis of the large joints
17. During the second spring of the life cycle of the *Ixodes* tick:
   a. Eggs are deposited and hatch into free-living larvae.
   b. Larvae feed once on the host's blood.
   c. Larvae molt and attach to the animal host and feed.
   d. Nymphs molt into adult stage, and ticks attach to larger animals.
18. Which of the following methods is recommended to diagnose Lyme disease?
   a. Two-tiered testing of culture on modified Kelly's medium and demonstration of antibody
   b. Single demonstration of patient antibody using IFA
   c. Two-tiered testing of demonstration of the patient's antibody using IFA or EIA, followed by Western blot
   d. Single-tiered testing of dark-field examination of erythema chronicum migrans and skin biopsy
19. Which statement is incorrect for *Leptospira interrogans*?
   a. Tightly coiled spiral with one or both ends hooked
   b. Primarily pathogenic on vertebrates other than humans
   c. Stains well with aniline dyes
   d. Infection may involve liver, kidney, or central nervous system

Bibliography

Aguero-Rosenfeld, M. E., Wang, G., Schwartz, I., & Wormser, G. P. (2005). Diagnosis of Lyme borreliosis. *Clinical Microbiology Reviews, 18*, 484–509.

Centers for Disease Control and Prevention. (2011). Lyme disease data. Retrieved from http://www.cdc.gov/lyme/stats/index.html

Centers for Disease Control and Prevention. (2011). Sexually transmitted diseases (STDs): Syphilis. Retrieved from http://www.cdc.gov/std/syphilis/default.htm

LaFond, R. E., & Lukehart, S. A. (2006). Biological basis for syphilis. *Clinical Microbiology Reviews, 19*, 29–49.

Levett, P. N. (2001). Leptospirosis. *Clinical Microbiology Reviews, 14*, 296–326.

Pope, V., Norris, S. J., & Johnson, R. E. (2007). Treponema and other human host-associated spirochetes. In P. R. Murray, E. J. Baron, J. H. Jorgensen, M. L. Landry, & M. A. Pfaller (Eds.), *Manual of clinical microbiology* (9th ed.). Washington, DC: American Society for Microbiology.

Singh, A., & Romanowski, A. E. (1999). Syphilis: Review with emphasis on clinical, epidemiologic, and some biologic features. *Clinical Microbiology Reviews, 12*, 187–209.

Wilske, B., Johnson, B. J. B., & Schriefer, M. B. (2007). *Borrelia*. In P. R. Murray, E. J. Baron, J. H. Jorgensen, M. L. Landry, & M. A. Pfaller (Eds.), *Manual of clinical microbiology* (9th ed.). (pp. 971–986). Washington, DC: American Society for Microbiology.

NEWS: LYME BORRELIOSIS—PREVALENCE AND CASE DEFINITION

Lyme disease, or Lyme borreliosis, is the most common vector-borne disease in the United States and was the sixth most common nationally notifiable disease in 2008, according to the CDC. Lyme disease was first described in 1977 after following analysis of a group of children who developed arthritis and who lived near Lyme, Connecticut. *B. burgdorferi* occurs naturally in many animal reservoir hosts, such as mice, squirrels, and other small vertebrates. Black-legged, or deer, ticks; *Ixodes scapularis*; and *I. pacificus* acquire the spirochete while feeding on the blood of these host animals. The infection is transmitted to incidental hosts, such as humans, if the infected ticks then take a blood meal on an incidental host.

Deer are not infected with *B. burgdorferi* but transport the ticks and maintain their population. During the colonization of North America, the New England woodlands were cleared for farming, and deer were extensively hunted, almost to extinction. During the 20th century, farmland reverted back to woodlands in the northeastern United States, which promoted the return of the deer population. White-footed mice were abundant, and the soil moisture and land cover found near rivers provided the necessary ecosystem for the deer tick. Later, these areas became very populated with both deer and humans, as the wooded suburbs became popular housing developments where hunting was prohibited. The infection has continued to spread throughout the northeastern United States, where the disease remains most concentrated, although cases also are found along the Pacific coast.

There were almost 30,000 confirmed cases of Lyme disease and 8,500 cases of probable Lyme disease reported to the CDC in 2009. In 2009, 95% of the cases of Lyme disease were reported from 12 states: Connecticut, Delaware, Maine, Maryland, Massachusetts, Minnesota, New Hampshire, New Jersey, New York, Pennsylvania, Virginia, and Wisconsin. Connecticut remains the state with the highest reported frequency of Lyme borreliosis. How are these cases identified and confirmed and these statistics reported?

In the United States, requirements for reporting diseases are mandated by state and local laws. The CDC, with the state agencies, has established a policy for uniform reporting on selected diseases. Health care providers, laboratories, and other public health personnel report to state and local public health agencies on these diseases. Lyme disease is one example of a reportable disease. Case definitions have been established for these diseases; these provide consistent and updated criteria for public health providers and include criteria for the person, time, location, and disease characteristics. Criteria for the person include age, gender, and ethnicity, and time criteria refer to the time period (specific months, seasons, or years) included in the report. Location criteria usually will include a geographic entity, such as a town, state, or country, but also may be defined as an institution, such as a school or hospital. Clinical characteristics include symptoms (cough, rash, and fever) and clinical tests (laboratory tests, X-rays). Case definitions also may be categorized into suspect, probable, and confirmed cases. Each case definition includes the clinical description of the disease, laboratory criteria for diagnosis, exposure, and case classification.

According to the CDC, the *clinical description* for Lyme disease is a systematic, tick-borne disease with protean manifestations, including dermatologic, rheumatologic, neurologic, and cardiac abnormalities. The most common clinical marker is erythema migrans (EM), which occurs in 60% to 80% of the patients. Other acute symptoms, such as fatigue, headache, fever, arthralgia, and myalgia, are included in the case definition. There are specific descriptions of the EM, as well as criteria for musculoskeletal, nervous, and cardiovascular manifestations. Laboratory confirmation is recommended for those who have symptoms but no known exposure. *Laboratory criteria for diagnosis* for surveillance requires one of the following:

- Positive culture for *B. burgdorferi*
- Two-tier testing interpreted using established criteria; a positive IgG is sufficient at any point during the illness. However, a positive IgM is sufficient only if it has been 30 days or less from the onset of the symptoms.
- Single-tiered IgG immunoblot that is seropositive
- Cerebrospinal fluid antibody positive for *B. burgdorferi* by EIA or IFA when the titer is higher than the titer of the serum

Exposure is defined as less than or equal to 30 days before the appearance of the EM in a wooded, brushy, or grassy area in a county where Lyme disease is endemic. A history of tick bite is not required. Endemic counties are those in which at least two confirmed cases of Lyme disease have been acquired or in which established populations of a known tick vector are infected with *B. burgdorferi*.

A *confirmed case* is one with an EM with known exposure, a case of EM with laboratory evidence of infection and without a known exposure, or a case with a least one late manifestation that has laboratory evidence of infection. A *probable case* is any other case of physician-diagnosed Lyme disease that has laboratory evidence of infection. A *suspected case* is a case of an EM where there is no known exposure and no laboratory evidence of infection or a case with laboratory evidence of infection but no clinical information available.

Thus, specific criteria must be met for a disease to be included in the statistics published by the CDC and *Morbidity and Mortality Weekly Report*. As with other diseases, consistent criteria have enabled public health agencies to provide statistical evidence of the occurrence, location, and populations affected with Lyme borreliosis.

BIBLIOGRAPHY

Centers for Disease Control and Prevention. (2011). Lyme disease (*Borrelia burgdorferi*): 2011 case definition. Retrieved from http://wwwn.cdc.gov/nndss/script/casedef.aspx?CondYrID=752&DatePub=1/1/2011%2012:00:00%20AM

Centers for Disease Control and Prevention. (2011). National Notifiable Diseases Surveillance System. Retrieved from http://wwwn.cdc.gov/nndss/

Steere, A. C., Coburn, J., & Glickstein, L. (2004). The emergence of Lyme disease. *Journal of Clinical Investigation, 113,* 1093–1101.

CHAPTER 16

Anaerobes

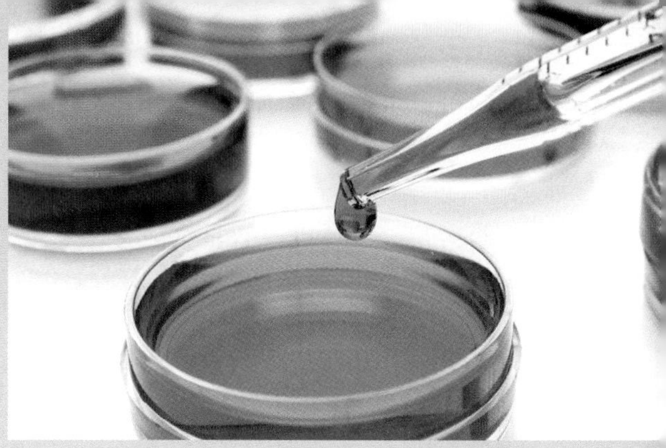

CHAPTER OUTLINE

KEY TERMS

Actinomycoses
Aerotolerance
Botulism
Facultative anaerobe
Gas-liquid chromatography
Microaerophilic
Moderately obligate anaerobe
Myonecrosis
Obligate anaerobe
Polymicrobic
Strict obligate anaerobe
Tetanospasmin
Tetanus

LEARNING OBJECTIVES

1. Define and differentiate among obligate, facultative, and obligate anaerobes.
2. Describe the types of anaerobic infections and differentiate endogenous infections from exogenous infections.
3. Identify three anaerobes that are normal flora of the body and identify the site(s) of each.
4. When given types of specimens submitted for anaerobic culture, indicate whether each specimen is acceptable. Explain why needle aspiration is preferred over collection by swab for anaerobes.
5. State the purpose of each of the following anaerobic media:
   a. Anaerobic blood agar
   b. Phenylethyl alcohol blood agar
   c. Kanamycin-vancomycin blood agar
   d. Paromomycin-vancomycin laked blood
   e. Thioglycollate
   f. *Bacteroides* bile-esculin agar
   g. Egg yolk agar
6. Explain how an anaerobic environment is obtained with the anaerobic jar, evacuation replacement, glove box, or other methods.
7. Explain how anaerobes are identified.
8. Perform and interpret Gram stains on at least four anaerobes.
9. Explain the clinical relevance and recite the important characteristics (Gram stain, colonial morphology, biochemical reactions) to identify each of the following gram-negative bacilli:
   a. *Bacteroides fragilis*
   b. *Prevotella intermedius*

c. *Porphyromorias asaccharolyticus*
d. *Fusobacterium nucleatum*
e. *Fusobacterium necrophorum*
f. *Fusobacterium mortiforum*

10. For each of the following *Clostridium*, discuss the disease process and explain how each is identified:
    a. *C. botulinum*
    b. *C. tetani*
    c. *C. perfringens*
    d. *C. difficile*
11. List those organisms categorized as gram-positive non–spore-forming anaerobic bacilli.
12. Describe the clinical relevance of isolation of the following gram-positive non–spore-forming bacilli:
    a. *Actinomyces israelii*
    b. *Propionibacterium acnes*
13. Discuss the relevance of the gram-negative anaerobic cocci.
14. Explain how the following anaerobic cocci are identified and relate the clinical significance of each.
    a. *Peptostreptococcus anaerobius*
    b. *Peptinophilus*
    c. *Finegolida*
    d. *Parvimonas*
    e. *Veillonella*
15. Inoculate the following media and interpret the results. State the principle of each.
    a. Anaerobic blood agar, PEA, KV
    b. Thioglycollate
    c. Egg yolk agar
    d. *Bacteroides* bile-esculin agar
16. Perform and interpret the antibiotic disk test and explain its use in the identification of anaerobes.
17. Discuss the use of antibiotic susceptibility testing for anaerobes.

Overview of Anaerobes

Anaerobes are prevalent throughout the environment and commonly found in soil, sediments, foods, and animals. These organisms also are present as a part of the normal flora in the human mouth, gastrointestinal tract, skin, and colon. Anaerobes are important human pathogens and may be isolated as the single infectious agent in a clinical site. However, anaerobes more frequently are involved in **polymicrobic** infections, which are infections involving more than one bacterial species. Further, both aerobes and anaerobes may be isolated from the same site of infection. Anaerobes cause many types of infections which are often fulminating and devastating. Anaerobic infections may follow trauma and be associated with vascular stasis or tissue necrosis. These situations offer a tissue environment that favors anaerobic growth. A list of anaerobic infections is shown in BOX 16-1.

Some anaerobic infections are **exogenous**, with an origin from an external source; however, most anaerobic infections are **endogenous** and arise from sources within the host. Sources of endogenous anaerobic infections include commensal anaerobes that are found as normal flora in the mouth, intestinal tract, or female genital tract. Anaerobes are the predominant normal flora in the lower intestine, where they outnumber aerobes by as much as 1,000 to 1 and are a constant source of endogenous infection when removed to other sites through surgery, disease, or trauma. For example, a major normal flora of the bowel, the anaerobe *Bacteroides fragilis*, is a significant cause of intra-abdominal abscesses. The upper respiratory

BOX 16-1 Anaerobic Infections

Brain abscess
Chronic otitis media
Dental infection
Aspiration pneumonia
Lung abscess
Liver abscess
Peritonitis
Appendicitis
Intra-abdominal abscess
Wound infections following surgery or trauma
Post-abortion sepsis
Gynecological infections
Cellulitis
Myonecrosis

tract, including the mouth, nasopharynx, oropharynx, and nasal passages, are inhabited by *Fusobacterium* and other anaerobic cocci and bacilli associated with aspiration pneumonia and lung abscesses. *Actinomyces* species normally may be found in the upper respiratory and gastrointestinal tracts and also may cause actinomycoses of the mouth, chest, and abdomen. Anaerobes, including *Propionibacterium acnes* and the anaerobic gram-positive cocci, are members of the normal flora of the skin, whereas anaerobic gram-positive non–spore-forming bacteria, such as *Lactobacillus*, are found as normal flora in the female genital tract. Examples of exogenous anaerobic infections include myonecrosis, tetanus, food-borne botulism, and infant botulism.

OXYGEN TOLERANCE

Anaerobes are defined as those bacteria that require a reduced oxygen tension for growth and fail to grow on solid media in the presence of oxygen. Obligate aerobes require oxygen as the final electron acceptor, whereas **obligate anaerobes** do not use oxygen and are inhibited by its presence. Bacteria classified as **facultative anaerobes** can grow either in the presence or absence of oxygen. **Microaerophilic** bacteria prefer reduced oxygen tension but can grow on solid media in 10% carbon dioxide (CO_2) in air. Obligate anaerobes are further differentiated on the level of oxygen tolerance. Bacteria have varying degrees of tolerance to oxygen and peroxides as well as differing limits of oxidation-reduction potentials, which are dependent on the organism's ability to produce superoxide dismutase, catalases, and peroxidases. These enzymes protect the organism against toxic oxygen products, such as the superoxide radical and hydrogen peroxide. The toxic products react to free hydroxyl radicals, which are very powerful oxidants. Superoxide dismutase catalyzes the conversion of superoxide radicals to less toxic hydrogen peroxide and molecular oxygen. Catalase converts hydrogen peroxide to water and oxygen. Anaerobes that produce some superoxide dismutase are thus more resistant to the toxic effects of oxygen. An example is *Clostridium perfringens*, which is classified as a **moderately obligate anaerobe** because it is able to grow at oxygen levels of 2% to 8%. Most anaerobes associated with human infection are moderately obligate anaerobes. Other anaerobes are classified as **strict obligate anaerobes** and cannot grow on the agar surface when exposed to as little as 0.5% oxygen.

Specimen Collection and Transport

Whenever possible, it is preferred to collect a specimen for anaerobic examination by needle aspiration instead of by a swab. Collection using a swab has several drawbacks, including contamination with normal flora, collection of a small amount of specimen, the danger of the swab drying out, and exposure of the swab to toxic oxygen. Although often difficult when culturing mucous membranes near a site of infection, the area should be properly disinfected with a surgical soap scrub, alcohol, and iodine to avoid normal flora contamination.

Blood culture media that sustain the growth of obligate anaerobes, aerobes, and facultative anaerobes should be inoculated. The skin over the venipuncture site must be cleansed using alcohol and povidone-iodine to avoid contamination from the normal flora of the skin, especially *Staphylococcus epidermidis* and the anaerobic *Propionibacterium acnes*. Today, automated systems are used to detect anaerobes in the blood; these systems signal when growth occurs. Manual blood cultures are checked twice daily for growth for the first 3 days, which may be evidenced through hemolysis, gas production, or turbidity. Cultures are then checked once daily and held for a total of 5 to 7 days until reported as negative. Tissue biopsies, serous body fluids, exudates, abscesses, and bone are other suitable anaerobic specimens. BOX 16-2 lists general guidelines for the collection of anaerobic specimens.

It also is important to maintain the specimen in an anaerobic state during transport to the microbiology laboratory. Transport systems include pre-reduced media, with cysteine (as a reducing agent) and a redox indicator, such as resazurin, which turns pink in the presence of oxygen. In the BBL™ Port-A-Cul™ (Becton Dickinson), the vials and jars contain a pre-reduced transport medium with reducing agents that will maintain both aerobes and anaerobes during transport to the laboratory. Swabs containing specimens are inserted into the pre-reduced soft agar. The swabs can later be removed from the tube with sterile forceps to inoculate culture media. There also are Port-A-Cul™ vials, which are used for transport of fluid specimens. Fluid specimens are injected directly through the rubber seal onto the soft agar surface. Reducing agents in the agar generates and maintains anaerobiosis. Upon arrival at the laboratory, the fluid is removed from the vial with a sterile syringe and needle and transferred to growth media. An indicator is present that changes color

BOX 16-2 **General Guidelines for Collection of Anaerobic Specimens**

Preferable Specimens

Abscesses of the liver, lung, brain, and abdomen

Necrotic tissue associated with poor vascular perfusion, trauma, or malignancy

Wound infections proximal to mucous membranes

Exudates from deep wounds or abscesses, especially when associated with the production of gas, necrosis, or a foul smell

Gram stain that indicates anaerobes

Serous fluid exudates from normally sterile sites, such as amniotic, pleural, peritoneal, and synovial fluids

Cerebrospinal fluid

Suprapubic urine

Transtracheal aspirate or bronchial washing

Infected human or animal bites

Food suspected of causing botulism

Specimen containing sulfur granules

Stool or feces for *Clostridium difficile* toxin

Specimens to Avoid or Reject

Nasal, pharyngeal, vaginal, cervical, and rectal swabs

Voided or catheterized urine

Swabs of surface skin ulcers and abscesses

Sputum

Feces (except as noted above), gastric contents, and intestinal contents

if oxygen has entered the system. The A.C.T.® transport systems (Remel) permit aerobic, facultative, and anaerobic culture transport with semisolid, nonnutritive medium. The systems can be used with swabs or fluid samples, which are introduced through a septum in the cap.

IDENTIFICATION

Direct Examination

Gram stain morphology is an important tool in the preliminary identification of anaerobes because of their unique appearances. Specimens should be fixed with methanol instead of heat to enhance the stained appearance of anaerobes. *Bacteroides*, *Porphyromonas*, and *Prevotella* species typically appear as pale, pleomorphic, gram-negative coccobacilli, with bipolar staining (**FIGURE 16-1**). *Fusobacterium* species are long, thin, filamentous gram-negative bacilli with tapered ends and often are arranged end to end (**FIGURE 16-2**). *Fusobacterium necrophorum* may appear as pale, irregularly staining, highly pleomorphic, and gram-negative bacilli with swollen areas. Clostridia are large gram-positive bacillus; the cells of *Clostridium perfringens* typically line up like boxcars of a train. *Actinomyces* species appear as branching gram-positive bacilli.

The presence and location of spores is also an important identifying characteristic, especially for the genus *Clostridium*. **Terminal spores** are located at the end of the organism, **central spores** appear in the middle, and **subterminal spores** are located between the end and the middle of the organism. *Clostridium tetani* has swollen terminal spores, whereas *C. botulinum* has subterminal spores.

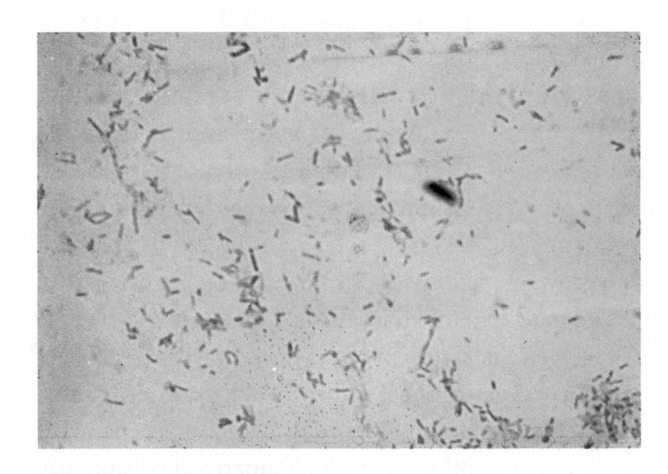

FIGURE 16-1 *Bacteroides fragilis* showing pale-staining pleomorphic bacillus. Appearance is also characteristic of *Prevotella*.

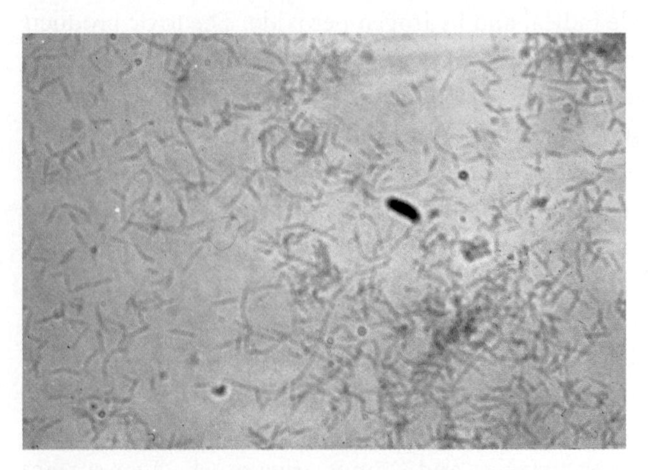

FIGURE 16-2 *Fusobacterium* Gram stain showing typical morphology of long, thin, filamentous gram-negative bacilli.

Anaerobic bacteria and cultures typically produce extremely putrid odors, which result from the production of volatile and nonvolatile fatty acids during metabolism. Broths may appear turbid and frothy with gas bubbles.

Anaerobic Culture Media and Incubation

CULTURE MEDIA

Anaerobic media contain supplements, including hemin, blood, and vitamin K, as well as sodium bicarbonate, which provides a source of CO_2. Reducing agents, such as thioglycollic acid, sodium thioglycollate, and L-cystine, are added to the media to absorb oxygen. For primary isolation of anaerobes, a nonselective anaerobic blood agar plate, anaerobic-selective media, and an enriched broth are inoculated. The enriched broth, usually thioglycollate, is used as a supplement, which may be needed if the anaerobic system fails or if the agar plates do not grow. Growth may occur in the thioglycollate broth, from which a second set of anaerobic agar plates can be inoculated and incubated. **TABLE 16-1** describes the more commonly used anaerobic plating media. Although anaerobic media do not need to be stored anaerobically, they are held in a reduced state 8 to 16 hours prior to inoculation.

TABLE 16-1 Anaerobic Media

Media	Description and purpose
CDC anaerobic blood agar (AnBAP)	Trypticase soy agar with 5% sheep blood. Supplements: yeast, hemin, vitamin K–reducing agent, L-cysteine. Nonselective plate for primary isolation of all anaerobes, including obligate anaerobes and facultative anaerobes.
Anaerobic phenylethyl alcohol blood agar (PEA)	CDC anaerobic blood agar plus phenylethyl alcohol. Selective isolation of anaerobes from specimens that likely contain more than one organism. Isolation of gram-positive and gram-negative obligate anaerobes Gram-positive facultative anaerobes, such as *Staphylococcus*, *Streptococcus*, *Bacillus*, and *Corynebacterium*, also grow on PEA. PEA inhibits swarming of *Proteus* and the growth of gram-negative facultative anaerobes, such as the Enterobacteriaceae.
Anaerobic kanamycin-vancomycin blood agar (KV)	CDC anaerobic blood agar plus the antibiotics kanamycin and vancomycin. Vancomycin inhibits facultative and obligate gram-positive anaerobes, and kanamycin inhibits most facultative gram-negative rods. However, *Porphyromonas* also may be inhibited. Isolation of gram-negative obligate anaerobes, especially *Bacteroides*, *Prevotella*, *Fusobacterium*, and *Veillonella*.
Anaerobic paromomycin-vancomycin laked blood agar (PVLB)	Similar to KV and can be used instead. Medium is "laked," which means the blood is frozen and then thawed. Isolation of gram-negative obligate anaerobes, especially *Bacteroides*, *Prevotella*, and some *Fusobacterium*; pigment production of *Prevotella* detected earlier because of laked blood.
Enriched thioglycollate broth	Enriched broth with hemin and vitamin K. Supplement to plating media for slower-growing and more fastidious bacteria. Supports growth of most anaerobes found in clinical specimens. Helpful in growing *Actinomyctes*.
Bacteroides bile-esculin (BBE) agar	Detects organism's ability to grow in 20% bile and to hydrolyze esculin. Interpret plate for growth and hydrolysis of esculin, which is indicated by a brown-black discoloration of the media. Important isolation characteristic of *Bacteroides fragilis* group, which grows on BBE and hydrolyzes esculin.
Cycloserine-cefoxitin fructose agar (CCFA)	Trypticase soy agar with fructose and phenol red indicator. Cycloserine and cefoxitin inhibit growth of intestinal flora. Selective isolation of *Clostridium difficile* from stool and intestinal specimens. *C. difficile* appears as yellow, rhizoid colonies, which show speckled opalescence.

INCUBATION

Once the specimen has been inoculated onto the appropriate media, the agar plates must be incubated in an anaerobic environment. Anaerobic systems for incubation include the anaerobic jar method, evacuation-replacement systems, the glove box, disposable anaerobic bags, and other systems.

The **anaerobic jar method** (**FIGURE 16-3**) is useful for laboratories that have a small to medium volume of anaerobic specimens. In this system, inoculated plates are placed into the jar, and a gas generator envelope that has been activated with water is added. Hydrogen gas generated from the envelope reacts with oxygen, forming water. This effectively removes oxygen from the system. Palladium catalyst pellets are placed in the lid of the jar. In the GasPak™ System (Becton Dickinson), a generator envelope is opened and activated by adding water. This activates the generation of hydrogen and CO_2. In the presence of the palladium catalyst, the following reaction occurs:

$$2H_2 + O_2 \rightarrow 2H_2O$$

Because palladium can be inactivated by the production of metabolic products of the bacteria, it must be replaced

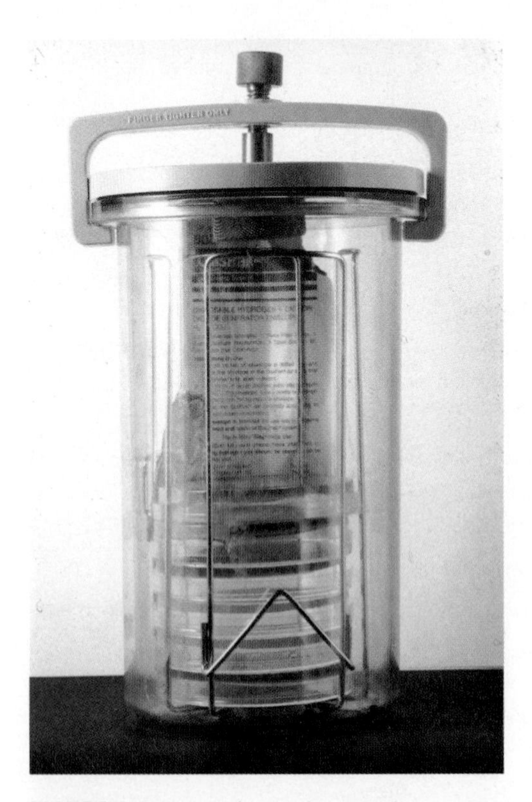

FIGURE 16-3 Anaerobic jar showing plates, generator envelope, indicator, and palladium catalyst.

or reactivated each time the anaerobic jar is used. The palladium is reactivated by heating the pellets in a dry-heat oven for 2 hours at 160°C to 170°C. The pellets must be stored in a desiccator until use.

To determine the effectiveness of the system, methylene blue or other oxidation-reduction indicator strips are used. When minimal anaerobic conditions are achieved, the indicator strip becomes white. If the strip remains blue or reverts back to blue, the system is failing, and an anaerobic environment has not been achieved. This is a sign that oxygen has entered the system.

In the **glove-box method,** or **anaerobic chamber**, a self-contained anaerobic environment of 85% nitrogen gas (N_2), 10% hydrogen (H_2), and 5% CO_2 is provided through external gas sources. This system is used by microbiology laboratories with a moderate to large volume of anaerobic specimens. Specimens and other materials are passed into the chamber through an entry lock system with either gloved or gloveless openings in front of the cabinet. Cultures are incubated in an incubator that is contained within the glove box. Most techniques necessary to isolate and identify anaerobes are performed within the glove-box chamber.

Disposable anaerobic bags provide a convenient anaerobic incubation system. The Bio-Bag™ Type A (Becton Dickinson) consists of a plastic bag with an ampule of weak hydrochloric acid solution and a gas-generating tablet. When the ampule is crushed, the acid reacts with the tablet, forming hydrogen and carbon dioxide gases. The hydrogen reacts with oxygen present in the bag to form water. A resazurin indicator monitors the system's effectiveness, changing from red to colorless to indicate that an anaerobic environment has been achieved. These bags can hold from one to three petri plates and are suitable for laboratories that handle a very small volume of anaerobic specimens.

The GasPak™ EZ Gas-Generating Pouch (Becton Dickinson) is a single-use system that operates without a catalyst. In this self-contained system, a reagent sachet is activated when exposed to air and placed in the incubation chamber with the culture plates. The container is sealed, and the sachet removes oxygen from the system, producing carbon dioxide. The pouches used in this system can hold one or two Petri plates. The AnaeroGen (Oxoid) is an anaerobic atmosphere–generating system for use in anaerobic jars for primary cultures and subcultures. The system enables oxygen in the air to be absorbed without the production of hydrogen or the addition of water. The sachet, when placed in a sealed jar, causes oxygen in the jar to be rapidly absorbed without the production of hydrogen. There is a simultaneous generation of carbon dioxide.

An anaerobic holding jar can be used to hold media, recently inoculated plates, or plates to be subcultured. This is a three-jar system in which the first jar holds uninoculated plates, the second jar holds plates with colonies for subculture, and the third jar holds freshly inoculated plates. Nitrogen or CO_2 gas is piped into the system to provide an anaerobic environment.

Anaerobic cultures are incubated at 35°C to 37°C for at least 48 hours. After examination, plates should be incubated for an additional 2 to 5 days to ensure that some of the slower-growing organisms, such as *Actinomyces*, are not missed. Broth cultures should be held for 7 days before reporting growth as negative.

There also are self-contained anaerobic agars that permit the examination of culture plates after 24 hours of incubation. AnaeroGRO™ (Hardy Diagnostics) is a pre-reduced anaerobic culture medium that is packaged in oxygen-free gas. The system includes gas-flushed foil pouches, an oxygen scavenger sachet, and a moisture-absorbing desiccant packet. Plates are quickly inoculated and returned to the pouch and incubated in an anaerobic chamber. They can be examined for growth at 24 hours without opening the bag, thus reducing the exposure to oxygen.

It is important to note that facultative anaerobes also can grow on anaerobic media. Thus, **aerotolerance** tests may need to be performed on any colony type found growing anaerobically. The colony is subcultured onto an aerobic chocolate agar plate, which is incubated in increased CO_2 and also onto an anaerobic blood agar plate, which is incubated anaerobically. Chocolate agar must be used for the aerobic growth so that fastidious facultative bacteria, such as *Hemophilus*, are able to grow. The growth patterns can be interpreted as shown in **TABLE 16-2**.

BIOCHEMICAL AND OTHER IDENTIFICATION METHODS

Biochemical reactions also are used to identify anaerobes. Commercially packaged systems are available and include the BBL™ Crystal™ Anaerobe ID Kit (Becton Dickinson) and the API® 20A System (bioMérieux). Some of the important characteristics and reactions used to identify anaerobes are summarized below.

1. **Colonial morphology and pigment production.** *Actinomyces israelii*, a gram-positive non–spore-forming bacillus, appears as rough, heaped, white colonies that are said to resemble a "molar tooth" on anaerobic blood agar. The pigmented *Prevotella* and *Porphyromonas* produce brown to black colonies on anaerobic blood agar because these bacteria can degrade hemoglobin present in the red cells to heme. The pigment is observed more readily on laked blood agar and usually is seen after 4 to 7 days of incubation.
2. **Fluorescence.** Those bacteria that degrade hemoglobin into heme produce porphyrins that exhibit red fluorescence when viewed with an ultraviolet light at 366 nm for 15 to 30 seconds. *Prevotella* and *Porphyromonas* produce a brick-red to rust-orange fluorescence. A yellow to green fluorescence may be observed with *Clostridium difficile* and other clostridia and *Fusobacterium*.
3. Susceptibility to **sodium polyanethol sulfonate** (SPS) can be used to differentiate *Peptostreptococcus anaerobius* from other gram-positive anaerobic cocci, such as *Staphylococcus asaccharolyticus* (formerly *P. asaccharolyticus*) and *Finegoldia magna* (formerly *P. magnus*). Anaerobic blood agar is inoculated with the test organism, and an SPS disk is placed on the inoculum. The plate is incubated anaerobically for 24 to 48 hours and then interpreted for susceptibility. A zone of 12 mm or more is considered susceptible or sensitive, which is characteristic of *P. anaerobius*. No

TABLE 16-2 Aerotolerance Interpretations

Colony type	Growth on chocolate agar at 35°C	Growth on anaerobic blood
Obligate aerobe	Growth	No growth
Obligate anaerobe	No growth	Growth
Facultative anaerobe	Growth	Growth
Microaerophile or aerotolerant anaerobe	Light growth	Enhanced growth

zones are expected with other gram-positive anaerobic cocci, such as *S. asaccharolyticus* and *F. magna*. SPS disks are commercially available through Becton Dickinson as BBL™ Taxo™ Differentiation Discs SPS.

4. **Catalase** activity is determined by suspending the suspected colony in one drop of 10% to 15% hydrogen peroxide. The test is performed in a manner similar to that of the aerobic catalase test. The higher concentration of peroxide increases the sensitivity of the reaction. A positive reaction is indicated by sustained bubbling. Because red blood cells contain catalase, false-positives can occur if red blood cells are picked up while selecting the colonies for testing.
5. **Nitrate** reduction can be determined by placing a nitrate disk onto the suspected colony, which has been grown on anaerobic blood agar. One drop each of sulfanilic acid and α-naphthylamine is dropped onto the nitrate disk; a pink to red color indicates the reduction of nitrates to nitrites. Zinc dust is sprinkled onto all negative reactions to ensure that nitrates were not totally reduced to nitrogen gas. A pink-red color after zinc application indicates the presence of nitrate or a negative reaction for the reduction of nitrates to nitrites.
6. **Indole** production is determined by rubbing growth from a pure culture grown on tryptophan medium or on anaerobic blood agar onto a piece of filter paper. Anaerobic blood agar contains tryptophan, which provides a suitable substrate. After the addition of 1% *p*-dimethylaminocinnamaldehyde reagent, the development of a blue to green color indicates a positive reaction and the degradation of tryptophan to indole. The test also can be performed by placing a sterile blank filter paper disk on the heavy growth area of a pure culture plate for 5 minutes. Next, the filter paper is removed and placed into an empty Petri dish. One drop of reagent is added, and the disk is observed for a blue to green color.
7. **Growth in 20% bile** is useful for classification of the anaerobic gram-negative bacilli. Thioglycollate medium containing 20% bile is inoculated with the test organism. A control tube without the bile is similarly inoculated, and growth is compared between the two tubes. Members of the *Bacteroides fragilis* group grow well in 20% bile, whereas other members of the genus *Bacteroides* are inhibited. The test also can be performed by placing a 20% bile disk in the primary growth area of the organism when streaked onto isolation agar. Growth up to the disk is interpreted as a positive reaction, whereas a zone of inhibition is interpreted as a negative reaction. *Bacteroides* bile-esculin (BBE) medium can be used as a primary inoculation plate to evaluate the ability of an organism to grow in 20% bile and hydrolyze esculin, producing a blackening of the medium. The *Bacteroides fragilis* group gives a positive bile-esculin reaction.
8. **Lipase.** Egg yolk agar can be used to demonstrate lipase activity. In a positive reaction, lipase degrades fat into fatty acids and glycerol, which is demonstrated by an oil on water, or shimmery, appearance. *Fusobacterium necrophorum*, *Prevotella intermedia*, and *Clostridium botulinum* are lipase positive.
9. **Lecithinase.** Lecithin is present in egg yolk, so egg yolk agar is used to demonstrate the presence of lecithinase. In a positive reaction, lecithinase breaks down the lecithin into water-insoluble diglycerides, forming opaque white halos around the bacterial colony. *Clostridium perfringens* is lecithinase positive.
10. **Antibiotic disks.** Antibiotic disks containing vancomycin (5 μg), kanamycin (1,000 μg), and colistin (10 μg) are used to differentiate anaerobic bacteria based on their susceptibility or resistance to the antibiotics. A pure culture of the organism is inoculated onto anaerobic blood agar, and the disks are placed on the plate. The plate is incubated anaerobically for 24 to 48 hours, and the zone diameters are measured. A zone of inhibition of over 10 mm is considered susceptible. *Bacteroides fragilis* is generally resistant to all three antibiotics, whereas *Fusobacterium* is resistant to vancomycin but susceptible to kanamycin and colistin. *Porphyromonas* is resistant to kanamycin and colistin but susceptible to vancomycin. *Clostridium perfringens* is resistant to colistin and susceptible to vancomycin and kanamycin. This method is used to identify anaerobes and should not be used as an antibiotic susceptibility test. Antibiotic disks are commercially available from Hardy Diagnostics and Becton Dickinson. Microring® AN and AC (Polysciences) are systems to determine the susceptibility pattern of the anaerobes. Microring® AN has six tips impregnated with a variety of antibiotics for the identification of species of anaerobic gram-negative bacilli and also can distinguish gram-positive cocci from gram-negative cocci. Microring® AC provides additional tests, including SPS and novobiocin, which also will assist with the identification of gram-positive anaerobic cocci.

Gas-liquid chromatography (GLC) involves the analysis of metabolic end products released into broth during anaerobic growth. Fermentative products produced by bacteria from organic compounds, primarily glucose, can be used to identify anaerobes. Certain organisms characteristically produce one or a pattern of end products. Short-chain volatile fatty acids can be identified through a gas chromatograph. The following volatile acids can be detected: acetic, propionic, butyric, isobutyric, isovaleric, valeric, caproic, and isocaproic. These volatile acids are identified by comparing unknown results with known standards. Nonvolatile acids identified include pyruvic, lactic, succinic, and phenylacetic. For example, the major end products of *Propionibacterium acnes* are acetic and propionic acid, and those for *Bacteroides fragilis* are acetic, lactic, succinic, and phenylacetic acids. GLC is considered to be the gold standard in the identification of anaerobes, especially gram-negative aerobic bacilli. However, the instrumentation is costly and complex and labor intensive to use, which limits its use in many clinical microbiology laboratories.

Clinically Relevant Anaerobes

This section discusses the clinical relevance and identification of some of the more clinically relevant anaerobes.

ANAEROBIC GRAM-NEGATIVE BACILLI

The anaerobic gram-negative bacilli are the major normal flora in the colon and oral cavity. The gram-negative bacilli are the most common clinically isolated anaerobes. Infections usually involve the presence of endogenous anaerobes that have moved to sterile sites. These infections may develop following surgery, trauma, or disease, which disrupts the normal mucosal surface of the bowel or oral cavity. The anaerobic gram-negative bacilli are identified using colonial morphology, Gram stain appearance, pigment production, antibiotic susceptibility, hemolysis, and biochemical testing. Gas-liquid chromatography (GLC), when available, also is used to identify these organisms.

Bacteroides

The *Bacteroides fragilis* group contains several species of *Bacteroides*, including *B. fragilis*, which is the most clinically relevant species. In fact, *B. fragilis* is the most commonly isolated anaerobe, although it makes up less than 1% of the normal flora of the colon. Other species included in the *B. fragilis* group include *B. nordii*, *B. ovatus*, *B. stercoris*, *B. thetaiotaomicron*, and *B. vulgatus*.

B. fragilis is extremely virulent and can cause widespread tissue necrosis. Its pathogenicity is related to the production of several compounds and virulence factors. Fimbriae and agglutinins act as adhesions and enable the organism to establish infection. There is a polysaccharide capsule that is believed to induce the formation of abscesses and also cause resistance to phagocytosis and complement-mediated killing. *B. fragilis* also produces several histolytic enzymes that cause tissue destruction and enable the infection to spread. These enzymes include hyaluronidase and chondroitin sulfatase, which attack the extracellular matrix of the host cells. Some strains also produce fibrinolytic enzymes and neuraminidase, which can alter the host's immune functions. Endotoxin LPS, which is released upon cell lysis through the gram-negative cell wall, induces many physiologic functions, including endotoxic shock.

Enterotoxin production is associated with diarrhea, and β-lactamase destroys the β-lactam ring in the penicillin and cephalosporin antibiotics, rending these antibiotics ineffective. Thus, a β-lactamase resistant penicillin, metronidazole, cefoxitin, carbapenems, or clindamycin must be used for treatment.

Bacteroides, especially the *B. fragilis* group, is associated with abdominal and urogenital abscesses, peritonitis, and appendicitis. Generally, the *Bacteroides* organisms have been displaced following surgery or trauma to the abdominal cavity or female genital tract. Other types of infections from *Bacteroides* include lower respiratory tract infections, skin and soft tissue abscesses, decubitus ulcers, chronic wound infections, and bone infections. *B. fragilis* is the most common *Bacteroides* species isolated from clinical infections, which accounts for approximately 50% of all *Bacteroides* infections. Other frequently isolated *Bacteroides* include *B. thetaiotaomicron* and *B. ovatus*.

Bacteroides organisms have rounded ends and may be pleomorphic with vacuoles or clear areas on Gram-stained smears. On anaerobic blood agar, colonies are large, gray, moist, and nonhemolytic with an entire margin and ring-like structures. Growth is enhanced in 20% bile, and the organisms are resistant to penicillin (2 U), kanamycin (1 mg), vancomycin (5 μg), and colistin (10 μg) but are susceptible to rifampin (15 μg). *Bacteroides* organisms are

BOX 16-3 Important Characteristics of *Bacteroides fragilis*

Growth in 20% bile (resistant to bile)
Bile-esculin hydrolysis: Positive
Catalase: Positive
Lipase: Negative
Lecithinase: Negative
Gelatinase: Negative
Indole: Negative
No pigment or spore production
Vancomyin (5 μg): Resistant
Kanamycin (1 mg): Resistant
Colistin (10 μg): Resistant

saccharolytic and speciated based on the specific fermentation pattern. Important characteristics of *B. fragilis* are shown in BOX 16-3.

B. vulgatus is the only member of the *B. fragilis* group that is bile-esculin negative, and *B. thetaiotaomicron* is the only *Bacteroides* species that is indole positive.

Prevotella

The pigmented saccharolytic gram-negative bacilli are included in the genus *Prevotella*. These organisms ferment glucose and other carbohydrates. Species included in this group include *Prevotella melaninogenica*, *P. oris*, *P. denticola*, *P. buccae*, and *P intermedia*. The organisms are one of the predominant commensal organisms in the oral cavity but also are the agents of a variety of oral infections. *Prevotella* also is normal flora of the upper respiratory tract, including the oropharynx and nose. They also can cause infections in the head, neck, and lower respiratory tract.

The bacteria are typically slow growing, requiring up to 3 weeks for growth. Young colonies are tan to buff in color, whereas older colonies develop a brown pigment on laked blood agar. An important characteristic is brick-red fluorescence when viewed under ultraviolet light at 365 nm. Other important reactions include:

- Inhibition by 20% bile
- Susceptible to rifampin (15 μg)
- Resistant to kanamycin (1 mg)

P. intermedia produces black colonies in 2 to 3 weeks on laked blood agar and is indole and lipase positive. It is resistant to vancomycin and kanamycin but susceptible to colistin and is associated with infections in the oropharynx and respiratory tract. *P. melaninogenica* is indole, esculin, and lipase negative; it is resistant to vancomycin and kanamycin. *P. melaninogenica* is an important cause of periodontal diseases, mouth abscesses, and endodontic infection. It also is associated with infections and abscesses of the ear, nose, throat, and urogenital tract. *Prevotella* produces β-lactamase, and infections can be treated with metronidazole, imipenem, and clindamycin.

Porphyromonas

The asaccharolytic pigmented gram-negative bacilli are contained in the genus *Porphyromonas*, which are normal flora of the oropharynx, nose, urogenital tract, and GI tract. The bacteria are associated with infections of the head, neck, oral cavity, and urogenital tract and with pleuropulmonary infections. Important species include *Porphyromonas asaccharolytica*, *P endodontalis*, and *P. gingivalis*. *P. gingivalis* and *P. endodontalis* are important causes of periodontal disease.

Similar to *Prevotella*, the bacteria are typically slow growing, requiring 48 hours to as long as 2 weeks to grow. Colonies characteristically show a brick-red fluorescence when viewed under ultraviolet light (365 nm). Older colonies develop a black to brown pigment. *Porphyromonas* is asaccharolytic and cannot ferment carbohydrates; it is indole positive. These bacilli do not grow on kanamycin-vancomycin anaerobic medium because they are inhibited by vancomycin. These bacteria also are inhibited by 20% bile and thus do not grown on *Bacteroides* bile-esculin agar. The organisms are inhibited by penicillin (2 U) and rifampin (15 μg) and susceptible to kanamycin (1 mg). *Porphyromonas* produces β-lactamase but can be treated with metronidazole, imipenem, and chloroamphenicol.

Fusobacterium

Fusobacterium is found as normal flora of the upper respiratory, gastrointestinal, and urinary tracts. Infections include serious pulmonary and blood infections, brain abscesses, and sinus and dental infections. Important species are *F. nucleatum* and *F. necrophorum*. The species isolated most frequently is *F. nucleatum*, which is an important pathogen in biofilms in periodontal disease, root canal infections, and dental abscesses. It also is associated with infections and abscesses of the genitourinary tract, blood, brain, lung, liver, abdomen, and joints; it also is a cause of aspiration pneumonia. Another important species is *F. necrophorum*, which causes particularly virulent infections, including septicemia and metastatic infections, such as lung and liver abscesses, arthritis, and osteomyelitis. *F. necrophorum* also is associated with abscesses in the tonsils and pharynx, sinusitis, and otitis media. It plays a role in Lemierre's syndrome, an invasive disease that occurs in young adults following bacterial infection of the throat. Peritonsillar abscesses occur, which penetrate the neck tissues and then enter the blood through the jugular vein. Blood clots may occur, which may disseminate to the lungs, liver, and other organs.

F. necrophorum, in the presence of commensal spirochetes, may cause Vincent's angina, commonly known as trench mouth. Vincent's angina is characterized by inflammation of the oral cavity, with a purulent discharge and ulcerating lesions. A direct methylene blue smear will reveal both bacilli and spirochetes.

Fusobacterium appears as spindle-shaped cells in long filaments with tapered or pointed ends. *F. necrophorum* is very pleomorphic and also may show coccobacillary forms with rounded ends. *F. necrophorum* grows on anaerobic blood agar as yellow to gray colonies. The organism is indole and lipase positive. An important characteristic is the colonial morphology, which is opalescent with speckles when viewed under a stereoscope. There is a yellow-green fluorescence when observed under ultraviolet light. Negative reactions are seen for catalase, esculin hydrolysis, 20% bile, gelatin, and lecithinase. The organism can ferment glucose and is resistant to vancomycin and susceptible to kanamycin and colistin.

F. nucleatum exhibits a variety of colonial morphologies and may resemble bread crumbs or coarse granules. It also may exhibit an opalescence, or ground-glass appearance, or grow as smooth gray colonies. *F. nucleatum* is quite inactive biochemically, yielding a positive indole reaction but negative reactions for catalase, esculin hydrolysis, growth in 20% bile, gelatin, lipase, and lecithinase. It cannot ferment glucose.

TABLE 16-3 outlines reactions used to identify some of the more important gram-negative anaerobes.

TABLE 16-3 Identification of Anaerobic Gram-Negative Bacilii

	Bacteroides fragilis	*Porphyromonas asaccharolyticus*	*Prevotella intermedia*	*Fusobacterium necrophorum*	*Fusobacterium nucleatum*
Indole	–	+	+	+	+
Esculin hydrolysis	+	–	–	–	–
H_2S	–	–	–	V	V
Catalase	+	–	–	–	–
Lecithinase	–	–	–	–	–
Lipase	–	–	+	+	–
Growth on 20% bile	E	I	I	I	I
Glucose fermented	+	–	+	+	–
Starch hydrolysis	–	–	+	–	–
Milk digested	–	+	+	V	–
DNase	–	–	+	–	–
Gelatin hydrolysis	–	+	+	V	–
Fermentation of					
Mannitol	–	–	–	–	–
Lactose	+	–	–	–	–
Rhamnose	–	–	–	–	–

+, most strains positive; –, most strains negative; V, variable reaction; E, growth on 20% bile equal to that without bile; I, growth on 20% bile inhibited

Anaerobic Gram-Positive Spore-Forming Bacilli: *Clostridium*

The *Clostridium* bacteria are found in soil, water, and dust, and some species are normal inhabitants of the intestinal tract of many animals, including humans. These organisms are anaerobic or aerotolerant gram-positive bacilli with large, swollen spores. Most clostridia are catalase negative, which is an important reaction to differentiate clostridia from *Bacillus* species, which are catalase positive. Bacilli form spores aerobically, whereas *Clostridium* sporulate anaerobically. The sporangia of clostridia may be located in a terminal, subterminal, or central position. The spores of *Clostridium tetani,* round and terminal, are said to resemble a drumstick or tennis racket, whereas those of *Clostridium botulinum* are oval and subterminal. Although spores can be seen using the Gram stain technique or a special spore stain, those of *Clostridium perfringens* (**FIGURE 16-4**) and *Clostridium ramosum* are often not observed because they do not sporulate in short-term cultures. Spore production enables the organism to remain dormant yet potentially infective upon germination when in a favorable environment.

Clostridia produce true **exotoxins**, which are toxins liberated by living bacterial cells. Examples include **tetanospasmin**, the toxin secreted by *C. tetani*, the agent of tetanus. **Botulism** toxin is produced by *C. botulinum*, the agent of botulism. *C. perfringens*, an important agent of myonecrosis and food poisoning, is known to produce several products, including hemolysins, lecithinase, protease, collagenase, and enterotoxin.

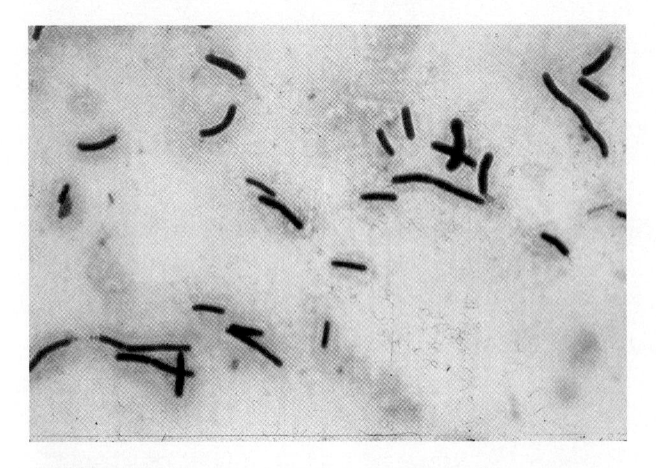

FIGURE 16-4 Microscopic appearance of *Clostridium perfringens*, showing large gram-positive bacilli. Spores are generally not seen in culture.

CLOSTRIDIUM TETANI

Clostridium tetani is the etiologic agent of **tetanus**, which results from entry of the organism or its spores through a puncture wound, gunshot, burn, or animal bite. The spores often are present in the environment, including in soil, dust, and animal feces. Once inside the body, the presence of necrotic cells, which are no longer receiving oxygen, provide an anaerobic environment that permits germination of the spores into active bacilli. Subsequently, tetanospasmin toxin is produced, released, and absorbed. Germination time is variable, and the spores can remain dormant for a few days to a few months before germination.

Tetanospasmin is a potent neurotoxin that travels along nerve fibers from the wound to the anterior horn cells of the spinal cord. Here it causes convulsive contractions of voluntary muscles. Because these spasms first involve the neck and jaw, the disease is commonly known as "lockjaw." The spastic contractions resulting from the toxin also produce a characteristic backward arching of the back muscles. Respiratory paralysis also may occur.

Diagnosis of tetanus is accomplished through the clinical picture and history of the injury. Untreated tetanus has a greater than 50% mortality rate. Therapy involves the administration of neutralizing antibodies to bind the free toxin and supportive therapy to assist in breathing and control the muscle spasms. Antibiotics, such as penicillin, metronidazole, or erythromycin can be given to prevent further bacterial growth.

Tetanus is rare in developed counties, where immunizations are routinely used. In the United States, children are vaccinated with five doses of the DTaP (diphtheria, tetanus, acellular pertussis) at 2, 4, 6, and 15 to 18 months and at 4 to 6 years. The Td is a tetanus, diphtheria vaccine, which is given to adolescents and adults as a booster every 10 years or after a possible exposure to tetanus.

Identification of *C. tetani* includes the observation of the gram-positive bacillus with round, terminal spores that resemble a drumstick or tennis racket. The organism produces gelatinase and indole but is negative for lecithinase and lipase. It is motile and unable to ferment most carbohydrates. However, the organism is usually not cultured from clinical specimens and rarely is seen clinically in wounds before autopsy.

CLOSTRIDIUM BOTULINUM

C. botulinum is the agent in food, wound, and infant **botulism.** The organism and its spores are found throughout the environment in soil and water and on vegetation. The effects of botulism result from the liberation of botulism toxin, which enters the blood at the peripheral site of the wound, lung, or gastrointestinal tract. Botulism toxin is a powerful neurotoxin that binds to the synapse of the cholinergic nerve fibers. The result is acute and flaccid paralysis involving first the muscles of the face, head, and throat and later those of the thorax, diaphragm, arms, and legs. Death usually occurs from respiratory paralysis.

Food-borne botulism was first reported in the United States in the late 18th century. Botulism is a concern in food production and as a possible cause of crib death, potential agent of bioterrorism, and risk for intravenous drug users. There are seven types of botulism toxin: A, B, C, D, E, F, and G. The most common types found in human botulism are types A (30%), B (50%), and E (12%).

Food-borne botulism is associated with the ingestion of preformed botulism toxin in improperly prepared home-canned foods and contaminated food products. Home-canned foods, such as beans, beets, fish, tuna, mushrooms, corn, and peppers are especially susceptible to botulism contamination. The spores are not inactivated because of an inadequate canning process that does not destroy the spores. The spores can then germinate under the anaerobic conditions produced during the canning process, when the jars are sealed. The incubation period of botulism ranges from 12 to 72 hours after ingestion, and symptoms may include nausea, vomiting, and constipation, in addition to the neurological symptoms. Administration of trivalent antitoxin against serotypes A, B, and E should be given to bind the neurotoxin. Once the neurotoxin enters the nerve endings, antitoxin is no longer effective. Thus, the prompt administration of the antitoxin is very important. The case fatality rate from food-borne botulism is 5% to 10% in developed countries.

Wound botulism is a rare type of botulism that occurs as the organism germinates in wounds or abscesses. This condition can result from improperly sterilized surgical dressings and contaminated casts. It also may occur following the use of needles contaminated with botulism spores by intravenous drug users.

The most common type of botulism is infant botulism, in which the organism grows in the gastrointestinal tract of infants who are less than 1 year of age. Infant botulism involves the ingestion of botulism spores from soil, dust, or honey that germinate in the infant's gastrointestinal tract, which has not yet established its normal flora. The germinating bacillus produces botulism toxin; infant botulism can range in severity from a subclinical state to sudden death. The infant first experiences constipation, which may be followed by difficulty in swallowing, muscle weakness, loss of head control, and eventually respiratory distress and failure.

Botulism is diagnosed through clinical symptoms and patient history. It is treated by administration of an antitoxin that binds to the botulism toxin; antitoxin must be released from the Centers for Disease Control and Prevention (CDC). Identification of the toxin is usually performed in public health laboratories. *C. botulinum* is lipase positive and lecithinase and indole negative. It ferments glucose but not lactose or xylose and is motile. The spores are oval and located subterminally. Botulism must be reported to the state health department and to the CDC.

CLOSTRIDIUM PERFRINGENS

C. perfringens is the most common species of *Clostridium* isolated from clinical specimens. It is a cause of **myonecrosis** (gas gangrene), food poisoning, post-abortion sepsis, intra-abdominal and pleuropulmonary infections, enterocolitis, and antibiotic-associated diarrhea. The organism is known to produce several toxins, including α-toxin, lecithinase (results in cell destruction), hemolysins, cardiotoxin, collagenase, fibrinolysin, DNase, ribonuclease (RNase), enterotoxin, and proteolytic enzymes.

C. perfringens is the most common cause of myonecrosis in the United States. Myonecrosis is characterized by severe muscle destruction and the production of gas pockets in the tissue. The tissue becomes more necrotic with a poorer blood supply, which promotes an anaerobic environment in the tissues. *C. perfringens* secretes both enzymes and exotoxins, which are the causes of additional tissue destruction and allow the organism and infection to spread to other tissues. The organism is very saccharolytic, and as carbohydrate fermentation occurs, gas is released, which accumulates in the tissue. This further restricts the blood flow to the tissue, increasing the necrosis. Gas gangrene is found in individuals with impaired circulation, diabetics, and others with poor oxygen perfusion to the tissues. *C. perfringens* also is a cause of uterine gangrene from induced abortion; it is normal flora in the female genital tract, providing a source for endogenous infection.

Treatment of gas gangrene includes surgical debridement or amputation of the necrotic tissue. The use of a hyperbaric oxygen chamber, a chamber of pure oxygen under pressure, can prevent the spread of gas gangrene. Antibiotics, including penicillin, vancomycin, and clindamycin, also are used as a part of the treatment regime.

C. perfringens also is a common cause of food poisoning in the United States and usually produces a mild and self-limiting condition lasting 2 to 3 days. However, the infection can be more severe in the very young, old, and immunosuppressed. The symptoms of *C. perfringens* foodborne disease result from the production of an enterotoxin released after the spores of the organism germinate. Implicated foods that may be contaminated with *C. perfringens* include beef, turkey, chicken, and processed meat products. Symptoms occur 7 to 15 hours after ingestion and include foul-smelling stools and diarrhea, but usually no vomiting occurs. The organism also causes a necrotizing bowel disease known as enteritis necroticans or necrotizing enteritis, which is characterized by abdominal cramps, vomiting, bloody diarrhea, and acute inflammation. Symptoms are related to the effects of a β-toxin. In severe cases, there may be extensive fluid and electrolyte loss and death. While the condition is rare in the United States, it occurs more frequently in other parts of the world.

The gram stain of *C. perfringens* shows large gram-positive bacilli that align end to end in a boxcar formation. Spores are round and subterminal but rarely demonstrated. An important identifying characteristic is a double zone of hemolysis on anaerobic blood agar. The inner zone is completely hemolyzed from the effects of θ-toxin, and the outer zone is incompletely hemolyzed from the effects of α-toxin and lecithinase activity. It is very saccharolytic, fermenting glucose, lactose, maltose, and fructose. Lecithinase and lipase activity can be demonstrated on egg yolk agar (EYA). *C. perfringens* is lecithinase positive as indicated by an opaque yellow halo on egg yolk agar. *C. perfringens* is lipase negative. The organism is nonmotile.

Lecithanase activity also can be demonstrated using a Nagler plate. Half the surface of the Nagler plate is streaked with a few drops of *C. perfringens* type A antitoxin. Then the suspected culture is streaked across the plate at a right angle to the antitoxin. A zone of precipitation around the colonies on the side without antitoxin, with little or no precipitation around colonies on the side with antitoxin, indicates a positive lecithinase test. A limited number of *Clostridium* species, including *C. perfringens*, *C. sordellii*, and *C. bifermentans*, give a positive Nagler reaction. Because the antisera are difficult to obtain commercially, the Nagler reaction is not usually performed in clinical laboratories.

The reverse CAMP procedure also can be performed to identify *C. perfringens*. In this technique the suspected clostridial species is streaked on a blood agar plate. Group B streptococcus (*Streptococcus agalactiae*) is streaked at a right angle to the first streak. After incubation, a positive reaction is indicated by the formation of an arrowhead at the intersection of the two streaks.

Although *C. perfringens* accounts for most cases, there are other species of *Clostridium* that cause myonecrosis. These include *C. novyi*, *C. septicum*, *C. histolyticum*, and *C. sordelli*.

CLOSTRIDIUM DIFFICILE

Clostridium difficile was first isolated in 1975 and was originally considered to be nonpathogenic until shortly later, when it was isolated as an important cause of antibiotic-associated pseudomembranous colitis. *C. difficile* is found in soil and water, intestinal contents of various animals, and stools of healthy infants. The organism also is found in the stools of approximately 5% of healthy adults and up to 30% of hospitalized adults. Today, *C. difficile* is an important cause of antibiotic-associated pseudomembranous colitis and is the most frequent cause of antibiotic-associated diarrhea acquired in the health care setting. As an important cause of hospital-acquired diarrhea and colitis, *C. difficile* is frequently found in patients who have received one or more broad-spectrum antibiotics, including the aminoglycosides, penicillins, second- and third-generation β-lactams, cephalosporins, erythromycin, clindamycin, and rifampin. It also has been associated as a cause of pseudomembranous colitis and diarrhea in patients who have not undergone antibiotic therapy. Complications of *C. difficile* infection may include colon perforations, sepsis, and death. The clinical signs of *C. difficile* infection include watery diarrhea, fever, nausea, and abdominal pain. Antibiotic use, especially broad-spectrum antibiotics; gastrointestinal surgery; long-term stays in a health care facility; serious underlying disease; advanced age; and immunosuppressive states are some of the risk factors for *C. difficile* infection. An individual can be colonized with *C. difficile* but not have infection. Those who are colonized have no clinical symptoms but may test positive for *C. difficile* on culture or for its toxins. Those with infection have clinical symptoms and also have positive test results.

Diagnosis of *C. difficile* is performed by testing liquid or semisolid fecal specimens, using culture techniques and demonstration of toxins. *C. difficile* produces toxin A, an enterotoxin (TcdA) and toxin B, a cytotoxin (TcdB). Several products are available that demonstrate the cytotoxin, which can confirm the identification. Methodologies to demonstrate the toxin include enzyme immunoassay, tissue culture, and latex agglutination. Some of the procedures currently available to identify toxin A include the Culturette CDT Kit (Becton Dickinson), which is a latex agglutination method; and the BD ColorPAC™ *C. difficile* Toxin A test kit (bioMérieux) and the Clearview™ *C. difficile* Toxin A test (Inverness Medical), which are immunochromatographic assays. There also are enzyme immunoassay tests that identify both toxins A and B, such as the Tox A/B Quik Chek™ (Inverness Medical), the Immuno*Card*® Toxins A&B (Meridian Bioscience), and the Xpect® *Clostridium difficile* Toxin A/B test (Remel).

Cell culture methods are known as the gold standard for toxin identification because of their high sensitivity and high specificity. Cytotoxicity testing on cell cultures is used to identify toxin B cytotoxin. TechLab offers the *C. difficile* Tox-B test. Antigen detection of glutamate dehydrogenase (GDH) can be used to screen stool samples for *C. difficile*. GDH is secreted by *C. difficile* and may be detected though enzyme immunoassay. GDH is not specific for *C. difficile* but may be used in combination with other methods to identify the organisms. There also are DNA methods to detect toxin A (tcdA) and toxin B (tcdB) genes.

Specimens also can be inoculated on either cycloserine cefoxitin fructose (CCF) agar or *Clostridium difficile* selective agar (CDSA), which are both selective agars for *C. difficile*. CDSA contains amino acids that when utilized by *C. difficile* cause an increase in pH, resulting in a color change of the agar from rose to yellow. Cefoxitin and cycloserine inhibit normal fecal flora. *C. difficile* will appear as yellow, umbonate colonies with a ground-glass appearance after 48 to 72 hours of anaerobic incubation. Biochemical reactions also may be used to identify *C. difficile*. The organism produces gelatinase but is negative for lecithinase, lipase, and indole. It ferments glucose and fructose but not lactose, maltose, or xylose. Spores are oval and subterminal. The organism is motile and fluoresces under ultraviolet light.

MISCELLANEOUS CLOSTRIDIA

Clostridium ramosum is a part of the normal flora of the large bowel and an important agent in intra-abdominal infections following trauma. It usually stains gram negative, which can lead to confusion in its identification. *C. ramosum* grows well on 20% bile agar, hydrolyzes esculin, and does not produce lecithinase, catalase, or lipase. It produces round to oval terminal spores that are difficult to demonstrate. The organism is highly fermentative and can utilize glucose, lactose, maltose, fructose, and mannitol.

Clostridium septicum is a cause of bacteremia in individuals who have malignancies, such as colon and breast cancer and leukemia. The organism is pleomorphic and may produce long filaments and has oval, subterminal spores. It is gelatinase positive and negative for lecithinase, lipase, and indole. *C. septicum* ferments glucose, lactose, maltose, and fructose but does not ferment mannitol. **TABLE 16-4** outlines biochemical reactions used in the identification of *Clostridium* species.

Anaerobic Gram-Positive Non–Spore-Forming Bacilli

The anaerobic gram-positive non–spore-forming bacilli are normal flora of the human urinary tract, oral cavity, bowel, and vagina and are rare causes of opportunistic infection. The organisms include *Bifidobacterium*, *Eubacterium*, *Lactobacillus*, *Actinomyces*, and *Propionibacterium*. *Actinomyces* may be normal flora of the mouth and urogenital tract and is the cause of opportunistic infections of endogenous origin. The most significant species is ***Actinomyces israelii***, which is usually isolated in mixed anaerobic infections and is an agent of pelvic **actinomycoses**. Cells are branching and diphtheroid in appearance. Actinomycoses is characterized by the presence of "sulfur granules" in the exudate of the infection. On agar, the organism grows heaped, rough, and white, and the colonies are described as resembling a "molar tooth."

Bifidobacterium is found as normal flora of the mouth and gastrointestinal tract and is a rare cause of pulmonary, dental, and wound infection. The bacteria are very pleomorphic gram-positive rods with branching ends. *Bifidobacterium* grows as small, smooth white colonies on anaerobic blood agar.

TABLE 16-4 Identification of *Clostridium* Species, Using Lombard-Dowell Medium

	C. Difficile	*C. Perfringens*	*C. Ramosum*	*C. Septicum*	*C. Sordellii*	*C. Tetani*
Indole	–	–	–	–	+	+
Esculin hydrolysis	+	V	+	+	–	–
H_2S	–	N/A	N/A	N/A	V	V
Catalase		–	–	–	–	–
Lecithinase	–	+	–	–	+	–
Lipase	–	–	–	–	–	–
Growth on 20% bile	E	E	E	E	E	E
Glucose fermented	+	+	+	+	+	–
Starch hydrolysis	–	V	–	–	–	–
Milk digested	–	–	–	V	+	–
DNase	V	+	–	+	–	+
Gelatin hydrolysis	V	+	–	+	+	+
Fermentation of:						
Mannitol	+	–	+	–	–	–
Lactose	–	+	+	+	–	–
Rhamnose	–	–	+	–	–	–

+, most strains positive; –, most strains negative; V, variable reaction; E, growth on 20% bile equal to that without bile; I, growth on 20% bile inhibited; N/A, not applicable

Propionibacterium acnes is the most frequent gram-positive non–spore-forming bacillus isolated from clinical cultures. It is a part of the normal flora of the skin, nasopharynx, oral cavity, and gastrointestinal tract. A rare pathogen, *P. acnes* is more often found as a skin contaminant in blood culture specimens. It also can cause infections associated with prosthetic devices, such as heart valves and prosthetic joints; bacteremia; and endocarditis. Proper disinfection of the skin in preparation for blood cultures, lumbar puncture, or aspiration of abscesses is important to reduce contamination from *P. acnes* and other skin contaminants.

P. acnes produces propionic acid as the major end product of glucose metabolism, which is detected using gas-liquid chromotography. Sometimes referred to as anaerobic diphtheroids, *P. acnes* resembles the corynebacteria and appear as "picket fences" in stained smears.

Eubacterium is a rare cause of infections in the female genital tract and from wounds and abscesses in mixed infections. It is pleomorphic, and its morphology may be that of either a bacillus or a coccobacillus in pairs or chains. *Lactobacillus* is the major normal flora in the female genital tact and also is a part of the normal flora in the mouth and gastrointestinal tract. *Lactobacillus* is aerotolerant and was discussed previously with the aerobic gram-positive bacilli.

Anaerobic Gram-Positive Cocci

The anaerobic gram-positive cocci have undergone significant changes in nomenclature based on DNA–DNA hybridization and 16S rRNA gene sequencing. In the past, most important human pathogens were classified as members of the genus *Peptostreptococcus*. There have been several new genera and species proposed, which are summarized in BOX 16-4.

The microscopic morphology of these bacteria includes cocci in chains and pairs and as single organisms. *Parvimonas micra* appears as small cocci arranged in packets or short chains. *Anaerococcus tetradus* and some of the other bacteria are larger cocci arranged in pairs and clusters.

The anaerobic gram-positive cocci are normal flora of the mouth, upper respiratory tract, female genitourinary tract, bowel, and skin. *Parvimonas micra* is the

BOX 16-4 **Anaerobic Gram-Positive Cocci**

Current Name	Former Name (if applicable)
Peptococcus niger	*Peptococcus niger*
Peptostreptococcus stomatis	Peptostreptococcus anaerobius,
Peptostreptococcus anaerobius,	Peptostreptococcus anaerobius
Parvimonas micra	Peptostreptococcus micros, Micromonas micros
Peptinophilus asacccharolyticus	Peptostreptococcus asaccharolyticus
Anaerococcus prevotii	Peptostreptococcus prevotii
Anaerococcus tetradus	Peptostreptococcus tetradus
Blaudia producta	Peptostreptococcus productus, Ruminococcus preductus
Finegoldia magna	Peptostreptococcus magnus
Staphylococcus sacchrolyticus	Peptostreptococcus saccharolyticus

predominant anaerobe found in the oral cavity, where *P. anaerobius* and *F. magna* also are found. *F. magna* and *P. asacccharolyticus* are found as normal flora on the skin, and *Peptostreptococcus*, *B. producta*, and *F. magna* are found as normal flora in the gastrointestinal tract. Many species of anaerobic gram-positive cocci are found as normal flora in the female genital tract, including *A. tetradus*, *P. anaerobius*, *P. asacccharolyticus*, and *F. magna*. These bacteria are associated with abscesses of the liver and brain, wound infections, and infections of the female genital tract, abdominal cavity, and respiratory tract. Gram-positive anaerobic cocci are involved in polymicrobic infections but also may be found as the single pathogen.

Peptostreptococcus anaerobius causes infections in the brain, ear, jaw, pleural cavity, and urogenital tract; it also is a cause of perodontitis, peritonsillar abscess, and abdominal abscess. *P. anaerobius* is the only gram-positive anaerobic cocci that is susceptible to sodium polyanethol sulfonate (SPS), producing a zone of inhibition of ≥ 12 mm to SPS. It also is resistant to kanamycin and colistin. *P. anaerobius* grows as small gray to white colonies on anaerobic blood agar, with a sweet, putrid odor.

Finegoldia magna is associated with skin and soft tissue infections; endocarditis; meningitis; pneumonia; breast abscesses; and infections of bones, joints, and prosthetic implants. *F. magna* produces small, grayish white colonies on anaerobic blood agar and may resemble *Staphylococcus* in the Gram stain, appearing as gram-positive cocci in clusters. It is resistant to SPS and both indole and catalase negative.

Parvimonas micra is an oral pathogen and an agent in polymicrobic infections, such as brain abscess, otitis media, human bite infections, septicemia, abdominal infections, and infections of prosthetic joints. *Peptinophilus asacccharolyticus* produces small, yellow colonies with a musty odor on anaerobic blood agar. It is SPS negative (resistant), catalase negative, and indole positive. In older cultures, it may appear gram negative.

Anaerobic Gram-Negative Cocci

The gram-negative anaerobic cocci include the following genera: *Veillonella*, *Megasphaera*, *Acidoaminococcus*, *Anaeroglobus*, and *Negativicoccus*. These bacteria account for only a small amount of human infection. *Veillonella* is found as commensal flora in the oral cavity and respiratory, genitourinary, and respiratory tracts of humans and other animals. There are currently 10 species of *Veillonella*, of which five are found in humans: *V. atypica*, *V. denticarius*, *V. dispar*, *V. parvula*, *and V. rogoase*. *Veillonella* appears as gram-negative cocci arranged in pairs, short chains, or irregular clumps. They grow as small, grayish white colonies on anaerobic blood agar and may produce a weak red fluorescence when viewed under ultraviolet light.

TABLE 16-5 Identifying Reactions for Anaerobic Cocci

Organism	Catalase	SPS susceptibility	Kanamycin	Colistin	Vancomycin	Nitrate reduction	Indole
Finegoldia magna	–	R	V	R	S	–	–
Pepto-streptcoccus anaerobius	–	S	R	R	S	–	–
Peptino-philus asacccharol-yticus	–	R	S	R	S	–	+
Veillonella	V	R	S	S	R	+	–

R, resistant; S, susceptible, V, variable

These bacteria are rare causes of osteomyelitis, meningitis, bacteremia, and infections of prosthetic joints. Because of its high sensitivity to oxygen, *Veillonella* usually is not isolated unless a glove box is used.

Infections of anaerobic cocci are generally treated with penicillins, cephalosporins, and carbapenems. Identifying reactions for some of the anaerobic cocci are found in **TABLE 16-5.**

Antimicrobial Susceptibility Testing for Anaerobes

Antimicrobial susceptibility testing for anaerobes remains controversial; once an anaerobe is isolated and identified, susceptibility testing may or may not be performed for a variety of reasons. First, the time required to perform susceptibility testing is much longer when compared to that for aerobes, which may hinder its clinical usefulness. In the past, many anaerobes had a predictable susceptibility pattern, and physicians often relied on this principle to prescribe empirical therapy without the aid of susceptibility testing. Other issues in anaerobic susceptibly testing include the lack of reproducibility, the failure of some anaerobes to grow because of their fastidious nature, the lack of comparison between methods, and difficulty in identifying end points. Also, there is no gold standard for susceptibility testing for anaerobes even though there are several testing methods available. The Clinical Laboratory Standards Institute (CLSI, 2012) recommends that agar dilution and broth microdilution testing be performed when appropriate and plausible. The recommended agar dilution method uses *Brucella* agar supplemented with hemin, vitamin K, and laked sheep blood. Broth microdilution and macrodilution methods using *Brucella* broth supplemented with hemin, vitamin K, and lysed horse blood also are recommended by CLSI. Broth microdilution is used extensively, but results may be inaccurate or inconsistent for fastidious bacteria that grow poorly from exposure to oxygen. These methods are labor intensive and may yield unreliable results. However, as more anaerobes develop antibiotic resistance, there will be a greater need for accurate susceptibility testing for anaerobes. Disk diffusion methods are not suitable for anaerobic susceptibility testing.

Currently, several circumstances exist when it is recommended that susceptibility testing should be performed on anaerobes. For example, susceptibility testing may be needed to determine the susceptibility pattern to a new antimicrobial agent in a specific health care setting. Another indication occurs when the usual treatment is failing or there is not a known effective treatment regime for a specific anaerobe. Other indications occur when there is a documented resistance of a species to the most commonly used antimicrobial agents. Long-term and recurrent anaerobic infections also may indicate the need for susceptibility testing. Severity of the infection is another important consideration; susceptibility testing should be performed in severe cases, including brain abcesses, endocarditis, infections of prosthetic devices, recurrent bacteremia, osteomyelitis, and joint infections.

As an adjunct to antibiotic susceptibility testing, the identification of the production of β-lactamase and cephalosporinase enzymes can be performed. Production of these enzymes inactivates the β-lactam ring of the β-lactam antibiotics. Members of the *Bacteroides fragilis* group are known to produce β-lactamase, as are certain species of *Clostridium* and *Fusobacterium*. Anaerobes also demonstrate different mechanisms for resistance to the β-lactam antibiotics as well as resistance to other antibiotic groups.

Laboratory Procedures

Procedure
CDC anaerobic blood agar

Purpose
CDC anaerobic blood agar is an enriched medium to isolate all anaerobic bacteria, including obligate, facultative, and fastidious anaerobes.

Principle
The medium contains 5% defibrinated sheep blood base, which is enriched with peptones, yeast, hemin, and vitamin K. The reducing agent L-cystine also is incorporated into the medium. The peptones provide nitrogenous growth factors, carbon, and sulfur, and yeast extract provides B vitamins.

Procedure

1. Streak plate for isolation and minimize exposure to air. Inoculate with one drop of liquid specimens. Mince and grind tissue specimens in sterile broth, such as enriched thioglycollate, before inoculation. For swab specimens, roll over first quadrant of plate and then inoculate thioglycollate broth. Swabs also may be vigorously mixed in a small volume of reduced broth and this broth used to inoculate, as for liquid specimens.
2. Incubate anaerobically at 35°C ± 2°C for a minimum of 48 hours.
3. Interpret plate at 48 hours for growth, colonial morphology, and hemolysis.
4. Plates are generally incubated for an additional 2 to 4 days.

Quality Control
Clostridium perfringens: Growth with double zone of hemolysis around colonies
Bacteroides fragilis: Growth

Notes

1. Medium must be pre-reduced immediately prior to inoculation by placing under anaerobic conditions for 18 to 24 hours.
2. An enriched broth, such as enriched thioglycollate, should be inoculated when the primary plates are inoculated.
3. The pigmented *Prevotella* and *Porphyromonas* will fluoresce orange to brick red under ultraviolet light prior to pigmentation.
4. Aerotolerance tests may be performed by inoculating an anaerobic blood agar plate and incubating it anaerobically and a chocolate agar plate inoculated aerobically under increased CO_2. Interpret as shown in Box 16-2.

Source: Becton, Dickinson and Company. (2009). *Manual of microbiological culture media*, 2nd ed. (pp. 110–112). Sparks, MD.

Procedure
Anaerobic blood agar with kanamycin and vancomycin

Purpose
Anaerobic blood agar with kanamycin and vancomycin is recommended for isolation of gram-negative anaerobes, particularly *Bacteroides*, *Prevotella*, and some *Fusobacterium*.

Principle
The medium is the CDC anaerobic blood agar base with the antibiotics kanamycin and vancomycin. Kanamycin inhibits facultative gram-negative bacilli. Vancomycin inhibits facultative and obligate gram-positive bacteria.

Procedure

1. Streak plate for isolation.
2. Incubate anaerobically at 35°C ± 2°C for a minimum of 48 hours.
3. Interpret plate at 48 hours for growth.
4. Plates are generally incubated for an additional 2 to 5 days.

Quality Control
Bacteroides fragilis: Growth
Clostridium perfringens: No growth

Notes

1. Laked blood agar with paromomycin or kanamycin and vancomycin is similar to anaerobic blood agar with kanamycin and vancomycin (CDC). Laked blood is prepared by freezing and then thawing whole blood.
2. Pigment production by *Prevotella melaninogenica* is enhanced on laked blood medium.

Source: Becton, Dickinson and Company. (2009). *Manual of microbiological culture media*, 2nd ed. (pp. 110–112). Sparks, MD.

Procedure
Anaerobic blood agar with phenylethyl alcohol

Purpose
Anaerobic blood agar with phenylethyl alcohol (PEA) isolates gram-positive and gram-negative obligate anaerobes.

Principle
The medium is an anaerobic blood agar base with PEA added. The medium inhibits the growth of gram-negative facultative anaerobes, such as the Enterobacteriaceae, and the swarming of *Proteus*. The medium permits the isolation of obligate anaerobes. Facultative gram-positive anaerobes, such as *Staphylococcus*, also can grow on PEA.

Procedure
1. Streak PEA plate for isolation.
2. Incubate anaerobically at 35°C ± 2°C for a minimum of 48 hours.
3. Interpret plate for growth.
4. Plates are generally incubated for an additional 2 to 5 days.

Quality Control
Peptostreptococcus anaerobius: Growth
Escherichia coli: No growth
Source: Becton, Dickinson and Company. (2009). *Manual of microbiological culture media*, 2nd ed. (pp. 110–112). Sparks, MD.

Procedure
Egg yolk agar

Purpose
Egg yolk agar is used in the primary identification of *Clostridium* and other obligate anaerobic bacilli based on production of lipase and lecithinase.

Principle
Digests of casein and soybean meal provide amino acids and other nitrogenous supplements, and yeast extract supplies B complex vitamins. Hemin is incorporated as a growth supplement and L-cystine is the reducing agent. An egg yolk suspension is incorporated into the medium to detect production of lipase and lecithinase. Lipase breaks down free fats present in the egg yolks, causing an "oil on water" iridescent sheen on the surface of the colony. Lecithinase degrades the lecithin in the egg yolks, forming an insoluble opaque precipitate surrounding the colony. Proteolysis is shown by clear zones in the medium surrounding the growth.

Procedure
1. Reduce the medium immediately before inoculation by holding it in anaerobic conditions for 18 to 24 hours.
2. Inoculate egg yolk agar plate for isolation.
3. Incubate anaerobically at 35°C ± 2°C for a minimum of 48 hours. If no growth occurs, incubate for up to 7 days.
4. Examine plates for lecithinase and lipase and proteolytic activity.

Quality Control
Clostridium perfringens: Lecithinase positive and lipase negative
Fusobacterium necrophorum: Lipase positive and lecithinase negative

Note
Hold plates for up to 7 days because lipase production may be delayed.
Source: Becton, Dickinson and Company. (2009). *Manual of microbiological culture media*, 2nd ed. (p. 209). Sparks, MD.

Procedure
Bacterioides bile-esculin agar

Purpose
Bacteroides bile-esculin (BBE) agar is used for the preliminary isolation of the *Bacteroides fragilis* group, which are frequently isolated anaerobes.

Principle
The medium contains gentamycin and oxgall, which inhibits most gram-negative anaerobes and most facultative anaerobes. *B. fragilis* group is bile resistant and able to grow on the medium. It is able to hydrolyze esculin, producing esculetin, which reacts with iron salts to form a dark brown to black complex, which surrounds the colonies of *B. fragilis*.

Procedure
1. Reduce the medium immediately before inoculation by holding it in anaerobic conditions for 18 to 24 hours.
2. Inoculate *Bacteroides* bile-esculin agar plate for isolation.
3. Incubate anaerobically at 35°C ± 2°C for a minimum of 48 hours. If no growth occurs, incubate for up to 7 days.
4. Examine plates for growth and hydrolysis of esculin.

Quality Control
B. fragilis: Colonies larger than 1 mm in diameter with a gray, circular, raised appearance with a brown to black discoloration
Fusobacterium: No growth

Note

1. Inoculate and incubate an anaerobic blood agar plate because some strains of *B. fragilis* are inhibited on *Bacteroides* bile-esculin agar.

Source: Becton, Dickinson and Company. (2009). *Manual of microbiological culture media*, 2nd ed. (pp. 70–71). Sparks, MD.

Procedure
Antibiotic disk tests

Purpose
The use of antibiotic disks to determine an anaerobe's inhibition can be a useful identification method. Most anaerobes have a characteristic susceptibility pattern to colistin (10 µg), vancomycin (5 µg), and kanamycin (1 mg).

Principle
After streaking an anaerobic blood agar plate to obtain a lawn of growth, each antibiotic disk is placed over the area of the streak. After incubation, the plates are interpreted by measuring the zone of inhibition.

Media and Material
5 µg vancomycin disk (Va)
1 mg (1,000 µg) kanamycin disk (K)
10 µg colistin disk (Co)
Anaerobic blood agar (ABA)

Procedure

1. Transfer a portion of one colony to the ABA plate and streak the first quadrant of the plate to produce a heavy lawn of growth.
2. Streak the other quadrants for isolation.
3. Place the Co, K, and Va disks in the first quadrant well, separated from each other.
4. Incubate the plates anaerobically for 48 hours at 35°C.

Interpretation
Observe for a zone of inhibition of growth. A zone of 10 mm or less indicates resistance, and a zone greater than 10 mm indicates susceptibility. Zone-size interpretation is not to be used as an indicator to predict clinical susceptibility.

Quality Control
Fusobacterium necrophorum: Susceptible to K and Co; resistant to Va
Bacteroides fragilis: Resistant to K, Co, and Va
Clostridium perfringens: Susceptible to Va and K; resistant to Co

Notes

1. Gram-positive anaerobes are usually susceptible to Va and K and resistant to Co.
2. Kanamycin can be used to separate *Fusobacterium*, which is susceptible, from *Bacteroides*, which is usually resistant.

Organism	Kanamycin (1,000 µg)	Colistin (10 µg)	Vancomycin (5 µg)
Bacteroides fragilis group	R	R	R
Other *Bacteroides* species	R	V	R
Prevotella and *Porphyromonas* species	R	V	V
Fusobacterium	S	S	R
Veillonella	S	S	R
Peptostreptococcus	V	R	S
Clostridium	S	R	S
Propionibacterium	S	R	S

R, resistant; S, susceptible; V, variable

Laboratory Exercises

1. Observe prepared Gram-stained smears of the following anaerobes and make a sketch of your findings.

Organism	Observations
Bacteroides fragilis	
Peptostreptococcus anaerobius	
Peptococcus niger	
Fusobacterium nucleatum	

2. Plate the following organisms on anaerobic blood agar, phenylethyl alcohol (PEA), and kanamycin-vancomycin (KV), and inoculate a thioglycollate (Thio). Incubate under anaerobic atmosphere for 35 ± 2°C. Observe each plate for growth after 48 hours of incubation. Gram stain the thioglycollate broth and record your findings. Incubate plates without growth for an additional 2 to 5 days. Describe your findings and record your observations.

Organism	Anaerobic blood	PEA	KV	Thio
Bacteroides fragilis				
Clostridium perfringens				
Peptostreptococcus anaerobius				
Peptococcus niger				
Fusobacterium nucleatum				

3. Explain the principle of the anaerobic jar method. Properly prepare the activator, catalyst, and indicator for incubation of cultures.
4. Plate the following organisms on the media listed. Incubate under anaerobic atmosphere for 35 ± 2°C. Observe each plate for growth after 48 hours of incubation. Incubate plates without growth for an additional 2 to 5 days. Describe your findings and record your observations.

Organism	*Bacteroides* bile esculin	Egg yolk agar
Bacteroides fragilis		
Clostridium perfringens		
Fusobacterium necrophorum		

How is lipase production interepreted on egg yolk agar? ______________________

____

How is lecithanase activity interpreted on egg yolk agar? ______________________

____

5. Perform the antibiotic disk tests on the organisms listed. Measure all zone diameters and interpret as susceptble (S) or resistant (R).

Organism	Zone diameters (mm) Va K Co	Interpretation
Bacteroides fragilis		
Clostridium perfringens		
Peptostreptococcus anaerobius		
Peptococcus niger		
Fusobacterium nucleatum		

Review Questions

Matching

Match each of the following anaerobic media with its purpose:

1. Enriched broth to supplement plating medium
2. Isolation of obligate and facultative anaerobes
3. Inhibition of gram-positive anaerobes and facultative gram-negative bacilli
4. Ability of organism to grow in 20% bile and hydrolyze esculin
5. Inhibition of Enterobacteriaceae and swarming of *Proteus;* allows for isolation of gram-positive and gram-negative obligate anaerobes
   a. Thioglycollate
   b. Anaerobic blood agar
   c. Anaerobic PEA
   d. Anaerobic KVBA
   e. BBE

   Match the *Clostridium* species with its infection:
6. *C. tetani*
7. *C. botulinum*
8. *C. difficile*
9. *C. perfringens*
   a. Pseudomembranous colitis
   b. Myonecrosis
   c. Tetanus
   d. Botulism

Multiple Choice

10. An organism that cannot use oxygen as the final electron acceptor and is inhibited by its presence is a(an):
    a. Obligate aerobe
    b. Obligate anaerobe
    c. Facultative anaerobe
    d. Microaerophile

For each of the following, indicate whether the specimen is acceptable (A) or unacceptable (U) for anaerobic culture:

11. Peritoneal fluid
12. Vaginal swab
13. Exudate from abscess
14. Feces

15. Necrotic tissue
16. Sputum
17. Tissue from liver abscess
18. Swab of wound
19. Which of the following is the environment achieved in the anaerobic glove box?
    a. 85% hydrogen, 5% carbon dioxide, 5% nitrogen
    b. 85% nitrogen, 10% hydrogen, 5% carbon dioxide
    c. 85% oxygen, 10% hydrogen, 5% carbon dioxide
    d. 75% nitrogen, 15% hydrogen, 10% carbon dioxide
20. After the incubation of cultures in an anaerobic jar, the methylene blue strip has reverted to its original blue color. This indicates:
    a. Anaerobiosis has been achieved.
    b. Oxygen may have entered the system.
    c. The system has failed.
    d. Both b and c are correct.
    e. All are correct.
21. An organism isolated from anaerobic blood agar was subcultured onto chocolate agar, which was incubated aerobically with increased CO_2, and anaerobic blood agar, which was incubated anaerobically. After 48 hours, growth was evident on only the anaerobic blood agar plate. This organism is most likely:
    a. An obligate aerobe
    b. An obligate anaerobe
    c. A facultative anaerobe
    d. Capnophilic
22. The group of anaerobes most frequently associated with human infection is the:
    a. Gram-positive spore-forming bacilli
    b. Gram-positive non–spore-forming bacilli
    c. Gram-negative bacilli
    d. Gram-positive cocci
    e. Gram-negative cocci
23. The pigmented saccharolytic gram-negative bacilli belong to the genus:
    a. *Bacteroides*
    b. *Prevotella*
    c. *Porphyromonas*
    d. *Clostridium*
    e. *Veillonella*
24. A gram-negative anaerobic bacillus produced nonhemolytic colonies on ABA. The following biochemical reactions were noted:
    BBE: Growth with positive hydrolysis
    Catalase: Positive
    Lecithinase: Negative
    Lipase: Negative
    Starch hydrolysis: Negative
    Milk digested: Negative
    DNase: Negative
    Fermentation of glucose and lactose: Positive
    Fermentation of mannitol and rhamnose: Negative
    This organism is most likely:
    a. *Porphyromonas asaccharolytica*
    b. *Fusobacterium nucleatum*
    c. *Prevotella intermedius*
    d. *Bacteroides fragilis*
    e. *Veillonella*
25. A gram-negative anaerobic bacillus with tapered or pointed ends and opalescent with speckles is most likely:
    a. *Porphyromonas asaccharolytica*
    b. *Fusobacterium nucleatum*
    c. *Prevotella intermedius*
    d. *Bacteroides fragilis*
26. The spores of *Clostridium tetani* are located:
    a. Centrally
    b. Subterminally
    c. Terminally
    d. *C. tetani* does not have spores.
27. Food poisoning from *Clostridium botulinum* is most often caused by:
    a. Contaminated poultry products
    b. Improperly home-canned foods
    c. Dairy products and custards
    d. Contaminated and poorly cooked seafood
28. Which of the following reactions is *incorrect* for *Clostridium perfringens*?
    a. Lecithinase positive
    b. Ferments glucose and maltose
    c. Motile
    d. Double zone of hemolysis on anaerobic blood agar
29. *Clostridium difficile* is most commonly identified by:
    a. Demonstration of cytotoxin
    b. Identification of *C. difficile* common antigen
    c. Isolation of organism from stool culture
    d. Demonstration of lecithinase
30. A gram-positive non–spore-forming bacillus isolated from an abscess in a patient recovering from a bone marrow transplant produced white, heaped colonies on anaerobic blood agar. The Gram stain of the abscess revealed branching, diphtheroid, gram-positive bacilli with sulfur granules. This organism is most likely:
    a. *Clostridium perfringens*
    b. *Bifidobacterium*
    c. *Streptococcus anaerobius*
    d. *Actinomyces israelii*
31. *Propionibacterium acnes* was isolated in one tube of a set of three blood cultures. The other two tubes revealed no growth, and no organisms were seen on the Gram stain. This most likely indicates:
    a. Septicemia from the organism
    b. Failure to inoculate the negative bottles properly with blood
    c. Skin contamination from improper disinfection before venipuncture
    d. None of the above

Bibliography

Baron, E. J. (2011). Approaches to identification of anaerobic bacteria. In J. Versalovic (Ed.), *Manual of clinical microbiology*, 10th ed. (electronic). Washington, DC: American Society for Microbiology.

Centers for Disease Control and Prevention. (2006). Surveillance for food borne disease outbreaks—United States. *Mortality and Morbidity Weekly Report, 58,* 609–615.

Centers for Disease Control and Prevention. (2007). Botulism associated with commercially canned chili sauce—Texas and Indiana. *Mortality and Morbidity Weekly Report, 56,* 96–97.

Centers for Disease Control and Prevention. (2013). *Clostridium difficile* infection. Retrieved from http://www.cdc.gov/HAI/organisms/cdiff/Cdiff_infect.html

Clinical and Laboratory Standards Institute. (2012). *Methods for antimicrobial susceptibility testing of anaerobic bacteria*, 8th ed. Wayne, PA.

Finegold, S. M., Rosenblatt, J. E., Sutter, V. L., & Attebery, H. R. (1976). *Scope monograph on anaerobic infections.* Kalamazoo, MI: Upjohn Co.

Lindström, M., & Korkeala, H. (2006). Laboratory diagnostics of botulism. *Clinical Microbiology Reviews, 19,* 298–314.

Murdach, D. A. (1998). Gram-positive anaerobic cocci. *Clinical Microbiology Reviews, 11,* 81–129.

Nucci, M., & Anaissie, E. (2007). *Fusarium* infections in immunocompromised patients. *Clinical Microbiology Reviews, 20,* 695–704.

Song, Y., & Finegold, S. M. (2011). *Peptostreptococcus, Finegoldia, Anaerococcus, Peptoniphilus, Veillonella* and other anaerobic cocci. In J. Versalovic (Ed.), *Manual of clinical microbiology*, 10th ed. (electronic). Washington, DC: American Society for Microbiology.

Stevens, D. L., Bryant, A. E., Berger, A., & von Eichel-Streiber, C. (2011). *Clostridium.* In J. Versalovic (Ed.), *Manual of clinical microbiology*, 10th ed. (electronic). Washington, DC: American Society for Microbiology.

Sutter, V. L., & Finegold, S. M. (1971). Antibiotic susceptibility tests for rapid presumptive identification of gram-negative anaerobic bacilli. *Applied Microbiology, 21,* 13–20.

Turton, L. J., Drucker, D. B., Hillier, V. F., & Ganguli, L. A. (1983). Effect of eight growth media upon fermentation profiles of ten anaerobic bacteria. *Journal of Applied Bacteriology, 54,* 295–304.

Wexler, H. M. (2007). *Bacteroides*: The good, the bad, and the nitty-gritty. *Clinical Microbiology Reviews, 20,* 593–621.

Winn, Jr., W., Allen, S., Janda, W., Koneman, E., Procop, G., Schreckenberger, P., & Woods, G. (2006). The anaerobic bacteria. In *Koneman's color atlas and textbook of diagnostic microbiology*, 6th ed. (pp. 309–391). Philadelphia, PA: Lippincott Williams & Wilkins.

NEWS: *CLOSTRIDIUM DIFFICILE* INFECTION (CDI)

Clostridium difficile colonizes the intestines of a small percentage of the healthy population. When individuals are placed on broad-spectrum antibiotics, especially the fluoroquinolones, clindamycin, broad-spectrum penicillins, or broad-spectrum cephalosporins, the normal intestinal flora is suppressed. *C. difficile* is resistant to the effects of these antibiotics, and overgrowth occurs with the production of two toxins. Toxin A is a an enterotoxin that attracts neutrophils and stimulates the production of cytokines, and toxin B is a cytotoxin that attacks the cells in the intestinal wall, causing increased permeability and diarrhea.

Spore formation by the organism allows it to remain in the physical environment and on patients, which enhances its transmission. Any surface or material that becomes contaminated with *C. difficile*–contaminated feces may be a source of infection. Spores also can be transmitted to patients through the contaminated hands of health care personnel and through contaminated medical devices.

To treat *C. difficile* infection, the antibiotic should be discontinued, and a new antibiotic treatment initiated. Possible choices include metronidazole or vancomycin. Unfortunately, the infection may reoccur, so multiple courses may be needed until the spores and infection are destroyed.

CDI can be prevented by judicious use of antibiotics and contact precautions for those patients with known or suspected *C. difficile* infection. Patients' rooms should be cleaned with soap and water because alcohol does not kill the spores, which are extremely difficult to remove. Thorough hand washing and appropriate glove use by health care personnel are also important. Personnel protective equipment should be used when necessary. Sporicidal disinfectants and dilute bleach also are useful agents to control the organism.

While most concern remains with hospital-associated *C. difficile* infections, there have been some cases of community-acquired *C. difficile*-associated diarrhea. Risk factors for the community-acquired infection include increasing age, underlying health problems, antibiotic exposure, and contact with persons who are infected with and shedding *C. difficile*.

A hypervirulent strain of *C. difficile* was reported in 2006 in the United States, Canada, and Europe. The strain, known as NAP1/BI/027, has a gene mutation that affects the regulation of enterotoxin and cytotoxin production. This results in excessive amounts of toxin production by the organism with a more severe disease, higher occurrence of relapse, and higher mortality. This strain also has enhanced sporulation and is resistant to the fluoroquinolone antibiotics.

BIBLIOGRAPHY

Centers for Disease Control and Prevention. (2007). Surveillance for community-associated *Clostridium difficile*—Connecticut, *57*(13), 340–343.

O'Donoghue, C., & Kyne, L. (2001). Update on *Clostridium difficile* infection. *Current Opinion in Gastroenterology, 27,* 38–47.

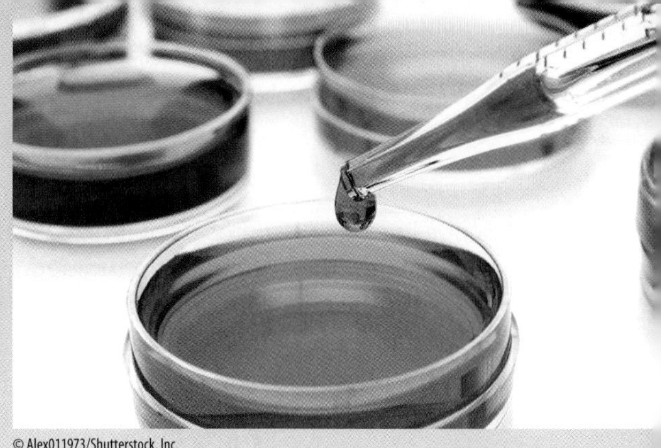
© Alex011973/Shutterstock, Inc.

CHAPTER 17
Mycobacterium

CHAPTER OUTLINE

Classification

Mycobacterium tuberculosis Complex

KEY TERMS

Acid-fast bacilli (AFB)
Hansen's disease
Multidrug-resistant tuberculosis
Mycobacterium tuberculosis complex
Mycobacteria other than tubercle bacilli
Nonchromogen
Nontuberculosis mycobacteria
Photochromogen
Rapid grower
Reactivation tuberculosis
Scotochromogen
Tuberculosis

LEARNING OBJECTIVES

1. Explain why mycobacteria are known as "acid-fast bacilli."
2. Discuss safety measures to be observed when working with mycobacteria.
3. Describe the processes of digestion and decontamination for mycobacteria.
4. a. Name and give examples of the three categories of media used to cultivate mycobacteria; compare the composition and use of each.
   b. Correctly inoculate and incubate mycobacterial media.
5. Contrast the Kinyoun and Ziehl-Neelsen stains. Perform and interpret at least three Kinyoun stains.
6. When given the number of acid-fast bacilli (AFB) seen per number of fields, state the CDC rating.
7. State the principle and purpose of the following assays:
   a. Photochromogenicity assay
   b. Niacin accumulation
   c. Nitrate reduction
   d. Heat-stable catalase
   e. Tween 80 hydrolysis
   f. Arylsulfatase
   g. Pyrazinamidase
   h. Urease
   i. Growth in 5% NaCL
   j. Iron uptake
8. Perform and interpret each of the following assays:
   a. Photochromogenicity
   b. Niacin accumulation
   c. Nitrate reduction
   d. Tween 80 hydrolysis
   e. Arylsulfatase
9. List the members of the *Mycobacterium tuberculosis* complex and describe their clinical relevance.
10. Discuss the nontuberculosis mycobacteria (NTM) and state their important characteristics.
11. Name the Runyon groups (non tuberculosis mycobacterium) and describe the characteristics of each.

12. Describe the infectious process of tuberculosis.
    a. Explain how the infection is transmitted.
    b. Describe the infectious process and relate the importance of cell-mediated immunity.
13. Discuss the principle and purpose of the tuberculin skin test and interferon gamma release assays.
14. State the important morphological and biochemical characteristics of *M. tuberculosis* and relate how it is identified.
15. Briefly discuss the molecular diagnostic techniques available for mycobacteria.
16. Discuss how tuberculosis is treated and list some first- and second-line drugs.
17. For each of the following mycobacteria, state the Runyon group (when applicable), briefly describe its clinical significance, and discuss its identification:
    a. *M. ulcerans*
    b. *M. bovis*
    c. *M. leprae*
    d. *M. kansasii*
    e. *M. marinum*
    f. *M. simiae*
    g. *M. scrofulaceum*
    h. *M. szulgai*
    i. *M. gordonae*
    j. *M. xenopi*
    k. *M. avium-intracellulare* complex
    l. *M. haemophilum*
    m. *M. fortuitum-chelonei* complex

Mycobacteria are the agents of **tuberculosis** and other chronic infections in humans. The organisms are slender, slow-growing bacilli, which are obligate aerobes. Growth is enhanced under increased carbon dioxide (CO_2). Cell division typically occurs by branching. More than 60% of the cell wall contains lipid, and numerous lipid-containing structures have been isolated from the mycobacterial cell wall, including **cord factor wax D** and **mycolic acid.** These organisms have the characteristics of a gram-positive cell wall, although the mycobacteria do not readily Gram stain. In fact, stains must be driven into the cell wall of the mycobacteria either through heating or the use of detergent. The bound lipid in the cell wall permits mycobacteria to bind to alkaline stains, such as carbolfuchsin. Once stained, the mycobacteria are difficult to decolorize, even when using acid-alcohol as a decolorizer. Thus, the *Mycobacterium* organisms are commonly referred to as **acid-fast bacilli** (AFB).

First isolated by Robert Koch as the cause of tuberculosis, the organism was originally named *Bacterium tuberculosis* by Zoppfin in 1886. It was later renamed *Mycobacterium tuberculosis* by Neumann because of its fungus-like characteristics ("myco"). Unlike most other bacterial infections, tuberculosis is classified as a chronic infectious disease because mycobacteria can remain chronically within the host. *Mycobacterium bovis* was identified as a cause of tuberculosis in cattle in the early 20th century, and *Mycobacterium avium* was identified as a pathogen for chickens. Today, there are over 130 species of *Mycobacterium*. Many are saprobes, which are distributed widely in the environment and in animals and are not considered to be pathogenic for humans. However, others are important human pathogens and the cause of serious infections.

Classification

There are different schemes to classify and categorize mycobacteria. Until the 1980s, mycobacteria were classified based primarily on phenotypic studies, including traditional culture and growth characteristics and biochemical analysis. Beginning in the 1990s, genotypic studies became increasingly important in the identification of mycobacteria. Currently, mycobacteria are categorized as either members of the ***Mycobacterium tuberculosis* complex** (MTBC) or as members of the **nontuberculosis mycobacteria (NTM)**. The *Mycobacterium tuberculosis* complex contains the most clinically significant human pathogens; all of these species are capable of causing tuberculosis. MTBC includes *M. tuberculosis*, *M. bovis*, *M. africanum*, *M. carnetti*, and *M. microti*. The NTM formerly have been known as the "atypical mycobacteria" and **mycobacteria other than tubercle bacilli** (MOTT). In 1959, Runyon classified the MOTT into the four **Runyon groups** based on production of pigment and growth characteristics. The NTM are found in the environment and may cause pulmonary, soft tissue, and lymphatic infections in those with predisposing medical factors, such as chronic obstructive pulmonary disease, in the immunosuppressed and the elderly.

Because many mycobacterial infections, especially tuberculosis, are spread through inhalation of contaminated droplets, laboratory safety measures are extremely important when performing any laboratory procedures to prevent laboratory-associated infections. BOX 17-1 lists safety measures to prevent laboratory infections that are associated with mycobacteria.

BOX 17-1 Safety Measures for Mycobacteria

- It is imperative to employ all measures to minimize the risk of aerosol production. Biosafety Level 3 (BSL 3) is recommended for all procedures that may involve *M. tuberculosis* or *M. bovis*. All procedures should be performed using a BSL 3 safety cabinet and centrifuge. The biological safety hood should have directional airflow, with the lowest pressure in the laboratory. The air is vented directly to the outside from the BSL space, using high-efficiency particulate air filters. All centrifuges must be BSL 3 and have carrier shields or aerosol-free tops.
- Laboratory personnel must use personal protective equipment (PPE), which includes respirators, caps, face masks, gloves, disposable gown over scrubs, and shoe covers for all procedures. These items must be bagged and autoclaved.
- Employees must be screened with a tuberculin skin test (TST), such as the purified protein derivative (PPD), and chest X-ray annually. Two-step testing may be used for those who will be retested periodically. There are also interferon-gamma release assay (IGRA) blood tests for TB infection, which may be used for annual screening.
- The mycobacterial laboratory should be housed in a room separate from other parts of the microbiology laboratory. The room must have impermeable walls and work surface. A germicide, such as phenol with soap, must be used to decontaminate the laboratory work station.

SPECIMEN COLLECTION

Tuberculosis most frequently involves the lung, although other body sites and organs may be infected. Respiratory specimens are submitted to diagnose pulmonary tuberculosis and include expectorated or nebulized sputum, secretions obtained through bronchoscopy, transtracheal aspirates, or laryngeal swabs. Sputum should represent lung secretions collected from a deep cough. Early morning specimens collected on three consecutive days are recommended to enhance the recovery of mycobacteria. For those who are unable to produce a specimen, sputum may be induced by having the patient inhale warmed aerosolized sodium chloride. Twenty-four-hour collections are discouraged because of the increased possibility of bacterial contamination. A gastric lavage may be collected for those who cannot provide a sputum sample, such as children.

Urine specimens should be collected on three consecutive mornings and centrifuged to concentrate the mycobacteria. Sterile specimens, such as cerebrospinal fluid, synovial fluid, pericardial fluid, and peritoneal fluid, also are centrifuged for concentration. The sediment is used for staining and inoculation onto suitable media.

Blood is prepared through lysis centrifugation, which will enhance the recovery of the organism. An anticoagulant and a lysing agent, such as saponin, are used in this method. The lysing agent ruptures the red and white blood cells, releasing the mycobacteria. A biphasic culture system with modified Middlebrook 7H11 and oleic acid and albumin as the agar phase and brain heart infusion used as the broth phase is recommended.

Tissue specimens, such as bone marrow, lymph node, and liver specimens, should be homogenized.

Fecal specimens are collected to isolate *Mycobacterium avium-intracellulare* (MAI) complex, a mycobacterial species found with increasing frequency in patients with acquired immunodeficiency syndrome (AIDS). The specimen is directly stained for acid-fast bacilli. If the slide is positive for AFB, the stool is decontaminated, concentrated, and suspended in Middlebrook 7H9 broth and then plated onto the appropriate isolation medium.

SPECIMEN PROCESSING

Specimens submitted for identification of mycobacteria that may be contaminated with normal flora bacteria or other bacterial contaminants must be **decontaminated**.

Mycobacteria are slow growing compared with other bacterial organisms and can be overgrown by contaminants, normal flora, or other pathogens in the specimen. Sputum may contain these bacterial contaminants, which requires decontamination of the specimen to enhance the recovery of the mycobacteria. There is no need to decontaminate sterile specimens, such as cerebrospinal fluid or blood. Unfortunately, decontamination also may destroy some of the mycobacteria, although the mycobacteria are more resistant to the effects of strong alkali than other organisms found in sputum. Suitable agents for decontamination are weak bases, such as 2% NaOH or benzalkonium chloride. Sputum samples also must be **digested**, which splits the disulfide bonds present in mucin, which may trap the mycobacteria. Agents for digestion include N-acetyl-L-cysteine and dithiothreitol. BOX 17-2 provides examples of methods for decontamination and digestion of mycobacteria.

Once decontaminated and digested, sputum specimens must be centrifuged using a high centrifugal force to concentrate the mycobacteria. Specimens should be centrifuged at either 3,000Xg for 15 minutes or 2,000Xg for 20 minutes.

BOX 17-2 **Methods for Digestion and Decontamination of Mycobacteria**

- N-acetyl-L-cysteine (NALC) and 2% NaOH

  NALC splits disulfide bonds, and 2% NaOH is antibacterial.

  Most common method used
- Trisodium phosphate and benzalkonium chloride (Zephiran)

  Recommended when *Pseudomonas* is present in sample
- Dithiothreitol and 2% NaOH

  Similar to NALC and 2% NaOH; commercially known as Sputolysin
- 4% NaOH

  Strong alkali acts as both a mucolytic and an antibacterial agent. Exposure time must be limited to 15 minutes because the strong alkali also may kill the mycobacteria.

STAINING

The **acid-fast stain** is an important tool in the preliminary identification of the mycobacteria. A positive smear provides a presumptive but vital clue for the clinician in the diagnosis of tuberculosis when combined with other clinical symptoms. However, a negative acid-fast stain does not eliminate the possibility of tuberculosis, because of limitations in its sensitivity. The acid-fast stain also is to be used to monitor the course of treatment. In the acid-fast stain method, **carbolfuchsin** binds to the mycolic acid in the cell wall of mycobacteria, using heat or detergent to drive the stain into the cell wall. The stain cannot be removed, even with acid alcohol, giving the mycobacteria the property of acid fastness. In the **Ziehl-Neelsen technique**, or the "hot method," fuchsin and hot phenol are driven into the cell wall of the organism. In the **Kinyoun technique**, or "cold method," detergent is used to force the carbolfuchsin into the mycobacterial cell wall. Methylene blue may be used as a counterstain in both methods, and stains the other bacteria a blue color. FIGURE 17-1 illustrates mycobacteria stained with carbolfuchsin.

Fluorochrome stains also may be used to directly stain specimens for acid-fast bacilli (AFB). **Auramine O** stains mycobacteria a yellow-green color, and **rhodamine** is used as the counterstain, which stains the other bacteria a red fluorescent color. Fluorochrome stains are more sensitive but are more labor intensive and costly to perform than are carbolfuchsin stains. A larger area of the smear is scanned in fluorochrome stains.

Smears that are prepared from concentrated specimens improve the sensitivity of staining for mycobacteria.

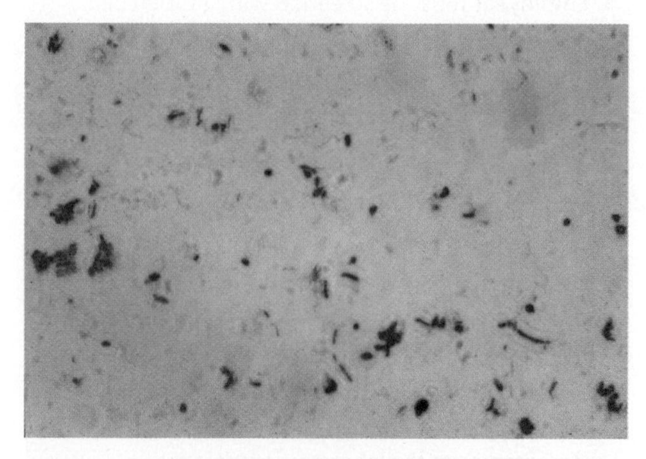

FIGURE 17-1 Carbolfuchsin stain showing red-staining acid-fast bacilli.

TABLE 17-1 CDC Method to Report Acid-Fast Bacilli (AFB)

Number of AFB seen carbolfuchsin (× 1,000)	Fluorochrome (× 250)	Report
No AFB/300 fields	No AFB/30 fields	No AFB seen
1–2 AFB/300 fields	1–2 AFB/30 fields	Doubtful—repeat test
l–9 AFB/100 fields	1–9 AFB/10 fields	Rare or 1+
l–9 AFB/10 fields	1–9 AFB/field	Few or 2+
1–9AFB/field	10–90 AFB/field	Moderate or 3+
More than 9 AFB/field	More than 90 AFB/field	Numerous or 4+

Data from Centers for Disease Control.

However, smears also can be prepared directly from clinical specimens. The Centers for Disease Control and Prevention (CDC) provides a semiquantitative method to report AFB (TABLE 17-1). Slides showing questionable results, such as doubtful, are repeated on a second slide.

CULTURE MEDIA

After digestion and decontamination, when needed, clinical specimens suspected of containing mycobacteria are plated onto culture media. Culture is needed for several reasons; it is more sensitive than microscopy. Growth is needed for biochemical identification and most susceptibility testing and cultured organisms are needed for genotyping. There are different types of nonselective culture media, including egg-based media, such as Lowenstein-Jensen; agar based, such as Middlebrook 7H10 and 7H11; and broth, such as Middlebrook 7H9. Each of these can be modified with antibiotics, which creates a more selective media. Most laboratories recommend the use of one of each type of media.

Mycobacterium species require whole egg for growth. Examples of **nonselective media** include **Löwenstein-Jensen, Petragnani**, and **American Thoracic Society**. These media, prepared as agar slants, contain coagulated whole egg, glycerol, salt, potato flour, and malachite green, which acts as an inhibitor. Petragnani contains a higher concentration of malachite green and is more inhibitory than are the other non-selective media. American Thoracic Society contains a lesser amount of malachite green, is less inhibitory, and may allow the growth of other bacterial contaminants. Nonselective media should be incubated for 6 to 10 weeks and examined weekly for growth.

Agar-based media include Middlebrook 7H10 and Middlebrook 7H11. These media are transparent, and growth can be detected earlier than on the nonselective media. For example, growth may be detected as early as 10 to 12 days on Middlebrook agar compared to 18 to 24 days on the Löwenstein-Jensen (LJ) slants. Middlebrook media contain salts, vitamins, catalase, biotin, cofactors, oleic acid, albumin, and glycerol. Middlebrook 7H10 also contains dextrose, and 7H11 contains casein hydrolysate. Both media contain malachite green as an inhibitory agent. Middlebrook 7H9 is a broth with a similar formulation.

Selective media may enhance the recovery of the mycobacteria but also may inhibit their growth. These media have antibiotics designed to inhibit bacterial or fungal contaminants. In the **Gruft modified Löwenstein-Jensen slant**, ribonucleic acid (RNA), penicillin, and nalidixic acid are incorporated into the LJ slant. In the **selective Middlebrook 7H11 agar**, carbenicillin, amphotericin B, polymyxin B, and trimethoprim sulfate are added to Middlebrook 7H11 agar.

BOX 17-3 summarizes mycobacterial media.

Mycobacterium species exhibit a variable temperature for optimal growth. Species that infect the skin, such as *M. marinum* and *M. ulcerans*, grow best at 30°C to 32°C, whereas those that are environmental contaminants, such as *M. xenopi*, prefer 42°C to 45°C. *M. tuberculosis*, which usually infects the lungs and other internal organs in humans, grows optimally at 35°C to 37°C. Thus, it is important to note the site of infection and incubate cultures at the appropriate incubation temperature. Media should be incubated with loosened caps for the first week of incubation for Middlebrook media and for the first three weeks for LJ slants to permit circulation of CO_2. After this time, the caps are tightened to prevent dehydration and then loosened briefly once per week. Culture plates are generally incubated for a total of 8 to 10 weeks before growth is reported as negative.

IDENTIFICATION

Because of newer methods in the identification of *Mycobacterium*, biochemical procedures have a diminished significance. Biochemical procedures are cumbersome to perform and often require a lengthy reaction or incubation period to determine the result. Molecular techniques, such as nucleic acid probes for *M. tuberculosis* complex and *M. avium-intracellulare* complex, *M. kansasii*, and *M. gordonae* are available. Molecular techniques permit a more rapid and accurate identification. Automated methods also

BOX 17-3 **Mycobacterial Media**

Nonselective: Egg Based

Löwenstein-Jensen: Coagulated whole eggs, salts, glycerol, potato flour, malachite green inhibitory agent (0.025 g/dl)

Petragnani: Coagulated whole eggs, egg yolks, whole milk, potato flour, glycerol, malachite green inhibitory agent (0.052 g/dl); more inhibitory than other nonselective media—use for heavily contaminated specimens

American Thoracic Society: Coagulated egg yolks, potato flour, glycerol, malachite green inhibitory agent (0.02 g/dl); less inhibitory than other nonselective media—use for sterile specimens

Nonselective Agar Based (Transparent)

Middlebrook 7H10: Salts, vitamins, cofactors, oleic acid, albumin, catalase, biotin, glycerol, glucose, malachite green inhibitory agent (0.0025 g/dl)

Middlebrook 7H11: Salts, vitamins, cofactors, oleic acid, albumin, catalase, biotin, glycerol, casein hydrolysate, malachite green inhibitory agent (0.0025 g/dl)

Selective Media

Gruft modified Löwenstein-Jensen: LJ slant with RNA, penicillin, and nalidixic acid

Selective Löwenstein-Jensen: LJ slant with cycloheximide, lincomycin, and nalidixic acid

Selective Middlebrook 7H10: Middlebrook 7H10 with cycloheximide, lincomycin, and nalidixic acid

Selective Middlebrook 7H11 (Mitchison's): Middlebrook 7H11 with carbenicillin, amphotericin B, polymyxin B, and trimethoprim lactate

can be used to decrease the time to isolate and identify mycobacteria from sputum and blood specimens. Thus, a combination of traditional microscopy, culture, biochemical methods, and molecular techniques may be used to identify mycobacteria. A brief summary of the traditional biochemical techniques follows.

Biochemical Reactions

1. **Growth rate.** Mycobacteria exhibit a wide range of growth times. The average time is 3 weeks but may range from 3 to 60 days. Those that grow within 7 days are known as **rapid growers**, and those that need longer than 7 days are known as slow growers. Growth is defined as visible colonies without the use of magnification.
2. **Pigment production.** Some *Mycobacterium* species have the ability to develop pigment because of the presence of carotenoids. Runyon described groups of the nontuberculosis mycobacterium (NTM) and categorized them into groups based on pigment production. Those mycobacteria that develop a yellow to orange pigment only when exposed to light are categorized as **photochromogens**. Mycobacteria that are pigmented in the light and dark are classified as **scotochromogens**. Scotochromogens have a yellow to deep orange pigment in the dark, which intensifies to an orange to red when exposed to a constant light source. Those mycobacteria that do not develop pigment are known as **nonchromogens**. Nonchromogens have an off-white, tan, buff, or very pale yellow color. Pigment production is determined through a **chromogenicity assay.** BOX 17-4 summarizes some of the more important mycobacteria based on the Runyon classification by pigment production.
3. **Colonial morphology.** Growth of young colonies is observed at approximately 5 to 14 days; the size, pigmentation, elevation (flat or raised), and consistency (smooth or rough) are noted.
4. **Growth temperature.** Because mycobacteria grow at a wide temperature range, it is important to determine the optimal growth temperatures. Most human pathogens grow optimally between 35°C ± 2°C, but some may grow at temperatures as low as 30°C ± 2°C. *M. marinum* grows optimally at 30°C, and *M. haemophilium* grows best at 25°C. *M. xenopi* prefers a higher temperature of 42°C.

BOX 17-4 Runyon Classification of Mycobacteria Other Than Tubercle Bacilli (MOTT) or Nontuberculosis Mycobacteria (NTM)

Group I: Photochromogens

Develop yellow pigment when exposed to constant light source; nonpigmented in dark

M. kansasii

M. marinum

M. simiae

M. asiaticum

Group II: Scotochromogens

Pigmented yellow to orange in dark. Pigment intensifies to orange or red when exposed to constant light source for 2 weeks.

M. scrofulaceum

M. szulgai (at 35°C–37°C)

M. xenopi (young cultures may be nonpigmented)

M. gordonae

M. flavescens

M. thermoresistible

Group III: Nonphotochromogens

White to tan in color; cannot develop pigment on exposure to light

M. avium

M. gastri

M. intracellulare

M. malmoense

M. haemophilum

M. terrae complex

M. triviale

M. ulcerans

Group IV: Rapid Growers

Grow in 3 to 5 days in culture media; saprophytes

M. fortuitum complex

M. chelonae

M. phlei

M. smegmatis

5. **Niacin accumulation.** All *Mycobacterium* species produce niacin, and most possess another enzyme that converts free niacin to niacin ribonucleotide. Only *M. tuberculosis*; *M. simiae*; and rare strains of *M. bovis*, *M. marinum*, and *M. chelonei* cannot convert free niacin to niacin ribonucleotide; this results in the accumulation of niacin. Commercially available reagent strips impregnated with cyanogen bromide are inoculated with the organism. In a positive reaction a yellow color indicates the accumulation of free niacin, which is useful in the identification of *M. tuberculosis*.
6. **Nitrate reduction.** Mycobacteria that possess the enzyme nitroreductase can convert nitrates (NO_3) to nitrites (NO_2). The test can be performed using broth or commercial filter paper strips impregnated with sodium nitrate. In a positive reaction the filter paper strip changes to a blue color. In the broth method, sodium nitrate broth is inoculated with the organism. Hydrochloric acid, sulfanilamide, and N-l-naphthylethylenediamine is added. A positive reaction is indicated by the development of a pink to red color. Mycobacteria that give a positive nitrate reaction include *M. tuberculosis*, *M. kansasii*, *M. szulgai*, *M. fortuitum*, and *M. flavescens*. Negative reactions are seen with *M. bovis*, *M. marinum*, *M. simiae*, *M. gastri*, and *M. avium-intracellulare* complex.
7. **Catalase and heat-stable catalase.** Most *Mycobacterium* species are catalase positive. However, not all are positive for heat-stable catalase. In this procedure the isolate is heated at 68°C for 20 minutes, cooled, and reacted with 30% hydrogen peroxide. Negative reactions are characteristic of all members of the *M. tuberculosis* complex, which include *M. tuberculosis*, *M. bovis*, *M. africanum*, *M. ulcerans*, *M. leprae*, and *M. microti*.
8. **Tween 80 hydrolysis.** Tween 80 (polyoxyethylene sorbitan monooleate) is converted to oleic acid by Tween 80 lipase. The test is most useful in the identification of *M. kansasii*, which gives a positive reaction as quickly as 6 hours. The test also is useful in differentiation of the similar *M. gordonae* (Tween 80 positive) from *M. scrofulaceum* (Tween 80 negative).
9. **Arylsulfatase.** Arylsulfatase splits the sulfate group from tripotassium phenolphthalein to form free phenolphthalein. The test is useful in the identification of the *M. fortuitum-chelonei* group, which produces a positive reaction in 3 days.

10. **Pyrazinamidase.** In this reaction, pyrazinamidase is converted to pyrazinoic acid and ammonia. Pyrazinoic acid is detected by reaction with 1% ammonium sulfate. *M. tuberculosis* and *M. marinum* are positive, whereas *M. bovis* and *M. kansasii* are negative.
11. **Urease.** Those mycobacteria that possess the urease enzyme can hydrolyze urea to ammonia and carbon dioxide. The presence of urease is most useful in the identification of *M. scrofulaceum*, *M. gastri*, and *M. bovis*, which are urease positive, and *M. gordonae* and *M. avium-intracellulare*, which are urease negative.
12. **Growth in 5% NaCl.** Most mycobacteria cannot grow in 5% sodium chloride (NaCl). The test is useful in the identification of *M. triviale*, which is the only slow grower that gives a positive reaction. *M. flavescens* also can grow in 5% NaCl.
13. **Iron uptake.** Only the rapid growers are able to grow in 20% ferric citrate. The test is most useful in the differentiation of the *M. fortuitum-chelonei* complex. *M. fortuitum* gives a positive iron uptake reaction, whereas *M. chelonei* gives a negative result.
14. **Growth on MacConkey agar.** The rapid-growing mycobacteria can grow on MacConkey agar that does not contain crystal violet. Most other mycobacteria are unable to grow on this agar.

Methods for the chromogenicity assay, niacin accumulation, nitrate reduction, arylsulfatase, and Tween 80 hydrolysis are found at the end of the chapter.

There are several automated systems to identify mycobacteria. Gas-liquid chromatography can be used to analyze the long-chain fatty acids. Automated methods include the BACTEC™ 460TB (Becton Dickinson), the BACTEC™ MGIT™ 960 (Becton Dickinson), the BACTEC™ Myco/F Lytic (Becton Dickinson), the ESP Culture System II (Trek Diagnostics), and the MB/BacT (bioMérieux).

Molecular diagnostic methods available include nucleic acid probes, which are used to identify mycobacteria in positive cultures. There are currently probes available for the *M. tuberculosis* complex, *M. avium-intracellulare*, *M. kansasii*, and *M. gordonae*. DNA sequencing permits the identification of specific genetic regions in clinically significant mycobacteria. Strain typing and DNA fingerprinting are useful for epidemiological studies. Molecular techniques are sensitive and specific but require complex laboratory skills and technology. As more molecular diagnostic tools become available, these methods will be used more frequently to identify the pathogenic mycobacteria.

TABLE 17-2 outlines morphological and biochemical characteristics of *M. tuberculosis* and other clinically significant mycobacteria.

Mycobacterium tuberculosis Complex

MYCOBACTERIUM TUBERCULOSIS AND TUBERCULOSIS

Most cases of tuberculosis are caused by *Mycobacterium tuberculosis*, which is found only in humans. Unlike most other bacterial diseases, tuberculosis is classified as a chronic infection. There are over 8 million new cases identified each year worldwide. Additionally, the World Health Organization estimates that there are over 3 million deaths each year from tuberculosis. There were approximately 11,500 cases of tuberculosis in the United States in 2009; the case count has continued to decline in the United States since 1993. However, there are higher rates in specific populations, who include foreign-born people, and U.S. borne blacks. In 2007, there were approximately 500 deaths from tuberculosis in the United States.

At the turn of the 20th century, tuberculosis was the second leading cause of death in the United States. Those with tuberculosis were sent to sanatoriums, health care facilities that provided therapy of bed rest, open air, and sunshine. The successful use of antibiotics, streptomycin and isoniazid (INH), as well as improvements in working conditions, had led to the decline of the disease. In fact, by the 1970s, most sanatoriums were closed. An increase in tuberculosis occurred in the 1980s and was related to the human immunodeficiency virus (HIV) epidemic, increased immigration from countries where tuberculosis is prevalent, and increased transmission in homeless shelters and prisons. There also has been an increased incidence of multidrug-resistant tuberculosis. Generally, a disease of impoverished persons who live in close quarters, the infection has been increasing in areas of crowding, poor ventilation, poverty, and poor nutrition. In addition, tuberculosis infections often are found in those individuals who have AIDS. Tuberculosis always has been and continues to be a disease that occurs disproportionately

TABLE 17-2 *M. tuberculosis* Complex

Test	*M. tuberculosis*	*M. bovis*	*M. africanum*		
Colonial morphology	**Rough nonpigmented**	**Rough nonpigmented**	**Rough nonpigmented**		
Niacin accumulation	+	–	–		
Nitrate reduction	+	–	–		
Heat-stable catalase	–	–	–		
Urease	V	+	+		
Tween 80 hydrolysis	V	–	–		
Arylsulfatase (3 days)	–	–	–		
5% NaCl (growth)	–	–	–		
Iron uptake	–	–	–		
Growth on MacConkey agar (without crystal violet)	–	–	–		
Pyrazinamidase	+	–	–		
Scotochromagens					
Test	***M. scrofulaceum***	***M. szulgai***	***M. gordonae***	***M. flavescens***	
Colonial morphology	**Smooth pigmented**	**Smooth or rough pigmented**	**Smooth pigmented**	**Smooth pigmented**	
Niacin accumulation	–	–	–	–	
Nitrate reduction	–	+	–	+	
Heat-stable catalase	+	+	+	+	
Urease	+	+	V	+	
Tween 80 hydrolysis	–	Slow +	+	+	
Arylsulfatase (3 days)	V	–	–	–	
5% NaCl (growth)	–	–	–	+	
Iron uptake	–	–	–	V	
MacConkey agar (without crystal violet)	–	–	–	–	
Pyrazinamidase	+	+	–	+	
Photochromogens					
Test	***M. kansasii***	***M. marinum***	***M. simiae***	***M. asiaticum***	
Colonial morphology	**Smooth or rough pigmented**	**Smooth or rough pigmented**	**Smooth pigmented**	**Smooth pigmented**	
Niacin accumulation	–	V	V	–	
Nitrate reduction	+	–	–	–	
Heat-stable catalase	+	–	+	+	
Urease	V	V	+	–	
Tween 80 hydrolysis	+	+	–	+	
Arylsulfatase (3 days)	–	V	–	–	
5% NaCl (growth)	–	–	–	–	
Iron uptake	–	–	–	–	
MacConkey agar (without crystal violet)	–	–	–	–	
Pyrazinamidase	–	+	+	–	

(*continues*)

TABLE 17-2 *M. tuberculosis* Complex (*continued*)

Nonchromogens					
Test	***M. avium-intracellulare***	***M. terrae* complex**	***M. malmoense***	***M. haemophilum***	***M. gastri***
Colonial morphology	**Smooth or rough nonpigmented**	**Smooth or rough nonpigmented**	**Smooth nonpigmented**	**Rough nonpigmented**	**Smooth or rough nonpigmented**
Niacin accumulation	–	–	–	–	–
Nitrate reduction	–	V	–	–	–
Heat-stable catalase	V	+	V	–	–
Urease	–	–	–	–	–
Tween 80 hydrolysis	–	+	+	–	+
Arylsulfatase (3 days)	–	–	–	–	–
5% NaCl (growth)	–	–	–	–	–
Iron uptake	–	–	–	–	–
MacConkey agar (without crystal violet)	–	–	–	–	–
Pyrazinamidase	+	V	+	+	–
Rapid Growers					
Test	***M. fortuitum***	***M. chelonei***	***M. phlei***	***M. smegmatis***	
Niacin accumulation	–	–	–	–	
Nitrate reduction	+	–	+	+	
Heat-stable catalase	+	+	+	+	
Urease	+	+	NA	NA	
Tween 80 hydrolysis	V	–	+	+	
Arylsulfatase (3 days)	+	+	–	–	
5% NaCl (growth)	+	–	+	+	
Iron uptake	+	–	+	+	
MacConkey agar (without crystal violet)	+	+	–	–	
Pyrazinamidase	+	+	–	NA	

+, most reactions positive; –, most reactions negative; V, variable reaction; NA, not applicable

in the impoverished community, including the homeless, malnourished, and overcrowded.

Transmission and Infectious Process

Tuberculosis is transmitted from person-to-person contact through the air by droplet nuclei that contain *M. tuberculosis.* These infected droplets are expelled in the respiratory secretions of infected individuals and also may be produced by sputum induction and aerosol treatments or in specimen collection or processing in the hospital or laboratory. The droplet nuclei contain two to three tuberculosis organisms, which are able to remain airborne for long periods of time because of their small size. These small particles are inhaled and then descend the bronchial tree and are deposited in the bronchiole or alveoli. Larger particles do not remain airborne and if inhaled, do not reach the alveoli but instead are trapped on mucous membranes of the upper respiratory tract and either swallowed or expectorated.

Cell-mediated immunity (CMI) is the primary host defense against tuberculosis. Thus, those individuals with diminished CMI are at increased risk of tuberculosis disease. If the organism can survive within the alveolar macrophage, it will multiply slowly with a doubling time of every 24 to 30 hours. *M. tuberculosis* does not produce any endotoxins or exotoxins, so there is no host response and very few clinical signs early in the infection. The organisms continue to multiply and eventually in 2 weeks to 3 months reach a high enough number to produce a cellular immune response. Primary tuberculosis usually begins in the middle or lower lung.

Before the development of CMI, the tubercle bacteria can spread through the lymph nodes and lymph vessels to other sites, where they may multiply. These sites include the regional lymph nodes in the hilum of the lung, the kidneys, and the brain. Hematogenous spread of the bacteria generally occurs 3 to 6 weeks after infection. Most often, mycobacteria spread to the apices of the lung because of the high oxygen tension there. Other areas for dissemination include the spine, long bones, heart, meninges, and genitourinary system. Delayed hypersensitivity usually develops 1 to 2 months after infection. Cellular immunity inhibits further multiplication of the bacteria.

In those with intact cell-mediated immunity, T cells and macrophages limit the multiplication and dissemination of the organism by forming granulomas. As phagocytosis proceeds, macrophages continue to engulf the mycobacteria, forming multinucleated cells, which are surrounded by epithelial cells and lymphocytes. These cells join to form granulomatous lesions, known as tubercles, which are characteristic of the infection. As the centers of the tubercles break down, cheese-like masses develop; this process is known as caseation. In those with a healthy immune response, a strong CMI will halt the multiplication and dissemination of the mycobacteria. The lesions may heal, but viable bacteria may still remain in these areas, which can serve as a source of reactivation tuberculosis. Lesions in the middle and lower lobes of the lung may become fibrotic and calcify.

Tuberculosis infection leads to tuberculosis disease in those individuals who have an inadequate cellular immune response. In this case, caseation proceeds to liquefaction from the hydrolytic enzymes of the macrophage. There is a tremendous multiplication of the organism within the lesions. As the caseous masses rupture, the organisms are disseminated to other areas of the lung. During this period, the host is highly infectious because the organism is easily spread to the environment through respiratory secretions via coughing and sneezing or even talking.

Tuberculosis infection does not lead to tuberculosis disease in individuals with an adequate cellular immune response. The organism is rapidly phagocytized and destroyed, multiplication is inhibited, and the lesions eventually begin to heal.

Reactivation tuberculosis, also known as secondary tuberculosis, may occur in those who have had primary tuberculosis. Reactivation may occur at any site where dormant mycobacteria remain, although it most frequently occurs in the apices of the lung. Factors that may contribute to reactivation include pulmonary disease; immunosuppression; malnutrition; alcoholism; being elderly; and hormonal factors, such as pregnancy, diabetes mellitus, and other pulmonary diseases.

Symptoms of pulmonary tuberculosis include fever, leukocytosis, and anemia. There is a cough, hemoptysis, dyspnea, and weight loss. The infection may disseminate to the lymph nodes, pleural cavity, genitourinary tract, bones, central nervous system, abdomen, and heart.

Diagnosis and Identification

The Mantoux tuberculin skin test (TST) is used to determine whether an indiviudal has been exposed to *Mycobacterium tuberculosis*. Purified protein derivative (PPD), which is a heat-killed, filtered, ammonium sulfate–precipitated organism, is injected intradermally into the forearm. The site is read at 48 hours for redness and induration. False-positive and false-negative TST reactions can occur if the test is not correctly administered. False-positives also may occur if there has been a prior bacillus Calmette-Guerin (BCG) vaccination or if there is infection with non-tuberculosis mycobacteria. False-negative reactions may occur in anergy, which is the inability of the individual to react to the skin test because of a suppressed immune system. Also, false-negatives may occur in recent infections and in very old infections. Infants less than 6 months of age in overwhelming tuberculosis disease and certain viral disease also may produce a false-negative result. A positive skin test indicates the presence of tubercle bacillus but not necessarily active disease.

Two-step testing is recommended for initial testing for those adults who are retested periodically, such as nursing home residents and health care workers. The ability to react to PPD may diminish with time, and there is a risk of a false-negative reaction. Two-step testing is done to diminish the possibility that a boosted reaction to a subsequent TST will be misinterpreted as a positive or recent infection. Giving the second TST after an initial negative is known as two-step testing. If the person's initial skin test is negative, a second skin test is given 1 to 3 weeks later. If the second test is positive, it is most likely because of a boosted reaction; if the second test is negative, the individual is most likely not infected.

The BCG is a vaccine for tuberculosis disease, which is administered to many foreign-born persons who come from countries that have a high incidence of tuberculosis. It is used to prevent or reduce the incidence of disease in these countries but is not recommended in the United States.

Interferon-gamma release assays (IGRAs) are blood tests to detect tuberculosis infection. Currently, there are two tests approved by the U.S. Food and Drug Administration: the QuantiFERON®-TB Gold In-Tube test (QFT-GIT) and the T-SPOT®.*TB* test (T-Spot). These tests measure the individual's immune response to *M. tuberculosis*. When white blood cells are infected with *M. tuberculosis*, interferon-gamma (IFN-γ) is released. The IFN-γ reacts with *M. tuberculosis* antigens in the test system. TST and blood tests are used with patient's clinical symptoms and other laboratory results to diagnose tuberculosis infection.

Identification

M. tuberculosis is a thin, slightly curved, strongly acid-fast bacillus. In Gram-stained cultures, it may appear as a beaded gram-positive bacillus. Mycobacteria may appear as a poorly staining or nonstaining bacillus with a clear halo. The bacteria tend to clump in cultures. *M. tuberculosis* produces nonpigmented, tan to buff colonies in 14 to 28 days when grown on Löwenstein-Jensen and Middlebrook media at 35°C to 37°C. The colonies have been described as rough, dry, warty, and granular (**FIGURE 17-2**). Colonies can be observed microscopically as early as 5 to 10 days on Middlebrook 7H10 or 7H11 medium. The organism fails to grow at 25°C and 42°C to 45°C.

The organism is positive for niacin accumulation and reduces nitrates to nitrites. It is heat-stable catalase negative and pyrazinamidase positive. As previously discussed, there are both automated and molecular methods available to assist in the identification of *M. tuberculosis*.

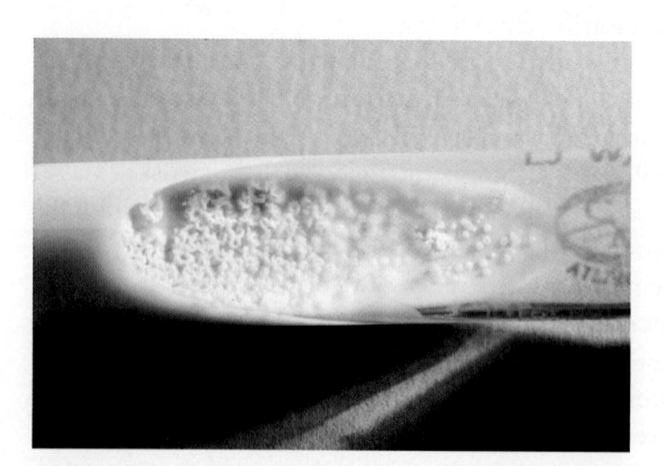

FIGURE 17-2 *Mycobacterium tuberculosis* on Löwenstein-Jensen (LJ) slant, showing characteristic nonpigmented, dry, granular colonies.

Treatment

Antibiotic therapy is extremely important in the treatment of both latent and active tuberculosis infections. Standard disk diffusion antibiotic susceptibility testing cannot be used for these slow-growing mycobacteria. Thus, automated susceptibility testing or modified testing with antibiotics incorporated into the media is used. There also are some molecular testing methods available to detect resistance.

Long-term multidrug therapy is needed because of the organism's slow doubling time and also to prevent the development of resistance. There are currently 10 drugs approved by the Food and Drug Administration for the treatment of tuberculosis. First-line drugs for tuberculosis are isoniazid (INH), rifampin, pyrazinamide, and ethambutol. The current recommendation is a therapy of several of the first-line drugs. Second-line drugs generally are incorporated when there is resistance to the first-line drugs. Second-line drugs include streptomycin, cycloserine, *p*-aminosalicylic acid, and ethionamide. Treatment regimes include an initial phase of 2 months, followed by a variety of options for an additional 4 to 7 months.

Drug-resistant tuberculosis refers to tuberculosis whereby the organism is resistant to at least one first-line antituberculosis drug. **Multidrug-resistant tuberculosis** (MDR TB) indicates that the organism is resistant to more than one antituberculosis first-line drug, which is isoniazid or rifampin or both.

Additional components of treatment include proper nutrition, well-ventilated and noncrowded housing, and improved personal hygiene.

Mycobacterium ulcerans

M. ulcerans produces rough, flat, pale-buff colonies with an irregular outline when grown at 32°C to 33°C. The organism requires 6 to 12 weeks to grow and fails to grow at 24°C and 35°C to 37°C. *M. ulcerans* can be described as biochemically inert because it produces very few positive reactions. It is positive for heat-stable catalase. The organism produces cutaneous lesions, known as Buruli ulcers, which appear as lumps under the skin that do not heal. *M. ulcerans* is primarily found in Central and Western Africa, Mexico, New Guinea, and Australia. It is believed that the organism is carried from the soil into the water in tropical regions. The infection is contracted by direct contact with the contaminated water sources.

Mycobacterium africanum

M. africanum is associated with pulmonary disease similar to tuberculosis, which may disseminate in immunocompromised hosts. Important reactions include positive niacin accumulation, nitrate reduction, and pyrazinamide.

Mycobacterium bovis

M. bovis is the agent of tuberculosis in cattle and other warm-blooded animals, including dogs, cats, swine, rabbits, primates, and humans. The disease has virtually been eliminated as a cause of human tuberculosis in industrialized countries as a result of the pasteurization of cows' milk and because of improved disease control in cattle herds. There have been occasional cases of human tuberculosis caused by *M. bovis* in the United States in the past several years, which most often are attributed to the consumption of unpasteurized cheese products. *M. bovis* grows at 35°C to 37°C but not at 24°C or 42°C. Growth is evident on Middlebrook medium in approximately 3 weeks, whereaws 6 to 8 weeks are necessary for growth to occur on LJ medium. The colonies are buff and small and may be rough or smooth. The organism resembles water droplets on Middlebrook medium. *M. bovis* may be differentiated from the similar *M. tuberculosis* by its negative niacin and nitrate reactions.

Mycobacterium leprae

M. leprae, the agent of **Hansen's disease**, or leprosy, cannot be cultured in vitro but has been grown on the foot pads of mice. Leprosy is an infection of the skin and mucous membranes, which is believed to be spread through direct contact with infected respiratory droplets. Leprosy has been virtually eliminated in the developed Western world, but it remains an important health concern in the southern hemisphere, especially in Asia, India, Africa, and Latin America. There were almost 800,000 new cases detected worldwide in 2002. Additionally, it is estimated that 1 to 2 million people are disabled permanently from leprosy. According to the World Health Organization, 90% of the cases are found in Brazil, Madagascar, Mozambique, Tanzania, and Nepal. In the United States, there has been a steady decline in the number of cases since 1985. Annually, there are approximately 70 to 100 cases reported in the United States from 20 states, although over 60% were reported from California, Hawaii, and Texas. It is believed that many of the cases are because of immigration from areas in which the disease is endemic.

Leprosy affects the skin, mucous membranes, and peripheral nerves. There are two types of disease: tuberculoid leprosy, or paucibacillary Hansen's disease, and multibacillary, or lepromatus Hansen's, disease. Tuberculoid leprosy, or paucibacillary Hansen's disease, is characterized by a few hypopigmented or red skin lesions. There is sensory nerve loss, and the lesions contain few if any acid-fast bacilli. Multibacillary, or lepromatus Hansen's, disease has more widespread skin involvement with many symmetric skin lesions and nodules and a thickening of the skin. There is less nerve involvement than in tuberuloid leprosy, but the nasal mucous membranes are infected with many acid-fast bacilli. Nerve damage from leprosy may affect sensory and motor nerves and lead to paralysis and deformities.

Identification is made through observation of acid-fast bacilli in characteristic skin lesions and clinical symptoms.

PHOTOCHROMOGENS

Mycobacterium kansasii

M. kansasii, or "yellow bacillus," produces a yellow pigment when exposed to light from the presence of β-carotene pigment. The color darkens to red with prolonged incubation and exposure to light (**FIGURE 17-3**). The organism grows best at 37°C, and growth is evident in 14 to 28 days. It grows slowly at 24°C but does not grow at 42°C. Important reactions to identify *M. kansasii* include its rapid Tween 80 hydrolysis (positive reaction in 3 days), strong reduction of nitrates to nitrites, rapid catalase activity, and negative

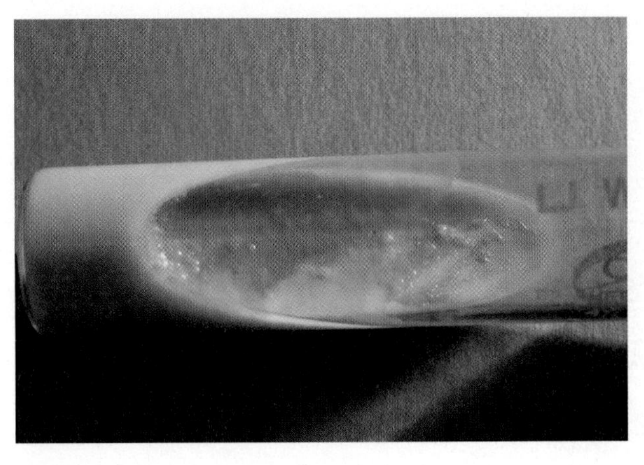

FIGURE 17-3 *M. kansasii* on LJ slant.

pyrazinamidase reaction. There is a nucleic acid probe available to identify *M. kansasii.*

The organism causes a chronic pulmonary disease, similar to tuberculosis, which rarely disseminates. *M. kansasii* also may cause soft tissue infections, lymphadenitis, and skin infections. Infections generally do not disseminate unless the host is severely immunosuppressed.

Mycobacterium marinum

M. marinum ("of the sea") grows optimally at 30°C to 32°C. Growth at 24°C and 32°C occurs in 2 weeks, whereas the organism grows poorly or fails to grow at 35°C to 37°C. The organism appears as nonpigmented colonies that develop a deep yellow pigment when exposed to a constant light source (**FIGURE 17-4**). Important reactions to identify *M. marinum* include positive niacin accumulation by some strains, positive hydrolysis of Tween 80, failure to reduce nitrates to nitrites, positive urease and pyrazinamidase activity, and failure to produce heat-stable catalase.

M. marinum is associated with skin infections occurring as red to blue lesions. Infection most often results from contact with poorly chlorinated or unchlorinated freshwater or saltwater. Water sources that may harbor *M. marinum* include swimming pools, fish aquariums, and water-cooling towers. Swimming pool granuloma, a more serious form of the infection, involves the formation of nodules on the elbows, knees, toes, or fingers, which may ulcerate. Those at increased risk of infection include fishermen and lifeguards.

Mycobacterium simiae

Mycobacterium simiae, a photochromogen, is nonpigmented when grown in the dark but pigmented yellow when exposed to a constant light source. Colonies usually grow within 2 to 3 weeks. Important reactions include a positive niacin accumulation, positive Tween 80 hydrolysis, and positive heat-stable catalase. *M. simiae* is a rare cause of pulmonary infections, which may disseminate.

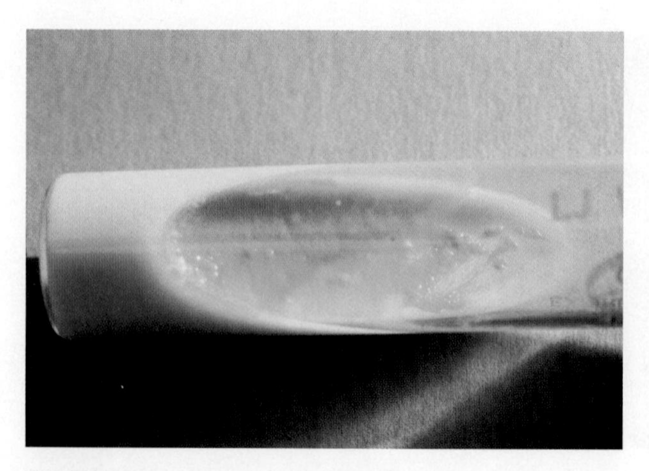

FIGURE 17-4 *M. marinum* on LJ slant.

Mycobacterium asiaticum

Mycobacterium asiaticum is a rare cause of pulmonary disease. Important reactions include positive heat-stable catalase and Tween 80 hydrolysis and negative urease and nitrate. It is similar to *M. simiae* but is niacin accumulation negative.

SCOTOCHROMOGENS

Mycobacterium scrofulaceum

M. scrofulaceum produces smooth, buttery yellow to orange colonies in 4 to 6 weeks. Pigment production occurs in both the absence and presence of light. Showing no temperature preference, *M. scrofulaceum* grows at 25°C, 32°C, and 37°C. Important reactions include negative results for Tween 80 hydrolysis and nitrate reduction and positive heat-stable catalase activity.

The organism is the cause of cervical lymphadenitis, particularly in children between 18 months and 7 years of age. It also causes lymphadenitis in older children and young adults with emerging molar teeth. It is believed that *M. scrofulaceum* colonizes the mouth and throat, which serve as the route of infection.

Mycobacterium szulgai

M. szulgai can be classified as both a photochromogen and a scotochromogen. When grown at 25°C, the organism is classified as a photochromogen but when grown at 35°C to 37°C, it is classified as a scotochromogen. The organism grows in 2 weeks at 35°C to 37°C and produces an orange pigment when exposed to constant light. Important reactions include positive nitrate reduction, positive heat-stable catalase, a slow positive reaction for Tween 80 hydrolysis, and failure to grow in 5% NaCl. The negative growth in 5% NaCl is important in its differentiation from *M. flavescens*, which shows positive growth in 5% NaCl.

M. szulgai is a rare cause of pulmonary infections.

Mycobacterium gordonae

M. gordonae, the "tap water bacillus," is found in a variety of water sources and is generally nonpathogenic. It frequently

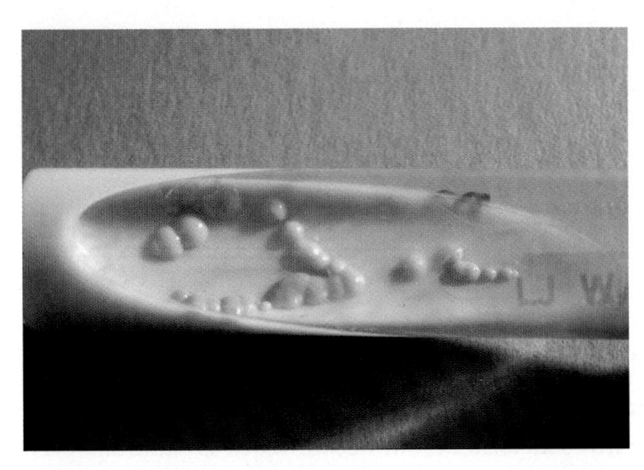

FIGURE 17-5 *Mycobacterium gordonae*, the "tap water bacillus," produces smooth, glistening yellow colonies in both the absence and presence of light.

is isolated, however, often as a contaminant from a water source. It has been associated with a variety of infections in the immunosuppressed host. The organism, previously known as *M. aquae*, grows in approximately 7 days at 37°C as smooth yellow to orange colonies (**FIGURE 17-5**). Notable reactions include positive results for Tween 80 hydrolysis and heat-stable catalase. It is urease negative and does not reduce nitrates.

Mycobacterium xenopi

M. xenopi, a slow-growing organism, produces small yellow colonies. Growth is optimal at 42°C. The organism also grows at 37°C but fails to grow at 25°C. *M. xenopi* produces branching colonies with aerial hyphae on cornmeal agar, which have been described as "birds' nests." Important reactions include negative reactions for niacin accumulation and nitrate reductions and positive reactions for catalase and arylsulfatase, which become positive within 2 weeks. The organism was first isolated from the African toad and also has been isolated from birds and several hot and cold water sources. It was considered to be nonpathogenic until recent years, when *M. xenopi* was identified as the agent of pulmonary infection in patients with preexisting lung pathologies. The organism also can disseminate into the bone marrow and lymph nodes.

Miscellaneous Scotochromogens

M. thermoresistible, a rare pulmonary isolate, is unique in its ability to grow at 52°C. The organism produces smooth yellow colonies. *N. flavescens*, considered to be normal flora, produces smooth yellow colonies and grows moderately at 37°C.

NONPHOTOCHROMOGENS

Mycobacterium avium and *Mycobacterium intracellulare* (*M. avium-intracellulare* complex)

M. avium-intracellulare complex is composed of the species *M. avium* and *M. intracellulare*, which are joined into a complex because of similar morphological and biochemical characteristics. These are slow-growing organisms that produce buff-colored colonies. The colonies are thin and transparent or smooth; asteroid margins may be present. Because of these variable morphologies, one may mistakenly conclude that it is a mixed culture. The organisms are found throughout the environment and have been isolated from air and water sources, natural and potable, including pools, and soil and plants. These mycobacteria grow at 35°C to 37°C and 42°C but not at 24°C. Most biochemical reactions are negative with the exception of heat-stable catalase and pyrazinamidase, which are positive. There is a nucleic acid probe available to identify *M. avium* and *M. intracellulare*. *M. avium-intracellulare* causes infections in swine, poultry, and other animals. These bacteria are opportunistic pathogens in humans, especially in those with acquired immunodeficiency syndrome (AIDS). In those with AIDS, *M. avium-intracellulare* may cause pulmonary, gastrointestinal, and disseminated diseases; it is isolated from the sputum, stool, or blood. The route of infection is believed to be through ingestion of contaminated food or water or through inhalation of aerosols.

The organism has been known as the "Battey bacillus," which refers to an outbreak of *M. avium-intracellulare* infection in Battey State Hospital in Rome, Georgia, in the 1950s.

Mycobacterium malmoense

M. malmoense produces gray to white, smooth, raised colonies in 2 to 3 weeks when grown at 37°C. Growth is slower at 22°C to 24°C and may require 7 to 12 weeks. Important reactions include negative niacin accumulation and nitrate reduction negative, and positive Tween 80 hydrolysis, pyrazinamidase, and heat-stable catalase. It is associated with pulmonary disease, often in those with an existing lung disease.

Mycobacterium haemophilum

M. haemophilum grows at 28°C to 32°C in 2 to 4 weeks but requires 4 to 8 weeks to grow at 25°C or 35°C. Colonies are nonpigmented. The organism cannot grow at 37°C. The organism is unique in its growth requirement for hemin, requiring chocolate agar or Mueller-Hinton agar with Fildes enrichment to grow. The organism is negative for many biochemical reactions.

M. haemophilum has been identified as the agent of subcutaneous lesions, ulcers, and abscesses in immunosuppressed patients.

Miscellaneous Nonchromogens

M. gastri is nonpathogenic and has been isolated from gastric lavage. *M. terrae* and *M. triviale* also are classified as the *M. terrae-M. triviale* complex. They are rare causes of arthritis and osteomyelitis. *M. terrae* is known as the "radish bacillus." The complex grows slowly at both 25°C and 37°C as a nonphotochromogen.

RAPID GROWERS: *MYCOBACTERIUM FORTUITUM-CHELONEI* COMPLEX

M. fortuitum and *M. chelonei* are similar morphologically and biochemically and thus may be classified as a complex. As rapid growers, these mycobacteria grow in less than 7 days and are not pigmented. *M. fortuitum* is found in water, soil, and dust and grows as smooth, waxy, heaped colonies in 2 to 4 days. Hyphae are present in young colonies at 1 to 2 days (**FIGURE 17-6**). The source of *M. chelonei* is not known; colonies are round, smooth, and colorless and do not produce hyphae. These organisms produce a positive arylsulfatase test and grow on MacConkey agar without crystal violet. The two species can be differentiated by the iron uptake and nitrate reactions. *M. fortuitum* reduces nitrates to nitrites, whereas *M. chelonei* does not. *M. fortuitum* is positive for iron uptake, whereas *M. chelonei* is negative.

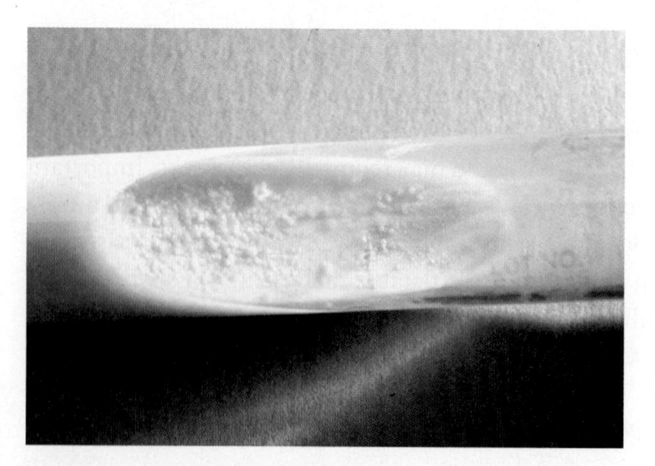

FIGURE 17-6 *Mycobacterium fortuitum* grows within 7 days, producing nonpigmented, smooth, and heaped colonies.

Laboratory Procedures

Procedure
Acid-fast stains: Carbolfuchsin

Principle
The mycobacteria do not decolorize after staining, even with the addition of acid or acid-alcohol, because of the mycolic acid in the cell wall. Heat, solvents, or detergents are needed to drive the stain into the cell wall of the mycobacteria.

Purpose
Mycobacteria, commonly known as acid-fast bacilli (AFB), are detected in clinical specimens and cultures through use of carbolfuchsin staining.

Ziehl-Neelsen Method Materials
Carbolfuchsin stain: Basic carbolfuchsin in 95% ethanol in 5% phenol
Decolorizer: 95% ethanol in concentrated hydrochloric acid
Counterstain: Methylene blue chloride in distilled water

Procedure
This procedure must be performed wearing gloves, mask, and gown in a class 2 biohazard hood.

1. Fix smears using an electric warmer at 65°C for 2 hours.
2. Place a small piece of filter paper over the smear.
3. Flood slide with carbolfuchsin and heat the electric warmer to steaming for 15 minutes.
4. Remover filter paper and rinse slides with distilled water.
5. Decolorize with acid-alcohol until no more color drains from the smear.
6. Rinse with distilled water.
7. Counterstain with methylene blue for 30 seconds.
8. Rinse with distilled water and allow to dry.
9. Examine using the oil-immersion objective (100X).

Interpretation
Acid-fast bacilli stain red, and the background should be blue.

Report number of organisms seen using the CDC recommendation (see Table 17-1).

Number of organisms seen	Report
1 or 2 per slide	Report number found and request another specimen
3 to 9 per slide	Rare (1+)
10 or more per slide	Few (2+)
1 or more per oil-immersion field	Numerous (3+)

1+, 2+, and 3+ results should be reported as a positive AFB smear.

Procedure

Kinyoun stain

Materials

Kinyoun carbolfuchsin stain (basic fuchsin in 95% ethanol with liquefied phenol)

Decolorizer: 95% ethanol in concentrated hydrochloric acid

Counterstain: Methylene blue chloride in distilled water

Procedure

This procedure must be performed wearing gloves, mask, and gown in a class 2 biohazard hood.

1. Prepare smear as described in the Ziehl-Neelsen method.
2. Stain with Kinyoun carbolfuchsin for 3 minutes. *Do not heat.*
3. Rinse with distilled water.
4. Decolorize with acid-alcohol until no more color drains from slide—approximately 2 minutes.
5. Rinse with distilled water.
6. Counterstain with methylene blue for 30 seconds.
7. Rinse with distilled water and allow to dry.
8. Examine under oil-immersion objective (100X).

Interpretation

See interpretation for the Ziehl-Neelsen method.

Procedure

Löwenstein-Jensen (LJ) medium

Principle

LJ medium contains whole egg, potato flour, and glycerol to support the growth of mycobacteria. Malachite green is added to inhibit the growth of contaminating bacteria. The medium can be modified with the addition of RNA, which has been shown to increase the percentage of positive results. In the Gruft modification, penicillin and nalidixic acid are added to suppress further the growth of contaminating bacteria.

Purpose

LJ medium is an egg-based medium used to isolate and cultivate mycobacteria. There are several modifications, which include:

Tubed slants: Semiquantitative catalase test

Gruft's modification: Selective medium used for isolation and cultivation of mycobacteria; contains penicillin and nalidixic acid, which inhibit other bacteria, and RNA, which increases recovery of mycobacteria.

Iron: Iron update for differentiation of slow-growing mycobacteria from rapid-growing bacteria. Rapid growing mycobacteria take up iron in the medium and produce rusty brown colonies and a tan color in the medium. *M. chelonae* and slow-growing species are negative for iron uptake.

Pyruvic acid: The addition of pyruvic acid to egg-based media enhances the recovery of mycobacteria.

5% NaCl: Most rapid growers, *M. triviale*, and some *M. flavescens* can grow on NaCl-containing media. *M. chelonae* subspecies *chelonae* cannot grow on NaCl media and thus can be differentiated from other members of the *M. fortuitum* complex, such as *M. chelonae* subspecies *abscessus*, which are NaCl positive.

Procedure

This procedure must be performed wearing gloves, mask, and a gown in a class 2 biohazard hood.

1. Select a single colony from medium or inoculate processed specimen onto medium. Streak for isolation.
2. Incubate 4 to 8 weeks at 35°C in 5% to 10% CO_2.
3. Interpret results by reading plates in 5 to 7 days after inoculation. Cultures are held for 6 to 8 weeks before being considered negative. Cultures should be examined weekly for growth and evaluated for bacterial and fungal contamination.
4. Record the following:
    a. Number of days for colonies to become visible macroscopically
       Rapid growers have mature colonies within 7 days.
       Slow growers require more than 7 days for mature colonies.
    b. Number of colonies
       1+ = 50–100 colonies
       2+ = 100–200 colonies
       3+ = 300–500 colonies (almost confluent)
       4+ = Over 500 colonies (confluent growth)
    c. Pigment production
       Nonchromogen = white, cream, or buff
       Chromogen = lemon, yellow, orange, or red

Notes

1. Following inoculation, keep plates from light.
2. Tubes should be incubated horizontally until the inoculum is absorbed.
3. Tubes and bottles should be incubated with screw caps loose for at least 3 weeks to permit circulation of CO_2. After this time, tighten caps to prevent dehydration and loosen caps briefly once per week.
4. Skin cultures suspected to be *M. marinum* or *M. ulcerans* should be incubated at 25°C to 33°C for primary incubation. Cultures suspected of containing *M. avium* or *M. xenopi* should be incubated at 40°C to 42°C. A second culture should be incubated at 35°C to 37°C in both cases.
5. Negative cultures do not rule out mycobacterial infection, because of a number of factors.
6. Mycobacteria are strict aerobes, but growth is stimulated by increased CO_2.

Source: Becton, Dickinson and Company. (2009). *Manual of microbiological culture media*, 2nd ed. (pp. 309–311). Sparks, MD.

Procedure
Middlebrook 7H9 broth

Principle
The medium contains vitamins, such as pyridoxine and biotin; salts; buffers; and other nutrients to support the growth of mycobacteria

Purpose
Middlebrook 7H9 broth is used to cultivate mycobacteria for use in biochemical procedures, such as arylsulfatase and niacin accumulation.

Procedure
This procedure must be performed wearing gloves, mask, and a gown in a class 2 biohazard hood.

1. Inoculate 7H9 broth using an isolated colony or a specimen.
2. Incubate 1 to 8 weeks at 35°C in 5% to 10% CO_2. The time will vary based on the procedure for which broth is to be used.
3. Perform acid-fast stain weekly. When positive, subculture to Löwenstein-Jensen slant.

Procedure
Middlebrook 7H10 and 7H11 agars

Principle
Middlebrook 7H10 medium contains inorganic salts, vitamins, cofactors, albumin, catalase, oleic acid, glycerol, and dextrose. Sodium citrate when converted to citric acid is able to maintain inorganic salts in solution, and glycerol serves as an energy and carbon source. Oleic acid and other long-chain fatty acids are needed by mycobacteria for metabolism, and albumin protects the organism against toxic agents, thus promoting its growth. Dextrose is a nutrient source, and catalase will inactivate toxic peroxides in the medium. The incorporation of malachite green will partially inhibit other bacterial growth.

Middlebrook 7H11 contains the same ingredients as does 7H10, with the addition of casein hydrolysate. Advantages of Middlebrook media include earlier growth detection than with egg-based media and earlier recognition of contaminants.

Purpose
Middlebrook 7H10 and 7H11 agars are used for the isolation of mycobacteria. Mitchison's selective 7H11 agar contains carbenicillin, polymyxin B, trimethoprim lactate, and amphotericin B and is useful in the isolation of mycobacteria from heavily contaminated cultures.

Procedure
This procedure must be performed wearing gloves, mask, and gown in a class 2 biohazard hood.

1. Inoculate medium and streak for isolation.
2. Incubate 4 to 8 weeks at 35°C ± 2°C under increased (5% to 10%) CO_2.
3. Interpret results by reading plates in 5 to 7 days after inoculation. Cultures are held for 6 to 8 weeks before being considered negative. Cultures should be examined weekly for growth and evaluated for bacterial and fungal contamination.
4. Record the following:
    a. Number of days for colonies to become visible macroscopically
    b. Number of colonies
       1+ = 50–100 colonies
       2+ = 100–200 colonies
       3+ = 300–500 colonies (almost confluent)
       4+ = Over 500 colonies (confluent growth)
    c. Pigment production
       Nonchromogen = white, cream, or buff
       Chromogen = lemon, yellow, orange, or red

Notes

1. Following inoculation, keep plates from light.
2. Tubes should be incubated in a slanted position at a 5° angle.
3. Tubes and bottles should be incubated with screw caps loose for at least 1 week to permit circulation of CO_2. After this time, tighten caps to prevent dehydration and loosen caps briefly once per week.
4. Skin cultures suspected to be *M. marinum* or *M. ulcerans* should be incubated at 25°C to 33°C for primary incubation. Cultures suspected of containing *M. avium* or *M. xenopi* should be incubated at 40°C to 42°C. A second culture should be incubated at 35°C to 37°C.
5. Negative cultures do not rule out mycobacterial infection, because of a number of factors.
6. Mycobacteria are strict aerobes, but growth is stimulated by increased CO_2.

Source: Becton, Dickinson and Company. (2009). *Manual of microbiological culture media*, 2nd ed. (pp. 356–358). Sparks, MD.

Procedure
Chromogenicity assay for mycobacteria

Principle
Photochromogens possess carotenoid pigments that are activated only in the light (yellow/orange). Scotochromogens produce carotenoids that are active in the dark (yellow/orange) and the light (orange/red). Nonphotochromogens may produce a tan or buff pigment that does not intensify on exposure to the light.

Purpose
The chromogenicity assay is used to categorize mycobacterial isolates into the appropriate Runyon classification: photochromogen, scotochromogen, or nonchromogen.

Materials
Löwenstein-Jensen (LJ) or American Thoracic Society (ATS) medium (do not use mycobacterial media containing antibiotics)
60-watt lamp
Aluminum foil

Procedure
This procedure must be performed with gloves, mask, and gown in a Class 2 biohazard hood.

1. Record the pigment of the isolate's colonies.
2. Streak two LJ (or ATS) slants with the isolate.
3. Wrap one of the slants with aluminum foil.
4. Incubate both slants at 37°C in increased CO_2 until visible growth appears on the unwrapped slant.
5. Remove foil from the other tube. If pigmentation occurs in this tube, the organism is a scotochromogen.
6. If the organism is nonpigmented, cover half the tube with foil and expose the other half to a 60-watt lamp at 8 to 10 inches for 1 hour. Loosen the cap during this time.
7. Cover the entire tube with the foil and incubate again at 37°C in increased CO_2 for 18 to 24 hours. Leave the cap loosened.
8. Compare the pigmentation of the colonies on the exposed half with those on the unexposed half.

Interpretation
Nonchromogen: No pigment production after exposure to light or in the dark
Scotochromogen: Pigmented colonies in dark. Pigmentation may intensify on exposure to light.
Photochromogen: Nonpigmented colonies in dark, which become pigmented on exposure to light

Quality Control
Incubate at 35°C under increased CO_2 for 2 weeks.
Nonphotochromogen: *M. ulcerans*
Scotochromogen: *M. gordonae* or *M. flavescens*
Photochromogen: *M. marinum*

Procedure
Niacin accumulation

Principle
Acidified potassium thiocyanate reacts with chloramine-T to release cyanogen chloride. In the presence of *p*-aminosalicylic acid, cyanogen chloride reacts with free niacin to produce a yellow color.

Purpose
The niacin test distinguishes *Mycobacterium tuberculosis* from other slow-growing nonchromogenic mycobacteria. Niacin is a metabolic by-product of all mycobacteria. Only those species that lack the enzyme necessary to convert free niacin to niacin ribonucleotide yield a positive result for accumulation of niacin.

Materials
Sterile water 3 ml syringes
13 mm × 75 mm capped plastic test tubes
Taxo™ TB Niacin Test Strips (available from Becton Dickinson)

Procedure

This procedure must be performed wearing a mask, gloves, and gown in a class 2 biohazard hood.

1. Layer 1.5 ml of sterile water over the suspected growth on a Löwenstein-Jensen (LJ) slant.
2. Stab the medium several times. This permits the extracting fluid to contact the culture media. Niacin is extracted from the medium, not from the growth.
3. Position the LJ slant so that the fluid is in contact with the medium for 20 to 30 minutes. Incubate at 36°C.
4. Add 0.5 ml of sterile water in a 13 mm × 75 mm plastic test tube to serve as a reagent control. This should give a negative result.
5. Remove approximately 0.5 ml of extracted liquid from the patient's slant. Add to a 13 mm × 75 mm test tube.
6. Using flamed forceps, drop a niacin test strip downward into the tube. Add a niacin test strip in the same manner to the tube containing sterile water. Cap immediately and shake gently.
7. Gently shake every 5 minutes for a total of 15 minutes.

Interpretation

Positive: Yellow color

Negative: No yellow color (clear)

Quality Control

Mycobacterium tuberculosis: Positive—yellow color*

Mycobacterium avium: Negative—clear

*TB niacin control disks that also produce a positive result are commercially available.

Procedure

Tween 80 hydrolysis

Principle

Tween 80 (polyoxyethylene sorbitan monooleate) is converted to oleic acid by Tween 80 lipase. Neutral red indicator takes on its red acidic color on the release of oleic acid.

Purpose

Tween 80 hydrolysis separates the clinically significant scotochromogens and nonphotochromogens from saprophytic members of these groups. It also may be used to confirm the identification of *Mycobacterium kansasii.*

Materials

Tween 80 hydrolysis substrate (available through Becton Dickinson)

Sterile deionized water

37°C incubator

1 ml sterile pipettes

16 mm × 125 mm sterile, glass screw-cap test tube

Procedure

This procedure must be performed wearing gloves, mask, and a gown in a class 2 biohazard hood.

1. Pipette 1 ml of sterile deionized water into 16 mm × 125 mm sterile, glass screw-cap test tube.
2. Add two drops of Tween 80 substrate to the tube.
3. Add one loopful of the organism to be tested.
4. Replace cap and incubate at 37°C for 10 days.
5. Observe fluid for color change to pink-red at 24 hours, 5 days, and 10 days. Do not shake tube while reading.

Interpretation

Positive: Development of pink to red color

Negative: No color change from original color

Quality Control

Mycobacterium kansasii: Positive—development of pink color

Mycobacterium chelonei: Negative—no color change

Procedure

Arylsulfatase

Principle

Arylsulfatase broth is Middlebrook 7H9 broth supplemented with tripotassium phenolphthalein. Arylsulfatase splits the sulfate group from tripotassium phenolphthalein to form free phenolphthalein, which is detected by adding a small amount of an alkaline solution, sodium carbonate. The 0.001 M arylsulfatase broth is used in a 3-day test and the 0.003 M arylsulfatase broth is used in the 14-day test.

Purpose

Arylsulfatase is an enzyme produced by certain mycobacteria. *Mycobacterium fortuitum-chelonaei* complex is unique in its ability to produce a positive result in 3 days.

Materials

Arylsulfatase broth (available from Remel)

Middlebrook 7H9 or 7H10 broth

Sodium carbonate 2 normal (2 N)

Sterile 1 ml pipettes

35°C to 37°C incubator

Procedure

This procedure must be performed wearing gloves, mask, and gown in a class 2 biohazard hood.

1. Inoculate Middlebrook 7H9 broth or 7H10 agar for the organism to be tested. Incubate for 7 days at 35°C to 37°C in 5% to 10% CO_2.

2. Inoculate the arylsulfatase broth with a 7-day culture either from the 7H10 agar or 7H9 broth.
3. Incubate at 35°C to 37°C without CO_2 for 3 days.
4. After incubation, add 1 ml of 2 N sodium carbonate solution.
5. Observe for a color change.

Interpretation

Positive: Development of pink color after addition of sodium carbonate, indicating presence of free phenolphthalein

Negative: No color change after addition of sodium carbonate

Quality Control

Mycobacterium fortuitum-chelonei: Positive—pink color after addition of sodium carbonate

Mycobacterium phlei: Negative—no color change after addition of sodium carbonate

Note

Substrate concentration, inoculum size, and time of incubation must be followed to avoid false-positive reactions. For 0.003 M arylsulfatase, incubate for 14 days and add 1 ml of 2 N sodium carbonate solution.

Procedure

Nitrate reduction

Principle

In the nitrate strip method (available from Becton Dickinson), the lower end of the strip is impregnated with sodium nitrate. Organisms that produce nitroreductase reduce the nitrate after 2 hours of incubation.

Purpose

Nitrate reduction may be used to differentiate *Mycobacterium* species. The test is useful in identification of slow-growing mycobacteria. Positive results are seen with *M. tuberculosis*, *M. kansasii*, *M. szulgai*, *M. fortuitum*, and *M. flavescens*. Negative results are characteristic of *M. bovis*, *M. marinum*, *M. simiae*, *M. avium-intracellulare* complex, and *M. gastri*.

Material

Nitrate test strips

20 mm × 110 mm glass test tubes with screw caps

Sterile water

Sterile 1 ml pipettes

37°C incubator

Procedure

This procedure must be performed wearing gloves, mask, and gown in a class 2 biohazard hood.

1. Add 0.5 ml of sterile water to a sterile glass screw-cap 20 mm × 110 mm test tube.
2. Make a turbid suspension of the organism to be tested.
3. Holding the tube vertical, add one nitrate test strip into the tube, using sterile forceps.
4. Incubate the tube at 37°C for 2 hours.
5. After incubation, tilt the tube gently to wet the entire strip.
6. Slant the tube at room temperature to cover the strip with liquid for 10 minutes.
7. Interpret color reaction.

Interpretation

Positive: Change of color of top portion of strip to a light or dark blue

Negative: No color change in top portion of strip

Quality Control

M. kansasii: Positive—light- to dark-blue color in top of strip

M. marinum: Negative—no color change in top of strip

Laboratory Exercises

1. Describe the safety measures required when working with mycobacteria.
2. Using the Kinyoun method, prepare and examine acid-fast smears for the following mycobacteria. Record your observations.

Organism	Observations
Mycobacterium gordonae	
Mycobacterium ulcerans	
Mycobacterium szulgai	

3. Perform the chromogenicity assay on the following mycobacteria using Löwenstein-Jensen slants. Record your observations and interpret your results.

Organism	Appearance in dark	Appearance in light	Classification
M. ulcerans			
M. kansasii			
M. szulgai			
M. gordonae			
M. fortuitum			

4. Perform the niacin test on the following mycobacteria. Record your observations and interpret your results. State the principle of this reaction.

Organism	Observation	Interpretation
M. gordonae		
M. marinum		

Principle: ______________________

5. Perform the nitrate reduction procedure on the following mycobacteria. Record your observations and interpret your results. State the principle of this reaction.

Organism	Observation	Interpretation
M. kansasii		
M. marinum		

Principle: ______________________

6. Perform the arylsulfatase procedure on the following mycobacteria. Which species is unique in its ability to produce a positive reaction in 3 days?

Organism	Observation	Interpretation
M. gordonae		
M. fortuitum		

7. Perform the Tween 80 hydrolysis procedure on the following mycobacteria. Record your observations and interpret your results. State the principle of this procedure.

Organism	Observation	Interpretation
M. kansasii		
M. szulgai		

Principle: ______________________

8. Identify an unknown mycobacterium. Indicate the medium inoculated, tests performed, and your observations and results.

Unknown number:

Medium inoculated	Observation	Result
Procedures performed	**Observation**	**Result**
Identification and explanation		

Review Questions

Matching

Match the description to the correct classification:

1. photochromogen
2. scotochromogen
3. nonchromogen
4. rapid growers
   a. Growth occurring in 3 to 5 days in culture medium
   b. Develop yellow pigment when exposed to constant light source
   c. Cannot develop pigment even with exposure to light
   d. Yellow pigment in the dark that intensifies to orange or red when exposed to light

Match the species of *Mycobacterium* with its common name:

5. *M. leprae*
6. *M. kansasii*
7. *M. marinum*
8. *M. gordonae*
9. *M. avium-intracellulare*
   a. "of the sea"
   b. Tap water bacillus
   c. Battey bacillus
   d. Yellow bacillus
   e. Hansen's bacillus

Match the species of *Mycobacterium* with its description or associated infection:

10. *M. szulgai*
11. *M. haemophilum*
12. *M. marinum*
13. *M. bovis*
14. *M. thermoresistible*
    a. Can grow at temperatures above 50°C
    b. Tuberculosis in cattle
    c. "Swimming pool granuloma"
    d. Photochromogen at 25°C and scotochromogen at 37°C
    e. Requires hemoglobin for growth

Multiple Choice

15. The mycobacteria are described as "acid fast" because:
    a. The organisms cannot be stained with acidic dyes.
    b. The organisms are rapidly decolorized with acid-alcohol.
    c. Once stained, the organisms cannot be decolorized with acid-alcohol.
    d. The organisms are easily stained with acidic dyes.
16. Sputum samples for tuberculosis are optimally collected:
    a. In the morning on 3 consecutive days
    b. In the evening on 3 consecutive days
    c. By collecting sputum for a 24-hour period for 1 day
    d. By collecting sputum for three 24-hour periods
17. Sputum samples may contain normal flora and other contaminating microorganisms, so samples must be:
    a. Digested with N-acetyl-L-cysteine
    b. Decontaminated with 2% NaOH
    c. Digested with trisodium phosphate
    d. Decontaminated with dithiothreitol
18. A required component in media for *Mycobacterium* is:
    a. Hemoglobin
    b. Lactose
    c. Potato flour
    d. Whole egg
19. Which of the following is an example of nonselective medium to isolate mycobacteria?
    a. Gruft modification of Löwenstein-Jensen
    b. Middlebrook 7H10
    c. Petragnani
    d. Mitchison's Middlebrook 7H11
20. Which statement correctly describes acid-fast staining?
    a. The Ziehl-Neelsen technique does not require heat.
    b. Mycobacteria stain blue with carbolfuchsin.
    c. The Kinyoun method uses hot phenol.
    d. Auramine O stains mycobacteria yellow-green in the fluorochrome method.
21. A sputum smear reveals an average of five acid-fast bacilli per 1,000X field. According to CDC guidelines, report this result as:
    a. Negative
    b. Rare
    c. 1 + or few
    d. 2 + or moderate
    e. 3 + or numerous
22. Which of the following is noted for a positive result for niacin accumulation?
    a. *M. tuberculosis*
    b. *M. avium-intracellulare*
    c. *M. fortuitum-chelonae*
    d. *M. gordonae*
23. Which of the following groups is characterized by a negative reaction for heat-stable catalase?
    a. *M. tuberculosis* complex
    b. Photochromagens
    c. Scotochromagens
    d. Rapid growers
24. In which reaction is free phenolphthalein detected using an alkaline indicator?
    a. Negative
    b. Rare or 1 +
    c. Few or 2 +
    d. Moderate or 3 +
    e. Numerous or 4 +
25. Tuberculosis is spread through:
    a. Contact with contaminated inanimate objects
    b. The fecal-oral route
    c. Contaminated blood products
    d. Contaminated respiratory droplets
26. Granulomatous lesions consisting of multinucleated cells with epithelial cells and lymphocytes are known as:
    a. Caseates
    b. Chancres
    c. Tubercles
    d. Sclerotic granules
27. Which of the following is *not* a member of the *M. tuberculosis* complex?
    a. *M avium*
    b. *M. africanum*
    c. *M. tuberculosis*
    d. *M. bovis*
28. Multidrug resistant (MDR) tuberculosis is:
    a. Resistant to all antitubercular medications
    b. Resistant to more than one antituberculosis medication, including isoniazid (INH) and/or rifampin
    c. Resistant only to INH
    d. Resistant to all second-line drugs for tuberculosis

Bibliography

American Thoracic Society. (2000). Diagnostic standards and classification of tuberculosis in adults and children. *American Journal of Respiratory and Critical Care Medicine, 161,* 1376–1395.

Centers for Disease Control and Prevention. (2010). Leprosy (Hansen's disease): Technical information. Retrieved from http://www.cdc.gov/nczved/divisions/dfbmd/diseases/hansens_disease/technical.html/#cli nical

Centers for Disease Control and Prevention. (2011). Summary of Notifiable Diseases—United States, 2009. *Morbidity and Mortality Weekly Report, 58*(53), 1–100. Retrieved from http://www.cdc.gov/mmwr/preview/mmwrhtml/mm5853a1.htm

Centers for Disease Control and Prevention. (2013). Tuberculosis. Retrieved from http://www.cdc.gov/tb/publications/factsheets/statisics/TBTrends.htm

Kwan, C. K., & Ernst, J. D. (2001). HIV and tuberculosis: A deadly human syndemic. *Clinical Microbiology Reviews, 24,* 351–376.

Parsons, L. M., Somoskovi, A., Gutierrez, C., Lee, E., Paramasivan, C. N., Abimiku, A., . . . Nkengasong, J. (2011). Laboratory diagnosis of tuberculosis in resource-poor countries: Challenges and opportunities. *Clinical Microbiology Reviews, 24,* 314–350.

Pfyffer, G. E. (2007). *Mycobacterium*: General characteristics, laboratory detection, and staining procedures. In P. R. Murray, E. J. Baron, J. H. Jorgensen, M. L. Landry, & M. A. Pfaller (Eds.), *Manual of clinical microbiology* (9th ed.). (pp. 543–572). Washington, DC: American Society for Microbiology.

Winn, Jr., W., Allen, S., Janda, W., Konemen, E., Procop, G., Schreckenberger, P., & Woods, G. (Eds.). (2005). Mycobacteria. In *Koneman's color atlas and textbook of diagnostic microbiology* (6th ed.). (pp. 1065–1124). Philadelphia, PA: Lippincott Williams & Wilkins.

Wolinsky, E. (1979). Nontuberculosis mycobacteria and associated diseases. *American Review of Respiratory Disease, 119,* 107.

Woods, G. L., Washington, J. A. (1987). Mycobacteria other than *M. tuberculosis*: Review of microbiologic and clinical aspects. *Reviews of Infectious Diseases, 9,* 275.

World Health Organization (2010). Global tuberculosis control. Geneva, Switzerland: World Health Organization.

NEWS: TRENDS IN TUBERCULOSIS

According to the World Health Organization, there were 9.4 million new cases of tuberculosis in 2009, and over 1.7 million people died from the disease in 2009. Most of the estimated number of cases in 2009 occurred in Asia (55%) and Africa (30%) and smaller proportions of cases occurred in the Eastern Mediterranean (7%), Europe (4%), and the Americas (3%).

Factors that favor the transmission of tuberculosis include the number of tubercle bacilli that are released into the air and the concentration of the organism in the air. Poor ventilation and overcrowded living conditions directly impact the number and concentration of mycobacteria in the air. Transmission also is affected by the length of time people are exposed to the contaminated air and their immune status, in particular, the cell-mediated immunity of the host.

Of the 9.4 million incident cases in 2009, 1.0 to 1.2 million people were positive for human immunodeficiency virus (HIV). In fact, of the over 33 million people living with HIV, over 30% were estimated to have latent or active tuberculosis infection. HIV-associated tuberculosis has a higher mortality, accounting for almost 30% of the deaths among those with tuberculosis. This relationship has been described as a syndemic, which is the convergence of two or more diseases that together magnify the impact of the disease.

There also were over 400,000 cases of multidrug resistant tuberculosis (MDR-TB) in 2008. MDR-TB is described as *M. tuberculosis* that is resistant to more than one antituberculosis medication, including at least one of the first-line drugs, including isoniazid or rifampin. The four countries that had the largest number of cases of MDR-TB were China, India, the Russian Federation, and South Africa. Drug-resistant tuberculosis may occur when there is noncompliance with people taking their medication and in those who have developed active tuberculosis after a past infection or who live in or immigrate into areas where drug-resistant tuberculosis is more common.

Extensively drug-resistant tuberculosis (XDR-TB) is a relatively new type of multidrug-resistant tuberculosis. XDR-TB is resistant to almost all drugs used to treat tuberculosis, including the two first-line medications—isoniazid and rifampin. XDR-TB also is resistant to second-line medications, such as the fluoroquinolones, and to at least one of the three available injectable drugs—amikacin, kanamycin, or capreomycin. By July 2010, 58 countries and territories had reported at least one case of XDR-TB. Patients with XDR-TB have limited treatment options. In the United States, there have been approximately 80 cases of XDR-TB reported between 1993 and 2008.

Strides are being made in tuberculosis control and prevention. While estimated rates of tuberculosis are dropping worldwide, rates continue to increase in Africa, the Eastern Mediterranean, and Southeast Asia. Many challenges remain, especially when it is reported that over 80% of all cases occur in countries with poor and inadequate resources for laboratory testing, diagnosis, and effective treatment.

BIBLIOGRAPHY

Kwan, C. K., & Ernst, J. E. (2011). HIV and tuberculosis: A deadly human syndemic. *Clinical Microbiology Reviews, 24,* 351–376.

World Health Organization. (2010). 2010/2011 Tuberculosis global facts. Geneva, Switzerland: World Health Organization.

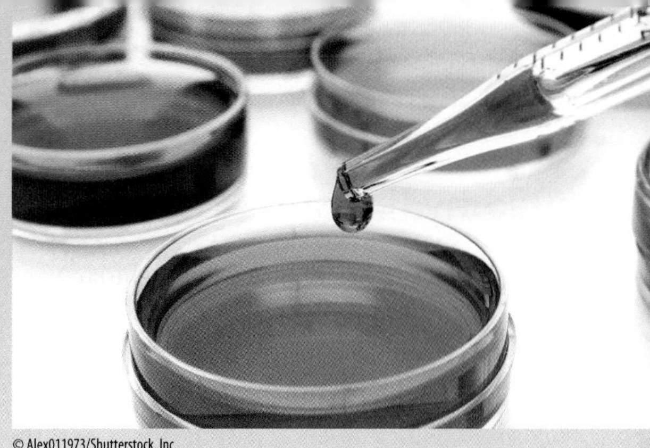

CHAPTER 18

Chlamydia, *Mycoplasma*, and *Rickettsia*

CHAPTER OUTLINE

Chlamydiaceae
Mycoplasma
Rickettsiaceae
Anaplasmataceae

KEY TERMS

Cold agglutinins
Lymphogranuloma venereum
Primary atypical pneumonia
Psittacosis
Trachoma
Weil-Felix reaction

LEARNING OBJECTIVES

1. State the distinguishing characteristics of the genus *Chlamydia*.
2. Describe the diseases and identification of:
   a. *Chlamydia trachomatis*
   b. *Chlamydophila pneumoniae*
   c. *Chlamydophila psittaci*
3. State the specific serovars of *Chlamydia trachomatis* that cause lymphogranuloma venereum (LGV) and nongonococcal urethritis.
4. Describe the life cycle of *Chlamydia*.
5. List the important characteristics of the genus *Mycoplasma*.
6. Discuss the infectious diseases associated with *Mycoplasma pneumoniae*.
7. Explain how *M. pneumoniae* infection is diagnosed.
8. List the clinically significant genital mycoplasmas and ureaplasmas and name the associated infections.
9. For each of the following diseases, name the etiologic agent, vector, and animal reservoir. Briefly describe the infection.
   a. Rocky Mountain spotted fever
   b. Rickettsialpox
   c. Endemic typhus
   d. Brill-Zinsser disease (recrudescent typhus)
   e. Scrub typhus
   f. Ehrlichiosis (human monocytic ehrlichiosis)
   g. Human anaplasmosis
   h. Q fever

Chlamydiaceae

Chlamydiaceae are obligate intracellular parasites originally thought to be viruses because they cannot produce adenosine triphosphate (ATP) or survive outside an animal host cell. In the past the organisms have been known as *Bedsonia*, which refers to a large virus and the trachoma inclusion conjunctivitis (TRIC) agent. Members of the Chlamydiaceae possess a gram-negative–like cell wall and multiply by binary fission. The organisms contain both deoxyribonucleic acid (DNA) and ribonucleic acid (RNA) and possess prokaryotic ribosomes. The Chlamydiaceae are also able to synthesize proteins, lipids, and nucleic acids, and they are susceptible to a variety of antibiotics. Because of these characteristics, the members of the Chlamydiaceae are classified as bacteria.

There are two important genera in the Chlamydiaceae: *Chlamydia* and *Chlamydophila*. The three species of Chlamydiaceae that cause human infection are *Chlamydia trachomatis*, *Chlamydophila psittaci*, and *Chlamydophila pneumoniae*. These organisms have a unique life cycle (**FIGURE 18-1**) and possess intracytoplasmic inclusions. The elementary body (EB) is an inactive, but infective, particle, which is able to bind to the host cell, and the reticulate body (RB) is metabolically active but not infective. The EBs bind to the host cells and are taken into the cell within the phagosome, where they are reorganized into RBs. Eventually the RBs reorganize into smaller elementary bodies and are released when the cell ruptures. The Chlamydiaceae use host ATP for energy and replicate through binary fission.

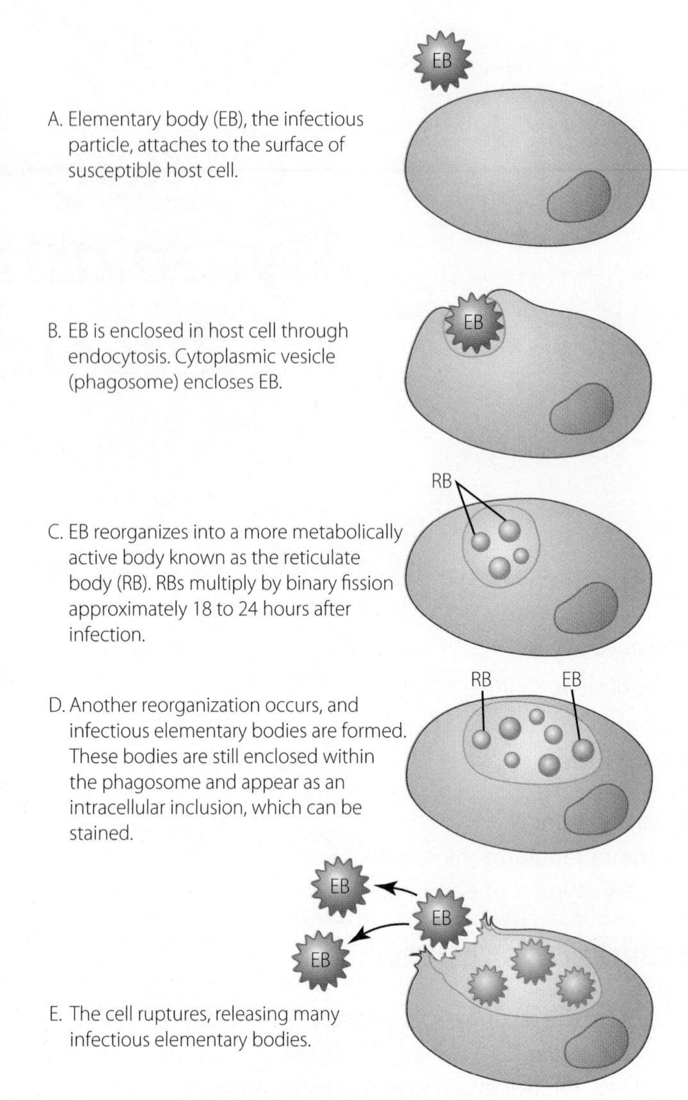

FIGURE 18-1 Life cycle of *Chlamydia*.

CHLAMYDIA TRACHOMATIS

Chlamydia trachomatis is an agent of lymphogranuloma venereum, endemic trachoma, nongonococcal urethritis, and infant pneumonitis. There are two biovars: trachoma and lymphogranuloma venereum. These biovars are further divided into serologic variants or serovars based on the composition of the major outer membrane protein (MOMP). Serovars are associated with specific diseases. For example, serovars A, B1, B2, and C are associated with endemic trachoma; serovars D through K are associated with urogenital infections; and serovars L1, L2, L2a, L2b, and L3 are causes of lymphogranuloma venereum. *Chlamydia* has a limited range of host cells for infection, which are nonciliated columnar, cuboidal, and transitional epithelial cells found on the mucous membranes of the cervix, endocervix, respiratory tract, and conjunctiva. *Chlamydia* attaches to the host cells, entering through minor breaks in the tissue or abrasions at the site of infection.

Trachoma is the leading cause of preventable blindness in the world. This disease is found in many areas of the world and is most prevalent in developing areas in the Middle East, Southern Asia, sub-Saharan and North Africa, and South America. Trachoma disease is more common in young children and is spread by close contact with infected individuals. Transmission may occur through direct contact with infected eye secretions and contaminated hands or indirectly through contaminated articles, such as clothing. Because there is a high carrier rate in children, trachoma also may be transmitted through infected respiratory secretions. The infection also may be spread by infected biting flies. Trachoma begins as a conjunctivitis, which may persist for months to years, spreading to the cornea. Conjunctival scarring and corneal vascularization may occur, which may lead to permanent scarring and blindness. Adult inclusion and newborn inclusion conjunctivitis are also caused by *C. trachomatis*.

C. trachomatis serovars D, E, F, G, H, I, J, and K cause diseases spread primarily by the venereal routes. These infections include nongonococcal urethritis, cervicitis, endometritis, epididymitis, proctitis, and salpingitis. Other types of diseases associated with serotypes D through K include neonatal pneumonitis and inclusion conjunctivitis. *Chlamydia* is the most common sexually transmitted disease in the United States and also the most common cause of nongonococcal urethritis. Chlamydial infections in females, such as pelvic inflammatory disease, may lead to severe damage to the fallopian tubes, infertility, and ectopic pregnancies. *Chlamydia* may be carried asymptomatically, especially in females, who serve as a significant reservoir for infection. The infection may be transmitted from an infected mother to the infant during delivery, which may lead to conjunctivitis or pneumonia.

C. trachomatis serotypes L1, L2, and L3 cause **lymphogranuloma venereum** (LGV), which is also transmitted through the venereal route. LGV is endemic in Asia, Africa, and South America and occurs rarely in the United States. The initial lesion of LGV is a small, painless genital ulcer, which may be unnoticed and spontaneously heal. This is followed in 2 to 6 weeks by lymphadenopathy of the inguinal lymph nodes, near the site of the initial infection. In the secondary stage of the infection, the lymph nodes enlarge and become inflamed and buboes develop. The lymph nodes rupture, and there is a high fever, chills, pain, and a severe headache. The infection can spread systemically, resulting in pneumonia, meningitis, conjunctivitis, or arthritis. The infection also may remain localized, causing granulomatous proctitis. In the chronic form of LGV, there is chronic ulceration with the development of genital ulcers and fistulas. Individuals can become re-infected with *Chlamydia* because lifelong immunity does not occur. Inflammation increases with each infection, which leads to scarring and permanent tissue damage.

Specimen Collection

Specimens that are collected to diagnose chlamydial diseases depend on the site of the infection. Scrapings are preferred over swabs whenever possible, and Dacron and rayon swabs are recommended because cotton is toxic to the organism. Swabs are placed in a suitable transport medium, which contains sucrose and phosphate buffer and antibiotics to inhibit other organisms. Two swab systems are commercially available and include a narrow swab for conjunctival and male urethral specimens as well as a second, larger swab for collection of the cervical specimen. Specimens include conjunctival, urethral, cervical, or rectal scrapings or swabs; endocervical and nasopharyngeal swabs; and biopsy samples from the lung.

Identification

Identification of *Chlamydia* includes cytological methods, cell culture, antigen detection, nucleic acid probes, and nucleic acid amplification tests. Cytological tests require epithelial cells, which have been scraped from the infected areas. The cells are stained with iodine solution or Giemsa stain and examined for the presence of cytoplasmic and perinuclear chlamydial inclusions. Glycogen in the inclusions stains light to dark brown with iodine stain, whereas the inclusions stain purple with Giemsa stain. The inclusions also can be detected using a fluorescein-labeled serum with antichlamydial antibodies. The specificity of the fluorescent technique can be improved with the use of monoclonal antibodies.

Cell cultures are needed to grow *Chlamydia* organisms; cell scrapings are collected and placed into a cell culture medium. The usual cell line is McCoy's heteroploid murine cells that have been pretreated with cycloheximide. Other suitable cell lines for chlamydia include HeLa-229 cells, L-929 cells, and BHK-21 cells. In this process, a monolayer of the cell culture is inoculated with the skin scrapings, and a coverslip is applied. The cell cultures are examined in 48 to 72 hours, at which time the coverslip is removed and stained with iodine and Giemsa and then examined for inclusion bodies. Alternatively, fluorescein-labeled chlamydial antibody can be added to the coverslip, which is then observed for fluorescent inclusion bodies. Although extremely sensitive, cell culture methods are complex and may be labor intensive.

Serological methods to detect antibody formation to *Chlamydia* include complement fixation, enzyme immunoassay, and immunofluorescence. The usefulness of serologic testing is limited because of a high prevalence of *C. trachomatis* antibody in the population, even in the absence of infection. Complement fixation is more valuable in the diagnosis of lymphogranuloma venereum and *C. psittaci* infections. Commercially available ELISA products, which use purified *Chlamydia* antigen, are used to detect chlamydial antibody in the patient's serum. Immunofluorescent procedures also can detect patient antibody in serum or secretions through reaction with specific serotypes of chlamydial antigen. Many methods are available that provide for serial dilutions of the patient serum so that the antibody titer can be determined.

Chlamydial antigen can be detected with a direct fluorescent antibody (DFA) technique in which antibodies to the outer membrane protein or lipopolysaccharides are bound to fluorescein-labeled isothiocyanate. The specimen is added, and in a positive reaction the fluorescein-labeled antibody binds to the elementary body in the organism. The antigen also can be detected by using a direct enzyme immunoassay: Antibodies are directed against the outer membrane protein, or lipopolysaccharides are used to detect these components of the organism.

Molecular methods, including nucleic acid amplification and polymerase chain reaction, have been shown to have high sensitivity and have become important diagnostic tools for *C. trachomatis*. Nucleic acid probes identify the specific 16S ribosomal RNA sequence. Because amplification is not required, these tests are rapid and cost effective; however, sensitivity may be low because of low levels of antigen in the specimen. Nucleic acid amplification methods are very sensitive because the specific nucleic acid sequence is amplified, which enhances its detection even when present in small amounts.

Treatment

Most *Chlamydia* infections can be treated with tetracycline, such as doxycycline; erythromycin, such as azithromycin; or the fluoroquinolones.

CHLAMYDOPHILA PSITTACI

Chlamydophila psittaci is the agent of psittacosis, a disease of psittacine birds, such as parrots, parakeets, and cockatoos. The infection also is known as **ornithosis**, because *C. psittaci* also can be carried by other birds, including turkeys, pigeons, and chickens. Humans may acquire the infection by inhalation of contaminated aerosols or fomites found in excrement or urine from infected birds. The infection incubates for 1 to 2 weeks and is characterized by chills, fever, and malaise. The severity of the infection can vary from a mild and subclinical respiratory infection to a severe and fatal pneumonia. After inhalation, the organism is deposited in the alveoli of the lungs and ingested by alveolar macrophages; it then enters the regional lymph nodes. This may be followed by dissemination to the reticuloendothelial system, where the liver and spleen may be infected. Necrosis may occur, and the infection also can spread to the lungs and other organs. The most common manifestation is a mild to moderately severe pneumonia with fever, headache, and a nonproductive cough. Jaundice and endocarditis may occur in the severe form of the disease. Ornithosis is an occupational hazard for poultry workers, zookeepers, veterinarians, and pet shop workers, and avian pet owners also are at increased risk of infection.

Ornithosis is usually diagnosed through the patient's history and through serological testing by the demonstration of a fourfold increase in antibody titer, using the complement fixation technique. Acute and convalescent sera are required.

The infection is treated with macrolides and tetracycline.

CHLAMYDOPHILA PNEUMONIAE

Chlamydophila pneumoniae is associated with mild respiratory tract infections, including pharyngitis and sinusitis. The organism also may cause more serious respiratory infections, such as bronchitis and pneumonia. It is believed that the organism is spread from human to human without an animal reservoir. The species, which was once known as "TWAR" (for the first two isolates, which were designated TW-183 and AR-39), is pear shaped with a large periplasmic space and round elementary bodies. The infection is diagnosed through tissue culture, using HeLa or Hep-2 cell lines; serological methods; and molecular amplification techniques. For serological diagnosis, micro-immunofluorescence is recommended; an IgM titer of over 1:16 or a fourfold increase in the IgG titer is diagnostic for infection.

C. pneumoniae infections are treated with macrolides, tetracyclines, or levofloxacin.

Mycoplasma

Mycoplasma species are classified as Mollicutes in the family Mycoplasmataceae. The *mycoplasma* are the smallest free-living organisms known and are found in several animals and plants. *Mycoplasma* organisms differ from bacteria because they do not have a cell wall and thus have a very pleomorphic morphology. These organisms contain both DNA and RNA and can replicate on their own and grow on artificial media. Mycoplasmas cannot synthesize cell wall components and are therefore resistant to all antibiotics that inhibit cell wall synthesis, such as the β-lactams. Mycoplasmas were originally known as "pleuropneumonia-like organisms" (PPLOs) because they were first discovered causing pleuropneumonia in cattle.

The family Mycoplasmataceae contains two genera: *Mycoplasma* and *Ureaplasma*. Several species of *Mycoplasma* and *Ureaplasma* exist, but only a few species are associated with human infection. These include the species *M. hominis*; *M. genitalium*; and *U. urealyticum*, which colonize and possibly infect the genital tract. *M. pneumoniae* is an important cause of respiratory infections, most notably primary atypical pneumonia. Several species, such as *M. orale*, *M. buccale*, *M. faucium*, and *M. salivarium*, are considered to be normal flora of the upper respiratory tract or oral cavity.

Mycoplasma organisms can be speciated on their ability to ferment glucose, utilize arginine, and hydrolyze urea. **TABLE 18-1** lists reactions for the significant pathogens.

Mycoplasma pneumoniae, previously known as the Eaton agent, is a frequent cause of community-acquired pneumonia and tracheobronchitis in children and young adults. The infection is spread through direct respiratory contact and attaches to the respiratory epithelium by adhesion proteins, which stimulate an inflammatory response. The organism injures the respiratory mucosal cells, impairing the function of the cilia. *Mycoplasma pneumoniae* also can colonize the nose, throat, and lower respiratory airways, and the infection can be spread by coughing. Infections may be either asymptomatic or manifest as a respiratory tract infection. After an incubation period of 2 to 3 weeks, the infection begins with mild respiratory symptoms, but later there may be a fever; a headache; malaise; and a persistent, dry nonproductive cough. The disease often is referred to as **primary atypical pneumonia** because it is accompanied by a dry cough instead of the typical exudate associated with bacterial pneumonia. In addition, because it lacks a cell wall, *M. pneumoniae* does not respond to traditional antimicrobial therapy, such as penicillin, for bacterial pneumonias.

Another common name for mycoplasma pneumonia is "walking pneumonia," so called because the individual may appear only moderately ill and is still well enough to participate in daily activities, despite the presence of widespread pulmonary infiltrates. The chest X-ray film usually shows a patchy infiltration of the hilar areas of the lungs; the middle and lower portions of the lobes may be involved later. The Gram stain of sputum usually shows mononuclear inflammatory cells with normal oropharyngeal flora. Infections are most common in the autumn and winter months and often seen in individuals who are in close contact, such as in military camps, schools, or dormitories.

M. pneumoniae also is associated with pharyngitis, rhinitis, and ear infections. Complications of *M. pneumoniae* infections include hemolytic anemia, skin rash, meningitis, and a temporary arthritis. Infections can be treated with erythromycin or tetracycline but not with the β-lactams or other cell wall–inhibiting antibiotics.

The genital mycoplasmas include *Mycoplasma hominis*, *Mycoplasma genitalium*, and *Ureaplasma urealyticum*. These organisms can colonize adults asymptomatically and also are a cause of nongonococcal urethritis in males. *M. hominis* also has been identified as an agent in salpingitis and postpartum fever in females.

Mycoplasmas may be identified through culture, antigen detection, serology, or polymerase chain reaction. For culture methods, blood, sputum, synovial fluid, vaginal discharge, urethral swabs, tissue washings, or amniotic fluid can be examined, based on the site of infection. Throat swabs may be used to isolate *M. pneumoniae* because the organism can colonize the throat.

Because the organisms are very prone to drying and osmotic changes, specimens should be placed into a transport medium. Usually, two media are inoculated to grow mycoplasmas. A diphasic liquid medium that contains fresh yeast extract, peptone, and horse serum is used. In addition, an agar, such as E-agar or Shepard's A7-B agar, should be inoculated. The agars may be supplemented with substrates, such as glucose, arginine, or

TABLE 18-1 Biochemical Reactions for Clinically Significant Mycoplasmas

Species	Glucose fermented	Arginine utilized	Urease produced
M. hominis	–	+	–
M. pneumoniae	+	–	–
U. urealyticum	–	–	+

urea. Incubation, either anaerobically or in 5% to 10% carbon dioxide (CO_2), is recommended. *M. hominis* and *U. urealyticum* grow within 1 to 5 days, whereas *M. pneumoniae* requires 1 to 2 weeks to grow. On E-agar, colonies of *M. pneumoniae* appear as a typical "fried egg" appearance, with a dense center and translucent periphery. The reactions for each substrate can be determined and used in the identification of the species. Culture has a low sensitivity, and because of the long incubation time, it has limited clinical utility.

However, because of the difficulty and lengthy process of culturing mycoplasmas, serological identification methods have been the primary method for identification. **Cold agglutinins**, which are nonspecific antibodies produced in response to *M. pneumoniae* infection, develop in approximately 50% of all patients. Cold agglutinins are γ-globulins of the immunoglobulin M (IgM) type, which agglutinate human group O erythrocytes at 4°C but not at 37°C. These antibodies can be detected in the patient's serum shortly after the onset of disease and peak during the convalescent period. A fourfold increase in antibody titer between the acute- and convalescent-phase specimens is diagnostic for current infection. A titer greater than 1:128 also is diagnostic for current infection.

Antibody production against *M. pneumoniae* can be detected using complement fixation, ELISA, or fluorescent antibody methods. Several of these methods are commercially available and able to detect IgG and IgM antibodies against *M. pneumoniae*. It is most useful to test acute and convalescent sera and show an increasing titer for diagnosis. Enzyme immunoassay tests are used most frequently to diagnose *mycoplasma* infection in the United States.

Antigenic testing has a low sensitivity and specificity and is thus not recommended. Polymerase chain reaction is useful in that it shows a higher degree of sensitivity in detecting the organism.

The mycoplasmas can be treated with erythromycin, doxycycline, or the fluoroquinolones.

Rickettsiaceae

Included in the family Rickettsiaceae are the genera *Rickettsia* and *Orienta*. The organisms are gram-negative, obligate intracellular bacteria that divide by binary fission and contain both RNA and DNA. *Rickettsia* infects a larger variety of wild animals, including birds, small mammals, rats, cattle, sheep, rodents, and flying squirrels. The infections are spread through insect vectors, such as lice, fleas, mites, and ticks. The *Rickettsia* cannot survive outside of the animal host or insect vector. **TABLE 18-2** summarizes the Rickettsiaceae, including group, species, disease, and insect vector.

TABLE 18-2 Clinically Significant *Rickettsia, Coxiella, Ehrlichia, Orientia,* and *Anaplasma*

Group	Species	Infection	Transmission
Spotted fever	*Rickettsia rickettsii*	Rocky Mountain spotted fever	Ticks: *Dermacentor*
	R. akari	Rickettsialpox	Mites: *Allodermanyssus*
	R. australis	Queensland typhus	Ticks: *Ixodes holocyclus*
	R. conorii	Boutonneuse fever Mediterranean spotted fever	Ticks: *Haemaphysalis*
Typhus	*R. prowazekii*	Epidemic typhus and sporadic typhus	Human body louse: *Pediculus humanus* Fleas from flying squirrels
		Brill-Zinsser disease (recrudescent typhus)	Reactivation of latent infection
	R. typhi	Murine typhus	Fleas (infected feces)
Scrub typhus	*Orientia tsutsugamushi*	Scrub typhus	Mites and chigger bites
Q fever	*Coxiella burnetii*	Q fever	Aerosols and ticks
Ehrlichiosis	*E. chaffeensis*	Human monocytic ehrlichiosis	Lone star tick: *Amblyomma americanum*
	E. ewingii	Canine granulocytic ehrlichiosis	Lone star tick: *Amblyomma americanum*
	Anaplasma phagocytophilum	Human granulocytic ehrlichiosis (human anaplasmosis)	Ticks: *Ixodes*

Rickettsial diseases are divided into the spotted fever group, of which there are several species, and the typhus group. The distribution of the type of disease depends on the geographic distribution of the vector. While some *Rickettsia* have a worldwide existence, others have a more limited geographic range.

Rickettsial organisms attach to the host by cell surface receptors. The host is needed for carbohydrate metabolism, amino acid synthesis, and nucleotide formation for the organism. The disease incubates for 3 to 14 days, and the organism multiplies in the endothelial cells of the blood vessels. *Rickettsia* are phagocytized by the host cells, forming a phagolysosome, where the *Rickettsia* multiply and are released after cell lysis. Signs of infection include fever, headache, and a characteristic maculopapular rash, which first appears on the wrists and ankles. The rash spreads to the chest and abdomen and may eventually become petechial in appearance. Cell injury and eventually death can occur from vascular changes as multiplication continues in the blood vessels. Other manifestations of infection include conjunctivitis, pharyngitis, and mild respiratory distress.

Rickettsial disease most often is diagnosed through clinical signs and the patient's medical history. Because these organisms are a Biosafety Level 3 biohazard, specific safety guidelines must be followed. Aerosols can release viable organisms from blood specimens, and laboratory-acquired infections can occur when appropriate safety precautions are not observed.

RICKETTSIA RICKETTSII

Rocky Mountain spotted fever is caused by *Rickettsia rickettsii*, which is the most common rickettsial infection in the United States. There are approximately 2,000 identified cases each year in the United States, with most occurring from April to September. The vector is the hard tick: *Dermacentor variabilis* (the dog tick) is found in the southeastern part of the United States, and *Dermacentor andersoni* (the wood tick) is found in the Rocky Mountain region and in southwestern Canada. The infection incubates for about 1 week following the tick bite. Symptoms include a high fever, severe headache, myalgia, nausea, vomiting, and abdominal pain. Eventually, a spotted or petechial rash may appear, which indicates a more severe infection. This may be followed by neurological, pulmonary, renal, or cardiac complications.

The organism may be visualized in Giemsa stains of tissue biopsies. Direct antigen testing and polymerase chain reaction also are used, generally through reference laboratories. Rocky Mountain spotted fever may be treated with doxycycline; control of the tick population is an important preventive measure.

RICKETTSIA AKARI

Rickettsia akari is the agent of rickettsialpox, which is transmitted through the mite vector. The major animal reservoir is rodents, and humans are an accidental host. This is a biphasic infection where there is first a papule at the area of the bite; the infection spreads, and an eschar form develops after a 1- to 3-week incubation. In the second phase, there is an abrupt onset of fever, severe headache, chills, perspiration, and photophobia. A papulovesicular rash occurs in 2 to 3 days, which eventually crusts over. The infection is generally mild and is treated with doxycycline.

RICKETTSIA PROWAZEKII

Rickettsia prowazekii is the agent of louse-borne or epidemic typhus, which is found most often in Central and South America and Africa and occurs less frequently in the United States. It is generally found in crowded, unsanitary, impoverished living conditions. The vector is the human body louse (*Pediculus humanus*). Sporadic cases occur in the southeastern United States, where infected squirrel fleas can transmit the organism from flying squirrels to humans. Recrudescent disease, or Brill-Zinsser disease, can occur after initial infection with *R. prowazekii*. There is no eschar with *R. prowazekii*; the disease is characterized by fever, headache, myalgia, arthralgia, and neurological symptoms. A petechial or macular rash may occur. Treatment is with tetracycline, and louse control is an important preventive measure.

RICKETTSIA TYPHI

Rickettsia typhi is the agent of endemic, or murine, typhus, which is found in warm, humid climates. In the United States, there are approximately 50 to 100 cases per year, with most cases occurring along the Gulf Coast and in Southern California. The disease also is found in Africa, Asia, Australia, Europe, and South America. Rodents are the primary animal reservoirs, and the vectors include the rat flea (*Xenopsylla cheopis*) and the cat flea (*Ctenocephalides felis*), which is found in cats, raccoons, and squirrels.

There is a 1- to 2-week incubation period, followed by an abrupt onset of fever, chills, headache, myalgia, and nausea. A rash may occur later, generally on the chest and abdomen. The infection is not very severe and is treated with tetracycline.

ORIENTIA TSUTSUGAMUSHI

Orientia tsutsugamushi, formerly known as *Rickettsia tsutsugamushi*, is the agent of scrub typhus, which is transmitted through mites. The main animal reservoir is rodents. The infection is found in Eastern Asia, Australia, and Japan; imported cases may occur in the United States. There is headache, fever, myalgia, and a maculopapular rash on the trunk. Complications may include splenomegaly and lymphadenopathy. Scrub typhus is treated with doxycycline and prevented through control of the rodent and mite populations.

Identification of *Rickettsia*

Some laboratories may still use the **Weil-Felix reaction** to identify *Rickettsia*. Serum from patients with suspected rickettsial infections agglutinate specific strains of *Proteus vulgaris*; the strains of *P. vulgaris* used are OX-19, OX-2, and OX-K. For example, with rickettsialpox, no agglutination occurs in any of the *Proteus* strains, whereas agglutination is observed with OX-19 and OX-2 but not with OX-K for Rocky Mountain spotted fever. The test is lacking in specificity, and several diseases yield variable results; thus the test is only presumptive. Confirmation with a more specific method, such as micro-immunofluorescence, is necessary to detect serum antibodies to *Rickettsia*. In this procedure, antigenic dots for rickettsial diseases are fixed on a microscopic slide, and the patient's serum is added. A fluorescein-conjugated antihuman globulin is added, which binds to the antigen–antibody complex in a positive reaction.

Tissue samples can be cultivated in embryonated eggs or tissue culture or can be stained directly with an immunofluorescent dye to detect *Rickettsia*. There also are polymerase chain reaction methods to identify some of the *Rickettsia*.

Anaplasmataceae

The family Anaplasmataceae includes the genera *Ehrlichia* and *Anaplasma*. These organisms can survive in cytoplasmic vacuoles and are able to grow in neutrophils, monocytes, platelets, and erythrocytes. They multiply by binary fission within the vacuoles of the host's cells. The organism has two forms: the elementary body and the reticulate body, which forms morulae within the host cell. The morulae can be visualized by staining tissue with Wright's or Giemsa stain.

EHRLICHIA

Ehrlichia chaffeensis is the agent of human monocytic ehrlichiosis, which is found in the Southeast, Midwest and South–Central areas of the United States. The lone star tick (*Amblyomma americanum*) is the primary vector, and white-tailed deer and dogs are significant animal reservoirs. The infection begins with an infected tick bite. Symptoms include flu-like symptoms, fever, headache, and myalgia. A rash occurs later in approximately a third of the patients. There also may be leukopenia and thrombocytopenia; however, the infection is generally mild.

Ehrlichia ewingii is the agent of granulocytic ehrlichiosis. *Amblyomma americanum* is the tick vector, and dogs are the main animal reservoir for *E. ewingii. E. ewingii* invades granulocytes, especially neutrophils. *Anaplasma phagocytophilum* is the agent of human anaplasmosis. The animal reservoir for *Anaplasma phagocytophilum* includes chipmunks and white-footed mice, as well as horses and dogs. *Ixodes* ticks serve as the vector; the infection is transmitted when the larva and nymph stages ingest blood from an infected host during a blood meal. Humans are accidental hosts, and the organism invades the neutrophils, eosinophils, and basophils. There are flu-like symptoms—headache, myalgia, and a rash in a small percentage of those infected. There is a leukopenia, thrombocytopenia, and an elevation in liver enzymes. Infection with *Anaplasma* is more severe than infection than with *Ehrlichia ewingii.*

Ehrlichia infections are diagnosed through patient history, clinical symptoms, and demonstration of the morulae within the host cells. DNA amplification techniques are available through reference laboratories. An increasing antibody titer also can be used to diagnose infection. *Ehrlichia* and *Anaplasma* infections are treated with doxycycline.

COXIELLA

Coxiella burnetii was previously classified with *Rickettsia* because of its gram-negative cell wall, its association with tick-borne disease, and its intracellular growth. However, it is now believed that *Coxiella* more closely resembles the gram-negative bacillus *Legionella*. *C. burnetii* is the agent of Q (query) fever. The organism has a small cell variant (SCV) form, which is resistant to the environment, and a large cell variant (LCV) form, which multiplies in host monocytes and macrophages after phagocytosis. There is an antigenic variation in the lipopolysaccharide of the cell wall; phase I antigens are able to block the host antibody with surface proteins, whereas phase II antigens expose the host antibody. Acute antibodies are formed against the phase II antigens, whereas antibodies are formed against both phase I and II antigens in chronic infection.

There are many animal reservoirs for *C. burnetii* including cats, dogs, birds, sheep, and cattle. *Coxiella* can survive in soil and the environment for months once it has been shed in animal stools, urine, or other products. Humans may acquire the infection through inhalation of the organism in contaminated soil and also by ingesting contaminated milk or other animal products. Those at increased risk of *Coxiella* infection include food handlers, veterinarians, and cattle ranchers.

Q fever is generally an asymptomatic or mild infection; however, there may be nonspecific flu-like symptoms. A small percentage of the cases may progress to affect the liver or lungs. There also is a slowly progressive form of the disease, which is chronic and has a higher mortality.

C. burnetii may be grown in culture or identified serologically with immunofluorescence or enzyme-linked immunoassay. In chronic Q fever, there are antibodies to both phase I and II antigens, with the titers of phase I antigens at a higher amount. In acute Q fever, there are IgM and IgG phase II antibodies. *Coxiella* infection is treated with doxycycline; chronic forms of the infection may require a combination therapy of doxycycline with rifampin or fluoroquinolones.

Review Questions

Matching

Match the correct species for each rickettsial infection listed. Then select the mode of transmission of the infection. List all responses that apply.

Species	Insect	Vector
1. Rocky Mountain spotted fever	a. *Orientia tsutsugamushi*	A. Tick bite
2. Rickettsialpox	b. *Rickettsia rickettsii*	B. Lice
3. Epidemic typhus	c. *Coxiella burnetii*	C. Chigger bite
4. Q fever	d. *Rickettsia akari*	D. Aerosols
5. Scrub typhus	e. *Rickettsia typhi*	E. Mite bite
	f. *Rickettsia prowazekii*	

Multiple Choice

6. Which statement correctly describes the genus *Chlamydia?*
   a. Classified as viruses
   b. Do not contain both DNA and RNA
   c. Obligate intracellular bacteria
   d. Smallest free-living organisms known
7. The agent in ornithosis is:
   a. *Mycoplasma pneumoniae*
   b. *Chlamydophila pneumoniae*
   c. *Chlamydia trachomatis*
   d. *Chlamydophila psittaci*
8. Each of the following conditions has been associated with *C. trachomatis* except:
   a. Lymphogranuloma venereum
   b. Nongonococcal urethritis
   c. Infant pneumonitis
   d. Atypical pneumonia
9. Which of the following serotypes are associated with *Chlamydia* diseases acquired through the venereal route?
   a. A, B, B-1, and D
   b. D through K
   c. L4, L5, and L6
   d. All the above
10. The iodine stain for identification of *C. trachomatis* stains:
    a. The glycogen in the inclusion brown
    b. The periplasmic space purple
    c. The cell membrane brown
    d. The DNA in the inclusion purple
11. The DFA technique for *Chlamydia trachomatis* detects:
    a. Patient's antibodies to *C. trachomatis*
    b. Elementary bodies of *C. trachomatis*
    c. Cold-agglutinating antibodies produced in response to *C. trachomatis* infection
    d. Febrile agglutinins
12. Each of the following statements correctly describes the mycoplasmas *except:*
    a. They contain both DNA and RNA.
    b. They do not have a cell wall.

c. They cannot replicate on their own.
d. They are the smallest free-living organisms known.

13. *Mycoplasma pneumoniae*:
    a. Responds well to penicillin therapy
    b. Is the etiologic agent of primary atypical pneumonia
    c. Is most often identified through culture and biochemical reactions
    d. All the above

14. Which of the following results for cold agglutinins would be indicative of current infection with *Mycoplasma pneumoniae*?
    a. Acute titer of 4 and convalescent titer of 32
    b. Acute titer of 4 and convalescent titer of 8
    c. Convalescent titer of 256
    d. Both a and c are correct.
    e. All are correct.

Bibliography

Bachmann, L. H., Johnson, R. E., Cheng, H., Markowitz, L., Papp, J. R., Palella, F. J. Jr., & Hook, E. W. 3rd. (2010). Nucleic acid amplification test for diagnosis of *Neisseria gonorrhoeae* and *Chlamydia trachomatis* rectal infections. *Journal of Clinical Microbiology, 48,* 1827–1832.

Barnes, R. C. (1989). Laboratory diagnosis of human chlamydial infections. *Clinical Microbiology Reviews, 2,* 199.

Centers for Disease Control and Prevention. (2005). *Mycoplasma pneumoniae.* Retrieved from http://www.cdc.gov/ncidod/dbmd/diseaseinfo/mycoplasmapneum_t.htm

Centers for Disease Control and Prevention. (2010). Chlamydial infections. Retrieved from http://www.cdc.gov/std/treatment/2010/chlamydial-infections.htm

Centers for Disease Control and Prevention. (2010). Ehrlichiosis. Retrieved from http://www.cdc.gov/Ehrlichiosis/

Corsaro, D., & Greub, G. (2006). Pathogenic potential of novel chlamydiae and diagnostic approaches to infections due to these obligate intracellular parasites. *Clinical Microbiology Reviews, 19,* 283–297.

Crosse, B. A. (1990). Psittacosis: A clinical review. *Journal of Infectious Diseases, 21,* 251.

Gaydose, C. A., Cartwright, C. P., Colaninno, P., Welsch, J., Holden, J., Ho, S. Y., Webb, E. M., . . . Robinson, J. (2010). Performance of the Abbott RealTime CT/NG for detection of *Chlamydia trachomatis* and *Neisseria gonorrhoeae. Journal of Clinical Microbiology, 48,* 3235–3243.

McTighe, A. G. (1982). *Chlamydia trachomatis:* Review of human chlamydial infections and laboratory diagnosis. *Laboratory Medicine, 13,* 638.

Nelson, J. A., & Bouseman, J. K. (1992). Human tick-borne illnesses: United States. *Clinical Microbiology Newsletter, 14,* 105.

Parola, P., Paddock, C. D., & Raoult, D. (2005). Tick-borne rickettsioses around the world: Emerging diseases challenging old concepts. *Clinical Microbiology Reviews, 18,* 719–756.

Rikihisa, Y. (1991). The tribe Ehrlichiae and ehrlichial diseases. *Clinical Microbiology Reviews, 4,* 286.

She, R. C., Thurber, A., Hymas, W. C., Stevenson, J., Langer, J., Litwin, C. M., & Petti, C. A. (2010). Limited utility of culture for *Mycoplasma pneumoniae* and *Chlamydophila pneumoniae* for diagnosis of respiratory tract infections. *Journal of Clinical Microbiology, 48,* 3380–3382.

Waites, K. B., & Talkington, D. F. (2004). *Mycoplasma pneumoniae* and its role as a human pathogen. *Clinical Microbiology Reviews, 17,* 697–728.

Walker, D. H. (1989). Rocky Mountain spotted fever: A disease in need of microbiological concern. *Clinical Microbiology Reviews, 2,* 227.

NEWS: ROCKY MOUNTAIN SPOTTED FEVER

Tick-borne rickettsioses are some of the oldest known vector-borne diseases. The first clinical description of Rocky Mountain spotted fever (RMSF) was in 1899. By 1906, Howard T. Ricketts determined that the wood tick played a role in the transmission of the disease. In 1919, *Rickettsia rickettsii*, which was then known as *Dermacentroxenus rickettsii*, was maintained in ticks. *R. rickettsii* was the only tick-borne *Rickettsia* associated with human infection in the western hemisphere for the next 90 years! Ricketts and von Prowazek were early researchers of rickettsial diseases, and unfortunately, both died of typhus. The agents of typhus and Rocky Mountain spotted fever, *R. prowazekii* and *R. rickettsii*, were named in their honor. Other *rickettsii* identified as human pathogens prior to the 1980s include *R. conorii* subspecies *conorii* (Mediterranean spotted fever), *R. sibirica* supspecies *sibirica* (Siberian tick typhus), and *R. australis* (Queensland tick typhus). Emerging pathogens identified more recently include *R. japonica* (Japanese spotted fever), *R. africae* (African tick bite fever), and *R. honei* (Flinders Island spotted fever).

Ticks in the genus *Ixodes*, also known as "hard" ticks, act as vectors or reservoirs of infection. The principal vectors of RMSF in the United States are *Dermacentor variabilis* and *D. andersoni*. *D. variabilis*, the dog tick, is found in the Great Plains region, along the Atlantic coast, and in California, southwestern Oregon, and southwestern Canada. *D. andersoni*, the Rocky Mountain wood tick, is found in the Rocky Mountain states and Canada. The adult ticks feed on large animals, such as cattle, horses, deer, bears, and sheep, whereas the immature forms feed on small mammals. The ticks are most active during the late spring and summer. Thus, most cases of RMSF occur during June and July.

RMSF is the most severe of all tick-borne rickettsioses. It has been a reportable disease in the United States since the 1920s, and the incidence has increased from 2002 to 2008, from 495 to 2,500 cases. During 2009, cases decreased almost 30% from the previous year.

However, because of improvements in diagnosis and treatment, the case fatality rate has decreased to less than 0.5%. RMSF occurs in many states, but five states account for over half of the cases: North Carolina, Oklahoma, Arkansas, Tennessee, and Missouri. Of special note is the increased number of cases in Arizona, where over 90 cases were reported in 2009. The tick identified in these cases was *Rhipicephalus sanguineus*, and the reservoir was found to be free-roaming dogs.

Most cases are found in rural areas, but some cases have been found in large urban centers, where *Rickettsia*-infected *D. variabilis* was found in vacant lots and parks.

The incubation period of RMSF is about 1 week; there is no eschar, but there is an abrupt onset of high fever, headache, malaise, myalgia, nausea, vomiting, abdominal pain, and diarrhea. These symptoms are nonspecific, which may delay the diagnosis. The rash typically does not occur until at least the third day of the fever; it first appears as small, pink macules on the wrist, ankles, and forearms that may later form papules or petechiae. The rash spreads to the trunk and the palms of the hands and soles of the feet. The spotted rash is apparent by the fifth day of infection and is an indication of a more severe disease. Almost 90% of those infected exhibit a rash during the course of the disease.

RMSF may result in neurological complications, such as convulsions or hearing loss. There also may be renal and pulmonary failure, necrosis and gangrene of the fingers or toes, and myocarditis. The case fatality rate is 10 % to 25%; higher fatality rates are seen in older patients and those who receive delayed or no antibiotic treatment. Death may occur in the first 8 days of infection when not treated. Tetracyclines, especially doxycycline, are the recommended antibiotic treatments.

BIBLIOGRAPHY

Centers for Disease Control and Prevention. (2011). Rocky Mountain spotted fever. Retrieved from http://www.cdc.gov/rmsf/index.html

Parola, P., Paddock, C. D., & Raoult, D. (2005). Tick-borne rickettsioses around the world: Emerging diseases challenging old concepts. *Clinical Microbiology Reviews, 18*, 719–756.

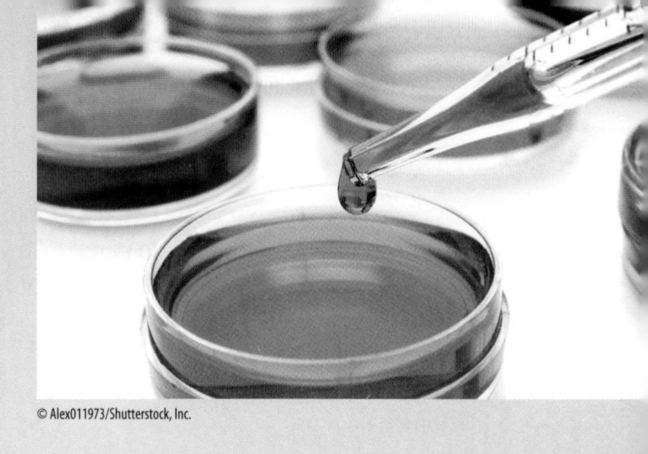

CHAPTER 19
Introduction to Virology

CHAPTER OUTLINE

Viral Structure and Characteristics

Seleted Medically Important Viruses

KEY TERMS

Acquired immunodeficiency syndrome
Adsorption
Capsid
Capsomer
Cytopathogenic effect
Diploid cell lines
Eclipse
Encephalitis
Envelope
Exanthem subitum
Hemagglutinin antigen
Hepatitis
Heteroploid cell lines
Latent viral infections
Mumps
Neuraminidase antigen
Nucleocapsid
Penetration
Polio
Primary cell cultures
Rabies
Retroviruses
Rubella
Rubeola
Smallpox
Uncoating
Varicella
Viremia
Virion

LEARNING OBJECTIVES

1. Define the terms "virion" and "capsid."
2. Discuss the general structural characteristics of viruses.
3. Classify medically important viruses as DNA or RNA viruses.
4. Describe the viral replication cycle.
5. Discuss important criteria in the selection, collection, and processing of specimens for virology.
6. Discuss the use of the following in viral identification:
   a. Cytological examination
   b. Electron microscopy
   c. Molecular diagnostics
7. Describe cell culture techniques used in clinical virology.
   a. Describe the various types of CPE (cellular changes or damage).
   b. Differentiate among primary, diploid, and heteroploid cell lines.
8. Name the methods for direct detection of viral antigens and genes.
9. Explain how viral antibodies can be detected serologically and describe the antibody response to a typical viral infection.

10. Discuss the important characteristics, route and type of infection, and identification of the following viruses:
    a. Adenovirus
    b. Herpes simplex 1 and 2
    c. Varicella-zoster virus
    d. Cytomegalovirus
    e. Epstein-Barr virus
    f. Human papillomavirus
    g. *Rubivirus*
    h. Poliovirus
    i. Influenza viruses
    j. *Morbillivirus*
    k. Pneumovirus
    l. *Rotavirus*
11. Compare the five hepatitis viruses with respect to epidemiology, identification, and infectious disease.
12. Name and describe the serological markers for hepatitis B virus.
13. Name the agents of the following viral infections and briefly describe the infection:
    a. Roseola
    b. Erythema infectiosum
    c. Smallpox
    d. Common cold
    e. Mumps
    f. Rabies
14. Discuss the important characteristics of the arboviruses.
15. Discuss the properties unique to the Retroviridae.
    a. List the subfamilies and associated viruses of this family.
    b. Describe the structure of human immunodeficiency virus (HIV).
    c. Discuss the transmission and clinical symptoms of acquired immunodeficiency syndrome.
    d. Name and describe the test methods used to identify HIV.

Virology is a rapidly expanding discipline in clinical microbiology. This expansion has occurred, in part, because of the development of modern technologies that have enhanced virus detection, including the use of genetic probes and the polymerase chain reaction (PCR). New antiviral agents have been developed to treat viral infections. There also has been an increased attention to specific viral agents, including influenza, West Nile virus, human immunodeficiency virus, and hepatitis viruses.

Viral Structure and Characteristics

Viruses are obligate intracellular parasites, which are unable to multiply by binary fission. Viruses lack ribosomal ribonucleic acid (RNA) and require host cell biochemical mechanisms for replication. Viruses contain either deoxyribonucleic acid (DNA) or RNA but never both. Because they lack ribosomal RNA, viruses are not able to make their own proteins. The viral RNA or DNA is transcribed into messenger RNA (mRNA) through use of the host cell ribosomes. Viruses cannot generate adenosine triphosphate (ATP) and thus depend on host cells to provide these missing components.

Viruses may be small with a simple structure or large with a complex structure. A virus may have a definite host range and may specifically infect animals, plants, or humans. The size of viruses ranges from 18 nm (parvovirus) to 300 nm (poxviruses), which is below the limits of light microscopy. Viruses may be classified by type of disease but are most commonly categorized based on the type of nucleic acid as either RNA-containing viruses or DNA-containing viruses. There are currently 21 viral families associated with human infection; 14 of these viruses are RNA-containing viruses, and the remaining seven are DNA-containing viruses.

The virus particle is known as the **virion**. The basic structure of the virion consists of a **capsid**, or protein coat, which encloses the genome or genetic material of either DNA or RNA. The capsid is composed of repeating, identical subunits arranged in a precisely defined fashion. Each protein subunit is known as a **capsomer**. The capsid functions to protect the nucleic acid and enables the virus to attach to and enter the host cell. Capsids vary in size and shape among the various types of viruses. Some capsomers assemble to form rod-like capsids, resulting in a helical structure. Other capsids that assemble in a cubic manner create an icosahedral arrangement.

The nucleic acid may be either DNA or RNA; DNA may be either single stranded or double stranded and arranged in either a linear or a circular form. RNA has either a positive sense (+), such as mRNA, or a negative sense (–) and is double stranded or ambisense, with both a positive and negative region. Considerable diversity exists in the genetic makeup and size of viruses. The nucleic acid may code for as few as four genes or as many as several hundred genes. Those viruses with larger genomes are able to carry more genetic information than those with smaller genomes.

The capsid and nucleic acid compose the **nucleocapsid**. Viruses that have an outer membrane, or **envelope**, surrounding the capsid are described as having **enveloped nucleocapsids**. The envelope is a phospholipid bilayer in which glycoproteins and matrix proteins are embedded. The matrix proteins serve to connect the envelope to the capsid, and the glycoproteins act as "spikes" to aid the attachment to host cells. Viruses with enveloped nucleocapsids are more resistant to unfavorable conditions, such as drying and pH changes; they are able to remain moist and are more readily transmitted via respiratory droplets, blood, and other tissues. All negative-sense RNA viruses are enveloped. Viruses that have only a protein coat and no outer envelope are described as having **naked nucleocapsids**. These viruses are more susceptible to drying and other environmental conditions. **FIGURE 19-1** illustrates some representative viral morphologies.

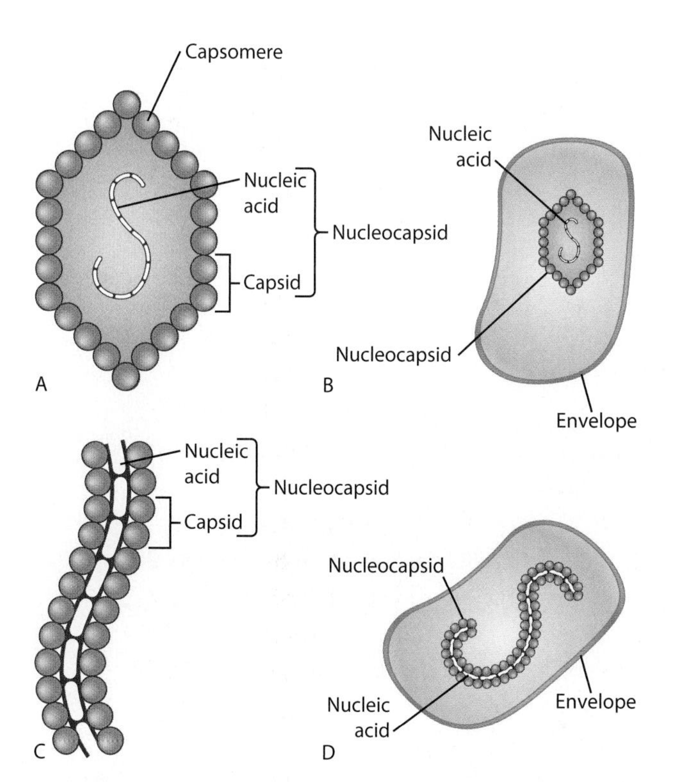

FIGURE 19-1 Viral morphology: (a) naked icosahedral nucleocapsid; (b) enveloped icosahedral nucleocapsid; (c) naked helical nucleocapsid; and (d) enveloped helical nucleocapsid.

Viruses are classified according to the type and arrangement of nucleic acid as well as by the shape of the capsid. The presence or absence of an envelope also is used in classification. **TABLE 19-1** lists viruses that infect humans and their important characteristics.

VIRAL REPLICATION

The host may be exposed to a virus through respiratory aerosols or contaminated food or water; through the congenital route; through contaminated body fluids, such as blood or plasma; through animal or insect bites; or through endogenous latent infections. After transmission of the virus, viral replication occurs in the host cell.

Establishment of viral infection and the intracellular development of a virus constitute a complex series of events. The first step is **adsorption**, which involves the attachment of the virus to the host receptor site. The next step is **penetration** of viral genetic material into the cell. Penetration can occur in various ways, including fusion, phagocytosis, or the injection of viral material into the host cell. The virus loses its capsid in a process known as **uncoating**, which exposes the viral nucleic acid. Replication and expression of genetic material are characteristics of the **eclipse** stage. In this stage, viral nucleic acid acts as a template for production of mRNA, which codes and directs the synthesis of viral proteins. Typically, protein synthesis occurs in the host cell cytoplasm, and the capsid is synthesized in the cytoplasm or nucleus. In the next stage the **assembly** of genetically material into the protein coat occurs. In this maturation stage, virions are assembled. Finally, mature virions migrate to the host nuclear or cytoplasmic membrane and are released. The release of viruses occurs by various means. In enveloped viruses, such as the influenza virus, the cytoplasmic or nuclear membrane surrounds the nucleocapsid to form an envelope. Next, the virus is released through "budding" as the virus is pinched off from the cell. Poliovirus is gradually leaked out of the host cell, while some other viruses enzymatically lyse the host cell after replication is completed and are then released.

Upon release, the virus may spread to local tissues or through the blood, which is known as **viremia**. Primary viremia involves viral invasion of cells of the reticuloendothelial system (RES). Replication in the RES system can result in a secondary viremia that spreads the virus to distal visceral cells.

TABLE 19-1 Classification of Medically Significant Viruses

DNA-containing viruses				
Family	**Genus or group**	**Common name**	**Nucleocapsid**	**Characteristics: shape and size (nm)**
Adenoviridae	*Mastadenovirus*	Adenovirus	DNA ds linear	Icosahedral, 70–90
Hepadnaviridae	*Hepadnavirus*	Hepatitis B virus (HBV)	DNA ds circular	Icosahedral, 42–47 Enveloped
Herpesviridae Subfamilies			DNA, ds Genome size varies with specific virus.	Icosahedral, 100–200 Enveloped
Alphaherpesvirinae	*Simplex virus*	Herpes simplex virus types 1 and 2 (HSV-1 and HSV-2)		
	Varicellavirus	Varicella-zoster virus (VZV) (chickenpox and shingles)		
Betaherpesvirinae	*Cytomegalovirus*	Cytomegalovirus (CMV)		
Gammaherpesvirinae	*Lymphocryptovirus*	Epstein-Barr virus (EBV)		
		Human herpesvirus type 6 (HHV-6) Human herpesvirus type 7 (HHV-7)		
Iridoviridae	*Iridovirus*	African swine fever virus	DNA ds	Icosahedral, 150–300
Papillomaviridae	*Papillomavirus*	Human papillomavirus (wart virus)	DNA ds circular	Icosahedral, 45–55
Polyomaviridae	*Polyomavirus*	*Polyomavirus* strains JC and BK	DNA ds circular	Icosahedral, 40 nm
Parvoviridae	*Parvovirus*	*Parvovirus* strains B-19 and RA-1	DNA ss linear	Icosahedral 20–25
Poxviridae	*Orthopoxvirus*	Variola virus (smallpox virus) Vaccinia virus Molluscum contagiosum Monkeypox virus	DNA ds linear	Complex, brick or oval shaped 225 × 300

RNA-containing viruses				
Family	**Genus or group**	**Common name**	**Nucleocapsid**	**Characteristics: shape and size (nm)**
Arenaviridae	*Arenavirus*	Lymphocytic choriomeninigitis (LCM) virus; Lassa fever virus, Machupo virus, Junin virus, Sabia virus	RNA ss linear + Sense	Helical, 100–130
Bunyaviridae			RNA ss linear + Sense	Helical, 80–110 spherical and pleomorphic
	Bunyavirus	La Crosse virus and California encephalitis viruses		
	Phlebovirus	Rift Valley fever virus		
	Nairovirus	Crimean-Congo hemorrhagic fever virus		
	Hantavirus	Hantaan virus (Korean hemorrhagic fever virus)		
Caliciviridae	*Calicivirus*	Norwalk virus, Sapporo virus	RNA ss linear – Sense	Icosahedral, 25–35
Coronaviridae	*Coronavirus*	Coronavirus strains	RNA ss linear + Sense	Helical, 80–200 spherical and pleomorphic
Filoviridae	*Filovirus*	Marburg virus, Ebola virus (hemorrhagic fevers)	RNA ss linear + Sense	Helical, 80 × 800 filamentous and pleomorphic
Flaviviridae			RNA ss linear + Sense	Icosahedral, 40–50
	Flavivirus	Yellow fever virus, Dengue fever virus, St. Louis encephalitis virus, Japanese encephalitis virus		

TABLE 19-1 Classification of Medically Significant Viruses (Continued)

RNA-containing viruses				
Family	**Genus or group**	**Common name**	**Nucleocapsid**	**Characteristics: shape and size (nm)**
	Hepacivirus	West Nile virus, hepatitis C virus, hepatitis G virus		
Orthomyxoviridae	*Orthomyxovirus*	Influenza viruses A, B, and C	RNA ss linear + Sense	Helical, 80–120 pleomorphic
Paramyxoviridae			RNA ss linear + Sense	Helical, 50–300 enveloped and pleomorphic
	Paramyxovirus	Paramyxoviruses Mumps virus		
	Morbillivirus	Measles virus		
	Pneumovirus	Respiratory syncytial virus (RSV) Human mentapneumovirus		
Picornaviridae			RNA ss linear – Sense	Icosahedral, 24–30
	Human enterovirus	Poliovirus Coxsackieviruses A and B, echoviruses		
	Hepatovirus	Hepatitis A virus (HAV)		
	Rhinovirus	Rhinoviruses (types A, B, C)		
Reoviridae	*Reovirus, Orbivirus, Rotavirus*	Reoviruses, Colorado tick fever Rotaviruses	RNA ds linear	Icosahedral, 60–80
Rhabdoviridae	*Lyssavirus*	Rabies virus	RNA ss linear + Sense	Bullet shaped, 75 × 180
Togaviridae	*Alphavirus*	Eastern, Western, and Venezuelan encephalitis viruses	RNA ss linear + Sense	Icosahedral, 60–70
	Rubivirus	Rubella		
Retroviridae Subfamilies			RNA ss	Icosahedral, 80–100
Oncornavirinae	*Oncornavirus*	Human T cell lymphotropic virus types 1 and 2 (HTLV-1 and HTLV-2)		
Lentivirinae	*Lentivirus*	Human immunodeficiency virus types 1 and 2 (HIV-1 and HIV-2)		

Clinical symptoms of viral infection may occur early in the disease, as is exhibited with rhinovirus, the cause of the common cold. In other types of viral infections, such as polio, the clinical signs may not be evident until the second viremic phase. Other viruses, such as hepatitis A virus (HAV) and hepatitis B virus (HBV), may incubate for weeks or months until clinical signs become apparent.

SPECIMEN SELECTION, COLLECTION, AND PROCESSING

Proper specimen selection and collection depend on good communication between the health care provider and the laboratory. Clinical and epidemiological considerations are important in the selection of specimen type and the determination of possible viral agents. In general, it is optimal to collect the specimen as early in the course of disease as possible. For most viral infections, the viral titer is highest during the first 4 days after the onset of symptoms. Exceptions include enterovirus, adenovirus, and cytomegalovirus (CMV) because prolonged shedding of enterovirus and adenovirus into the stool and CMV into the urine occurs.

It is best to sample the infected site directly. For example, for skin infections, the vesicles or rash should be sampled; for upper respiratory tract infections, the throat, nasal secretions, or nasal washing is cultured. In patients with disseminated viral infections or nonspecific clinical findings, it may be necessary to culture multiple sites. An exception is certain viral infections of the central nervous system (CNS), when it may be recommended to culture the stool or throat instead of the cerebrospinal fluid (CSF). In these patients the virus is typically shed in the stool or found in the throat.

A viral transport medium is recommended for most specimens. This medium contains buffered saline; a protein stabilizer; and antibiotics, such as penicillin, vancomycin, bacitracin, streptomycin, and amphotericin B, to suppress bacterial or fungal overgrowth. Several media are suitable for viral transport and commercially available, including Hank's balanced salt solution, veal infusion broth, sucrose-phosphate-glutamate broth, and Leibovitz-Emory medium. Collection systems consisting of a swab with a viral culture medium, such as Viral Culturettes (Becton Dickinson), are also available. Bacterial culturettes that contain Stuart transport broth also have been found to be suitable for viral transport. Swabs with cotton, rayon, or Dacron on plastic shafts should be used because wood is toxic to viruses. Calcium alginate may bind and inactivate the virus, and charcoal is toxic to several viruses, and thus neither should be used to collect viral specimens.

Prompt transport enhances the detection of the virus, but if a delay in processing the specimen is anticipated, specimens should be held at 4°C but not frozen. Freezing can destroy the infectivity of some viruses quickly and is recommended only when a prolonged delay of 24 hours or more after collection is expected. When freezing is required, viral specimens should be snap frozen to at least –70°C and transported in dry ice or with liquid nitrogen. Conventional freezing to –20°C is not suitable for storing specimens for virology.

For viral infections of the respiratory tract, including pharyngitis and the common cold, nasopharyngeal secretions, aspirates or swabs, sputum, throat swabs, or bronchial washings are collected. Viral agents associated with upper respiratory tract infections include rhinoviruses, influenza viruses, parainfluenza viruses, respiratory syncytial virus (RSV), Epstein-Barr virus (EBV), Herpes simplex virus types 1 and 2 (HSV-1 and HSV-2), and coronavirus. Viral agents associated with croup and bronchiolitis include the influenza and parainfluenza viruses, RSV, and adenovirus. Agents of pneumonia in children include RSV, the parainfluenza viruses, adenovirus, measles, and varicella-zoster virus (VZV). For adults, viral agents of pneumonia include the influenza viruses, HSV, VZV, CMV, and RSV.

For suspected cases of aseptic meningitis, CSF, a throat swab, and stool cultures should be collected. Viral agents associated with aseptic meningitis include the enteroviruses, echoviruses, HSV-2, VZV, mumps virus, and lymphocytic choriomeningitis virus (LCM). Urine also should be cultured if mumps virus is suspected. Serum for serological testing should be collected in addition to cultures for HSV, VZV, LCM, and mumps.

Encephalitis may result from infection with HSV-1, VZV, and the arboviruses. Brain biopsy and blood should be submitted for analysis, and serum also should be collected when arbovirus, HSV, or VZV are suspected.

Exanthems include vesicular rashes and maculopapular rashes. Vesicular rashes may be associated with HSV, VZV, coxsackievirus, and echovirus. Maculopapular rashes may result from infection with measles, rubella, the enteroviruses, CMV, EBV, parvovirus B-19, and human herpesvirus type 6 (HHV-6). Throat swabs or washings and stool cultures also may be collected to isolate these viral agents. If CMV is suspected, urine, EDTA-anticoagulated blood, and serum for acute-phase serology also should be collected. Acute and convalescent sera are recommended for the diagnosis of EBV, rubella, and measles.

HSV is an important viral pathogen in the genitourinary tract. Diseases include urethritis, cervicitis, vulvovaginitis, and penile lesions. For HSV, vesicular fluid collected using a needle aspirate or cells collected from the base of the lesion are recommended. Endocervical swabs are also acceptable.

Stool specimens should be collected in cases of viral gastroenteritis. Viral agents of gastroenteritis include rotavirus, Norwalk-like agent, adenovirus types 40 and 41, and calcivirus. Rectal swabs also may be submitted, although stool specimens are preferred. Direct antigen testing using enzyme-linked immunosorbent assay (ELISA) can be performed if rotavirus or adenovirus types 40 and 41 are suspected. Norwalk agent and calcivirus must be examined through electron microscopy.

Ophthalmic viral infections include conjunctivitis and keratitis. Viral agents associated with these infections include HSV, adenovirus, and VZV conjunctival swabs; corneal or conjunctival scrapings are suitable specimens.

Congenital or neonatal viral pathogens include rubella, HSV, and CMV. CMV is isolated from the urine or throat. When rubella is suspected, throat swabs placed into viral transport media are recommended for collection. Serum also should be collected during the acute phase of the illness for CMV and rubella.

In cases of disseminated diseases, throat, nasal, or eye swabs; urine; blood; or skin scrapings may be collected. Swabs or scrapings should be placed into viral transport media, and 5 ml to 10 ml of urine should be collected into a sterile screw-cap tube. Blood should be collected into an EDTA-anticoagulated blood collection tube. Viruses that may be associated with disseminated diseases include the enteroviruses (coxsackieviruses, echovirus), CMV, HSV, VZV, and HBV. HBV may be diagnosed through serological testing, and acute-phase serum should be collected for HSV, VZV, CMV, and HBV.

Viral agents associated with lymphadenopathy include EBV, CMV, and HIV. Urine or throat swabs should be collected for CMV, and serum for serology should be collected for HBV and HIV. Viral agents associated with immunosuppressed individuals include CMV, HSV, and VZV. Urine and throat swabs are recommended for CMV, and swabs of vesicular fluid should be submitted for HSV and VZV.

Blood is generally not cultured in suspected viremia because of the low virus yield and because the detectable viremic phase is usually gone by the time that symptoms become present. Blood should be collected, however, from patients with suspected viral hemorrhagic fevers caused by adenovirus and with arboviral infections. In these patients, 5 ml to 10 ml of blood should be collected into either an EDTA-, acid-citrate-dextrose–, or heparin-anticoagulated blood collection tube.

LABORATORY METHODS IN VIROLOGY

Laboratory methods for the detection of virus infections include cytological or histological examination; electron microscopy; virus isolation in cell or tissue culture; shell vial centrifugation–enhanced virus detection; direct detection of viral antigens or genes; molecular methods, such as target gene amplification (PCR); and serological detection of viral antibody.

Cytological or Histological Examination

Cytological or histological examination requires properly fixed and stained cells from an appropriate specimen. The presence of multinucleate giant cells or cytoplasmic or nuclear inclusions may aid in the diagnosis of a particular viral infection. DNA viruses usually are assembled in the nucleus and thus produce intranuclear inclusions, whereas RNA viruses, which are usually assembled in the cytoplasm, typically produce cytoplasmic inclusions. HSV and VZV produce intranuclear inclusions, which can be observed in cells from the cutaneous lesions. CMV may produce the characteristic "owl eyes" inclusions. In general, however, cytological examination is insensitive and nonspecific.

Electron Microscopy

Electron microscopy is a sensitive tool, although it is often not available in many microbiology laboratories. In negative staining using electron microscopy, clinical material is placed on a carbon-coated grid and then stained with potassium phosphotungstate or uranylacetate. Stain surrounds the virus, and the electron beam cannot pass through the metallic background. However, the beam can pass through the virus. The virus is seen as a light structure against a dark background. The virus particle can be examined for size and shape. Electron microscopy is the only way to detect Norwalk agent, astroviruses, caliciviruses, and coronaviruses because these viruses do not grow in conventional cell cultures and tests for viral antigens are either unavailable or inaccessible.

Virus Isolation in Cell or Tissue Culture

Virus isolation in culture remains the gold standard for the isolation of many viruses. When performed correctly, few, if any, false-positive results occur because infected target cells definitely indicate that the infectious agent is present in the specimen. Three types of cell cultures exist, including traditional cell cultures, shell vial centrifugation–enhanced (SVCE) cultures, and multiwell microplate cultures.

Cell cultures are animal or human cells grown in vitro that have lost their differentiation. The cells are grown as a single layer on the internal surface of glass or plastic containers to form a cell monolayer. As an alternative, the cells also can be grown in multiwell microtiter plates. These cells are sensitive to the effects of viruses, and after inoculation and incubation with the specimen are examined for **cytopathogenic effect** (CPE), which refers to cellular damage or changes in the cellular structure. Examples of CPE include a rounding of the cells, forming giant multinucleate cells, or other injurious effects to the original culture cells.

The selection of the type of cell culture depends on the particular virus to be isolated. **Primary cell cultures** are derived directly from parent tissue. The tissue is minced, treated with a proteolytic enzyme, filtered, and added to a nutrient medium. The cells are transferred next to a container with a flat surface, which permits the cell to multiply, forming a monolayer. In a primary culture the cells have the same karyotype and chromosome number as the original tissue. Examples of primary cell cultures include human embryonic kidney (HEK), rabbit kidney (RK), primary monkey kidney (PMK), Rhesus monkey kidney

(RMK), cynomolgus monkey kidney (CMK), and African green monkey kidney (AGMK).

Once a primary cell culture is subcultivated, it is known as a **cell line.** **Diploid cell lines** must have at least 75% of cells with the same karyotype as the normal cells of the tissue from which they were derived. Diploid cell lines can retain the diploid karyotype for approximately 20 to 50 subcultures before losing their viability. Examples of diploid cell lines include WI-38 and MRC-5, which are both derived from human embryonic lung, and human diploid fibroblasts (HDFs), which may be derived from human kidney or lung fibroblasts.

Cell lines with less than 75% normal cells are known as **heteroploid**, or immortal, **cell lines**. More than 25% of the cells have an abnormal karyotype when compared with the normal cells of the tissue type of the primary cell culture. Immortal cell lines are generally derived from malignant tissue or other transformed cells. These cell lines can undergo continuous or unlimited subcultures or passages in vitro. Examples of heteroploid cell lines include HeLa, derived from human cervical carcinoma and named for the individual from whom the cells were isolated; Hep-2, derived from carcinoma of the human larynx; KB, derived from nasopharyngeal carcinoma; A-549, derived from human lung carcinoma; and Vero, derived from AGMK.

In practice, virology laboratories generally select one type of cell culture from each type of cell line. Primary cell lines have a broad sensitivity to a number of human viruses, including influenza viruses, parainfluenza viruses, mumps viruses, enteroviruses, and adenoviruses.

HDFs are sensitive to HSV, VZV, CMV, adenovirus, and rhinovirus. Heteroploid cell lines are useful in the detection of HSV and the enteroviruses and adenoviruses.

Inoculated cell monolayers are usually incubated at 35°C to 37°C for the recovery of most viruses, although respiratory viruses are optimally recovered at 33°C. The cultures are generally incubated for 2 weeks because recovery is variable and dependent on the type of virus. HSV may be detected in as early as 5 to 7 days, while CMV may need up to 21 days for detection.

Cultures are examined for CPE using an inverted light microscope or a phase-contrast microscope with the low-power objective (4X or 10X magnification). The type of CPE depends on the infecting virus and type of cell line used. Examples of CPE include cells rounding, clumping, vacuolation, granulation, giant multinucleate cells, cell fusion or syncytial formation, cell destruction, and lysis. CPE may be observed in discrete cells or may involve the entire monolayer.

CPE is quantitated based on the percentage of cells showing cellular changes or damage on a scale of +/– to 4 +. CPE that is rated 2 + or more (50% of cell monolayer exhibiting CPE) requires identification of the virus through an immunological technique.

Viruses, such as the influenza, parainfluenza, and mumps viruses (orthomyxovirus and paramyxovirus), that produce little or no detectable CPE may be identified through **hemadsorption**. These viruses produce virus-specific hemagglutinins in the cell monolayer, which can combine with erythrocytes of certain animals. This permits the detection of the virus in the infected monolayers. Hemadsorption is characterized by the presence of plaques of red blood cells (RBCs), which adhere to the cell monolayer, and hemagglutination is visible as a clumping of RBCs. Influenza A and B viruses are able to hemadsorb and hemagglutinate guinea pig RBCs, whereas parainfluenza and mumps viruses produce only hemadsorption.

Shell Vial Centrifugation–Enhanced (SVCE) Virus Detection

SVCE virus detection involves centrifugation of the specimen onto virus-sensitive cells, which are grown on coverslips at the bottom of shell vials. SVCE produces a more rapid result than conventional cell culture because incubation time can be decreased to 1 to 5 days, depending on the virus. After incubation the cells are fixed, and a fluorescein-labeled monoclonal or polyclonal antibody specific for antigens of the virus is added. Detection of the antigen–antibody binding is accomplished through fluorescence microscopy The detection time is shortened because viral gene products, or antigens, rather than viral CPE are detected. SVCE was originally developed to detect CMV early antigens, and methods are currently available for HSV, adenovirus, VZV, influenza A and B viruses, and RSV.

Direct Detection of Viral Antigens or Genes

This method can identify a virus through the detection of specific antigens present in patient cells. A sufficient number of cells must be recovered from the specimen. The specimen is fixed onto a microscopic slide and then stained with a virus-specific fluorescein-labeled monoclonal or polyclonal antibody. This process is known as direct fluorescent antibody (DFA) and is used to detect viruses in patient specimens. Alternatively, viral antigens may be detected in specimens through antigen capture techniques. In these methods, viral antigen is captured through complexing with specific antibodies; ELISA is used to detect the reaction end point.

Latex agglutination methods also are available for the direct detection of viruses in clinical specimens. One example is the latex agglutination products that are available to detect rotavirus in stool specimens. Latex beads are coated with antibodies to the virus, and agglutination indicates a positive reaction.

Antigen detection is limited by the range of detection because the antibodies are highly specific and the range depends on the antibody used.

Molecular Diagnostic Methods

Viruses also can be directly identified through the detection of viral DNA or RNA in specimens. Molecular diagnostic test methods continue to expand in both the variety of methods and the types of viruses that can be identified. These methods include restriction fragment length polymorphism (RFLP), DNA and RNA genetic probes, polymerase chain reaction (PCR), reverse transcriptase polymerase chain reaction (RT-PCR), and real-time polymerase chain reaction (real-time PCR).

Commercially available viral gene probe kits can be used for the in vitro detection of HSV and CMV. Gene amplification techniques, including the application of the principle of target amplification in a PCR, are now available. Target amplification can increase the sensitivity of the method by amplifying one viral genome into several genomes. The viral DNA or RNA can be amplified 1 million times or more, thus enhancing the detection of the virus. **TABLE 19-2** summarizes the use of molecular techniques in virology.

SEROLOGICAL DETECTION OF VIRAL ANTIBODIES

Serological detection of antibodies to a virus is an indirect indicator that infection or exposure to the virus has occurred in the individual's past. Serological methods are useful when the virus will not grow in cell cultures; when viral antigen, nucleic acid probes, or amplification methods are not available; or when the virus is in a site that cannot be readily cultured, such as in brain tissue.

Within 1 to 2 weeks after a primary viral infection, virus-specific immunoglobulin M (IgM) antibodies will begin to appear. The first appearance of IgG occurs 1 to 2 days later. IgM levels peak in 3 to 6 weeks and drop to undetectable levels in 2 to 3 months. IgG levels peak in 4 to 12 weeks and remain for several months. In some types of viral infections, IgG may remain for years or life.

Paired sera are recommended for serological detection of viral infections. The first specimen, known as the **acute-phase specimen**, is collected when the clinical signs first appear. The second specimen, known as the **convalescent-phase specimen**, is collected 2 to 3 weeks later, depending on the virus. Traditionally, a fourfold increase in antibody titer indicates a seropositive reaction and strongly supports a diagnosis of current infection.

False-positive and false-negative reactions are important points to consider in serological diagnosis. Antibody detection is not useful in the diagnosis of chronic or recurrent viral infections, such as HIV and CMV. Antibodies may be produced indefinitely in such patients and do not necessarily indicate a current infection.

The specific method(s) chosen for viral detection depends on the virus suspected, host factors, and laboratory capabilities.

TABLE 19-2 Molecular Techniques in Virology

Method	Principle	Purpose
Restriction fragment length polymorphism (RFLP)	Comparison of DNA	Distinguish different strains of same virus, such as HSV-1 and HSV-2
Gene probes in situ hybridization	Detect and locate specific genetic sequences	Viral probes for CMV and human papilloma virus–infected cells
Polymerase chain reaction (PCR)	Amplifies a single copy of viral DNA millions of times to enhance sensitivity of detection	Detect DNA viruses
Reverse transcriptase polymerase chain reaction (RT-PCR)	Converts viral RNA to messenger RNA to DNA prior to PCR amplification; amplifies RNA viruses	Detect RNA viruses
Real-time polymerase chain reaction (real-time PCR)	Quantification of DNA and RNA virus in samples	Quantitate HIV genomic viral load

Selected Medically Important Viruses

ADENOVIRUS

Adenovirus is a member of the family Adenoviridae and the genus *Mastadenovirus*. The virus has linear double-stranded DNA, icosahedral symmetry, and a size of 70 nm to 90 nm. Adenovirus does not have an envelope, but each capsomer possesses a long fiber for attachment to the host cell.

Adenovirus was first isolated from spontaneous degeneration, which occurred in adenoid tissue. The virus is commonly isolated in children, and most individuals have antibody to adenovirus by 5 years of age. It is generally transmitted by the respiratory or fecal–oral route. Adenovirus is associated with sporadic or epidemic respiratory tract infections, urinary tract infections (UTIs), gastrointestinal tract (GI) infections, and eye infections, primarily in newborns and immunosuppressed patients. Adenovirus also causes an exudative pharyngitis in children and a severe diarrheal disease in newborns and immunosuppressed persons. Adenovirus may remain latent, without causing infection, and can be isolated from the tonsils, eyes, or respiratory secretions.

Specimens to be collected include throat swabs, nasal washings, conjunctival swabs or scrapings, or feces. The virus can be isolated in tissue culture, and serological detection of antibody production also is available.

HEPATITIS VIRUSES

Currently, there are five recognized hepatitis viruses: hepatitis A virus (HAV); hepatitis B virus (HBV); hepatitis C virus (HCV), previously known as non-A, non-B (NANB); hepatitis D virus (HDV); and hepatitis E virus (HEV). Viral hepatitis, or infectious disease from the hepatitis viruses, may range from mild and self-limiting disease to acute fulminating cirrhosis; chronic disease and asymptomatic carriage also are possible. The severity and course of the disease depend on the particular virus and the state of the host.

Hepatitis is diagnosed serologically through the identification of specific antigens or antibodies. Also, liver enzymes, including alanine aminotransferase (ALT), aspartate aminotransferase (AST), lactate dehydrogenase (LD), and alkaline phosphatase may be increased up to 10 times the normal value in hepatitis. The serum bilirubin level also is increased in symptomatic patients.

Hepatitis A Virus (HAV)

Hepatitis A virus (HAV) is a member of the family Picornaviridae in the genus *Enterovirus*. The virus possesses single-stranded RNA, + sense, icosahedral symmetry, and no envelope and ranges in size from 24 nm to 30 nm. HAV is a very stable virus, can withstand temperatures of 56°C to 60°C for 1 hour, and is acid stable. However, HAV is destroyed by autoclaving for 30 minutes, boiling for 20 minutes, or using dry heat (160°C) for 1 hour.

HAV infection is spread through the fecal–oral route via ingestion of the virus present in infected food or drinks or on contaminated objects. A common route of infection is through food contaminated by an infected food handler. Infections are facilitated by poor sanitation, international travel, crowded conditions, and poor personal hygiene practices. Another route of infection is through the ingestion of contaminated shellfish, such as clams, oysters, and mussels. Raw or improperly treated sewage that enters the water supply is another source of infection. The virus can be spread through the congenital route, from mother to baby at birth, if the mother is acutely infected at this time. Children in school and day care, prisoners, and those with poor personal hygiene are at an increased risk.

There were over 2,500 cases of acute HAV reported to the CDC in 2008 and almost 2,000 acute cases reported in 2009. There were approximately 1,000 deaths attributed to HAV in the United States in 2009. The HAV vaccine is credited with having decreased the number of cases of HAV in the United States; for example, there were approximately 30,000 cases of HAV reported in 1990.

HAV enters the blood through oropharyngeal or intestinal epithelial cells and replicates in hepatocytes and Kupffer cells. After exposure, the virus incubates asymptomatically for 15 to 40 days, with an average incubation period of 25 days. HAV infection may be asymptomatic or symptomatic; jaundice may or may not be present. Individuals become infectious during the latter part of the incubation period and remain so until 2 weeks after the appearance of symptoms. In fact, individuals are infectious 10 to 14 days prior to symptoms, and many exhibit no symptoms but are infectious. After incubation, a period of nausea, weakness, anorexia, and vomiting occurs; the individual also may have pain in the area of the liver. Chronic carriage of HAV and chronic HAV infection do not seem to occur. However, relapse is possible. In acute and symptomatic cases, classic symptoms include jaundice and elevated liver enzymes. However, many cases are asymptomatic. Acute disease lasts for about 1 week, and the disease is often self-limited. The severity of the disease depends on the host's age and health; less than 1% of cases result in mortality. Outbreaks generally arise from a common source, such as contaminated water or food or at a particular facility.

HAV particles can be detected in the stool 10 to 30 days after infection. However, viral shedding is greatest before clinical signs. Diagnosis most frequently is accomplished through clinical signs and serological testing. If acute hepatitis is suspected, a differential diagnosis must be made to identify the type of hepatitis virus. Most often, serology to detect hepatitis B surface antigen and hepatitis B core antibody, as well as antibodies to HAV, is performed. Anti-HAV is a measure of the total antibody to HAV, which includes antibodies to both IgM and IgG. It is a measure of past infection to HAV. Antibody to IgM (HAV IgM) is a measure of IgM-specific antibody to HAV. Anti-HAV IgM is present in acute HAV infection. If anti-HAV is present and anti-HAV IgM is absent, a past HAV infection is indicated.

Hepatitis A vaccine is available for long-term protection to HAV. Immune globulin may be given for short-term protection during the early incubation period.

Hepatitis B Virus (HBV)

Hepatitis B virus (HBV) is a member of the family Hepadnaviridae and is a DNA-containing virus with a complex capsid and icosahedral arrangement. HBV is a 42-nm to 47-nm envelope with circular DNA, which is partially double stranded and partially single stranded. The virus is very stable and resists freezing, heating, and acidic conditions, which facilitates its transmission. In 2008, there were over 4,000 new cases of HBV reported to the CDC in the United States and over 3,000 new cases reported in 2009. There were almost 2,000 deaths reported to the CDC from HBV in 2009. The CDC estimates that there are between 700,000 and 1.4 million persons infected with HBV in the United States.

HBV has a complex structure; the double-shelled form, known as the **Dane particle,** is recognized as the whole-virus particle. The Dane particle consists of a core that is surrounded by a lipid envelope. Hepatitis B surface antigen (HBsAg) is the outer lipid component. This outer envelope circulates in the blood as a viral particle either bound to protein or as a free, noninfectious protein, which is spherical or tubular. There are several antigenic variants or subtypes of HBsAg, such as adr, adw, ayr, and ayw. The inner core of the virus contains HBV core antigen (HBcAg), which surrounds the partially double-stranded DNA and DNA polymerase, which is needed for viral replication. Hepatitis B e antigen (HBeAg) also is a component of the core antigen.

HBV causes acute and chronic and symptomatic and asymptomatic disease; it is transmitted by the sexual, perinatal, or parenteral routes. The original name for HBV infection was "serum hepatitis" because of the contamination of vaccines in World War II with serum that contained HBV. This name is no longer valid because HBV is isolated from body fluids other than blood and blood products, including urine, amniotic fluid, semen, tears, saliva, feces, and CSF. Routes of infection include transmission through the transfusion of contaminated blood or blood products, accidental needlesticks, tattoos, ear piercing, sharing of contaminated razors, intravenous (IV) drug abuse, and hemodialysis. Actively infected mothers can transmit the virus to their infants through the congenital route. Individuals at risk include nonimmunized health care personnel, including laboratory workers, physicians, dentists, and medical personnel in hemodialysis units. Others at risk include those living in crowded quarters; intravenous drug users; institutionalized persons, including prisoners and the mentally disabled; those who receive frequent intravenous procedures; and homosexuals.

After exposure, HBV may incubate for 50 to 180 days, with an average incubation time of 90 days. The virus replicates in the liver. The infection can be mild and asymptomatic, symptomatic, fulminant, or chronic. HBV disease has an insidious onset, with initial signs of fever, rash, or arthritis. Jaundice may occur shortly after initial signs and usually may persist for 4 to 6 weeks. Fulminant, fatal hepatitis and chronic hepatitis are possible complications of primary infection. An individual may test positive for HBsAg for years without evidence of liver disease, whereas other chronic carriers may develop hepatitis. HBV also is associated with primary hepatocellular carcinoma if the HBV genome is incorporated into the cancerous cells, which then express the HBV antigen.

Patients with HBV infection typically have abnormal liver function, as evidenced by increased levels of the liver enzymes. Serum bilirubin level also is elevated. Diagnosis is made through clinical signs and serological testing. Currently, six HBV markers can be used in the diagnosis of infection. Tests for HAV also may be necessary if a differential diagnosis is to be made. The serological tests available for the diagnosis of HBV infection currently are as follows:

- **HBsAg.** HBsAg is present at the onset of infection. It is the first serological marker to appear and can be detected 30 to 60 days after exposure. HBsAg disappears as the liver enzymes return to normal and the patient recovers. Persistence of HBsAg for more than 6 months may indicate chronic infection. HBsAg is present in acute, active, chronic, and carrier states of HBV infection.
- **HBeAg.** HBeAg is present in acute and chronic hepatitis and is a marker of infectivity. Persistence of HBeAg usually indicates chronic liver disease. It usually appears soon after HBsAg.
- **Anti-HBsAg.** Anti-HBsAg is the total antibody to HBsAg. It appears 2 to 6 weeks after HBsAg is gone and usually persists for life. The presence of anti-HBsAg generally indicates recovery or immunity after the HBV immunization.
- **Anti-HBcAg-IgM.** Anti-HBcAg-IgM is an indicator of recent acute infection; it is usually present for 6 months. Acute infection is indicated when anti-HBcAg-IgM is present with HBsAg.
- **Anti-HBcAg.** Total antibody to HBcAg (IgG and IgM) appearing after HBsAg but before anti-HBsAg appears; thus it sometimes is referred to as the "core window." It is present in high levels at the onset of symptoms but drops to low levels, and levels may persist for 5 to 6 years. Anti-HBcAg indicates current or previous infection and is not associated with recovery or immunity.
- **Anti-HBeAb.** Anti-hepatitis Be antibody does not appear until HBeAg disappears; it is usually associated with a favorable outcome, recovery, and reduced infectivity.
- **HBV-DNA** demonstrates the presences of virus particles in the specimen. It is an indicator of infectivity.

Before the screening of blood donors for HBV, the virus was the major cause of post-transfusion hepatitis. Today, HBV transmission through donor blood is very rare in the United States. Hepatitis B infection is controlled through carefully screening blood donors, sterilization of dental and medical instruments, practice of blood-borne or standard precautions, and passive immunization through the HBV vaccine. The HBV vaccine is a series of three intramuscular (IM) doses of synthetic HBV. It is included in the childhood vaccination schedule and also required for most health care occupations. Newborns are vaccinated with the hepatitis B vaccine at birth, with the second dose given at 1 or 2 months, and the third dose given at around 6 months of age. In adults, after the initial injection, immunizations are given at 1 month and then at 6 months. Hepatitis B immune globulin may be given following suspected exposure. Other preventive measures include adherence to blood and body fluid precautions; the use of personal protective equipment, including gloves and eye protection; and precautions when exposed to blood or body fluids, needles, and other sharps. Disinfection of surfaces with 10% bleach is a suitable surface disinfectant.

Hepatitis C Virus (HCV)

Hepatitis C virus (HCV) is an RNA-containing virus with a lipid envelope, positive (+) sense, and a size of 30 nm to 60 nm. HCV is in the viral family Flaviviridae and in the genus *Hepacivirus*. Formerly known as non-A, non-B (NANB) hepatitis, HCV was first isolated in 1984. The genome encodes for a large protein, which is cleaved into structural and nonstructural proteins. There are different HCV variants, which are classified as types 1 through 6, and then further subtyped. HCV may be acquired parenterally through contaminated blood products, organ transplantation, hemodialysis, or intravenous drug use. Other possible routes of infection include the perinatal route and through sexual contact. HCV has a variable incubation rate, which ranges from 2 to 26 weeks after exposure, with an average incubation of 6 to 8 weeks. Disease is usually milder than with HBV, and many infected persons are asymptomatic, although persistent chronic infection may occur. There is a high level of chronic asymptomatic infection with HCV, which increases its rate of transmission. In fact, approximately 70% of those infected with HCV become chronic carriers; the CDC estimates that there are between 2.7 and 3.9 million persons living in the United States with chronic HCV infection.

Before the development of a marker for its detection, HCV was the most frequent cause of post-transfusion hepatitis, responsible for approximately 90% of all cases. Before 1990, elevation of the liver enzyme ALT and the presence of anti HBcAg were used as markers for HCV infection. In 1990, the first ELISA test to detect antibody to HCV was made available. This test has subsequently been modified to detect earlier antigens. The serological marker is anti-HCV, which detects antibody to HCV but cannot distinguish between acute, chronic, or resolved infection. This antibody does not usually appear until 8 weeks after initial infection. The use of HCV-RNA tests is helpful in monitoring antiviral therapy and to confirm an active or resolved infection following a positive anti-HCV test.

Hepatitis D Virus (HDV)

Hepatitis D virus (HDV), or delta virus, is a small virus with a size of 35 nm to 37 nm, which possesses single-stranded RNA and is infective only in the presence of HBV. It is an incomplete virus, which can cause acute or chronic hepatitis only when HBV also is present. It is transmitted through routes similar to those of HBV, such as percutaneous or mucosal contact with infectious blood or body fluids, and is acquired through coinfection or superinfection in those who are infected with HBV. Serological testing to detect HDV antigen, IgM antibody to HDV, and total antibody to HDV is available. HDV is uncommon in the United States. Hepatitis B vaccination can prevent HDV in those persons who are not infected with HBV.

Hepatitis E Virus (HEV)

Hepatitis E virus (HEV) possesses single-stranded RNA and has a size of 32 nm to 34 nm. It is associated with enterically transmitted NANB hepatitis, which is spread through the fecal–oral route. HEV is uncommon in the United States, and most cases that are identified in the United States are attributed to foreign travel to a developing country. HEV is most prevalent in developing countries with poorly developed sanitation and contaminated water supplies. HEV has been associated with hepatitis outbreaks in several parts of the world, including Asia, the Middle East, Africa, and Central America. Natural disasters and living in refugee camps are other risk factors. The disease resembles HAV, and symptoms include fever, fatigue, loss of appetite, nausea, vomiting, abdominal pain, and jaundice. The infection is diagnosed clinically and through demonstration of HEV RNA or by identifying antibodies to HEV. HEV also should be considered in cases of hepatitis that cannot be attributed to serologic markers for hepatitis A, B, or C in someone who has traveled to an endemic area for HEV. Other laboratory diagnostic methods include Western blot assays, PCR, and electron microscopy. Characteristics of the hepatitis viruses are summarized in **TABLE 19-3**.

HERPES VIRUSES

The Herpetoviridae (herpesviruses) are enveloped, DNA-containing viruses with icosahedral symmetry of approximately 100 nm in size. This viral family produces lytic, persistent, and **latent viral infections**, which can be reactivated and cause disease months and even years later. These viruses may remain latent in various body sites, including the white blood cells (WBCs) and peripheral

TABLE 19-3 Characteristics of the Hepatitis Viruses

	HAV	HBV	HCV	HDV	HEV
Viral type	Picornavirus RNA	Hepadnavirus DNA Enveloped	Flavivirus RNA Enveloped	Deltavirus (covirus) RNA Enveloped	Calicivirus RNA
Route of infection	Fecal–oral	Parenteral, sexual	Parenteral, sexual	Parenteral, sexual	Fecal–oral
Incubation period (days)	15–50	45–160	14–180	14–64	15–50
Characteristics	Abrupt onset, milder disease, < 0.5% mortality	Insidious onset, occasionally severe, 1%–2% mortality, chronic carriers	Insidious onset, often subclinical, 70% become chronic carriers, ~4% mortality	Abrupt onset, coinfection with HBV, high mortality fulminant hepatitis, chronic carriers	Abrupt onset, mild disease, more severe infection in pregnant females
Laboratory diagnosis	Anti-HAV (IgM)	HBsAg, HBeAg, anti-HBcIgM	Anti HCV HCV-RNA	Anti-HDV	Anti-HEV HEV-RNA
Vaccine available	Yes	Yes	No	No	No

nerves. Reactivation generally occurs from physical stresses, such as immunosuppression, chemotherapy, and other medical disorders. Infections of the herpesviruses generally are more severe in adults than in children. Asymptomatic infection is common, and patients may unknowingly carry and shed the virus.

There are currently seven recognized herpes viruses: The subfamily Alphaherpesvirinae includes herpes simplex virus-1 (HSV-1) and herpes simplex virus-2 (HSV-2) and varicella-zoster virus (VZV). Subfamily Betaherpesvirinae includes cytomegalovirus (CMV), and the subfamily Gammaherpesvirinae includes Epstein-Barr virus (EBV), human herpes virus type 6 (HHV-6), and human herpes virus type 7 (HHV-7).

Herpes Simplex Virus (HSV-1 and HSV-2)

HSV infections occur throughout the world. HSV-1 infection is common in childhood, and most adults have antibody to this virus. HSV-1 generally produces more mild infections and is less resistant to treatment when compared with HSV-2. Transmission of the virus is through active ulcerations of the mucous membranes or the genitalia.

HSV-1 causes oral herpes, gingivostomatitis, ulcerative mouth lesions, and fever blisters. The virus may spread to the lips and cheeks. Primary lesions may be accompanied by fever, malaise, and cervical lymphadenopathy. Most cases are mild or asymptomatic and resolve without treatment. Approximately 90% of all cases of primary herpes gingivostomatitis are attributed to HSV-1.

HSV-2 produces 80% to 90% of all cases of genital herpes, a common sexually transmitted disease (STD). It is transmitted through sexual contact or from autoinoculation. Early signs of infection include fever, malaise, and inguinal lymphadenopathy, although some primary infections are asymptomatic. Primary lesions typically appear on the vagina, cervix, glans, or penile shaft. Recurrent lesions may occur. There is an association between HSV-2 and cervical carcinoma.

Neonatal HSV-2 infections may result if the infant acquires infection during delivery from an actively infected mother. The virus typically attacks the infant's central nervous system, and developmental difficulties may be seen. Other infections associated with HSV include herpetic keratitis, which can lead to corneal scarring and blindness; herpetic whitlow, which infects the fingers of those who have contact with others who excrete the virus; and central nervous system infections, including sporadic encephalitis.

Specimens that may be collected for diagnosis of HSV include aspirates or swabs of lesions or vesicles and conjunctival scrapings. The virus can be isolated using cell culture or shell vial (SVCE) with HeLa cells, human embryonic fibroblasts, and rabbit kidney cells with CPE observed within 1 to 7 days. CPE is typically observed as round, clumping, syncytial, giant cells. Direct examination for the virus also can be accomplished through electron microscopy and in the Pap smear. Viral antigen can be demonstrated using immunofluorescent or immunoperoxidase techniques. Serological testing is not very helpful because uninfected individuals may possess antibody and because antibody against HSV-1 and HSV-2 cannot be differentiated. There are HSV-specific DNA probes and DNA primers that differentiate HSV-1 and HSV-2.

There is no vaccine currently available for HSV-1 and HSV-2. Infections may be treated with a variety of antiviral agents, such as acyclovir, valacyclovir, penciclovir, and famciclovir.

Varicella-Zoster Virus (VZV).

VZV is the agent of **varicella**, or chickenpox, and herpes zoster, or shingles, which is the reactivation of a latent varicella infection. Chickenpox is generally a childhood disease, with most cases occurring in children less than 10 years of age. The infection is characterized by a generalized skin rash with raised, fluid-filled lesions. VZV infection is transmitted through the respiratory route or fluid from the lesions; the virus may incubate for 10 to 20 days. VZV multiplies in the respiratory tract and regional lymph nodes and is then disseminated through the blood to the skin. In addition to the rash, there also may be headache and fever. The lesions first appear on the scalp and trunk and other warm areas of the body and later on the arms and legs. Lesions pass through several stages before healing. The lesion first appears as a vesicle with clear fluid, resembling a "dewdrop on a rose petal." The lesions then develop into pustules with purulent fluid, which eventually rupture. In the final stage, the lesions form scabs or crusts. Individuals are contagious 24 to 48 hours before the eruption of the rash and remain infectious until all lesions have scabbed. Chickenpox is very contagious and may be transmitted through the respiratory route and also through skin vesicles. Primary varicella is more serious in immunosuppressed children, including those with leukemia or solid tumors and transplant recipients. In these individuals, the rash may be more severe, and pneumonitis, hepatitis, and encephalitis may occur. Primary varicella often is more serious in adults than in children, and complications such as pneumonitis may occur.

Reactivation of VZV occurs in the form of herpes zoster. It is believed that the virus remains latent in the dorsal root ganglia of peripheral or cranial nerves after the primary infection. Reactivation occurs during periods of physical or emotional stress. Shingles occurs in the elderly, immunosuppressed patients, patients with transplants, and those individuals with other illnesses. Factors involving reactivation are not entirely understood, but trauma and an altered host immune system seem to play a role. Herpes zoster is accompanied by fluid-filled skin vesicles and pain along the areas of the rash. Complications include neuralgia, keratitis, ophthalmia, hearing loss, facial paralysis, and aseptic meningitis.

Diagnosis of VZV infections is usually made from clinical signs. The vesicular lesions can be examined directly for the appearance of intranuclear inclusions and multinucleate giant cells. Cell culture and serological tests to determine prior immunity to VZV also are available. Serological tests to detect antibody to VZV are mainly used to determine an individual's immune status and not to diagnose infection.

A live attenuated vaccine for VZV is available and given on the same schedule as the measles-mumps-rubella (MMR) for infants and children. The first dose is given at 12 to 15 months and the second dose given at 4 to 6 years of age. For those older children and young adults who have not had chickenpox or the vaccine, two doses administered 28 days apart is recommended. There also is a vaccine for shingles, which is recommended for those over 60 years of ages and is administered to prevent herpes zoster. Vaccination with VZV immune globulin is also available.

Varicella infections are treated with acyclovir, famciclovir, and valacyclovir.

Cytomegalovirus

A member of the subfamily Betaherpesvirinae, cytomegalovirus (CMV) is an opportunistic infection, which can be transmitted through direct contact with saliva, via blood transfusions, and through organ transplants. It typically produces asymptomatic or mild infection in healthy individuals, and approximately half of the population is seropositive by age 30. Formerly known as "salivary gland virus," CMV has been isolated from saliva, urine, feces, milk, and semen. Repeated contact with the virus is necessary for infection. The virus can remain latent in white blood cells, endothelial cells, and other organs.

CMV is the most common congenital viral pathogen. Congenital CMV may occur as a primary infection during pregnancy if the mother has CMV infection and lacks immunity to the virus. Reactivation of a latent viral infection in the mother also may result in congenital CMV. Although some infants are asymptomatic at birth, developmental abnormalities, mental retardation, or deafness may occur later. Symptoms of congenital CMV include jaundice, hepatosplenomegaly, growth retardation, mental retardation, microencephaly, and lung disease. Perinatal CMV may occur during delivery if the mother is infected, or the virus may be acquired through the mother's breast milk.

CMV is an important pathogen in transplant patients. The virus can be acquired if a seronegative recipient receives a transplanted organ positive for CMV. Post-transplant CMV infection manifests as a pneumonia more than 1 month after the transplant and thus is known as the "40-day fever."

CMV also can be acquired through transfused blood when the donor is CMV positive and seropositive and the recipient is seronegative. For this reason, blood products are screened for CMV, and only CMV-negative units are given to those at an increased risk of infection, such as newborns, the immunosuppressed, and patients with transplants. In immunocompromised hosts, CMV may lead to pneumonia, retinitis, and esophagitis.

Specimens for the identification of CMV include urine, saliva, tears, milk, and semen, and vaginal secretions also can be collected. Direct cytological examination reveals the characteristic "owl eyes"—large cells with large intranuclear, basophilic staining inclusions. These inclusions are found in all body tissues but are generally identified in urine specimens and visualized with the Pap or hematoxylin-eosin staining. The virus can be isolated in cell culture, such as diploid fibroblasts, and in shell vials. CPE is typically observed in 4 to 6 weeks and appears as the rounding of cells. Viral antigens can be detected using immunofluorescence or enzyme-linked immunoassay on blood, urine, and bronchial or other biopsy specimens. There also are polymerase chain reaction methods available to identify CMV.

Serological tests often are not very helpful because they cannot differentiate among primary, reactivated, and persistent infections. The use of paired sera is more useful;

latex agglutination and ELISA are available to detect CMV antibody.

Prevention of CMV infection is through the screening of blood donors and organ donors. Seropositive products should not be transfused into seronegative recipients. CMV infections are treated with ganciclovir, valganciclovir, and foscarnet.

Epstein-Barr Virus

Epstein-Barr virus (EBV), or HHV-4, is a member of the subfamily Gammaherpesvirinae and was first isolated from malignant Burkett's lymphoma cells in African children. The virus also is the cause of infectious mononucleosis.

EBV is shed in the saliva and transmitted through oral contact. The virus incubates for 1 to 2 months, during which time it disseminates to the reticuloendothelial system, including the liver, spleen, and lymph nodes. The most common signs of infectious mononucleosis are lymphadenopathy, splenomegaly, and exudative pharyngitis. Other symptoms include high fever, sore throat, enlarged tonsils, hepatomegaly, malaise, and elevated liver enzymes. Recovery usually occurs in 2 to 3 weeks; however, complications may occur and include rupture of the spleen, hemolytic anemia, and encephalitis. EBV infection can recur and cause recurrent tiredness, fever, and headache.

Infectious mononucleosis is diagnosed clinically and through hematology and serological testing. The differential WBC count typically shows a lymphocytosis with over 50% lymphocytes and the appearance of several reactive or atypical lymphocytes. The presence of heterophile antibody can be detected using one of several commercially available slide tests. Heterophile antibodies are defined as those antibodies that occur in one species but that react with antigens of different species. This antibody may be present in the serum of those individuals with infectious mononucleosis or in those with serum sickness, as well as in some healthy individuals or nonaffected individuals, where they are known as Forssmann antibodies. Heterophile antibodies will agglutinate sheep and horse red blood cells in cases of infectious mononucleosis and serum sickness and in those who are not affected. Guinea pig cells are used to absorb human serum and will remove the agglutinins of serum sickness and Forssmann antibodies, leaving the agglutinins of infectious mononucleosis. There also are serological tests that detect IgM antibodies to EBV.

African Burkett's lymphoma is a monoclonal B cell lymphoma of the jaw and face, which may also involve the kidneys, liver, and adrenal glands. It is endemic in children in Africa, where malaria is prevalent. It is believed that the malaria parasite acts to promote EBV involvement with the lymphoma.

EBV also is associated with some types of nasopharyngeal cancer.

Human Herpesvirus Type 6 (HHV-6)

Another member of the subfamily Gammaherpesvirinae, HHV-6 was originally known as "human lymphotropic virus" because it first was detected infecting B cells in vitro. The virus was first isolated in saliva and mononuclear cells of peripheral blood in 1986. It is now known that the virus primarily infects T lymphocytes, where it remains latent. The route of infection is most likely through respiratory contact.

HHV-6 is the agent of **exanthem subitum**, or **roseola**, also known as **sixth disease**. Roseola is a benign childhood disease most often seen in children ages 6 months to 3 years. Symptoms of HHV-6 include a sore throat and high fever, which persist for 3 to 5 days. A nonspecific maculopapular rash of the trunk and neck develops 24 to 48 hours after the fever subsides. The virus rarely produces infections in adults, which include lymphadenopathy and a mononucleosis-type disease.

Other Human Herpesviruses

Human herpesvirus 7 (HHV-7) also is the cause of exanthem subitum. Human herpesvirus 8 (HHV-8) is known as the Kaposi's sarcoma virus; it is associated with Kaposi's sarcoma, a cancer found in AIDS patients, and also is the cause of primary effusion lymphoma.

TABLE 19-4 summarizes the herpesviruses.

PAPILLOMAVIRIDAE

Papillomavirus

Human papillomavirus (HPV) has double-stranded circular DNA and an icosahedral structure, with a size of 45 nm to 55 nm. There are over 30 genetic types of HPV, which are causes of a variety of cutaneous lesions and benign growths, including plantar warts, common warts, and sexually transmitted venereal warts. Sexually transmitted diseases from HPV may be associated with neoplastic lesions, including cervical carcinoma. HPV is an oncologic agent for squamous cell carcinoma.

TABLE 19-4 Characteristics of the Herpes Viruses

Virus	Target cell	Site of latency	Route of infection	Other properties
HSV-1 or HHV-1	Mucosal cells	Neurons	Oral contact; sharing glasses, utensils, or other items contaminated with saliva; autoinoculation	Lytic infections of fibroblasts and epithelial cells; latent infections of neurons. Most cases of oral herpes are a result of HHV-1.
HSV-2 or HHV-2	Mucosal cells	Neurons	Sexual contact, autoinoculation, perinatal from mother to child	Lytic infections of fibroblasts and epithelial cells; latent infections of neurons. Most cases of HSV-2 are sexually transmitted.
Varicella zoster virus (VZV) or HHV-3	Mucosal cells and T cells	Neurons (trigeminal and dorsal root ganglia)	Respiratory secretions or direct contact with draining lesions	Primary infection is chickenpox, or varicella; reactivation occurs in those over 50 years as shingles, or herpes zoster, which appears as a rash along the involved sensory ganglion. Shingles usually appears on one side of the body—on the torso, face, or neck.
Epstein-Barr virus (EBV) or HHV-4	B lymphocytes and epithelial cells in the oropharynx	B lymphocytes	Oral contact through saliva, sharing of items contaminated with saliva	Peripheral blood shows lymphocytosis and reactive lymphocytes. Positive heterophile antibody test.
Cytomegalovirus (CMV) or HHV-5	Monocytes, lymphocytes, epithelial cells	Monocytes and lymphocytes	Transfusions, tissue and organ transplants, congenital, close contact	Virus is reactivated by immunosuppression; many infections are asymptomatic, but the virus remains latent and can be shed in the urine, saliva, and nasopharynx and through other secretions.
HHV-6	Monocytes, lymphocytes, epithelial cells, neurons	Monocytes and T lymphocytes	Saliva and respiratory secretions	Sixth disease or roseola (exanthem subitum).
HHV-7	Monocytes, lymphocytes, epithelial cells, neurons	Monocytes and T lymphocytes	Saliva and respiratory secretions	Also identified as a cause of roseola (exanthem subitum).
HHV-8 Kaposi's sarcoma–associated herpesvirus	Lymphocytes	B lymphocytes		Associated with Kaposi's sarcoma, a rare opportunistic skin malignancy found in immunosuppressed persons, especially those with AIDS.

HPV was identified as the cause of genital warts in 1907, and in 1984 HPV strain 16 was identified in some cervical carcinoma tumors; HPV strain 18 also was identified in cervical tumors in 1985. Using polymerase chain reaction, HPV-DNA was found in almost all cervical cancers in 1999. By 2003, a screening test using hybrid capture assay to identify HPV DNA in cervical specimens was available. Today, diagnostic methods are available to detect high-risk HPV types, which are those genetic types of HPV that present the highest risk for developing high-risk squamous dysplasia. The Hybrid Capture 2 (Digene) uses a nucleic acid hybridization assay probe to detect the DNA of 13 of the high-risk HPV types. There also are polymerase chain reaction techniques, which utilize a pool of 14 of the high-risk HPV serotypes, and there are specific probes for HPV 16 and 18. It is estimated that HPV strains 16 and 18 cause approximately 70% of cervical carcinoma and that strains 6 and 11 are associated with approximately 90% of genital warts.

There is a licensed quadrivalent vaccine that protects against HPV 6, 11, 16, and 18. It is highly protective and recommended for the prevention of genital warts, persistent HPV infection, and cervical carcinoma.

PAPOVAVIRUSES

The family Papovaviridae is characterized by having double-stranded DNA, icosahedral symmetry, no envelope, and a size of 45 nm to 55 nm. Included in the Papovaviruses are polyoma strains JC and BK, which produce mild or asymptomatic infections. These infections are most likely spread through respiratory secretions.

Parvovirus

Parvovirus is a small (18 nm to 26 nm), DNA-containing, nonenveloped virus with icosahedral symmetry. Parvoviruses are known to infect mice, hamsters, cats, and dogs; however, only parvovirus B-19 is known to cause human infection. The virus is the agent of erythema infectiosum, or fifth disease (after measles, rubella, varicella-zoster, and roseola), a childhood illness. The virus is spread through the respiratory route and characterized by fever and a unique "slapped-cheek rash." The virus has an affinity for red blood cell precursors, which may lead to a mild anemia; those with malignancies or other hematologic abnormalities may develop aplastic crisis or chronic anemia when infected with parvovirus B-19.

POXVIRUSES

The poxviruses are the largest viruses known, with a size of 225 nm × 300 nm. These are DNA-containing viruses that are enveloped with complex coats with a brick shape and complex morphology. The family includes variola, the smallpox virus, and vaccinia virus, as well as the agents of cowpox, monkeypox, and canarypox.

Variola Virus: Smallpox Virus

Smallpox is an ancient disease, which has killed millions throughout recorded history. The virus is spread through direct respiratory contact and multiplies in the lymph nodes. This is followed by the viremic phase, with dissemination to various organs and the development of pox lesions. The rash occurs in a single crop, in contrast to chickenpox.

Vaccinations were administered to those who lived or worked in potentially hazardous areas. The vaccine was produced using vaccinia virus as the carrier; because variola virus is a single serotype, the vaccine is very effective. The disease was considered to be eradicated, and in 1980 the World Health Organization (WHO) declared that the world was free of smallpox. All reference stocks of the virus were destroyed by WHO in 1996. However, some countries did maintain stocks of variola virus, which were stockpiled for believed intended use as agents of biowarfare. Today, smallpox virus is listed as a category A bioterrorism agent by the CDC.

Other Pox Viruses

The other pox viruses are primarily pathogenic for animals other than humans and humans becoming infected as incidental hosts. The orf virus is a pox virus that infects goats and sheep; vaccinia virus infects cattle and causes cowpox. There also is the monkeypox virus, which infects monkeys and squirrels, with its origin in Africa. All of these viruses pose occupational hazards to those with contact with animal pox lesions. After direct contact with infected lesions, humans develop nodular lesions on their hands or fingers, which form vesicles.

ARBOVIRUSES

The arthropod-borne viruses, or arboviruses, include the families Togaviridae, Flaviviridae, and Bunyaviridae. Most members of these families include viruses that require an arthropod vector. All three viral families have positive sense, single-stranded RNA and are enveloped. The alpha viruses, or group A togaviruses, are the agents in various types of encephalitis, which is an inflammation and infection of the brain, most often as a result of a viral infection. The arboviruses include the togaviruses and the flaviviruses.

Arbovirus infections are acquired from an arthropod bite, most often mosquitoes but also from ticks and mites. The mosquito vector takes a blood meal from an infected vertebrate host, and the virus multiplies in the midgut of the mosquito. The virus circulates to the mosquito's salivary glands, where it replicates in large numbers. Now, when the mosquito bites another host, such as humans, it is able to transmit the virus. The virus circulates in the blood and contacts susceptible target cells, such as monocytes, macrophages, and the endothelial cells of blood vessels.

These diseases range from a mild systemic disease, encephalitis, to arthrogenic disease and hemorrhagic fevers. Infection is characterized by fever, chills, headache, backache, and flu-like symptoms. After 3 to 7 days, primary viremia occurs, which leads to a mild systemic disease. There is a second viremia during which additional virus copies are made, which then attach to target organs, such as the liver, brain, skin, or blood vessels. Flaviviruses generally attach to monocytes and macrophages.

Humans are usually an accidental host, with birds, small mammals, reptiles, and amphibians serving as the reservoir hosts. Humans are the "dead end" host for many arboviruses because the virus cannot spread back to the vector unless there is significant viremia. Thus, the life cycle of the virus ends within the human host.

Western equine encephalitis (WEE) is found in the western United States and Canada, eastern equine encephalitis (EEE) is found in the eastern and southern United States, and Venezuelan equine encephalitis (VEE) is found in South and Central America. All of these viruses are transmitted to animals, including horses and birds, by the mosquito vector; humans serve as accidental hosts. In most cases, the virus usually dead ends in the human host.

The flavivirus of the family Flaviviridae is the agent of St. Louis encephalitis (SLE), which is found sporadically in the southern and south–central United States. Birds constitute the major reservoir, and mosquitoes are the vector in SLE. Epidemics seem to occur every 10 years in Texas or in the Gulf Coast area.

Flaviviruses also are the cause of Japanese B encephalitis, a severe form of the disease, found in the Far East, Korea, and Japan, as well as yellow fever and dengue fever. The vector in yellow fever is the mosquito, and the disease is severe and systemic. Symptoms of yellow fever include headache, backache, nausea, jaundice, and extensive damage to the liver, kidney, and heart. The disease gets its name from the jaundice; severe gastrointestinal hemorrhages also may occur. Dengue fever, found in the Caribbean and Southeast Asia, is characterized by fever, headache, severe bone pain, backache, fatigue, and chills. Rash and arthritis also may occur. Dengue fever also is known as "break bone disease." Hemorrhagic fever and dengue shock syndrome also may occur. In these diseases, the blood vessels rupture, and there is internal bleeding of the blood vessels and other tissues, which may lead to shock.

West Nile virus (WNV) was first detected in the western hemisphere in 1999, and it quickly spread across North America. The virus is transmitted by infected mosquitoes, which have fed on infected birds, including crows, blue jays, and other wild birds. Humans are an incidental host. In 2007, there were 3,600 cases of WNV reported in the United States; this number declined to approximately 1,300 cases in 2008. WNV infection can range from a mild fever to a fatal encephalitis. Because WNV causes a significant viremia, the infection does not dead end in the human host but instead can be transmitted to the mosquito vector during the blood meal. There have been increased isolate serotypes, which are associated with a more severe neurological disease. WNV is identified by detecting IgM or IgG antibodies, using enzyme immunoassay or immunofluorescence. Viral RNA also can be detected through reaction with viral-specific IgM.

Arboviruses can be identified serologically by demonstrating the specific viral IgM antibody through hemagglutination, enzyme-linked immunoassay, and latex agglutination. A fourfold increase in the IgM titer is generally diagnostic for infection. There also are polymerase chain reaction methods that identify viral RNA in blood or tissue. Animal inoculation or cell culture also may be used to isolate the arboviruses.

Arboviruses are controlled by controlling the insect vector to reduce the breeding of mosquitoes. Infections are highest in the spring and summer months, when there are increased numbers of mosquitoes.

The arboviruses are summarized in **TABLE 19-5**.

Rubivirus, also a togavirus, is unique in this viral group because it is a respiratory virus with no arthropod vector. The virus is the agent of **rubella**, or **German measles**, an acute febrile disease first discovered by German physicians. Rubella once was responsible for epidemics every 6 to 8 years, with cases occurring each spring in school-age children. The virus has single-stranded RNA; icosahedral symmetry; a diameter of 60 nm to 70 nm; and surface projections, including hemagglutinins. Humans are the only host for rubella. Rubella infection is spread through respiratory secretions, incubates for 2 to 3 weeks, and then invades the nasopharyngeal mucosa. The virus multiplies in the lymph nodes, followed by viremia and dissemination through the blood. Other symptoms include fever, lymphadenopathy, and a maculopapular rash, which has a duration of 3 to 4 days. Hence, the name "3-day measles" is commonly used to describe rubella infection. The virus is shed for approximately 1 week before clinical signs of infection and for up to 2 weeks following onset of the rash. The disease is more serious in adults, who may experience bone or joint pain also.

Pregnant women who have rubella infection may infect the baby in utero. The virus multiples in the placenta and enters the fetal blood, where it can infect most tissues in the fetus. Congenital infection may be mild and asymptomatic or severe, causing cataracts, glaucoma, deafness, heart abnormalities, mental retardation, or even death.

The rubella vaccine is given to children at 15 months of age and the second dose at 4 to 6 years of age as a part of the MMR (measles-mumps-rubella) immunization. Unvaccinated adults also should get the rubella vaccine if they have negative antibody titers for rubella and were born after 1957. Immunization is especially important for college students, those who work in health care facilities and travel

TABLE 19-5 Arboviruses

Alpha viruses			
Disease	**Vector**	**Reservoir host**	**Distribution and other characteristics**
Eastern equine encephalitis virus (EEE)	*Aedes* and *Culisetta* mosquitoes	Birds	North, South, and Central America; eastern and southern United States Mild encephalitis; dead ends in humans
Western equine encephalitis virus (WEE)	*Culex* and *Culiseta* mosquitoes	Birds	North and South America, Canada, western United States Mild encephalitis; dead ends in humans
Venezuelan equine encephalitis (VEE)	*Aedes* and *Culex* mosquitoes	Rodents and horses	South and Central America Mild to severe encephalitis; dead ends in humans
Chikungunya	*Aedes* mosquito	Humans and monkeys	Fever, arthralgia
Flaviviruses			
Dengue fever	*Aedes* mosquito	Humans and monkeys	Worldwide but especially in the tropics Mild systemic disease; "break-bone fever," dengue hemorrhagic fever, dengue shock syndrome
Yellow fever	*Aedes* mosquito	Humans and monkeys	Africa and South America Hepatitis, jaundice, hemorrhagic fever
Japanese B encephalitis	*Culex* mosquito	Pigs and birds	Asia Encephalitis
West Nile virus	*Culex* mosquito	Birds	Africa, Europe, North and Central America Fever, encephalitis, hepatitis; does not dead end in human host
St. Louis encephalitis	*Culex* mosquito	Birds	North America Encephalitis

internationally, and for women of child-bearing age. The vaccine is live and attenuated and confers lifelong immunity in approximately 95% of those immunized. There is only one serotype of rubella virus, so immunization is very effective. Before the 1962 to 1965 global pandemic, there were over 12.5 million rubella cases in the United States, with over 2,000 cases of encephalitis. In 1969, the live attenuated rubella vaccine was licensed in the United States, and the number of cases of rubella in the United States has declined from over 50,000 cases in 1969 to 10 cases in 2005, according to the CDC.

Tests to identify rubella include viral cultures and serologic testing. Acute infection is confirmed by the presence of rubella IgM or a significant increase in the rubella IgG titer between the acute and convalescent specimens. Serologic methods include enzyme immunoassay, hemagglutination inhibition, and immunofluorescent antibody. Rubella also may be isolated from nasal, throat, blood, urine, or cerebrospinal fluid specimens and grown in tissue cultures.

There also is molecular typing, which assists in determining the origin of the virus and its frequency of isolation in the United States.

Bunyaviridae

The family Bunyaviridae includes the genera *Bunyavirus*, *Phlebovirus*, *Nairovirus*, and *Hantavirus*. *Bunyavirus* includes the La Crosse virus, or California encephalitis virus. *Bunyavirus* infection is characterized by a fever and rash and encephalitis. It is spread by the mosquito vector, and vertebrate hosts include rodents, birds, and other small mammals. *Phlebovirus* is the agent of Rift Valley fever, which is spread through the fly vector. Vertebrate hosts include sheep, cattle, and domestic animals. Rift Valley fever is associated with encephalitis, conjunctivitis, and hemorrhagic fever. Hemorrhagic fevers are characterized by a petechial rash and ecchymosis, which occurs as the blood passes from ruptured blood vessels into the subcutaneous tissue.

There also is epistaxis, or bleeding from the nose; hematemesis, or the vomiting of blood; and bleeding gums. *Nairovirus* is the agent of Crimean–Congo hemorrhagic fever. It is transmitted through the tick vector, and animal reservoirs include cattle, goats, and hares. *Hantavirus*, the agent of Korean hemorrhagic fever and Hantaan virus, does not require an arthropod vector. The animal reservoir is the deer mouse. Hantavirus infection causes a severe pulmonary syndrome with high fever and muscle aches. The infection may lead to pulmonary edema, respiratory fever, and shock.

FILOVIRIDAE

Filoviruses include Marburg and Ebola viruses. These are negative sense, single-stranded RNA viruses, which are enveloped and filamentous and vary in length from 800 nm to 1,400 nm with a diameter of 80 nm. They are causes of severe hemorrhagic fevers and are endemic in Africa. Ebola virus is named for the river in the Democratic Republic of Congo, where it was first discovered. Marburg virus was first discovered in laboratory workers in Marburg, Germany, who had contracted the disease from infected green monkeys. The filoviruses are endemic in wild monkeys and bats, and disease is transmitted to humans by direct contact with infected blood or secretions. Humans also may acquire the infection through contaminated needles. These hemorrhagic fevers begin with flu-like symptoms but then quickly develop into severe hemorrhages from many body sites, especially the gastrointestinal tract.

Filoviruses require Biosafety Level 4 isolation techniques, which are not always readily available. The viruses may be grown in tissue culture or through animal inoculation. There also are direct immunofluorescent techniques available to detect viral antigen. Polymerase chain reaction can detect the viral genome in specimens. Serological testing also can be performed.

PICORNAVIRIDAE

The Picornaviridae are a large, diverse viral family, which includes the enteroviruses and rhinoviruses. The family is characterized by the presence of single-stranded RNA, icosahedral symmetry, and absence of an envelope. The viruses have a very small size of 20 nm to 30 nm, which is described by the prefix "pico" in their names. The Picornaviridae cause a variety of infections, which include central nervous system disorders, such as aseptic meningitis and polio; myocarditis; and mild or asymptomatic respiratory disease. Often, poor personal hygiene, overcrowding, or substandard sanitation are factors in the acquisition of these infections. Widespread vaccination against poliovirus has dramatically decreased the number of cases of polio from the wild poliovirus in the United States, as well as in many other parts of the world.

Enteroviruses

The enteroviruses include poliovirus, echovirus, the coxsackieviruses, and hepatitis A virus (HAV), which has been discussed previously under the hepatitis virus section.

Poliovirus

Poliovirus occurs naturally only in humans and is disseminated through the fecal–oral route and through respiratory secretions. The virus is shed in oral secretions prior to symptoms and for approximately 1 month after symptoms are noted. Primary infection occurs in the respiratory tract, followed by viremia to various parts of the body, including the skin, heart, and meninges. The virus is cytolytic and infects skeletal muscle. The most common type of **polio** is known as asymptomatic, or abortive, poliomyelitis. Abortive polio, which is mild or asymptomatic, with a rapid recovery, accounts for approximately 90% of all cases of polio. Symptoms include headache, fever, and sore throat. Poliovirus also may cause an aseptic meningitis or nonparalytic poliomyelitis in about 1% to 2% of those affected. Polio also may extend into the central nervous system in 1% to 2% of these cases. The virus travels through the blood to the anterior horn cells in the spinal cord and motor cortex in the brain. The virus is cytolytic and attacks skeletal muscle cells as it travels along neurons to the brain, resulting in paralytic poliomyelitis, the most severe type of polio infection. It is characterized by destruction of large motor neurons in the spinal cord and is usually accompanied by paralysis of the limbs and the respiratory center.

Polio vaccination began in the United States in 1955, when the first polio vaccine was approved. There are two formulations of the vaccine, both of which contain three strains of the poliovirus and induce an antibody response. The inactivated polio vaccine (IPV), first prepared by Salk, is formalin-killed virus and stimulates antibody production in the serum but not in the mucosa. The oral polio vaccine (OPV), first created by Sabin, is a live, attenuated vaccine given orally, which stimulates the production of both IgA and IgG. The OPV was recommended in the United States until 2000 because of the benefits of secondary spread and intestinal immunity. However, OPV presents a rare risk for vaccine-associated paralytic poliomyelitis (VAPP), which occurred in one child out of every 2.4 million, according to the CDC. Also, live poliovirus is shed in the stool of those vaccinated, which also presents a risk of infection for susceptible persons. Thus, the current recommendation for polio vaccination in the United States is the IPV, which is given as an injection to children at 2, 4, and 6 to 18 months, with a booster given at 4 to 6 years of age.

There have not been any cases of wild polio in the United States in over 20 years, but the disease remains common in other parts of the world. OPV is used in other parts of the world, where the disease is endemic and where there is a high risk of transmission.

Enteroviruses may be isolated from throat swabs, feces, CSF, urine, blood, and conjunctival swabs, depending on the site of the infection. Direct detection and serological testing are not recommended, and identification most often is accompanied through clinical signs and virus isolation in cell culture.

Coxsackie and Echo Viruses

Coxsackieviruses are named for Coxsackie, New York, where the viruses were first isolated. Coxsackieviruses A and B are associated with aseptic meningitis, paralysis, pharyngitis, myocarditis, and rash. Coxsackievirus A also is the agent of hand-foot-and-mouth disease and hepangina, which has symptoms of fever, sore throat, anorexia, and ulcerated lesions in the mouth.

Echovirus has been isolated in cases of aseptic meningitis, fever, respiratory infections, and paralysis.

Rhinovirus

Rhinovirus is the most frequent cause of the common cold. Other viruses that cause the common cold include coronavirus, adenovirus, respiratory syncytial virus, and parainfluenza virus. Rhinovirus infections are usually self-limiting, with symptoms of a mild respiratory illness, including nasal congestion. The virus incubates for 8 to 10 hours, and symptoms generally appear within 1 to 3 days following exposure. There are over 100 serotypes, and the virus is grouped into species, which are designated as species A, B, and C. Species A is found most often.

Rhinovirus can survive at room temperature for 24 hours, and because it prefers a growth temperature of 33°C, the virus does not usually infect the lower respiratory tract. If rhinovirus does invade the lower respiratory tract, severe pneumonia may occur; this is more common in immunosuppressed persons.

Rhinovirus is transmitted through contaminated hands and also through contaminated respiratory aerosol droplets. Those infected develop mucosal immunity, which doesn't reach the blood; thus, immunity is short lived. Because there are so many serotypes and there is short-term immunity, individuals can be repeatedly infected. Because of the large number of serotypes, immunizations have not been developed. Diagnosis is generally based on clinical symptoms, and identification is not attempted because of the large number of serotypes and the infections are most often mild. Rhinovirus infection is prevented through practicing thorough hand washing, avoidance of contact with those who have a cold, and good personal hygiene.

ORTHOMYXOVIRIDAE

The family Orthomyxoviridae includes the orthomyxoviruses and the genus *Influenza*, which has as its members influenza viruses A, B, and C. The viruses contain positive sense, single-stranded RNA and helical symmetry and are enveloped. Influenza viruses range in size from 80 nm to 120 nm. Important characteristics of this family include the presence of **hemagglutinin antigen** (HA) and **neuraminidase antigen** (NA). HA allows the virus to attach to sialic acid glycoproteins on the surface of the host red blood cells and respiratory epithelial cells. HA also promotes the fusion of the viral envelope to the host cell membrane and can hemagglutinate human, chicken, and guinea pig red blood cells. HA also elicits the neutralizing antibody response. NA permits virus entry into the host cell and also cleaves the sialic acid on the viral particle, which helps to release the virus from the host cells.

Influenza viruses are spread through aerosols and respiratory droplets and incubate for 1 to 4 days. The infections are characterized by an abrupt onset, fever, chills, headache, muscle aches, and a dry cough. Typical types of infections include influenza, upper respiratory tract infections, tracheobronchitis, and pneumonia. Individuals generally recover within 1 week, but complications, including secondary bacterial pneumonia, may occur.

The surface antigens of influenza A virus are constantly changing. Minor antigenic changes are known as **antigenic drift**, and these occur every 2 to 3 years. Drifts are a result of minor mutations in HA or NA and account for local influenza outbreaks. Major antigenic changes are known as **antigenic shift** and involve a reassortment of genomes among different strains. Antigenic shift is generally associated with a pandemic. Influenza A pandemics occur approximately every 10 years. Antigenic shifts occur because of the diversity of influenza A virus in its ability to infect and replicate in a variety of hosts, including humans, birds, pigs, and other animals. Because influenza B is primarily a human virus, there is no antigenic shift.

Regional or national influenza outbreaks occur in the winter and are named for the viral structure and location of the outbreak. Strains of influenza A virus are named for the virus type, place and date of original isolation, and HA and NA antigens. Strains of influenza B virus are named for type, location, and date of isolation.

H1N1 was first identified in 1947, and both antigens shifted, resulting in the Pandemic of 1957, known as A_2 Asian H2N2. Other pandemics included H3N2 in 1968, known as A_3 Hong Kong, and the Aj outbreak of 1978, which mutated to H1N1. Complications of type A infections include secondary bacterial pneumonia.

In the 2009–2010 year, there was a special concern because in addition to the seasonal influenza A strains, there also was a new strain identified as 2009 H1N1 influenza A and commonly referred to as the swine flu. This strain was believed to cause the majority of influenza in 2009–2010, which was declared a pandemic by the World Health Organization because of the many outbreaks that occurred worldwide during this period. Swine flu viruses usually infect pigs; the main virus types found in U.S. pigs recently are the swine triple reassortment (tr) H1N1 influenza virus, trH3N2 virus, and trH1N2 virus. There was an extensive vaccination effort to combat the H1N1 strain. Person-to-person transmission of swine influenza viruses does not seem to readily occur, and most confirmed infections are believed to be related to exposure to infected live pigs.

An annual influenza vaccine offers protection against influenza. Each year, the vaccination is developed against the three viruses that are believed to be the most common. This is based on the virus type isolated in the previous year, as well as on other researched factors. Vaccinations for high-risk people, including young children, pregnant women, those with chronic health conditions, and those older than 65 years, is recommended as well as for health care workers and those who work with those in high-risk groups. In recent years, public health officials have recommended the influenza A immunization for the general population.

Specimens collected for identification of influenza viruses include throat swabs and nasal aspirates or nasopharyngeal specimens. Rapid testing, direct immunofluorescence, and polymerase chain reaction can be performed on nasopharyngeal washings. The virus also can be isolated in cell culture and hemadsorption assay. There are rapid influenza diagnostic tests to detect the virus in nasal secretions, which can detect influenza A, influenza B, or both viruses. These are rapid tests that can be performed in the physician's office but suffer from low sensitivity and may have up to 30% false-negative results. Direct fluorescent antibody (DFA) stains detect influenza A or B virus in nasal secretions. These tests have higher sensitivity and specificity than rapid test methods.

Viral culture is the gold standard for diagnosing influenza but requires from 3 to 10 days for results. It is useful in confirming positive rapid tests and can differentiate influenza A from influenza B, as well as from other respiratory viruses. Shell vial culture can reduce the incubation time to 24 to 48 hours.

Reverse transcription polymerase chain reaction (RT-PCR) is a molecular method used to detect viral genetic material in nasal secretions. It is the most sensitive influenza test currently available. There also are serological tests to identify the immune response to influenza infection. Acute and convalescent samples are most helpful, and a fourfold titer is usually diagnostic for infection. Serological diagnosis through hemagglutination inhibition, a measure of the patient's antibody titer against the HA, also can be used. Antibodies to NA also may be detected. Both antibodies appear 1 to 2 weeks after infection and may persist for up to 4 months. Indirect immunofluorescent methods to detect IgG and IgM in influenza A and B also are available.

PARAMYXOVIRIDAE

The paramyxoviruses include the genera *Paramyxovirus*, *Morbillivirus*, and *Pneumovirus*. The family possesses negative sense, single-stranded RNA, helical symmetry, an envelope, and an average size of 150 nm to 300 nm.

Paramyxovirus

Paramyxovirus includes the parainfluenza viruses, mumps virus, and New Castle virus. Parainfluenza viruses cause mild upper respiratory tract infections as well as pneumonia, hepatitis, and meningitis. Infections are found worldwide. Parainfluenza virus type 1 produces laryngotracheobronchitis and croup, an infection seen in infants and characterized by difficulty in breathing and a hoarse, barking cough. These infections may cause subglottal swelling, which may block the airway. Parainfluenza infections are spread by direct contact from infected persons or through respiratory droplet infection.

Respiratory tract specimens are collected for identification of the parainfluenza viruses. Direct immunofluorescence and polymerase chain reaction can be performed on nasopharyngeal washings, and the virus can be isolated in cell culture. Hemadsorption is recommended for cell culture techniques because not all the viruses produce CPE. Serological diagnosis is not recommended because of recurrent infections.

Mumps virus causes parotitis, a painful infection of the parotid glands characterized by swelling behind the ears and difficulty swallowing. Mumps virus possesses both HA and NA antigens and a hemolysin. The virus is extremely contagious and transmitted through respiratory secretions in contaminated saliva. Mumps virus is most contagious just before and immediately after the parotid glands swell. The virus multiplies in the upper respiratory tract and in the adjacent lymph nodes. This is followed by a viremic phase, where the virus spreads through the blood to the testes, ovaries, thyroid gland, pancreas, and meninges. A complication that may be seen in adult males affected with mumps is inflammation of the gonads, which may lead to sterility.

Once a common childhood disease, mumps infections are rare in those countries where there has been consistent immunization. The mumps vaccine was first introduced in 1967; today the MMR is given to infants at 15 months of age, with a second dose given at 4 to 6 years. Most cases today are seen in those parts of the world and in communities where immunizations are not available or where there are compliance problems. There also have been cases of mumps in young adults and college students whose immune status has waned or who were not immunized.

Specimens collected to diagnose mumps infection include saliva, urine, and pharyngeal secretions. Mumps virus can be isolated in cell culture. Serological detection of IgM and IgG antibodies through enzyme immunoassay, immunofluorescence, and hemadsorption also are available. A fourfold increase in IgM antibody for mumps is considered to be diagnostic for mumps infection.

Morbillivirus

Morbillivirus, the cause of **rubeola** (measles), possesses hemagglutinin antigen (HA) and a hemolysin but does not possess neuraminidase antigen. Once a severe, acute, highly contagious childhood disease with epidemics seen every 2 to 3 years, the incidence has dramatically decreased because of successful vaccination. The virus is spread via respiratory secretions, nasal secretions, or coughing. Measles virus incubates in approximately 7 to 13 days, multiplying in the respiratory tract, before the first symptoms of fever, nasal drainage, headache, cough, and sore throat occur. A primary viremia occurs, and the virus is spread to the RES and viscera, where it multiples a second time. This is followed by a secondary viremia and the appearance of a characteristic maculopapular rash, initially behind the ears and then on other parts of the head. The rash characteristically moves down the body and heals in the order in which it first appeared.

Measles vaccination is a part of the MMR given to infants at 15 months of age and to children at 4 to 6 years of age. Prior to the vaccine, almost all children had measles by age 15, and there were almost 500 deaths from measles each year. Because of vaccination, measles is seen much less frequently; in fact, on average there are about 50 cases each year in the United States, with most cases originating in another country. Sporadic cases of measles occur in the United States, with most associated with traveling abroad or from visitors to the United States from other countries. The CDC estimates that worldwide there are 20 million cases of measles and almost 200,000 deaths each year.

Complications of measles infection are common and include pneumonia and encephalitis. Measles is diagnosed through clinical signs and usually not cultured because the virus is shed very early in the infection. The virus may be isolated in cell culture. Serological testing is available to determine whether an individual is seropositive to the virus.

Pneumoviruses: Respiratory Syncytial Virus

Respiratory syncytial virus (RSV), a member of the genus *Pneumovirus*, is a small virus with single-stranded RNA. RSV is pleomorphic and enveloped and does not contain hemagglutinin antigen (HA). Types of infections range from mild respiratory tract and ear infections to pneumonia and other severe respiratory diseases. RSV is a leading cause of pneumonia and bronchiolitis in infants and young children. RSV is spread through droplets of contaminated respiratory secretions, which enter through the eyes or nose. The virus attaches to the respiratory epithelial cells, and following cell-mediated immunity the bronchi are damaged. Necrosis and fibrin deposits clog the airways in the lung, leading to a severe respiratory infection. This acute respiratory tract infection may be fatal in infants and young children. RSV is a leading cause of hospitalization in infants and children less than 2 years old. RSV is very contagious and more common in the winter months. Almost all children have had RSV by the age of 4 years. The CDC estimates that there are between 75,000 and 100,000 hospitalizations related to RSV each year.

Diagnosis is achieved by clinical signs and cultures, including nasal aspirates, throat swabs, nasopharyngeal specimens, or sputum. The RSV antigen can be detected directly using molecular assays and immunofluorescence on the specimens or in cell culture. Serological testing methods include immunofluorescence or complement fixation; the IgM antibody is present within 1 to 2 days. A fourfold increase in titer is considered to be significant.

Treatment relies most on supportive care, including respiratory therapy. There is no vaccine for RSV.

RHABDOVIRIDAE

Lyssavirus in the family Rhabdoviridae is the agent of **rabies**. The virus is enveloped, bullet shaped, and ranges in size from a diameter of 60 nm to 95 nm and a length of 130 nm to 350 nm. The genetic material is negative sense, single-stranded RNA, with helical symmetry. Rabies is found in both wild and domestic animals, including skunks, foxes, coyotes, raccoons, bats, dogs, and cats. Infection is transmitted through contaminated respiratory secretions, most frequently from the bite of an infected animal. Cutaneous transmission from infected secretions and inhalation of aerosolized virus are other routes of infection. Once introduced into the host, the virus binds to neurons, where it may remain for days or months. The virus next travels to the central nervous system, where the brain becomes rapidly infected. Next, the virus is disseminated from the central nervous system through neurons to those tissues that are highly innervated, such as the skin of the head and neck, salivary glands, and eye and nasal mucosa. Symptoms include fever, headache, pain, or itching at the site of infection and fatigue and anorexia in the prodromal period. Neurological symptoms appear within 2 to 10 days and include seizures, disorientation, hallucinations, and eventually paralysis. When in the central nervous system, severe encephalitis, accompanied by coma, convulsions, and death, occurs within 1 to 2 weeks following infection.

Diagnosis is usually made through clinical signs and the medical history of a bite or direct contact with secretions of a possibly infected animal. The virus can be detected using direct immunofluorescence to detect viral antigen. Characteristic Negri bodies are found in the cytoplasm of infected brain cells. However, once rabies is apparent, the disease is often fatal.

The rabies vaccine is administered in animal bite cases when it cannot be determined whether the bite or contact occurred with a rabid animal or from a domestic animal that has not had the proper immunizations. Prevention of rabies requires control of rabies in wild and domestic animals. The use of attenuated oral vaccinations in the United States, which are dropped into areas where rabies is a concern, have been an effective control measure.

REOVIRIDAE

The family Reoviridae includes the genera ***Reovirus***, ***Rotavirus***, and ***Orbivirus***. Characteristics of the family include double-stranded RNA, icosahedral symmetry, no envelope, and a diameter of 60 nm to 80 nm.

Rotavirus is a common cause of gastroenteritis and is associated with both sporadic and epidemic outbreaks. Infants ages 6 months to 2 years are most frequently affected. In fact, rotavirus is the most common cause of gastroenteritis in this age group, and almost all children have been infected by 5 years of age.

Rotavirus is named for its appearance under electron microscopy as a double-shelled capsule that resembles a wheel (Latin *rota*). The virus is spread through the fecal–oral route and also may be associated with food- or water-borne infections. It is stable at room temperature and resistant to treatment with detergents and pH and temperature changes. *Rotavirus* also can survive in the stomach's acidic environment.

In the past, electron microscopy was needed to identify *Rotavirus*. However, rapid latex agglutination and ELISA are now commercially available for detection of the viral antigen in the stool.

CALICIVIRUSES

Calicivirus, commonly known as **Norwalk or Norwalk-like viruses**, is in the family Caliciviridae. Characteristics of the Caliciviridae include single-stranded RNA, icosahedral symmetry, no envelope, and a diameter of 25 nm to 35 nm. The virus is named for Norwalk, Ohio, where an outbreak of diarrhea occurred in 1968 in schoolchildren and their teachers and families. The virus is associated with epidemics of mild gastroenteritis, predominantly in children 6 years of age or older. Calicivirus infection is spread by the fecal–oral route, with virus shedding occurring in the stool as well as through contaminated food and water. Infectious outbreaks have occurred in hospitals, nursing homes, schools, restaurants, and on cruise ships. Often, the source of infection is a food handler who has contaminated foods with the virus. Caliciviral antigens can be detected using enzyme-linked immunoassay or the polymerase chain reaction technique to identify the virus. Electron microscopy also can be used.

RETROVIRIDAE

The family Retroviridae includes the subfamilies Oncornavirinae and Lentivirinae. The Retroviridae viruses possess single-stranded RNA, icosahedral symmetry, an envelope, and a diameter of 80 nm to 130 nm. The **retroviruses** possess the enzyme **reverse transcriptase**, or **RNA-dependent DNA polymerase**, which can transcribe RNA into DNA. This is the "reverse" of the normal transcription of DNA into RNA. There also is an integrase enzyme, which enables the viral genome to be incorporated into the host cell.

Oncornavirus

Oncornavirus includes the genus ***Oncornavirus***, of which human T cell lymphotropic virus type 1 (HTLV-1) and human T cell lymphotropic virus type 2 (HTLV-2) are members. HTLV-1, the first human retrovirus to be identified, is an oncogenic virus and the cause of adult T cell leukemia, lymphoma, and tropical spastic paraparesis. T cell leukemia is a malignancy of specific subtypes of T lymphocytes, which is characterized by dermal and bone involvement, including lesions of the bone. The second retrovirus to be isolated, HTLV-2, was originally isolated from a patient with hairy cell leukemia. Prevalence of both viruses is low in the United States but higher in other areas of the world. Transmission of the HTLV viruses is believed to occur through contaminated blood or blood products or through sexual contact.

Lentivirinae and Human Immunodeficiency Viruses

The **Lentivirinae** (Latin *lenti*, or "slow") include human immunodeficiency viruses types 1 and 2 (HIV-1 and HIV-2), which are characterized by slow viral diseases with neurological manifestations. The viruses were first named HTLV-3 and LAV (lymphadenopathy virus) by researchers who discovered the virus in the United States and France in 1983, respectively. Later, the virus was named HIV-1, and a second HIV virus (HIV-2) was subsequently isolated. HIV has a complex structure and possesses an envelope, viral core, and other proteins, including the following:

- **Group-specific antigen (Gag) proteins**, which code for retroviral core proteins and structural proteins. These are a part of the viral nucleocapsid and provide stability for the capsule. Gag proteins are p24, p17, and p7/p9.
- **Polymerase (Pol) proteins**, which are important in the viral life cycle. These include RNA-dependent DNA polymerase (reverse transcriptase), integrase, and protease.
- **Envelope (env) proteins**, which are glycoproteins in the retroviral coat that adhere to target cells and produce cytopathic cell fusion. The envelope includes cell wall components of the host as the virus "buds." Env proteins include gp120 and gp142.

Infection with HIV-1 can lead to **acquired immunodeficiency syndrome** (AIDS), which is characterized by loss of immune competency, opportunistic infections, and unusual neoplasms.

After being infected with HIV, some people develop a flu-like syndrome, which may occur 6 to 8 weeks after infection and persist for a few weeks, while others may have no symptoms. Circulating virus is present at this time, and antibodies develop within a few months of infection. This is followed by a long, asymptomatic phase, which may range from months to years. However, the virus may be multiplying within the host and affecting many organs in the body. Untreated early HIV can lead to kidney, liver, or cardiovascular disease and cancer. AIDS is the late stage of HIV infection, at which time the host immune system is severely devastated.

HIV attacks the CD4-positive T lymphocytes, which decreases T helper cell activity and diminishes delayed type hypersensitivity. As the level of CD4-positive T cells declines, the characteristic symptoms of AIDS infection become apparent. These include opportunistic infections, such as *Pneumocystis carinii* pneumonia, CMV infections, cryptosporidiosis or isosporiasis diarrhea, candidiasis, toxoplasmosis, and mycobacterial infections. Other symptoms include fever, night sweats, loss of weight, and lymphadenopathy. The development of unusual neoplasms, in particular Kaposi's sarcoma, as well as anal carcinomas and B cell lymphomas, also may occur. Neurological damage, including encephalopathies, also may be present.

The clinical disease now known as AIDS was first described in 1981; HIV was identified as the cause of AIDS in 1986. Routes of infection include sexual contact with an infected individual, intrauterine infection from an infected mother to the baby, and contaminated needles used in intravenous drug use. There also is the risk of transmission for health care workers through contaminated needle-sticks and other sharps and contact with mucous membranes through splashing. Many early cases of HIV-AIDS were diagnosed in homosexual males; however, today the infection is prevalent also in heterosexual populations. No evidence indicates that the virus is spread through the aerosol route or through casual contact. Standard precautions for blood-borne pathogens have been established and must be adhered to to decrease the incidence of HIV-acquired infections in the health care setting.

Before 1985, HIV was transmitted through contaminated blood; blood products, such as antihemophiliac factor (Factor VIII); and organ transplants. All donor products are screened for HIV; in addition, blood donor screening includes a rigorous donor history, which probes lifestyle activities that make an individual more likely to acquire HIV. All HIV-positive donors are notified of their status and all blood products discarded.

Diagnosis of HIV infection is based on clinical symptoms, patient history, and serological testing. Several commercially available ELISAs are available as screening tests. The confirmatory test for HIV, however, is the **Western blot**, which identifies antibodies for various HIV antigens. Antibodies to HIV p24, a Gag protein, and either gp41 or gp160, envelope antigens, usually confirm HIV infection. In the dot blot procedure, the patient's serum is added to a nitrocellulose sheet to which are bound HIV antigens. In a positive test, the patient's HIV antibodies bind to the HIV antigens. Next a labeled antihuman antibody is added, which will bind to the antigen–antibody complex. A positive reaction appears as a dot on the nitrocellulose sheet.

HIV-reverse transcriptase PCR is used to determine viral loading and the number of copies of HIV present. Molecular diagnostic methods continue to be developed and are available to identify and quantify HIV.

Treatment of HIV infections involves the use of several types of therapies. These include reverse transcriptase inhibitors, nucleotide/nucleoside analogues, and protease and fusion inhibitors. Treatment of the secondary opportunistic infections also is an important part of treatment.

HIV-2 infections, although rare in the United States, are found more frequently in West Africa, South America, and certain parts of Europe. HIV-2 produces an infection similar to HIV-1, with different opportunistic pathogens seen and a milder disease course.

Review Questions

Matching

For the following serological markers of HBV infection, match the marker with its correct description:

1. HBsAg
2. HBeAg
3. Anti-HBcAg
4. Anti-HBsAg
    a. Total antibody to hepatitis B surface antigen is associated with immunity or recovery.
    b. Marker of infectivity and persistence usually indicates chronic liver disease.
    c. Total antibody to hepatitis B core antigen appears between HBsAg and anti-HBsAg.
    d. Recent acute infection is indicated.
    e. First serologic marker to appear; persistence may indicate chronic infection.

Match the virus with its associated infection:

5. VZV
6. EBV
7. HHV-6
8. HSV-1
9. Human papillomavirus
10. Parvovirus
11. Togavirus
12. Variola
13. Flavivirus
14. *Rubivirus*
15. Enterovirus
16. *Morbillivirus*
17. Pneumovirus
18. *Lyssavirus*
19. Human T cell lymphotropic virus

20. HIV
    a. Adult T cell leukemia
    b. Gingivostomatitis
    c. Chickenpox
    d. Warts
    e. Rabies
    f. Measles (rubeola)
    g. Rubella
    h. AIDS
    i. Infectious mononucleosis
    j. Smallpox
    k. Respiratory syncytial virus
    l. Roseola
    m. Erythema infectiosum
    n. Equine encephalitis
    o. Polio
    p. Yellow fever

Multiple Choice

21. Properties of viruses include:
    a. Presence of both DNA and RNA
    b. Presence of an ATP-generating system
    c. Multiplication of binary fission
    d. Obligate intracellular parasites
22. The protein coat of the virus is known as the:
    a. Virion
    b. Capsid
    c. Nucleocapsid
    d. Envelope
23. Although dependent on the virus to be isolated, optimal specimen collection time to detect most viral infections is:
    a. Early in the course of the disease
    b. During the convalescent phase
    c. During the latent phase
    d. 1 week after the onset of symptoms
24. When specimen delay is anticipated, virology specimens are optimally maintained:
    a. At room temperature
    b. Incubated at 35°C
    c. Frozen immediately at –20°C
    d. Held at 4°C and snap frozen to ~70°C
25. Each of the following groups of viruses may be associated with aseptic meningitis *except*:
    a. Enterovirus
    b. Echovirus
    c. Influenza viruses
    d. Varicella-zoster virus (VZV)
    e. Mumps virus
26. Viral agents of gastroenteritis include:
    a. Cytomegalovirus (CMV), rotavirus, and Epstein-Barr virus (EBV)
    b. Rotavirus, calicivirus, and Norwalk agent
    c. Herpes simplex virus (HSV), human immunodeficiency virus (HIV), and enterovirus
    d. Parvovirus, rhinovirus, and echovirus
27. "Owl's eye" cytological inclusions are characteristic of infection caused by:
    a. HIV
    b. CMV
    c. HSV
    d. VZV
28. Heteroploid cell lines:
    a. Contain at least 75% of cells with the same karyotype as that of the normal original cells
    b. Include such examples as HEK and RMK
    c. Are directly derived from parent tissue
    d. Are usually derived from malignant or transformed cells
29. Which statement best describes normal antibody response to viral infection?
    a. IgG appears within 2 weeks of primary infection.
    b. IgM peaks in 3 to 6 weeks.
    c. IgG is usually undetectable by 6 weeks.
    d. None of the above is correct.
30. Which of the following hepatitis viruses is *not* transmitted through contaminated blood or blood products?
    a. HAV
    b. HBV
    c. HCV
    d. HDV
31. Which of the following viral families are associated with reactivation of latent infections?
    a. Hepatitis viruses
    b. Influenza viruses
    c. Parvoviruses
    d. Herpesviruses
32. A positive ELISA test for HIV-1 and a Western blot test with bands at p24 and gp41 most likely indicate:
    a. False-positive ELISA and inconclusive Western blot
    b. False-positive ELISA and Western blot
    c. Positive ELISA and Western blot, indicating HIV infection
    d. Lack of HIV infection
33. Which of the following are characteristic of EBV infection?
    a. Failure to agglutinate sheep RBCs after absorption with guinea pig cells

b. Presence of greater than 50% lymphocytes and atypical lymphotyces on WBC differential
c. Presence of heterophile antibody
d. b and c are correct.
e. a, b, and c are correct.

Arrange the sequence of steps of viral replication in the correct order. Number the responses 1 through 5.

34. Assembly
35. Adsorption
36. Penetration
37. Release
38. Uncoating

For each of the following viruses, indicate whether the nucleic acid is DNA or RNA:

39. HAV
40. HBV
41. HSV-1
42. Adenovirus
43. HIV
44. Influenza virus
45. VZV
46. CMV

Bibliography

Calisher, C. H. (1994). Medically important arboviruses of the United States and Canada. *Clinical Microbiology Reviews, 7,* 89.

Centers for Disease Control and Prevention. (2008). Rubella. In *Manual for the surveillance of vaccine-preventable diseases* (4th edition).

Centers for Disease Control and Prevention. (2009). Rubella. Retrieved from http://www.cdc.gov/rubella/index.htm

Centers for Disease Control and Prevention. (2011). HIV/AIDS. Retrieved from http://www.cdc.gov/hiv/default.htm

Centers for Disease Control and Prevention. (2011). Viral hepatitis. Retrieved from http://www.cdc.gov/hepatitis/index.htm

Centers for Disease Control and Prevention. (2013). HIV and Viral Hepatitis. Retrieved from http://www.cdc.gov/hiv/pdf/library_factsheets_HIV_and_viral_Hepatitis.pdf

Chou, S., & Scott, K. M. (1988). Latex agglutination and enzyme-linked immunosorbent assays for cytomegalovirus serologic screening of transplant donors and recipients. *Journal of Clinical Microbiology, 26,* 2116.

Dennehy, P. H., Gauntlett, D. R., & Tente, W. E. (1988). Comparison of nine commercial immunoassays for the detection of rotavirus in fecal specimens. *Journal of Clinical Microbiology, 26,* 1630.

Dock, N. L. (1991). The ABC's of viral hepatitis. *Clinical Microbiology Newsletter, 13,* 17.

Falsey, A. H., & Walsh, E. E. (2000). Respiratory syncytial virus in adults. *Journal of Clinical Microbiology, 26,* 1630–1634.

Feitelson, M. (1992). Hepatitis B virus infection and primary hepatocellular carcinoma. *Clinical Microbiology Reviews, 5,* 275–301.

Gallo, R. C. (1991). Retroviruses: A decade of discovery and link with human disease. *Journal of Infectious Diseases, 164,* 235.

Hamilton, J. R. (1988). Viral enteritis. *Pediatric Clinics of North America, 35,* 89.

Heilman, C. A. (1990). Respiratory syncytial and parainfluenza viruses. *Journal of Infectious Diseases, 161,* 402.

Henchal, E. A., & Pytnak, J. R. (1990). The dengue viruses. *Clinical Microbiology Reviews, 3,* 376–396.

Ho, M. (1990). Epidemiology of cytomegalovirus infections. *Reviews of Infectious Diseases,* 12, S701.

Hojvat, S. A. (1989). Diagnostic tests for viral hepatitis. *Clinical Microbiology Newsletter,* 11, 33.

Johnson, F. B. (1990). Transport of viral specimens. *Clinical Microbiology Reviews, 3,* 120.

Jones, C. (2003). Herpes simplex virus type 1 and bovine herpesvirus I latency. *Clinical Microbiology Reviews, 16,* 79–85.

Kinney, J. S., Onorato, I. M., Stewart, J. A. et al. (1985). Cytomegaloviral infection and disease. *Journal of Infectious Diseases, 151,* 772.

Leland, S. E., & Ginoccho, C. C. (2007). Role of cell culture for virus detection in the age of technology. *Clinical Microbiology Reviews, 20,* 49–78.

Mahony, J. B. (2008). Detection of respiratory viruses by molecular methods. *Clinical Microbiology Reviews, 21,* 716–747.

Malike Peiris, J. S., de Jong, M. D., & Guan, Y. (2007). Avian influenza virus (H5N1): A threat to human health. *Clinical Microbiology Reviews, 2,* 243–267.

Martina, B., Koraka, P., & Osterhaus, A. (2009). Dengue virus pathogenesis: An integrated view. *Clinical Microbiology Reviews, 22,* 464–581.

Marymont, J. H., & Herrman, K. L. (1982). Rubella testing: An overview. *Laboratory Medicine, 13,* 83.

Minnich, L. L., & Ray, C. G. (1987). Early testing of cell cultures for detection of hemadsorbing viruses. *Journal of Clinical Microbiology, 25,* 421.

Murray, P. R., Rosenthal, K. S., & Pfaller, K. S. (2009). Human herpesviruses. In *Medical microbiology,* 6th ed. (pp. 517–540). Philadelphia, PA: Mosby Elsevier.

Nainan, O. V., Xia, G., Vaughn, G., & Margolis, H. S. (2006). Diagnosis of hepatitis A virus infection: A molecular approach. *Clinical Microbiology Review, 19,* 63–79.

Palese, P., & Young, J. F. (1982). Variation of influenza A, B, and C viruses. *Science, 215,* 1468.

Reynolds, J. P. (2011). HPV: A look into new methods for high risk testing. *Medical Laboratory Observer, 43,* 10–14.

Sabin, A. B. (1981). Paralytic poliomyelitis: Old dogmas and new perspectives. *Reviews of Infectious Diseases, 3,* 543.

Salk, J. (1987). Commentary: Poliomyelitis vaccination—choosing a wise policy. *Pediatric Infectious Disease Journal, 6,* 889.

Shamberger, R. J. (1984). ELISA on the trail of viral diseases. *Diagnostic Medicine,* October, 52–57.

Silverman, A. L., & Gordon, S. C. (1993). Clinical epidemiology and molecular biology of hepatitis C. *Laboratory Medicine, 24,* 656.

Smith, T. J. (1994). Introduction to virology. In B. J. Howard (Ed.), *Clinical and pathogenic microbiology,* 2nd ed. St. Louis, MO: Mosby.

Tsoukas, C. M., & Bernard, N. F. (1994). Markers of predicting progression of human immunodeficiency virus-related disease. *Clinical Microbiology Reviews, 7,* 14.

Vainionpaa, R., & Hyypia, T. (1994). Biology of parainfluenza viruses. *Clinical Microbiology Reviews, 7,* 265.

Winn, Jr., W., Allen, S., Janda, W., Konemen, E., Procop, G., Schreckenberger, P., & Woods, G. (Eds.). (2005). Diagnosis of infections caused by viruses, *Chlamydia,* Rickettsia, and related organisms. In *Koneman's color atlas and textbook of diagnostic microbiology* (6th ed.). (pp. 1327–1419). Philadelphia, PA: Lippincott Williams & Wilkins.

Zein, N. N. (2000). Clinical significance of hepatitis C virus genotypes. *Clinical Microbiology Reviews, 13,* 223–235.

NEWS: UNCONVENTIONAL SLOW VIRUS—PRIONS AND SPONGIFORM ENCEPHALOPATHIES

Unconventional slow viral agents cause spongiform encephalopathies. Like other viruses, these agents can transmit disease and are filterable. However, unlike viruses, these infectious units have no genome or virion structure. They are mutated or distorted forms of a host protein known as a prion, which is a small infectious particle. These infectious agents incubate for long periods of time, even as long as 30 years.

Prions have no detectable nucleic acid and are composed of protease-resistant glycoproteins, known as PrP^{Sc}. Humans and other animals code for a similar protein, known as cellular prion protein, or PrP^{C}. These two proteins are very similar; however, PrP^{Sc} is resistant to protease, forms aggregates of amyloid fibrils, is found in cytoplasmic vesicles in the cell, and is secreted. By contrast, PrP^{C} is found on the cell surface and is susceptible to protease. In spongiform diseases, the abnormal PrP^{Sc} directs the conversion of PrP^{C} to the abnormal protein. It is believed that the protein molecule folds in an arrangement that alters its biological properties. The cell continues to replenish the PrP^{C}, providing the necessary protein for the cycle to continue. The PrP^{Sc} is taken up by neurons and accumulates, giving the cell the spongiform appearance.

Prions do not promote an immune response or stimulate an inflammatory reaction from the host. Spongiform encephalopathies occur in humans and other animals. Examples of human infection include kuru, classic Creutzfeldt-Jakob disease (CJD), and variant Creutzfeldt-Jakob disease (vCJD). Diseases in animals include bovine spongiform encephalopathy (BSE), or mad cow disease; scrapie in goats and sheep; and chronic wasting disease in mules, deer, and elks.

Classic CJD is a neurodegenerative disorder with rapid progression and death, occurring within 1 year after onset of the symptoms. There is diminished muscle control, tremors, progressive dementia, and loss of coordination. Classic CJD was first recognized in the 1920s, and the disease occurs worldwide, with most cases occurring sporadically with approximately 1 to 2 cases per million population. According to the CDC, there are fewer than 300 cases of CJD reported in the United States each year. Symptoms include dementia and neurologic signs early in the onset of symptoms. There also are inherited forms of the disease, known as Gerstmann-Straussler-Scheinker syndrome and fatal familial insomnia.

In the 1980s, there have been cases of individuals who developed CJD after receiving pituitary-derived human growth hormone (hGH) in the 1960s and 1970s. The association between hGH and CJD led to the discontinuation of hGH use by the National Hormone and Pituitary program. Transmission of CJG via dura mater grafts also was reported in the 1980s.

Variant CJD was first described in 1996 in the United Kingdom; it differs clinically and pathologically from classic CJD. Those affected with variant CJD are younger, with an average age of 28 years, compared to those with classic CJD, who have an average age of 68 years. Duration of illness is 13 to 14 months with variant CJD but only 4 to 5 months with classic CJD. Symptoms include psychiatric or behavioral symptoms, with the onset of neurological symptoms occurring later in the disease.

Bovine spongiform encephalopathy (BSE), or mad cow disease, is another prion disease found in cattle. The first cases occurred most likely in the 1970s, with others occurring in the 1980s. BSE is believed to have originated in the United Kingdom as a result of feeding calves meat and bone meal that contained BSE-infected products from sheep. There were almost 1,000 new cases a week of BSE in the United Kingdom in 1993, when the epizootic peaked. The number of cases has dropped significantly in the United Kingdom, however, from approximately 14,000 cases in 1995 to only 11 new cases in 2010. Still, there are over 184,000 cases of confirmed BSE in the United Kingdom in over 35,000 herds. Over a half million BSE-infected cattle have been slaughtered between 1980 and 1996 and potentially consumed in the United Kingdom. In the United States, there have been 22 cases of BSE identified through early 2011.

There is evidence that bovine spongiform encephalopathy (BSE) is caused by the same prion as vCJD. However, the risk of vCJD seems to be low even after consumption of contaminated beef products. The epizootic of BSE and cases of vCJD have led to legislation to ban animal products in livestock in the United Kingdom. Enhanced feed bans have been instituted in the United States and Canada.

BIBLIOGRAPHY

Belay, E. D., & Schonberger, L. B. (2005). The public health impact of prion diseases. *Annual Review of Public Health, 26,* 191–212.

Centers for Disease Control and Prevention. (2010). Prion diseases. Retrieved from http://www.cdc.gov/ncidod/dvrd/prions/

CHAPTER 20

Introduction to Medical Mycology

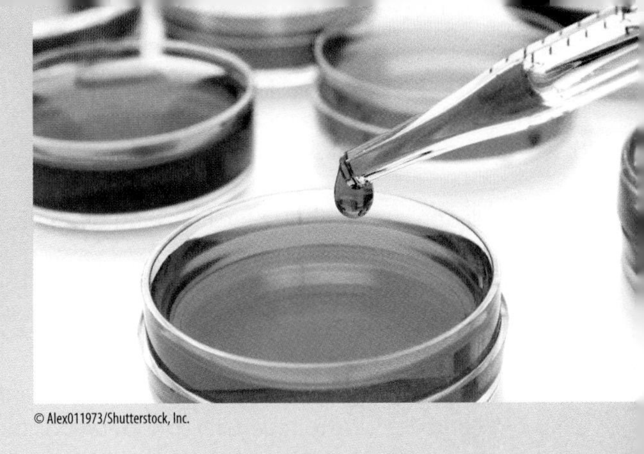

CHAPTER OUTLINE

Introduction to Mycology

Fungal Infections

KEY TERMS

Ascospores
Assimilation
Basidiospores
Black piedra
Blastomycosis
Chromoblastomycosis
Coccidioidomycosis
Conidia
Conidiogenesis
Dematiaceous fungi
Deuteromycetes
Dimorphic fungi
Ectothrix infection
Endothrix infection
Fungi imperfecti
Germ tube
Histoplasmosis
Hyphae
Macroconidia
Microconidia
Mold phase
Mycelium
Mycetoma
Mycoses
Oospore
Opportunistic mycoses
Paracoccidioidomycosis
Penicilliosis
Phaeohyphomycosis
Pityriasis versicolor
Sporangiospores
Sporotrichosis
Subcutaneous mycoses
Superficial (cutaneous) mycoses
Systemic mycoses
Thallophytes
Tinea
Yeast phase
Zygomycosis
Zygospores

LEARNING OBJECTIVES

1. Discuss the characteristics of the fungi.
2. Correctly define and describe the following:
    a. Hyphae
    b. Mycelium
    c. Septate hyphae
    d. Aseptate hyphae
3. Describe and recognize the following types of asexual reproductive structures:
    a. Blastoconidia
    b. Chlamydoconidia
    c. Arthroconidia
    d. Sporangiospores

4. Describe and recognize the following types of sexual reproductive structures:
   a. Ascospores
   b. Basidiospores
   c. Zygospores
5. Describe typical colonial textures and topographies.
6. List and describe four general considerations for proper fungal specimen collection.
7. Justify the importance of the direct examination of clinical specimens for fungi.
8. State the purpose, perform the procedure, and interpret the following microscopic techniques:
   a. Saline wet mount
   b. Lactophenol cotton blue
   c. Potassium hydroxide (KOH) preparation
9. List at least three types of primary fungal isolation media and state the purpose of each.
10. Describe, perform, and interpret the following laboratory techniques:
    a. Tease mount
    b. Slide culture
    c. Germ tube
    d. Carbohydrate assimilation
    e. Rapid urease
11. Identify the following dermatophytes from prepared slides, pictures, or cultures:
    a. *Microsporum audouinii*
    b. *Microsporum canis*
    c. *Microsporum gypseum*
    d. *Epidermophyton floccosum*
    e. *Trichophyton mentagrophytes*
    f. *Trichophyton rubrum*
    g. *Trichophyton tonsurans*
12. Describe the types of tinea and the dermatophytes associated with each.
13. Discuss the clinical significance and identify the following yeasts and yeast-like fungi from prepared slides, pictures, biochemical reactions, or cultures:
    a. *Candida albicans*
    b. *Candida glabrata*
    c. *Geotrichum candidum*
    d. *Rhodotorula*
    e. *Cryptococcus neoformans*
14. Discuss the clinical significance and identify the following subcutaneous mycoses from prepared slides, pictures, or cultures:
    a. *Cladosporium carrionii*
    b. *Fonsecaea pedrosoi*
    c. *Phialophora verrucosa*
    d. *Sporothrix schenckii*
15. Discuss the clinical significance and identify the following systemic mycoses from pictures:
    a. *Blastomyces dermatitidis*
    b. *Coccidioides immitis*
    c. *Histoplasma capsulatum*
    d. *Paracoccidioides brasiliensis*
    e. *Penicillium marneffie*
16. Describe the significance of infections attributed to the yeasts, phaeohyphomycetes, and hyalohyphomycetes.
17. Based on microscopic appearance on cornmeal Tween 80 agar, carbohydrate assimilation patterns, germ tube results, and biochemical reactions, identify a yeast or yeastlike fungi.
18. Discuss the significance and identify the following opportunistic fungi from prepared slides, pictures, or cultures:
    a. *Rhizopus*
    b. *Absidia*
    c. *Mucor*
    d. *Aspergillus*
    e. *Penicillium*

Introduction to Mycology

Mycology is the study of the fungi. Although more than 50,000 species of fungi are recognized, fewer than 100 have been identified as human pathogens. The fungi are present as saprobes in the environment, relying on decaying vegetation and plants for sources of nitrogen. Humans acquire fungal infections, or **mycoses**, through inhalation or direct contact with spores or inoculation by trauma into the skin. Person-to-person or animal-to-person contact occurs in some cases. Increases in opportunistic mycoses occur in individuals with underlying medical disorders. These disorders and predisposing factors include diabetes mellitus, infection with human immunodeficiency virus (HIV), prolonged corticosteroid or antibiotic therapy, and chemotherapy. Fungi previously considered to be saprobic or contaminants are now important opportunistic pathogens.

The fungi are classified as **thallophytes** because the organisms have true nuclei and are heterotrophic members of the plant family that lack stems and roots. The fungi do not contain chlorophyll and are larger, with a more complex morphology, than the bacteria. Fungi absorb nutrients through the environment.

Fungi demonstrate two phases: the mold phase and the yeast phase. The multicellular **mold phase** consists of a cottony mycelial mass and grows at 25°C. The unicellular **yeast phase** is creamy, resembling a bacterial colony, and grows from 35°C to 37°C. Some fungi demonstrate both a yeast phase, growing at 35°C to 37°C, and a mold phase, growing at 25°C, and are known as **dimorphic fungi**.

The **mycelium** is an intertwining structure composed of tubular filaments, known as **hyphae**, which are the microscopic units of the fungi. **Septate hyphae** contain cross-walls, whereas **aseptate hyphae** are continuous, without cross-walls. The mycelium consists of a vegetative portion, or **thallus**, which grows in or on a substrate and absorbs water and nutrients, and a reproductive, or aerial, part, which contains the fruiting bodies that produce the reproductive structures, known as conidia and spores. The aerial part extends above the agar surface.

Conidia and spores may remain dormant in the air or environment or may be transported through the air to other locations. The spores of pathogenic molds can be inhaled and enter the respiratory tract. This is a common route of infection, and because of this, it is imperative to practice good laboratory safety when working in the mycology laboratory. All laboratory analysis, including the preparation of slides, plating and transferring cultures, and any biochemical procedures, must be performed in a biological safety cabinet. Airborne conidia and spores are readily released from a fungal culture, so one should never smell a fungal culture. Screw-cap test tubes should be used in place of test tubes with a cotton, metal, or plastic lid. In addition, Petri plates, when used must be sealed tightly with either an oxygen-impermeable tape or with Parafilm. As always, gloves should be worn and any breaks or cuts in the skin covered to prevent the transmission of the fungal infection.

Fungi may reproduce either sexually or asexually. Fungi that exhibit a sexual phase are known as the **perfect fungi**. Sexual reproduction requires the formation of special structures so that fertilization or nuclear fission can occur. In sexual reproduction, meiosis, or reduction division of two fertile cells, followed by a merging of the cells and nuclear fusion, occurs. Types of specialized spores involved in sexual reproduction include **ascospores**, which are contained in a saclike ascus; **zygospores**, which involve the fusion of two identical cells arising from the same hypha; **oospores**, which involve the fusion of cells from two separate, nonidentical hyphae; and **basidiospores**, which are contained in a club-shaped basidium.

The **imperfect fungi**, or **fungi imperfecti**, do not exhibit a sexual phase, and spores are produced asexually from the mycelium. Asexual reproduction involves only mitosis, with nuclear and cytoplasmic division. **Conidiogenesis**, or conidia formation, can occur blastically or thallically. In **blastic conidiogenesis** the parent cell enlarges, a septum forms, and the enlarged portion splits off to form a daughter cell. In **thallic conidiogenesis** the septum forms first, and new growth beyond the septum becomes the daughter cell.

Conidia are asexual spores produced either singly or multiply in long chains or clusters by specialized vegetative hyphae, known as **conidiophores**. Conidiophores may branch into secondary segments, known as **phialides**, which then produce the conidia. Some fungi can produce conidia of two sizes. **Macroconidia** are large; usually septate; and club, oval, or spindle shaped. Macroconidia may be thick or thin walled and have either a spiny, or **echinulate**, or smooth surface. Usually the entire hyphae element becomes a multicellular conidium, known as the macroconidium. **Microconidia** are small and unicellular with a round, elliptical, or **pyriform** (pear) shape. Microconidia borne directly on the hyphae are known as **sessile microconidia**, and those borne on the end of a short conidiophore are known as **pedunculate microconidia**.

Other spores develop directly from the vegetative mycelium, including blastoconidia, chlamydoconidia, and arthroconidia. **Blastoconidia**, or **blastospores**, develop as the daughter cell buds off the mother cell and is pinched off. Yeasts, including *Candida*, produce blastospores. Blastoconidia may elongate to form **pseudohyphae**, which can align in an end-to-end manner, resembling true hyphae. Pseudohyphae can be differentiated from true hyphae because pseudohyphae are constricted at the septa; as a result, branches form at the septation. True hyphae are not constricted at the septa. **Chlamydoconidia**, or **chlamydospores**, are thick-walled, resistant, resting spores produced by "rounding up" and enlargement of the terminal hyphal cells. The spores germinate into a new organism when favorable environmental conditions exist. Chlamydoconidia may form at the hyphal tip in a terminal arrangement; on the hyphal sides in a sessile arrangement; or within the hyphal strand, which is an intercalary arrangement. It is important to differentiate chlamydoconidia from **conidiospores**, which are produced by yeast, such as *Candida*. Although conidiospores are thick-walled structures, they are not considered to be conidia because condiospores do not germinate. **Arthroconidia**, or **arthrospores**, involve the simple fragmentation of the mycelium at the septum into rectangular-, cylinder-, or cask-shaped spores. The spores are thick walled and may be adjacent or alternate in arrangement. In the alternate arrangement, empty spaces, or **disjunctor cells**, appear between each arthrospore. This is a useful identification characteristic of the dimorphic fungus *Coccidioides immitis* and *Geotrichum candidium*, a yeast.

Sporangiospores are asexual spores that are contained in sporangia, or sacs, and produced terminally on sporangiophores or aseptate hyphae. Sporulation results when the sporangial wall ruptures with the release of sporagiospores. Sporangiospores are unique to the group of fungi known as the Zygomycetes.

FIGURE 20-1 provides diagrams with definitions of basic structures, including hyphae, conidia, and spores.

The fungi can be classified in several ways, including the botanical taxonomy, which contains four divisions: Zygomycota (Zygomycetes), Ascomycota (Ascomycetes), Basidomycota (Basidomycetes), and Deuteromycota (Deuteromycetes). *Mucor, Absidia*, and *Rhizopus* are medically important genera of the Zygomycota, whereas most other medically important fungi are classified as **Deuteromycetes** and have the characteristics of septate hyphae and asexual reproduction. The fungi also can be classified according to the type of mycoses; using this method, the four categories follow:

- **Superficial and cutaneous mycoses**, including the dermatophytes, tinea versicolor, and piedra
- **Subcutaneous mycoses**, which usually do not disseminate, including *Sporothrix*, mycetoma, chromoblastomycosis, and phaeohyphomycosis
- **Systemic mycoses**, which often involve the lungs and disseminate, including *Blastomyces, Coccidioides, Histoplasma, Paracoccidioides*, and *Penicillium*
- **Opportunistic mycoses**, which are an ever-increasing group of fungi that attack immunocompromised individuals and include *Aspergillus*, zygomycosis, candidiasis, other yeast infections, and several other infections

SPECIMEN COLLECTION

General guidelines for specimen collection for fungal infections are very similar to those for bacterial infections. These guidelines include the use of sterile collection methods and containers to avoid contamination. Sufficient quantity and an accurate and complete label are also important requirements. The specimen should be from the actual infection site to avoid normal flora-contaminating bacteria. Of utmost importance is prompt delivery to the laboratory to avoid the danger of overgrowth of bacterial or fungal contaminants, which may hinder the recovery of the fungal pathogen. It also is helpful if the physician includes the suspected diagnosis so that any special procedures or specimen treatments can be used.

TABLE 20-1 summarizes specific guidelines for specimen collection and processing.

IDENTIFICATION METHODS

Laboratory methods in mycology include direct microscopic methods and specific stains. Macroscopic cultural characteristics on both general and differential media also are used for fungal isolation and identification.

Microscopic Methods

Microscopic methods include the saline mount, potassium hydroxide (KOH) preparation, India ink preparation, and lactophenol cotton blue. Microscopic methods must always be confirmed with cultures or antigen testing when available. Because these methods can be preformed quickly, they can provide valuable information to facilitate the identification of the fungi.

The **saline mount** is a quick and simple method to observe fungal elements, including budding yeast, hyphae, and pseudohyphae. The specimen is added to one drop of sterile physiological saline, a coverslip is applied, and the mount is examined under low and high magnification. A major disadvantage of this method is the lack of contrast, which makes identification of fungal elements somewhat difficult.

The **KOH preparation** is used to dissolve keratin in skin, hair, or nail specimens. The keratin may obscure the fungal elements in these specimens, and KOH facilitates the examination. Chitin in the fungal cell wall is resistant to the effects of KOH. One drop of KOH is added to the

Arthroconidia

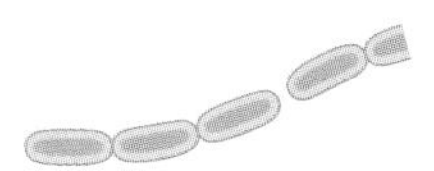

Asexual spores formed by fragmentation of mycelia into rectangular, barrel-shaped, or cask-shaped, thick-walled spores.

Ascospores

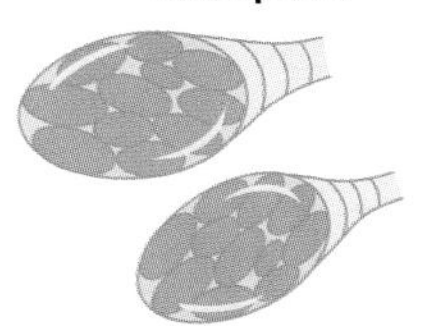

Sexual spores produced in a round, saclike ascus that usually contains two to eight ascospores.

Blastoconidia

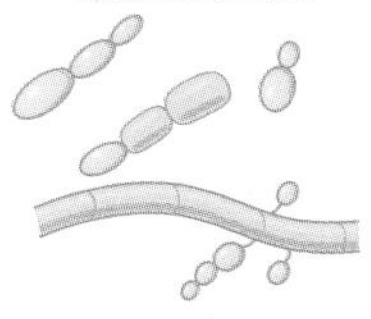

Asexual conidia produced by formation of conidia by simple budding from mother cells, hyphae, or pseudohyphae; budding is characteristic of yeasts and yeastlike fungi.

Chlamydoconidia

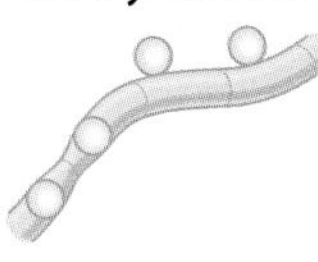

Thick-walled asexual conidia that are formed during unfavorable conditions and germinate when environment improves; greater in diameter than hyphae and may be observed at hyphal tip (**terminal**), within hyphal strand (**intercalary**), or on the sides of hyphae (**sessile**).

Cleistothecium

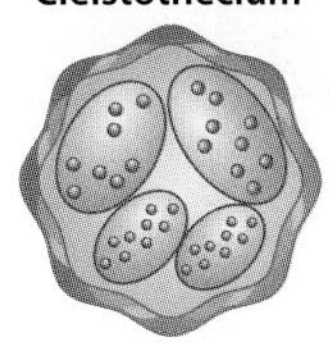

Large, round, multicellular structure that surrounds the asci and ascopores until the structure ruptures, releasing the ascopores.

Columella

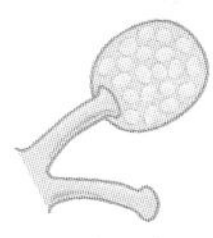

Dome-shaped, swollen sporangiophore tip that extends into the sporangiophore.

Conidiophore

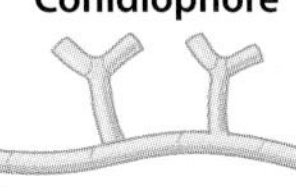

Specialized, vegetative hyphae that act as stalks on which conidia are found.

Conidia

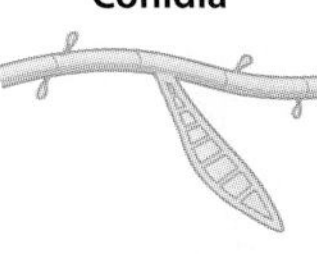

Asexual structures that form on the sides of hyphae or conidiophores; may be produced singly or in groups; **macroconidia** are large and multicelled, whereas **microconidia** are usually small and unicellular.

Fusiform

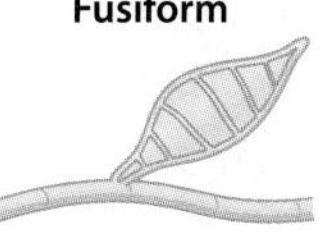

Spindle-shaped conidium that is wider in the middle and narrows toward either end.

Germ tube

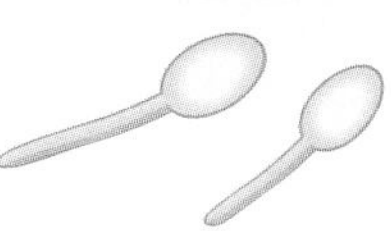

Outgrowth of a conidium or spore that is the beginning of a hypha; no constriction is observed at the point of attachment. Germ tubes are usually three to four times the length of the original yeast cell.

Hyphae

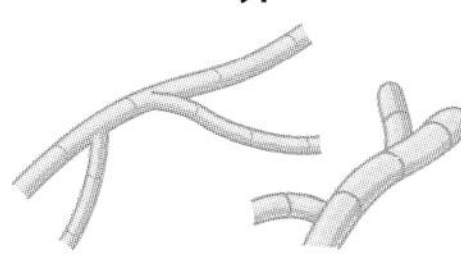

Tubelike structures that are the fundamental units of the fungus; many hyphae join to form the **mycelium**, which forms the colony of the fungus. **Septate hyphae** contain cross-walls or septa, whereas **aseptate hyphae** lack cross-walls.

Phialide

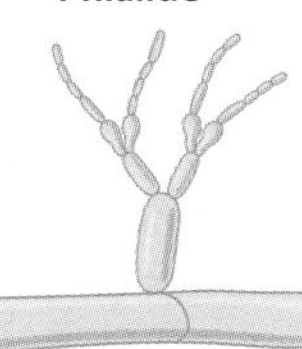

Flask-shaped or vase-shaped structure that produces phialoconidia.

Pseudohyphae

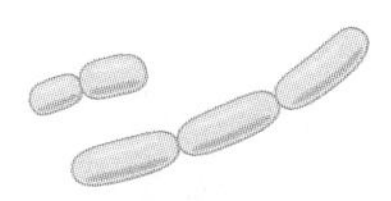

Chains of cells produced by budding that may resemble true hyphae. Pseudohyphae are constricted at the septa and form branches that begin at the septation. A mass of pseudohyphae is a **pseudomycelium**.

Piriform

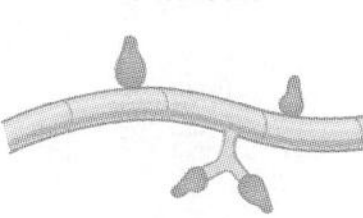

Pear-shaped conidia

Spherule

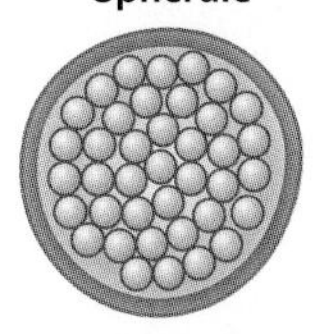

Large, round, thick-walled structure that contains spores characteristic of *Coccidioides immitis* in tissue.

Sporangiospore

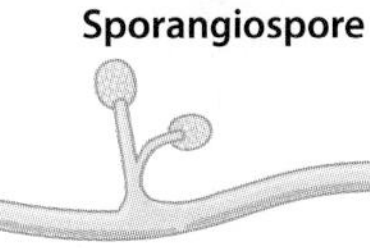

Asexual spore contained in a saclike structure (**sporangium**) in which spores are formed and held. The sporangium is borne on a specialized hyphal stalk, or **sporangiophore**.

Tuberculate

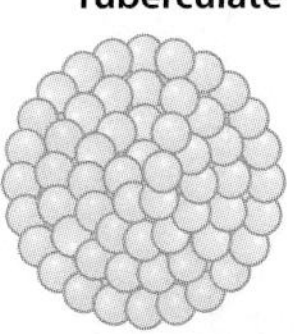

With knoblike projections.

Vesicle

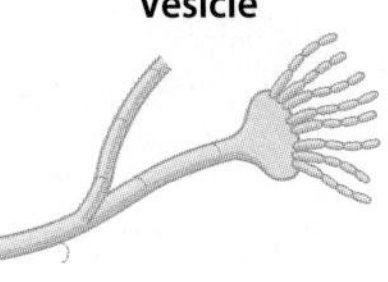

Enlarged structure at the end of a conidiophore or sporangiophore that may bear phialides.

FIGURE 20-1 Common structures and terms for medical mycology.

TABLE 20-1 Collection and Processing Guidelines for Fungal Specimens

Specimen	Normal fungal flora	Possible pathogenic fungi	Collection notes	Primary isolation media
Blood	None	*Histoplasma capsulatum* *Cryptococcus neoformans* *Candida albicans* *Blastomyces dermatitidis*	Wright's or Giemsa stain bottles are used frequently; India ink or direct antigen test for *Cryptococcus*; 5 ml blood to 20 ml broth	Sodium polyanethol sulfonate (SPS), brain-heart infusion (BHI) medium, vented biphasic culture without agar. Tilt daily.
Bone marrow	None	See under Blood.	Aspirate 0.5 ml marrow with sterile syringe in heparin anticoagulant	BHI broth, Sabouraud dextrose agar (SDA)
Cerebrospinal fluid	None	*C. neoformans* *Coccidioides immitis* *H. capsulatum*, *Candida* species, *Nocardia* species, *Actinomyces*	Collect in sterile tube(s). If volume is more than 2 ml, centrifugation and membrane filtration are recommended. Use sediment for slides and plating. If volume is less than 2 ml, prepare smears and plates from uncentrifuged specimen.	SDA, BHI with blood, anaerobic BHI with blood for *Actinomyces*
Cutaneous hair	Contaminants	*Trichophyton* or *Microsporum* species *Piedraia* or *Trichosporon*	Pluck by roots with sterile forceps. Select hairs that fluoresce or are broken and scaly.	SDA, SDA with cycloheximide and chloramphenicol (CC)
Nail	None	*Trichophyton* or *Epidermophyton* species *Candida* *Aspergillus*	Clean nails with 70% alcohol. Scrape discolored or hyperkeratotic areas: dispose of outer layer and collect inner, infected nail; also may collect using sterile nail clipper. Place nail in sterile Petri plate. Cut nail into small pieces, and examine microscopically using KOH.	SDA, SDA-CC
Skin	Few *Candida* and contaminants	Moderate to heavy growth of *Candida* *Trichophyton*, *Microsporum*, and *Epidermophyton* *Malassezia furfur*, *Fonsecaea*, *Phialophora*, *Cladosporium*, *Nocardia*, and *Actinomyces*	Clean skin with 70% alcohol. Scrape outer edge of ring in cases of suspected ringworm; scrape area of active infection if no ring. Place in sterile Petri plate, and examine microscopically using KOH.	SDA, SDA-CC, BHI with blood, SDA with oil for Malessezia
Mucocutaneous	None	Any growth of *C. albicans* *Paracoccidioides brasiliensis*	Collect by scraping plaque with tongue depressor if *Candida* is suspected. Transport in sterile saline.	SDA, SDA-CC

Subcutaneous tissue: lesions and abscesses	None	*Candida, Fonsecaea, Cladosporium* (chromoblastomycosis), *Nocardia, Actinomyces, Streptomyces,* and *Exophiala* (mycetoma) *Sporothrix schenckii* *C. immitis* *B. dermatitidis* *H. capsulatum* *C. neoformans*	Perform biopsy or needle aspiration. Examine for presence of granules. Tissue must be minced or ground. Place scrapings of lesions in sterile saline for transport. Use anaerobic processing if *Actinomyces* is suspected.	SDA, SDA-CC, anaerobic BHI with blood
Sputum, bronchial washings, transtracheal aspirates	None	Moderate to heavy growth of *Candida albicans* Moderate to heavy growth of *Aspergillus, Rhizopus, Mucor,* or *Penicillium* Less often with *Nocardia, Actinomyces, B. dermatitidis, C. immitis, P. brasiliensis, H. capsulatum,* and *S. schenckii*	Sputum should be collected during early morning on 3 consecutive days to enhance recovery. Avoid 24-hour collections because of contamination and overgrowth. Collect washings using a sterile saline aspirate.	SDA, BHI with blood and CC, anaerobic BHI with blood for bronchial washes and transtracheal aspirates
Throat	Few yeast, few contaminants	Moderate to heavy growth of *C. albicans* Less often with *Geotrichum candidum*	Collect with two sterile swabs. Scrape off and collect material with tongue depressor if *Candida* is suspected.	SDA, SDA-CC
Urine	None if clean-catch midstream or catheterized specimen	*Candida* with colony count >100,000/ml Less often with *B. dermatitidis, C. immitis, H. capsulatum,* and *C. neoformans*	Collect clean catch midstream of first morning void into a sterile container; place catheterized specimens into sterile container. Avoid 24-hour collections. Centrifuge and use sediment for microscopic examination and plating. Examine microscopically for fungal elements. Process within 2 hours or refrigerate to avoid bacterial overgrowth.	SDA, SDA-CC
Vaginal, cervical	Few to moderate colonies of *Candida*	Heavy growth of *Candida*	Collect two swabs and place in transport media. Prepare slide from one swab, and examine microscopically with KOH. Plate second swab.	SDA, SDA-CC

SDA = Sabouraud Dextrose agar; SDA-CC = Sabouraud Dextrose agar with cycloheximide and chloroamphenicol; BHI = Brain Heart Infusion specimen; after one hour, alternatively, the slide can be heated slightly briefly to dissolve the keratin. The preparation is allowed to clear and is then examined for hyphae, budding yeast, and spherules. Hair also can be examined to determine whether the infection is an **endothrix infection**, which is a fungal invasion within the hair shaft, or an **ectothrix infection**, which is an infection outside the hair shaft. KOH preparations are rapid and simple to perform but also have the disadvantage of poor contrast.

Cellufluor, a chemofluorescent brightening agent, can be added to the KOH solution. Cellufluor binds to the chitin in the fungal cell wall and provides excellent contrast in the preparation when examined with a fluorescent microscope. Fungi fluoresce intense apple green when stained with Calcofluor white stain and viewed with a fluorescent microscope.

The **India ink**, or **nigrosin**, preparation is used to identify the hyaline capsule of the yeast *Cryptococcus neoformans*. India ink is a colloidal suspension of carbon particles in an aqueous solution. Cerebrospinal fluid (CSF) can be examined directly for the presence of a capsule by adding one drop of fluid to one drop of India ink, mixing to form an emulsion, and adding a coverslip. The preparation is examined microscopically under the low power and then the high dry objective, using low light. Capsules do not stain with India ink and appear as clear halos against a dark background. Although a rapid method, the India ink preparation has been largely replaced by direct antigen testing for the cryptococcal capsular protein. India ink preparations may be difficult to interpret, and white blood cells (WBCs) and artifacts can be mistaken for yeast or capsules. However, not all *Cryptococcus* have a capsular and thus, capsular antigen is not always present or detectable. For example, the *Cryptococcus* may be capsule negative in those with immunodeficiency, such as acquired immunodeficiency syndrome (AIDS).

Lactophenol cotton blue (LPCB) may be used to visualize microscopic fungal morphology by imparting a blue color to the cell walls. One drop of LPCB is added to the specimen, a coverslip is applied, and the preparation is examined microscopically. Slides can be permanently sealed for later study with either Permount or clear nail polish. LPCB also can be used in the **tease preparation (wet mount)** and **slide cultures**, in which a small portion of an actively growing fungal culture can be examined.

The **Hucker modification of the Gram stain** is recommended for mycology. Fungi generally stain gram positive but may often stain poorly. For example, *C. neoformans* may appear pale lavender with blue inclusions because its capsule prevents adequate staining. Fungi are two to three times the size of gram-positive cocci, with the hyphae often two to three times wider than gram-positive bacilli. Oval or budding yeast, hyphae, and arthrospores generally stain well and can be observed with the Gram stain.

Giemsa or **Wright's stain** is used for the detection of intracellular *Histoplasma capsulatum* in blood smears, lymph nodes, lung, liver, or bone marrow. The organism appears as a small, oval yeast cell staining light to dark blue in color. *C. neoformans* also stains quite well with Giemsa or Wright's stain.

Methenamine silver nitrate stain is useful for the screening of clinical specimens. Chitin in the fungal cell wall is oxidized to aldehyde groups, which react with silver nitrate to form metallic silver. The stain provides good contrast and staining for the fungal elements. Fungi appear outlined in black, with an inner dark rose to black color, against a pale green background. Both viable and nonviable fungi stain using this method. The Gomori methenamine silver (GMS) nitrate modification of this stain is used in histology and can be used to detect fungi in histological specimens.

Periodic acid-Schiff (PAS) stains the hyphae of molds and also some yeasts. Periodic acid oxidizes the hydroxyl in the carbohydrates of the cell walls of the organisms to form aldehydes. The aldehydes react with basic fuchsin dye to form a pink-purple complex. A counterstain of fast green can be used to provide contrast. PAS is useful for staining tissue in histology.

The laboratory procedure for the KOH preparation is found at the end of the chapter.

CULTURE MEDIA

Media for the cultivation of fungi must include a source of nitrogen, such as nitrite, nitrate, amino acids, or urea and a carbon source, which is usually glucose. Vitamins, minerals, and other supplements also may be added.

Primary Isolation Media

Primary isolation for fungi generally includes a combination of media that may incorporate red cells and antibiotics, in addition to a general isolation media. Fungi require a carbon source and thus can grow on any compound that contains carbon. That is why these organisms are so prevalent in the environment. **Sabouraud dextrose agar** (SDA) is the main general isolation medium and contains peptone and glucose. **SDA with cycloheximide and chloramphenicol** (SDA-CC) contains cycloheximide, which inhibits many saprophytic, contaminating fungi, and the chloramphenicol is inhibitory for most bacteria. Since the cycloheximide also inhibits *C. neoformans*, some *Candida* species, and some *Aspergillus*, a medium free of these agents should also be used for initial cultures. SDA-CC is available commercially as Mycosel or Mycobiotic medium. **Dermatophyte test medium** (DTM) can be substituted for SDA-CC for the recovery of the dermatophytes from specimens contaminated with fungi or bacteria. **Brain-heart infusion** (BHI) **medium** is useful for the isolation of agents of systemic mycoses. BHI is a nutrient-rich medium and thus will grow bacteria, contaminants, saprobic fungi, and pathogenic fungi also. BHI can be supplemented with blood; there also are formulations of BHI that contain cycloheximide and chloramphenicol. BHI is most useful in the isolation of pathogenic fungi from sterile specimens.

Differential Media

Differential media are used to differentiate various groups or species of fungi. For example, **birdseed agar** (Niger seed agar) can be used for the differential recovery of *C. neoformans*, which forms brown to black colonies on birdseed agar in 4 to 7 days. **Cornmeal with Tween 80 agar** is used for the differentiation of *Candida* and other yeasts based on the production of chlamydospores, hyphae, pseudohyphae, and arthroconidia.

TABLE 20-2 summarizes primary and differential media for clinical mycology.

MICROSCOPIC EXAMINATION OF GROWTH

When the culture first begins to grow, microscopic examination is used to observe conidia and spores for identification. Several methods are available to observe the microscopic growth agar, including the tease mount, slide culture, and cellophane tape mount.

In the tease mount a drop of lactophenol cotton blue (LPCB) stain is placed on a microscopic slide, and a small portion of the colony from the agar surface is removed, using a bent dissecting needle, and placed into the LPCB. The mycelium is teased apart using dissecting needles, a coverslip is added, and the preparation is observed under the low power and high power objectives. The method, which is described at the end of the chapter is rapid but often disrupts the original arrangement of the spores and conidia.

The slide culture is the optimal examination method for preservation of fungal morphology. The method requires more skill and time than the tease mount but allows the fungus to be preserved in its original state. In this method a small block of agar is inoculated with the suspected organism and placed on a microscope slide, which is laid on a bent glass rod in a sterile Petri plate with a piece of filter paper. The growth is examined microscopically using LPCB. **FIGURE 20-2** illustrates the slide culture technique, and the procedure is described at the end of the chapter.

The cellophane tape mount involves the application of double-sticky tape or cellophane tape looped back on itself to the surface of the fungal colony. Aerial hyphae will adhere to the tape, which can be examined using LPCB.

INCUBATION AND MACROSCOPIC MORPHOLOGY

Most fungi grow optimally and more rapidly at an incubation of 30°C; room temperature, or 25°C, is acceptable if a

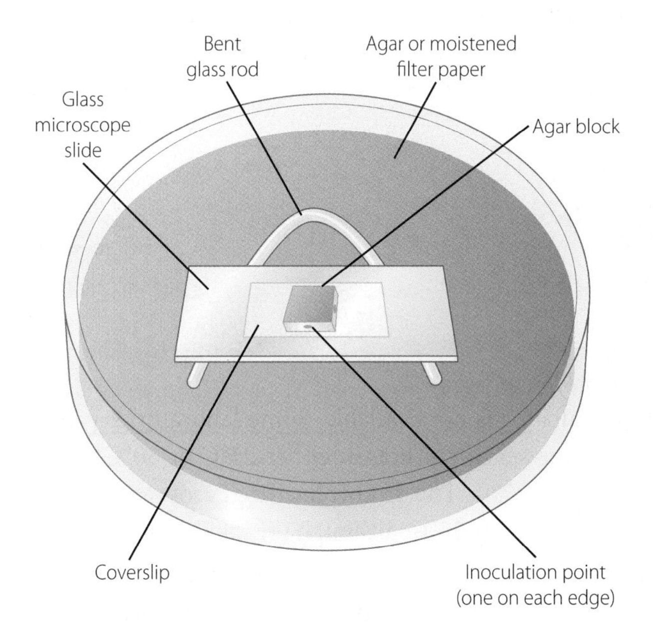

FIGURE 20-2 Slide culture procedure.

TABLE 20-2 Fungal Culture Media

Medium	Indication
Primary isolation media	
Brain-heart infusion (BHI) agar	Isolation of saprophytic and pathogenic fungi from sterile sites. However, bacteria may also grow in BHI.
BHI agar with antibiotics, cycloheximide, and chloramphenicol	Isolation of pathogenic fungi exclusive of dermatophytes; useful for specimens that may be contaminated with bacteria or saprophytic fungi
BHI biphasic blood culture bottles	Recovery of fungi from blood or bone marrow
Dermatophyte test medium (DTM)	Isolation of dermatophytes from hair, skin, and nail specimens. Dermatophytes produce alkaline metabolites, which raise the pH and change the color of the indicator from yellow to red. Antibiotics inhibit saprophytic fungi and bacteria.
Mycosel or Mycobiotic agar	Isolation of dermatophytes from hair, skin, and nail specimens. Contains the inhibitory agents, cycloheximide and chloramphenicol; similar to DTM
Sabouraud dextrose agar (SDA)	Primary recovery of saprobic and pathogenic fungi; primary agar for initial culture
SDA with cycloheximide and chloramphenicol	Recovery of pathogenic fungi; bacteria and saprophytic fungi inhibited
Differential test media	
Birdseed (Niger seed) agar	Isolation of *Cryptococcus neoformans*, which produces phenol oxidase, breaking down the medium and resulting in the production of melanin (black-brown colonies); similar to caffeic acid agar
Cornmeal agar with Tween 80	Stimulation of conidiation and chlamydospore production in *Candida* species; useful for species differentiation of *Candida*
Cottonseed agar	Conversion of mold phase of *Blastomyces dermatitidis* to its yeast phase
Nitrate reduction medium	Confirmation of nitrate reduction in *C. neoformans*
Potato dextrose agar	Stimulation of conidia production in fungi; useful in slide cultures; also demonstrates pigment production of *Trichophyton rubrum*
Rice medium	Identification of *Microsporum audouinii*
Trichophyton agars No. 1: casein agar base (vitamin free) No. 2: casein agar base and inositol; No. 3: casein agar base, inositol, and thiamine; No. 4: casein agar base and thiamine; No. 5: casein agar base and nicotinic acid; No. 6: ammonium nitrate agar base; No. 7: ammonium nitrate agar base and histidine	Nutritional requirement tests for the differentiation of *Trichophyton*. Seven media contain various growth factor requirements for *Trichophyton* species.
Urea agar	Detection of urease production by *C. neoformans* and differentiation of *Trichophyton mentagrophytes* from *T. rubrum*
Yeast assimilation media (carbon or nitrogen)	Detection of carbohydrate assimilation through utilization of carbon (or nitrogen) by yeast in the presence of oxygen
Yeast fermentation broth	Identification of yeasts by fermentation reactions with various carbohydrates

30°C incubator is not available. Some laboratories prefer to grow one set of cultures at either 25°C or 30°C and a second set at 37°C. The dimorphic fungi grow as yeasts at 37°C and molds at 25°C, although initial isolation at 30°C is recommended.

Most of the fungi are aerobic and thus can be incubated in a standard incubator. The fungi prefer moisture and increased humidity for growth. All plates must be sealed with Parafilm or oxygen-permeable tape to prevent infectious aerosols and also to provide increased humidity. A pan of water placed in the incubator can provide the necessary humidity. Fungal cultures are incubated for 2 to 4 weeks and examined periodically. Plates should be held for 4 weeks until reported negative for growth. Yeast usually grows within 24 to 72 hours, whereas *H. capsulatum* may require 10 to 12 weeks for growth.

The macroscopic examination of colonies includes the rate of growth, general topography, texture, and pigmentation, as well as characteristics on differential media.

Topography is best observed on the reverse side of the agar because it may be obscured by aerial hyphae. The topography may be flat, heaped, or folded. Rugose topography contains deep furrows that radiate from the center, and umbonate colonies are elevated in the center. Colonies also may be wrinkled or verrucose.

The **texture** of the colony is best determined through observation of a cross section of the colony; texture is usually related to the length of the aerial hyphae. Dense, high aerial mycelia produce a cottony or woolly texture, whereas dense, low aerial mycelia produce a velvety or silky texture. Flat, rough, crumbly colonies are described as powdery or granular. Yeasts typically produce glabrous, or smooth, colonies that are wet, waxy, creamy, or pasty, because no significant aerial mycelia are produced.

Surface pigmentation and pigmentation on the reverse side also are important gross colonial characteristics. Description of color should be specific. For example, pigmentation should be described as salmon or peach instead of orange.

Fungal Infections

SUPERFICIAL MYCOSES

Superficial fungal infections are noninvasive and involve the top, or outermost, layer of the skin, the stratum corneum. These organisms also may infect the hair and nails. While most dermatophyte infections are mild and superficial, others are more severe, affecting the dermis. These deeper infections may evoke an immune response, producing pain and ulcerating lesions.

Dermatophytes

The dermatophytes that cause superficial fungal infections include the genera *Microsporum*, *Trichophyton*, and *Epidermophyton*. The dermatophytes cause tinea, or ringworm. Ringworm has a ring-like appearance and is red and scaly with a distinct margin. There are cord-like bumps beneath the skin, which have been described as resembling a worm. As the infection spreads, there is a central clear area of healing. Tinea may be caused by **anthropophilic fungi**, which infect humans; **zoophilic fungi**, which are parasitic on animals other than humans; or **geophilic fungi**, which are free-living soil saprophytes. Tinea infections occur frequently in many animals, including dogs and cats, which serve as a route of infection for humans, especially children. BOX 20-1 lists the types of tinea and dermatophytes most frequently associated with each type of infection.

The diagnosis of dermatophytic infections is made on the clinical symptoms of the infection, including a KOH preparation. KOH preparations can be performed by the physician, who looks for hyphae, conidia, or other identifying features. Skin, hair, or nail biopsies are stained with PAS or Giemsa to identify the presence of fungal infection. The specimen or biopsy is cultured if appropriate.

FIGURE 20-3 shows a GMS stain of a biopsy of skin containing a dermatophyte.

Hairs for examination should be broken, twisted, or scaly. The hair can be examined to determine whether the infection is an endothrix or ectothrix infection.

Specimens are inoculated onto SDA, with and without antibiotics, or onto DTM. The indicator of DTM will turn from yellow to red with room temperature incubation within 14 days if a dermatophyte is growing. Plates should be examined at least once weekly and held for 1 month.

The dermatophytes are identified by the microscopic appearance of conidia and hyphae, as well as by colonial characteristics, particularly pigmentation. The organism's

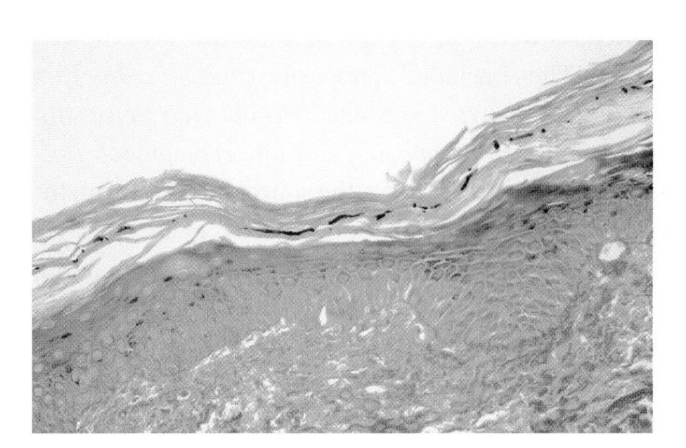

FIGURE 20-3 GMS stain of a biopsy of skin containing a dermatophyte infection.

BOX 20-1 Common Tinea Infections and Associated Organisms

Tinea barbae: Ringworm of the beard and mustache

Usually zoophilic and an occupational hazard for farm workers; most often caused by *T. mentagrophytes*, *T. verrucosum*, and *Microsporum canis*

Tinea capitis: Ringworm of the scalp, eyebrows, eyelashes

Gray-patch ringworm: common in children; typically caused by *Microsporum canis* and *Microsporum audouinii*

Black-dot ringworm: endothrix infections caused by *Trichophyton tonsurans*

Inflammatory: ectothrix infections caused by *Trichophyton mentagrophytes*

Tinea corporis: Ringworm of the body, especially the trunk

Typically caused by *Trichophyton rubrum* and *T. tonsurans*, *Epidermophyton floccosum*; geophilic infections associated with *Microsporum canis* and *M. gypseum*

Tinea cruris: Ringworm of the groin

Common infection in athletes, military personnel, and others who share towels or clothing; most frequently caused by *Epidermophyton floccosum*, *Trichophyton rubrum*, and *T. mentagrophytes*

Tinea favosa: Ringworm of the hair follicle at its base; *T. schoenleinii*

Tinea manuum: Ringworm of hands, palms, and between fingers; most frequently caused by *Trichophyton rubrum*

Tinea pedis: Ringworm of the foot, or "athlete's foot"

Common infection found on soles of feet and between toes characterized by itching, scales, and possible seeping; most often caused by *T. mentagrophytes*, *T. rubrum*, and *E. floccosum*

Tinea unguium: Ringworm of the nails; onychomycosis

Infection typically begins at edge of the nail, with nail eventually becoming thick and brittle; onychomycosis refers to nondermatophytic fungal nail infections attributed to the yeast and other fungi; most frequently caused by *T. rubrum*, *T. mentagrophytes*, and *E. floccosum*

ability to fluoresce when examined with an ultraviolet lamp, known as the Wood's light, also may be used.

More than 50 species of dermatophytes have been identified; however, only a few account for most human infections. These include *Microsporum canis*, *Microsporum gypseum*, *Trichophyton rubrum*, *Trichophyton tonsurans*, *Trichophyton mentagrophytes*, and *Epidermophyton floccosum*. BOX 20-2 summarizes the sources of the dermatophyte infections.

Microsporum species may infect the hair and skin but rarely the nails. The genus has large, spindle-shaped, thick-walled, multiseptate macroconidia, which contain over six cells. The macroconidia are rough and spiny and occur at the end of the hyphae. Microconidia are few in number or absent; when present, they are small and club shaped, occurring on the end of the hyphae. Aerial mycelium produces powdery or velvety colonies. **FIGURE 20-4** is an LPCB preparation of *Microsporum* illustrating the typical large, spiny, multiseptate macroconidia that predominate.

Microsporum canis is zoophilic and causes ringworm in cats, dogs, and other animals. Children may become infected through an infected pet. The organism

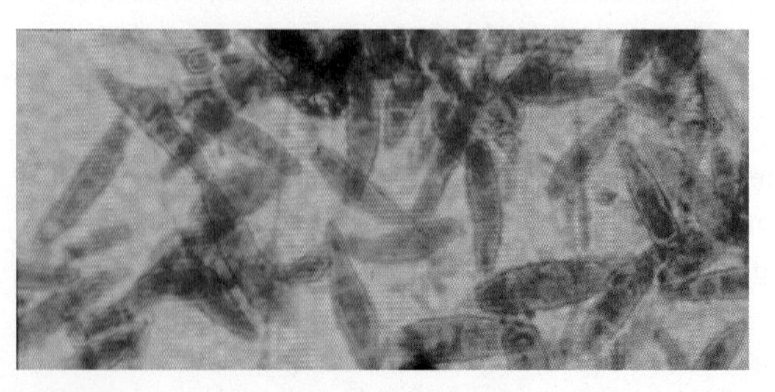

FIGURE 20-4 A microscopic LPCB stain of *Microsporum* showing predominance of macroconidia and rare microconidia.

BOX 20-2 **Sources of Dermatophyte Infections**

Geophilic: Soil, animal infected through contaminated soil

Microsporum gypseum

M. manum (swine from contaminated soil)

M. fulvum

Trichophyton terrestre

T. ajelloi

Anthropophilic: Through human sources, such as contaminated clothing, towels, brushes, locker room facilities, showers

Epidermophyton floccosum

Microsporum audouinii

Trichophyton rubrum

T. tonsurans

T. violaceum

T. schoenleinii

Zoophilic: Direct contact with an infected animal

Microsporum canis (dogs, cats)

Trichophyton mentagrophytes (dogs, cats, cattle, rodents)

T. verrucosum (cattle, horses)

fluoresces under the Wood's light. *Microsporum gypseum* is geophilic and associated with various types of tinea, including tinea corporis. Colonies are flat and tan to cinnamon-brown in color with a granular consistency; the reverse side is rose-brown to cinnamon in color. **FIGURE 20-5** shows a microscopic LPCB stain of *M. gypseum* with its typical thick-walled, cigar-shaped macroconidia with spiny surfaces, rounded tips, and rare microconidia. **FIGURE 20-6** shows *M. gypseum* on SDA. The organism does not fluoresce under the Wood's light. *Microsporum audouinii*, once a leading cause of tinea capitis in children, is now only rarely found in the United States. Colonies are tan to brown and velvety with a salmon underside. Macroconidia are the predominant form seen microscopically and show bizarre forms that are club or spindle shaped, thick walled, and multiseptate with a rough surface. **FIGURE 20-7** shows an LPCB microscopic view of *M. audouinii*. The organism is anthrophilic and fluoresces with the Wood's light.

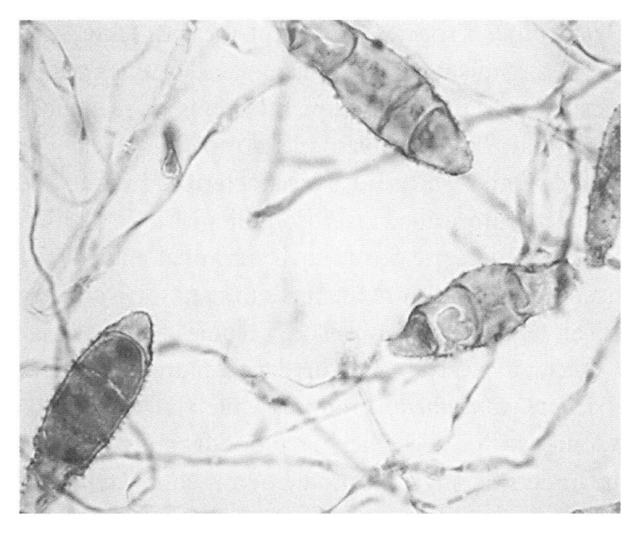

FIGURE 20-5 Microscopic view of *M. gypseum* with LPCB stain thick-walled, cigar-shaped macroconidia with spiny surfaces.

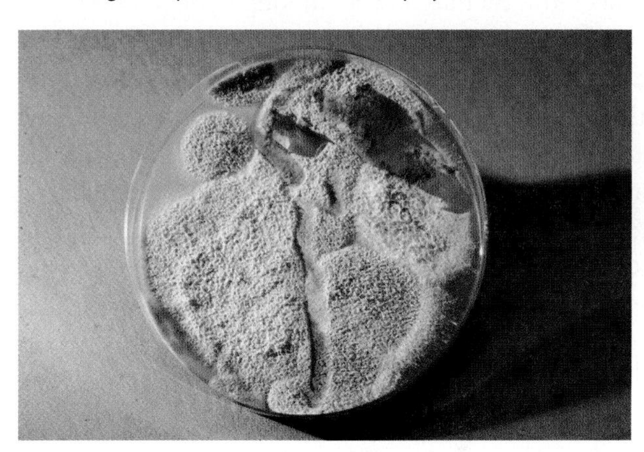

FIGURE 20-6 *M. gypseum* on SDA showing granular to cinnamon-colored colonies.

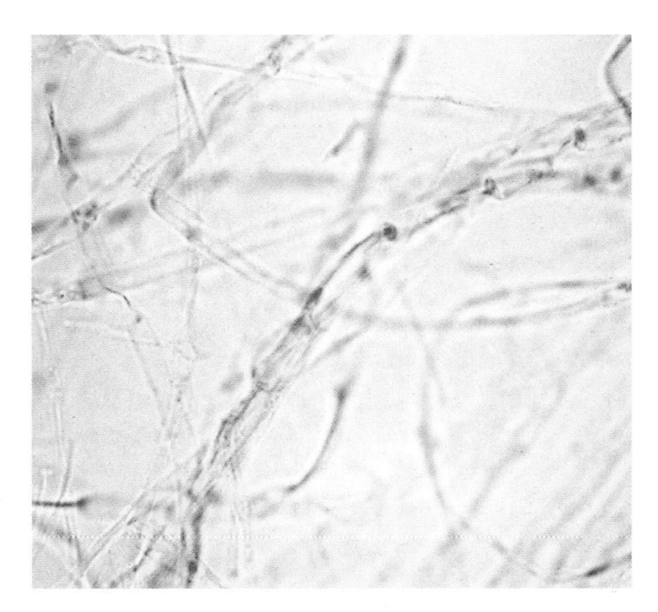

FIGURE 20-7 Microscopic view of *M. audouinii* with LPCB stain showing club-shaped, thick-walled, multiseptate macroconidia.

Trichophyton species can infect the hair, skin, and nails. The organism is a significant cause of tinea pedis, tinea capitis, and tinea unguium. Infections are seen more often in adults. *Trichophyton* species do not fluoresce under the Wood's light. The genus is characterized by smooth, club-shaped, thin-walled macroconidia with 8 to 10 septa. The macroconidia are borne at the terminal ends of the hyphae. Microconidia are the predominant form and are spherical, tear shaped, or clavate. Colonies may be powdery, waxy, or velvety. Macroconidia are more rarely seen.

Trichophyton rubrum produces white, fluffy or granular colonies with a deep cherry red or burgundy pigment on the underside. Pigment production is enhanced when the organism is grown on cornmeal or potato dextrose agar. Microscopically, there are numerous tear-shaped microconidia that are borne on long hyphal strands, as shown in **FIGURE 20-8**. The organism is urease negative and does not perforate hair in the hair-baiting procedure. In this technique a lock of hair is placed into a sterile Petri plate with water, and the colony to be tested is added. The hair shaft is invaded or perforated, which can be observed microscopically, in a positive test. *Trichophyton mentagrophytes*, an agent of tinea barbae, tinea pedis, and tinea unguium, produces flat and white, cream, or colored colonies with a rose or red-brown underside. Concentric rings may be seen. *T. mentagrophytes* causes ectothrix infections and gives a positive hair-baiting test within 7 to 10 days; it also hydrolyzes urea within 48 hours. Microscopically,

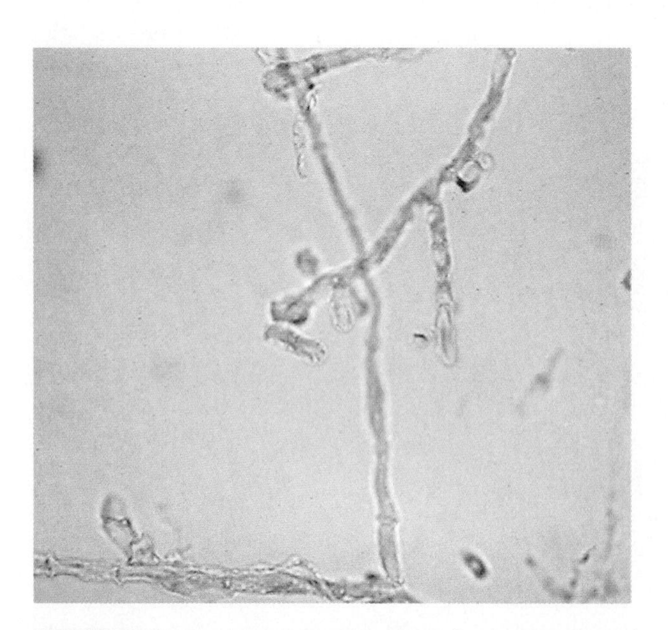

FIGURE 20-8 Microscopic view of *T. rubrum* showing tear-shaped microconidia borne on long hyphae.

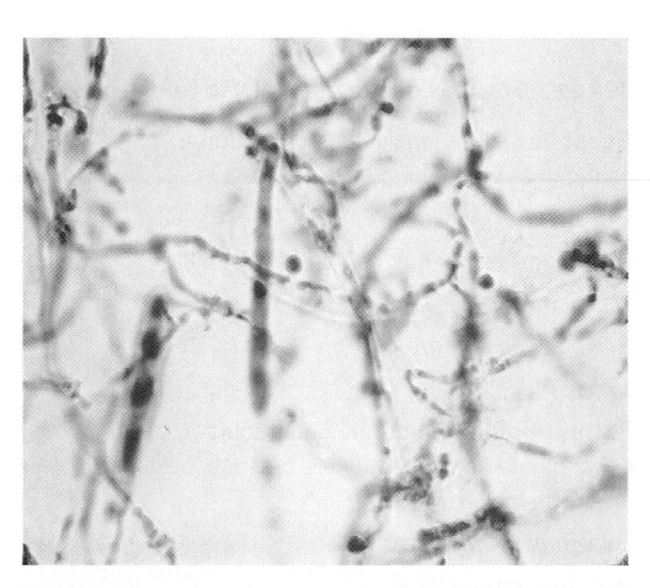

FIGURE 20-9 Microscopic view of *T. mentagrophytes* showing round microconidia arranged in coils and clusters.

T. mentagrophytes shows an abundance of small, round microconidia, which are arranged coils and clusters, as shown in **FIGURE 20-9**. *Trichophyton tonsurans*, an agent of epidemic tinea capitis in children, produces endothrix infections of the hair. Colonies are tan or yellow-rose with rugose with crater-like folds, wrinkled centers, and deep fissures (**FIGURE 20-10**). Abundant club-, tear-, or balloon-shaped microconidia (**FIGURE 20-11**) are predominant in the microscopic appearance of *T. tonsurans*.

Epidermophyton floccosum can infect the skin and nails but rarely the hair. The organism is an agent of tinea cruris, tinea pedis, and tinea unguium. Colonial appearance is velvety or powdery with a suede-like texture and

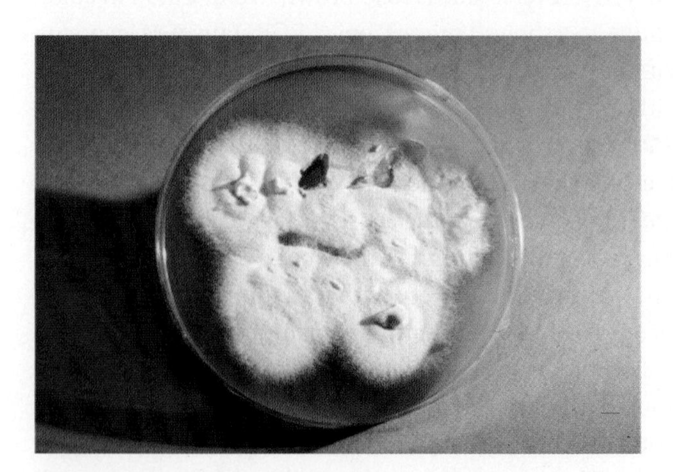

FIGURE 20-10 *T. tonsurans* on SDA showing tan or yellow-rose with crater-like folds and wrinkled centers.

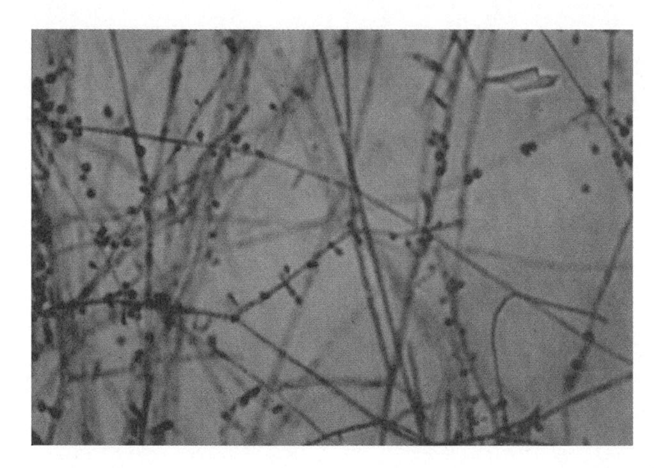

FIGURE 20-11 Microscopic view of *T. tonsurans* showing numerous club and tear-shaped microconidia.

yellow-green or khaki-green pigmentation. Microscopically, the macroconidia are smooth and club shaped with two to four cells; microconidia are absent, as shown in **FIGURE 20-12**.

TABLE 20-3 lists important morphological and microscopic characteristics of these fungi.

Tinea Versicolor

The **superficial mycoses** also include **tinea versicolor**, also known as **pityriasis versicolor**, which exhibits superficial brownish or scaly areas on light-skinned individuals. Irregular patches of nonpigmented or untanned skin may be seen on darker-skinned individuals. The organism requires lipid, or fat, for growth; thus, it grows in areas of the body where sebum and skin oil accumulate. Tinea versicolor infection is seen in individuals who live in warm, humid environments, including the tropics; in those with excess perspiration; and in those with oily skin. The infection typically involves the skin of the chest, back, and upper arms. The agent of tinea versicolor is *Malassezia furfur*, which is observed in skin scrapings and fluoresces under the Wood's light. Microscopically the organism appears as tight clusters of spherical, budding, yeast-like cells with short, unbranched hyphae or hyphal fragments. This has been described as having a "spaghetti and meatballs" appearance when observed in a direct microscopic preparation. The organism grows on SDA with olive oil or sterile mineral oil in 2 to 4 days at 30°C as smooth, cream-colored yeast-like colonies (**FIGURE 20-13**). With age, the colonies become tan to brown with a dull appearance. Microscopically, in smears prepared from artificial media, broadly budding yeast cells with a collarette are seen; no hyphae are observed.

Systemic and pulmonary infections and septicemia have been attributed to *M. furfur* in patients receiving parenteral therapy, which has a high lipid content.

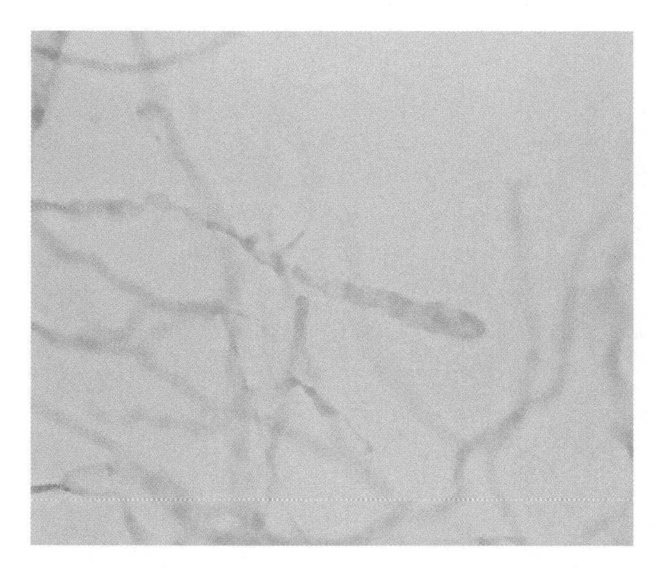

FIGURE 20-12 Microscopic view of *E. floccosum* showing typical smooth, club-shaped macroconidia with two to four cells.

Tinea Nigra Palmaris

Tinea nigra palmaris is a tropical infection, usually occurring in Africa, Asia, and South and Central America; it is rarely found in the United States. This superficial phaeohyphomycosis generally involves the palms of the hand and the soles of the feet. It is characterized by a single brown to black scaly patch with a distinct border. It is believed that the infection is acquired by direct contact

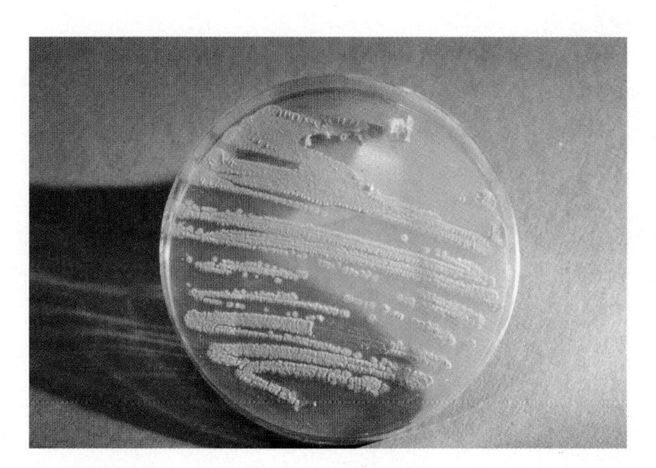

FIGURE 20-13 *Malassezia furfur* on SDA showing cream to tan yeast-like colonies.

TABLE 20-3 Morphology of Frequently Isolated Dermatophytes

Organism	Natural Habitat	Type of Disease	Colonial Appearance*	Microscopic Appearance	Comments
Microsporum audouinii	Humans	Tinea capitis, tinea corporis	Cream, tan, buff, or light brown, flat, velvety colony. Reverse side is salmon pink or orange-brown.	Bizarre-shaped macroconidia: thick walled, club or spindle shaped, and multiseptate, with rough surface; microconidia rare; terminal chlamydospores	Fails to grow on sterile, polished rice grains 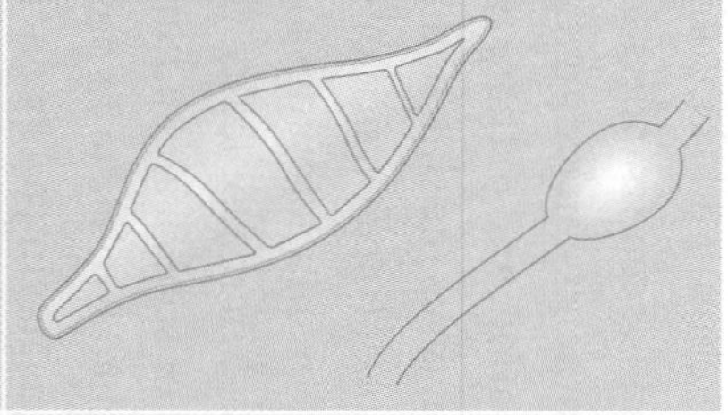
Microsporum canis	Cats, dogs	Tinea capitis, tinea corporis	White to buff granular or cottony surface, which develops bright yellow periphery. Reverse side is bright yellow or yellow-orange.	Thick-walled, spindle-shaped, large, multiseptate, rough-walled macroconidia with curved tip and knobby projections; sparse microconidia: clavate, smooth walled, and laterally attached to hyphae	Grows well on sterile, polished rice grains 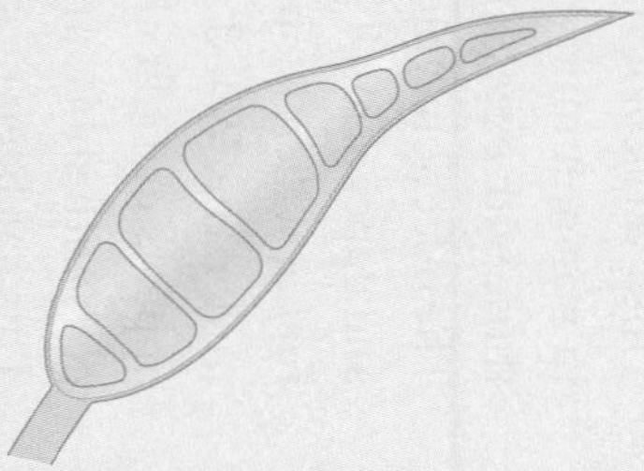
Microsporum gypseum	Soil	Tinea capitis, tinea corporis, tinea unguium	Flat, tan to brown or cinnamon-brown, granular or powdery colony. Reverse side is rose-brown, red-brown, or cinnamon.	Numerous, thick-walled, cigar-shaped multiseptate macroconidia with spiny surfaces and rounded tips; sparse, clavate, smooth-walled microconidia	Grows well on sterile, polished rice grains 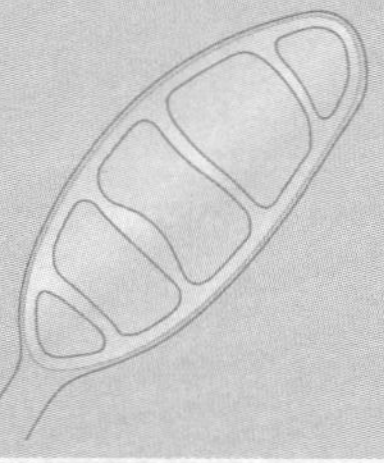
Epidermophyton floccosum	Humans	Tinea corporis, tinea pedis	White to tan colonies, which become yellow, mustard-yellow, or khaki-green with age; flat, suede-like texture with folded center. Reverse side is yellow-brown or dark orange with folds.	Numerous club-shaped, smooth-walled macroconidia with two to four cells occurring singly or in clusters of three to four; microconidia absent	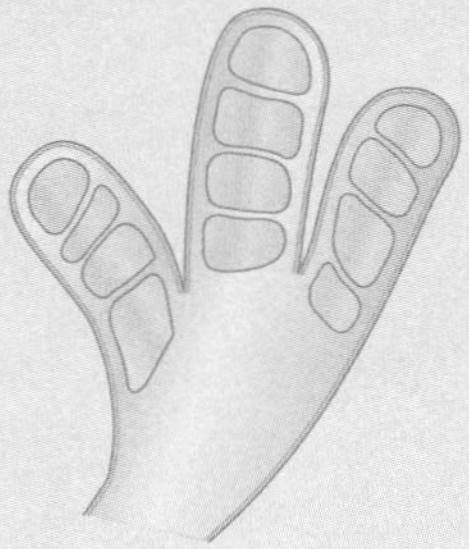

Trichophyton mentagrophytes	Humans, other animals	Tinea capitis, tinea corporis, tinea pedis, tinea unguium	Colonial types may be velvety and fluffy or granular and flat. Color is white or tan to pink. Reverse side is white, rose, or red-brown.	Microspores: numerous, small, globose, and arranged in grape-like clusters; coiled, spiral hyphae may be observed; macroconidia: rare, thin walled, smooth, and cigar shaped	Urease positive in 48 hours; positive hair-baiting test produces wedge shapes in hair; grows on *Trichophyton* agars Nos. 1, 2, 3, and 4
Trichophyton rubrum	Humans	Tinea capitis, tinea corporis, tinea unguium	Fluffy or granular white to pink colonies. Reverse side is cherry red or wine red when grown on cornmeal agar.	Tear-shaped microconidia borne laterally from long strands of hyphae; resemble "birds on a fence"; rare, thin-walled, smooth, pencil-shaped macroconidia	Rarely hydrolyzes urea; requires 7 days for observable reaction; negative hair-baiting test; grows on *Trichophyton* agars Nos. 1, 2, 3, and 4
Trichophyton tonsurans	Humans	Tinea capitis, tinea corporis, tinea pedis, tinea unguium	Flat, powdery, granular, and cream, tan, yellow-rose, or rust-colored colony. Colonies become heaped or sunken with folds. Reverse is yellow to tan.	Abundant tear-, club-, or balloon-shaped microconidia; rare smooth-walled, cylindrical macroconidia	Requires thiamine; fails to grow on *Trichophyton* agars Nos. 1 and 2; grows well on *Trichophyton* agars Nos. 3 and 4

*Colonial appearance based on growth on Sabouraud dextrose agar (SDA) at 2 weeks with incubation at 25°C to 30°C.

Trichophyton agars: No. 1—basal; No. 2—inositol; No. 3—thiamine and inositol; No. 4—thiamine.

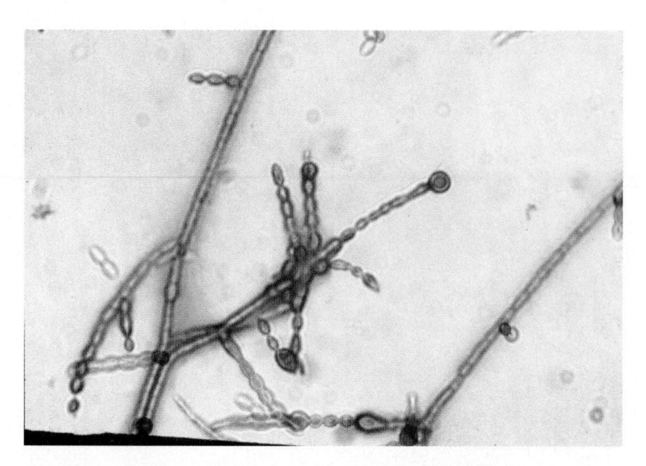

FIGURE 20-14 Microscopic view of *Hortaea werneckii* showing septate, branching hyphae and elongated budding yeast cells.

with contaminated decaying vegetation. The agent of tinea nigra palmaris is *Hortaea werneckii*, formerly known as *Phaeoannellomyces werneckii* and *Cladosporium werneckii*. In direct skin scrapings with 10-10% KOH, there are brown, septate, branching hyphae and elongated budding yeast cells. Gray, shiny, moist yeast-like cells with an olive-green mycelium are observed on SDA after incubation for up to 7 days at room temperature. The colonies become olive-green to black upon aging. Microscopically, from culture, there are brown, septate, branching hyphae, which are one- to two-celled blastoconidia. **FIGURE 20-14** shows the typical microscopic appearance of *Hortaea werneckii* in an LPCB stain.

Black Piedra

Black piedra, caused by the organism *Piedraia hortae*, results in hard brown-black crusts on the outside of the hair shaft, usually on the scalp. This infection is found most commonly in the tropical climates of South America, Africa, and eastern Asia. Direct examination of the infected hair shaft will show hard black nodules and ascospores from sexual reproduction. There are two to eight spindle-shaped spores per cell. Velvety, green-black heaped colonies are observed on SDA when incubated at room temperature. Microscopically, dark, thick-walled hyphae with intercalary chlamydocondia within the hyphae, appearing as swellings, are observed.

White Piedra

White piedra is caused by *Trichosporon beigelii*, which is also known as *Trichosporon cutaneum*. There are light brown, soft nodules on the beard, axillae, scalp, or mustache, which are less firmly attached than those of black piedra. In a direct microscopic examination with KOH, there are light-colored septate hyphae and round to rectangular arthroconidia. Moist, white to cream-colored colonies are seen on SDA in 5 days when incubated at room temperature. The colonies become darker yellow to gray and wrinkled with age. Hyaline hyphae, blastoconidia, and arthrospores are seen microscopically when grown on cornmeal with Tween 80 agar.

SUBCUTANEOUS MYCOSES

Subcutaneous fungal infections often result from a traumatic skin puncture from thorns or vegetation contaminated with fungi. These fungi are found as saprobes in the soil or as plant pathogens. Because the subcutaneous tissue is affected, there is a host immune response from macrophages, neutrophils, lymphocytes, and other cells. Subcutaneous mycoses may disseminate to other sites, and these infections often become chronic. There are four major groups of subcutaneous fungal infections: chromoblastomycosis, mycetoma, phaeohyphomycosis, and sporotrichosis.

Chromoblastomycosis

Chromoblastomycosis is caused by infection with **dematiaceous fungi**, a group of dark, slow-growing fungi that are found on vegetation and in the soil. Clinically significant fungi in this group include *Fonsecaea pedrosoi*, *Fonsacaea compactum*, *Phialophora verrucosa*, *Cladosporium carrionii*, *Exophiala jeanselmi*, *Exophiala spinifera*, and *Wangiella dermatitidis*. Infection is initiated through a puncture wound or trauma to the skin involving fungally contaminated vegetation. A local infection in the underlying tissue results, with the development of chronic, nonhealing, hard, warty, tumor-like lesions. The infection most frequently involves the feet and lower legs. Although chromoblastomycosis has a worldwide prevalence, it is seen most often in the tropics. Identification begins with a biopsy and histological examination of the lesions for the presence of sclerotic bodies, which are copper-colored, septate cells present in chromoblastomycosis. The fungi associated with chromoblastomycosis typically produce heaped, folded, and darkly pigmented (gray, olive, or black) colonies with a velvety black underside.

Fonsecaea pedrosoi is the species most frequently found worldwide as an agent of chromoblastomycosis. The colonies are very slow growing with olive, gray, or black colonies that have a velvety texture. *Fonsecaea* shows mixed sporulation, with a predominance of primary conidia forming at the tips of conidiophores arising from dark, septate hyphae. Another important species is *Phialophora verrucosa*, which rapidly grows producing olive-gray to black cottony or wooly colonies. Microscopically, *Phialophora* has septate hyphae with short conidiophores with flask-shaped phialides with collarettes; oval to cylindrical conidia form clusters at the ends of the phialides. The phialides and collarettes are described as resembling a vase with the conidial clusters resembling flowers, as is seen in **FIGURE 20-15**.

Phaeohyphomycosis

Phaeohyphomycosis refers to infections caused by any dematiaceous fungi, excluding chromoblastomycosis and mycetoma. These fungi are darkly pigmented with septate hyphae; a yeast phase may be observed in tissue. Phaeohyphomycosis may be superficial, local, subcutaneous, or systemic and may include endocarditis, sinusitis, mycotic keratitis, and pulmonary and systemic infections. Subcutaneous and brain abscesses also may be seen. Infections are usually opportunistic. Fungi associated with phaeohyphomycosis include *Bipolaris*, *Curvularia*, *E. jeanselmi*, *Phialophora richardsiae*, and *W. dermatitidis*. A direct examination of clinical material and a histological examination reveal yellow-brown septate hyphae with or without budding yeast cells. *Curvularia* rapidly grows white to pink woolly colonies, which darken in color to brown or black with age. Microscopically, there are brown septate hyphae and branched or straight conidiophores with pyriform, brown multiseptate conidia. Each cell is divided into multiple cells by the septum, and because the central cell is darker and larger, *Curvularia* has a curved shape (**FIGURE 20-16**). **FIGURE 20-17** is a microscopic view of *Wangiella*, which is a dark, budding yeast and later develops tube-like phialides and groups of single-celled hyaline conidia.

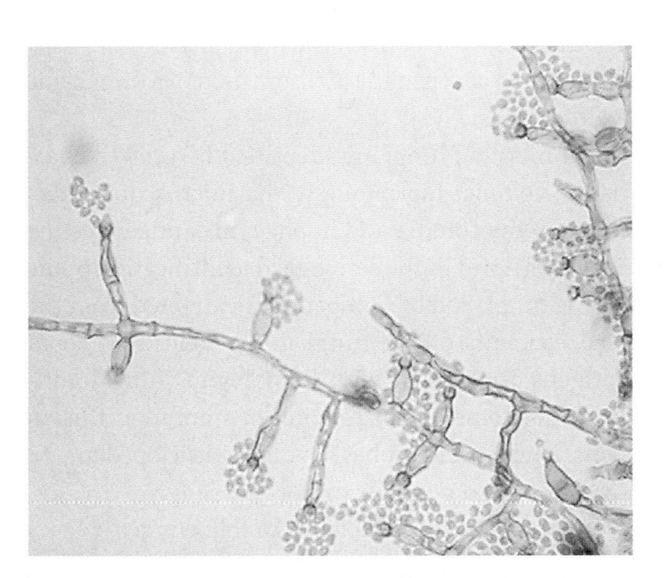

FIGURE 20-15 *Phialophora verrucosa* showing flask-shaped phialides with collarettes and oval, clustering conidia.

Mycetoma

Mycetoma is a chronic granulomatous infection of the cutaneous and subcutaneous tissue and bone. There are tumor-like deformities of the subcutaneous tissue with abscesses, draining sinuses, and granulomatous pus. Yellow, red, white, or black granules may be observed in the pus. The infection can occur worldwide but is seen most

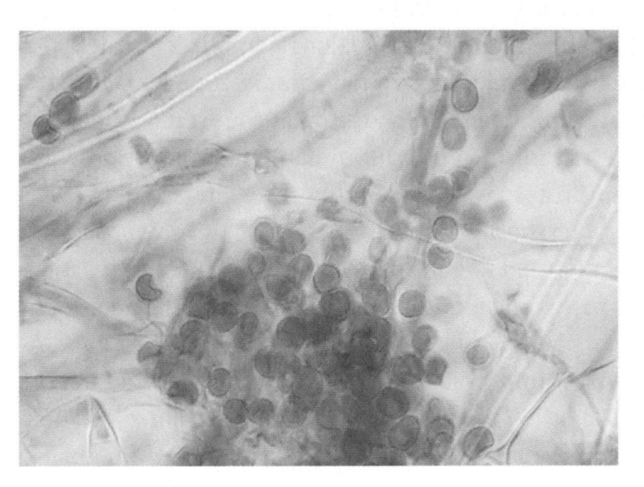

FIGURE 20-16 *Curvularia* showing curve-shaped conidia.

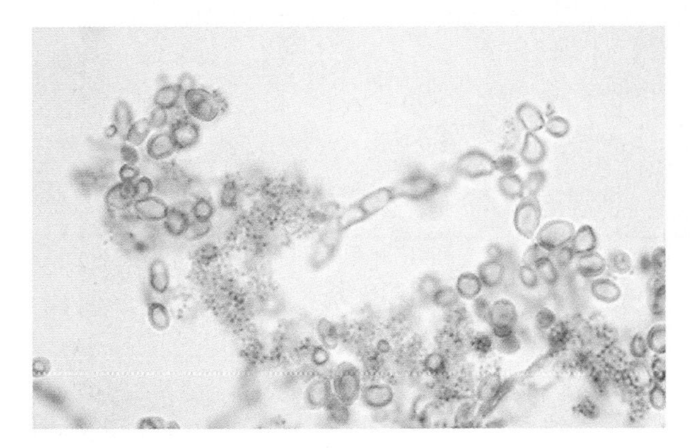

FIGURE 20-17 *Wangiella* showing tube-like phialides and groups of single-celled hyaline conidia.

frequently in the tropics and subtropics, including Africa and the Arabian peninsula. Mycetoma may be acquired as an occupational infection from the environment from contaminated vegetation or the soil. The infection can occur anywhere on the body but most frequently affects the feet.

Actinomycotic mycetoma results from infection with the aerobic *Actinomyces*, such as *Nocardia*, *Actinomadura*, and *Streptomyces*. **Eumycotic mycetoma** is associated with several fungal species that have septate hyphae, including *Pseudoallescheria*, *Aspergillus*, *Exophiala* (**FIGURE 20-18**), *Acremonium*, *Curvularia*, and *Madurella*.

Sporotrichosis

Sporothrix schenckii, the agent of **sporotrichosis**, a subcutaneous infection, is categorized as a dimorphic fungus and exhibits both a yeast phase and a mycelial phase. Sporotrichosis most often occurs from a skin trauma caused by a finger prick from thorny plants, such as roses. The infection may remain local or cutaneous but is usually subcutaneous. Local and regional lymphadenopathy also may occur, and the infection can disseminate. Although usually acquired through the cutaneous route, inhalation of the organism can result in pulmonary infections. The organism has a worldwide prevalence. Those working with woody or thorny plants and individuals in contact with vegetation and soil, including foresters, gardeners (particularly rose gardeners), horticulturists, masons, and miners, are particularly susceptible.

As a dimorphic fungus, *S. schenckii*, grows as a mold on SDA at 25°C as small, cream- to white-colored colonies, which are moist and pasty. The colonies become black, wrinkled, and leathery with age. This black pigmentation is enhanced on potato dextrose or cornmeal agar. Microscopically, the mold phase shows thin hyphae that are septate, branching, and hyaline in color. Oval, elliptical, or pyriform conidia, which are hyaline in color, also are seen. The conidia gather to form the pedals of a flower, or a "rosette" appearance. The yeast phase, which is inhibited on antibiotic media, grows on BHI (with or without blood) at 37°C as soft, white, cream- to tan-colored colonies. The microscopic yeast form that occurs in vitro shows oval, spherical, or fusiform yeast cells, which may produce multiple buds. The organism may be observed intracellular in polymorphonuclear neutrophils; an "asteroid body," a small, snail-shaped yeast cell with a single bud and a narrow attachment to the mother cell, may be observed on biopsy.

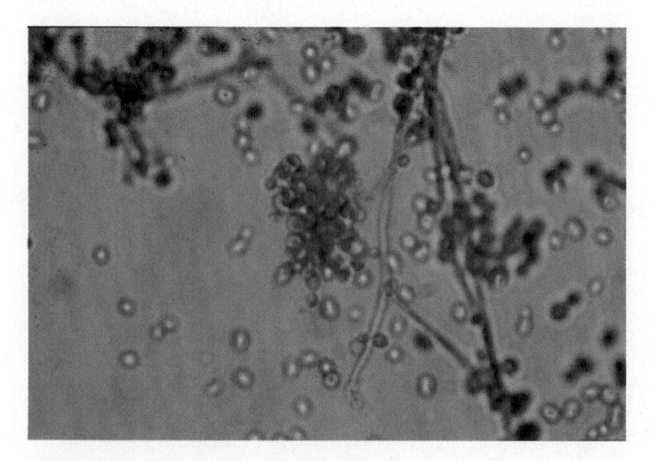

FIGURE 20-18 Microscopic view of *Exopohilia* showing one-celled conidia gather at tip of annelids.

TABLE 20-4 summarizes the morphological and microscopic characteristics of organisms typically associated with subcutaneous mycoses.

SYSTEMIC MYCOSES: DIMORPHIC FUNGI

The systemic fungal agents are dimorphic fungi, which exhibit both a yeast phase and a mycelial phase. The yeast phase is found within the host tissues and also is known as the tissue or invasive phase. The mycelial, or mold, phase is saprophytic and exists in nature on vegetation or decaying material; it is usually observed in vitro. The mycelial phase usually is observed in vitro on SDA when incubated from 25°C to 30°C. The yeast phase is grown on enriched media, usually supplemented with blood, at 35°C to 37°C. It may be necessary to convert the mold phase to the yeast phase in vitro to confirm the identification of a dimorphic fungal infection.

The dimorphic fungi are identified by growth characteristics, colonial morphology, and microscopic characteristics of the conidia and hyphae. Exoantigen testing also may be helpful in the serological identification of the dimorphic fungi. Soluble antigens are extracted from the mycelial elements of the fungi to be identified. Next, the antigens are reacted with homologous fungal antibodies, using complement fixation or immunodiffusion reactions. Nucleic acid probes have been developed for the identification of some of the dimorphic fungi.

The dimorphic fungi include the following:

- *Blastomyces dermatitidis*, the agent of **blastomycosis**
- *Coccidioides immitis*, the agent of **coccidioidomycosis**

TABLE 20-4 Morphology of Frequently Isolated Agents of Subcutaneous Mycoses

Organism	Colonial appearance	Microscopic appearance	Clinical significance
Cladosporium carrionii	Rapidly growing, velvety or cottony, olive to black colony; only saprophytic *Cladosporium* that cannot grow above 37°C	Dark, long-branching conidiophores, which give rise to chains of blastoconidia; septate hyphae	Chromoblastomycosis
Exophiala jeanselmi	Moderately fast-growing, gray to black, moist, yeast-like colony with black woolly mycelium; grows at 37°C but not at 40°C	Pale, brown conidiophores that form cylindrical annelids; one-celled hyaline conidia gather at tip of annelids	Mycetoma, phaeohyphomycosis
Fonsecaea pedrosoi	Very slow-growing, black-brown, gray-black, or olive-gray colony with black aerial mycelium; velvety to cottony texture	Mixed sporulation; predominant form is dark, septate hyphae with primary mycosis conidia developing at conidiophore tip. Secondary and tertiary conidia also are formed and result in a loosely organized conidial head. Branching conidiophores with chains of conidia and flask-shaped phialides also are seen.	Chromoblastomycosis
Phialophora verrucosa	Rapidly growing, olive-gray to black, dome-shaped, woolly or cottony colony	Septate hyphae with short conidiophores that give rise to flask- or cup-shaped phialides; with collarettes; oval to cylindrical conidia in clusters at ends of phialides	Chromoblastomycosis

(*continues*)

TABLE 20-4 Morphology of Frequently Isolated Agents of Subcutaneous Mycoses (Continued)

Organism	Colonial appearance	Microscopic appearance	Clinical significance
Pseudoallescheria boydii (telemorph or sexual form) *Scedosporium apiospermum* (anamorph or asexual form)	Rapidly growing, cottony, white to gray colony with black reverse side	*Teleomorph*: sac-like cleistothecia- (ascocarp-) containing asci and ascospores, which are oval, pointed, and released when ascus ruptures *Anamorph*: golden-brown, elliptoid, single-celled conidia on tips of conidiophores	Mycetoma; opportunistic infections, including nasal sinus infections, meningitis, brain abscesses, and arthritis
Sporothrix schenckii	Rapidly growing, white, pasty, moist colony that later becomes brown, black, wrinkled, or leathery	Dimorphic fungus; mycelial form (25°C): narrow, septate hyphae with pyriform conidia arranged singly or in floweret arrangement; yeast form (35°C–37°C): small, elliptoid budding, cigar-shaped yeast	Sporotrichosis
Wangiella dermatitidis	Rapidly growing, moist, shiny, yeasty colony that later develops black, olive, velvety mycelium; grows well at 40°C but other dematiaceous fungi do not	Dark, budding yeast that later develops tube-like phialides that lack both collarettes and annelations; bails of one-celled, hyaline conidia located at openings of phialides	Phaeohyphomycosis

- *Histoplasma capsulatum*, the agent of **histoplasmosis**
- *Paracoccidioides brasiliensis*, the agent of **paracoccidioidomycosis**
- *Penicillium marneffei*, the agent of **systemic penicilliosis**.

Blastomyces dermatitidis and Blastomycosis

Blastomyces dermatitidis infections may be mild and asymptomatic or severe and chronic. The infection is acquired through inhalation of the conidia or hyphae. Sporadic cases are usually observed, although common exposures leading to outbreaks also have been noted. Person-to-person transmission does not seem to occur. A mild respiratory infection most often results, but the infection can disseminate to the skin and bone also. Chronic infection is characterized by lesions or ulcerations in any part of the body but most frequently in the lungs, skin, and bone. Blastomycosis occurs in North America, from Canada to the Mississippi, Missouri, and Ohio River Valleys, and in Mexico. However, it is found most often in the southeastern United States, the area south of the Ohio River and east of the Mississippi River. Other names for blastomycosis include North American blastomycosis and Gilchrist's disease.

The organism appears in tissue or body fluids on direct microscopic examination as round to oval yeast cells with thick-walled, broad-based, single budding.

Coccidioides immitis and Coccidioidomycosis

Coccidioides immitis may cause an acute, benign, self-limiting respiratory infection or a chronic, malignant infection of the bones, joints, skin, lymph nodes, adrenal glands, and central nervous system. The geographic distribution of the organism includes the southwestern United States and the semiarid areas of Mexico and Central and South America. The infection has a high incidence in the San Joaquin Valley in California and may be commonly known as "desert fever" or "valley fever." Infection is acquired through inhalation of arthrospores that are present in the soil or environment. Many individuals exhibit no clinical signs, but others develop a mild respiratory infection characterized by cough, fever, chest pain, and malaise. Most patients recover within 2 to 6 weeks; however, the infection may disseminate in a small percentage of patients to the bones, joints, skin, brain, or meninges.

Large, thick-walled, round spherules that contain endospores are observed in direct preparations of tissue or body fluids. *C. immitis* is an extremely dangerous biohazard requiring Biosafety Level 3 containment; it may be considered the most infectious of all fungi.

Histoplasma capsulatum and Histoplasmosis

Histoplasma capsulatum is found in the midwestern and southern United States and is endemic in the Mississippi and Ohio River Valleys and the Appalachian Mountains. Cases also have been found in other areas of North America and in South America. The organism is saprobic in soil and multiplies in decaying chicken or pigeon droppings or bat guano. Histoplasmosis is acquired through inhalation of spores from the environment. Outbreaks have been associated with human contact with bird roosts, chicken houses, barns, and bat caves.

The primary infection involves the respiratory tract and may result in acute, chronic, or fatal pulmonary disease. The chronic, cavitary form may resemble tuberculosis and is characterized by coughing and fever. The infection may remain localized in the pulmonary tract but may disseminate also to the spleen, lymphatics, liver, kidneys, meninges, or heart.

Yeast cells are difficult to observe in direct sputum specimens. However, small, round to oval yeast cells may be observed within monocytes or neutrophils on bone marrow or peripheral blood smears, using Wright's or Giemsa stain.

Paracoccidioides brasiliensis and Paracoccidioidomycosis

Paracoccidioides brasiliensis causes a chronic granulomatous disease of the lungs, lymphatics, skin, and mucous membranes. The organism is found most often in South and Central America and Mexico, especially in Brazil, Venezuela, and Colombia. It is rarely found in the United States. Infection may be acquired through inhaling spores or chewing fungally contaminated food, which may invade the mucous membranes in the mouth. Symptoms of paracoccidioidomycosis include chronic mucocutaneous or cutaneous ulcers that spread to the liver and spleen.

Multiple budding yeast cells, which are said to resemble a "mariner's wheel," are observed on direct microscopic examination.

Penicillium marneffei and Systemic Penicilliosis

Penicillium marneffei causes systemic penicilliosis, an acute infection of the lungs, bone marrow, and other organs seen in immunocompromised hosts. The infection has been found in Southeast Asia, China, India, and Hong Kong, and the organism has been isolated from the intestines of the bamboo rat.

Oval yeast cells that may resemble *Histoplasma* are observed within histiocytes on direct examination. The yeast cells elongate when observed outside of histiocytes. *P. marneffei* grows as a *Penicillium* mold at 25°C as bluish green, powdery, velvety colonies. Microscopically, the mycelial phase is observed as septate hyphae with brush-like conidiophores.

TABLE 20-5 summarizes the morphological and microscopic characteristics of the dimorphic fungi.

YEAST AND YEAST-LIKE FUNGI

The yeast and yeast-like fungi are present throughout the environment on plants and as normal microbiota of humans and other animals. Most yeast infections are opportunistic and found in persons in immunosuppressive states and in individuals who are on prolonged antibiotic therapy, corticosteroids therapy, and parenteral nutrition, as well as persons with HIV, lymphomas, and leukemia.

The yeasts are the fungi most frequently isolated from clinical specimens. Their role as pathogens in nonsterile body sites is often difficult to interpret because the yeasts are normally found in small numbers on the skin and mucous membranes. Usually, yeast isolated in small numbers from the sputum, urine, vagina, or stool is not considered to be pathogenic. However, large numbers of yeast isolated from a nonsterile site or several sites are generally considered to be pathogenic. Any yeast isolated from a sterile or closed site is considered to be pathogenic and must be identified.

Yeasts are eukaryotic unicellular, budding, and round to oval organisms that multiply asexually through the production of blastoconidia. Blastoconidia are produced linearly from the mother cell without separation. With decreased levels of oxygen in tissue, yeast cells may form septate hyphae or pseudohyphae. Most yeasts grow on bacterial media in 48 to 72 hours as smooth, and moist colonies with a creamy, pasty, or membranous consistency. Yeasts that form capsules may appear mucoid on solid media; aerial hyphae are usually not produced. Growth at 37°C is an important identification tool because most pathogens are able to grow within the temperature range of 25°C to 37°C, whereas saprobes cannot grow at 37°C.

The yeasts are identified through microscopic and macroscopic features, carbohydrate assimilation and fermentation, and other biochemical reactions. Reproductive structures observed microscopically, such as and the presence of a germ tube, pseudohyphae, blastoconidia, chlamydospores, and capsules, and cell wall thickness provide useful information. Macroscopic growth characteristics, including presence or absence of growth with cycloheximide and chloramphenicol, are also helpful. For example, *Candida albicans* can grow on antibiotic media, but *Cryptococcus neoformans* cannot. Cornmeal agar can be inoculated to enhance the microscopic morphology of the pseudohyphae, blastoconidia, and chlamydospores used in identification.

The germ tube test, urease reaction, reduction of nitrates to nitrites, production of phenol oxidase on Niger seed agar, and carbohydrate assimilation and fermentation patterns also are helpful to identify the yeasts. Carbohydrate **assimilation** refers to the organism's ability to use a particular carbohydrate to grow. Carbohydrate-free medium is inoculated with the organism, and filter paper disks containing various carbohydrates are placed onto the inoculum on the agar. Growth surrounding a disk indicates that the organism can utilize or assimilate that carbohydrate.

Nomenclature of the yeast can be confusing, and some of the organisms have been reclassified based on DNA analysis. There is an anamorph, or asexual, name and also a teleomorph, or sexual, name. The teleomorph name is usually the recommended name and is the preferred name in DNA sequencing databases. The anamorph name is used when a teleomorph stage cannot be demonstrated. Taxonomy of the clinically relevant yeast is summarized in **BOX 20-3**.

BOX 20-3 Taxonomy of Clinically Relevant Yeast

Class Saccharomycetes

Subphylum: Ascomyctes

Genus: *Candida*

Subphylum: Basidiomycetes, Tremellomycetes

Genera: *Trichosporon* and *Cryptococcus*

TABLE 20-5 Morphology of Frequently Isolated Dimorphic (Systemic) Fungi

	Colonial appearance		Microscopic appearance		
Organism	**Mycelial phase**	**Yeast phase**	**Mycelial phase**	**Yeast phase**	**Clinical significance**
Blastomyces dermatitidis	On Sabouraud dextrose agar (SDA), colony first white, waxy, yeast-like and later cottony with white aerial mycelium; turns tan to brown with age	On brain-heart infusion (BHI) agar with blood, colony cream to tan, waxy, and heaped or wrinkled; inhibited by chloramphenicol or cycloheximide	Delicate, septate hyphae with round or pyriform conidia borne singly on conidiophores or directly on hyphae, resembling "lollipops"	Thick-walled, large yeast cells with single bud on a broad base; broad isthmus at constriction	Blastomycosis
	Growth rate: 7–28 days				
Coccidioides immitis	Moist, gray membranous colony that develops white, cottony aerial mycelium; turns tan to brown with age	Similar to mycelial phase	Coarse, septate, branched hyphae that produce thick-walled, barrel-shaped, rectangular arthroconidia that alternate with empty disjunctor cells	Large, round, thick-walled spherules with endospores observed in tissue and direct examination; not a true yeast	Coccidioidomycosis
	Growth rate: 5–14 days. Growth may occur as early as 3–5 days. Arthroconidia may need 1–2 weeks to form.				
Histoplasma capsulatum	On SDA, white to brown or pink mold with fine, dense, fluffy texture; white, yellow, or tan reverse side	On BHI, moist, white to cream, heaped colony; may be inhibited by cycloheximide or chloramphenicol	Septate hyphae with round to pyriform microconidia on short branches or directly on hyphal stalk; later, large, round, thick-walled knobby tuberculate macroconidia forms	Small, budding, round to oval yeast cells; intracellular to mononuclear cells with Giemsa or Wright's stain	Histoplasmosis
	Growth rate: Slow growing; usually requires 2–4 weeks at 25°C or 30°C				
Paracoccidioides brasiliensis	On SDA, white, glabrous, leathery colony; turns tan-brown with age; short aerial mycelium	On blood agar, cream to tan, moist, wrinkled colony; turns waxy with age	Small, septate, branched hyphae with intercalary and terminal chlamydoconidia; few pyriform microconidia	Large, round to oval, thick-walled yeast cells with multiple buds that attach to mother cell by narrow constrictions; resembles a "ship's wheel"	Paracoccidioidomycosis
	Growth rate: Very slow growing; usually requires 21–28 days				

CANDIDA

Candida is a heterogeneous genus with many species that are ubiquitous in the environment, being found on plants and vegetation. *Candida* is also found normally in the human alimentary canal and gastrointestinal tract and on the mucocutaneous membranes. These organisms show round to oval cells, with multilayer budding. The most frequently isolated yeast is *Candida albicans*, which normally is found in small amounts in the gastrointestinal tract and on mucocutaneous areas. Infections may occur in healthy individuals but more commonly occur in the immunocompromised host; candidiasis can involve almost any organ in the body, and infections range from mild to severe. *C. albicans* has a low degree of pathogenicity but causes the most severe infections in the immunosuppressed or debilitated host.

Candidiasis may involve the mucous membranes of the mouth (thrush) or vagina (vulvovaginitis). Cutaneous infections, including diaper rash, nail infections (onychomycosis), and cuticle infections (paronychomycosis), also are common *Candida* infections. Systemic infections include endocarditis, meningitis, urinary tract infections (UTIs), pulmonary infections, and fungemia.

Predisposition to *Candida* infection can be attributed to several host factors, including an altered skin barrier (burns, wounds, intravenous catheters); altered mucosal membranes caused by diabetes mellitus; prolonged antibiotic therapy, chemotherapy, corticosteroid therapy, and smoking; hormonal or nutritional imbalance in pregnancy; diabetes mellitus; malnutrition; leukopenia or defective leukocyte activity (leukemia, radiation therapy, chemotherapy, viral infections); and defective cell-mediated immunity (transplant recipients, immunosuppression).

Prolonged antibiotic therapy with broad-spectrum antibiotics, such as tetracycline, can suppress the host's normal flora and thus allow the "normal flora" *Candida* to overgrow into large numbers. *C. albicans* produces several virulence factors, including proteases and adhesions. Superficial infections are treated with a variety of creams, such as nystatin. Systemic infections are treated with oral ketoconazole or fluconazole.

C. albicans appears in direct microscopic examination from specimens as budding yeast with blastoconidia or pseudohyphae, showing no signs of constriction. The organism stains gram positive in the Gram stain preparation (**FIGURE 20-19**). *C. albicans* grows readily on blood agar and SDA in 48 to 72 hours at 35°C to 37°C, producing white-, cream-, or tan-colored colonies with a pasty, creamy appearance. Characteristic colonies with spiderlike projections are observed on eosin-methylene blue (EMB) agar.

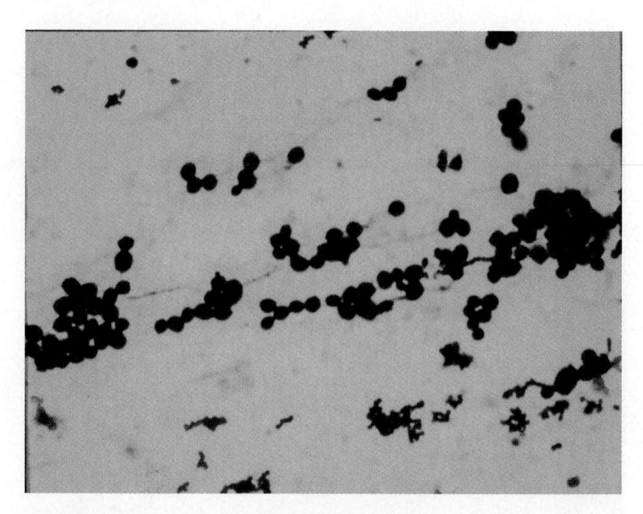

FIGURE 20-19 *Candida albicans* Gram stain.

C. albicans is the only yeast that produces a **germ tube** (**FIGURE 20-20**) when incubated with sterile serum for 1 to 3 hours at 35°C to 37°C. A germ tube is a hypha-like extension of the yeast cell, with no constriction at the point of origin. Rare strains of *Candida tropicalis* may produce a germ tube.

C. albicans produces chlamydioconidia on cornmeal agar when incubated at room temperature for 24 to 48 hours. It is urease negative and negative for nitrate reduction and does not produce a capsule. **TABLE 20-6** summarizes specific patterns for assimilation and fermentation of carbohydrates for various yeasts.

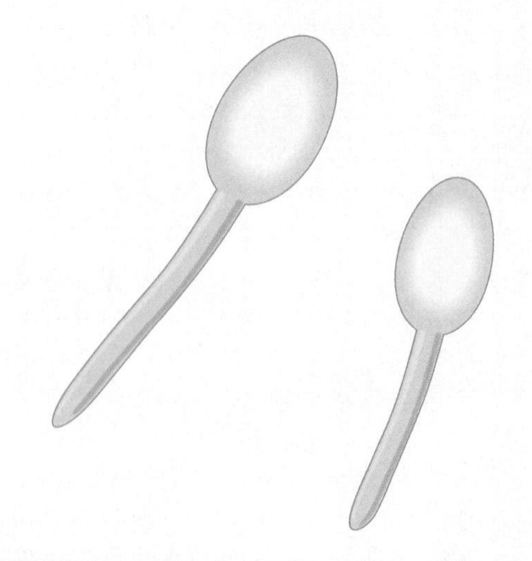

FIGURE 20-20 Germ tube, a hypha-like extension of the yeast cell, with no constriction.

TABLE 20-6 Assimilation and Fermentation Reactions of Clinically Significant Yeasts

	Assimilations												Fermentations							
Organism	Glucose	Maltose	Sucrose	Lactose	Galactose	Melibiose	Cellobiose	Inositol	Xylose	Raffinose	Trehalose	Dulcitol	Glucose	Maltose	Sucrose	Lactose	Galactose	Trehalose	Urease	Nitrate reduction
Candida albicans	+	+	V	–	+	–	–	–	+	–	+	–	+	+	–	–	+	+	–	–
Candida glabrata	+	–	–	–	–	–	–	–	–	–	+	–	+	–	–	–	–	+	–	–
Candida krusei	+	–	–	–	–	–	–	–	–	–	–	–	+	–	–	–	–	–	V	–
Candida parapsilosis	+	+	+	–	+	–	–	–	+	–	+	–	+	–	–	–	–	–	–	–
Candida tropicalis	+	+	+	–	+	–	+	–	+	–	+	–	+	+	+	–	+	+	–	–
Cryptococcus neoformans	+	+	+	–	+	–	+	+	+	+	+	+	–	–	–	–	–	–	+	–
Geotrichum candidum	+	–	–	–	+	–	–	–	+	–	–	–	–	–	–	–	–	–	–	–
Trichosporon beigelii	+	+	+	+	+	V	+	+	+	V	V	V	–	–	–	–	–	–	+	–

+, most strains positive; –, most strains negative; V, variable reaction

Other species of *Candida* associated with human infection include *C. tropicalis*, *C. parapsilosis*, *C. krusei*, and *C. glabrata*. These organisms have been isolated in a wide range of infections, frequently involving immunosuppressed patients. *Candida tropicalis* is associated with vaginitis and urinary tract, intestinal, pulmonary, and systemic infections. It is especially virulent in individuals with leukemia. *Candida parapsilosis* has been isolated as the causative agent in endocarditis, otitis externa, and nail infections. *Candida krusei* is a rare cause of endocarditis, urinary tract infections, and vaginitis. It produces spreading colonies on SDA and sheep blood agar.

Candida glabrata (formerly *Torulopsis glabrata*) is a budding yeast but with cells smaller than those of other *Candida species*. *C. glabrata* does not produce well-developed pseudohyphae or a germ tube. It is normal flora of the gastrointestinal tract, skin, and upper respiratory tract and an opportunistic pathogen. *C. glabrata* is an important cause of fungal urinary tract infections and should be suspected when small, glossy yeast colonies are isolated on blood agar. The organism has been isolated from cases of fungemia and kidney, lung, genitourinary, and central nervous system infections involving immunosuppressed, diabetic, and cancer patients. Tiny yeast cells are observed in preparations made from growth on cornmeal agar. *C. glabrata* rarely may produce red-colored colonies and thus must be differentiated from *Rhodotorula*. *C. glabrata* assimilates both glucose and trehalose, a characteristic that is useful in its identification.

Candida dublinensis is an important cause of oral candidiasis in those with the human immunodeficiency virus (HIV). It also is associated with infections of the blood and urine and infections in other sites in those who are immunocompromised. It resembles *C. albicans* because it can produce a germ tube and chlamydioconidia. *C. dublinensis* can be differentiated from *C. albicans* by its inability both to grow at 45°C and to assimilate xylose. The organism is believed to be more virulent than *C. albicans*.

Cryptococcus

Cryptococcus neoformans is an encapsulated, round to oval yeast. There is typically a single bud with a narrow neck between the parent and daughter cell. The organism is present in pigeon, bat, and bird droppings, as well as in decaying vegetation, fruit, plants, and milk. Humans exposed to dust or dirt containing bird droppings, including farmers and poultry workers, are at risk of infection. Cryptococcosis is acquired through inhalation of the yeast into the lungs, where it may spread hematogenously to the brain, meninges, bones, joints, and skin, especially in immunodeficient individuals. Others at risk of severe *Cryptococcus* infections include persons with lupus erythematosus, sarcoidosis, leukemia, and lymphoma.

A very striking characteristic of the organism is the appearance, on direct microscopic examination, of irregularly sized, spherical yeast cells, surrounded by a capsule. The capsule may be visualized by the India ink preparation, although demonstration of capsular cryptococcal antigen is recommended because the capsule may not be seen in all cases of cryptococcosis. Antigen typing for the capsule can be performed on cerebrospinal fluid, serum, or latex, using a latex agglutination method. Not all *C. neoformans* produce a capsule.

Cryptococcus grows on primary isolation as mucoid colonies, which are cream, tan, or pink in color. The colonies become darker and drier with age. On cornmeal agar, *C. neoformans* does not form pseudohyphae but instead appears as encapsulated yeast cells of various sizes. *C. neoformans* produces maroon to brown-black colonies on Niger seed agar, which is a unique identifying characteristic.

Important reactions to identify *C. neoformans* include positive urease and phenol oxidase, assimilation of inositol, and negative nitrate reduction.

Miscellaneous Yeasts

Saccharomyces cerevisiae species are ubiquitous in the environment and rare causes of a variety of human infections, including thrush and vulvovaginitis, in individuals with underlying medical conditions, including HIV, burns, and side effects from prolonged corticosteroid therapy. The organisms produce large yeast cells on cornmeal agar and ascospores when grown on an ascospore medium. The asci typically have 1 to 4 smooth ascospores.

Rhodotorula is found on human skin and in the environment. It is a rare cause of transient blood infections, peritonitis, and septicemia, especially in peritoneal dialysis patients. The organism produces an orange or orange-red pigment and round to oval, multilayer budding yeast cells. It is urease positive and unable to ferment carbohydrates. *Rhodotorula* cannot assimilate inositol, which is useful in its differentiation from *Cryptococcus neoformans.*

Geotrichum candidum is the agent of geotrichosis. It has been isolated as an agent in a variety of opportunistic fungal infections, including bronchitis, skin infections, colitis, conjunctivitis, wound infections, and oral infections such as thrush. *Geotrichum* infections rarely disseminate. The organism is found in the soil and on decaying foods. Morphologically, the organism exhibits round, oval, or rectangular yeast cells, which are paired or in chains, as shown in **FIGURE 20-21**. The organisms grows rapidly as smooth, moist, white- to cream-colored colonies. Fragmented hyphae with rectangular arthroconidia with rounded ends when grown on cornmeal agar are characteristic for *G. candidum.* The organism doesn't form blastoconidia, pseudohyphae, or chlamydioconidia.

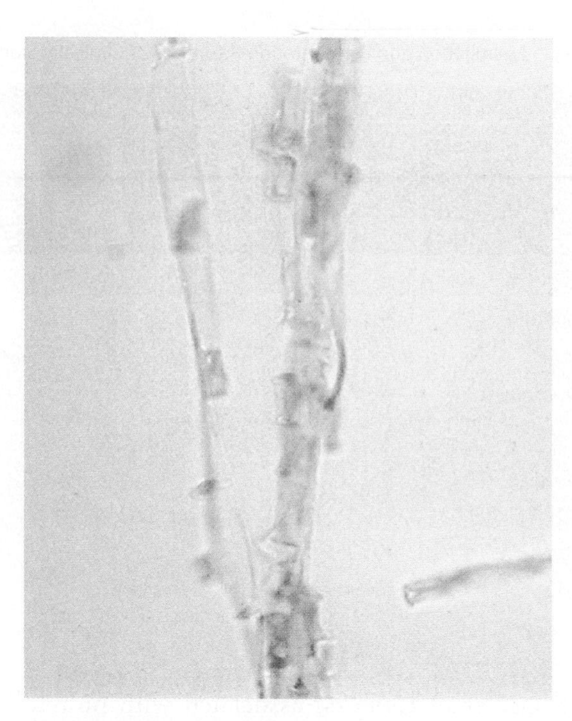

FIGURE 20-21 Microscopic view of *Geotrichum* showing rectangular yeast cells in chains.

Trichosporon beigelii (*T. cutaneum*) was previously discussed with the superficial mycoses. It is a basiodomycete with no sexual stage. It is unable to ferment carbohydrates but can assimilate a variety of carbohydrates. *Trichosporon* produces smooth, moist, cream-colored colonies on SDA, which become drier and folded with age. Its blastoconidia are enhanced when grown in malt extract broth at room temperature for 48 to 72 hours. In addition to superficial skin infections, *Trichosporon* can cause more severe infections in burn patients and those with intravenous catheters or those on corticosteroid therapy. Other important species of *Trichosporon* include *T. asahii*, *T. asteroides*, *T. mucoides*, *T. ovoides*, and *T. inkin*.

Several commercially available packaged systems are available for the identification of yeast. The API 20C AUX (bioMérieux) consists of 20 microcupules of carbohydrates, from which the assimilation pattern of the organism can be determined. A profile number is then determined and compared with a large database and index for identification. There also are the Uni-Yeast-Tek yeast identification system, from Remel, and the MicroScan Yeast Identification panel, from MicroScan. There also are automated identification systems to identify the clinically relevant yeasts, including the Yeast Biochemical Cards, from bioMérieux. Chromogenic agars, such as CHROMager™

TABLE 20-7 Characteristics of Clinically Significant Yeasts*

Organism	Capsules	Germ tubes	Blastoconidia	Arthroconidia	Chlamydoconidia
Candida albicans	–	+	+	–	+
Candida glabrata	–	–	+	–	–
Candida krusei	–	–	+	–	–
Candida parapsilosis	–	–	+	–	–
Candida stellatoidea	–	+	+	–	+
Candida tropicalis	–	–	+	–	V
Cryptococcus neoformans	+	–	+	–	–
Geotrichum candidum	–	–	–	+	–
Trichosporon beigelii	–	–	+	+	–

*Using cornmeal with Tween 80 agar; +, most strains positive; –, most strains negative; V, variable reaction

(Becton Dickinson), are differential agars that aid in the isolation and differentiation of *Candida* species. Characteristic colors are produced by the different species of yeast.

Table 20-6 and **TABLE 20-7** summarize important characteristics and biochemical reactions used in the identification of the clinically important yeasts. Procedures for germ tube production, cornmeal agar with Tween 80, carbohydrate assimilation, and urease production are described at the end of the chapter.

OPPORTUNISTIC SAPROBIC FUNGI

The opportunistic saprobic fungi, which were once considered to be contaminants, saprobes, or plant pathogens, are now important agents in opportunistic mycoses. This group of fungi includes the Zygomycetes and the genus *Aspergillus*, as well as the **Hyphomycetes** (hyaline molds) and the **Phaeohyphomycetes** (darkly pigmented, or dematiaceous molds), which have already been discussed.

Zygomycetes

The **Zygomycetes** are found on decaying vegetation and in the soil and are common laboratory contaminants but may produce mycoses in immunocompromised patients. **Zygomycosis** is acquired most often through inhalation of the spores. Patients with diabetes mellitus; those receiving prolonged antibiotic therapy, corticosteroid therapy, and immunosuppressive therapy; and those with chronic vascular problems seem to be at particular risk. The Zygomycetes cause infections of the nasal mucosa, palate, sinuses, face, lung, liver, spleen, kidney, and brain. These organisms have a propensity to attack the vascular system and can penetrate the arteries, often resulting in necrosis, vascular invasion, and thrombosis. These infections are rapidly spreading, may disseminate, and are often fatal.

A zygomycete should be suspected if branching, ribbon-like, nonseptate hyphae are observed on the direct microscopic examination. These organisms grow as fluffy white to gray molds with brown hyphae, which can cover the agar surface in 1 to 4 days and are thus given the designation "lid lifters." Coarse hyphae with brown or black spores are observed microscopically. The Zygomycetes include the genera *Rhizopus*, *Mucor*, and *Absidia*, which are differentiated by the presence and arrangement of horizontal runners, or **stolons**, and rootlike structures, or **rhizoids**.

Aspergillus, another common laboratory contaminant, is found in soil and on decaying vegetation and may colonize grains, leaves, or plants. Humans acquire aspergillosis through inhalation of the conidia in dust or direct, cutaneous inoculation. Aspergillosis, an opportunistic infection, may involve a variety of organs, including the lungs, CNS, eyes, heart, and skin. Pulmonary aspergillosis includes allergic bronchopulmonary aspergillosis of the bronchi and aspergillomas, or "fungus ball infections." Aspergillomas consist of a tangled mass of hyphae and may invade the lung or paranasal sinuses.

Aspergillus is a rapidly growing mold. The species isolated as human pathogens include *A. fumigatus*, *A. flavus*, *A. niger*, and *A. terreus*. The species are differentiated on the basis of pigmentation of the colonies and microscopically by the morphology of the organism's phialides.

TABLE 20-8 Opportunistic Saprobic Fungi and Fungal Contaminants

Organisms	Colonial appearance	Microscopic appearance	Comments
Aspergillus species	Rapid growth within 2 days; fluffy, granular, or powdery texture; pigment depends on species: *A. fumigatus*: white to blue-green, *A. niger*: black, *A. flavus*: yellow to green, *A. terreus*: tan to cinnamon	Branching, septate hyphae that terminate in a conidiophore, which expands into a large, spherical vesicle. Vesicle is covered with sterigmata (stalks), and parallel chains of conidia cover the sterigmata.	Widespread in nature; *A. fumigatus* most frequently isolated; pulmonary, eye, CNS, and systemic infections
Zygomycetes	Coarse, woolly, fluffy, white to gray or brown mycelium with black or brown sporangium. Hyphae grow within 1–3 days and rapidly cover agar surface.	*Rhizopus*: Large, broad, nonseptate hyphae that produce horizontal runners, or stolons, which attach at contact points by rootlike structures, or rhizoids. Sporangiophores arise in clusters at rhizoids and terminate in sporangia. *Absidia*: Similar to *Rhizopus*; however, sporangiophores arise between nodes, from which rhizoids are formed. *Mucor*: No rhizoids	Widespread in nature; vascular invasion, thrombosis, and necrosis; common laboratory contaminant

TABLE 20-8 describes the differentiation of the Zygomycetes and *Aspergillus*. **FIGURE 20-22** is a microscopic view of *A. fumigatus*.

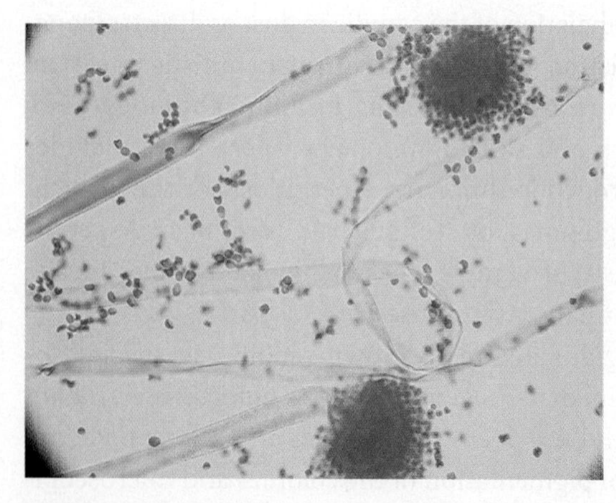

FIGURE 20-22 Microscopic view of *Aspergillus fumigatus*.

Hyalohyphomycetes and Phaeomycetes

Clinically important **Hyalohyphomycetes** include the genera *Acremonium*, *Fusarium*, *Penicillium*, *Scopulariopsis*, and *Pseudoallescberia*. *Pseudoallescberia* may have hyaline or light black hyphae and thus may be considered to be darkly pigmented. **FIGURE 20-23** illustrates the characteristic violet colonies of *Fusarium*, and **FIGURE 20-24** is a microscopic preparation of *Penicillium*, showing septate, hyaline to blue-green hyphae with brushlike conidiophores, phialides, and chains of conidia.

Phaeohyphomycetes that are isolated in human infection include *Alternaria*, *Bipolaris*, *Curvularia*, *Exserohilum*, *Aureobasidium*, and *Xylohypha*. **TABLE 20-9** lists important features of the Hyalohyphomycetes and Phaeohyphomycetes. **FIGURE 20-25** illustrates the black pigmentation of the fungus *Aureobasidium*, and **FIGURE 20-26** depicts the microscopic appearance of *Alternaria*. The

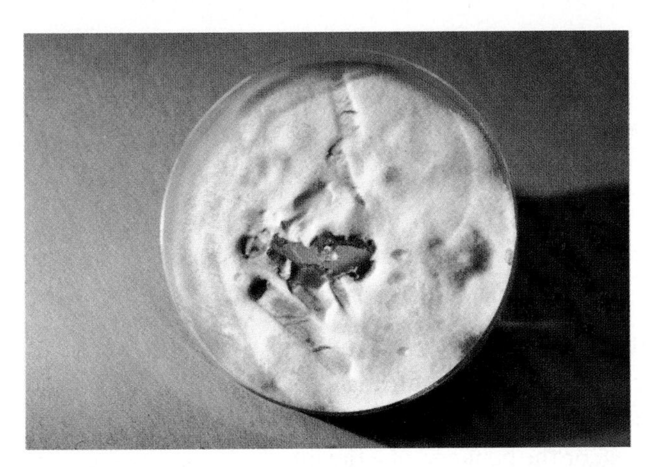

FIGURE 20-23 *Fusarium* illustrating its violet pigmented mycelium.

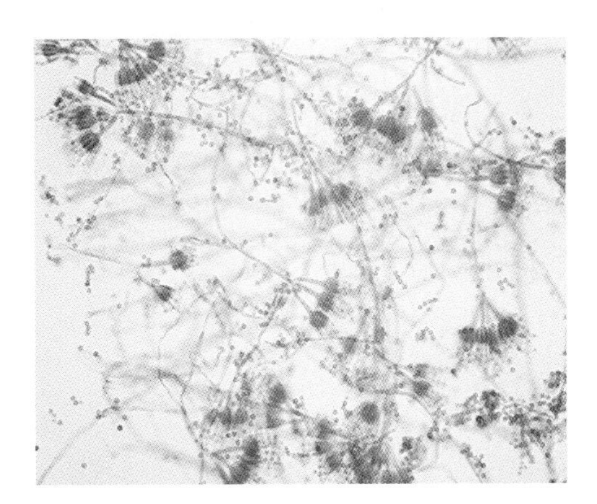

FIGURE 20-24 Microsopic view of *Penicillium* showing brushlike conidiophores, phialides, and chains of conidia.

Hyalohyphomycetes and Phaeohyphomycetes are associated with a variety of opportunistic infections, including keratitis; mycetoma; pulmonary disease; and cutaneous, nail, and sinus infections. These fungi are found in the environment in soil and organic matter, on vegetation, and also as laboratory contaminants.

SEROLOGICAL TESTING

Fungal serological testing may be performed to supplement microscopic or culture methods for identification. Antigen detection may be hampered by cross-reacting components, thus requiring the testing of multiple antigens for a definite interpretation.

TABLE 20-9 Characteristics of Some Hyalohyphomycetes and Phaeohyphomycetes

Genus	Characteristics
Hyalohyphomycetes (hyaline molds)	
Acremonium	White, spreading, moist, colorless colonies that become cottony with a gray top and a yellow or rose reverse side with age Small, hyaline, septate hyphae with phialides of hyaline phialoconidia; elliptical single-ceiled conidia
Fusarium	Rapidly growing, white then pink to violet, fluffy, cottony growth; hyaline, two-celled or multicelled, smooth-walled fusiform macroconidia, resembling a sickle or banana; small, septate, hyaline hyphae; unicellular microconidia in balls or short chains
Penicillium	Rapid, blue-green, velvety, powdery growth Septate, hyaline, or dark to blue-green hyphae that produce brushlike conidiophores that give rise to phialides, from which chains of conidia arise
Scopulariopsis	Moderately rapid growth with white, granular, glabrous colonies that later become gray and powdery Septate, hyaline hyphae with annelides that are produced singly or in groups on a conidiophore Thick-walled, spiny, hyaline annelconidia arranged in a chain
Phaeohyphomycetes (darkly pigmented molds)	
Alternaria	Rapidly growing, cottony, gray to black colonies Septate, dematiaceous conidiophores, which may branch with chains of brown conidia, which are muriform and tapered
Bipolaris	Rapid grower with gray-green to dark brown powdery, woolly, or cottony colonies Septate, dematiaceous hyphae, which are simple or branching, single or grouped conidiophores with multicelled, oblong to cylindrical conidia
Curvularia	Rapidly growing, woolly, fluffy, black colonies Dematiaceous, septate hyphae with conidiophores twisted at point of attachment to conidia, which are two-celled or multicelled and curved, with central, darkly staining, swollen cell

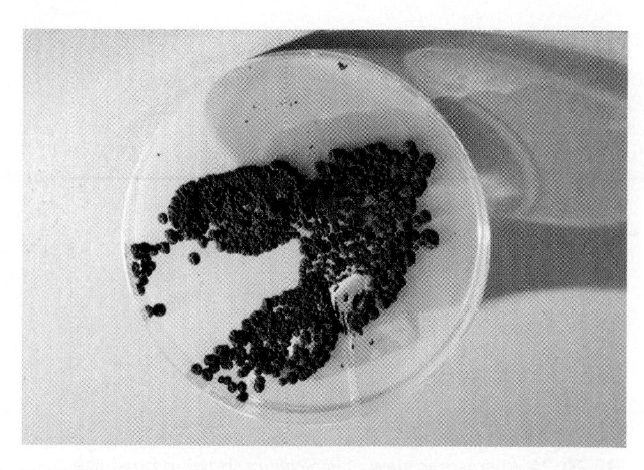

FIGURE 20-25 *Aureobasidium*. a dematiaceous fungi showing its typical black pigment on SDA.

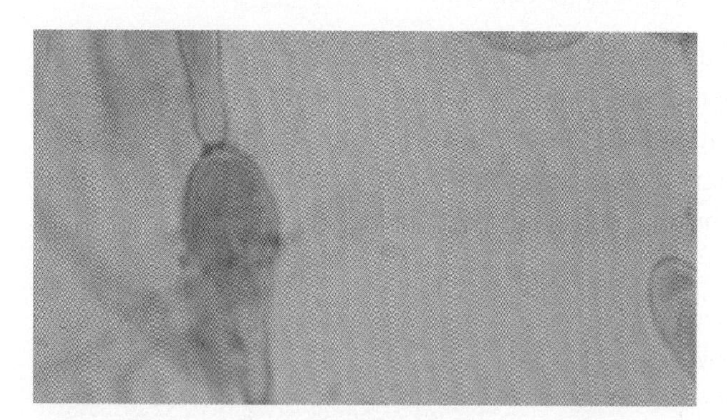

FIGURE 20-26 *Alternaria* showing and tapered conidia.

A very useful test is the cryptococcal antigen test for *Cryptococcus neoformans*, which detects the presence of cryptococcal polysaccharide in body fluids, such as CSF. This method uses latex particles coated with hyperimmune anticryptococcal globulin to detect cryptococcal antigen. The method is simple and reliable and has virtually replaced the India ink method for detection.

Fungal serology to detect antibody relies on correct timing of blood specimens. Antibody detection methods for blastomycosis, coccidioidomycosis, histoplasmosis, and sporotrichosis can detect active infections, but cross-reacting antigens and false-negative results are problems.

Tests also are available for the diagnosis of aspergillosis and candidiasis. Methodologies for serological testing include immunodiffusion, complement fixation, and latex agglutination.

Laboratory Procedures

Procedure
Slide culture

Purpose
The slide culture is the most accurate method to preserve and observe fungal microstructure.

Materials
Sterile Petri plate containing 2% agar or filter paper and two applicator sticks (a bent glass rod, two pieces of plastic tubing, or the bent end of a flexible drinking straw can be substituted for the applicator sticks)
Clean microscope slide and coverslip
Lactophenol cotton blue (LPCB) stain
Sabouraud dextrose agar (SDA) or other suitable agar
Sterile scalpel or sterile test tube without a lip

Procedure
A wet (tease) mount should be performed before the slide culture. Work should be done under a biological safety cabinet. This procedure should not be performed on organisms suspected of being *Coccidioides, Histoplasma*, or *Blastomyces.*

1. Cover the bottom of a Petri plate with filter paper if this method is being used. Place a bent glass rod (or two sterile applicator sticks, flexible straw, or plastic tubing) in the Petri plate.
2. Place a clean microscope slide onto the bent glass rod or, alternatively, onto the surface of the agar in the Petri plate.
3. Using a sterile scalpel, cut a 2 mm deep section of agar that measures approximately 1 mm × 1 mm. Alternatively, cut the block using a sterile test tube that has no lip.
4. Transfer the block of agar to the microscope slide.
5. Using either a sterile applicator stick or a heavy wire, inoculate the fungus into the center of the four sides of the agar square. If using a circular block, inoculate the four quadrants of the block.
6. Gently place a sterile coverslip over the block.
7. If using the filter paper method, add approximately 1.5 to 2.0 ml of sterile water to the bottom of the Petri plate.
8. Incubate at room temperature (25°C to 30°C).
9. Examine periodically for growth. Growth is usually seen on the slide's surface and underneath the

coverslip. If the filter paper dries out, add additional sterile water.

10. When structures are visible, gently remove the coverslip, using sterile forceps if needed. Place the coverslip on a microscope slide containing one drop of LPCB.
11. The agar plug can be further incubated after the addition of a second coverslip if desired.
12. Slides can be sealed with clear nail polish or Permount for later analysis if desired.

Procedure
Potassium hydroxide (KOH) preparation

Purpose
KOH preparations are used in the initial examination of keratinized tissue suspected of fungal infection.

Principle
Fungal elements may be obscured by skin, hair, or nail tissue. KOH dissolves keratin in these specimens but does not dissolve the chitin in the fungal cell wall, which facilitates observation of the organism's morphology.

Materials
KOH solution is prepared by slowly adding 10 g of KOH to 80 ml of distilled water and then adding 20 ml of glycerol. Mix until completely dissolved and store in the refrigerator. Glycerol prevents crystallization of KOH, so preparations can be examined for up to 2 days without drying.

Procedure

1. Into one drop of KOH reagent on slide, place a small portion of the material (skin scrapings, hair, nail) to be examined.
2. Press coverslip down on sample.
3. Warm slide gently to dissolve keratinized cells. Do not boil. Alternatively, allow to react at room temperature for one hour.
4. Allow specimen to clear, approximately 20 minutes.
5. Examine under low (100×) and high-dry (430×) magnification.

Interpretation
Observe for the presence of characteristic fungal elements, including hyphae, budding yeast, and spherules. For hair specimens, determine whether the infection is ectothrix or endothrix.

Notes

1. Do not use cotton swabs to collect specimens because cotton fibers may resemble hyphae.
2. For nail and hard skin scrapings, it may be necessary to add dimethyl sulfoxide (DMSO) to the KOH reagent. To prepare KOH-DMSO reagent, add 40 ml of DMSO with caution to 60 ml of distilled water. Then carefully add 10 g of KOH and mix until completely dissolved. Follow the procedure previously outlined.

Procedure
Tease mount

Purpose
The tease mount allows for the rapid examination of conidia, spores, and other microscopic fungal structures.

Materials
Bent dissecting needle or wire bent at 90° degree angle
Lactophenol cotton blue (LPCB) stain
Clean microscope slide and coverslip
Two dissecting needles

Procedure

1. With the bent dissecting needle or wire, remove a small portion of the colony from the agar surface. Select a portion midway between the center and the periphery.
2. Place a drop of LPCB on the microscope slide and place the culture into the stain.
3. Place a coverslip over the culture, and using a pencil eraser, press down gently to disperse the mycelium. Alternatively, using two dissecting needles, gently tease apart the mycelium and then add the coverslip.
4. Observe microscopically under low (100×) and high-dry (430×) magnification for fungal characteristics.

Note
Although this is a rapid method, preservation of the original arrangement of spores may be disrupted as a result of teasing or pressure in applying the coverslip.

Procedure
Germ tube test

Purpose
Candida albicans can be presumptively identified based on the production of a germ tube.

Principle
When incubated with serum at 37°C for 1 to 3 hours, *C. albicans* will form a germ tube.

Materials
Germ tube solution (bovine serum albumin), commercially available from Becton Dickinson

Procedure

1. Pipette 0.5 ml of serum into a test tube.
2. Inoculate the tube with a small amount of the organism to be tested. A large inoculum may produce false-negative results.
3. Incubate at 37°C for 1 to 3 hours.
4. Place a drop of the suspension on a slide, apply a coverslip, and examine for the presence of germ tubes.

Interpretation

A germ tube is approximately half as wide and three to four times as long as the yeast cell. No point of constriction should exist where the germ tube arises from the mother cell.

Quality Control

C. albicans: Positive control; produces germ tube within 2 hours

C. tropicalis: Negative control; fails to produce germ tube within 3 hours

Procedure

Cornmeal Agar with Tween 80

Purpose

Cornmeal agar with Tween 80 is used to distinguish the various species of *Candida* and other yeasts through examination of hyphae, blastoconidia, chlamydoconidia, and arthroconidia.

Principle

Cornmeal agar stimulates conidiation. Tween 80 (polysorbate) reduces surface tension and enhances the formation of hyphae, blastoconidia, chlamydoconidia, and arthroconidia.

Materials

Cornmeal agar with Tween 80
Inoculating wire
Coverslip

Procedure

1. Using approximately a third of the plate, streak the center of the area with the organism to be identified.
2. While holding the inoculating wire at about a 45° degree angle, make three or four parallel cuts about 5 mm apart into the agar.
3. Place a coverslip on the surface of the agar, covering a portion of the parallel cuts.
4. Incubate at room temperature for 24 to 72 hours.
5. Examine by placing the plate, with its lid, on the microscope stage using the low-power (10×) and high-power (43×) objectives. The most characteristic morphology is found near the end of the coverslip.

Interpretation

Note the presence and morphology of hyphae, blastoconidia, chlamydoconidia, and arthrospores.

Presence of pseudohyphae (absence of true hyphae) and blastoconidia indicates the genus *Candida*.

C. albicans: Numerous chlamydospores with several tight clusters of blastoconidia evenly spaced along hyphae

C. tropicalis: Fewer numbers of blastoconidia, which are arranged singly or irregularly in small clusters along the hyphae; no chlamydospores present

C. parapsilosis: Colonies that appear as "spiders" or "sagebrushes" along streak lines on agar; delicate mycelium with occasional blastoconidia observed singly or in short chains

C. pseudotropicalis: Elongated blastoconidia that break away from the pseudohyphae and arrange in a parallel fashion, described as "log in a stream" arrangement

Presence of true hyphae and arthroconidia may indicate *Trichosporon* or *Geotrichum*. The arthroconidia of *Geotrichum* may have a hyphal extension from one corner and are said to resemble "hockey sticks." The urease test is used to further differentiate these organisms: *Trichosporon* is urease positive, and *Geotrichum* is urease negative.

Procedure

Carbohydrate assimilation test for yeast

Purpose

Carbohydrate assimilation of various carbohydrates can provide a definite identification for yeast and yeastlike organisms.

Principle

The yeast's ability to utilize a particular carbohydrate is determined by using a carbohydrate-free (nitrogen-based) agar and filter paper disks that are impregnated with various carbohydrates. Growth around the disk indicates the yeast can utilize that carbohydrate.

Materials

Sterile saline tubes

Yeast nitrogen-based agar, available commercially, or prepare as follows:

1. Dissolve 6.5 g of yeast nitrogen-based agar in 100 ml of distilled water. Adjust pH to 6.2 to 6.4 by adding 1 *N* of NaOH. Sterilize by filtration, and add 88 ml of agar to 100 ml of filtered bromcresol purple indicator to 1 L of 2% agar solution. Pour approximately 20 ml into sterile, plastic Petri plate. Prepare 2% agar by adding 20 g of agar to 1 L of distilled water.

Carbohydrate-impregnated filter paper disks, commercially available, or prepare as follows:

2. Soak 10 mm of filter paper disks in 1% carbohydrate solution. Allow to dry.

Carbohydrates tested may include glucose, maltose, sucrose, lactose, galactose, melibiose, cellobiose, inositol, xylose, raffinose, trehalose, and dulcitol.

Procedure

1. Prepare a McFarland standard No. 4 with the yeast to be tested in a sterile tube of saline.
2. Using a sterile pipette, flood the surface of the yeast nitrogen-based agar plate with the entire suspension and allow it to soak into the medium. Remove and discard any excess suspension from the plate. Allow surface of plate to dry (approximately 5 minutes).
3. Place carbohydrate disks onto agar surface, pressing down gently with flamed forceps. For optimal results, place the disks on the four corners of the plate and in the center to form a cross.
4. Incubate plate at 30°C for 24 hours. Plates should be re-incubated for another 24 hours and read again if growth is insufficient.

Interpretation

Growth surrounding a disk indicates the carbohydrate has been assimilated by the yeast, indicating a positive test.

Quality Control

Each new batch of agar and new set of carbohydrate disks should be tested with positive-reacting and negative-reacting yeasts for each carbohydrate tested.

Procedure

Rapid urease test for yeast

Purpose

The production of the enzyme urease is useful in the preliminary identification of *Cryptococcus neoformans*, which is urease positive.

Principle

Urease converts the substrate urea to ammonia and carbon dioxide, which produces an alkaline environment in the medium and is detected by a color change from yellow to pink in the phenol red indicator.

Matcrials

Urea R broth (commercially available from Hardy Diagnostics)

Microdilution plates

Procedure

1. Reconstitute a vial of Urea R broth by adding 3 ml of sterile distilled water. Reagent should be prepared the day it is used.
2. Add three or four drops of the broth into the appropriate number of microtiter wells for the yeast to be tested.
3. Inoculate the broth, using a heavy inoculum of a pure culture of the yeast to be tested.
4. Seal the plate with plastic tape. Incubate for 4 hours at 37°C.

Interpretation

Positive: Pink to purple color, indicating urease production

Negative: No pink to purple color

Quality Control

C. neoformans: Positive control—pink to purple color observed after 4 hours

Candida albicans: Negative control—yellow color observed after 4 hours

Note

Procedure is not reliable for pink-colored yeasts, such as *Rhodotorula*, because of interference from the pigment.

Laboratory Exercises

All procedures should be performed using a biological safety cabinet.

Use the following organisms for exercises 1 and 2, which have been previously plated on Sabouraud dextrose agar (SDA): *Microsporum gypseum, Trichophyton rubrum, Epidermophyton floccosum, Rhizopus, Aspergillus fumigatus,* and *Fusarium.*

1. Examine the colonial morphology of each of the following organisms. Record the pigmentation on top and reverse side, texture, and topography.

Organism	Pigment top	Pigment reverse	Texture	Topography
M. gypseum				
T. rubrum				
E. floccosum				
Rhizopus				
A. fumigatus				
Fusarium				

2. Prepare a tease preparation (wet mount) of each of the following organisms. Examine your slides and make a sketch of your findings; label all significant structures.

M. gypseum
T. rubrum
E. floccosum
Rhizopus
A. fumigatus
Fusarium

3. Inoculate an unknown mold onto SDA and incubate at room temperature. Observe daily for growth, and perform the slide culture when sufficient growth is present.
Unknown Number ________________

Colonial morphology	
Pigment top	
Pigment reverse	
Texture	
Topography	
Microscopic description	

Preliminary Identification: ________________

4. Perform the germ tube test on the following organisms. Draw a picture of your results, labeling the germ tube, hyphae, or pseudohyphae as appropriate.

Yeast	Drawing/Description
Candida albicans	
Candida tropicalis	
Rhodotorula	
Candida glabrata	

5. Inoculate a section of cornmeal with Tween 80 plate for each of the following yeasts. After incubation at 24 or 48 hours, draw a picture of your results, labeling all significant structures.

Organism	Sketch/Description
C. albicans	
C. tropicalis	
Rhodotorula	
T. glabrata	

6. Perform the rapid urease test on *C. albicans* and *T. glabrata*. Record your observations and results.

Organism	Observations	Interpretation
C. albicans		
C. glabrata		

7. Perform carbohydrate assimilation tests on the following organisms. Record your observations and interpret the results.

	C. albicans	*C. tropicalis*	*Rhodotorula*	*T. glabrata*
Glucose				
Maltose				
Sucrose				
Lactose				
Galactose				
Cellobiose				
Raffinose				
Inositol				
Xylose				
Trehalose				
Melibiose				
Dulcitol				

8. Plate an unknown yeast on SDA. Perform the germ tube, cornmeal agar, rapid urease, and carbohydrate assimilation tests on the organism once it has grown.

SDA colonial morphology	
Cornmeal with Tween 80 agar morphology	
Germ tube	
Urease	
Microscopic description	
Carbohydrates assimilated	

Review Questions

Matching

Match the dimorphic fungus with its description:

1. Thick-walled, large-celled, single-budding yeast cells at 37°C and pyriform conidia attached to septate hyphae at 25°C
2. Small, budding yeast cells at 37°C and large, thick-walled tuberculate macroconidia at 25°C
3. Large, round, multibudding yeast cells at 37°C and small, septate, branched hyphae with chlamydoconidia at 25°C
4. Thick-walled, round spherules on direct examination and thick-walled, septate, barrel-shaped arthroconidia at 25°C
5. Small, cigar-shaped yeast cells at 37°C and small, oval conidia arranged singly or as flowerets
   a. *Blastomyces dermatitidis*
   b. *Sporothrix schenckii*
   c. *Coccidioides immitis*
   d. *Paracoccidioides brasiliensis*
   e. *Histoplasma capsulatum*

Match the yeast or yeastlike fungus with its significant characteristics:

6. Germ tube produced
7. Encapsulated and urease positive
8. Orange-red pigment
9. Fragmented hyphae and rectangular arthroconidia on cornmeal agar
10. Small budding yeast that assimilates glucose and trehalose
    a. *Geotrichum candidum*
    b. *Candida albicans*
    c. *Cryptococcus neoformans*
    d. *Candida glabrata*
    e. *Rhodotorula*

Multiple Choice

11. The type of asexual spore produced by simple budding off from the mother cell is a (an):
    a. Ascospore
    b. Blastospore
    c. Chlamydospore
    d. Sporangiospore
12. The fundamental unit of the fungus is the:
    a. Hypha
    b. Conidium
    c. Mycelium
    d. Capsule
13. The vegetative hyphae:
    a. Absorb nutrients and water for the fungus
    b. Extend into the air
    c. Are known also as the reproductive hyphae
    d. Contain the spores or conidia
14. Using the botanical taxonomy, the division of fungi that causes the majority of fungal infections is the:
    a. Zygomycota
    b. Ascomycota
    c. Basidomycota
    d. Deuteromycota
15. Which microscopic method is preferred to examine nails, skin, or hair?
    a. Saline mount
    b. KOH preparation
    c. India ink
    d. Giemsa stain
16. Small, oval intracellular yeast cells appearing in Giemsa-stained preparations of bone marrow or peripheral blood should most likely be worked up as:
    a. *Candida albicans*
    b. *Microsporum gypseum*
    c. *Blastomyces dermatitidis*
    d. *Histoplasma capsulatum*
17. Fungal cultures should be held and observed for growth for at least:
    a. 72 hours
    b. 1 week
    c. 1 month
    d. 2 months
18. Which of the following techniques best maintains the microscopic morphology of the fungus?
    a. Tease mount
    b. Cellophane preparation
    c. Slide culture
    d. India ink
19. An organism cultured from a case of tinea capitis in a 5-year-old child produced woolly colonies with a bright yellow rim and reverse side. Macroconidia predominated and appeared spindle shaped and multiseptate, with thick walls, warty projections, and curved tips. The most likely identification is:
    a. *Trichophyton tonsurans*
    b. *Epidermophyton floccosum*
    c. *Microsporum canis*
    d. *Microsporum gypseum*
20. A case of tinea unguium produced green-brown, velvety colonies that were gently folded. Microscopically, the fungus produced numerous thin-walled macroconidia with three and four cells. Microconidia were absent. The organism is most likely:
    a. *Trichophyton tonsurans*
    b. *Epidermophyton floccosum*
    c. *Microsporum canis*
    d. *Trichophyton mentagrophytes*

21. A group of darkly pigmented fungi found on vegetation and in the soil are the:
    a. Dermatophytes
    b. Dematiaceous fungi
    c. Dimorphic fungi
    d. Hyalohyphomycetes
22. Dimorphic fungi exhibit:
    a. A mycelial phase at 25°C to 30°C and a yeast phase at 35°C to 37°C
    b. A yeast phase at 25°C to 30°C and a mycelial phase at 35°C to 37°C
    c. Both a mycelial phase and a yeast phase at 25°C to 30°C, depending on the isolation medium
    d. A yeast phase only in vivo and a mycelial phase only in vitro
23. An agent of chromoblastomycosis that is a very slow-growing, black-olive or gray mold and that microscopically produces dark, septate hyphae with primary conidia forming at the tip of the conidiophore with secondary and tertiary conidia is most likely:
    a. *Cladosporium carrionii*
    b. *Exophiala jeanselmi*
    c. *Fonsecaea pedrosoi*
    d. *Pseudoallescheria boydii*
24. A saprobic fungus with branching, aseptate hyphae that grows as fluffy, white to gray molds with brown hyphae in 4 days is most likely a member of the:
    a. Genus *Aspergillus*
    b. Zygomycetes
    c. Phaeohyphomycetes
    d. Hyphomycetes
25. A laboratory contaminant that produced blue-green growth and microscopically showed branching septate hyphae; large, flask-shaped vesicles; phialides; uniserated heads; and parallel chains of conidia covering the upper half of the vesicle is most likely:
    a. *Rhizopus*
    b. *Absidia*
    c. *Aspergillus fumigatus*
    d. *Aspergillus flavus*
    e. *Penicillium*
26. Which of the following is characterized by aseptate hyphae, stolons with rhizoids, and sporangiophores giving rise to sporangia in an internodal attachment?
    a. *Aspergillus*
    b. *Mucor*
    c. *Rhizopus*
    d. *Absidia*

Bibliography

Brummer, E., Castaneda, A., & Restreppo, A. (1993). Paracoccidioidomycosis: An update. *Clinical Microbiology Reviews, 6,* 89–117.

Cox, R. A., & Magee, D. M. (2004). Coccidioidomycosis: Host response and vaccine development. *Clinical Microbiology Reviews, 17,* 804–839.

Elewski, B. E. (1998). Onychomycosis: Pathogenesis, diagnosis, and management. *Clinical Microbiology Reviews, 11,* 415–429.

Fidel, P. L., Vazquez, J. A., & Sobel, J. D. (1999). *Candida glabrata*: Review of epidemiology, pathogenesis, and clinical disease with comparison to *C. albicans*. *Clinical Microbiology Reviews, 12,* 80–96.

Forbes, B. A., Sahm, D. F., & Weissfeld, A. S. (2007). Laboratory methods in basic mycology. In *Bailey and Scott's diagnostic microbiology*, 12th ed. (pp. 629–713). St. Louis, MO: Mosby.

Fridkin, S. K., & Jarvis, W. R. (1996). Epidemiology of nosocomial fungal infections. *Clinical Microbiology Reviews, 9,* 499–511.

Guarner, J., & Brandt, M. E. (2011). Histopathologic diagnosis of fungal infections in the 21st century. *Clinical Microbiology Reviews, 24,* 247–280.

Guarro, J., Gene, J., & Stchigel, A. M. (1999). Developments in fungal taxonomy. *Clinical Microbiology Reviews, 12,* 454–500.

Kojic, E. M., & Darouiche, R. O. (2004). *Candida* infections of medical devices. *Clinical Microbiology Reviews, 17,* 255–267.

Koneman, E. W., & Fann, S. E. (1971). *Practical laboratory mycology*, 3rd ed. Baltimore, MD: Williams & Wilkins.

Latge, J. P. (1999). *Aspergillus fumigatus* and aspergillosis. *Clinical Microbiology Reviews, 12,* 310–350.

Marcon, M. J., & Powell, D. (1992). Human infections due to *Malassezia* species. *Clinical Microbiology Reviews, 5,* 101–119.

McGinnis, M. R. (1980). *Laboratory handbook of medical mycology*. New York, NY: Academic Press.

Merz, W. (1990). *Candida albicans* strain delineation. *Clinical Microbiology Reviews, 3,* 321–324.

Musial, C. E., Cockerill, II, F. R., & Roberts, G. D. (1988). Fungal infections of immunocompromised hosts: Clinical and laboratory aspects. *Clinical Microbiology Reviews, 1,* 349–364.

Nucci, M., & Anaissie, E. (2007). *Fusarium* infections in immunocompromised patients. *Clinical Microbiology Reviews, 20,* 695–704.

Pappagianis, D., & Zimmer, B. L. (1990). Serology of coccidioidomycosis. *Clinical Microbiology Reviews, 3,* 247–268.

Rippon, J. W. (1988). Medical mycology—the pathogenic fungi and pathogenic actinomycetes (3rd ed.) Philadelphia, PA: Saunders.

Saccente, M., & Woods, G. L. (2010). Clinical and laboratory update on blastomycosis. *Clinical Microbiology Reviews, 23,* 367–381.

Salkin, I. F., Land, G. A., Hurd, N. J., Goldson, P. R., & McGinnis, M. R. (1997). Evaluation of Yeastident and Uni-Yeast-Tek yeast identification systems. *Journal of Clinical Microbiology, 25,* 624–627.

Singh, N., & Paterson, D. L. (2005). *Aspergillus* infections in transplant recipients. *Clinical Microbiology Reviews, 18,* 44–69.

Trofa, D., Gacser, A., & Nosanchuk, J. D. (2008). *Candida parapsilosis,* an emerging fungal pathogen. *Clinical Microbiology Reviews, 21,* 606–625.

Weems, J. J. (1992). *Candida parapsilosis*: Epidemiology, pathogenicity, clinical manifestations, and antimicrobial susceptibility. *Clinical Infectious Diseases, 14,* 75.

Yeo, S. F., & Wong, B. (2002). Current status of nonculture methods for diagnosis of invasive fungal infections. *Clinical Microbiology Reviews, 15,* 465–484.

CHAPTER 21

Introduction to Medical Parasitology

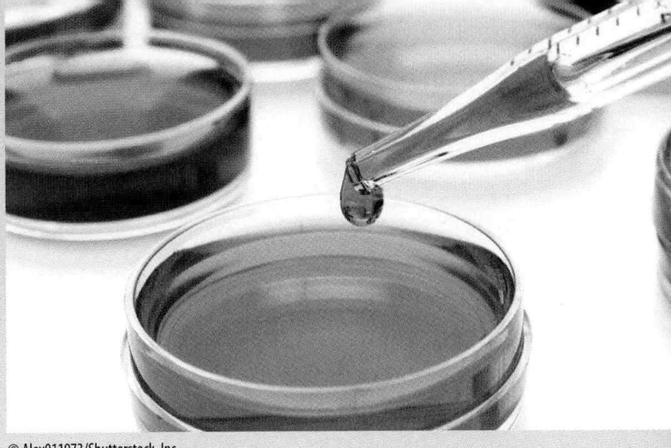

CHAPTER OUTLINE

Introduction and Definitions
Specimen Collecting, Processing, and Examining of Stool Specimens
Protozoa
Nematodes
Cestodes
Trematodes

KEY TERMS

Accidental host
Amastigote
Bradyzoites
Cercaria
Coracidium
Cyst form
Cysticercus
Definitive host
Digenetic
Ectoparasite
Endoparasite
Epimastigote
Exoerythrocytic schizogony
Facultative parasites
Gravid proglottids
Hermaphroditic
Incidental host
Intermediate host
Macrogametes
Merogony
Merozoites
Metacercaria
Microgametes
Miracidium
Obligate parasites
Oocysts
Parasitism
Plerocercoid
Procercoid
Proglottids
Promastigote
Redia
Rostellum
Schizogony
Schizont
Scolex
Sporogony
Sporozoites
Strobila
Tachyzoites
Trophozoite form
Trypomastigote
Vectors

LEARNING OBJECTIVES

1. Describe the requirements for suitable collection of stool specimens for parasitic examination.
2. Describe and contrast the flotation and sedimentation methods for the concentration of stool specimens.
3. Perform at least two flotation or sedimentation procedures for stool concentration.
4. Describe the use of the following stains in the examination of parasites:
   a. Iodine and merthiolate-(thimerosal-)iodine-formalin (MIF)
   b. Trichrome
   c. Modified acid-fast
5. Describe how thick and thin blood smears are prepared and stained.
   a. State the purpose of each smear.
   b. Interpret at least two blood smears for blood parasites, identifying any parasites.
6. Describe the important characteristics of the cyst and trophozoite forms of the following amoebas. Identify each from stained smears, pictures, or microphotographs and discuss the clinical significance of each.
   a. *Entamoeba histolytica*
   b. *Entamoeba coli*
   c. *Iodamoeba butschlii*
7. Describe the important identifying characteristics of the following flagellates and ciliate. Identify each from stained smears, pictures, or images and discuss the clinical significance of each.
   a. *Giardia lamblia*
   b. *Trichomonas vaginalis*
   c. *Trichomonas hominis*
   d. *Chilomastix mesnili*
   e. *Dientamoeba fragilis*
   f. *Balantidium coli*
8. Discuss the clinical significance and identification of the following:
   a. *Toxoplasma gondii*
   b. *Cryptosporidium parvum*
   c. *Cystoisospora belli*
   d. *Cyclospora cayetanensis*
9. Recite the life cycle of *Plasmodium*, indicating the infective stage for humans and mosquitoes.
10. Recognize and discuss the important morphological characteristics of the following *Plasmodium* species:
    a. *P. falciparum*
    b. *P. vivax*
    c. *P. malariae*
    d. *P. ovale*
11. Discuss the life cycle of *Babesia* and explain how the infection is diagnosed.
12. Differentiate *Trypanosoma brucei* subspecies *rhodesiense* from *Trypanosoma brucei* subspecies *gambiense*, including the following:
    a. Clinical significance and course of disease
    b. Identifying characteristics
13. List the agent of Chagas disease and explain how it is identified and transmitted.
14. Discuss the life cycle of *Leishmania*, listing the important species and the infections associated with each.
15. Recite the life cycle, indicate and identify the infectious and diagnostic stages, and state the common name of each of the following nematodes:
    a. *Strongyloides stercoralis*
    b. *Necator americanus*
    c. *Ancylostoma duodenale*
    d. *Enterobius vermicularis*
    e. *Ascaris lumbricoides*
    f. *Trichuris trichiura*
16. Examine at least two cellulose acetate or paddle preparations for the presence of pinworm.
17. Differentiate the microfilariae of the clinically important filarial worms and briefly discuss the infection associated with each organism.
18. Recite the life cycle, identify the infectious and diagnostic stages, and state the common name of each of the following cestodes:
    a. *Diphyllobothrium latum*
    b. *Hymenolepsis nana*
    c. *Hymenolepsis diminuta*
    d. *Taenia saginata*
    e. *Taenia solium*
19. Recite the life cycle, identify the infectious and diagnostic stages, and state the common name of each of the following trematodes:
    a. *Fasciolopsis buski*
    b. *Fasciola hepatica*
    c. *Paragonimus westermani*
20. Discuss the life cycle and identification of the schistosomes and differentiate *Schistosoma japonicum*, *S. haematobium*, and *S. mansoni* based on the location of infection and characteristics of the egg.

Introduction and Definitions

Human parasites are found worldwide, with most infections occurring in the tropics. Estimates of the number of parasitic infections is inaccurate because reporting of morbidity and mortality in many of the endemic areas is poor or nonexistent. Medical parasitology has become increasingly important in the clinical microbiology laboratory in the United States in recent years. This can be attributed to a number of factors, including the increased incidence of isolation of medically significant parasites in the immunosuppressed population, which includes those afflicted with acquired immunodeficiency syndrome (AIDS). The influx of immigrants from parts of the world with endemic levels of parasites and the increase in travel to foreign lands where parasites are more common have also increased the incidence of parasitic infections in the United States. Traveling to tropical areas, where insect bites can transmit malarial parasites, or swimming in fresh tropical waters, where schistosomal infections may be acquired, illustrates these modes of transmission. Drinking contaminated water and eating contaminated foods, such as raw or uncooked fruits, vegetables, and meats, are other routes of acquiring parasitic infections in foreign countries. This chapter serves as an introduction to medical parasitology, with emphasis on the major types of parasitic infections and their life cycles and microscopic identification.

The classification of human parasites can follow various schemes. BOX 21-1 summarizes clinically significant parasites, using the major subdivisions for classification.

Parasitism is a relationship in which one organism, the **host**, is injured through the actions of the other organism, or **parasite**. The host is an animal or plant in which the parasite lives and grows. In a symbiotic relationship, there is a close and lengthy association between two or more organisms of different species. This relationship may benefit one but not necessarily both of the organisms. In the case of parasitism the relationship is beneficial to the parasite but injurious to the host. **Obligate parasites** cannot survive without their designated host, whereas **facultative parasites** may exist in a free-living state as a commensal or a parasite. In the commensal state, the relationship is beneficial to the parasite without harming the host.

Parasites may have a simple or complex life cycle, requiring one or more hosts. An **accidental**, or **incidental, host** refers to infection of a host that is not the usual

BOX 21-1 Classification of Medically Significant Parasites

I. Protozoa
- **A.** Amoebas—Intestinal
  1. *Entamoeba histolytica*
  2. *Entamoeba coli*
  3. *Entamoeba hartmanni*
  4. *Entamoeba polecki*
  5. *Iodamoeba butschlii*
  6. *Endolimax nana*
- **B.** Flagellates—Intestinal
  1. *Giardia lamblia*
  2. *Trichomonas hominis*
  3. *Trichomonas vaginalis* (vaginal parasite)
  4. *Dientamoeba fragilis*
  5. *Chilomastix mesnili*
- **C.** Ciliate—Intestinal
  Balantidium coli
- **D.** Coccidia—Intestinal
  1. *Cryptosporidium parvum*
  2. *Cystoisospora belli*
  3. *Cyclospora cayetanensis*
- **E.** Amoebas from other body sites
  1. *Naegleria fowleri*
  2. *Acanthamoeba*
- **F.** Miscellaneous protozoa
  1. *Toxoplasma gondii* (coccidia)
  2. Microsporidians
  3. *Blastocystis hominis*
- **G.** Sporozoa from blood and tissue
  1. Malarial parasites: *Plasmodium* species
     - **a.** *P. falciparum*
     - **b.** *P. vivax*
     - **c.** *P. malariae*
     - **d.** *P. ovale*
  2. *Babesia species*
- **H.** Hemoflagellates from blood and tissue
  1. *Trypanosoma* species
     - **a.** *T. brucei* subspecies *gambiense*
     - **b.** *T. brucei* subspecies *rhodesiense*
     - **c.** *T. cruzi*

(continues)

BOX 21-1 Classification of Medically Significant Parasites (Continued)

2. *Leishmania* species
    a. *L. tropica*
    b. *L. donovani*
    c. *L. braziliensis*
    d. *L. mexicana*

II. Nematodes (roundworms)

A. Intestinal nematodes
1. *Necator americanus*
2. *Ancylostoma duodenale*
3. *Ascaris lumbricoides*
4. *Enterobius vermicularis*
5. *Trichuris trichiura*
6. *Strongyloides stercoralis*

B. Tissue nematodes
1. *Trichinella spiralis*
2. *Toxocara canis*

C. Blood and tissue nematodes—Filarial worms
1. *Wuchereria bancrofti*
2. *Brugia malayi*
3. *Loa loa*
4. *Onchocerca volvulus*
5. *Mansonella* species

III. Cestodes (flatworms)

A. *Taenia saginata*
B. *Taenia solium*
C. *Diphyllobothrium latum*
D. *Echinococcus granulosus*
E. *Hymenolepsis nana*
F. *Hymenolepsis diminuta*
G. *Dipylidium caninum*

IV. Trematodes (flukes)

A. Blood flukes
1. *Schistosoma mansoni*
2. *Schistosoma haematobium*
3. *Schistosoma japonicum*

B. Intestinal, liver, or lung flukes
1. *Fasciolopsis buski*
2. *Fasciola hepatica*
3. *Clonorchis (Opisthorchis) sinensis*
4. *Paragonimus westermani*

host for the parasite. The parasite may or may not complete the life cycle in the accidental host. The adult and sexual reproductive phases of the parasite occur in the **definitive host**. The larval, or asexual reproductive phase, occurs in the **intermediate host**. Some parasites need one or two intermediate hosts to complete their life cycles, while other parasites do not require an intermediate host. A host also can serve as a **carrier**, in which case the parasite is present in the host, but there are no signs of infection. Carriers can transmit the parasite to other animal and plant hosts. **Vectors** are arthropod or other carriers of certain parasites that serve as modes of transmission to the host.

Ectoparasites are found on the outside, or surface, of the body, and **endoparasites** live within the host.

Specimen Collecting, Processing, and Examining of Stool Specimens

COLLECTION AND PROCESSING OF STOOL SPECIMENS

Because many parasitic infections are diagnosed through recovery of the egg or larva in feces, proper collection and processing methods are essential for identification. Fecal specimens should be collected before any radiologic procedures that use barium sulfate are conducted because such procedures may obscure the visualization of the parasite. Medications that may interfere with detection include certain antibiotics, such as tetracycline; antimalarial medications; antidiarrheal products that are not absorbed; mineral oil; and bismuth. During collection, contact with water that may have free-living parasites should be avoided. Contact with urine, through collection with a bedpan or through the toilet bowl, is discouraged because urine may destroy motile parasites in the specimen.

The stool specimen is collected into a clean, waxed, cardboard container, with a wide opening and tight-fitting lid.

The number of specimens required to diagnose a parasitic infection depends on the type and severity of infection, quality of the sample submitted, and the examination performed. A general rule is that before therapy, a minimum of three fecal specimens should be collected. Castor oil or mineral oil laxatives should be avoided because oil decreases the motility of the trophozoite form of intestinal protozoa. Increasing the number of samples collected will enhance positive findings. Specimens collected on alternate days instead of those collected daily may also enhance the recovery. The specimen is accurately and completely labeled.

Freshly passed stools are needed for the detection of the trophic forms of amoebas and flagellates. The cyst form is more readily found in formed stools, whereas the trophozoite form is more readily found in liquid stools. Liquid samples should be examined within a half hour of collection, and soft or semisoft stools should be examined within 1 hour of collection. If this is not possible, the stool can be refrigerated at 3°C to 5°C for up to 4 hours. Stools must not be left at room temperature, incubated, or frozen. When examination within these time constraints is not possible, the stool should be placed into a preservative, such as polyvinyl alcohol (PVA), to maintain the morphological characteristics needed to identify the organism. PVA, which is a combination of Schaudinn's fixative (mercuric chloride and ethyl alcohol), polyvinyl alcohol, glycerin, and glacial acetic acid, preserves protozoan cysts and trophozoites. One part fecal material is mixed with three parts PVA directly on a slide. The mixture is spread and allowed to air-dry for several hours at 35°C or overnight at room temperature.

A gross macroscopic examination of the feces includes examination for proglottids and adult worms, which may be visible on the specimen's surface. Areas containing mucus and blood should be examined more carefully because the parasite may be concentrated in these areas of the specimen.

MICROSCOPIC EXAMINATION

A quality binocular microscope with a calibrated micrometer is necessary for the identification of parasitic eggs, cysts, and trophozoites. Oculars of both 5× and 10× magnification are recommended, as well as high-dry (40× or 43×) and oil-immersion (100×) objectives.

The identification of parasites depends on the accurate measurement of the organism, which requires a calibration of the microscope. A micrometer disk, which is generally calibrated into 50 units, is placed into the ocular of the microscope. These units are compared with those on a known calibrated scale, most often a stage micrometer with a scale divided into 0.1 mm and 0.01 mm divisions. Each objective must be calibrated on the microscope.

DIRECT SMEARS

The primary purpose of the direct wet mount is to detect the motile trophozoite amoebas and flagellates. The smear is prepared by mixing a small amount of feces with 1 drop of physiological saline, adding a coverslip, and examining the slide for trophozoites. The mount should be thin enough so that newsprint can be read through the slide. When using a 22 mm × 22 mm coverslip, the entire area under the coverslip should be scanned using the 10× objective with low-intensity light. Next, the 40× objective is used to examine any material resembling a parasite. The smear should be prepared by sampling various parts of the fecal sample, especially those areas that contain blood or mucus. The smear also is observed for the presence of helminth eggs, larvae, and protozoan cysts as well as for the type of motility. Protozoan trophozoites and flagellates are pale and transparent in the direct preparation.

One drop of iodine is then placed at the edge of the coverslip so that it may diffuse into the smear. Weak iodine solutions of a 1% concentration highlight the internal structures of the parasites. Suitable solutions include D'Antoni's, Lugol's, and Dobell and O'Connor's. D'Antoni's iodine solution is prepared by adding 1.0 g of potassium iodide to 1.5 g of powdered iodine crystals in 100 ml of distilled water. Gram's iodine in full strength is *not* suitable for parasitic staining; diluted Gram's iodine, however, may be used for staining. Protozoan cysts have yellow cytoplasm, brown glycogen inclusions when present, and pale nuclei when observed using the iodine mount.

CONCENTRATION METHODS FOR STOOL SPECIMENS

Fecal concentration methods enhance the detection of smaller amounts of parasites that may not be detected in the direct mount. Thus, concentration methods should be performed on all stool specimens submitted for the examination of ova and parasites. Two types of concentration methods, flotation and sedimentation, can be used to separate intestinal protozoa and helminth eggs from fecal debris. Flotation methods separate protozoan cysts and helminth eggs through use of a high-specific gravity solution, usually zinc sulfate. The parasitic forms float to the top of the solution and can be skimmed from the surface film, while the debris forms a sediment at the bottom of the tube. Flotation provides a very clean concentrate, but certain operculated eggs and protozoa do not float well and thus would not be detected. Thus, sedimentation methods, which rely on gravity or centrifugation, are preferred because all protozoa, eggs, and larvae can be sedimented. A drawback of sedimentation is the presence of additional fecal debris, which decreases the smear's clarity. In sedimentation methods, formalin is frequently used as a fixative for the eggs, larvae, or cysts. Fecal debris is extracted into the ether phase of the reaction, which frees the sediment parasitic forms from the fecal material.

The zinc sulfate flotation procedure and formalin-ether sedimentation procedure are found at the end of this chapter.

PERMANENTLY STAINED MOUNTS

Permanently stained mounts are recommended for stool samples submitted for the identification of ova and parasites. These mounts provide a permanent record of the organisms identified. Permanently stained smears can be prepared from fresh or PVA-preserved material.

For fresh stools, a small amount of the fecal material is smeared with an applicator stick onto two clean slides. Next, the slide is immersed immediately into Schaudinn's fixative for 30 minutes, which fixes the material to the slide and preserves the morphology. Liquid stools are first mixed with PVA by mixing 1 or 2 drops of the stool with 3 or 4 drops of PVA. Then, the mixture is spread on the slide and allowed to air-dry for several hours at 35°C or overnight at room temperature.

For PVA-fixed material, slides are prepared by thoroughly mixing the specimen and straining through gauze to remove any large particles. After sedimentation, a portion of the feces is removed with applicator sticks and placed on blotting paper or another absorbent material to remove any excess PVA. The material is then streaked onto slides and allowed to airdry at room temperature for 2 hours or at 37°C for 1 hour. The slides are stained or can be stored for later staining.

Merthiolate-iodine-formalin (MIF) stain is a combination preservative, fixative, and stain for direct examination of feces. The solution contains Lugol's iodine solution and merthiolate (thimerosal) as staining agents and formaldehyde as the fixative. MIF is suitable for fixation and staining of trophozoites and cysts.

The Wheatley adaptation of the trichrome stain can be used to stain both fresh material and PVA-preserved material. Properly fixed and stained smears produce green background debris with blue-green to purple cytoplasm with red or red-purple nuclei and inclusions. Helminth eggs and larvae stain dark red or purple but often are distorted and difficult to identify. The color of white blood cells (WBCs), yeast, and other tissue cells may resemble those of the parasites, which may present identification problems.

Iron hematoxylin stain can be used with fresh or PVA-preserved material. Background debris and the parasites stain gray-blue to black, with the nuclei and other inclusions stained darker than the cytoplasm. The modified acid-fast stain is used to identify *Cryptosporidium* and other coccidia-like organisms.

There also are qualitative immunochromatographic assays for specific parasites, such as *Giardia* and *Cryptosporidium*, which are two frequent causes of parasitic infection. One example is the ColorPAC Giardia/Cryptosporidium assay (Becton Dickinson), which detects *Giardia* and *Cryptosporidium* antigens simultaneously in stool specimens.

BLOOD SPECIMENS

Blood specimens are collected to detect blood parasites, such as *Plasmodium*, the agent of malaria. Both thick and thin blood smears are used. The thick blood smear allows for the examination of a larger volume of blood and is used to screen the specimen for parasites. The thin blood smear is used to identify the parasite if the screen is positive. Blood is collected at 6- to 18-hour intervals on 3 successive days. Free-flowing earlobe or finger stick collections are preferred. Ideally, no anticoagulant is recommended because the viability and morphology of the parasites can be affected. EDTA anticoagulated blood specimens can be used if necessary.

The procedures for preparing and staining thin and thick blood films are found at the end of this chapter.

Protozoa

The protozoa are divided into four groups:

- Amoebas, which are motile by pseudopods
- Flagellates, which are motile by one or more flagella
- Ciliates, which are covered with short hairlike structures known as cilia
- Coccidia

The protozoan parasites are unicellular, and most, with the exception of the flagellate *Trichomonas vaginalis*, inhabit the small intestine. Most protozoans have two developmental stages: the cyst form and the trophozoite form. The rigid **cyst form** is nonmotile and usually found in the formed stool and is the infectious form of the parasite. The pleomorphic **trophozoite form** is usually found in loose or watery stools and is motile. The cyst form usually indicates inactive infection or the carrier state, whereas the trophozoite stage, the active feeding form, is associated with active disease. The trophozoite form is more sensitive to environmental changes, especially temperature, and rapidly deteriorates in the specimen, while the cyst form is more resistant to environmental changes. The transformation of the cyst form to the trophozoite form is known as encystation. This occurs after the cyst is ingested by the host.

INTESTINAL AMOEBAS

The amoebas include free-living and parasitic organisms that are found as pathogens and nonpathogens in the intestinal tract. The amoebas are motile through cytoplasmic extensions known as pseudopods. Important characteristics to identify the amoebas include size, shape, motility, the number of nuclei, size and location of the karyosome (nucleolus), and presence or absence and characteristics of peripheral chromatin. Cytoplasmic characteristics useful in identification include granularity of the cytoplasm; delineation of the ectoplasm and endoplasm; and the presence of vacuoles, ingested materials (red blood cells, bacteria, yeast, debris), glycogen, and chromatoidal bodies.

Entamoeba histolytica, a human pathogen, is an agent of amoebic dysentery. Its life cycle is summarized in BOX 21-2. The cyst form is ingested, and each cyst produces eight small trophozoites in the small intestine. The trophozoites invade the tissue and multiply and then encyst as they enter the lower intestinal tract as water is concentrated from the feces. The cyst form is passed from the body through the feces in formed or semisolid stools.

> **BOX 21-2 Life Cycle of *Entamoeba histolytica***
>
> 1. Ingest infective cysts in/on contaminated food, water, fomites, contaminated hands
> 2. Encystation in small intestine and cyst form is transformed into trophozoite form
> 3. Trophozoite in large intestine multiplies asexually by binary fission
> 4. Cyst (diagnostic and infectious stage) passed in stool and ingested

The primary infection, intestinal amoebiasis, which may be subclinical, occurs in the gastrointestinal tract. Intestinal amoebiasis may be characterized by abdominal pain, anorexia, weight loss, and bloody diarrhea. Trophozoites may spread through the blood or lymphatic vessels to the liver, lungs, or brain, where secondary infections or extraintestinal amoebiasis may occur. The infection is found most often in underdeveloped, tropical countries, although intestinal amoebiasis exists worldwide. The most common source of infection is food or water contaminated with stools containing cysts.

Intestinal amoebiasis is diagnosed through the identification of the cyst or trophozoite stage in the stool specimen. However, the presence of cysts in the stool does not always indicate active infection.

There are other intestinal amoebas of which are nonpathogens or of limited pathogenicity. Including *Entamoeba coli*, *E. hartmanni*, *E. polecki*, *Endolimax nana*, and *Iodamoeba butschlii*. These are generally considered to be nonpathogenic and are found in the large intestine. *Entamoeba gingivalis* also is considered nonpathogenic and is found in the human oral cavity within the gingival pockets of the teeth. *Entamoeba hartmanni* also is considered to be of low pathogenicity and may be a smaller variant of *E. histolytica*. *Iodamoeba butschlii* is nonpathogenic and characterized by a large glycogen mass, which appears reddish brown with iodine stain in the cyst form.

TABLES 21-1 and **21-2** summarize important characteristics used to identify amoebas. **FIGURE 21-1** illustrates cyst and trophozoite forms of clinically significant amoebas. **FIGURE 21-2** illustrates the trophozoite form of *E. histolytica*.

FREE-LIVING AMOEBAS

Naegleria, *Acanthamoeba*, *Balamuthia*, and *Sappinia* are free-living amoebas found in water, such as rivers, lakes, air-conditioner systems, humidifiers, and cooling towers. Some of the organisms also are found in vegetation, sewage, dust, air, and compost. Infections may be acquired through direct contact with contaminated water, such as by swimming in nonchlorinated lakes. These organisms

TABLE 21-1 Characteristics to Identity Intestinal Amoebas—Cyst Form

Characteristic	*Entamoeba histolytica*	*Entamoeba coli*	*Entamoeba hartmanni*	*Endolimax nana*	*Iodamoeba butschlii*
Pathogenicity	Pathogenic	Commensal	Commensal	Commensal	Commensal
Size diameter or length (µm)	10–20	10–35	5–10	5–10	8–20
Usual range (µm)	12–15	15–12	6–8	6–8	10–12
Shape	Spherical	Usually spherical; may be oval or triangular	Spherical	Spherical, oval, or ellipsoid	Oval, ellipsoid, or bean shaped
Nucleus	Young cyst has 1 nucleus, which increases to 4 nuclei in mature cyst.	Young cyst has 1 to 8 nuclei; mature cyst has 8 nuclei.	Young cyst has 1 or 2 nuclei; mature cyst has 4 nuclei.	One to 4 nuclei. Mature cyst usually contains 4 nuclei.	Usually 1 nucleus and occasionally 2 nuclei are located eccentrically on nuclear membrane.
Karyosome	Small, compact, centrally located	Large; may be compact and eccentric	Small, compact, central	Smaller than in trophozoite form	Large and central and surrounded by retractile granules
Cytoplasm					
Chromatoidal bodies	Two or more blunt-ended, sausage-shaped bodies with smooth, rounded edges	Slender, splinter-shaped bodies with rough, pointed ends	Cigar-shaped, long bodies with blunt smooth ends	None seen. Small, spherical, or elongated granules may be seen.	None usually seen. Occasionally, small granules may be seen.
Glycogen	Diffuse; may be seen in young cysts; usually absent in older cysts	May be present and diffuse or absent	May or may not be present	Diffuse when present	One large mass that stains red-brown with iodine

TABLE 21-2 Characteristics to Identify Intestinal Amoebas—Trophozoite Form

Characteristic	*Entamoeba histolytica*	*Entamoeba coli*	*Entamoeba hartmanni*	*Endolimax nana*	*Iodamoeba butschlii*
Size diameter or length (µm)	10–60	15–50	5–12	6–12	10–20
Usual range (µm)	15–20	20–25	8–10	8–10	12–15
Cytoplasm	Hyaline, finely granular, "ground-glass" appearance; ectoplasm and endoplasm well defined	Granular, "junky"; ectoplasm and endoplasm not well delineated; usually vacuolated	Finely granular	Granular, vacuolated	Coarsely granular with many vacuoles
Nucleus	Single and central or pushed to one side; difficult to see in unstained preparations. Fine peripheral chromatin is usually evenly distributed or beaded.	Single; readily visible in unstained preparations. Chromatin is coarse, irregular, and peripheral.	Single; usually not seen in unstained preparations. Chromatin may appear as solid ring, not beaded.	Large, lobulated; no peripheral chromatin	Large; usually not visible in unstained preparations; no peripheral chromatin
Karyosome	Single, tiny, central, compact	Large, irregular, diffuse, usually eccentric	Small, compact, central, rarely eccentric	Large, irregular, may be round or various other shapes	Large; central, surrounded by retractile granules
Motility	Rapid amoeboid with fingerlike pseudopods	Sluggish, nonprogressive movement with multiple broad, blunt pseudopods	Nonprogressive by single pseudopod	Sluggish, nonprogressive	Sluggish, nonprogressive
Comments	Ingested red blood cells (RBCs) and bacteria may be seen.	May contain bacteria, yeast, and debris. RBCs are never ingested.	May ingest bacteria, yeast, and debris; no RBCs are seen; may be a small variant of *E. histolytica*	May contain bacteria	May contain bacteria, yeast, debris

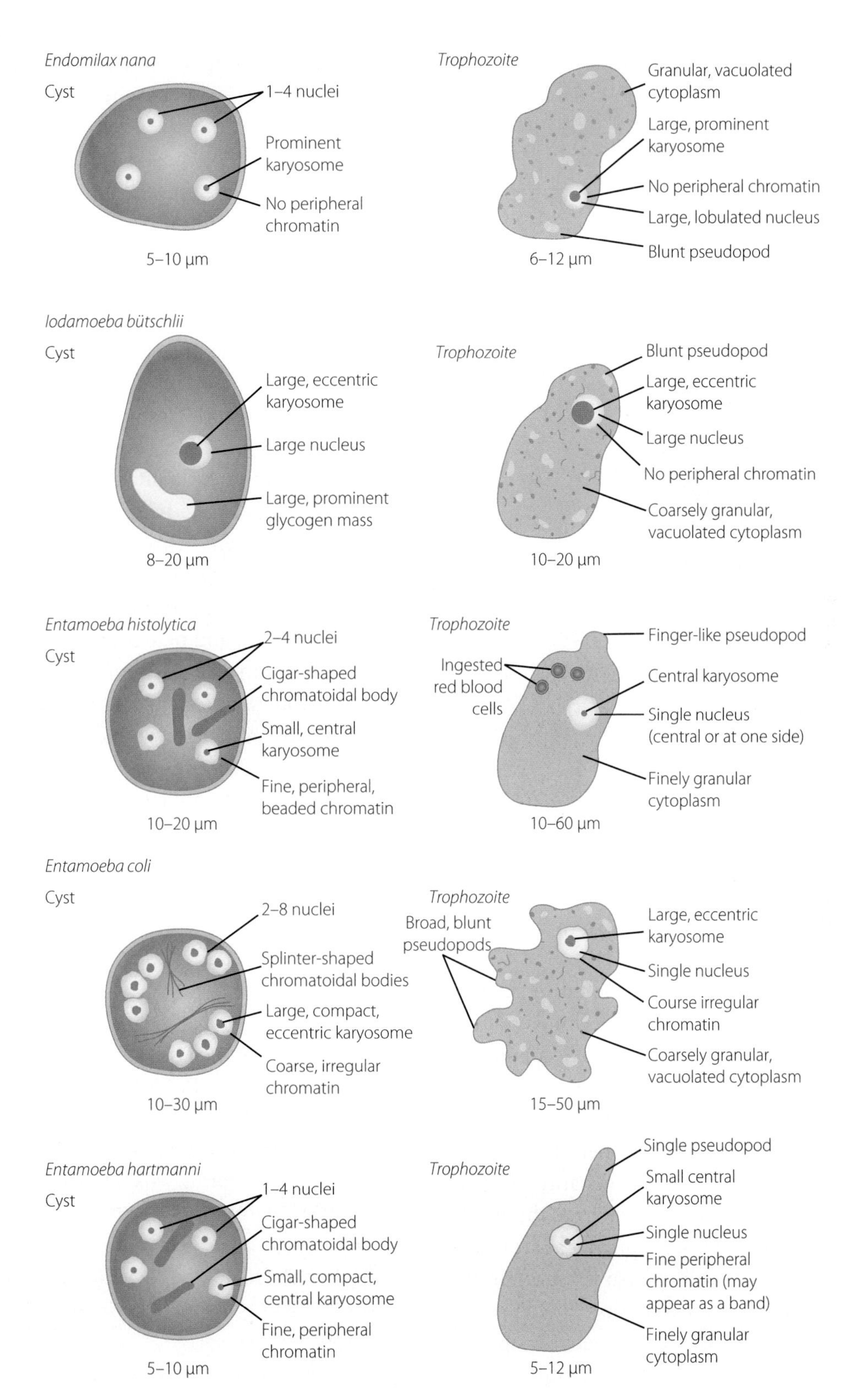

FIGURE 21-1 Cyst and trophozoite forms of common intestinal amoebas.

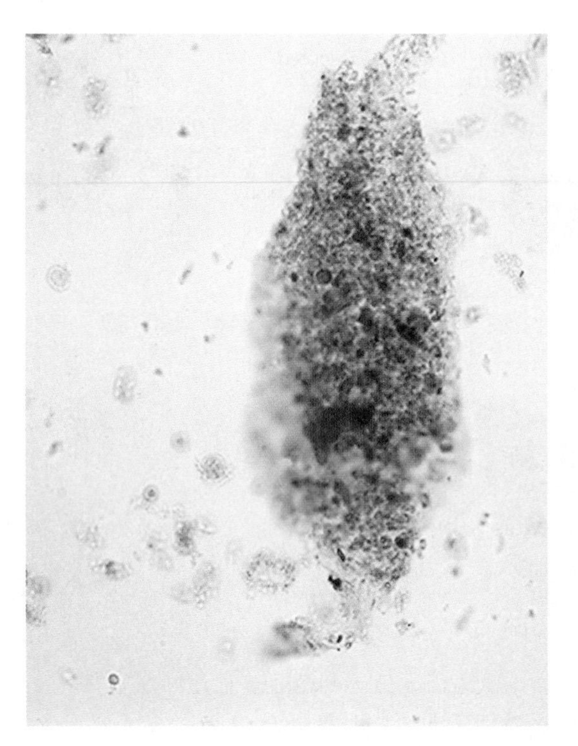

FIGURE 21-2 Trophozoite of *Entamoeba histolytica* showing finely granular cytoplasm and ingested red blood cells.

also may be inhaled in contaminated dust or aerosols or enter the host through breaks in the skin. These free-living amoebas are generally opportunistic pathogens that cause severe infections in the immunocompromised but mild infections, with few if any symptoms, in immunocompetent hosts.

Infections are found worldwide, including in the southern and southeastern regions of the United States. *Acanthamoeba* and *Balamuthia* are causes of granulomatous amoebic encephalitis (GAE) in those who are immunocompromised. *Naegleria* is the cause of an acute and generally fatal infection of the central nervous system known as primary amoebic meningoencephalitis (PAM). The free-living amoebas have been isolated from the lungs, sinuses, eyes, ears, and skin lesions. *Sappinia* is a rare cause of amoebic encephalitis. *Balamuthia* also is found in the environment and has been found as a cause of GAE.

Naegleria fowleri is a cause of PAM, which may appear to be bacterial meningitis because of the predominance of neutrophils in the cerebrospinal fluid. The organism enters the upper respiratory tract through inhalation, often as a result of swimming in contaminated water. The parasite infects the nasal mucosa and spreads along the nerves to the brain and central nervous system. *Naegleria* possesses broad, lobed pseudopods and exhibits active, progressive motility. The organism has a hexagonal, thin-walled cyst that lacks pores and may encyst in tissue. Of note is the organism's ability to transform temporarily into a pear-shaped flagellate when placed into water and its ability to survive in temperatures up to 45°C. *Naegleria* infection is diagnosed by examining the cerebrospinal fluid, which shows an abundance of neutrophils but no bacteria. Diagnosis often is not made until autopsy. BOX 21-3 summarizes characteristics of the life cycle of *Naegleria*.

There are six species of *Acanthamoeba*. These parasites are found in soil, freshwater and saltwater, sewage, swimming pools, dialysis equipment, heating and air-conditioning systems, contact lens solutions, and vegetation. They also have been isolated from human skin and lung specimens, throats, and nostrils. *Acanthamoeba* causes subacute or chronic granulomatous amoebic encephalitis (GAE). Clinical symptoms include headaches, mental confusion, and neurologic deficit, which progress and often result in death. *Acanthamoeba* species can cause granulomatous skin lesions and ulcerative, vision-threatening keratitis, associated with corneal contact with contaminated water. Keratitis occurs most often in those who wear extended-wear contact lenses when the lenses are not properly disinfected or when worn while swimming.

Acanthamoeba organisms are larger in size and more sluggish than are *Naegleria*. *Acanthamoeba* has spiny

BOX 21-3 **Characteristics of *Naegleria***

- *Naegleria fowleri* is found in water, soil, swimming pools, hydrotherapy pools, and aquariums.
- Trophozoites can transform into nonfeeding flagellated forms, which can then revert back into the trophozoite form.
- Trophozoites can penetrate the nasal mucosa of humans, enter the nasal cavity, and then migrate along the olfactory nerves to the brain, infecting the cortex.
- The trophozoites, but not the cysts, are seen in brain tissue and cerebrospinal fluid. Flagellated forms also may be seen in cerebrospinal fluid. The cysts are not observed in brain tissue.
- Cause primary amoebic meningoencephalitis.

pseudopods, known as acanthapodia, and exhibit well-defined ectoplasm and endoplasm. There is no flagellar phase, and the nuclei and cyst forms resemble those of *Naegleria*. *Acanthamoeba* may encyst in tissue. The cysts may be resistant to chlorination and drying. Characteristics of *Acanthamoeba* are summarized in BOX 21-4.

INTESTINAL FLAGELLATES

The flagellates, or Mastigophora, are motile through long extensions of cytoplasm known as flagella. When compared with the amoebas, which have variable shapes, the flagellates are more rigid and maintain their shape. Infections may occur in the intestinal tract and blood and in other tissues. The medically significant flagellates include *Giardia lamblia*, *Trichomonas vaginalis*, *T. hominis*, *Chilomastix mesnili*, and *Dientamoeba fragilis*, which was formerly classified as an amoeba.

Giardia (intestinalis) lamblia

Giardia intestinalis, or *Giardia lamblia*, the agent of giardiasis, is the most frequent parasite associated with gastroenteritis in the United States. Although more commonly known by *G. lamblia*, it is believed that the more correct name is *G. intestinalis*. *Giardia* is found in unfiltered water and untreated lake or pond water and most often infects campers, infants and children in day care, and homosexual males. Infections are contracted after exposure to contaminated food or water. The trophozoite form, found in soft or liquid stools, contains two nuclei with large central karyosomes that may resemble eyes. There is a large, ventral sucking disk in the upper one half of the body. *G. lamblia* is bilaterally symmetrical, with a pointed anterior end and a rounded posterior end, a parallel pair of axonemes, and a parabasal body that is said to resemble a mouth. *G. lamblia* has four pairs of flagella and is motile, with a smooth, rapid motion that has been described as a falling leaf or leaf tumbling in a stream. When observed microscopically, the trophozoite form may give the appearance of a monkey face. **FIGURE 21-3** shows *Giardia* cysts stained with trichrome.

G. lamblia causes an inflammation of the intestinal mucosa that results in acute diarrhea, bloating, nausea, vomiting, and abdominal pain. The infection incubates for 1 day to 2 weeks, and symptoms last for 1 to 3 weeks. More serious or chronic infections can lead to weight loss, malabsorption, and malnutrition. There usually are no red blood cells or white blood cells found in the stool with *Giardia* infection.

Trichomonas

The trophozoite form of *Trichomonas vaginalis* is a pear-shaped, motile parasite approximately 10 to 20 μm in length. The organism has an undulating membrane that extends for half of the length of the organism. There are four anterior flagella, and the organism shows a jerky motility when observed in fresh preparations. There is no cyst form. It is the cause of vaginitis, urethritis, and prostatitis and is generally transmitted through sexual contact.

BOX 21-4 **Characteristics of *Acanthamoeba***

- There are both cyst and trophozoite stages.
- The trophozoites multiply by mitosis and enter the body through breaks in the skin, through inhalation, or through the eye. Cysts also can enter, but only the trophozoites are infective.
- Causes chronic granulomatous amoebic encephalitis (GAE).
- In the eye, ulcerative keratitis occurs. When entering the respiratory system or skin, the organism is spread hematogenously to the central nervous system.
- Both cysts and trophozoites are found in the tissue.

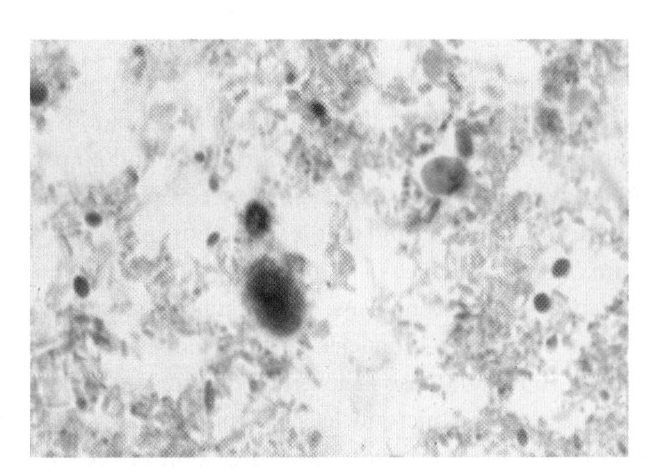

FIGURE 21-3 Cysts of *Giardia lamblia*.

T. vaginalis is found in urine, urethral fluid, and vaginal discharge.

Trichomonas hominis resembles *T. vaginalis* and also is pear shaped; however, it is considered to be nonpathogenic. The trophozoite form has four anterior flagella and an undulating membrane that extends over the whole body of the organism. There is no cyst form.

Other Flagellates

Chilomastix mesnili has a pear-shaped, elongated trophozoite form. A prominent, curved, cytostomal fibril borders the cytostome, resembling a shepherd's crook. It is 6 μm to 10 μm in diameter. The arrangement of fibrils may give the trophozoite form the appearance of an open safety pin. The cyst form is rounded with a clear knob on one end, a single nucleus, and a cytostome. The cyst form may be ingested, but the organism is considered to be nonpathogenic.

Dientamoeba fragilis is the only binucleate flagellate that infects humans. Although classified as a flagellate, the flagella are rarely, if ever, visible. The trophozoite form is 5 to 20 μm in diameter with broad-lobed pseudopods and usually two nuclei ("di"). *Dientamoeba fragilis* has a sluggish, nondirectional motility. The parasite produces a diarrheal syndrome characterized by abdominal pain, nausea, fatigue, malaise, and anorexis. It is transmitted by the fecal–oral route through ingestion of fecally contaminated materials. The infective form is the trophozoite; no cyst form has been demonstrated. The trophozoite multiply asexually by binary fission in the large intestine. It is diagnosed by observing the binucleated forms in stools.

FIGURE 21-4 provides descriptions and figures of the clinically important intestinal flagella.

INTESTINAL CILIATE

The only member of the Ciliophora, or ciliates, that infects humans is *Balantidium coli.* The largest protozoan, this trophozoite measures 50 μm to 100 μm long and 40 μm to 70 μm wide. It is oval shaped, covered completely with cilia of uniform length, and motile with a boring or rotary motion. The organism has a kidney-shaped macronucleus and a spherical micronucleus, which appears as a crescent dot within the macronucleus. The cyst form measures 40 μm to 50 μm and also is covered with cilia and has a macronucleus and a micronucleus. Balantidiasis is a severe diarrheal disease that results from ingestion of the cyst form in fecally contaminated food or water. Encystation occurs in the small intestine; the trophozoites colonize the large intestine. Here they replicate by binary fission and then produce cyst forms. Some of the trophozoites multiply in the lumen of the colon or bowel wall, resulting in the formation of lesions. Mature cyst forms are passed in the stool.

The infection is seen worldwide but more often in the tropics. Because pigs are an important animal reservoir for *B. coli*, balantidiasis is found more often in areas where there is pig farming. Infections in humans may be asymptomatic but in heavy infestations may cause bloody dysentery. Diagnosis is achieved by observation of the cysts in formed stools or the trophozoites in liquid stools.

FIGURE 21-5 provides an image of *B. coli.*

INTESTINAL COCCIDIA

The coccidia are obligate, intracellular parasites that have both sexual and asexual phases in their life cycles. Clinically important intestinal coccidia include *Cryptosporidium* species, *Cystoisospora belli* (formerly known as *Isospora belli*) and *Cyclospora* (formerly known as cyanobacteria-like or coccidia-like bodies, or CLBs).

Cystoisospora belli (Isospora belli)

Cystoisospora belli (*Isospora belli*) is the agent of cystoisosporiasis (isosporiasis), an infection that is either asymptomatic or associated with diarrhea and malabsorption. The infection is most serious in immunosuppressed individuals; AIDS patients have particularly severe infections. Cystoisosporiasis is acquired through the ingestion of infective oocysts in fecally contaminated food or water. Each oocyst contains two round sporoblasts that contain four oval-shaped **sporozoites**, which are released in the small intestine. The sporozoites develop into trophozoites, which then multiply asexually to form a **schizont**, which is a group of immature trophozoites. When the schizont ruptures, merozoites are released, which invade epithelial cells and continue the asexual reproduction. These organisms also may enter a sexual reproductive stage, known as **sporogony**, by forming microgametocytes (male gametes) and macrogametocytes (female gametes). Fertilization between the **microgametes** and **macrogametes** occurs in the intestinal lumen. After fertilization the macrogametes develop into **oocysts**, which are passed in the feces. Because both the sexual and asexual forms occur in the human gastrointestinal tract, no secondary host is needed.

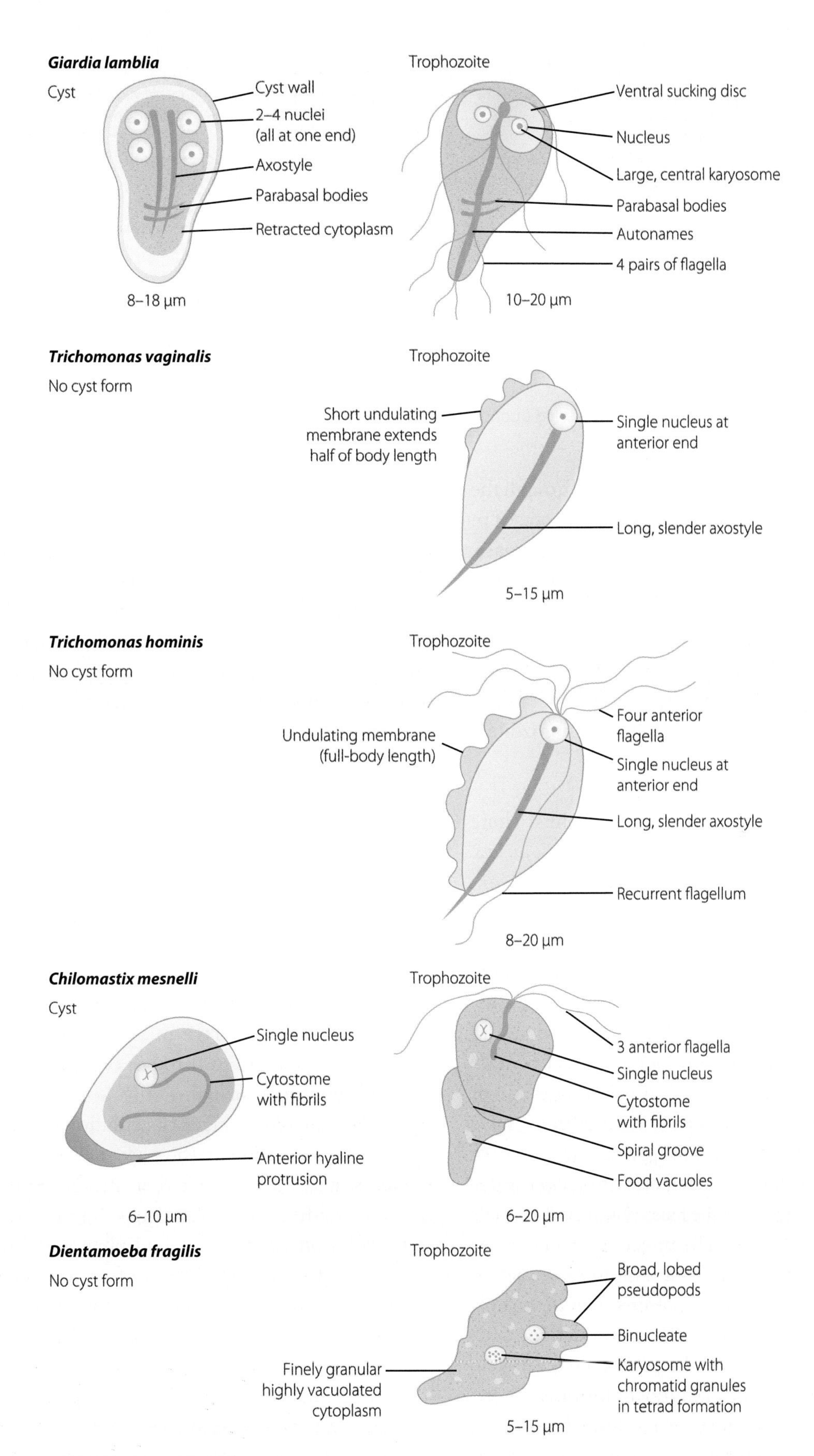

FIGURE 21-4 Clinically important intestinal flagella.

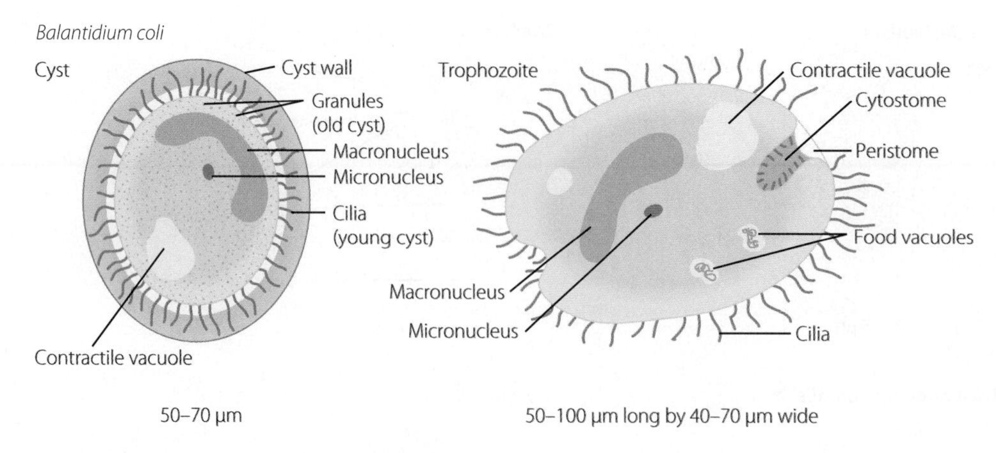

FIGURE 21-5 *Balantidium coli* cyst and trophozoite.

Diagnosis of infection with *C. belli* is made through the observation of either the immature or the mature oocyst in the stool. Immature cysts contain a single granular mass, the sporoblast, which will develop into two sporozoites in the mature cyst. The mature oocyst is ellipsoidal and measures 20 μm to 30 μm by 10 μm to 20 μm in size. The oocysts may be observed in iodine preparations, although detection is enhanced by the modified acid-fast stain, in which the oocysts stain pink with bright red sporozoites.

Cryptosporidium

Cryptosporidium species are agents of enterocolitis. There are several species: *C. parvum*, *C. hominis*, *C. felis*, *C. meleagridis*, *C. canis*, and *C. muris*. *Cryptosporidium parvum* and *C. hominis* are the species that most frequently infect humans. The oocysts of *Cryptosporidium* are resistant to the effects of chlorine and other disinfectants. These infections are found worldwide, with many documented outbreaks, including contaminated water, apple cider, and chicken salad. Routes of infection include direct contact with another infected individual or animal or ingestion of fecally contaminated water or food. Other outbreaks have been linked to community swimming pools, day care centers, and water parks. Exposure to infected animals or water that has been contaminated by the feces of infected animals is another source of infection. The infection incubates for about 1 week and is usually mild in an immunocompetent host, lasting for 1 to 2 weeks. Symptoms include a cholera-like, watery diarrhea, with mucous production, nausea, vomiting, malabsorption, and a low-grade fever. The infection is more severe in the immunocompromised host, especially in AIDS patients, who may develop a devastating, chronic and sometimes fatal diarrheal disease. Other sites of infection may include the lungs and conjunctiva of the eye.

After ingestion or inhalation of the infective oocysts, the infection may incubate for 1 to 2 weeks. Excystation, the release of the infective sporozoites, is followed by their penetration into host cells of the respiratory or gastrointestinal tract or other tissues. Asexual reproduction (**merogony**, or **schizogony**) occurs in the host cells, forming **merozoites**, which develop through the process of gametogony into microgametes and macrogametes. Mating of the microgametes and macrogametes forms zygotes, which in turn form two types of oocysts: thick walled and thin walled. The thick-walled oocysts undergo sporogony, forming sporozoites in the oocysts, which subsequently rupture, releasing the sporozoites to complete the life cycle. The thin-walled oocysts are believed to be involved in autoinfection.

Cryptosporidiosis is diagnosed through observation of the small (4 μm to 5 μm), oval or spherical oocysts in the stool. The oocysts have smooth outer walls, and four sporozoites may be seen within the oocyst. Observation of the oocysts is enhanced through concentrating the stool either through the formalin-ethyl acetate sedimentation method or Sheather's sugar flocculation method. Sheather's sugar flocculation method uses a heavy suspension of the feces in saline, which is then strained through gauze into a centrifuge tube. An equal amount of Sheather's sugar solution (sucrose, melted phenol, distilled water) is added to the strained stool to float the oocysts to the top of the solution. A direct mount is prepared from the coverslip, which is examined using the phase-contrast microscope.

The modified acid-fast method stains the oocysts bright pink to red (**FIGURE 21-6**). An indirect fluorescent procedure, using monoclonal antibodies, also is commercially available.

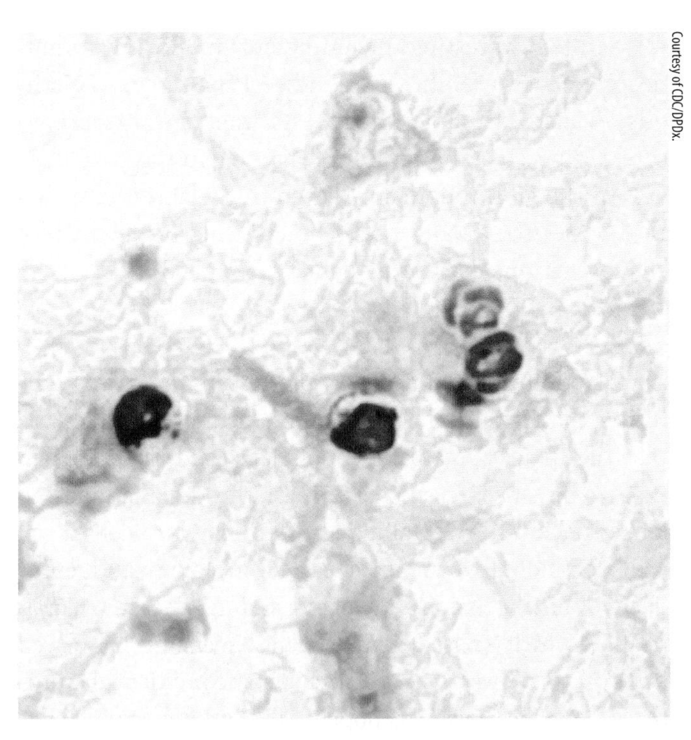

FIGURE 21-6 Modified acid-fast stain of oocysts of *Cryptosporidium parvum.*

Cyclospora cayetanensis

Cyclospora cayetanensis is found worldwide but most often in the tropical and subtropical climates. There have been several food- and water-borne outbreaks in North America in recent years. Fecal–oral transmission does not occur because the oocyst is not infective. Spores form in the environment after days or weeks of incubation in temperatures ranging from 22°C to 32°C. Two sporocysts develop from each oocyst, and each sporocyst contains two long-shaped sporozoites. Water and fresh fruits or vegetables are the typical vehicles for transmission. The oocysts are ingested in the contaminated food or water and then encyst in the gastrointestinal tract. This releases the sporozoites, which then attack the epithelial cells in the small intestine. The sporozoites multiply asexually and also undergo a sexual reproductive phase, which results in the production of oocysts, which are then shed in the stool.

The infection incubates for about 1 week. Symptoms include a severe, watery diarrhea; abdominal pain; nausea; vomiting; weight loss; myalgia; fever; and anorexia. Infections may be mild but are more severe in immunosuppressed individuals. Symptoms can persist for as long as 2 to 3 months when the infection is not treated.

Using the modified acid-fast stain, *Cyclospora* oocysts appear as pink to red cells, but the color may range from clear to purple. The oocysts are not completely round and may be collapsed on one side. The oocyst wall doesn't stain as well when compared to *Cryptococcus* and also shows a wrinkled, granular, or bubbly appearance within the oocyst. A modified safranin stain, which includes heating in a microwave during the staining process, improves the staining quality of *Cyclospora*. The oocysts stain more uniform, appearing red to red-orange, with a more distinct structure when using the modified safranin stain.

MISCELLANEOUS PROTOZOA

Toxoplasma gondii

Toxoplasma gondii is a protozoan parasite that infects the tissue of the human central nervous system. This parasite has worldwide existence, and humans serve as accidental hosts. Classified as a coccidian parasite, the organism has both sexual and asexual life cycles. The sexual cycle, also known as the enteric cycle, occurs in the intestinal cells of domestic cats and felines, which are the only definitive hosts. The asexual, or extraintestinal, cycle involves the multiplication of trophozoites outside of the intestinal tract of felines, cats, and other carnivorous and herbivorous animals, including humans. The enteric cycle is typically completed in cats that ingest the oocysts of *T. gondii*, which have been shed in the feces of another cat or animal, or through ingestion of the trophozoite or cyst form of the parasite in the tissues of a reservoir host. Common reservoir hosts include rodents and birds. After introduction into the feline gastrointestinal tract, asexual multiplication occurs, resulting in the formation of additional trophozoites. Sporogony, the sexual form of the life cycle, then leads to the formation of microgametocytes and macrogametocytes in the intestinal tract of cats. Oocysts are formed and passed in the cat's feces. Although shed for only a few weeks, the oocysts are shed in large numbers. The oocysts are not infective when passed but mature into infective forms in the soil or other suitable environment in 1 to 5 days. Intermediate hosts, such as birds, rodents, and other small mammals, become infected by ingesting water, plants, or soil that are contaminated with the oocysts.

The extraintestinal phase refers to the asexual multiplication of the trophozoites in host cells of the brain, eye, lymph nodes, and heart. Infection begins with the ingestion of oocysts or trophozoites in food or on unwashed hands after contact with infected cat feces. After penetration of the intestinal wall, host cells, most often white blood cells, are directly infected by the parasite. **Tachyzoites** are rapidly forming, crescent-shaped forms of the parasite, which form within the host cells. Two daughter cells are produced in each tachyzoite, and the tachyzoites spread quickly through the body in the blood. The infected cells rupture, releasing the tachyzoites, which can then infect other cells. The replication eventually slows as the host immune system responds to the parasite. Next, **bradyzoites**, formed from this slower replication, accumulate in large numbers in the infected host cells. The bradyzoites become encysted in tissue cysts, where the parasite remains dormant unless the host is immunocompromised. In this case the bradyzoites are released from the cysts, resulting in a new extraintestinal life cycle.

Humans may acquire the infection by several routes. One such route is through the ingestion of tissue cysts in undercooked or raw meat from domestic animals, including cattle, sheep, chicken, and pigs. Another route of infection is the ingestion of food or water that has been contaminated with oocysts passed in cat feces. The oocysts also can be ingested by direct contact with soil or litter box material that has been contaminated with cat feces. Transplacental contact, or congenital infection, may result if a pregnant woman acquires toxoplasmosis during pregnancy. The infection also may be transmitted via blood transfusion or through organ transplant. There has been an increase in toxoplasmosis in immunosuppressed patients, including in those who have AIDS.

Primary infection with *T. gondii* is generally asymptomatic or mild in immunocompetent persons. Lymphoadenopathy, fever, fatigue, and hepatosplenomegaly may be noted. Rare but serious consequences of toxoplasmosis include encephalitis, pneumonitis, and myocarditis.

The parasites form tissue cysts in skeletal muscle and in the heart, brain, and eyes, which may remain dormant for long periods of time. Congenital infection is a serious concern for seronegative mothers who do not have antibody to *T. gondii*. Infections acquired in the third trimester may mildly affect the baby; however, those infections acquired early in the pregnancy can have very damaging effects on the baby, including damage to the central nervous system and eyes. In immunosuppressed adults, including AIDS patients and those with hematologic abnormalities, toxoplasmosis often results in severe disseminated disease.

Toxoplasmosis is diagnosed through demonstration of the pear-shaped or crescent-shaped tachyzoites in tissue sections stained with Wright-Giemsa, periodic acid-Schiff (PAS), or hematoxylin-eosin stains.

Serological testing, including enzyme-linked immunosorbent assay (ELISA) and indirect fluorescence methods, is also available. Such tests must be interpreted carefully because antibodies are observed in approximately half of the adult population, even in the absence of disease. Molecular diagnostic methods, including polymerase chain reaction, also are available.

Blastocystis hominis

The taxonomic classification of *Blastocystis hominis* is confusing; the organism has been reclassified several times as a yeast; a fungus; and an amoeboid, flagellated, or sporozoan protozoan. Once classified as a yeast, this designation is no longer believed to be valid because *B. hominis* lacks a cell wall, does not grow on media used for mycology, and reproduces by binary fission and not by budding. The latest classification, which is based on molecular sequencing, has placed this organism in a group of unicellular and multicellular protists known as the stramenopiles. This group also includes water molds, slime molds, brown algae, and diatoms.

The infection, which is usually gastrointestinal, is acquired via the fecal–oral route through ingestion of food or water contaminated with the infective form, which is the thick-walled cyst. The cysts infect the epithelial cells of the gastrointestinal tract, where asexual multiplication occurs. Vacuolar forms of the parasite develop into amoeboid and multivacuolar forms. The amoeboid form develops into a precyst form, which then forms the thick-walled cyst form, which is excreted in the feces. The multivacuolar form is believed to form a precyst that develops into a thin-walled cyst, which is thought to be involved in autoinfection.

B. hominis is not readily observed in concentrated wet mount stool preparations. *B. hominis* is round and 6 μm to 40 μm in diameter, with a large central body, resembling a vacuole surrounded by many small nuclei. In trichrome stains, the large central body stains gray to green, with bright red inclusion bodies in the cytoplasm.

Infection is frequently associated with immunosuppressed hosts, in particular AIDS patients, and in those who travel abroad.

SPOROZOA FROM BLOOD AND TISSUE

Plasmodium

Parasites of the genus *Plasmodium* are agents of malaria. The four species of *Plasmodium* infectious to humans are *P. falciparum*, *P. vivax*, *P. malariae*, and *P. ovale*.

Plasmodium organisms have a sexual cycle of reproduction, known as sporogony, which occurs in the intestinal tract of the *Anopheles* mosquito—the definitive host. An asexual cycle, known as schizogony, occurs in humans, which are the intermediate hosts.

The *Plasmodium* life cycle begins with the bite of an infective *Anopheles* mosquito whose salivary fluid is filled with infective sporozoites. The sporozoites enter through the wound produced in humans while the mosquito is taking its blood meal. The sporozoite form is motile, spindle shaped, and 10 μm to 15 μm in length. The sporozoite enters the blood within 30 to 60 minutes and then enters the parenchymal cells of the liver, where the first asexual cycle occurs. This is known as **exoerythrocytic schizogony**, or the preerythrocytic cycle, because it does *not* occur within the host erythrocytes but does occur before the erythrocytic cycle. The parasitic nucleus divides repeatedly, and the sporozoite enlarges and then fragments into several daughter cells, which are smaller forms of sporozoites known as merozoites. The duration of this phase and the number of merozoites produced depend on the species. For example, the cycle may last from 5 to 7 days, producing approximately 40,000 merozoites for *P. falciparum*; for *P. vivax*, however, the cycles last 6 to 8 days, producing only 10,000 merozoites. The duration of this cycle is the longest for *P. malariae*, with approximately only 2,000 merozoites produced.

The merozoites then are released into the blood and invade the erythrocytes; this is known as the **intraerythrocytic cycle**. As the merozoites invade the RBCs, early stages known as ring forms develop. These young trophozoites grow in the RBCs, utilizing their hemoglobin and partially metabolizing it to malarial pigment known as **hemozoin**, which stains as black granules in Giemsa- or Wright-stained smears. As the chromatin becomes divided throughout the organism, the cytoplasm divides and arranges with the nuclear fragments, forming mature schizonts, which are composed of individual merozoites. The infected RBCs rupture, releasing the parasites and metabolic toxins into the blood. The merozoites now can invade uninfected RBCs, releasing toxic compounds. If several RBCs rupture at the same time, a malarial paroxysm, with an abrupt onset and characterized by high fever, shaking chills, and sweating, occurs. A periodicity of either 48 or 72 hours is established in several days. The paroxysm is believe to be the host's allergic reaction to the malarial antigens and toxins. In early infections an asynchronous rupture results in either a continuous or a daily fever.

Many generations of merozoites form; some enter into the asexual reproductive cycles, but others enter into a sexual reproductive cycle. The sexual cycles lead to the formation of gametocytes instead of the development of schizonts. The gametocytes circulate in the blood, and the sexual cycle is initiated if the gametocytes are ingested during the blood meal of an infected host with an uninfected *Anopheles* mosquito. The gametocytes mature in the intestines of the mosquito to male, sperm-like, flagellated microgametocytes, which fertilize the female macrogametocytes. Once fertilized, the macrogametocytes produce embryos that mature into round oocysts, or zygotes. The zygotes enter the wall of the mosquito's stomach, where sporogony occurs, resulting in the development of thousands of infective sporozoites that burst from the oocysts. The sporozoites next travel to the salivary glands of the mosquito, awaiting injection into the next human host during the blood meal. **FIGURE 21-7** shows the *Plasmodium* life cycle.

Clinical symptoms of malaria begin with a prodromal period of headache, myalgia, anorexia, and a low-grade fever. As the erythrocytes periodically burst, the paroxysm of shaking chills begins, lasting for 10 to 15 minutes. As the chills subside, the fever spikes, and there is skin flushing, a severe headache, pain in the limbs and back, and disorientation. As the fever declines, the patient sweats profusely and falls asleep until the next paroxysm begins.

The periodicity of the fever is classified as either quartan or tertian. Tertian periodicity occurs every 48 hours, with each paroxysm occurring on the third day. Quartan periodicity occurs every 72 hours, with each paroxysm occurring on the fourth day. As the host's immune system responds, each paroxysm becomes less and less severe.

Malaria may lead to anemia because of the hemolysis of RBCs and the host's response to toxins released. Impaired utilization of hemoglobin and hemoglobinuria occur, commonly known as "black water fever" as the hemozoin pigment is released into the urine. Splenomegaly is a common complication, but there is no lymphoadenopathy. Leukocytosis and eosinophilia also are observed in the complete blood count and differential.

P. vivax and *P. ovale* tend to infect younger red cells, whereas *P. malariae* infects older red cells. *P. falciparum* causes the most severe form of malaria and infects red cells of all ages, with rapid multiplication and the production of the greatest number of merozoites of all of the *Plasmodium* species. In addition, *P. falciparum* can adhere

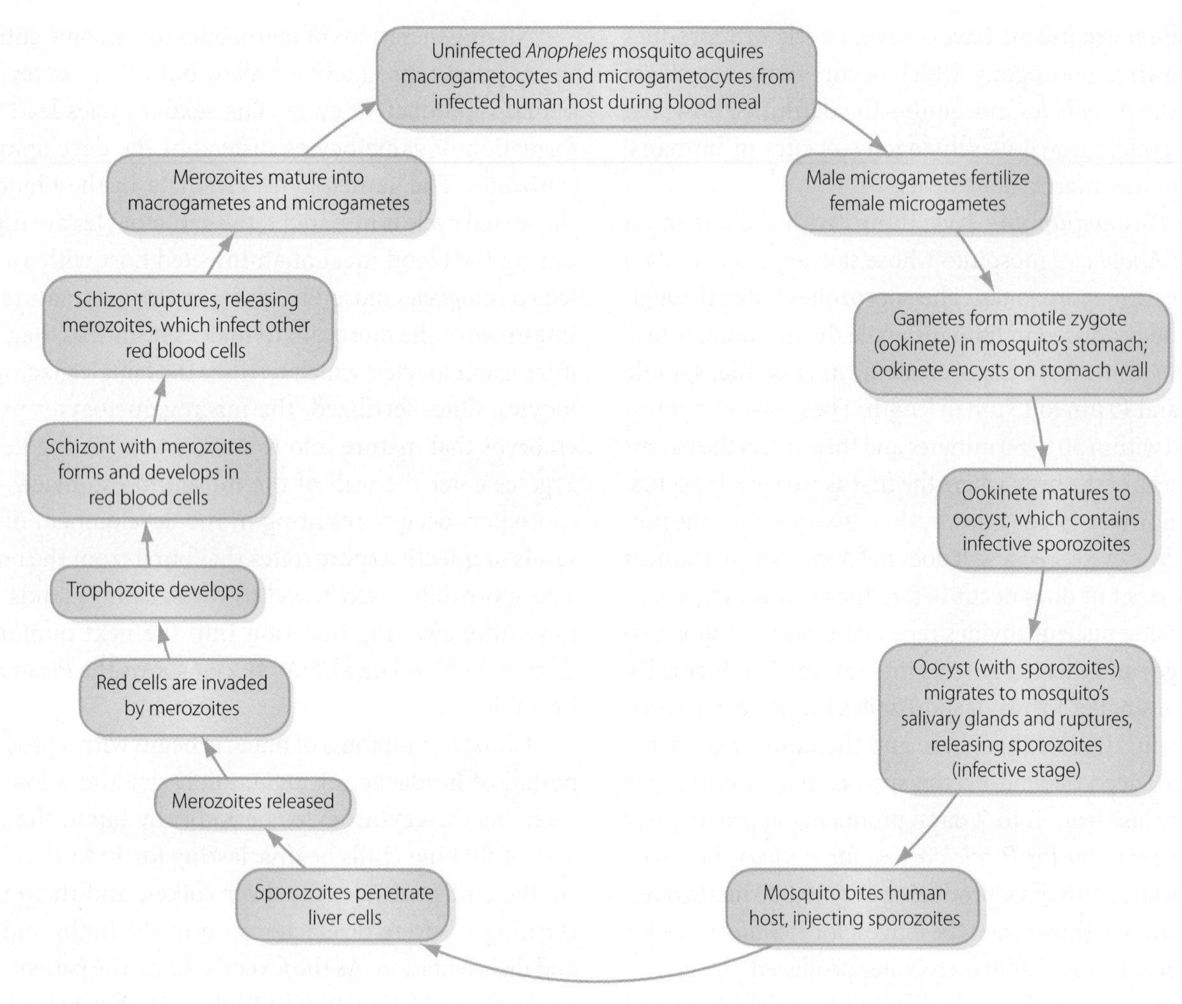

FIGURE 21-7 Life cycle of *Plasmodium.*

to the vascular epithelium of internal organs, resulting in capillary thrombosis and leading to tissue hypoxia of the brain, liver, lungs, or kidneys. Because it produces the most devastating form of malaria and paroxysms occur on each third day, *P. falciparum* infection is referred to as "malignant tertian" malaria. By contrast, *P. vivax* infection is known as "benign tertian" malaria because the infection is generally less severe than that of *P. falciparum*.

Malaria is present in more than 100 countries, and 100 million cases occur annually worldwide. Malaria most often is found in the tropics and subtropics, especially in sub-Saharan Africa, which accounts for 98% of all global malaria deaths. The World Health Organization estimates that there were between 200 and 300 million clinical episodes of malaria and between 700,000 and 1 million deaths from malaria in 2008. Malaria is the fifth-leading infectious disease in the world, following respiratory infections, HIV/AIDS, diarrheal disease, and tuberculosis. In the United States, approximately 1,500 cases of malaria are reported per year, although the disease had been eradicated in the 1950s. First- and second-generation immigrants from countries where malaria is endemic and those who travel to their home countries where *Plasmodium* is endemic are more likely to contract malaria. There have been 63 local malaria outbreaks in the United States between 1957 and 2009, which occured when local mosquitoes became infected by taking a blood meal from a person carrying the malaria parasite (who had previously acquired the parasite in an endemic area). Then, it is possible for malaria to be transmitted within the community. Between 1963 and 2009, there were almost 100 cases of transfusion-transmitted malaria. Donor deferrals would have prevented many of these individuals from donating blood, as most cases had been acquired during foreign travel or found in students and other individuals from foreign countries or in refugees.

TABLE 21-3 Characteristics of *Plasmodium* Species

Characteristic	*P. falciparum*	*P. vivax*	*P. malariae*	*P. ovale*
Periodicity	Tertian 36–48 hr	Tertian 48 hr	Quartan 72 hr	Tertian 48 hr
Disease	Malignant malaria	Tertian malaria	Quartan malaria	Ovale malaria
Red blood cell (RBC) size	Normal	1.5–2 times normal	Normal	1.5 times normal; oval with irregular edges
Dots/clefts	Maurer's clefts (comma shaped, red) seen rarely	Schuffner's dots present in all stages except early ring forms	No dots or clefts	Schuffner's dots present in all stages, including early rings; stains darker than *P. vivax*
Early ring stage	Small rings, multiple rings per cell; double-nuclei, accole (appliqué), and signet-ring forms seen	Usually single parasite per cell; rings with two nuclei possible	Usually single parasite per cell	Usually single parasite per cell
Mature ring stage	Small and round; rarely seen in blood	Large, amoeboid, with cytoplasm-filling cell	Ribbon, band, or basket forms; not amoeboid	Similar to *P. malariae* but larger in size; many large, dark-staining granules
Schizonts	8–16 merozoites per schizont; rarely seen in peripheral blood	12–24 merozoites per schizont; finely granular, golden brown malarial pigment	6–12 merozoites per schizont, which may form rosette; coarsely granular malarial pigment	8 merozoites, usually arranged around 1 large pigment aggregated
Gametocytes	Crescent or banana shaped	Large, round, almost filling cell; coarse malarial pigment	Round, RBCs not enlarged; coarse, unevenly distributed pigment	Similar to *P. malariae*
Comments	Stages other than early ring and gametocyte rarely seen; multiple infected RBCs common	Generally infects young RBCs; all stages found in peripheral blood	Low levels of parasitemia when compared with other species; all stages found but generally few rings and gametocytes in peripheral blood	Difficult to identify because *P. ovale* resembles *P. vivax* and *P. malariae*; all stages found in peripheral blood found

Malaria is diagnosed through clinical symptoms and the demonstration of the organism in thick and thin Wright- or Giemsa-stained smears. It is best to collect the blood specimen before the fever because the parasites are most concentrated in the red cells at this time. In examination of the blood smears, the clinician must first recognize the presence of malarial parasites, using the thick smear. The organisms are intracellular, with a red nucleus and blue cytoplasm. Next, each species has trademark characteristics that are used for identification, using the thin smear. **TABLE 21-3** summarizes important characteristics of each *Plasmodium* species. The first step in speciation is to identify *P. falciparum* because it causes the most fatal and progressive form of malaria and it is becoming increasingly resistant to chloroquine. If *P. falciparum* has been ruled out, the possibility of *P. vivax* is next investigated. *P. malariae* often is diagnosed through exclusion. **FIGURES 21-8** through **21-11** show various forms of *P. falciparum*, **FIGURE 21-12** shows *P. vivax*, and **FIGURE 21-13** shows *P. malariae*. **FIGURE 21-14** illustrates the morphology of the malarial parasites.

Babesia

Babesia is a tick-borne sporozoan parasite that generally infects animals other than humans. Species include *Babesia microti*, which infects rodents; *Babesia equi*, which infects horses; *Babesia canis*, which infects dogs; and

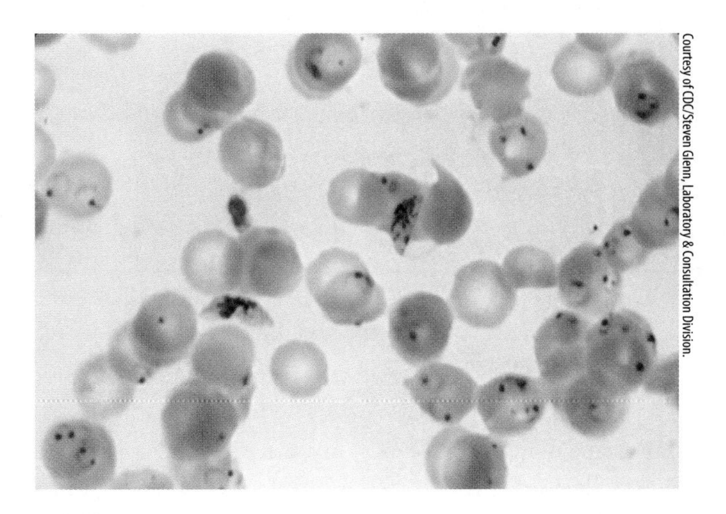

FIGURE 21-8 *P. falciparum*—multiply infected red blood cells.

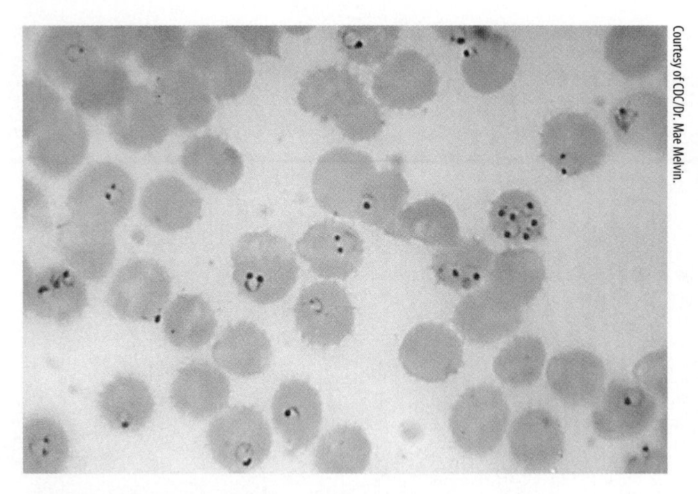

Courtesy of CDC/Dr. Mae Melvin.

FIGURE 21-9 *P. falciparum*—ring forms.

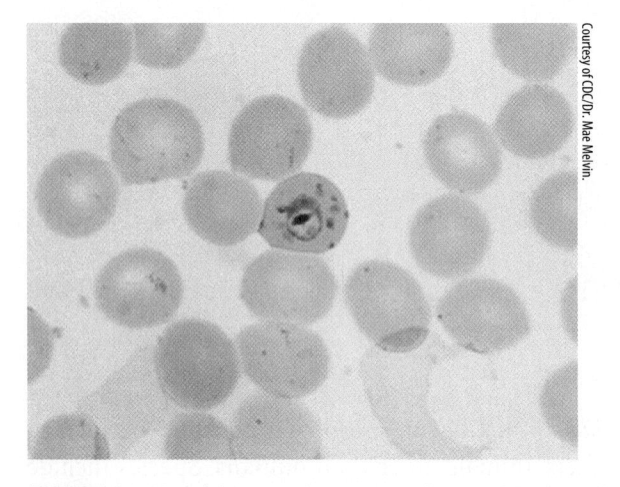

Courtesy of CDC/Dr. Mae Melvin.

FIGURE 21-10 *P. falciparum* showing ring form and Maurer's dots.

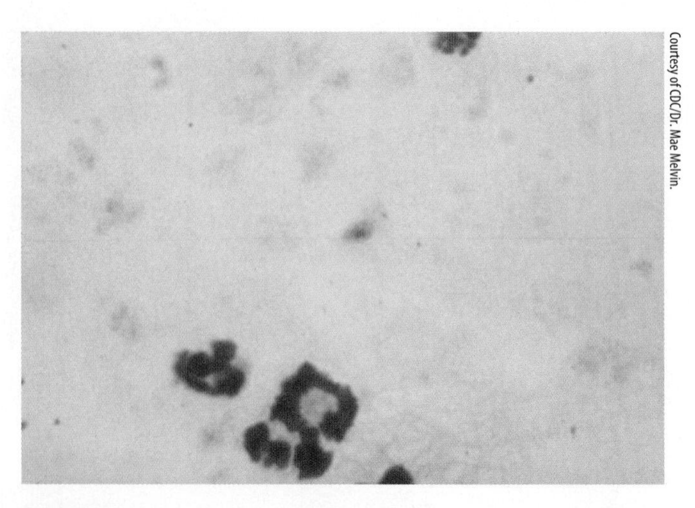

Courtesy of CDC/Dr. Mae Melvin.

FIGURE 21-11 *P. falciparum* showing hemozoin pigment within red blood cells.

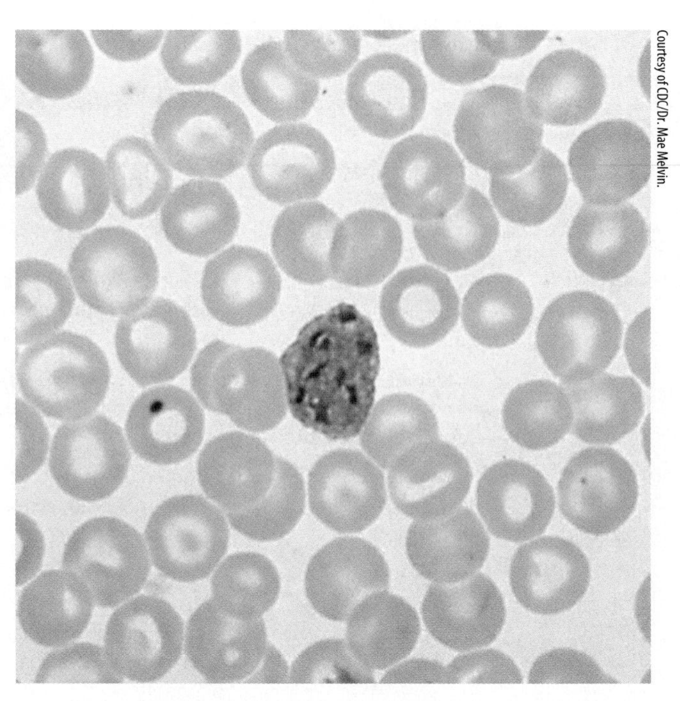

Courtesy of CDC/Dr. Mae Melvin.

FIGURE 21-12 *P. vivax* showing ring form filling entire red blood cell.

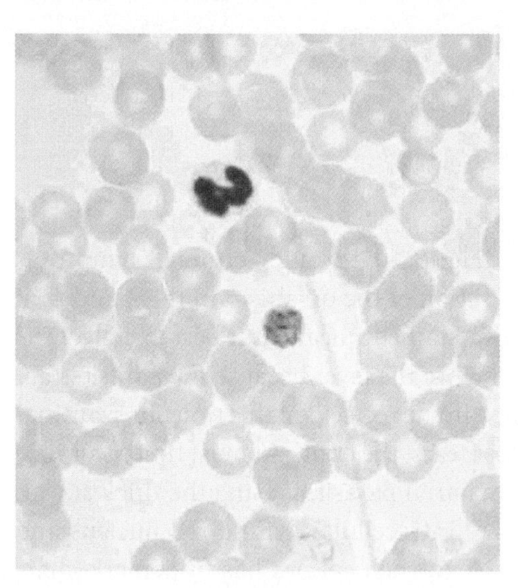

FIGURE 21-13 *P. malariae* showing merozoites in red blood cells.

Babesia bovis and *Babesia divergens*, which infect cattle. Humans serve as an accidental host, with individuals who have had splenectomies at an increased risk of babesiosis. *B. microti* is endemic in southern New England, Texas, and other parts of North America. It also is the cause of Texas cattle fever. Most human infections in North America from *B. microti* occur in the coastal areas of southern New England and the eastern coastal areas, including Nantucket Island. *B. equi* is found in Europe, Russia, Africa, Asia, India, and North and South America.

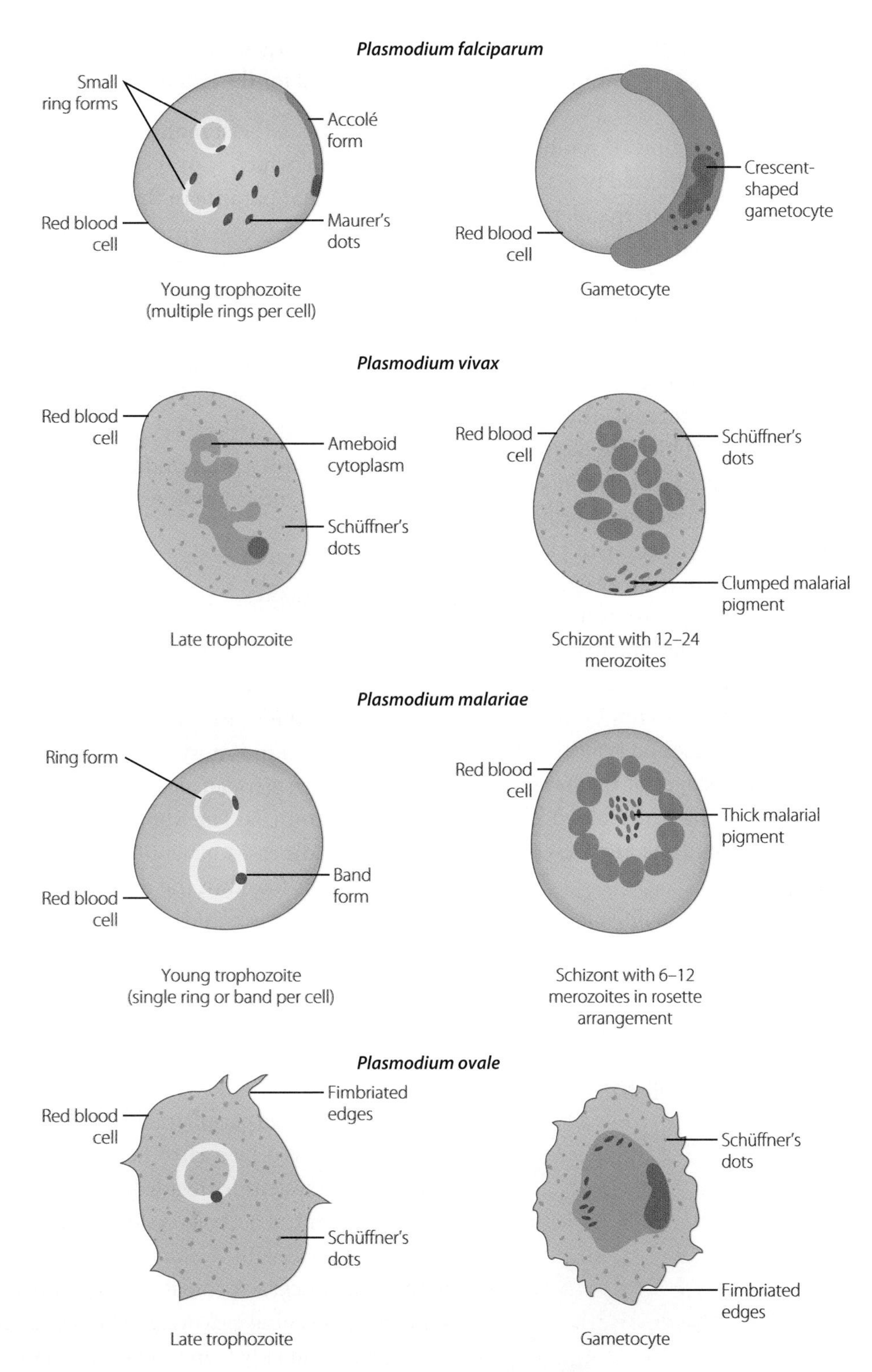

FIGURE 21-14 Morphology of malarial parasites (diagnostic forms).

Ticks are the arthropod intermediate host for *Babesia* species that occur in domestic and wild animals. Ticks may become infected by either taking a blood meal from an infected mammal or having the parasite transmitted from an infected female to her progeny. In the animal host the parasite is inoculated during the blood meal into the host, and invasion of the RBCs occurs. The trophozoite form develops, and schizogony—in this case a form of asexual reproduction resembling budding—results in the formation of a tetrad arrangement of four merozoites.

Upon rupture of the infected erythrocytes, the merozoites are released, infecting other RBCs and continuing the life cycle.

Many *Babesia* infections are subclinical; symptoms occur 2 to 3 weeks after the bite of an infected tick. Clinically, babesiosis resembles malaria, with an irregular fever, chills, sweats, nausea, vomiting, and fatigue. Patients also may have hemolytic anemia, jaundice, and an enlarged liver and spleen. The disease is most severe and often fatal in splenectomized individuals.

Diagnosis is made by demonstration of the parasites in stained blood films. Within the erythrocyte the organism most often appears as a pleomorphic ringlike structure, which may resemble the ring stages of *Plasmodium*. Piriform, round, oval, elongate, and amoeboid forms are possible. The piroplast form is pear shaped, with packets of two or four organisms seen and may be described as resembling rabbit ears. The piriform parasites may form a cross after division into four organisms, said to resemble a Maltese cross. The red cells are not enlarged, and there is hemozoin or pigment deposited, as occurs in malaria. Babesiosis is suspected by the small size and typical shape of the organism, the lack of other stages of the parasite, normal RBC size, and lack of pigment. Thick blood films are preferred because very few organisms are present in the early stages of the infection.

FIGURE 21-15 shows a stained smear of *Babesia microti*.

HEMOFLAGELLATES

The blood and tissue flagellates include the trypanosomes and leishmania. These parasites may infect the blood, lymph nodes, muscles, and reticuloendothelial cells of the hematopoietic organs. Four morphologies or stages have been described for the hemoflagellates:

- Amastigote (Leishman-Donovan body), or **leishmanial form**, which is oval and found in humans as an intracellular parasite in the reticuloendothelial cells
- Promastigote, or **leptomonal form**, which is long and thin and found in the intermediate (arthropod) host as an extracellular form
- Epimastigote, or **crithidial form**, which is also long and thin, has an undulating membrane, and is an extracellular form found in the arthropod host
- Trypomastigote, or **trypanosomal form**, which is long and thin, has an undulating membrane and free flagellum, and is found extracellularly in the arthropod host

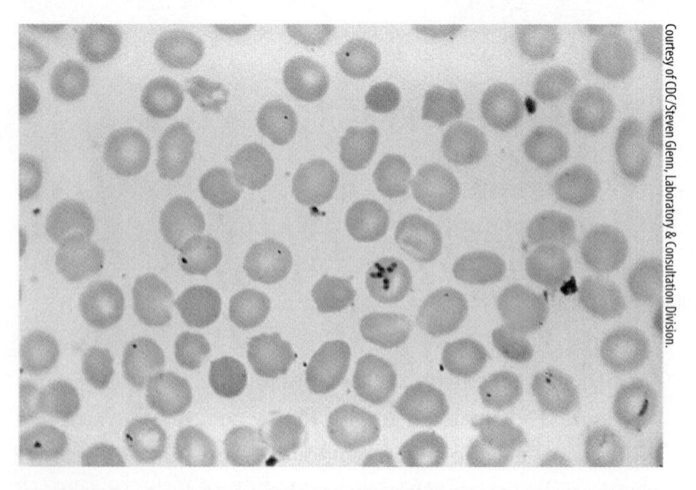

FIGURE 21-15 *Babesia microti* showing Maltese cross appearance in red blood cell.

TRYPANOSOMES

Trypanosoma brucei subspecies *rhodesiense* and *Trypanosoma brucei* subspecies *gambiense* have similar morphologies and are the causes of African sleeping sickness. *T. rhodesiense* is found most often in eastern Africa as the agent of eastern African sleeping sickness, with its reservoir in wild animals. The Rhodesian form is found in isolated or sporadic cases, generally in hunters and herdsmen. *T. gambiense* is found in the dense vegetation near rivers and lakes in western and central Africa, with its reservoir in the human population. African trypanosomes are transmitted by the bite of infected tsetse flies of the genus *Glossina*. The Gambian form is more prevalent and found in epidemic numbers.

African sleeping sickness is characterized by an acute phase in which the peripheral blood and lymph nodes are invaded, followed by a chronic phase in which the central nervous system is invaded, resulting in meningoencephalitis. Central nervous system involvement occurs in 6 months to 1 year with *T. gambiense* and as early as 1 month with *T. rhodesiense*. A comatose state develops, commonly known as "sleeping sickness." The Rhodesian form progresses more quickly to meningoencephalitis, whereas the Gambian form may incubate for months or years before the development of meningoencephalitis.

The life cycle of *T. brucei* begins when the infectious trypomastigotes exit the fly's salivary glands during a blood meal. The trypomastigote forms a thin, spindle-shaped flagellate, which multiplies asexually in the bite wound and then enters the human host's peripheral blood and lymphatic circulation, where division continues. When another fly ingests a blood meal, the trypomastigote enters the midgut of the fly, migrates to its salivary glands, and develops into the epimastigote form. Division continues, resulting in the formation of the metacyclic trypanomastigotes.

A hard nodule develops at the area of the bite, with regional lymphoadenopathy. As the disease progresses, the patient has an intermittent fever and hyperplasia of the lymphoid tissue as the reticuloendothelial organs are invaded. A high fever, night sweats, and joint and muscle pain also are seen. As the host produces immunoglobulin M (IgM) antibody to the parasite, a generalized lymphoadenopathy develops. Then, as new antigenic strains of the parasite emerge, the host continues to mount an immune response, producing antibody until the immune system is eventually overwhelmed. Lymph nodes may eventually atrophy or become fibrotic.

The trypomastigotes are identified in peripheral blood smears during febrile episodes and in lymph node aspirates in the early stages of infection. The two species are usually not differentiated. Wet mounts can be performed to observe the motile trypomastigote, and confirmation is made through Giemsa-stained smears, in which the characteristic spindle-shaped organism, ranging in size from 12 μm to 40 μm long, is observed. The trypanosome has a central nucleus and a small red kinetoplast near the rounded posterior end. Other important characteristics include an undulating membrane and a free flagellum that extends forward, exiting the body at the anterior end. Broad, stumpy forms also may be observed. Serologically, *T. brucei* infection is characterized by marked increases in serum IgM levels, which may reach eight times the normal level. The IgM to IgG ratio may increase to as high as 3:1.

Trypanosoma cruzi is the agent of American trypanosomiasis, or Chagas disease. Triatomid or reduviid bugs serve as the intermediate host, and the bugs are infected when they feed on animals, including humans, that have infective trypomastigotes in their blood or amastigotes in their macrophages or other cells. Reduviid bugs infect various wild and domestic animals, including dogs, cats, and raccoons, in addition to humans.

In contrast to African trypanosomiasis, in American trypanosomiasis the intracellular amastigote form multiplies in the human host. The life cycle begins when the metacyclic trypomastigote is passed onto the host's skin in the feces of the infected reduviid or triatomid bugs during a blood meal. Typically the bugs bite the face of the individual at night, and the trypomastigotes are rubbed into the skin or mucous membranes when the area of the bite is scratched. The metacyclic form enters various host cells, in particular phagocytes, where transformation into the round amastigote form occurs. The amastigote forms, which are not flagellated, multiply asexually. The host cells rupture, releasing new generations of amastigotes, which continue to infect other cells. The amastigote forms infect the lymph nodes and later various internal organs, including the heart, reticuloendothelial system (RES), and central nervous system. Transformation into a trypomastigote form, which is able to circulate in the blood, also may occur. The trypomastigotes do not divide in the peripheral blood, as is the case in African trypanosomiasis. Insect vectors may become infected when they ingest a blood meal of the circulating trypanomastigotes. Transformation into the epimastigote form occurs in the midgut of the insect vector, followed by transformation into the metacyclic trypanomastigote. The life cycle continues as the metacyclic trypanomastigotes travel to the hindgut of the vector and await the next blood meal for injection into a host.

Clinically, Chagas disease involves an acute phase, lasting 1 to 4 months, with symptoms of facial swelling, redness, and edema over the area of the bite. Although bites occur anywhere on the body, the most common site is on the face and over the eyelid. Because bites most often occur on the face, reduviid bugs are commonly known as "kissing bugs." The acute phase also may be accompanied by fever, headache, muscle aches, hepatosplenomegaly, cardiac abnormalities, and lymphoadenopathy. The infection may subside after the acute phase or continue into a chronic phase, which causes prolonged cellular damage, particularly to muscle and nerve cells. Complications include the loss of muscle tone in the heart, esophagus, and intestine.

Laboratory diagnosis of the acute phase of Chagas disease relies on the demonstration of C-shaped trypomastigotes in thin and thick blood smears prepared from peripheral blood or from the spinal fluid. The rapid, progressive, snakelike motility of the trypomastigotes can be observed in wet mounts of peripheral blood. Confirmation is achieved through thick and thin Giemsa-stained smears, in which the trypomastigotes are C shaped and 15 μm to 20 μm in length. An undulating membrane the full length of its body, a free flagellum, and a large kinetoplast located

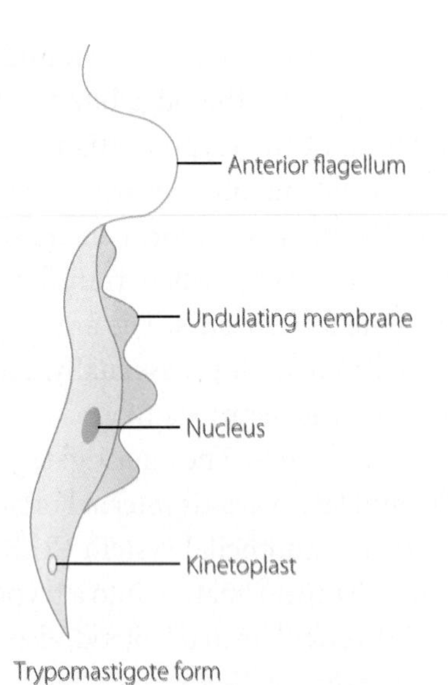

FIGURE 21-16 Trypomastigote form for *Trypanosoma* species.

in the posterior pointed end are also important identifying characteristics. Xenodiagnosis, which uses parasitic free triatomids that are raised in the laboratory, is an unusual method of diagnosis. The insects are allowed to feed on the blood of a patient suspected of having Chagas disease. The intestinal contents of the insect are later examined for the presence of the epimastigote form of the parasite. Serum IgM is normal in Chagas disease, in contrast to infection with *T. brucei*, where it is significantly elevated.

The diagnostic stage for trypanosomal infections is the trypomastigote form in blood, as illustrated in **FIGURE 21-16**. **FIGURE 21-17** shows *T. cruzi* in a Giemsa stain from ascitic fluid.

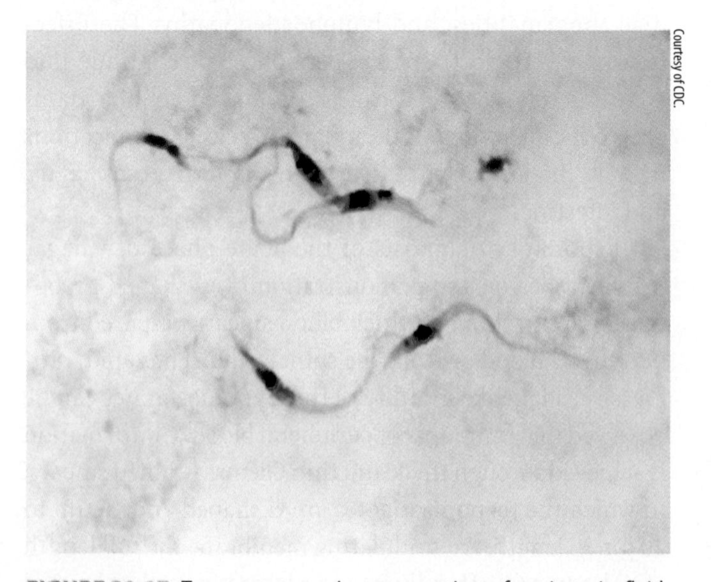

Courtesy of CDC.

FIGURE 21-17 *Trypanosoma cruzi*—trypomastigote form in ascite fluid.

Leishmania

Leishmania species are the agents of cutaneous and visceral leishmaniasis. Visceral leishmaniasis, or kalaazar, is caused by the *Leishmania donovani* complex, with the disease occurring in the Mediterranean, India, eastern Africa, China, and South and Central America. Old World cutaneous leishmaniasis, or Oriental sore, is caused by *Leishmania tropica* and is found in the Near East and Middle East, Mediterranean countries, India, and Africa. New World cutaneous leishmaniasis is caused by *Leishmania mexicana* and is found in rural South and Central America. Mucocutaneous leishmaniasis of the New World is caused by *Leishmania braziliensis* and is found in the rural and forested areas of South and Central America.

The life cycle of *Leishmania* begins with the bite of an infected sand fly from the genus *Phlebotomus*, which injects the promastigote form into the human host. After biting the host, the sand fly regurgitates promastigotes, which enter through the site of the bite wound. Conversion to the amastigote form occurs, with multiplication occurring within the macrophages in the host's skin. The bite of another sand fly continues the life cycle, with ingestion of the infective macrophages occurring during the blood meal. Shaking chills, profuse sweating, weight loss, and hepatosplenomegaly may be observed as the parasites disseminate throughout the reticuloendothelial system. Cutaneous leishmaniasis is generally confined to the skin and lymphatics. Visceral leishmaniasis invades the visceral organs following primary infection in the skin. The liver, spleen, bone marrow, and other organs of the RES may be involved.

The diagnostic stage is the amastigote form, which is found in the macrophages of the skin lesion, for *L. tropica* and *L. mexicana*. The amastigotes of *L. braziliensis* can be isolated at the edge of the skin lesion. *L. donovani* is identified through the observation of the amastigote form in young skin lesions and Leishman-Donovan bodies in tissue samples of the spleen, lymph node, bone marrow, or liver. **FIGURE 21-18** illustrates the amastigote form of *Leishmania*, and **FIGURE 21-19** shows *Leishmania* in ascitic fluid.

Nematodes

The Nematoda are known as roundworms because they appear round when viewed in a cross section. **TABLE 21-4** lists common intestinal nematodes.

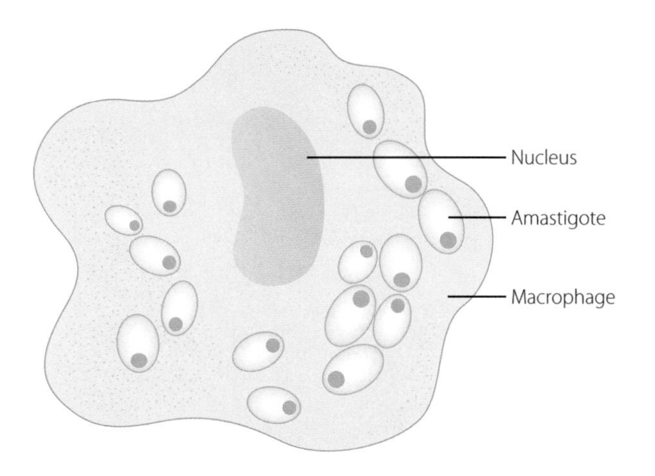

FIGURE 21-18 Amastigote form for *Leishmania* species.

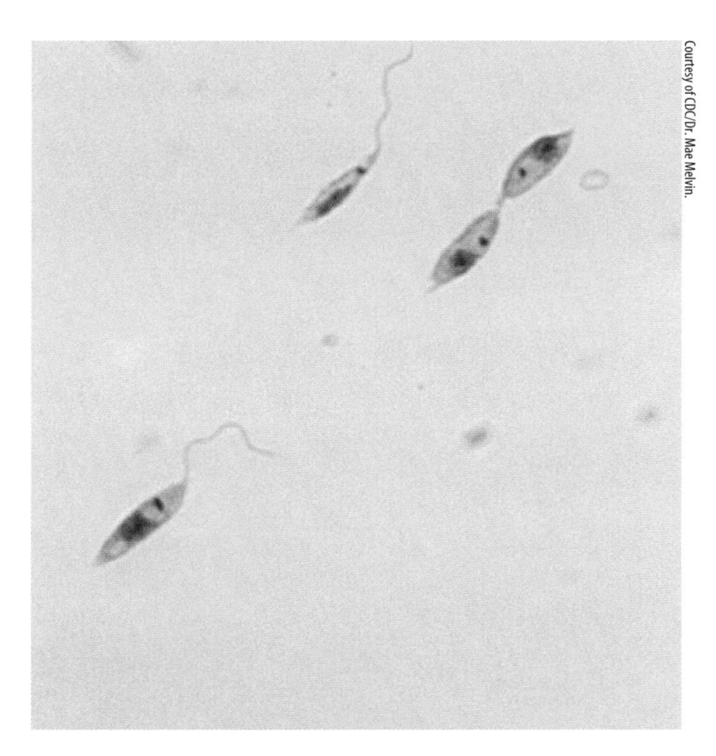

FIGURE 21-19 *Leishmania* in ascite fluid.

TABLE 21-4 Intestinal Nematodes

Scientific Name	Common Name
Enterobius vermicularis	Pinworm
Trichuris trichiura	Whipworm
Ascaris lumbricoides	Large intestinal roundworm
Necator americanus	New World hookworm
Ancylostoma duodenale	Old World hookworm
Strongyloides stercoralis	Threadworm

STRONGYLOIDES STERCORALIS

Strongyloides stercoralis, threadworm, has both parasitic and free-living generations. **FIGURE 21-20** illustrates the life cycle of *S. stercoralis*.

The rhabditiform larvae are the diagnostic form for *S. stercoralis* because the eggs are generally not found in the stool. The eggs, when found, resemble the eggs of hookworm. If larvae are found in the feces, it is most likely that the parasite is *S. stercoralis* and not hookworm. Threadworm larvae must be differentiated from hookworm larvae. Important criteria include the length of the buccal cavity, which is much shorter in *Strongyloides*. *Strongyloides* has a bulge or notch, known as the genital primordium, in its buccal cavity, which is either indistinct or absent in hookworm larvae.

Threadworm infections more often are found in the tropics and subtropics, including in South America and southeast Asia. The infection also is found in the United States in the rural southeast in lower socioeconomic and institutional settings. The life cycle is perpetuated by the presence of organic material in the moist soil, which provides a favorable environment for the free-living adult parasite forms. Symptoms produced are determined by the location of the larva and may include a cutaneous phase, a pulmonary phase, and an intestinal phase, which may be mild and asymptomatic or severe with abdominal pain, diarrhea, or constipation. The cutaneous phase may include urticarial rashes along the waist, while pulmonary symptoms may be exhibited while the filariform larvae migrates to the lungs. The infection can disseminate in those who are immunosuppressed, in which case there may be neurologic or respiratory complications, septicemia, or shock. Eosinophils are increased in the peripheral blood during the acute phase of infection. Infections are treated with ivermectin or albendazole.

HOOKWORMS: *NECATOR AMERICANUS* AND *ANCYLOSTOMA DUODENALE*

Necator americanus, New World hookworm, and *Ancylostoma duodenale*, Old World hookworm, are the agents of human hookworm infestations. The organisms possess similar life cycles, and their eggs are almost identical and thus are not differentiated. The diagnostic stage, the egg, is passed in the feces and hatches into rhabditiform larvae in the external environment. Larvae are generally not seen in the feces. **FIGURE 21-21** illustrates the life cycle and eggs of hookworm.

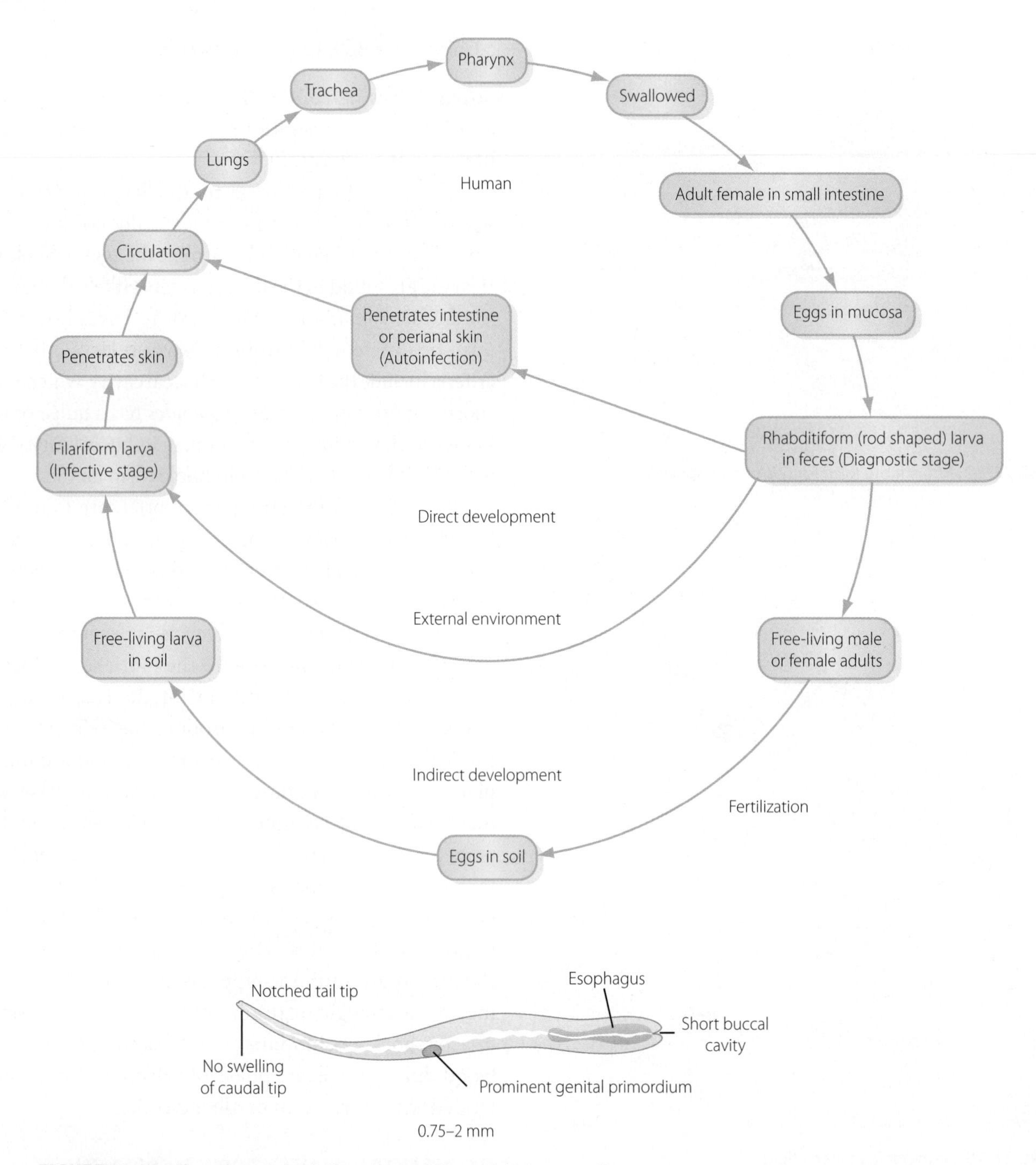

FIGURE 21-20 Life cycle and rhabidiform larva of *Strongyloides stercoralis.*

Hookworm infections are found throughout the world but generally where the climate is warm and humid. These infections occur most frequently in the tropical farming areas of Africa, Asia, South America, and Caribbean countries. Infections in the United States are most often seen in the southern states. *N. americanus* is the predominant hookworm in North and South America and in Australia, and *A. duodenale* is more often found in southern Europe, the Mediterranean countries, the Middle East, and North Africa. Infections are associated with poor sewage disposal, which allows the eggs to remain and hatch in the soil.

Once the eggs are passed in the stool, the rhabditiform larvae hatch in 1 to 2 days and grow in the soil or feces, developing into filariform larvae, which are the infective form. The filariform larvae can survive for up to a month in favorable conditions. The filariform larvae penetrate human skin and are carried in the blood to the heart and lungs, where they travel up the bronchial

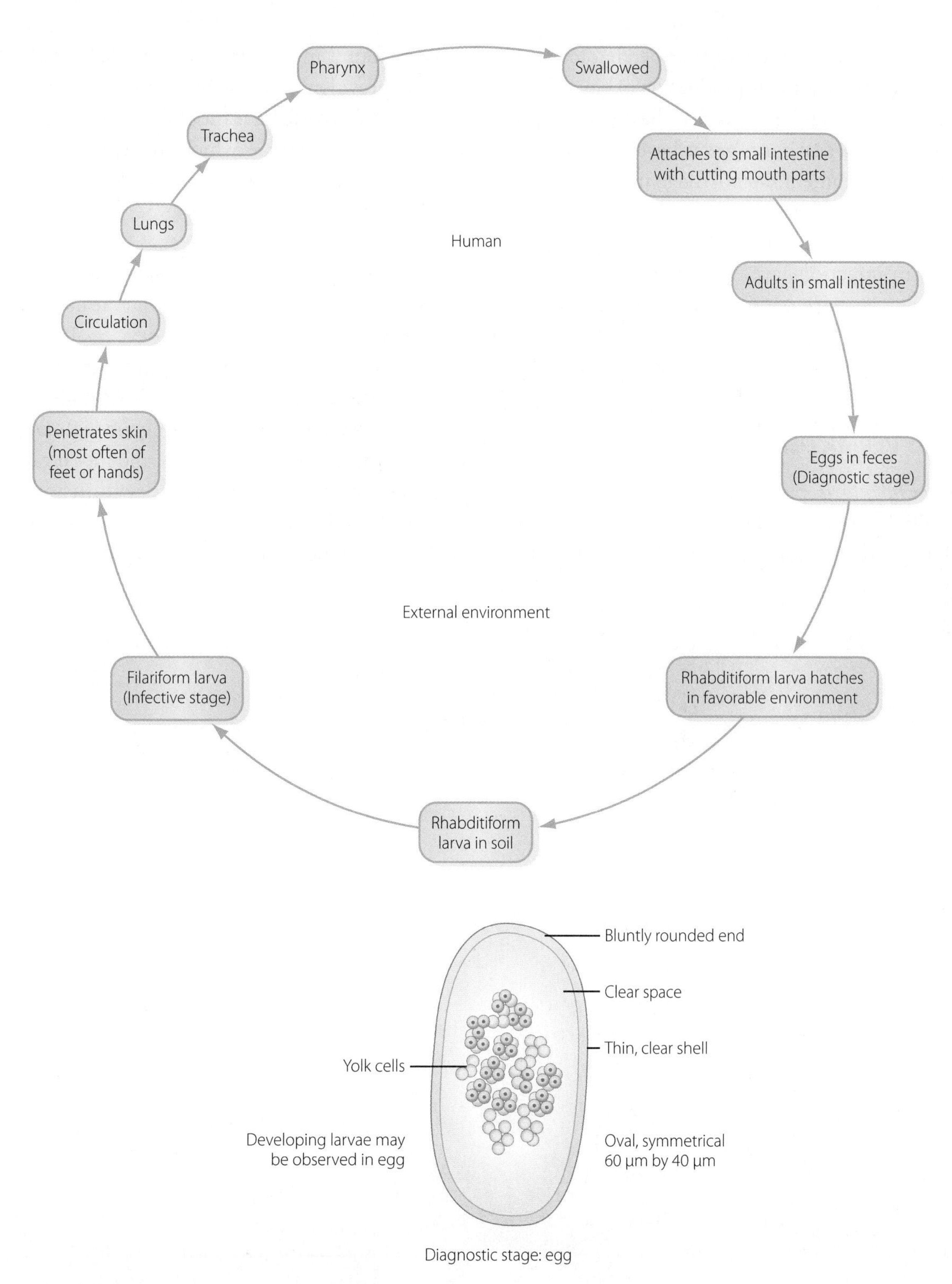

FIGURE 21-21 Life cycle and egg of hookworm.

tree to the pharynx. Here the larvae are swallowed and travel to the small intestine, where they mature into adult forms, attaching to the intestinal wall. The adult worms can remain in the intestines indefinitely; however, many are eliminated in 1 to 2 years.

Symptoms are related to the type of infection and include a cutaneous phase known as cutaneous larva migrans, or "ground itch," a local dermatitis with redness and swelling at the site of penetration. These symptoms are attributed to the migration of the hookworm larvae to the dermis. The pulmonary phase may be characterized by pharyngitis, a cough, and the production of bloody sputum. The intestinal stage involves diarrhea, nausea, and vomiting. Because the filariform larvae have sharp-cutting mouthparts for attachment, hemorrhage may occur, and there also may be iron deficiency anemia, fatigue, weakness, edema, and congestive heart failure.

Hookworm infections are treated with albendazole or mebendazole. Because reinfection occurs in countries where the parasite is more common, light infections may not be treated.

ENTEROBIUS VERMICULARIS

Enterobius vermicularis, pinworm, is the agent of enterobiasis, which is present worldwide but occurs more frequently in temperate or colder climates. The infection most often is found in school-age and preschool children and is more prevalent in those living in crowded conditions.

The infective form is the embryonated egg, which contains third-stage larvae, which are ingested by mouth. The life cycle continues as noted in **FIGURE 21-22**.

Eggs are deposited on the perianal folds, and self-infection occurs by ingesting eggs that have been deposited on the hands while scratching the perianal area. After ingestion of the infective eggs, the larvae hatch in the small intestine, where the adult forms develop. It takes approximately 1 month for the infective eggs to mature into gravid adult female forms. Adult worms live for about 2 months. The gravid female migrates during the night outside of the anus, where she deposits the eggs, and the larvae within the eggs develop and become infective within hours. Retroinfection, whereby the hatched larvae can crawl back into the rectum from the anal area, also may occur.

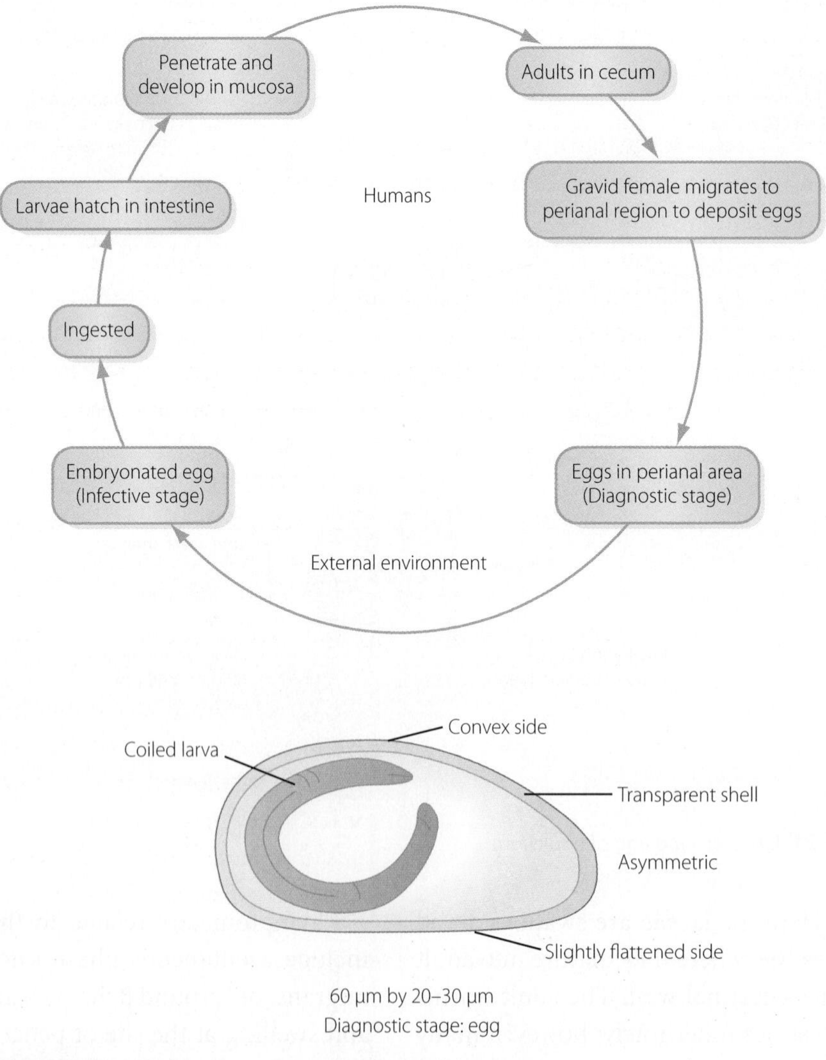

FIGURE 21-22 Life cycle and egg of *Enterobius vermicularis*.

The adult worms do not have to pass through the circulatory system, as is the case for threadworm and hookworm. The mature adults are not very long, measuring approximately 5 mm to 10 mm in length. There is a winglike bulge at the anterior end and a long pointed tail, and thus the worm is said to resemble a pin.

Pinworm eggs are present on the perianal folds but may not be observed in the feces. Because, the female generally deposits the eggs at night, the best specimen is obtained in the morning. The cellophane test, which employs a strip of cellophane tape placed on the anus, with its sticky side out to collect any eggs, may be used to collect the perianal specimen. The tape is next pressed onto a microscope slide with a glass coverslip and examined for the presence of eggs. The use of sticky paddles and commercially available swatches also may be used to collect the eggs. It is important to collect the specimen before bathing or a bowel movement to enhance recovery of the eggs.

The egg is the diagnostic stage (**FIGURE 21-23**) for pinworm infection. The adult worms are generally not recovered.

Pinworm infection is found worldwide and transmitted through ingestion of infected food or contaminated hands. Children may scratch the perianal region at night, gathering eggs or larvae under their fingernails, and then transmit the parasite by person-to-person contact to other individuals. Pinworm infection also may be acquired after handling contaminated clothing, bedding, or other articles of the infected person. Eggs also can be inhaled, swallowed, and ingested. Pinworm infection is generally a mild, self-limiting infection, with minimal symptoms of perianal, nocturnal itching. In heavy infestations the scratching may result in bleeding of the perianal region, nausea, abdominal pain, and irritability and nervousness. Children 5 to 10 years old most often are infected. Pinworm infections are treated with pyrantel pamoate. Attention to preventive measures, such as good personal hygiene and laundering of bedding and other contaminated articles, also is important to avoid reinfection.

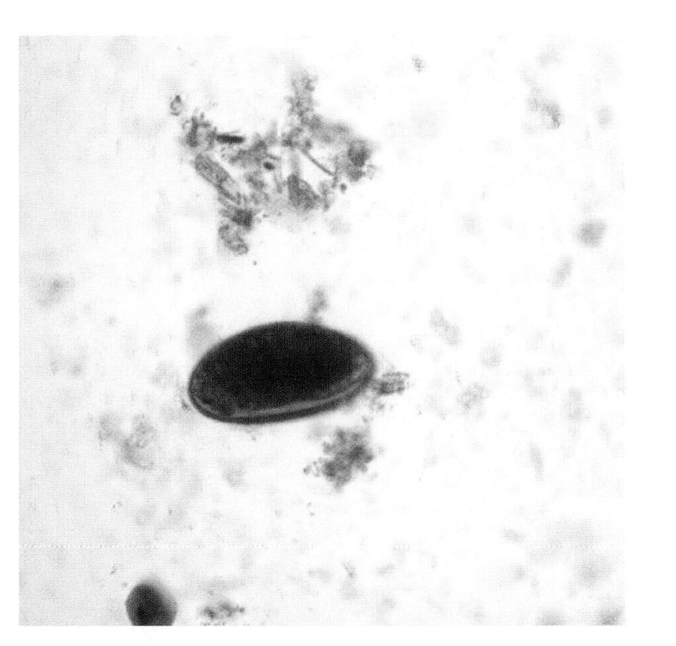

FIGURE 21-23 *E. vermicularis* egg in an iodine mount.

ASCARIS LUMBRICOIDES

Ascaris lumbricoides, large intestinal roundworm, is acquired through ingestion of the embryonated eggs, which contain the second-stage larvae. **FIGURE 21-24** illustrates its life cycle and egg.

The diagnostic form is the egg, which is oval and may be observed in four forms. A cortical layer, or albuminous coat, may or may not surround the egg, and the egg may be fertilized or unfertilized. The form generally observed is fertilized and unembryonated, with a thick, bile-stained albuminous coat and small, rounded projections measuring 60 μm × 45 μm. The unfertilized form is longer, with an undifferentiated protoplasm, brown color, and distorted coat. **FIGURE 21-25** illustrates typical *Ascaris* eggs.

The adult worms are found in the small intestine, and the gravid female may produce as many as 200,000 eggs each day. The eggs are passed in the feces; however, the unfertilized form does not develop and is not infectious. The fertilized egg embryonates in 2 to 3 weeks when present in a favorable environment of warm, moist soil. After the infective fertilized egg is swallowed, the larvae hatch and travel to the intestinal mucosa. Next, the larvae enter the portal circulation and travel through the blood to the lungs. Additional maturation occurs in the lungs, where the larvae reach the bronchi and enter the pharynx, where they are swallowed. Finally, the larvae travel to the small intestine, where they mature into adult worms and the gravid female produces eggs. It takes approximately 2 to 3 months to go from the initial ingestion of the infective eggs to the production of eggs by the adult female. Adult worms generally live for 1 to 2 years. Adult *Ascaris* worms measure 200 mm to 300 mm in length with a diameter of 3 mm to 5 mm. Male forms are shorter than females' and have a curved tail.

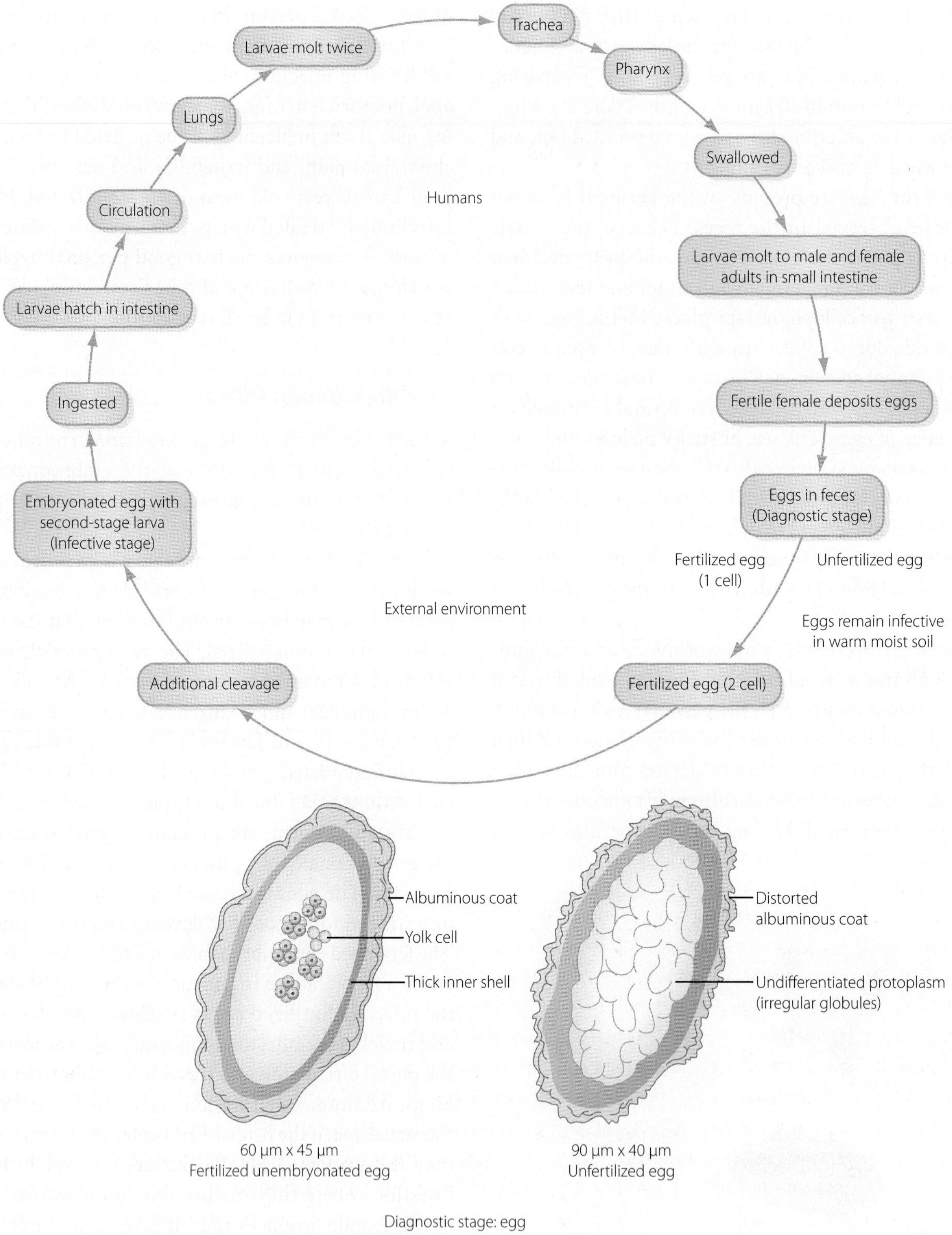

Trachea
Larvae molt twice
Pharynx
Lungs
Swallowed
Humans
Circulation
Larvae molt to male and female adults in small intestine
Larvae hatch in intestine
Fertile female deposits eggs
Ingested
Eggs in feces (Diagnostic stage)
Embryonated egg with second-stage larva (Infective stage)
Fertilized egg (1 cell)
Unfertilized egg
External environment
Eggs remain infective in warm moist soil
Additional cleavage
Fertilized egg (2 cell)

Albuminous coat
Yolk cell
Thick inner shell
60 µm x 45 µm
Fertilized unembryonated egg

Distorted albuminous coat
Undifferentiated protoplasm (irregular globules)
90 µm x 40 µm
Unfertilized egg

Diagnostic stage: egg

FIGURE 21-24 Life cycle and egg of *Ascaris lumbricoides*.

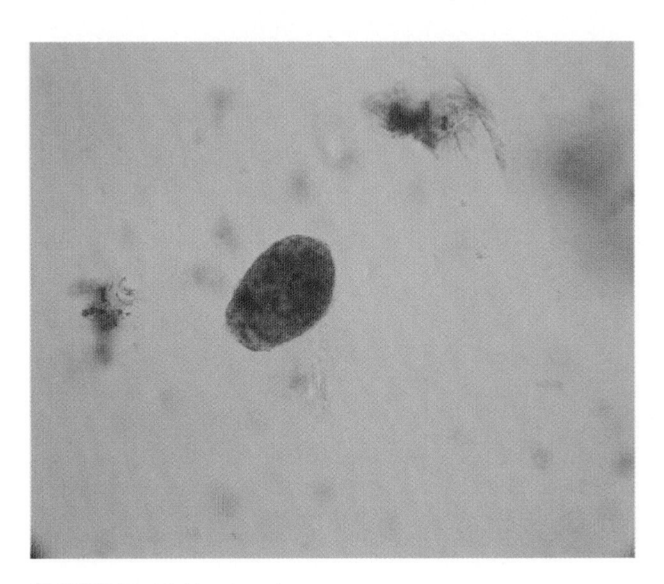

FIGURE 21-25 Egg *Ascaris.*

Because *Ascaris* eggs are too heavy to float in zinc sulfate solution, sedimentation concentration methods are recommended for recovery.

Ascariasis, the most common helminth infection, has a worldwide prevalence and is most frequently seen in the tropics and subtropics; infections also are seen in the southeastern part of the United States in rural areas. Infections most often are seen in young children and may be attributed to ingesting dirt or placing contaminated fingers in the mouth. Infection may result from the ingestion of raw foods that may be contaminated with soil containing human feces that contains *Ascaris.* Infections are generally mild and self-limiting, and the mortality rate is low. In more severe infections the lungs may be affected. Intestinal signs include abdominal pain and diarrhea. In large infestations the host may experience weight loss and malnutrition as the adult worms feed in the intestine; intestinal obstruction is a possible complication of high worm burdens. While the parasite is in the lung, there may be respiratory symptoms, such as cough, dyspnea, and hemoptysis. Ascariasis may be treated with albendazole with mebendazole.

TRICHURIS TRICHIURA

Trichuris trichiura, whipworm, infections are acquired through the ingestion of food or water contaminated with eggs that contain the first-stage larval form. The infection is found worldwide, most often in tropical areas, and associated with poor sanitation methods. It also is found in the southern United States, and most infections occur in children.

The life cycle is shown in **FIGURE 21-26.** Unembryonated eggs are passed in the stool and develop into a two-cell form in the soil. The eggs then embryonate and become infectious within 2 to 4 weeks. The infective eggs are ingested and travel to the small intestine, where larvae are released, which then migrate to the cecum, where the larvae mature into adult forms. Gravid females produce eggs approximately 2 months after infection, releasing between 2,000 and 20,000 eggs each day. Adult worms live for approximately 1 year.

The adult worms are said to resemble a whip, with a long, thin esophagus and thick end resembling a handle, where the intestinal and reproductive organs are located.

The diagnostic form is the egg, which is characteristically elongated or lemon shaped, resembling a football or barrel (**FIGURE 21-27**). There are very few eggs in the stool, which leads to difficulty in their detection.

Trichuriasis is most often seen in warm, humid climates, including in the southeastern portion of the United States. The infection most frequently occurs in children and is related to poor hand-washing practices and poor sanitary measures. Trichuriasis is usually asymptomatic or mild but also may be accompanied by abdominal pain, diarrhea, dysentery, and nausea. Malabsorption may be seen in heavy infestations. *Trichiura* infections are treated with mebendazole.

TRICHINELLA SPIRALIS

Trichinella spiralis is the agent of trichinosis. Humans are considered to be accidental hosts who acquire the infection through the ingestion of contaminated raw or undercooked meat. Trichinosis is an infection of pigs and other carnivores, such as bears, and the life cycle is completed in these animals as depicted in **FIGURE 21-28.** After ingestion of the infective cysts, the larvae are released in the stomach because of the effects of stomach acid and pepsin. The larvae travel to the small bowel and mature into adult forms. After about 1 week, the females release larvae, which migrate to striated muscles, where they encyst. The larvae can lodge in the myocardium, nervous tissue, or other tissue, but further development occurs only in striated muscle tissue. In striated muscle the larvae grow and molt, developing into the characteristic spiral form for which the species is named.

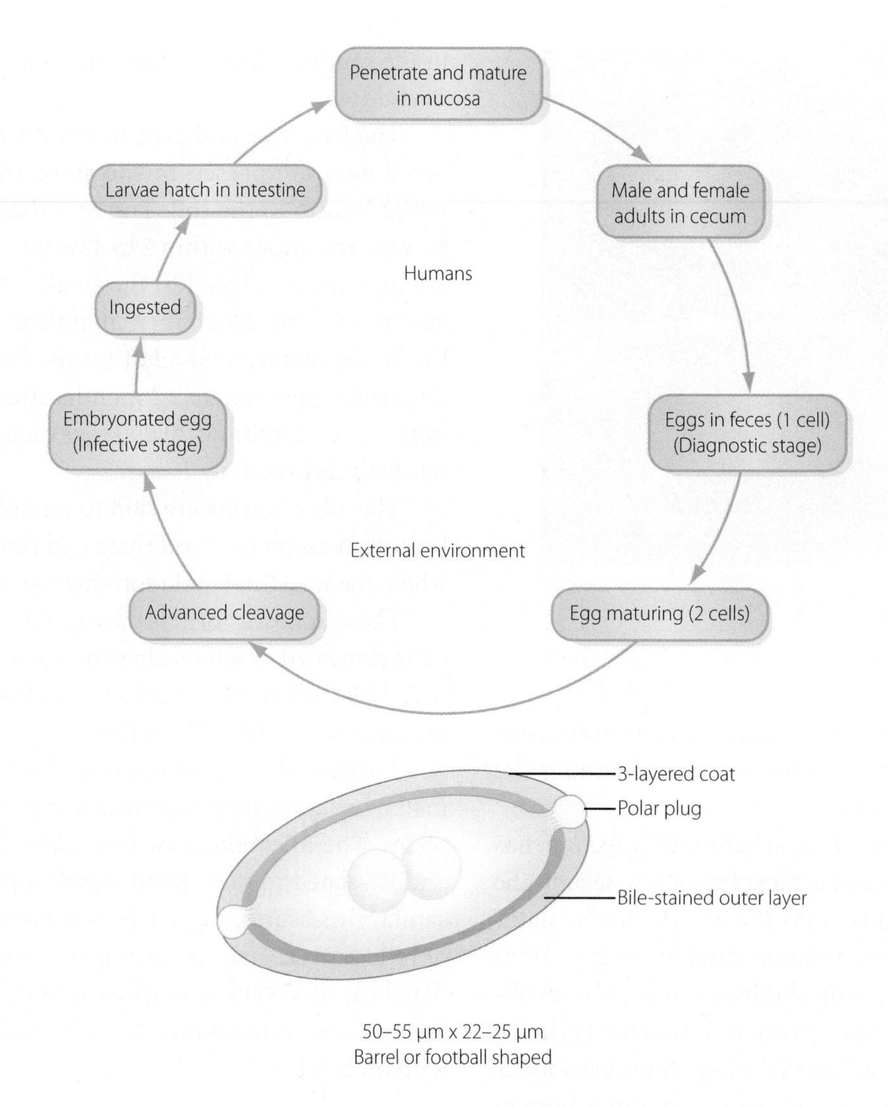

FIGURE 21-26 Life cycle and egg of *Trichuris trichiura*.

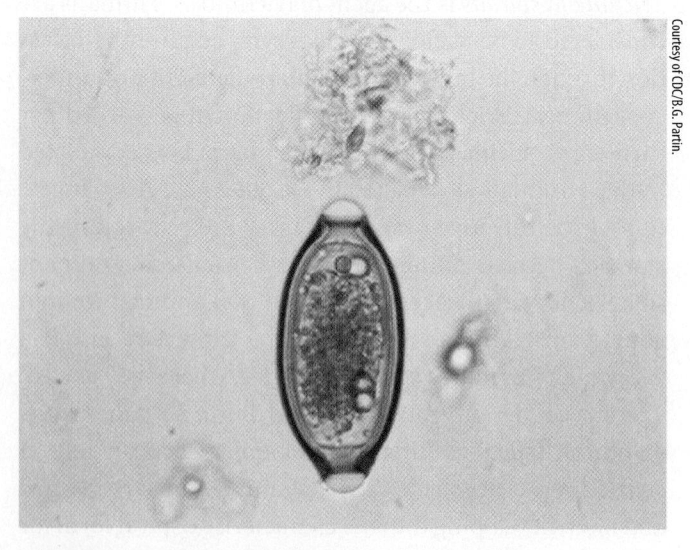

FIGURE 21-27 *Trichuris trichiura* egg in an iodine mount.

A host's reaction occurs in the muscle cells, where a cyst forms around the larvae. The encysted larvae may remain in the muscle until ingested by a new host or may become calcified. Thus, the parasitic life cycle is ultimately completed and dead ends in the human host. The life cycle follows the same pathway in other carnivorous animals, with its continuance through the ingestion of contaminated meat by another animal.

The prevalence of trichinosis depends on the dietary habits of the population, as well as on prevention and control measures. The infection has a worldwide existence, and cases are especially found in North America and Europe, with life cycles existing in bears, walruses, pigs, dogs, cats, and rats. Measures for prevention include the use of irradiation and improved agricultural control

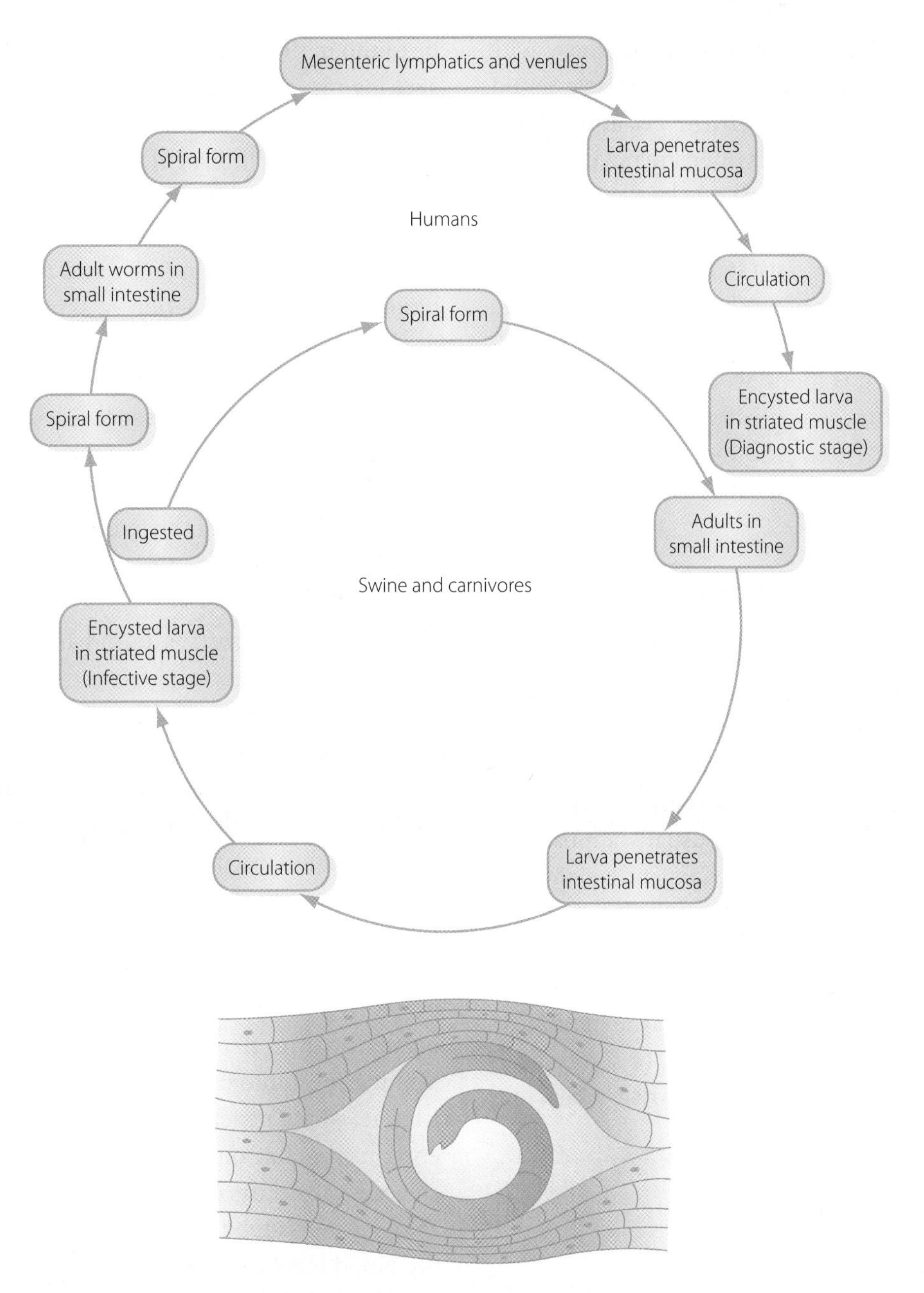

FIGURE 21-28 Life cycle and encysted larva of *Trichinella spiralis*.

measures. There are government regulations that prohibit the use of garbage as pig feed.

The infection has a low mortality rate, and symptoms may mimic those of other diseases. Symptoms may be absent or very severe depending on the number of encysted larvae. The intestinal phase may be characterized by abdominal cramps and diarrhea as the toxic metabolites are released by the worms. As the parasites enter the tissue, an eosinophilia develops, with the eosinophil count ranging from 10% to 90% in the first month of infection, which then tapers off. The larvae can penetrate various muscle tissues, initially in the eye, which leads to periorbital swelling and edema. Headache, muscle pain, and swelling occur as the larvae penetrate the muscles of the neck, tongue, arms, legs, chest, and back. The convalescent phase may be associated with cardiac, pulmonary, or neurological symptoms.

Clinical diagnosis is made through muscle biopsy, with observation of the encysted larvae in the muscle tissue. Enzyme immunoassay that detects *Trichinella* antibodies is available; however, antibody levels often are not detectable until 1 month after infection. Antibody levels peak in the second or third month after infection and then decline. A skin test also can be used to assist in the diagnosis.

There are other species of *Trichinella* with particular animal reservoirs and geographic locations. These include *T. pseudospiralis*, which is found worldwide in mammals and birds, and *T. nativa*, which is found in Arctic bears. Another species, *T. nelsoni*, is found in African predators, and *T. britovi* is associated with carnivores native to Europe and western Asia.

BLOOD AND TISSUE NEMATODES: FILARIAL WORMS

The filarial worms are long, thin nematodes that parasitize the circulatory and lymphatic systems; serous cavities; and subcutaneous and deep connective tissues, including the muscles. These nematodes are agents of filariasis, which requires an arthropod vector, usually a mosquito, to complete the life cycle. There are currently eight species of filarial parasites that cause the majority of human infections. These are summarized in BOX 21-5.

The life cycle begins as the infected arthropod takes a blood meal on the human host. The parasite matures in the circulatory system, connective tissue, or serous body cavity. The adult worms produce microfilariae, which may be found in the blood or on the skin. Ingestion by a bloodsucking insect perpetuates the life cycle.

The clinically important filarial worms include *Wuchereria bancrofti*, *Brugia malayi*, *Brugia timori*, *Loa loa*, *Onchocerca volvulus*, *Mansonella persans*, and *Mansonella ozzardi*. Diagnosis is made through observation of the motile microfilariae in fresh and thin and thick stained blood smears. Examination of skin snips may be used to diagnose infection by those worms that infect the skin and subcutaneous tissue. Important identifying characteristics include the presence or absence of a sheath on the microfilaria, the shape of the tail, and the distribution of nuclei in the tail region. The sheath is an envelope over the worm, which is a remnant of the ovum membrane.

BOX 21-5 Filarial Parasites

Filarial Parasite Disease

Wuchereria bancrofti—Lymphatic filariasis (Bancroft's filariasis)

Brugia malayi—Lymphatic filariasis (Malayan filariasis)

Brugia timori—Lymphatic filariasis

Dracunculus medinensis—Dracunculias, guinea worm disease

Onchocerca volvulus—Onchocerciasis (river blindness)

Loa loa—Filariasis (eye worm)

Mansonella perstans—Filariasis

M. ozzardi—Filariasis

Wuchereria bancrofti

Wuchereria bancrofti is found in the tropics, subtropics, Caribbean, central Africa, the southwestern Pacific Islands, Turkey, Hungary, Brazil, and the West Indies. The life cycle begins as infected mosquitoes take a blood meal, injecting the third-stage larval form into the host's skin. Maturation to adult forms occurs in several months to a year, and adult worms can survive for 10 to 15 years within coiled masses in the lymphatics. The adult male fertilizes the female, which releases hundreds of microfilariae into the peripheral blood. The microfilariae have a nocturnal periodicity, with the greatest yield in the peripheral blood occurring from 10 P.M. to 2 A.M. The life cycle continues if a female mosquito takes a blood meal, ingesting the microfilariae, which penetrate the gut wall of the mosquito and enter its thoracic muscles, where maturation to the third-stage larvae occurs in 10 days. Migration to the proboscis, the mosquito's tubular feeding organ, follows, and during the blood meal the larvae escape into the host's skin.

The infection is known as Bancroft's filariasis or elephantiasis, and the adult worms live in the host's lymphatic channels, primarily in the arms, legs, and pelvis. An acute tissue reaction occurs, with the accumulation of lymphatic fluid, swelling, and later fibrosis. Eosinophilia is often present.

The microfilariae are sheathed and measure 250 μm to 300 μm. The nuclear column is arranged in parallel rows of nuclei, which do not extend into the tip of the tail. A clear, cephalic space develops at the tip of the tail. The body is slightly curved with a tail that tapers to a point. Microfilaria may be absent from the blood and found in pulmonary vessels and other organs during the day.

Brugia malayi and *B. timori*

Brugia malayi, the cause of Malayan filariasis and elephantiasis, is found in southeast Asia, Korea, India, Indonesia, and China. *Brugia timori* is restricted to some of the islands of Indonesia; it also is associated with lymphatic filariasis. The vectors are mosquitoes within the genera *Mansonia* and *Aedes*. The infected mosquito injects third-stage larvae into the human host during the blood meal. Here, the larvae penetrate the wound and mature into adult forms in the lymphatic vessels. The life cycle is similar to that of *W. bancrofti*, with the adult worms living primarily in the lymphatics but also sometimes in the blood vessels. Adult worms are smaller in size than those of *Wuchereria*, with females measuring 40 mm to 55 mm long by 130 μm to 170 μm wide. Males measure 10 mm to 25 mm by 70 μm to 80 μm wide.

Sheathed microfilariae are produced by the adult female and found in the blood during evening hours. The microfilariae migrate into the lymph, enter the blood, and reach the peripheral blood. During a blood meal, the mosquito ingests the microfilariae, which now lose their sheaths. Within the thoracic area of the mosquito, they develop into first-stage larvae and mature into third-stage larvae. The microfilariae eventually travel to the mosquito's proboscis, where they can infect another person when the mosquito takes a blood meal.

Microfilariae of *Brugia malayi* measure 180 μm to 250 μm by 5 μm to 6 μm. The two distinct nuclei are isolated in the tip of the tail, one subterminally and the other terminally. The tail is tapered, with a constriction separating the terminal nucleus from the remaining nuclei. The microfilaria of *B. timori* have a longer cephalic space and more nuclei arranged in a single row toward the tail compared to those of *B. malayi*. The sheath of *B. timori* does not stain with Giemsa.

Loa loa

Loa loa, eye worm, initiates infection when the bloodsucking tabanid fly (in the genus *Chrysops*) takes a blood meal, injecting the third-stage larvae into the host's skin. The adults mature in the subcutaneous tissue within 6 months but can survive for up to 17 years. The adult female measures 40 mm to 70 mm long by 0.5 mm wide, and the male measures 30 mm to 35 mm long by 0.4 mm wide. The fertilized female releases sheathed microfilariae, which measure 250 μm to 300 μm into the blood. The microfilariae also may be found in the lungs. The life cycle continues if a fly takes a blood meal from an infected host. Following ingestion, the microfilariae lose their sheaths and travel from the midgut of the fly to its thoracic muscles. Here they develop into first-stage larvae and then into third-stage larvae. The third-stage larval form travels to the fly's proboscis, where infection can continue if the fly takes a blood meal.

Loiasis occurs as the adult worms migrate through subcutaneous tissue, releasing their toxic metabolites and resulting in inflammation. The worms typically migrate to the conjunctiva, across the bridge of the nose, and into the cornea of the eye.

Diagnosis is achieved through clinical signs and the demonstration of sheathed microfilariae in peripheral blood. The highest yield is found in specimens obtained between 11 A.M. and 1 P.M. The microfilariae measure 250 μm to 300 μm in length and have a gradually tapered tail that does not draw to a point. The nuclei extend all the way into the tip of the tail, with the last several nuclei irregularly spaced.

FIGURE 21-29 shows *Loa loa* in a Giemsa-stained blood smear.

Onchocerca volvulus

Onchocerca volvulus is the agent of onchocerciasis, or river blindness. The disease is found in South and Central America and Africa, where areas for the breeding of the black fly vector in the genus *Simulium* are abundant. Black flies inject larvae into the wound during their blood meal. The larvae migrate to the subcutaneous tissue and mature to adults within 3 to 15 months but can survive for up to 15 years. The mature female releases unsheathed

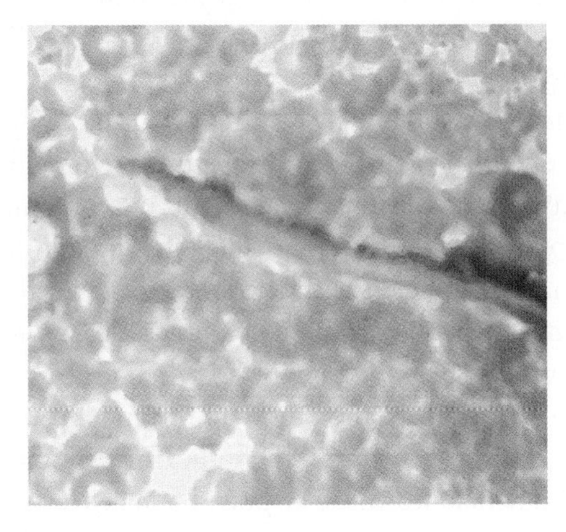

FIGURE 21-29 *Loa loa* in a blood smear.

microfilariae, which are found primarily in the lymphatics of connective and cutaneous tissues. Adult worms survive in coiled masses in the host's subcutaneous tissue. The host's inflammatory response results in the formation of an encapsulated nodule, or onchocercoma, which can be felt in the large bones of the arm, leg, and scalp and also in deeper tissues.

Diagnosis is made through clinical signs and demonstration of the microfilariae in skin snips; the microfilariae are usually not found in the blood. During heavier infestations, the microfilariae may invade the eye, causing river blindness. The microfilariae are large and unsheathed, measuring 300 μm to 345 μm, with a sharply pointed tail. The tail may appear sharply bent. There are no nuclei in the tip of the tail, and a cephalic space is present.

Mansonella ozzardi and *M. perstans*

Mansonella infections may be asymptomatic or have symptoms, which include fever; headache; arthralgia; and skin irritations, such as pruritus and pigmentation changes. There also may be lymphoadenopathy, pulmonary and neurological symptoms, and hepatosplenomegaly. The life cycle follows that of the other filarial worms. The microfilariae of *M. ozzardi* are unsheathed and measure 160 μm to 250 μm and have a tail that tapers to a point. The nuclei do not extend into the tip of the tail; the tail may be bent to form a small hooklike appearance. The microfilariae of *M. perstans* have a tail that tapers to a point, and the nuclei end well before the end of the tail. Microfilariae of *Mansonella* circulate in blood. *Mansonella perstans* is found in Africa and South America, and the vector is the infected midge from the genus *Culicoides. M. ozzardi* is found in South America, and its vectors are midges in the genus *Culicoides* and black flies in the genus *Simulium*.

Dracunculus medinensis

Dracunculus medinensis, the guinea worm, is the cause of dracunculiasis, also known as guinea worm disease. Humans acquire the infection by drinking contaminated, unfiltered water that contains small crustaceans or copepods that are infected with the larvae of *D. medinensis*. After ingestion, the copepods die and release the parasitic larvae, which penetrate the host's stomach and intestinal wall. The larvae then move to the abdominal cavity and retroperitoneal space, where they mature into adult male and female worms. The gravid female travels to the subcutaneous tissues of the arms and legs, near the skin's surface. Approximately 1 year after initial infection, the female worm migrates to the surface of the skin, causing a blister and releasing its larvae. The infected host may seek relief from the painful blister by wading in water, which permits the female worm to emerge and release its rhabditiform larvae into the water. Next, the larvae are ingested by copepods, which perpetuate the life cycle when humans ingest the contaminated water.

The infection is characterized by a painful blister, generally on the leg of the infected host, in the area where the female worm emerges. Other symptoms of dracunculiasis prior to the emergence of the worm include nausea, vomiting, and urticaria. There may be secondary bacterial infections and inflammation if the worm is broken when removed.

Diagnosis is made through observation of the characteristic skin lesion; the infection is treated with metronidazole. Dracunculiasis is found in rural, isolated areas in parts of Africa, the Middle East, and India. The infection is found in areas where step-down wells are used; an eradication program has reduced the incidence of the infection.

FIGURE 21-30 provides diagrams and descriptions of the microfilariae.

Cestodes

The members of the class Cestoda are commonly known as tapeworms because of their long, ribbonlike bodies, which appear flat in a cross section. The anterior end of the worm, or **scolex**, is used for attachment to the host through suckers and, in some parasites, hooklets. The **rostellum**, crown of the scolex, may be armed and fitted with hooklets or unarmed and smooth without hooklets. The body of the worm is composed of segments known as **proglottids**, which form by budding at the posterior end of the worm. The chain of developing proglottids is known as the **strobila**. Each mature proglottid is **hermaphroditic**, which means that it contains both male and female reproductive organs. The organs gradually mature, and eventually the proglottids at the posterior end of the worm, known as **gravid proglottids**, have fully developed reproductive organs with a uterus filled with fertilized eggs. The embryo, which may be visible in the tapeworm eggs, is known as the **oncosphere**, or **hexacanth embryo**. The first-stage larvae are motile and usually contain six

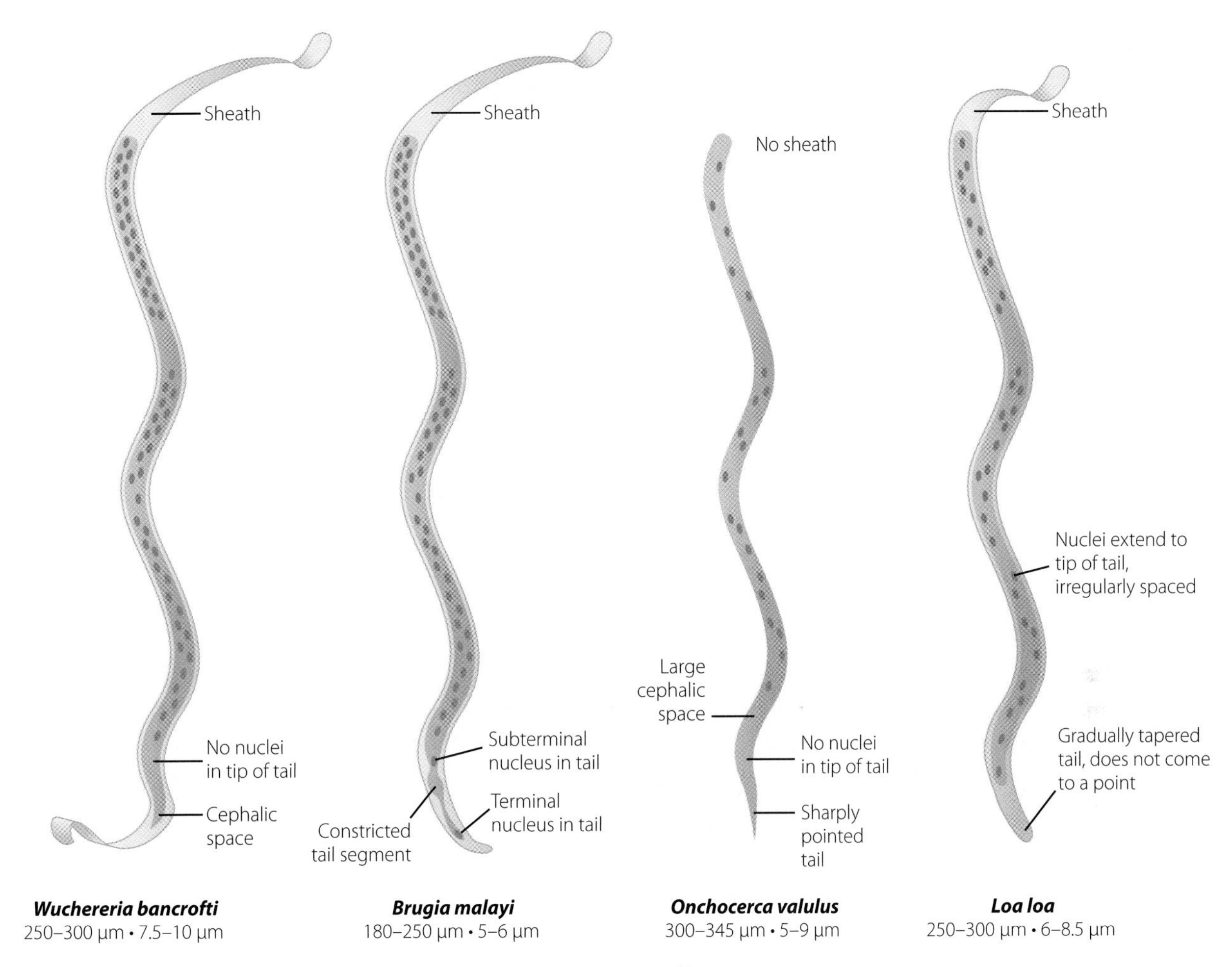

FIGURE 21-30 Diagrams and descriptions of clinically important microfilariae.

hooklets, which enable them to enter the intestinal tract of the intermediate host. Tapeworms do not have mouths, digestive tracts, and vascular systems and must absorb all nutrients and release all waste products through their outer body surface.

TABLE 21-5 summarizes the medically significant tapeworms.

TABLE 21-5 Cestodes-Tapeworms

Scientific name	Common name
Dipylidium caninum	Cat and dog tapeworm
Diphyllobothrium latum	Broad fish tapeworm
Echinococcus granulosus	Dog tapeworm (hydatid cyst)
Taenia saginata	Beef tapeworm
Taenia solium	Pork tapeworm
Hymenolepsis nana	Dwarf tapeworm
Hymenolepsis diminuta	Rat tapeworm

DIPHYLLOBOTHRIUM LATUM

Diphyllobothrium latum, broad fish tapeworm, is the largest tapeworm known to infect humans, with mature adults measuring up to 10 m in length. Crustaceans serve as the first intermediate hosts, and humans and other mammals are the definitive hosts. The definitive hosts are infected by ingesting the **plerocercoid**, or second, larval form. This is the second intermediate host which is raw or uncooked, contaminated freshwater fish. The scolex of the larva, which is shaped like a rounded spatula ("phyllo," meaning leaf) and has a pair ("di") of longitudinal shallow grooves or plates ("both-ria") for sucking on its ventral surface, attaches to the intestine. The individual proglottids are broader than long, and thus the organism is known as "broad tapeworm." The uterus of the gravid proglottid resembles a rosette, or flower petals, with the eggs clustered around the central opening or pore of the uterus. The adult worms develop in the host's small intestine, growing

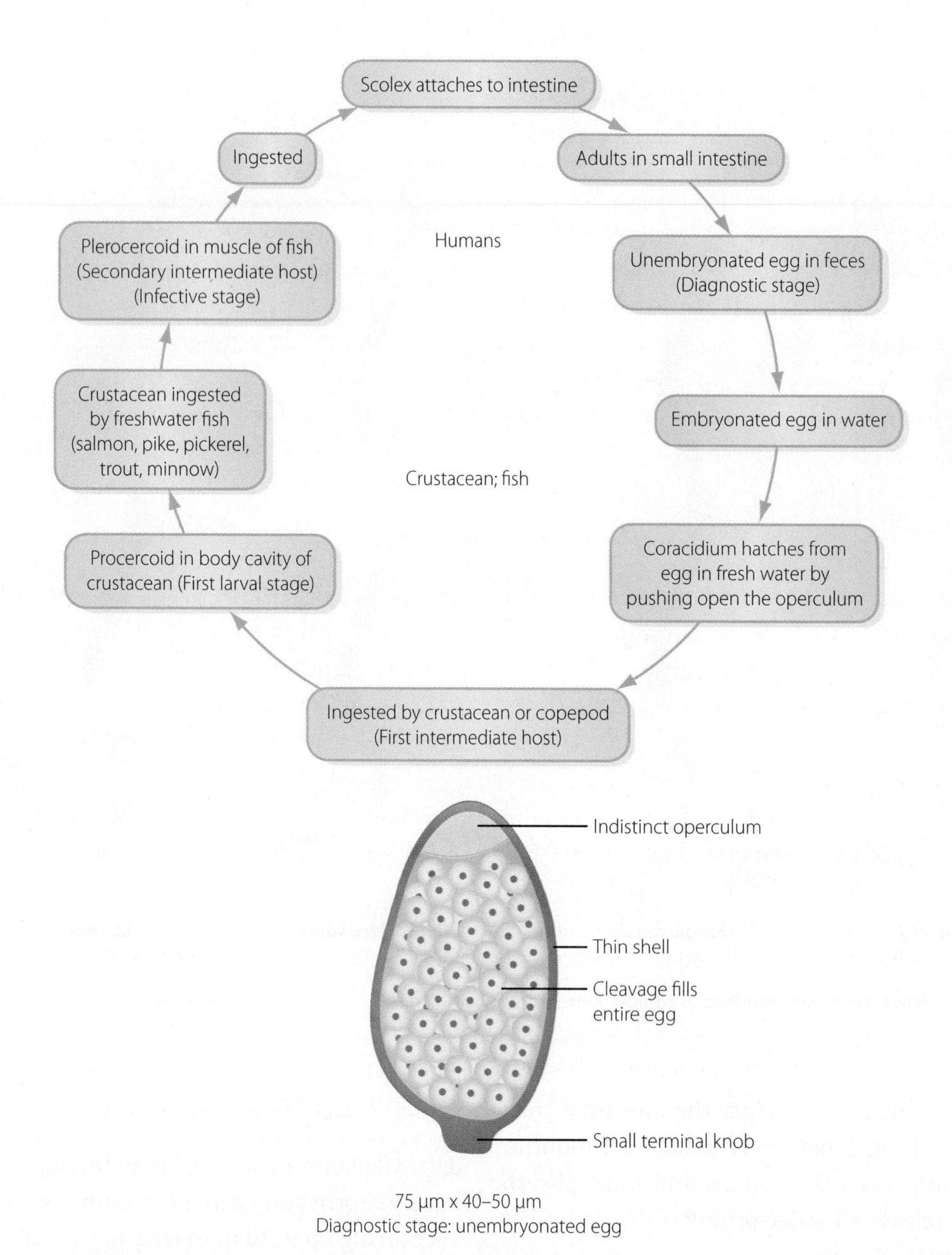

FIGURE 21-31 Life cycle and egg of *Diphyllobothrium latum.*

up to 10 m with over 3,000 proglottids per worm. The unembryonated eggs, which are the diagnostic stage, are passed in the feces of infected humans; up to 1 million eggs per day per worm may be released from the proglottids. **FIGURE 21-31** illustrates the life cycle and egg.

The eggs are passed in the feces 4 to 6 weeks after infection and must reach freshwater for the life cycle to continue. In freshwater the embryos, or oncospheres, develop in the egg and are released from the egg by pushing open the operculum, or lid, of the egg. This free-living larval stage, or **coracidium**, further develops in water and is then ingested by the first intermediate hosts, crustaceans or copepods of the genus *Diaptomus*. **Procercoid larvae**, the first larval stage, develop in the body cavity of the first intermediate host, which are eventually ingested by freshwater fish, usually salmon, trout, pickerel, or pike. Minnows also may ingest the infected crustaceans, which may in turn be ingested by the larger freshwater fish. Within these larger fish, the procercoid larvae develop into the plerocercoid larvae, which are the infective form for humans and other mammals. The life cycle continues, as seen in Figure 21-31.

Infections from *D. latum* are endemic in colder climates in the northern hemisphere, where there are freshwater lakes. These areas include Russia, Europe, northern Asia, China, and Scandinavia, as well as Chile and Argentina. In North America, infections are found in Canada, Alaska, Michigan, and Minnesota. An increased incidence is associated with the consumption of raw fish, especially smoked, pickled, and kippered freshwater fish. Other mammals, including seals and bears, also are known to harbor the parasite.

The diagnostic form is the egg (Figure 21-31). Because each worm may contain thousands of proglottids, which can release up to 1 million eggs daily. Thus the eggs may be observed even in unconcentrated stools in wet mount preparations. The eggs resemble those of *Paragonimus westermani*. However, *D. latum* eggs are shorter and widest in the middle, with an indistinct knob and rounded operculum. *P. westermani* eggs are the widest near the operculum, with no knob, and measure 80 μm to 120 μm. The characteristic morphology of the gravid proglottid and scolex also can be used in identification when isolated.

Diphyllobothriasis may cause infections that last for years and decades. While many infections are asymptomatic, there may be abdominal pain, diarrhea, vomiting, and weigh loss. In severe infections, vitamin B_{12} deficiency, with pernicious anemia and intestinal obstruction, may occur.

Infections are treated with praziquantel or niclosamide.

There are other *Diphyllobothrium* species known to cause infections in humans. These are found less frequently than are *D. latum* and include *D. pacificum*, *D. cordatum*, *D. ursi*, and *D. dendriticum*.

HYMENOLEPSIS NANA

Hymenolepsis nana, dwarf tapeworm, possesses a scolex with four rounded suckers. Along with *H. diminuta*, it is the cause of hymenolepiasis. Infections may be asymptomatic, but there may be weakness, anorexia, abdominal pain, and diarrhea with more heavy infestations. Infections are treated with praziquante.

The infective form is the egg, which is ingested by humans in food or water contaminated with the embryonated egg. The eggs are immediately infectious when passed but don't survive for longer than a week to 10 days in the external environment. The egg contains the oncosphere, or hexacanth embryo, in a double-walled structure, which penetrates the intestinal wall and matures into cysticercoid larvae. Once the intestinal villa rupture, the cysticercoid larvae attach to the intestinal lumen and mature into adult forms. These live in the small intestine and produce gravid proglottids, which then release eggs into the environment, thus continuing the cycle.

Adult worms can live for 4 to 6 weeks. A route of autoinfection also is possible.

The scolex of *H. nana* is an armed rostellum with a ring of 20 to 30 spines and hooks, which resemble a beaklike structure. The scolex has a single row of hooklets, or sucking organs, and is very small, measuring less than 0.4 mm. The gravid proglottids may be passed in the feces and have a narrow neck region, which broadens at the distal end. The gravid uterus is a small, saclike cluster near the center of each segment, and the uterine pore is central but usually not visible.

H. nana does not need a separate intermediate host, and humans serve as both the intermediate and the definitive host. However, eggs also may be ingested by intermediate arthropod hosts, such as fleas and beetles. Within these arthropods, cysticercoid forms develop, which then can infect humans or rodents upon ingestion and mature into adults in the gastrointestinal tract.

The infection is acquired through the ingestion of food or water contaminated with the feces of rats or mice. The infection is seen worldwide but most often occurs in the warmer climates, including Central America and the southeastern parts of the United States. It is the most common cestode infection in the world and is found most often in children and in institutionalized settings. Children also can acquire the infection from the hand-to-mouth route.

The diagnostic form is the egg, which is hexacanth or lancet shaped, with six hooklets (**FIGURE 21-32**). It is round to oval, measuring 30 μm to 50 μm, with a thin, smooth membrane ("hymen") and outer shell ("lepsis") surrounding the membrane. The oncosphere is enclosed within the thin membrane, leaving a clear space between it and the shell. Four to eight filaments emerge from the inner membrane of the egg.

HYMENOLEPSIS DIMINUTA

Hymenolepsis diminuta, the cause of rat tapeworm infection, very rarely is found in humans. The organism requires an intermediate host of arthropods, such as fleas or grain beetles, for the life cycle to be completed. The definitive hosts may be humans, rats, or mice. Humans may acquire the infection through ingestion of arthropods in contaminated foods, such as cereals or grains, or directly through

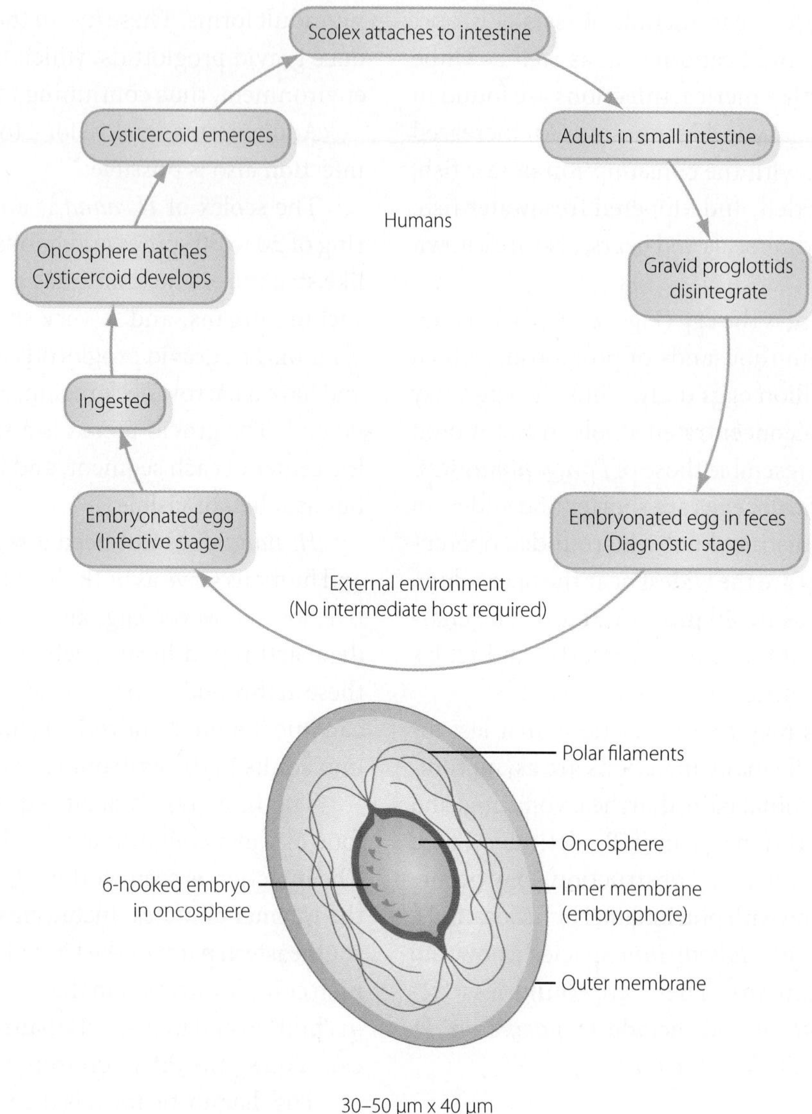

FIGURE 21-32 Life cycle and egg of *Hymenolepsis nana.*

the environment. Grain beetles or fleas may ingest the eggs and serve as the intermediate host. The oncosphere hatches within the arthropod, and if the arthropod is ingested by humans, the adult worm may develop in the intestinal tract. The eggs are passed in the feces of the infected definitive hosts, which are rodents or humans. The eggs may be ingested by the intermediate hosts, and oncospheres are released, which penetrate the intestinal tract of the host. The cysticercoid larvae develops, and mature adults form in the intermediate host. The definitive host frees the parasite by ingesting the intermediate host; the cysticercoid larvae are released in the stomach and small intestine.

The parasite attaches to the wall of the small intestine by four suckers on its scolex. It takes about 3 weeks for the maturation of the parasite; adult worms grow to approximately 30 cm. The gravid proglottid releases eggs in the small intestine, which are passed into the environment through the stool.

To differentiate *H. nana* from *H. diminuta*, the eggs and rostellum are examined. The eggs of *H. diminuta* are slightly larger (50 μm–70 μm) and more oval, with no filaments (**FIGURE 21-33**). In contrast to the armed rostellum of *H. nana*, *H. diminuta* has an unarmed rostellum.

DIPYLIDIUM CANIUM

Dipylidium canium, the double-pored tapeworm, is a common tapeworm of dogs and cats but also may cause

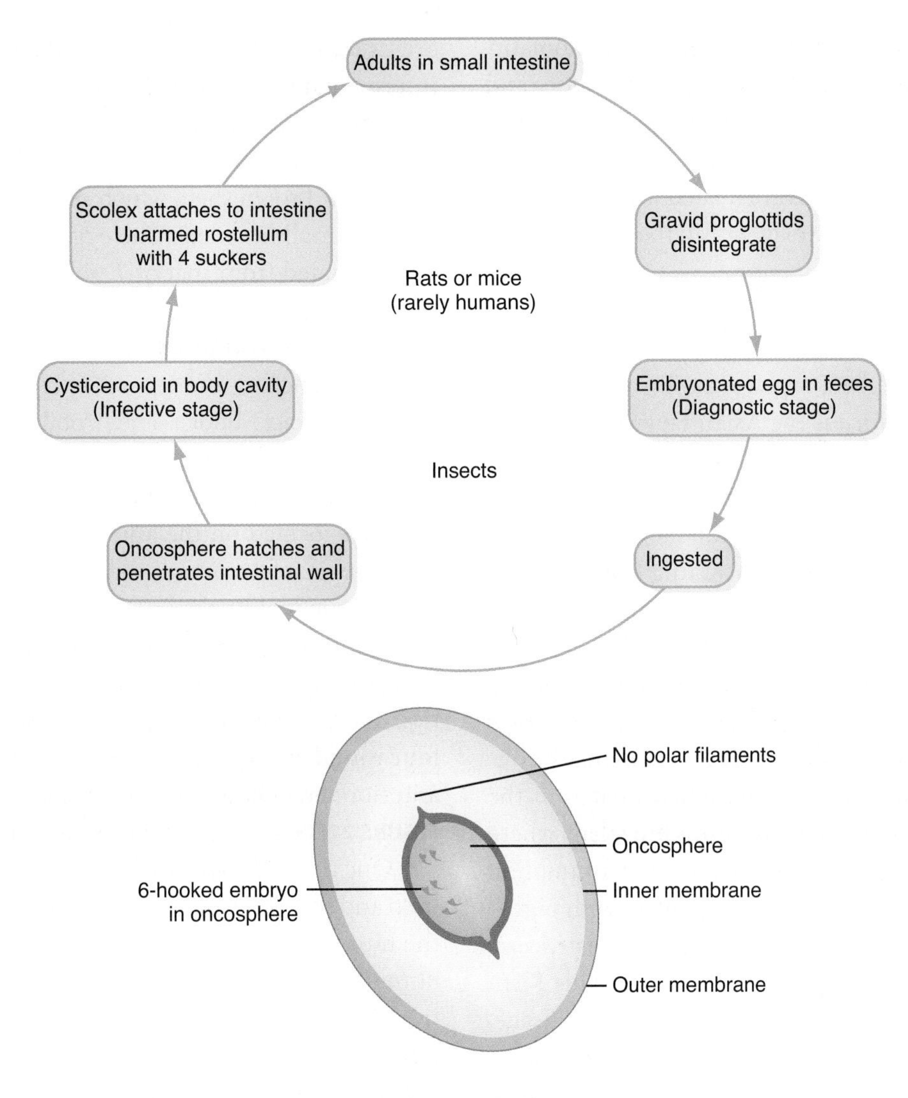

FIGURE 21-33 Life cycle and egg of *Hymenolepsis diminuta.*

infections in children and household pets. Humans may acquire the infection by ingesting food or water contaminated with dog or cat fleas. The infection is found worldwide, with human infections occurring in Europe, the United States, China, Japan, and Argentina.

The stroblia measure 15 cm to 75 cm long, with 50 to 150 proglottids. The scolex is conical rhomboidal, with an armed rostellum. The proglottids may detach and then migrate from the anus of the animal, appearing as small grains of rice in the external environment. Cysticercoid larvae develop in the feces after ingestion of embryonated egg packets. The infection is diagnosed by observation of the egg packets or gravid proglottids in the feces or on the genital hair. Each egg packet is large and irregular, containing 15 to 25 globular eggs, each with a diameter of 35 μm to 60 μm, with an oncosphere with six hooklets.

Humans acquire the infection by ingesting cysticercoid-contaminated fleas through contact with infected pets. The cysticercoid form develops into the adult tapeworm in the intestinal tract of the mammalian host approximately 1 month after infection. Adult worms, which can grow up to 50 cm in length, attach by the scolex to the small intestine. Here they produce proglottids that have two genital pores ("double pored"). As the proglottids mature, they break off of the tapeworm and migrate to the anus, where they are passed in the stool with the characteristic egg packets.

Infections with *Dipylidium* are usually asymptomatic; however, there may be mild abdominal pain and nausea and pruritus in the anal area, exhibited by dogs and cats. The presence of proglottids in the stool is a remarkable finding in pets and children. Infections are treated with praziquantel, which dissolves the tapeworm within the intestines.

TAENIA SAGINATA, *T. SOLIUM*, AND *T. ASIATICA*

Taenia saginata is the beef tapeworm, *T. solium* is pork tapeworm, and *T. asiatica* is the Asian tapeworm. All are causes of taeniasis; *T. solium* also is a cause of cysticercosis. *T. saginata* and *T. solium* are found worldwide, including in Central and South America, Russia, and Africa. *T. asiatica* mostly is found in Asia, including Korea, China, Indonesia, and Thailand. Humans are the only definitive host for all three parasites.

Eggs or gravid proglottids are passed in the stool and remain infective in the environment for months. Pigs (*T. solium* and *T. asiatica*) or cows (*T. saginata*) ingest contaminated vegetation, and the oncospheres hatch in the animal's intestine. Infections are more prevalent where there is substandard disposal of human feces, consumption of raw pork or beef, and close human contact with pigs.

The intestinal walls are attached, and the cysticerci form develops within striated muscle tissue. This form can survive for many years in the animal's muscle tissue. Humans acquire the infection by consuming raw or undercooked infected beef or pork. Once in the human intestine, the cysticercus matures into the adult worm within 2 months. Here the adult worms attach by the scolex. The adults form proglottids, which become gravid, break off of the tapeworm, and travel to the anus, where they are passed in the stool. The eggs also are released from the proglottids when passed in the stool. *T. solium* has approximately 1,000 proglottids and produces about 50,000 eggs per proglottid, whereas *T. saginata* has from 1,000 to 2,000 proglottids and produces up to 100,000 eggs per proglottid.

Taenia saginata, beef tapeworm, infection occurs from the ingestion of the cyst form in contaminated rare or uncooked beef. The infective form is the **cysticercus** in the muscle tissue of cattle and other herbivores. The cysts hatch in the intestinal tract and attach by four rounded suckers to the mucosa in the small intestine. The worm has hooklets and an unarmed rostellum. The life cycle continues, as seen in **FIGURE 21-34**. The adult worm measures 4 m to 10 m in length but can grow as long as 25 m. There are usually 1,000 to 2,000 proglottids per tapeworm. The intermediate hosts, usually cattle, ingest the proglottids on contaminated grass. Both the eggs and the gravid proglottids are the diagnostic stages (Figure 21-34). The egg has a dark brown shell, which surrounds the oncosphere, and six small hooklets. The egg of *T. saginata* cannot be differentiated from that of *T. solium*, and thus the gravid proglottid should be examined for a definitive identification. The gravid proglottid of *T. saginata* has 15 to 20 uterine branches, and its scolex is very small, with four suckers and lacks hooks. The strobila of *T. solium* measures 2 m to 4 m, with up to 1,000 proglottids. Its gravid proglottid has 5 to 12 major uterine branches, with two rows of hooks located on the anterior scolex, which is armed. *T. solium* is referred to as the "armed tapeworm" because of this crown of hooks.

T. solium, pork tapeworm, has a life cycle similar to that of *T. saginata*. Humans are infected through the ingestion of cysts in uncooked pork. The scolex of *T. solium* has four round suckers and two rows of hooks, located at the anterior end. The adult worm measures from 2 m to 6 m. **FIGURE 21-35** depicts the life cycle and egg of *T. solium*.

One major distinction between the life cycle of *T. saginata* and that of *T. solium* is *T. solium*'s ability to autoinfect the human host. The eggs are infective for both pigs and humans. Once the eggs are produced by the gravid proglottids, the oncospheres may hatch in the small intestine, penetrate the intestinal wall, and enter the circulation. This can lead to cysticercus, the development of the extraintestinal encysted larval form in various organs, including the brain, lungs, eye, or connective tissue. This does not happen with *T. saginata* because the eggs are not believed to be infectious.

Those who are infected usually harbor one adult worm and have few clinical manifestations. *T. solium* infections are usually more serious because the entire encystment may occur in the brain or muscle, which may result in paralysis and mental disorientation. A striking characteristic of the infection is the presence of the proglottids in the stool. *Taenia* infections are treated with praziquantel.

ECHINOCOCCUS GRANULOSUS

Echinococcus granulosus is the agent of echinococcosis, or hydatid cyst disease. The infection occurs worldwide and most frequently is found in rural areas, where dogs eat organs from infected animals.

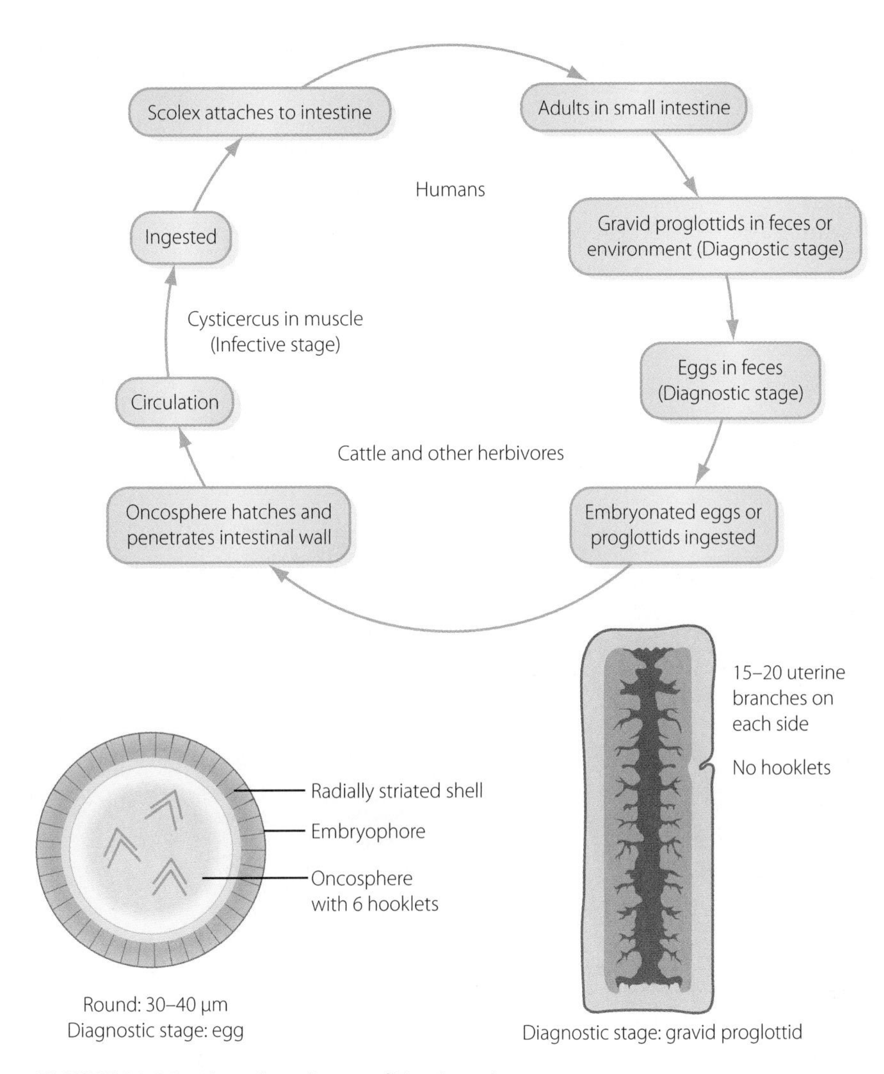

FIGURE 21-34 Life cycle and eggs of *Taenia saginata.*

Infection results from ingestion of embryonated eggs in the feces of dogs and other carnivores, which serve as the definitive hosts. After ingestion in humans, the oncosphere hatches, penetrates the intestinal wall, enters the circulation, and forms hydatid cysts in the liver, lungs, or other tissues, where the life cycle ends. The cysts may have a longevity up to 30 years in humans and require surgical removal.

If the embryonated eggs are ingested by sheep, pigs, or cattle, the cycle results in the formation of hydatid cysts in the viscera, which may be ingested by carnivores, such as dogs or wolves. The scolex from the cyst attaches to the intestine, and adults develop in the small intestine. The gravid proglottids then produce eggs, which are released in the animal's feces. If ingested by the intermediate hosts, including humans, sheep, pigs, or cattle, then the life cycle continues.

Hexacanth eggs, resembling those of *Taenia*, are passed in dog feces and embryonate in the soil. The eggs are ingested by intermediate hosts, such as sheep, cattle, or pigs. Larvae are released from eggs in the intestine of the intermediate host, bore through the bowel wall with hooklets, and then enter the circulation. Humans are accidental hosts and can acquire the infection through ingestion of vegetation or soil contaminated with dog feces that contain the eggs.

Diagnosis is made by demonstration of the fluid-filled cysts, which contain the worm, in biopsy. Small cysts, commonly known as "bladder worms," also may be observed in tissue biopsy.

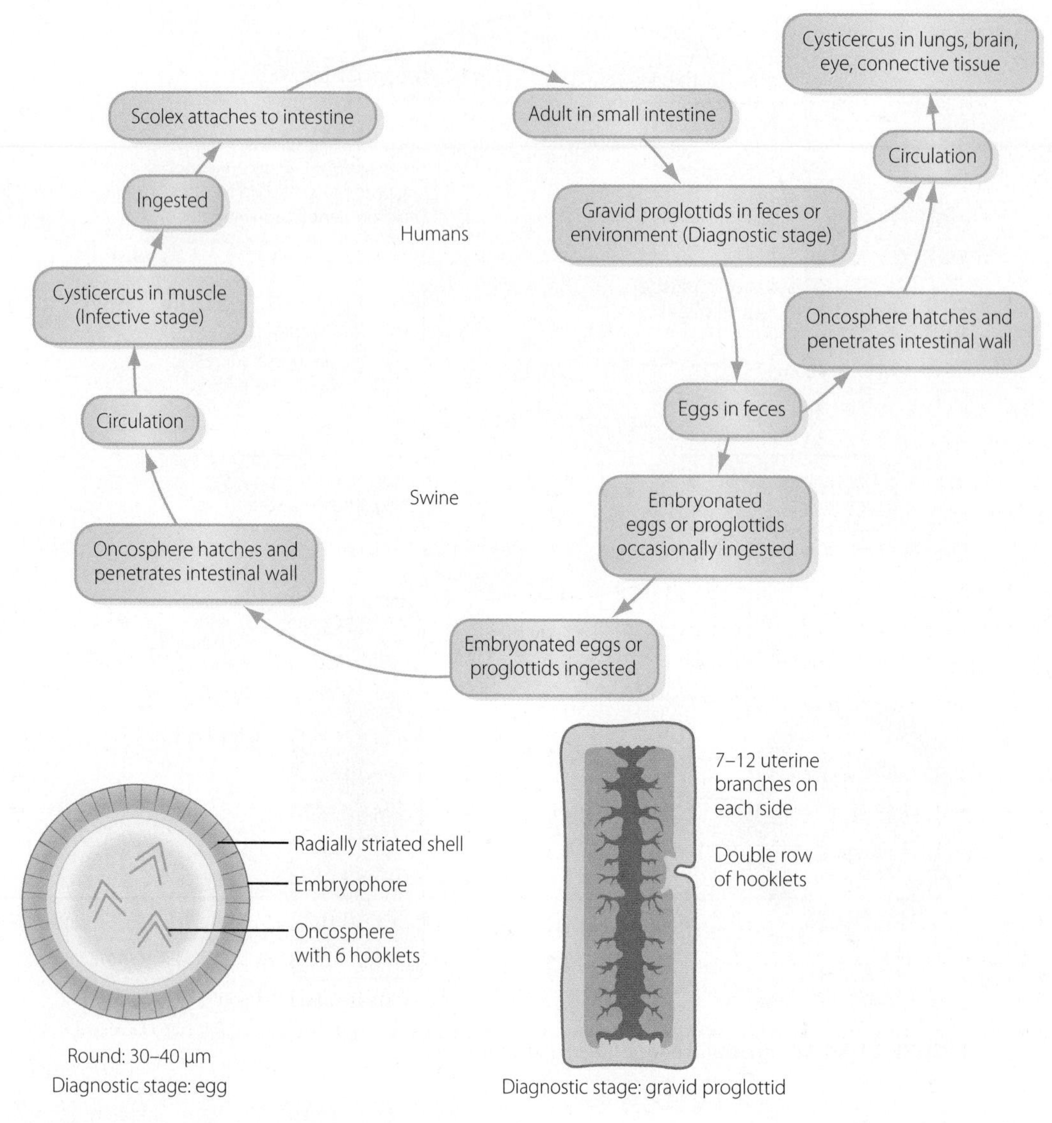

FIGURE 21-35 Life cycle and egg of *Taenia solium.*

Hydatid cyst disease is a disease of those whose lifestyles are closely associated with sheep or dogs. Herdsmen who slaughter animals and feed the organs to dogs may cause the disease in dogs. Humans then may be infected by ingesting the eggs. These infections may remain latent for many years until the cysts are large enough to cause symptoms. Organs involved include the liver, where there may be bile duct obstruction and abdominal pain, and the lungs, where there may be chest pain, coughing, and hemoptysis. If the cysts rupture, there is fever, urticaria, and eosinophilia. The brain, heart, and bones also may be affected, and the cysts can disseminate, causing shock.

Surgical removal of the cyst is necessary to prevent its rupture and reinfection when the scoleces and daughter cysts are released. Albendazole also is given to prevent recurrence of the cyst.

Trematodes

The trematodes, or flatworms, belong to the class Digenea and commonly are known as flukes. Flukes are **digenetic**, which means that they are able to multiply through both sexual and asexual cycles. The worms appear flat in cross section and are nonsegmented and leaf shaped. Adult flukes possess one oral sucker, which opens to the digestive tract, and one ventral sucker for attachment. The suckers are cup shaped and muscular. The digestive system consists of the oral cavity in the middle of the oral sucker and the intestinal tract, which terminates in one or two sacs. Waste products are regurgitated because there is no anal opening. The body surface absorbs nutrients and releases wastes.

Two types of flukes parasitize humans: hermaphroditic and blood flukes. The hermaphroditic flukes, which infect the intestinal tract and other organs, have a complex reproductive system with both male and female structures. Blood flukes have unisexual male and female forms and infect the blood vessels of the definitive host. The male and female forms coexist as adults in the blood vessels, and the male wraps around the female during copulation. BOX 21-6 summarizes the life cycle of the flukes, and **TABLE 21-6** summarizes the medically important flukes.

The flukes possess a complex life cycle that involves several stages and at least two intermediate hosts. The adult flukes lay eggs, which are deposited in the feces, urine, or sputum of the host depending on the species of the fluke. The first larval stage, the **miracidium**, hatches from the egg in freshwater and enters the first intermediate host, the freshwater snail. The species of snail infected depends on the specific fluke. The miracidium is ciliated and free swimming and must be able to penetrate the snail. Several stages of asexual reproduction occur in the snail, and the final larval stage, known as the **cercaria**, leaves the snail. This is the stage of the life cycle that develops from germ cells in a sporocyst, which is a saclike structure with germinal cells, or rediae. **Redia** is the name given to a series of maturation stages that occur within the snail. This stage is the larval stage, characterized by the development of the pharynx and tail and early intestinal development. Hundreds of cercaria form from each miracidium that enters the snail. The hermaphroditic cercariae then encyst as metacercariae on freshwater vegetation, such as water chestnuts, or can enter a second intermediate host, usually a freshwater fish or crustacean. Humans acquire the infection through ingestion of vegetation or fish, crab, or crayfish that contain encysted metacercariae. The **metacercaria** is the stage of the hermaphroditic fluke that occurs after the cercaria sheds its tail, secretes a protective wall, and encysts on water plants or the second intermediate host. This is the infective stage for humans. The motile schistosomes of the blood flukes directly penetrate the host tissues. The metacercariae then encyst in the human intestinal tract and migrate to various sites, depending on the species, and mature to the adult stage. Eggs are then released, which can be detected in either the feces, urine, or sputum.

TABLE 21-6 Medically Important Flukes

Scientific name	Common name
Hermaphroditic flukes	
Fasciolopsis buski	Large intestinal fluke
Fasciola hepatica	Sheep liver fluke
Clonorchis (Opisthorchis) sinensis	Chinese liver fluke
Paragonimus westermani	Oriental lung fluke
Blood flukes: Schistosomes	
Schistosoma mansoni	Manson's blood fluke
Schistosoma japonicum	Blood fluke
Schistosoma haematobium	Bladder fluke

BOX 21-6 **Life Cycle of Flukes**

1. The adult flatworm produces eggs, which are released in the feces, urine, or sputum of the host.
2. Miracidium is the first larval stage; it hatches from the egg in freshwater.
3. Miracidium is a free-swimming form and penetrates the first intermediate host (snail, copepod).
4. Several stages of sexual reproduction occur in the first intermediate host: the sprorocyst, rediae, and cercariae forms.
5. Cercaria are released from the snail and penetrate the flesh of freshwater fish. Here they encyst and develop into the metacercariae form.
6. Metacercariae excyst in the small intestine and travel up the biliary tract, where they mature in about 1 month.
7. Adult flukes live in biliary ducts and produce eggs.

INTESTINAL FLUKES

Fasciolopsis buski

Fascioloposis buski is known as the large intestinal fluke, with humans and hogs serving as the definitive hosts, and snails and water vegetation as the intermediate hosts. The infection most frequently is seen in the Far East, including Vietnam, Thailand, and Bangladesh, where pigs may serve as the definitive host, with nuts and roots of water plants, such as bamboo and water chestnuts, serving as the second intermediate host. **FIGURE 21-36** depicts the life cycle of *F. buski*.

Immature eggs are shed from the intestinal tract into the stool. While in the water, the eggs embryonate and release miracidia, which attack the intermediate host (snails or water vegetation). The maturation stages that occur in the intermediate host are the sporocyst, rediae, and cercariae, which are released from the snail and then encyst in the metacercariae form on water plants. The metacercariae form is ingested on the water plants by humans or hogs, the definitive hosts. Here they attach to the intestinal wall and grow into adult flukes, which measure 20 mm to 80 mm in length. The egg is the diagnostic form for *F. buski* and is very large, measuring 130 μm to 160 μm long by 50 μm to 70 μm wide (Figure 21-36). The eggs are very similar to those of *Fasciola bepatica* and cannot be differentiated.

Symptoms of infection may be minimal or absent and include abdominal pain, fever, and diarrhea. Intestinal obstruction may occur in heavier infestations, and children may experience edema. The infection is treated with praziquantel.

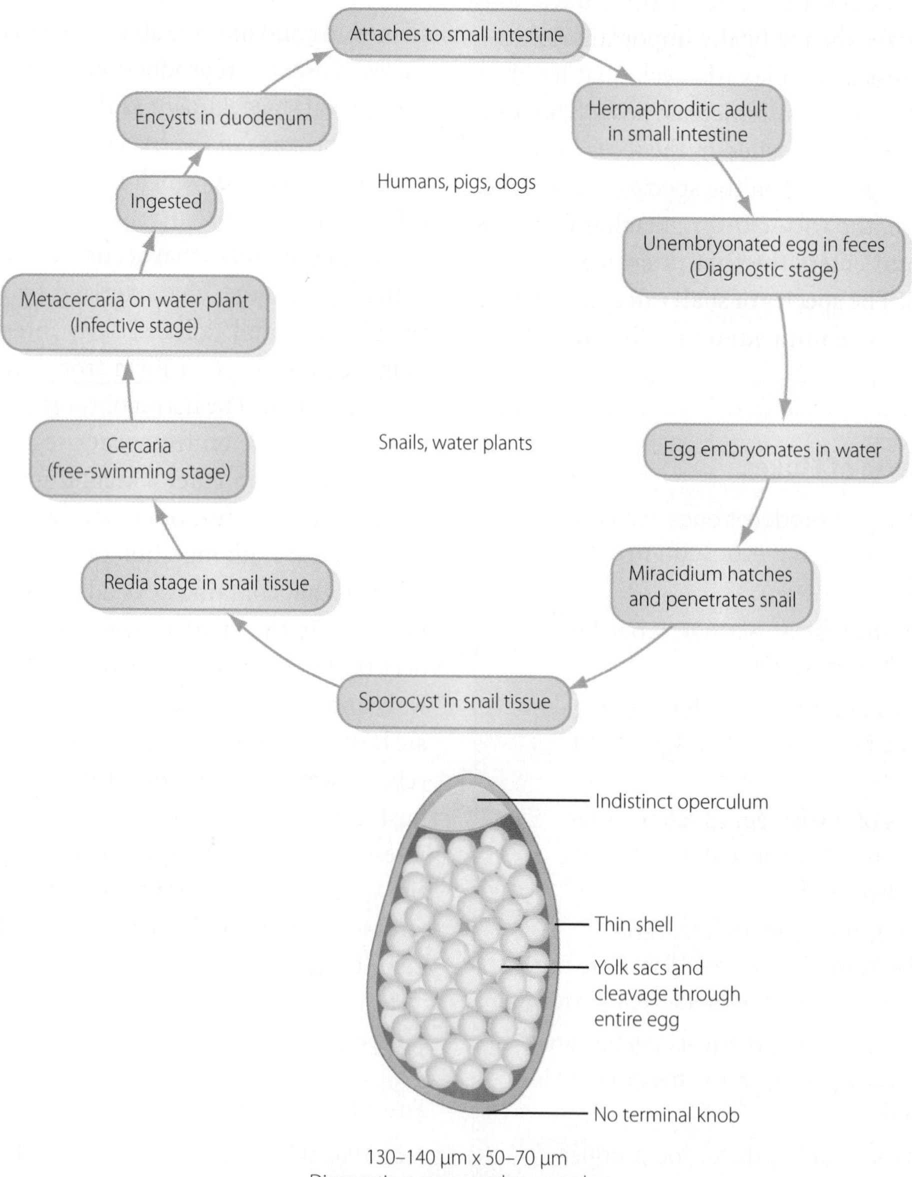

FIGURE 21-36 Life cycle and egg of *Fasciolopsis buski.*

Fasciola hepatica

Fasciola hepatica, the sheep liver fluke, has a life cycle similar to that of *Fasciolopsis buski*. Sheep, cattle, goats, horses, and humans serve as the final definitive host, and snails and water plants serve as the first and second intermediate hosts. Although human infections are rare, cases most often are found in Central, South, and Latin America; the Mediterranean countries; southern France; the United Kingdom; the Middle East; and Algeria. Infections usually are associated with those raising sheep and cattle and where raw watercress is eaten. Infection in the United States is very rare, but cases have been found in southwestern regions, associated with infections acquired from cattle or sheep.

When the immature flukes migrate through the liver, there may be abdominal pain, fever, vomiting, diarrhea, hepatosplenomegaly, urticaria, and eosinophilia. There is a chronic stage of the disease, when the adult fluke is in the bile duct, which may be associated with transient bile duct obstruction and inflammation. *Fasciola hepatica* infections are treated with triclabendazole because praziquantel may not be effective.

The egg is the largest operculated egg isolated from human infections (**FIGURE 21-37**). Differentiation from

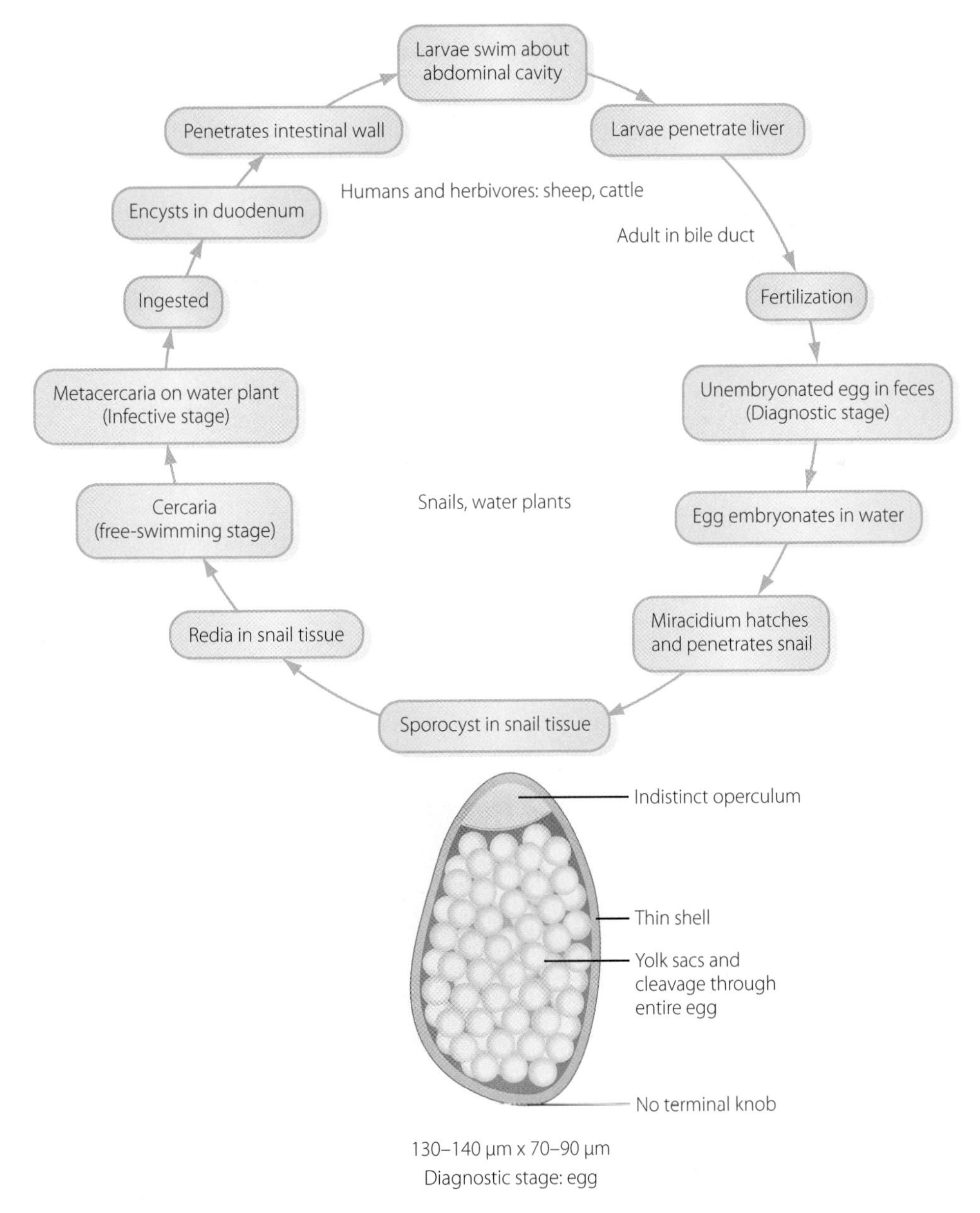

FIGURE 21-37 Life cycle and egg of *Fasciola hepatica*.

Fasciolopsis buski is usually not made, and "*Fasciolopsis/Fasciola* eggs" generally is reported when either of the eggs is isolated.

Clonorchis (Opisthorchis) sinensis

Clonorchis (*Opisthorchis*) *sinensis*, the Chinese or Oriental liver fluke, is found only in those populations that frequently eat raw fish. Infections generally are limited to the Far East, including Japan, China, and Taiwan. The infection has been reported in other areas of the world and is believed to have been brought here through Asian immigrants or following ingestion of imported, undercooked freshwater fish that contains the metacercarial form. Humans, pigs, and cattle may serve as the final, definitive hosts, and the first and second intermediate hosts are snails and fish. **FIGURE 21-38** depicts the life cycle of *C. sinensis*. The life cycle is perpetuated through the use of human or animal feces as fertilizer, which reaches ponds where freshwater fish are caught for food.

Symptoms are generally mild and include indigestion, abdominal pain, nausea, diarrhea, and eosinophilia. Severe infections may result in bile duct obstruction, pancreatitis, and jaundice. Infections are treated with praziquantel or albendazole.

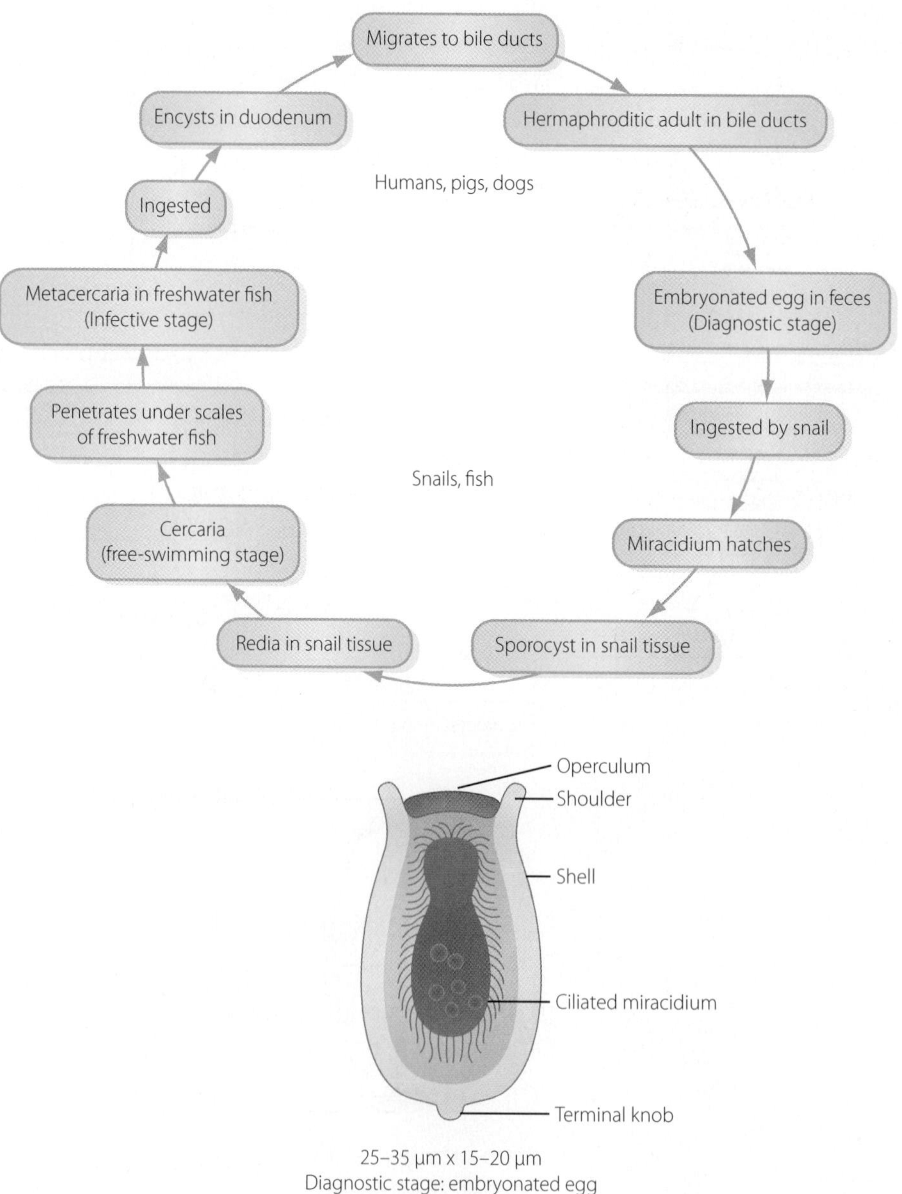

FIGURE 21-38 Life cycle and egg of *Clonorchis* (*Opisthorchis*) *sinensis*.

Paragonimus westermani

Paragonimus westermani, the lung fluke, most frequently is found in the Far East and thus is also known as the Oriental lung fluke. Infections are generally found in the Far East (China, Japan, Vietnam, Korea, Thailand), India, Africa, and South and Central America, where raw or improperly cooked freshwater crab or crayfish is eaten. Humans and other mammals, such as sheep, dogs, and pigs, serve as the final, definitive hosts, and snails and crustaceans serve as the first and second intermediate hosts.

The unembryonated eggs are excreted in the sputum or may be swallowed and then passed in the stool. The eggs embryonate in the environment, hatching miracidia, which penetrate the tissue of the first intermediate host—the snail. Within the snail, the miracidia form sporocysts, rediae, and then cercariae forms, which are released. The cercaria attack the second intermediate host—crabs, crayfish, or other crustaceans—where they develop into metacercariae. The metacercaria is the infectious form for humans and other mammals who ingest the parasite in undercooked crab or crayfish. The metacercariae excyst in the small intestine, penetrate the intestinal wall, and enter the peritoneal cavity. Next, they travel through the abdominal wall and diaphragm and enter the lungs, where they encapsulate and mature into adults. The adult worms also can travel to the brain and striated muscle tissue; however, the life cycle cannot be completed in these tissues. It takes approximately 2 to 3 months to go from infection to egg production; infections can remain in humans for up to 20 years.

The unembryonated egg is typically found in the sputum or feces if it has been swallowed. **FIGURE 21-39** shows the life cycle of *P. westermani*.

The diagnostic form for *P. westermani* is the egg, which is oval and measures 70 μm to 110 μm long by 40 μm to 60 μm wide (Figure 21-39). There are more than 30 species of *Paragonimus*, and over 10 cause human infection. *P. westermani* is the most common species causing human infection. There may be diarrhea, abdominal pain, fever, coughing, hepatosplenomegaly, and pulmonary symptoms during the acute phase of infection. Pulmonary abnormalities become more severe during the chronic phase and include severe cough and hemoptysis. If the brain is involved, there are serious neurologic abnormalities. The infection is treated with praziquantel or bithionol.

SCHISTOSOMES: BLOOD FLUKES

Schistosoma japonicum, S. haematobium, and *S. mansoni*

Schistosomes, or blood flukes, are the agents of schistosomiasis, bilharziasis, and swamp fever. The three species that cause most infections in humans are *S. japonicum*, *S. haematobium*, and *S. mansoni*. There are two less frequent human pathogens: *S. mekongi* and *S. intercalatum*.

Eggs are released in the stool or urine of the infected host. Under favorable conditions, the life cycle begins when the miracidium hatches in freshwater and swims to and penetrates the tissue of the snail, the intermediate host. The sporocyst and redia stages occur in the snail tissue, and eventually the free-swimming cercaria is released. The cercaria, the infective stage, penetrates the skin of humans or other mammals, losing its tail during penetration. The cercariae migrate to the liver through the blood and mature in the portal circulation. The adult worms, which are unisexual, then migrate to the blood vessels, where the female is fertilized by the male. *S. mansoni* is concentrated in the mesenteric vessels of the lower intestine, *S. japonicum* concentrates around the small intestine, and *S. haematobium* is most concentrated around the bladder. The eggs are released into small blood vessels, with the vessels first dilating to allow the egg to enter and then snapping shut tightly to trap the egg. The eggs then are released through the bladder wall into the urine (*S. haematobium*) or through the intestinal wall into the feces (*S. mansoni* and *S. japonicum*).

The diagnostic stage is the egg, which is yellow, elongated, and embryonated, with no operculum. The eggs can be differentiated by the location found, as well as by their size and the location of an extension known as the spine, as shown in **FIGURE 21-40**.

The schistosomes are located worldwide, with certain species predominating in various geographic locations. *S. mansoni* is the most frequently isolated species and is found in South America, Africa, the West Indies, the Middle East, and the Caribbean countries. *S. haematobium* most often is found in Africa, including the Nile Valley; Egypt; India; and Spain. *S. japonicum* infections occur most often in the Far East (Japan, China, Asia) and the Philippines. *S. mekongi* is found in Southeast Asia, and *S. intercalatum* is found in West Africa.

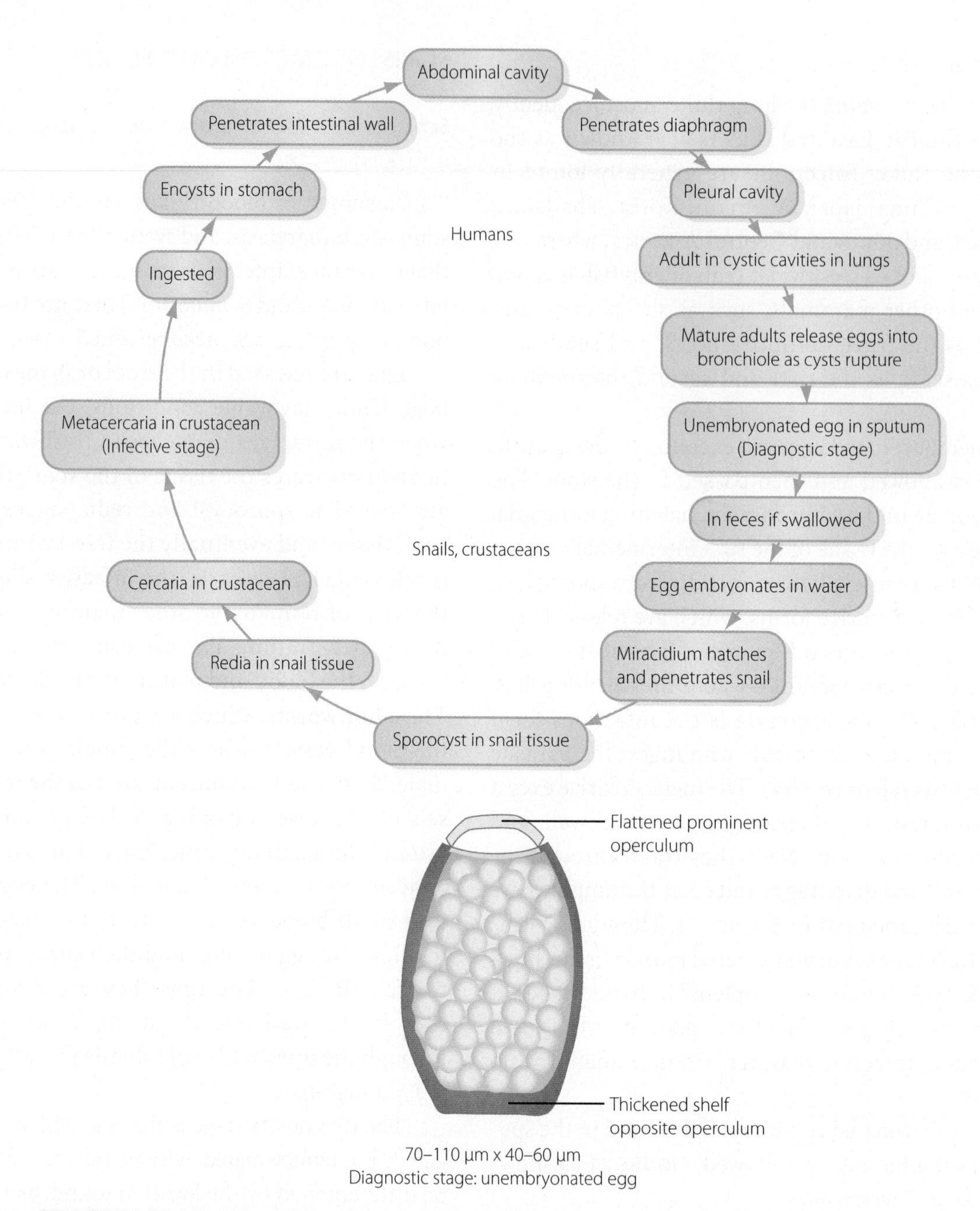

FIGURE 21-39 Life cycle and egg of *Paragonimus westermani.*

The early stages of infection are characterized by a local dermatitis as the cercariae penetrate the skin. As the eggs are deposited in the blood, a serum-like sickness occurs, with allergic symptoms, including eosinophilia and fever, abdominal pain, diarrhea, and hepatosplenomegaly. Later, jaundice may develop, with a hepatitis-like syndrome and bloody diarrhea. Hyperplasia and fibrosis may occur as the host forms granulomas around the eggs, which can travel to various organs, including the liver, bladder, brain, or lung. This may result in intestinal obstruction, impaired urinary function, or other organ damage. *S. mansoni* and *S. japonicum* infections also can cause portal hypertension, egg granulomas in the sinuses of the liver, Katayama fever, and egg granulomas in the brain. *S. haematobium* infections also may cause hematuria, scarring, calcification, squamous cell carcinoma, and egg granulomas in the brain.

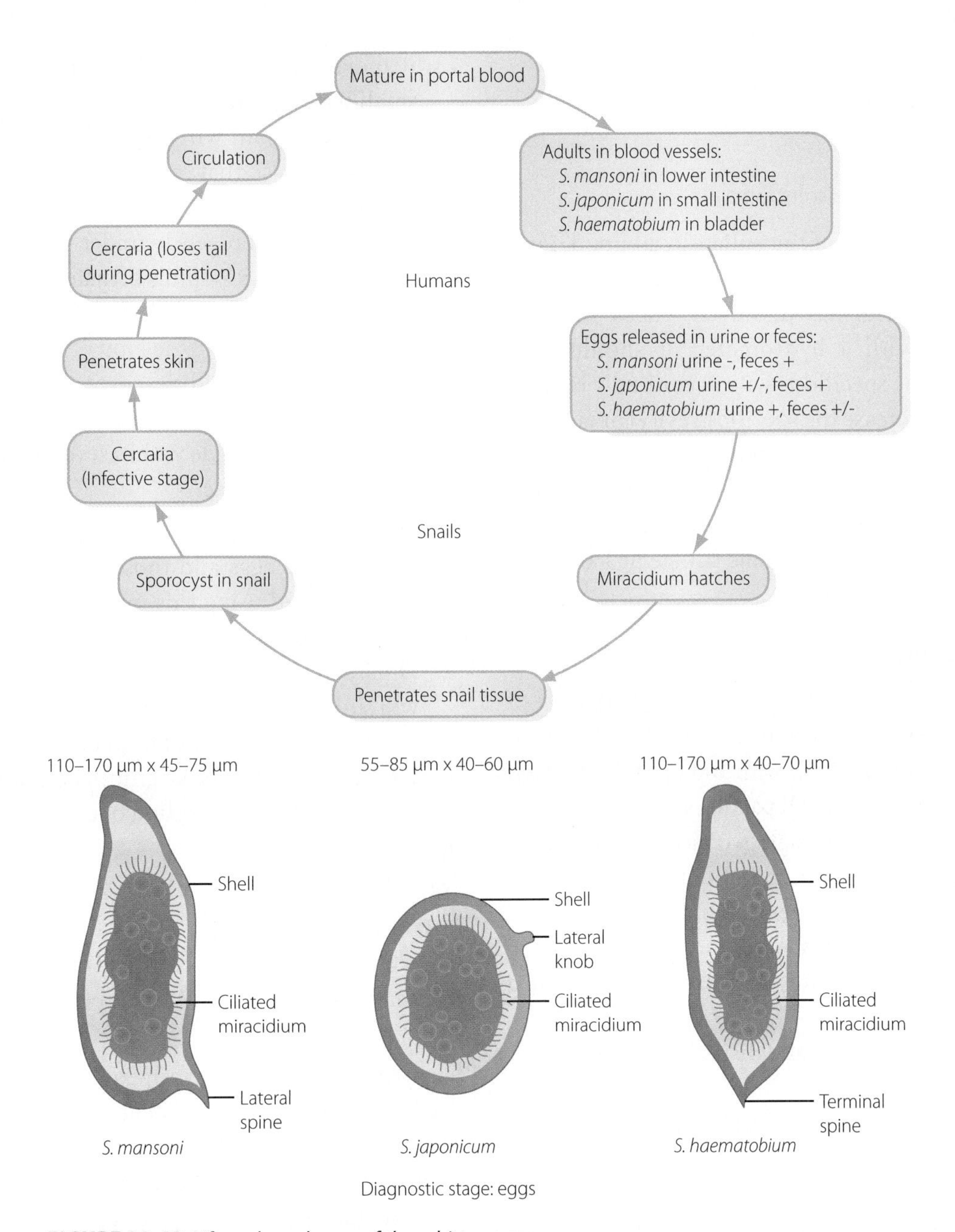

FIGURE 21-40 Life cycle and eggs of the schistosomes.

Laboratory Procedures

Procedure

Modified zinc sulfate concentration

Purpose

Flotation is one method of concentrating feces to enhance the recovery of parasitic elements in fecal specimens.

Principle

Protozoan cysts and helminth ova will float to the surface in solutions that have higher specific gravities than that of the egg or cyst. Zinc sulfate, with a final specific gravity of 1.180, is used to float the eggs or cysts, which can then be skimmed from the surface.

Materials

USP-grade zinc sulfate
Hydrometer
Applicator sticks
100 mm × 13 mm test tubes
Centrifuge
Woven, pressed gauze, one layer thick

Small wire loop
Microscope slides and coverslips

Procedure
Preparation of zinc sulfate solution

1. Prepare a 33% solution of zinc sulfate by adding 331 g of zinc sulfate to 1 L of warm water. Mix until dissolved.
2. After the chemical has dissolved, check the specific gravity with a hydrometer; it should read 1.180. Adjust the specific gravity accordingly by adding water (to decrease the specific gravity) or zinc sulfate (to increase the specific gravity).
3. When using a formalinized fecal specimen, the specific gravity of the solution should be adjusted to 1.120 by dissolving 400 g of zinc sulfate in 1 L of distilled water.

Flotation Procedure

1. Using two applicators, place a fecal sample the size of a pea in a 100 mm × 13 mm test tube that has been half filled (10 ml to 15 ml) with water. Make an even suspension, breaking up all particles.
2. Filter the suspension through two pieces of the single-layered gauze into a small, round-bottomed test tube.
3. Add additional water to the filtrate until the test tube is approximately two-thirds full.
4. Centrifuge for 1 minute at approximately 500 g (1,500 rpm).
5. Pour off the supernatant and dispose of, using proper techniques.
6. Refill the tube with water and resuspend the sediment, stirring with an applicator stick. Centrifuge again for 1 minute at 500 g.
7. The washing procedure can be repeated if the stool is very oily.
8. Decant water and add enough zinc sulfate (2 ml to 3 ml) to fill the tube approximately half full.
9. Using an applicator, break up the sediment thoroughly and resuspend it in the zinc sulfate.
10. Add additional zinc sulfate to fill the tube to within 0.5 inch of the top of the test tube.
11. Centrifuge the suspension for 1 to 2 minutes at 500 g. Do not use a break on the centrifuge and allow the tube to come to a stop without agitation.
12. Without shaking or spilling, carefully place the tube in a rack. This step also may be performed by leaving the tube in the centrifuge. Allow the tube to stand undisturbed for 1 minute.
13. Remove the material in the surface layers by using a small wire loop or pipette.
    a. Make a small wire loop, approximately 7 mm in diameter, so that the loop is at a right angle to the stem.
    b. Slide the loop gently under the surface film and remove 2 or 3 loopfuls of material. Do not go below the surface of the film. Transfer the film to a microscope slide, using the loop of a capillary pipette.
    c. Add 1 drop of iodine, cover with a clean 22 mm × 30 mm coverslip and seal.
    d. Examine the slide within several minutes for eggs, cysts, and larvae.

Notes

1. Operculated eggs and those of the schistosomes are not recovered using this method, and sedimentation should be used.
2. Organisms that rise to the surface of the zinc sulfate will sink in about 1 hour. Thus, slide mounts should be made as soon as the flotation technique is completed. Background debris is eliminated using flotation, enhancing the observation of eggs and cysts.

Procedure
Formalin-ether concentration

Purpose
Parasitic elements are concentrated through sedimentation to enhance the recovery in fecal specimens.

Principle
Formalin acts as both a fixative and preservative of protozoan eggs, larvae, and cysts. The specific gravity of protozoan cysts and helminth eggs is greater than that of water. Fecal debris is extracted into the ether phase so that the parasitic forms can be separated and then sedimented by centrifugation.

Materials
10% formalin
Ether substitute
Pointed paper cup or funnel
Gauze or cheesecloth
15 ml centrifuge tube
Saline
Centrifuge

Procedure

1. Mix a small portion of the stool, about the size of a marble, in 10 ml of 5% to 10% formalin or saline in a flat-bottomed waxed paper cup, carton, or 16 mm × 125 mm test tube. Allow to stand 30 minutes for fixation.

2. Strain about 10 ml of this suspension through a small funnel (or pointed paper cup with the end cut off) containing wet gauze or cheesecloth into a 15 ml centrifuge tube. Use two layers of wide-mesh gauze or one layer of narrow-mesh gauze.
3. Add physiological saline or 5% to 10% formalin to within 0.5 inch of the top of the test tube. Centrifuge for 10 minutes at 500 g.
4. Decant supernatant, leaving 0.5 to 1.5 ml of sedimented material.
5. Resuspend the sediment in saline to within 0.5 inch of the top of the tube. Centrifuge again for 10 minutes at 500 g. This second wash is not needed if the first supernatant wash is light tan or clear in color.
6. About 1 ml of sediment should remain. If the amount is much larger or smaller, adjust to the correct quantity as follows:
   a. Amount too large: Resuspend the sediment in saline and pour out a portion. For example, if the amount is twice that needed, pour out slightly less than half of the suspension. Then, add saline to bring the volume up to 10 ml and centrifuge again.
   b. Amount too small: Pour off the supernatant and strain a second portion of the original fecal suspension into the tube. The amount to be strained depends on the amount of sediment. For example, if it is about half the amount obtained from the first centrifugation, strain another 10 ml into the tube. Centrifuge again.
   c. After adjustment, if necessary, decant and resuspend the sediment in 5% to 10% formalin, filling the tube about half full.
7. Add approximately 3 ml of ethyl acetate, insert stopper, and shake vigorously for a minimum of 30 seconds. Carefully remove the stopper by holding tube away from yourself to avoid spraying as the stopper is removed and pressure is released.
8. Centrifuge at 500 g for 10 minutes. Four layers should result:
   - Top layer of ethyl acetate
   - Plug of fecal debris
   - Layer of formalin
   - Sediment with parasitic eggs, cysts, or larvae
9. Free the plug of debris from the sides of the tube with an applicator stick. Carefully decant the three layers. Use a cotton swab to clean debris from the walls of the tube to prevent it from settling down into the sediment.
10. Using a pipette, mix the remaining sediment with a small amount of the fluid that drains from the sides of the tube.
11. Mix the sediment well and prepare a wet mount for examination.

Procedure for PVA-Preserved Specimens

1. Fixation time with polyvinyl alcohol (PVA) should be for at least 30 minutes. Mix one part stool to two to three parts PVA.
2. Pour 2 ml to 5 ml of this suspension into a flat-bottomed waxed paper cup, carton, or 16 mm × 125 mm test tube. Add 10 ml of saline. Filter suspension through funnel or paper cup with the end cup off, lined with gauze or cheesecloth.
3. to 11. Follow as previously described.

Examination of Sediment

1. Prepare a saline mount by adding 1 drop of sediment to 1 drop of saline. Add a 22 mm × 22 mm coverslip. Scan the entire area under the coverslip under the 10× objective for eggs or larvae.
2. Add 1 drop of iodine to the edge of the coverslip to assist in the observation of cysts. Examine under the high-dry objective (40× to 45×).

Procedure

Thick and thin blood films

Purpose

Thick and thin blood films stained with Giemsa hematological stain permit the detection of blood parasites, including malarial parasites, trypanosomes, and microfilariae.

Principle

The thick blood film permits the examination of a large amount of blood for the presence of parasites. Because the smear is not fixed with methanol, the red blood cells (RBCs) lyse, permitting better visualization of the organisms. The thin film allows for the observation of RBC morphology, inclusions, and intracellular and extracellular parasites. A larger area of the slide must be examined in the thin smear, although there is less distortion when compared with the thick smear.

Materials

Microscope slides
Triton-buffered water
Absolute methanol disodium phosphate
Giemsa stock stain
Giemsa buffers 1 and 2

Procedure

Stain Preparation

1. Giemsa stain may be purchased as a concentrated stock or prepared by grinding 1 g of powdered Giemsa with 5 ml to 10 ml of glycerol in a mortar. Add additional glycerol, to a final total volume of 66 ml, and heat to 55°C in a water bath until the stain is dissolved. Cool and add 66 ml of absolute methanol. Allow to stand for 2 to 3 weeks. Filter and store in a brown bottle, protected from the light.
2. Prepare working Giemsa stain by mixing one part stock Giemsa stain to 10 to 50 parts triton-buffered water. The dilution chosen will determine the staining time. For example, if using a 1:50 dilution, stain for 50 minutes.
3. To prepare buffer 1, add 9.5 g of 0.067 M Na_2HPO_4 (disodium phosphate) to 1,000 ml of distilled water.
4. To prepare buffer 2, add 9.2 g of 0.067 M NaH_2PO_4: H_2O to 1,000 ml distilled water.
5. Working buffer is prepared weekly and filtered before each use. Prepare the working buffer by adding 61.1 ml of stock buffer 1 and 38.9 ml of stock buffer 2 to 900 ml of distilled water.

Thick Film

1. Prepare thick blood film by applying a free-flowing drop of blood, preferably without an anticoagulant, to a microscope slide cleaned with alcohol to remove any oil present.
2. Using the corner of a second slide, spread the film in a circle about the size of a dime. Avoid the formation of fibrin strands by spreading rapidly in a circular motion.
3. Allow to air-day overnight.
4. Place smears in a 1:50 dilution of stock Giemsa stain for 50 minutes. The lack of methanol fixation allows lysis or laking of the RBCs.
5. Rinse gently three times with triton-buffered water.
6. Drain slides in a vertical position and air-dry.

Thin Film

1. Clean a microscope slide with alcohol to remove any oil.
2. Touch the slide to 1 drop of free-flowing blood toward one end of the slide.
3. Holding a second slide at a 30° angle to the first slide, draw back into the drop and allow it to spread into the edge of the spreader slide. Then quickly and evenly push the spreader slide forward, allowing the blood to spread out. There should be a "feathered edge" at the end of the smear and no holes, and the smear should cover half to two-thirds of the slide.
4. Allow the slide to air-dry.
5. Fix the thin smear in absolute methanol for 30 seconds.
6. Place in working Giemsa stain for 50 minutes if using a 1:50 dilution. Staining time can be reduced by reducing the dilution of the stain. For example, when using a 1:20 dilution, staining time is reduced to 20 minutes.
7. Rinse gently with buffer for 2 minutes.
8. Dry vertically and examine under the 100× objective.

Examination of Smears

1. Thick smear: Examine 200 to 300 oil-immersion fields for the presence of blood parasites.
2. Thin smear: Examine the slide for a minimum of 30 minutes and examine a minimum of 100 fields under the oil-immersion objective.
3. Giemsa stains blood components as follows:
   Erythrocytes: Pale gray-blue
   White blood cells: Nuclei—purple
   Cytoplasm—pale purple
   Granules—Eosinophils—bright red-purple
   Neutrophils: Dark pink-purple
   Parasites stain blue to purple with red nuclei.

Quality Control

Stain known positive blood smears or control slides periodically with patient samples.

Procedure

Cellophane (cellulose acetate) tape preparation

Purpose

To collect the eggs of pinworm, *Enterobius vermicularis*, as the female deposits the eggs at night on the perianal folds.

Principle

Pinworm eggs will adhere to cellophane tape placed against the perianal folds. The tape is fixed to a microscope slide and examined microscopically.

Materials

Cellophane tape
Microscope slides
Toluene or xylene

Procedure

1. Place a strip of cellophane tape around the end of a tongue depressor by looping the tape around the top edge of the depressor so that the sticky side is out.
2. Spread the buttocks and apply the tape to the perianal folds. Press tape firmly against the left and right perianal folds and anal opening.
3. Remove the tape from the tongue depressor and place it sticky side down onto a microscope slide. Press firmly to remove all trapped air bubbles.
4. Lift one side of the tape and apply 1 small drop of toluene or xylene to clear the tape. Press the tape down onto the slide.
5. Examine under low power (10×) with low light intensity. The entire area under the tape must be examined. Eggs are colorless and football shaped with one side flattened.
6. Generally, specimens should be collected on five consecutive mornings before a pinworm infection can be ruled out. The specimen is optimally collected before a bowel movement or bathing because the eggs may not be detected otherwise.

Laboratory Exercises

1. Perform the modified zinc sulfate concentration procedure on the two stool specimens provided. Examine the slide and make a sketch of any significant findings, labeling it appropriately.

Specimen identification	Observations

   a. State the principle of this procedure: ____________

   ____

   b. Indicate which parasites this method is not suitable for: ____________

   ____

2. Perform the formalin-ether concentration procedure on the two specimens provided. Examine your slides and make a sketch of any significant findings, labeling appropriately.

Specimen identification	Observations/Sketch

   a. State the principle of this procedure: ____________

   ____

   b. Indicate what is present in the four layers that form after the addition of ethyl acetate:

   Top layer (first layer): ____________
   Second layer: ____________
   Third layer: ____________
   Bottom layer of sediment (fourth layer): ____________

3. Examine the cellulose acetate preparation for the presence of pinworm eggs. Record your findings.

Specimen identification	Observations

4. Examine the prepared Giemsa- or Wright-stained smears for the presence of blood parasites. Make a sketch of each, labeling the significant findings.

Specimen identification	Observations
Plasmodium falciparum	
Plasmodium ovale	
Trypanosoma species	
Babesia species	

5. Examine fixed iodine- or trichrome-stained mounts of each of the following parasites. Sketch your findings.

Specimen identification	Observations
Entamoeba histolytica	
Giardia lamblia	
Trichomonas species	
Hookworm	
Ascaris lumbricoides	
Trichuris trichiura	
Taenia species	
Hymenolepsis nana	
Schistosoma mansoni	
Fasciolopsis or fasciola	
Paragonimus westermani	

Review Questions

Matching

Match the parasite with its common name (responses may be used once or not at all):

1. *Strongyloides stercoralis*
2. *Necator americanus*
3. *Enterobius vermicularis*
4. *Ascaris lumbricoides*
5. *Trichuris trichiura*
6. *Taenia saginata*
7. *Taenia solium*
8. *Fasciolopsis buski*
9. *Clonorchis sinensis*
10. *Ancylostoma duodenale*
    a. Large intestinal fluke
    b. Old World hookworm
    c. Pinworm
    d. Whipworm
    e. Broad fish tapeworm
    f. Threadworm
    g. Chinese liver fluke
    h. Lung fluke
    i. Large roundworm
    j. Dwarf tapeworm
    k. New World hookworm
    l. Pork tapeworm
    m. Sheep liver fluke
    n. Beef tapeworm

Correctly identify the parasitic eggs and proglottids shown. Use each response once. Choose from the list on page 491:

11. 60 μm by 25 μm

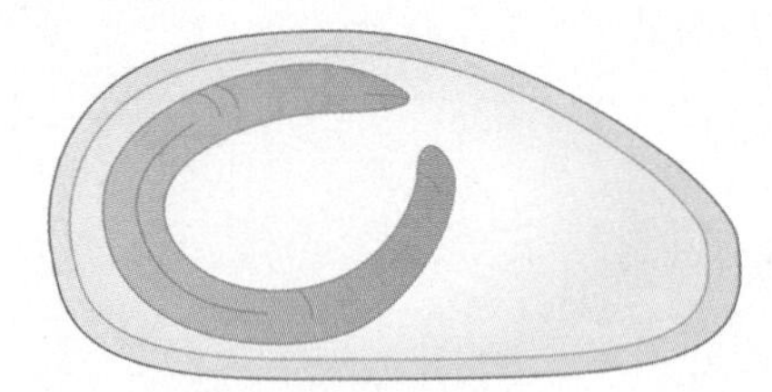

12. 60 μm by 40 μm

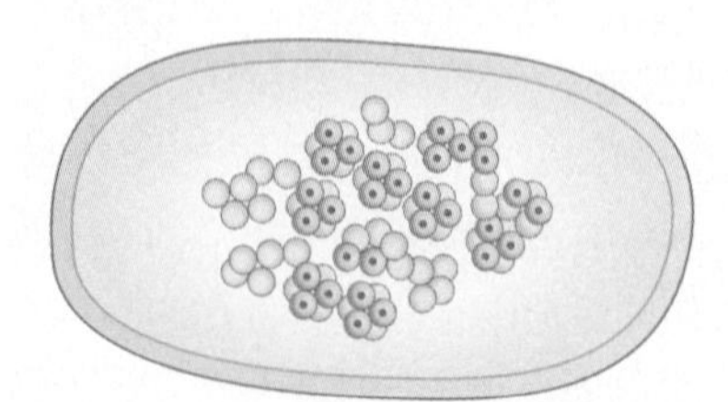

13. 75 μm by 40 μm

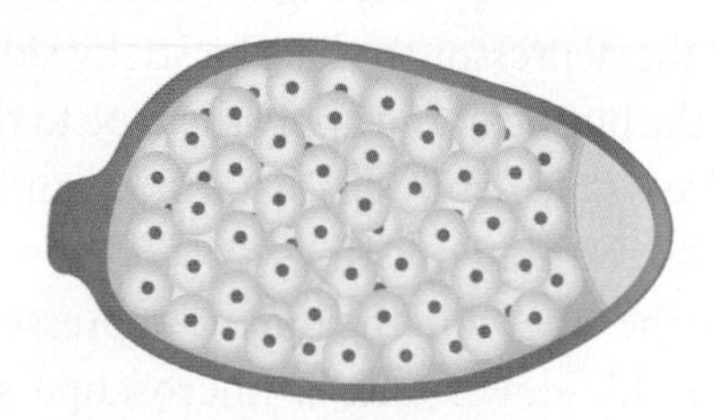

14. 50 μm by 40 μm

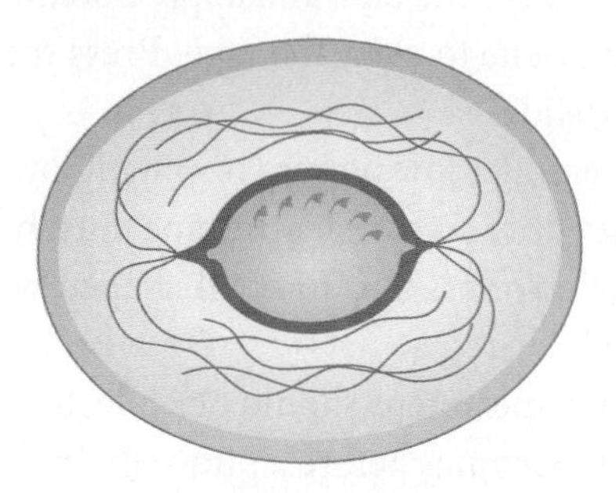

15. 100 μm by 50 μm

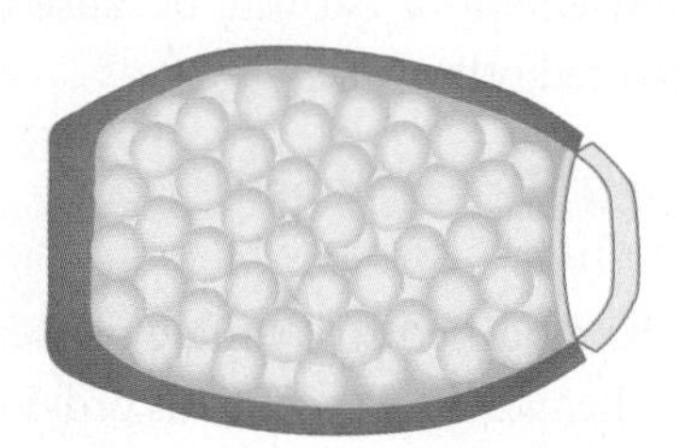

16. 60 μm by 45 μm

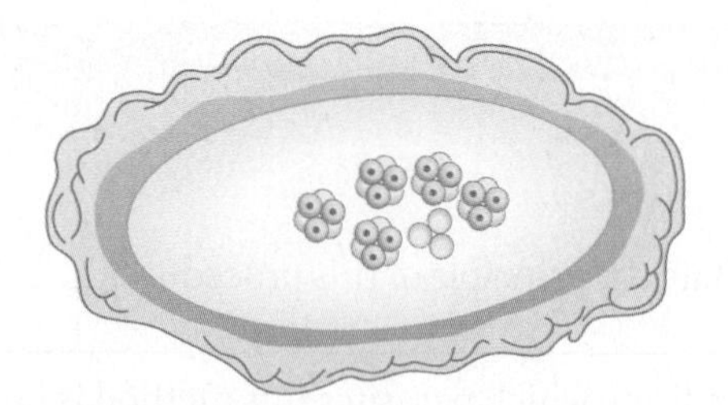

17. 55 μm by 20 μm

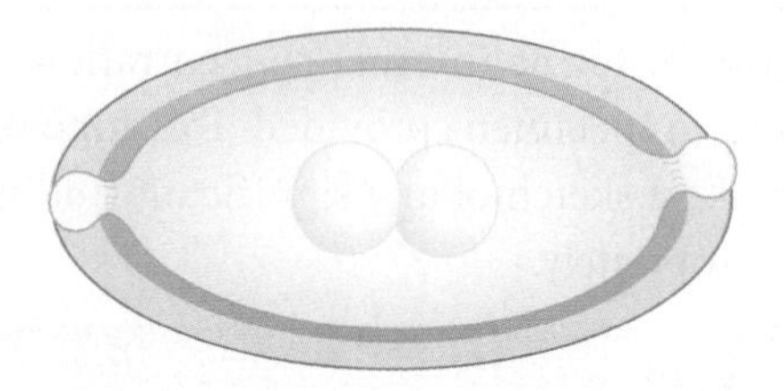

18. 35 µm diameter

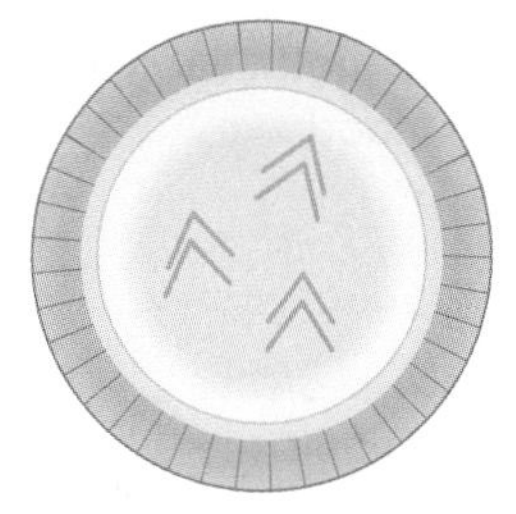
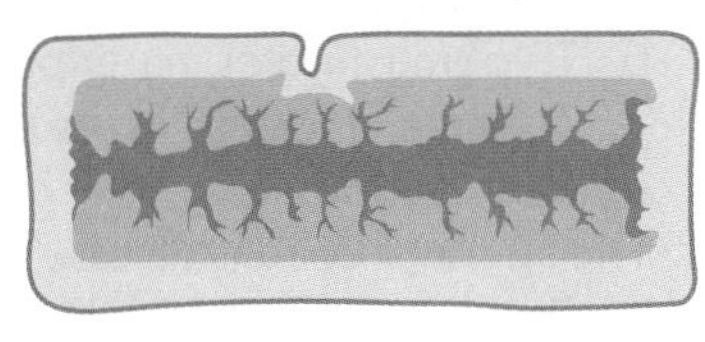

19. 160 µm by 65 µm

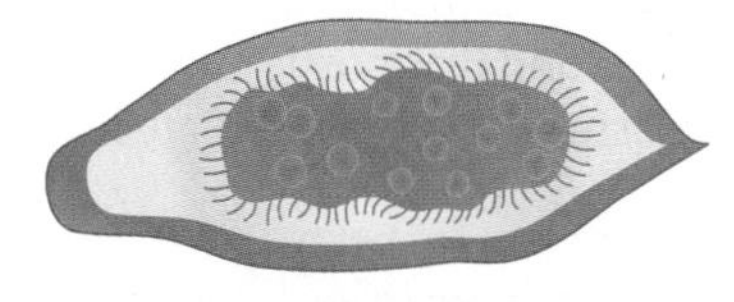

20. 140 µm by 80 µm

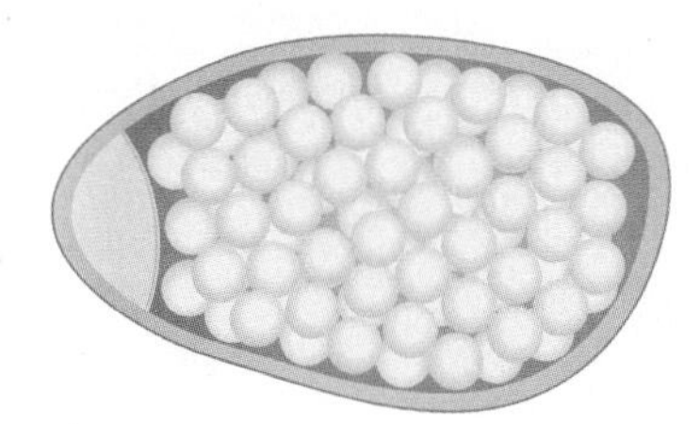

21. 120 µm by 50 µm

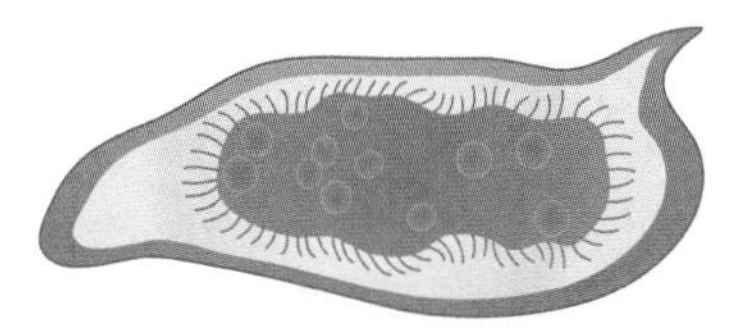

22. 60 µm by 70 µm

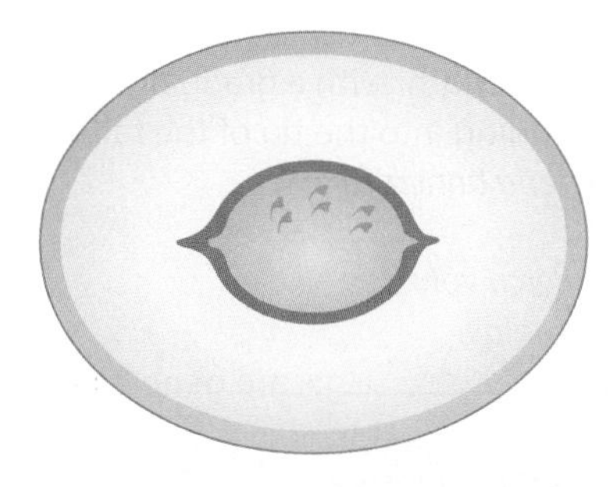

23. 35 µm diameter

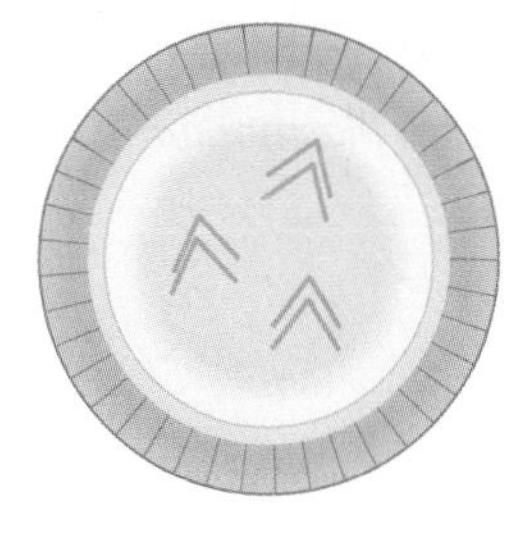
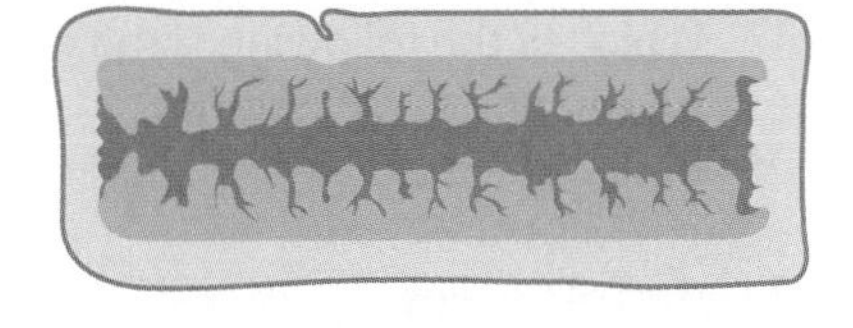

a. *Trichuris trichiura*
b. *Fasciola hepatica*
c. *Hymenolepsis diminuta*
d. *Enterobius vermicularis*
e. *Ascaris lumbricoides*
f. Hookworm
g. *Diphyllobothrium latum*
h. *Schistosoma mansoni*
i. *Taenia solium*
j. *Taenia saginata*
k. *Hymenolepsis nana*
l. *Schistosoma haematobium*
m. *Paragonimus westermani*

Multiple Choice

24. The host where the asexual or larval phase of the parasite occurs is known as the:
    a. Incidental host
    b. Intermediate host
    c. Definitive host
    d. Carrier
25. If a semisolid stool specimen cannot be examined within 1 hour of collection:
    a. Freeze the specimen for up to 4 hours.
    b. Refrigerate the specimen for up to 4 hours.
    c. Allow the specimen to remain at room temperature for up to 4 hours.
    d. Preserve the specimen with polyvinyl alcohol (PVA).
    e. Both b and d are suitable actions.
26. In the flotation method for concentration of stool specimens:
    a. Parasitic forms float to the top of the solution.
    b. Fecal debris floats to the top of the solution.
    c. All protozoan eggs and larvae are concentrated in the sediment of the tube.
    d. Additional fecal debris may distort the clarity of the smear.
27. The modified acid-fast stain most often is used in parasitology to identify:
    a. Protozoan cysts and trophozoites
    b. Helminth eggs
    c. *Plasmodium*
    d. *Cryptosporidium* and other coccidia
    e. Hemoflagellates
28. Which statement is *incorrect* for thick blood films?
    a. Use 2 to 4 drops of blood.
    b. Spread blood to an area about the size of a dime.
    c. The smear is fixed in methanol.
    d. The smear is used to determine tentatively if blood parasites are present.

29. An amoeba isolated from a patient with keratitis has spiny pseudopods, well-defined ectoplasm and endoplasm, and no flagellar phase noted. It is most likely:
    a. *Iodamoeba butschlii*
    b. *Acanthamoeba*
    c. *Cryptosporidium*
    d. *Naegleria*
30. A pear-shaped flagellate with an undulating membrane extending half the length of its body with four recurrent flagella but no anterior flagellum is:
    a. *Giardia lamblia*
    b. *Trichomonas hominis*
    c. *Trichomonas vaginalis*
    d. *Chilomastix mesnili*
    e. *Dientamoeba fragilis*
31. Sporogony refers to:
    a. The asexual life cycle of the *Plasmodium* parasites
    b. The sexual life cycle of the *Plasmodium* parasites
    c. The life cycle of *Plasmodium* that occurs in the intermediate host
    d. Both a and b
    e. Both b and c
32. Which of the following statements is *incorrect* for *Plasmodium falciparum*?
    a. Infection is commonly known as malignant tertian malaria.
    b. Tiny ring forms, multiple infected red cells, and accole rings may be seen on the blood smear.
    c. Schuffner's dots are present in most stages of infection.
    d. Gametocytes are crescent shaped.
33. Which species of *Plasmodium* is characterized by enlarged red blood cells, Schuffner's dots, amoeboid-like cytoplasm, and 12 to 14 merozoites per schizont?
    a. *P. falciparum*
    b. *P. vivax*
    c. *P. malariae*
    d. *P. ovale*
34. The observation of piroplasts in packets of two to three or a Maltese cross formation in stained blood films most likely indicates:
    a. *Plasmodium ovale*
    b. *Babesia microti*
    c. *Trypanosoma brucei* subspecies *gambiense*
    d. *Leishmania donovani*
35. The hemoflagellate form characterized by an oval shape, nucleus, and kinetoplast, which is found intracellularly in human macrophages, is the:
    a. Amastigote form
    b. Promastigote form
    c. Epimastigote form
    d. Trypomastigote form
36. Diagnosis of African sleeping sickness is based on the observation of:
    a. The amastigote form in reticuloendothelial cells
    b. Trypomastigotes in peripheral blood
    c. A marked increase in serum IgG
    d. Xenodiagnosis
37. The agent of Chagas disease is:
    a. *Trypanosoma brucei subspecies rhodesiense*
    b. *Trypanosoma brucei subspecies gambiense*
    c. *Trypanosoma cruzi*
    d. *Leishmania tropica*

For questions 38 to 44, complete the chart, indicating the intermediate host(s) and diagnostic and infective stages for each parasite listed. If no intermediate host exists, write "None."

	Parasite	Intermediate hosts		Infective stage	Diagnostic stage
		First/ Primary	Secondary		
38.	*Strongyloides stercoralis*				
39.	*Necator americanus*				
40.	*Trichuris trichiura*				
41.	*Diphyllobothrium latum*				
42.	*Hymenolepsis nana*				
43.	*Taenia saginata*				
44.	*Paragonimus westermani*				

45. The microfilaria of ____________ is sheathed, 230 μm to 300 μm in length, with a gradually tapered tail and nuclei extending into the tip of the tail.
    a. *Wuchereria bancrofti*
    b. *Loa loa*
    c. *Onchocerca volvulus*
    d. *Brugia malayi*
46. The eggs of ____________ are generally found only in the urine.
    a. *Schistosoma mansoni*
    b. *Schistosoma haematobium*
    c. *Schistosoma japonicum*
    d. *Paragonimus westermani*
47. Which of the following is the vector for *Plasmodium*?
    a. *Anopheles* mosquitoes
    b. Sand flies
    c. Ticks
    d. Tsetse flies

Bibliography

Bern, C., Kjos, S., Yabsley, M. J., & Montgomery, S. P. (2011). *Trypanosoma cruzi* and Chagas' disease in the United States. *Clinical Microbiology Review, 24,* 655–681.

Bouzid, M., Hunter, P. R., Chalmers, R. M., & Tyler, K. M. (2013). Helminth infections and host immune regulation. *Clincal Microbiology Review, 26,* 115–134.

Bruckner, D. A. (1992). Amebiasis. *Clinical Microbiology Review, 5,* 356–369.

Clark, D. P. (1999). New insights into human cryptosporidiosis. *Clinical Microbiology Review, 12,* 554–563.

Centers for Disease Control and Prevention. (2012). Parasites—*Blastocystis* spp. infection http://www.cdc.gov/parasites/blastocystis/

Centers for Disease Control and Prevention. (2009). Parasites—Dracunculiasis (also known as Guinea Worm Disease). http://www.cdc.gov/parasites/guineaworm/index.html

Collins, W. E., & Jeffery, G. M. (2007). *Plasmodium malariae*: Parasite and disease. *Clinical Microbiology Review, 20,* 579–592.

Cox, F. E. G. (2002). History of human parasitology. *Clinical Microbiology Review, 15,* 595–612.

Forbes, B. A., Sahm, D. F., & Weissfeld, A. S. (2007). Laboratory methods for diagnosis of parasitic infections. In *Bailey and Scott's diagnostic microbiology* (12th ed.). St. Louis, MO: Mosby Elsevier.

Gangneus, F. R., & Darde, M. L. (2012). Epidemiology of and diagnostic strategies for toxoplasmosis. *Clinical Microbiology Review, 25,* 264–296.

Keiser, P. B., & Nutman, T. B. (2004). *Strongyloides stercoralis* in the immunocompromised population. *Clinical Microbiology Review, 17,* 208–217.

Lindsay, D. A., Upton, S. J., & Weiss, L. M. (2007). Isospora, cyclospora, and sarcocystis. In P. R. Murray, E. J. Baron, J. H. Jorgensen, M. L. Landry, & M. A. Pfaller (Eds.), *Manual of clinical microbiology* (9th ed.). Washington, DC: American Society for Microbiology.

Marshall, M. M., Naumovitz, D., Orega, Y., & Sterling, C. R. (1997). Waterborne protozoan pathogens. *Clinical Microbiology Review, 10,* 67–85.

McSorley, H. J., & Maizels, R. M. (2012). *Cryptosporidium* pathogenicity and virulence. *Clinical Microbiology Review, 25,* 585–608.

Nanduri, J., & Kazura, J. W. (1989). Clinical and laboratory aspects of filariasis. *Clinical Microbiology Reviews, 2,* 39–50.

Neafie, R. C., & Marty, A. M. (1993). Unusual infections in humans. *Clinical Microbiology Reviews, 6,* 34–56.

Orega, Y. R., & Sanchez, R. (2010). Update on *Cyclospora cayetanensis*, a food-borne and waterborne parasite. *Clinical Microbiology Review, 23,* 218–234.

Rogers, W. O. (2007). *Plasmodium* and *Babesia*. In P. R. Murray, E. J. Baron, J. H. Jorgensen, M. L. Landry, & M. A. Pfaller (Eds.), *Manual of clinical microbiology*, 9th ed. Washington, DC: American Society for Microbiology.

Scholz, T., Garcia, H. H., Kuchta, R., & Wicht, B. (2009). Update on the human broad tapeworm (Genus *Diphyllobothrium*), including clinical relevance. *Clinical Microbiology Reviews, 22,* 146–160.

Schuster, F. L. (2002). Cultivation of *Babesia* and *Babesia*-like blood parasites: Agents of an emerging zoonotic disease. *Clinical Microbiology Review, 15,* 365–373.

Smith, J. W. et al. (1984). Vol. 1: Blood and tissue parasites, Vol. 2: Intestinal protozoa, and Vol. 3: Intestinal helminths. In *Atlas of diagnostic medical parasitology.* Chicago, IL: American Society of Clinical Pathologists.

Stark, D., Barratt, J. L. N., van Hall, S., Marriott, D., Harkness, J., & Ellis, J. T. (2009). Clinical significance of enteric protozoa in the immunosuppressed human population. *Clinical Microbiology Reviews, 22,* 634–650.

Tanyuksel, M., & Petri, W. A. (2003). Laboratory diagnosis of amebiasis. *Clinical Microbiology Reviews, 16,* 713–729.

Tanowitiz, H. B., Kirchhoff, L. V., Simon, D., Morris, S. A., Weiss, L. M., & Wittner, M. (1992). Chagas' disease. *Clinical Microbiology Review, 5,* 400–419.

Teixeira, A. R. L., Hecht, M. M., Guimaro, M. C., Sousa, A. O., & Nitz, N. (2011). Pathogenesis of Chagas' disease: Parasite persistence and autoimmunity. *Clinical Microbiology Reviews, 24,* 592–630.

Wolfe, M. S. (1992). Giardiasis. *Clinical Microbiology Reviews, 5,* 93–100.

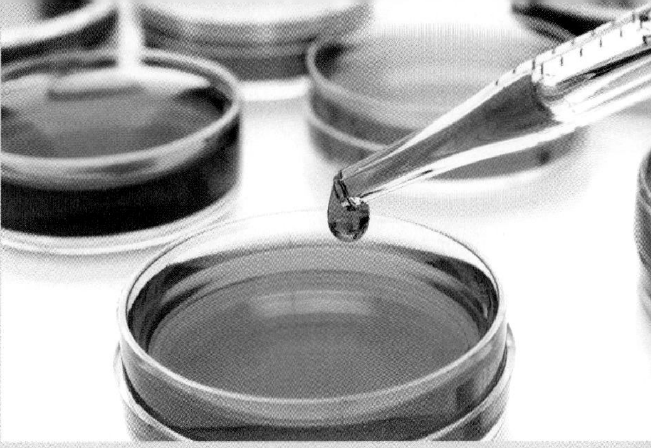

© Alex011973/Shutterstock, Inc.

CHAPTER 22
Clinical Specimens

CHAPTER OUTLINE

Introduction
Primary Plating of Specimens
Blood Cultures and Bacteremia
Cerebrospinal Fluid—Meningitis and Central Nervous System Infections
Respiratory Tract Specimens and Infections
Eye and Ear Specimens and Infections
Urinary Tract Specimens and Infections
Gastrointestinal Tract Specimens and Infections
Genital Tract Specimens and Infections
Skin and Wound Specimens and Infections
Pleural, Peritoneal, Pericardial, and Synovial Fluids

KEY TERMS

Arthrocentesis
Bacteremia
Bacteriuria
Bronchitis
Cellulitis
Cervicitis
Effusion
Encephalitis
Erysipelas
Erysipeloid
Exudates
Fungemia
Gastroenteritis
Impetigo
Meningitis
Paracentesis
Pneumonia
Septicemia
Thoracentesis
Transudates
Tympanocentesis
Urethritis

LEARNING OBJECTIVES

1. Select and streak the appropriate media for primary plating of frequently requested cultures.
2. Discuss and practice proper skin preparation techniques for collection of blood cultures.
3. Discuss the aspects of blood culture collection, including timing and number of specimens, volume of blood, and anticoagulants.
4. List the microorganisms usually associated with septicemia.
5. Collect at least one set of blood cultures using the proper technique.
6. Correctly process, subculture, and stain at least one set of blood cultures and identify any pathogens present.
7. List the microorganisms most frequently associated with bacterial and viral meningitis.
8. Perform one cerebrospinal fluid analysis, including gross examination, Gram stain, primary plating, and identification of any pathogens.

9. Collect at least one throat culture using proper technique.
   a. Correctly process, inoculate, and interpret at least one throat culture and identify any pathogens present.
   b. Differentiate normal oropharyngeal flora from pathogenic organisms.
   c. Accurately perform and interpret a rapid antigen test for group A *Streptococcus*.
10. Screen a minimum of three sputum samples to evaluate the acceptability of the specimen through examination of the Gram stain.
    a. Correctly process, inoculate, and interpret at least three sputum samples.
    b. Identify all pathogens and note the presence or absence of normal flora.
11. List the microorganisms most often associated with lower respiratory tract infections.
12. Correctly process, inoculate, and interpret at least three urine specimens, including the colony count, and identify all pathogens present.
13. List the microorganisms most frequently associated with urinary tract infections.
14. Correctly process, inoculate, and interpret at least three stool specimens.
    a. Screen specimens using the Gram stain for the presence of neutrophils.
    b. Differentiate normal flora coliforms from pathogens and identify all pathogens.
15. List the bacteria most often associated with infections of the lower gastrointestinal tract.
16. Examine Gram-stained urogenital smears for the presence of gram-negative diplococci and segmented neutrophils.
17. Name the major sexually transmitted diseases and indicate the etiologic agent of each.
18. List the major pathogens associated with wound or abscess infections.
19. Briefly discuss infections of the normally sterile body fluids, the eye, and the ear.

Introduction

This chapter describes the basic laboratory methods used in the plating and interpretation of clinical specimens, the identification of any pathogens, and the recognition of normal flora. The material in this chapter is presented for the clinical laboratory student as a summary and not as a comprehensive identification scheme, which would be used in the clinical setting. The reader is referred to more comprehensive textbooks or to each facility's laboratory procedure manuals for more detailed specimen workup guidelines.

Primary Plating of Specimens

Each microbiology laboratory establishes guidelines as to selection of agars and broths for primary plating. On receipt of a specimen in the microbiology laboratory, the specimen collection guidelines presented in **BOX 22-1** should be reviewed. Any concerns should be discussed with the physician and health care team so that appropriate specimen collection methods may be observed. The selection of media for primary plating depends on the source of the specimen and the species of bacteria most frequently isolated as pathogens from the source. **TABLE 22-1** presents an example of such guidelines that are suitable for the student microbiology laboratory.

Blood Cultures and Bacteremia

Blood is a normally sterile site and should not contain any microorganisms. The presence of bacteria in the blood, or **bacteremia**, may be transient, intermittent, or continuous. In transient bacteremia, the bacteria are spontaneously released into the blood. This may result from brushing the teeth, contaminated mucosal surfaces, the incision or drainage of an abscess, colonization of indwelling catheters, or insertion of a urinary catheter. Intermittent bacteremia refers to the periodic release of bacteria into the blood from other sites, such as an abscess, meningitis, septic arthritis, infections from the genitourinary tract, gastrointestinal tract, tissue, or the lung. In continuous bacteremia, there is a constant release of bacteria into the blood; this may occur from endocarditis, septic shock,

BOX 22-1 Specimen Collection and Processing Guidelines

1. Log the specimen into the laboratory, using the laboratory information system or log book. Record the time that the specimen is received in the laboratory. Verify that the specimen has the correct patient information, including name and identification number, room number, date and time of collection, and source. Check the specimen label against the requisition for any errors or discrepancies. Bring any concerns to the instructor's or supervisor's attention.
2. Evaluate the specimen collection method, noting whether the container is appropriate (sterile, without leakage) and if the quantity is sufficient. Bring any concerns to the instructor's or supervisor's attention.
3. Perform any required or requested microscopic methods, such as the Gram stain, methylene blue stain, or acid-fast bacilli stain. Record all results.
4. Select and correctly inoculate primary plating media. Incubate at the correct temperature and atmosphere. Most aerobic cultures are examined for growth at 24 and 48 hours. Most anaerobic cultures are incubated for up to 5 or 7 days.

or endovascular infections. **Septicemia** is a systemic disease caused by the multiplication of the microorganism and the associated harmful effects of the microorganisms and their products to the host. The bacteria multiply more rapidly than they can be cleared by the host's immune mechanisms. Signs of septicemia include increased pulse, hyperventilation, fever, chills, changes in mental status, and respiratory alkalosis. Endotoxin derived after breakdown of the gram-negative cell wall may activate complement and the clotting factors and decrease the amount of circulating granulocytes. Other effects of bacterial products include disseminated intravascular coagulation, which may lead to septic shock. Septic shock is accompanied by hypotension, metabolic acidosis, disseminated intravascular coagulation (DIC), congestive heart failure, hyperventilation, toxicity, oliguria, and respiratory failure.

TYPES AND CAUSES OF BACTEREMIA

Bacteremia may have either an intravascular or extravascular source. Intravascular bacteremia begins in the blood and includes infective endocarditis and intravenous catheters. Those with congenital valve disorders, intravenous catheters, and damaged surface to the endothelium of the heart are predisposed to infective endocarditis. Platelets and fibrin adhere to the heart endothelium, and bacteria can stick to this surface, causing colonization. Vegetation occurs, which can then seed the bacteria. Species most frequently associated with endocarditis are *viridans streptococcus*, especially *S. mutans* and *S. sanguis*. These bacteria are normal flora of the oral cavity and can travel to the heart following dental procedures and periodontitis. Intravenous catheters, arterial lines, and vascular prosthetic devices are other sources of intravascular bacteremia. *Staphylococcus epidermidis*, which is normal flora of the skin; other coagulase negative staphylococci; and *Staphylococcus aureus* are the bacteria most often found in these cases.

Extravascular sources of bacteremia occur when bacteria enter the blood from another source, including the lymphatic system. These sources include the genitourinary and respiratory tracts, abscesses, and wound infections. The severity of the infection depends on several host factors, including age, immune status, and other underlying medical conditions. Bacteria most often associated with extravascular bacteremia include the Enterobacteriaceae, *Streptococcus pneumoniae*, *Staphylococcus aureus*, anaerobic cocci, *Bacteroides fragilis* group, *Clostridium* species, *Pseudomonas aeruginosa*, and *Listeria monocytogenes*.

BLOOD CULTURE SPECIMEN COLLECTION

It is imperative to avoid the normal skin flora and contaminants while collecting blood for culture to avoid confusion in the diagnosis of bacteremia. Some commensal bacteria of the skin, such as *Staphylococcus epidermidis*, other coagulase-negative staphylococci, *Propionibacterium acnes*, and *Corynebacterium* species also may be agents of bacteremia. Thus proper skin disinfection is essential to help differentiate contamination from true infection. The intended venipuncture site should be located below any intravenous lines that are present. The venipuncture site is first cleaned with 70% isopropyl alcohol or ethanol and allowed to air-dry. This is followed by swabbing the area with 1% to 2% tincture of iodine or 10% povidine

TABLE 22-1 Gram Stain and Primary Plating Media for Clinical Specimens

Site	Gram	SBA	CNA	MAC	CHOC	MTM	HE	GN	THIO	AB	PEA	KV
Abscess/boil	X	X	X	X					X	X	X	X
Abscess/throat	X	X	X	X	X							
Bone	X	X	X	X					X	X	X	X
	Homogenize bone in nutrient broth with tissue grinder. For anaerobes, first homogenize in THIO											
Bone marrow	X	X	X	X								
Brain/liver abscess	X	X		X	X				X	X	X	X
Breast fluid		X		X								
Burn	X	X	X	X						X	X	X
Catheter site	X	X	X	X								
Catheters (central venous)		X										
	Role catheter tip for colony count.											
Cerebrospinal fluid shunt tip		X			X							
	Roll shunt tip on plates.											
Bone marrow	X	X		X	X				X			
Catheter (intravenous)		X							X	X		
Decubitus ulcer	X	X		X	X							
Dialysis fluid		X										
	Use 100 µl loop for colony count.											
Ear—inner	X	X		X	X							
Ear—outer	X	X		X								
Eye—conjunctiva	X	X	X		X							
Fine needle lung aspirate	X	X	X	X	X							
Fluids	**Gram**	**SBA**	**CNA**	**MAC**	**CHOC**	**MTM**	**HE**	**GN**	**THIO**	**AB**	**PEA**	**KV**
	Centrifuge fluids if volume is over 1 ml at 2,500 rpm for 15 minutes. Culture and Gram stain from sediment after resuspending in 0.5 ml of supernatant.											
Amniotic	X	X	X	X	X				X	X	X	X
Bile	X	X	X	X					X	X	X	X
Cerebrospinal	X	X	X	X	X							
	Report all positive smears on CSF to nursing unit and physician immediately.											
Gastric	X	X		X								
Gastric biopsy	X	X		X	X							
	Place chocolate in *Campylobacter* bag in increased CO_2; hold 7 days.											
Liver biopsy	X	X	X	X					X	X	X	X
Lung aspirate	X	X	X	X	X							
Pericardial	X	X		X					X	X	X	X
Peritoneal or ascitic	X	X		X	X				X	X	X	X
Pleural	X	X		X	X				X	X	X	X
Synovial	X	X		X	X				X	X	X	X
Genital—Female	**Gram**	**SBA**	**CNA**	**MAC**	**CHOC**	**MTM**	**HE**	**GN**	**THIO**	**AB**	**PEA**	**KV**
Bartholin cyst		X		X		X				X	X	X
Gonorrhea screen	X				X	X						

TABLE 22-1 Gram Stain and Primary Plating Media for Clinical Specimens (Continued)

Genital—Female	Gram	SBA	CNA	MAC	CHOC	MTM	HE	GN	THIO	AB	PEA	KV
Cervix or endocervix	X	X			X	X				X	X	X
Screen—group B *Streptococcus*	Todd Hewitt broth with CNA											
Cul-de-sac	X	X	X	X						X	X	X
Endometrium	X	X	X	X	X	X				X	X	X
Fallopian tube	X	X	X	X	X	X				X	X	X
Urethra	X	X			X	X						
Vagina		X			X	X						
Placenta	X	X	X	X								
Genital—Male	**Gram**	**SBA**	**CNA**	**MAC**	**CHOC**	**MTM**	**HE**	**GN**	**THIO**	**AB**	**PEA**	**KV**
Epididymis biopsy	X	X	X	X	X							
Penis, penile drainage	X	X		X	X	X						
Prostatic fluid	X	X		X	X				X			
Semen	X	X		X	X	X			X	X	X	X
Urethra	X	X				X						
Respiratory	**Gram**	**SBA**	**CNA**	**MAC**	**CHOC**	**MTM**	**HE**	**GN**	**THIO**	**AB**	**PEA**	**KV**
Bronchial biopsy or brush	X	X	X	X								
Bronchial lavage	X	X	X	X								
Epiglottis	X	X	X	X								
Lung	X	X	X	X								
Mouth (dental/oral surgery)	X	X		X					X	X	X	X
Nares (screen for staphylococcus)	MRSA agar											
Nasopharyngeal		X		X	X							
	For *Bordetella pertussis*, do DFA and Reagen Lowe or Bordet Gengou media.											
Nasal sinus	X	X		X	X				X	X	X	X
Sputum	X	X	X	X	X							
	Screen sputum for acceptability before setup.											
Thoracentesis	X	X	X	X					X	X	X	X
Throat		X			X++							
	Perform group A *Streptococcus* screens on all throat cultures. If screen is negative, set up the culture. Add chocolate agar if *Haemophilus* is suspected.											
Transtracheal aspiration	X	X		X	X				X	X	X	X
Gastrointestinal	**Gram**	**SBA**	**CNA**	**MAC**	**CHOC**	**MTM**	**HE**	**GN**	**THIO**	**AB**	**PEA**	**KV**
Rectal swab	X	X					X	X				
	Add sorbitol MacConkey agar for verotoxic *E. coli* and Campy blood agar for *Campylobacter*											
Rectal abscess	X	X	X	X		X	X	X	X	X	X	X
Stool		X		X			X	X				
	Add sorbitol MacConkey agar for verotoxic *E. coli*, Campy blood agar for *Campylobacter*, and CIN media for *Yesinia.* Add TCBS for *Vibrio.*											
Stool or swab for VRE	Use VRE media (bile esculin with 6 µg/ml of vancomycin)											

(*continues*)

TABLE 22-1 Gram Stain and Primary Plating Media for Clinical Specimens (Continued)

Tissue	Gram	SBA	CNA	MAC	CHOC	MTM	HE	GN	THIO	AB	PEA	KV
	Homogenize tissue before setting up.											
Appendix	X	X	X	X					X	X	X	X
Cardiac valve	X	X	X	X								
Gall bladder	X	X	X	X					X	X	X	X
Pancreas	X	X	X	X					X	X	X	X
Spleen	X	X	X	X					X	X	X	X
Urine	**Gram**	**SBA**	**CNA**	**MAC**	**CHOC**	**MTM**	**HE**	**GN**	**THIO**	**AB**	**PEA**	**KV**
Catheter (straight or indwelling)	X	X		X								
	Do colony count with 1 ml (0.001 ml) calibrated loop on SBA.											
Clean catch	X	X		X								
	Do colony count with 10 ml calibrated loop for clear specimens and 1 ml calibrated loop for cloudy specimens.											
Suprapubic aspiration	X	X		X						X	X	X
	Do colony count with 10 ml calibrated loop on SBA.											
Urine for VRE	Use VRE media (bile esculin with 6 μg/ml of vancomycin).											
Wounds	**Gram**	**SBA**	**CNA**	**MAC**	**CHOC**	**MTM**	**HE**	**GN**	**THIO**	**AB**	**PEA**	**KV**
Jaw or mouth	X	X	X	X					X	X	X	X
Bite wound	X	X	X	X					X	X	X	X
Nonsurgical	X	X	X	X								
Surgical—deep or incision/drainage	X	X	X	X					X	X	X	X
Pelvic or abdominal wound	X	X	X	X					X	X	X	X
Wound for VRE	Use VRE media (bile esculin with 6 μg/ml of vancomycin).											

Key: SBA, 5% sheep blood agar; CNA, colistin-nalidixic acid agar; MAC, MacConkey agar (may substitute with eosin-methylene blue); CHOC, chocolate agar; MTM, modified Thayer-Martin agar (may substitute with Martin-Lewis); HE, hektoen enteric agar; GN, gram-negative broth (may substitute with selenite broth); THIO, thioglycollate broth; AB, anaerobic blood agar; PEA, phenylethyl alcohol agar; KV, kanamycin-vancomycin laked blood agar; SAB, Sabouraud dextrose agar; BHI, brain-heart infusion medium; CIN, cefsulodin-irgasan-novobiocin agar; TCBS, thiosulfate-citrate-bile salts-sucrose agar

iodine. The area should be swabbed in a circular motion, working outward from the site of collection. There are commercially available skin preparation kits that can be used to prepare the skin to collect peripheral blood culture specimens.

Ideally, blood should be collected before the administration of antimicrobial agents. However, most blood culture bottles contain substances that can absorb antibiotics. Timing is not critical in cases of endocarditis, uncontrolled infections, typhoid fever, and endarteritis when bacteremia is continuous. However, in cases where bacteria are intermittently shed into the blood, collection before the febrile episode is recommended. Bacteria are in the highest concentration before the spike of the fever, and because this cannot be predicted, multiple samples from separate venipunctures often are required to confirm a case of bacteremia. A set includes one aerobic bottle (which grows aerobes and facultative bacteria) and one anaerobic bottle. Two or three separate samples from different venipuncture sites, spaced at least 1 hour apart, are recommended during a 24-hour period. The maximal number of culture sets that may be ordered in a 24-hour period is determined by each microbiology laboratory; most facilities set a maximum of three or four sets of blood cultures per 24 hours unless a unique situation exists. A single blood culture is generally considered insufficient to detect bacteremia. A single blood culture will usually detect 90% to 95% of blood infections; adding a second culture increases the detection rate to 98%. Adding a third set is said to increase the detection to 99.6%. Collection over three sets per 24 hours doesn't provide significant positive detections.

Volume is the major factor for detection of bacteria in blood cultures. A minimum of 20 ml to 30 ml per culture set for adults is advised, which means that at least 10 ml of blood is inoculated into each culture bottle. Because bacterial counts in infants and children may be as high as 100 colony-forming units per milliliter (CFU/ml) and the volume of blood collected becomes a concern, lesser quantities are needed. In small children, 1 ml to 5 ml per culture set is recommended, and 0.5 ml to 1 ml per culture set is advised for small infants. Usually a single blood culture is ordered for infants and children for these reasons.

The culture bottles ideally are inoculated directly, without changing the collection needle to prevent accidental needle stick. Prior to inoculation, the tops of the bottles are disinfected with alcohol or iodine solution, allowed to dry, and then wiped off with alcohol. Using iodine alone will cause cracks in the bottle tops, which can introduce contamination. Sufficient sample is needed to inoculate two bottles per venipuncture: one to be incubated anaerobically and the second vented to permit oxygen from the environment to enter. Most blood culture bottles have 5% to 10% carbon dioxide (CO_2) in the headspace to permit the fastidious bacteria and those requiring increased CO_2 to grow. Collection and transport in blood collection tubes containing the anticoagulant sodium polyanethol sulfonate (SPS) for later inoculation in the laboratory is also acceptable.

Several media are commercially available for the culture of blood. These include soybean casein digest agar (tryptic or trypticase soy broth), Columbia broth, thiol broth, thioglycollate broth, brain-heart infusion (BHI) agar, and supplemented peptone broth (SPB). It is recommended that a blood culture set be composed of two different systems; for example, two different types of broth media might be used. **FIGURE 22-1** shows typical blood culture bottles.

Most blood culture media also contain the anticoagulant sodium polyanethol sulfonate (SPS). In addition to preventing blood from clotting, SPS inactivates neutrophils and the antibiotics streptomycin, kanamycin, gentamycin, and polymyxin and inhibits certain components of complement and the coagulation cascade. However,

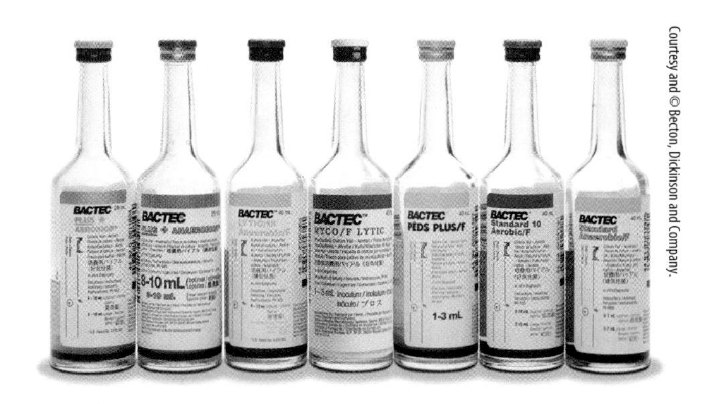

FIGURE 22-1 Blood culture bottles.

SPS also may inhibit certain bacteria, including *Neisseria gonorrhoeae*, *Neisseria meningitidis*, and *Gardnerella vaginalis*. The addition of 1% gelatin to the medium can neutralize these effects.

The dilution factor of blood to culture medium is important because of the bactericidal components of human serum and cells. In most cases a 1:10 dilution of blood in broth is sufficient to reduce these bactericidal effects.

MANUAL BLOOD CULTURES

Using manual methods, blood culture bottles are incubated at 35°C to 37°C, with agitation. The bottles are examined daily for signs of growth for a total of 7 days, including on the day of collection. Signs of growth include cloudiness, color change in the broth, hemolysis of the red blood cells, gas bubbles, turbidity, or the appearance of small colonies in the broth or on the surface of the red blood cell (RBC) layer. Examination is aided by viewing bottles against fluorescent bulbs or transmitted incandescent light. All suspected positive cultures are stained using either the Gram stain or the acridine orange method. **FIGURES 22-2** and **22-3** show positive Gram stains performed from positive blood culture bottles.

Blind subcultures should be performed at 6 to 17 hours and then every 2 days by removing a few drops of the well-mixed blood culture medium and spreading over the entire surface of a chocolate agar plate. The plate is incubated at 35°C ± 2°C at 5% to 10% CO_2 for 48 hours. The culture bottles are reincubated for 5 to 7 days. A second subculture or stain (Gram or acridine orange) can be performed at 48 hours of incubation on the original culture if desired.

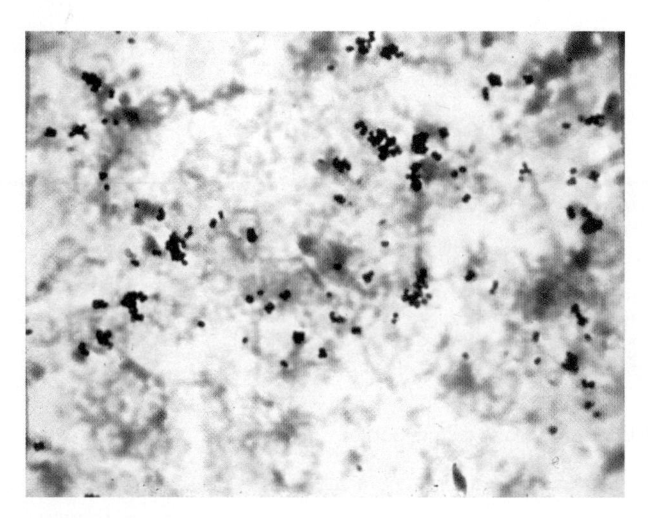

FIGURE 22-2 Blood culture Gram stain showing Gram positive cocci in clusters.

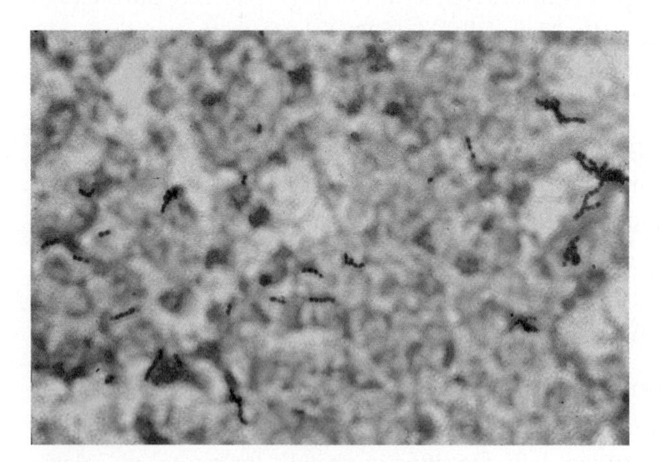

FIGURE 22-3 Blood culture Gram stain showing Gram positive cocci in chains.

After this time, a routine microscopic examination of blood culture bottles is not recommended because the limits of detection are similar to those attained through the macroscopic observation of the bottles for visible changes in the broth. All suspected positive results from subcultures should be inoculated onto media that support the growth of most aerobes and anaerobes. This would include chocolate agar, 5% sheep blood agar, MacConkey agar if a gram-negative organism is suspected, and anaerobic blood when anaerobes are suspected. All aerobic bottles should be subcultured before disposal. Performing blind subcultures on anaerobic bottles is generally not recommended.

Any positive reaction, either from a slide or culture bottle, must be reported immediately to the physician. Manual blood cultures are time consuming and labor intensive; however, modifications of the manual method can improve the timely detection of bacteria in blood. For example, the use of a biphasic blood culture system may increase the sensitivity of blood cultures. In the BBL™ SEPTI-CHEK™ Blood Culture System (Becton Dickinson), the bottles contain a paddle of agar, such as chocolate agar, MacConkey agar, or fungal media. The bottles are inoculated with blood and tilted so that the specimen contacts the agar and then incubated at 35°C ± 2°C for a 7-day period. The broth is observed for turbidity, color change, hemolysis, or gas formation. The slide is examined daily for growth, and the bottle is inverted periodically. Because selective and differential media are present on the paddle, isolates can be differentiated based on their growth patterns.

Another manual system is the Thermo Scientific™ Oxoid™ SIGNAL Blood Culture System (Thermo-Fisher Scientific), which provides for the detection of aerobic and anaerobic organisms. The top of the blood culture bottles has a chamber with a plastic locking sleeve attached. The chamber has a long needle and a clear plastic compartment with a narrow cylinder at the bottom and a large upper reservoir. The chamber needle is inserted through the rubber stopper at a position below the surface of the culture medium. If organisms grow in the bottle, gas is produced. The system also creates pressure in the sealed bottle when organisms are growing. As a sign of growth, positive pressure is detected by a growth indicator device when pressure in the bottle displaces a quantity of blood/broth mixture. A positive result is indicated when the blood/broth mixture rises above the locking sleeve of the growth indicator device. The bottles also should be inspected visually for signs of bacterial growth, such as hemolysis, turbidity, or colonies on the interface of the blood layer.

The lysis centrifugation method (Isolator from Wampale Laboratories) uses a stoppered tube with saponin to lyse cells, propylene glycol to decrease foaming, and SPS (sodium polyanethol sulfonate) as an anticoagulant and agent to inactivate certain antibiotics. There also is a fluorochemical that provides cushion during centrifugation and also concentrates the microorganisms. The tubes are inoculated with the blood specimen and centrifuged; then the supernatant is removed. The sediment, which contains the cells and microorganisms, is vortexed and then used to inoculate media. This system is believed to provide better recovery of fragile bacteria and some fungi; however, it also is believed that this system is more prone to contamination and aerosol production.

AUTOMATED BLOOD CULTURE SYSTEMS

Automation in the detection of bacteria in the blood has significantly improved the detection of bacteremia. The BACTEC™ (Becton Dickinson) was the first automated blood culture system. The early models, such as the BACTEC 460, used a radiometric principle and relied on the release of $^{14}CO_2$ from ^{14}C radioactively labeled substrates. These models were replaced by newer versions, such as the BACTEC 660 and BACTEC NR 860, which detect the release of CO_2 directly with an infrared spectrophotometer. The newer models alleviate the disadvantages associated with radioactivity, including safety hazards and strict disposal guidelines. The BACTEC 860 is fully automated and includes incubators, shakers, and detectors.

In the BACTEC 860 model, blood culture vials are injected with the patient's blood sample. Media are available for aerobic and anaerobic bacteria, as well as for fungi and some species of *Mycobacterium*. Trays with the vials are incubated in the appropriate atmosphere: 2.5% CO_2 with air for aerobes and 5% CO_2 with nitrogen for anaerobes. The vials are agitated periodically by a rotary shaker that is part of the system. Periodically, the vials enter the monitoring module, where they are moved by a detector. The detector penetrates the rubber stopper at the top of the vial with two needles, removing any gas that has accumulated above the liquid medium. This gas is known as the headspace gas. The headspace gas is replaced with a fresh mixture of the appropriate aerobic or anaerobic gaseous mixture. The amount of CO_2 in each vial is measured with an infrared spectrophotometer. Any level of CO_2 above a preset threshold is monitored and processed by the microbiologist. A computer handles the data and interprets and records the results.

The newest versions of the BACTEC, the 9240 and 9120, are fully automated and use fluorescence to measure released CO_2 or consumed oxygen. There is a gas-permeable CO_2 sensor on the bottom of each vial. When released from bacterial metabolism, the CO_2 dissolves in water and forms hydrogen ions (H^+), which causes the pH to decrease, initiating a fluorescent signal. There is continuous monitoring with repeated measurements every 10 minutes in the 9000 series, and detection is external to the bottle, which decreases the risk of contamination. Thus, bacterial growth is detected as a consequence of production of carbon dioxide or utilization of oxygen.

The BacT/ALERT® 3D (bioMérieux) uses colorimetric technology and measures microbial-produced CO_2 photometrically. The system is fully automated and noninvasive and utilizes a colorimetric CO_2 sensor, which is placed at the bottom of each blood culture bottle. A CO_2-permeable membrane separates the sensor from microbial growth. CO_2 generated from microbial metabolism diffuses across the membrane into the sensor and dissolves in a pH-sensitive water solution. This results in the production of hydrogen ions, which lowers the pH, changing the color of the sensor from dark green to yellow. Light reflected from the sensor is detected and measured photometrically. Changes in reflectance are determined, and a voltage signal proportional to the intensity of the reflected light is generated. The voltage signal is analyzed by a computer, which determines whether growth is present based on changes in absorbance, rate of change, and the color threshold produced. A significant advantage of the BacT/ALERT® 3D is continuous monitoring of each vial. Because the vials remain in one place during incubation, the time necessary to detect a positive result is decreased.

The VersaTREK® System (Trek Diagnostic Systems) monitors pressure changes in the bottle headspace created from bacterial metabolism. Changes are monitored every 24 minutes. Advantages of the VersaTREK® System include its adaptability to small- or large-volume laboratories and using a smaller amount of blood. Because it detects all gasses produced or consumed by microorganisms, the system is not limited by organisms that produce low CO_2 concentrations.

MICROORGANISMS ASSOCIATED WITH BLOOD INFECTIONS

Septicemia may result from bacteria entering the blood through the genitourinary, respiratory, or biliary tract and from abscesses, contaminated intravenous catheters, burns, and infected surgical wounds. Predisposing conditions to bacteremia include surgery, trauma, diabetes mellitus, renal or hepatic failure, corticosteroid therapy, and malignancies.

The bacteria most often isolated from blood infections are the gram-positive cocci, including *Staphylococcus aureus*, coagulase-negative *Staphylococcus*, the viridans streptococci, *Streptococcus pneumoniae*, and *Enterococcus*. Also isolated as the agents of bacteremia or septicemia are gram-negative bacilli, including *Escherichia coli*, *Klebsiella*, *Pseudomonas*, *Enterobacter*, *Proteus*, *Salmonella*, and *Haemophilus*. Many of these bacteria are found in the hospital environment or as normal flora and may colonize in patients, including on the skin or in the oropharynx or gastrointestinal tract. *Bacteroides fragilis* is the anaerobe most often isolated from blood cultures. Other important anaerobes isolated from blood cultures include *Clostridium perfringens* and *Clostridium septicum*.

Candida albicans is the most common cause of **fungemia**, being found frequently in immunosuppressed hosts. The saprobic fungus *Rhizopus* and *Malassezia furfur* and *Fusarium* also have been found with more frequency in blood cultures. Standard blood culture bottles that are vented and incubated at 30°C are sufficient to isolate most fungi. Biphasic systems also are acceptable.

It may be difficult to differentiate contaminants from pathogens in blood cultures. Organisms that normally colonize the skin can be presumed to be contaminants because of poor skin disinfection unless found in multiple cultures. These organisms include *Bacillus*, *Corynebacterium*, *Propionibacterium*, and coagulase-negative staphylococci. When found in more than one culture, the organisms should be considered pathogenic. With an increase in opportunistic infections, it is important to realize that these colonizers can be pathogenic in certain situations. BOX 22-2 is a guide in differentiating contaminated blood cultures from true infections.

Circulating antigens can be detected directly in blood cultures. Latex agglutination methods to detect antigens of *Streptococcus agalactiae*, *Haemophilus influenzae* type b, *Streptococcus pneumoniae*, *Neisseria meningitidis*, and certain yeasts are available commercially. These rapid methods serve as an adjunct in the diagnosis of bacteremia.

FIGURE 22-4 shows a scheme for the identification of common blood culture pathogens. The procedure for collection and analysis of blood cultures is outlined at the end of the chapter.

BOX 22-2 Differentiation of Positive Blood Cultures from Contaminated Blood Cultures

Microorganism isolated:

Coagulase-negative staphylococci (CoNS), *Corynebacterium* species, *Bacillus* other than *B. anthracis*, *Propionibacterium acne*, *Micrococcus* species, viridans streptococci, *Enterococcus*, and *Clostridium perfringens* may be associated with contamination; however, these also can be agents of bacteremia.

Staphylococcus aureus, *Streptococcus pneumoniae*, *E. coli* and other Enterobacteriaceae, *Pseudomonas aeruginosa*, *Cryptococcus neoformans*, and *Candida albicans* are generally considered to be pathogenic.

Number of positive blood culture sets:

Proportion of positive culture sets that grow organisms. If only one is positive, suspect contamination.

If multiple sets grow the same organism, it is more likely a true bacteremia.

Number of positive bottles in a blood culture set:

There is a greater likelihood of contamination when only one bottle shows growth in a blood culture set.

Time to growth:

There is a greater likelihood of contamination if growth occurs over 3 to 5 days.

Clinical clues:

Clinical signs of sepsis

Symptoms of true blood infections include:

Fever (body temperature >40°C) or hypothermia (body temperature <36°C)

White blood cell count either <4,000/ml or >20,000/ml; hypotension

Source of culture and collection method

Catheters can be colonized or contaminated because microorganisms can grow on the surface of the catheter and therefore in the blood specimen.

Correctly collected peripheral venipuncture specimens are less likely to be contaminated.

Contamination rates are lower in those facilities where there is a dedicated and well-trained phlebotomy team.

Cerebrospinal Fluid—Meningitis and Central Nervous System Infections

Cerebrospinal fluid (CSF) supports and surrounds the brain and spinal cord. CSF also protects and cushions the soft tissue of the brain and brings nutrients to and removes waste from the area.

Meningitis is the inflammation of the meninges, which are three thin membranes that cover the brain and spinal cord. There are four fluid-filled spaces in the brain, which are known as ventricles. Choroid plexus, located in

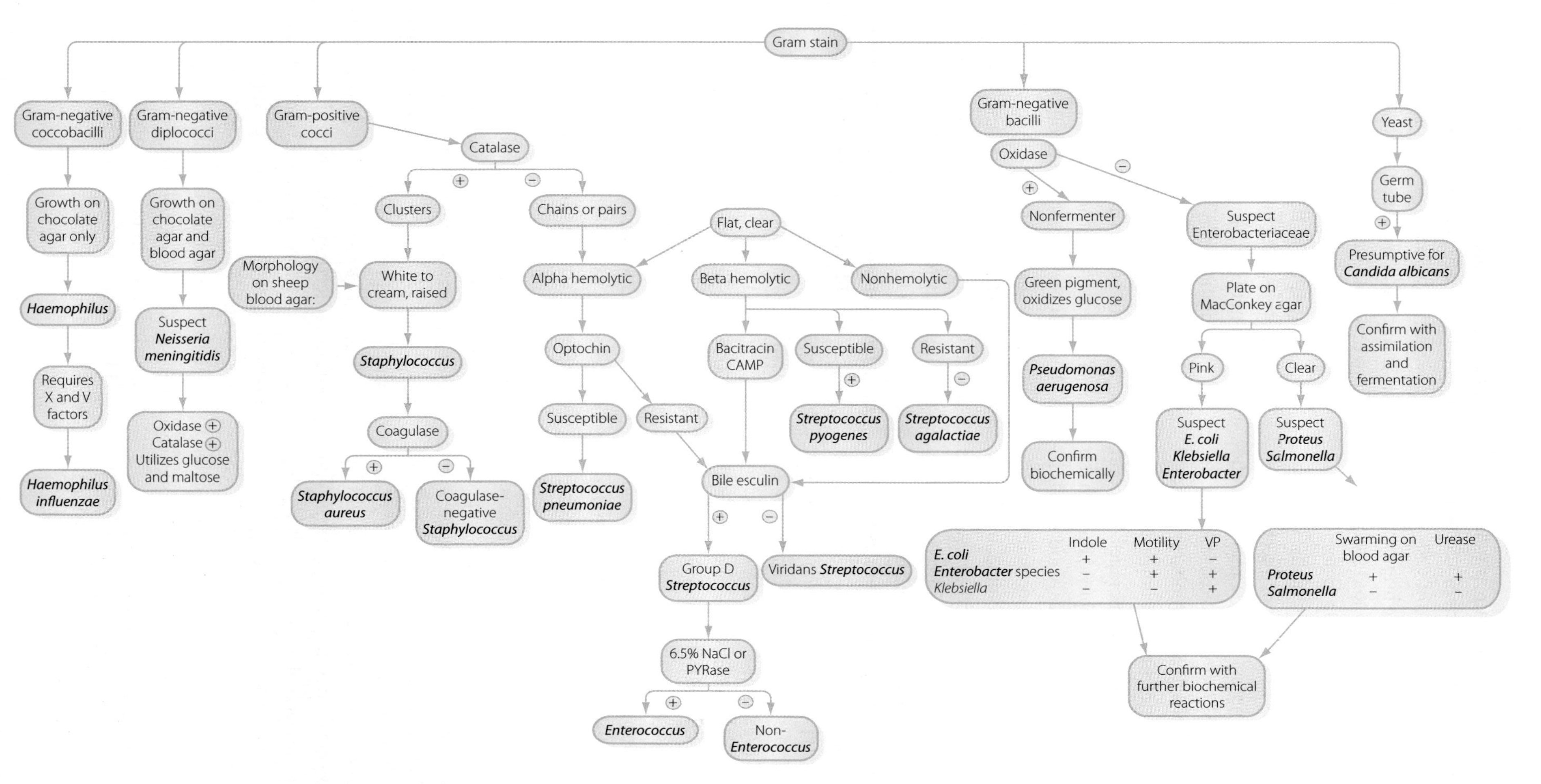

FIGURE 22-4 Identification scheme for common blood pathogens.

the third and fourth ventricles in the brain, produces CSF. Normally, approximately 20 ml to 25 ml of CSF is in the ventricles. Changes in the composition of CSF provides useful information about diseases in the brain and spinal cord. Meningitis occurs in the subarachnoid space, which is located between the arachnoid and pia mater.

Different mechanisms may lead to meningitis. The infectious agent may spread directly from a site of infection, such as from the middle ear or sinuses. Bacteria may enter the central nervous system (CNS) through colonization of the mucosal surfaces of the nasopharynx or oropharynx. Bacteria that have mechanisms for attachment, known as pili, can attach to the epithelial cells of mucous membranes. A second mechanism of infection is hematogenous spread through the blood into the subarachnoid space or other blood vessels in the brain. The presence of anatomical abnormalities in the CNS structure from congenital defects, trauma, or surgery provides another mechanism of meningitis. Finally, some infectious agents, such as the rabies virus or herpes simplex virus, can invade the brain by traveling along nerves.

Bacteria that possess antiphagocytic capsules are some of the most frequent causes of meningitis. These include *Haemophilus influenzae* type b, *Streptococcus pneumoniae*, and *Neisseria meningitidis*. After multiplication at the site of attachment, the organism either enters the blood directly or is carried to the blood by the lymphatic system. Dissemination throughout the host occurs, and the organism enters the CSF as the capillary integrity and tight junctions of the blood-brain barrier are damaged and no longer effective. Once in the CSF, the organism can multiply relatively easily because there are few if any white blood cells or antibodies present.

CSF is an ultrafiltrate of plasma formed through selective secretion and absorption. CSF glucose is approximately 60% to 70% of the patient's serum glucose level, and the normal CSF protein concentration ranges from 15 mg/dl to 50 mg/dl. The blood-brain barrier serves as a mechanical and osmotic barrier between blood and CSF. Thus, certain components do not normally enter the CSF unless the blood-brain barrier is altered as a result of infection, trauma, or other abnormal states.

Normally, there are relatively few cells in the CSF. The total in adults should not exceed five white blood cells (WBCs) per microliter (μl). During infection the total WBC count increases.

There are different types of meningitis based on the symptoms of the infection, the microorganism causing the infection, and host factors. Acute meningitis is a severe infection characterized by fever, stiff neck, headache, nausea, vomiting, neurologic disorders and altered mental status, and an increase in neutrophils. Chronic meningitis has a slow onset of fever, headache, nausea, vomiting, and stiff neck. There may be confusion and mental deterioration. In chronic meningitis, the predominant cell is generally the lymphocyte. Acute, purulent meningitis is characterized by many neutrophils and bacteria in the CSF. In bacterial meningitis the WBC count usually exceeds 1,000/μl, with a predominance of neutrophils, and the total protein increases to more than 100 mg/dl. The glucose level is decreased to values that may be less than 40 mg/dl.

Those at risk of meningitis include neonates; those with respiratory tract infections, which serve as a portal of entry into the CNS; the immunosuppressed; those with prosthetic CNS shunts; and those with anatomical defects in the CNS. The species of bacteria that causes meningitis differs with host factors. The most common causes of bacterial meningitis include *H. influenzae* type b, *S. pneumoniae*, *N. meningitidis*, *Streptococcus agalactiae*, *Escherichia coli*, *Listeria monocytogenes*, *Staphylococcus aureus*, and *Mycobacterium* species. *S. pneumoniae* is currently the most common etiologic agent of bacterial meningitis in the United States. Also, children less than 2 years of age have a high incidence of developing invasive pneumococcal disease. Before the *Haemophilus influenzae* type b conjugate vaccinations were available and licensed in the United States, this organism accounted for 45% to 48% of cases of bacterial meningitis. Most of these cases were found in infants and children less than 6 years of age; the peak incidence was found in infants who were 6 to 12 months of age. Today, *H. influenzae* type b accounts for approximately 7% of the cases of bacterial meningitis in the United States; most of these cases are found in adults. Worldwide, *H. influenzae* is still widespread where vaccination is not prevalent.

Most cases (over 90%) of *Neisseria meningitidis* are sporadic infections. Subgroup B and subgroup C each accounts for approximately 32% of the cases in the United States, and group Y accounts for approximately 24% of the cases. Group Y accounts for most (53%) of endemic cases of meningococcal meningitis. The quadrivalent meningococcal vaccine, which has been licensed in the United States since 2005, protects against serogroups A, C, Y, and W-135. Meningococcal meningitis is most prevalent in neonates and young adults who have not been immunized.

Risk factors also include living in the same household as a patient or carrier, which places those living in college dormitories and military recruits at a high risk when not immunized. Meningococcal meningitis may range from mild symptoms to a severe bacteremia (meningococcemia) and fulminant meningitis. Individuals with terminal complement component deficiencies also are at increased risk of meningococcal meningitis.

Approximately 70% of *Streptococcus agalactiae* (group B streptococcus, GBS) meningitis is found in newborns and infants up to 3 months of age. In the 1990s, the incidence of GBS infection in newborns was 1.7 cases per 1,000, which has declined greatly because of the use of screening and penicillin. All pregnant women are screened for colonization of *S. agalactiae* at 35 to 37 weeks gestation, and antibiotics, such as penicillin, are given prophylactically to carriers.

Neonates during the first week of life have the highest prevalence of meningitis; there is also a high mortality. The most common agent of early onset neonatal meningitis is *S. agalactiae*, followed by *E. coli* and other gram-negative bacilli and *Listeria monocytogenes*. Early onset meningitis is generally acquired from the mother during birth. Late-onset neonatal meningitis occurs from the first week of life until the infant is 2 to 3 months old. Bacterial species that cause late-onset neonatal meningitis include staphylococci, *L. monocytogenes*, and gram-negative bacilli. Less frequent causes include *Chryseobacterium meningosepticum*; coagulase-negative *Staphylococcus*, *Klebsiella*, and *Enterobacter*; *Listeria* organisms; and *Mycobacterium tuberculosis*.

H. influenzae type b was once the leading cause of meningitis in older infants and young children. Widespread vaccination has greatly decreased its incidence in these populations. Today, *S. pneumoniae* and *N. meningitidis* are the most common causes of bacteria meningitis in this age group. Other causes of bacterial meningitis in this age group include *S. agalactiae*, *E. coli*, nontypeable *H. influenzae* (other than group b), *L. monocytogenes*, and *Streptococcus pyogenes* (group A streptococci). Young adults who may be at risk of developing meningitis include those who live in close quarters, such as in college dormitories or military barracks, especially when poor nutrition and insufficient rest also are contributing factors.

Immunocompromised adults are at a higher risk of meningitis. The most common etiologic agents are *S. pneumoniae*, *L. monocytogenes*, *E. coli*, and *Staphylococcus aureus*. Other predisposing factors for meningitis include infections of the upper respiratory tract, such as sinusitis and otitis; subdural abscesses; surgery or trauma; ventricular shunts; diabetes mellitus; and immunosuppression.

Recurrent meningitis accounts for 1% to 6% of the cases of meningitis. In children, this most commonly is a result of an anatomic defect in the CNS, whereas in adults it may occur because of a head trauma or CSF leakage. Immunodeficiency also is a risk factor for recurrent meningitis. *S. pneumoniae*, *N. meningitidis*, and *H. influenzae* are causes of recurrent meningitis.

In aseptic meningitis, there is a predominance of lymphocytes and other mononuclear cells, which is known as pleocytosis. The cultures for bacteria are negative, and most cases are a result of viral infections. In early viral infections, neutrophils may be present, but lymphocytes are the predominant WBCs later in the infection. Glucose may be normal or slightly decreased, whereas the total protein is normal or slightly increased to values less than 100 mg/dl. Symptoms include fever, stiff neck, headache, nausea, and vomiting. The WBC count increases in viral meningitis but generally remains less than 500 WBC/μl.

Agents of fungal meningitis include *Cryptococcus neoformans*, an opportunistic pathogen, and *Candida* species.

Encephalitis is an inflammation of the brain, which is usually the result of viral infection. When meningitis also occurs, the infection is known as meningoencephalitis. Viruses also can directly enter the CNS via the nerves.

Agents of viral meningitis, encephalitis, or meningoencephalitis include the enteroviruses (Coxsackie viruses A and B, echovirus), mumps virus, herpes simplex virus, and the arboviruses (togavirus, bunyavirus, West Nile virus, St. Louis encephalitis virus, eastern equine encephalitis virus). Less common agents of viral meningitis include cytomegalovirus (CMV), measles virus, Epstein Barr virus (EBV), rabies virus, myxovirus, paramyxovirus, and varicella-zoster virus.

COLLECTION AND ANALYSIS OF CSF

CSF is collected through lumbar puncture of the subarachnoid space. In adults, three or four separate tubes are collected for analysis. The last tube collected is usually used for the cell count and differential because it is least likely to be contaminated with capillary blood. The other tubes can be used for microbiology, chemistry, and other testing. Some facilities prefer to use tube 3 or 4 for microbiology for the Gram stain and culture because these tubes should be free from skin contaminants that might be present in tubes 1 and 2. The tube used and the test selection vary with the facility and the volume of fluid available.

Spinal fluids must be processed immediately. In most cases, CSF should not be refrigerated and should be held at room temperature or at 37°C. Some fastidious bacteria, such as *S. pneumoniae*, *N. meningitis*, and *H. influenzae* may lose their viability when refrigerated. If viral studies are requested, CSF can be refrigerated for up to 23 hours or frozen at –70°C.

The CSF is concentrated by centrifuging for at least 15 minutes at 1,500 × g by using a cytospin or a membrane filter. This will increase the yield of microorganisms, which increases the sensitivity of the stain and culture. The sediment is used for staining and plating of primary media; the supernatant can be used for chemical tests.

A Gram, methylene blue, or acridine orange stain is performed on the concentrated specimen. Membrane filtration uses a filter with minute pores through which the CSF is filtered onto a chocolate agar plate. **FIGURE 22-5** shows a Gram stain of a positive CSF specimen, and **FIGURE 22-6** shows a Wright's stain hematology smear of the same specimen. **FIGURE 22-7** shows gram-negative diplococci in a CSF specimen. Any positive results from the Gram stain or other direct examination methods must immediately be reported to the physician or health care provider.

Rapid methods of examination for CSF include Neufeld quellung reaction, which may be used to detect capsular polysaccharide. Bacterial or fungal antigens also can be detected and identified because capsular polysaccharides are released into the surrounding body tissue and CSF as the bacteria multiply. Methods to detect capsular polysaccharide to *H. influenzae* type b, *S. agalactiae*, and *N. meningitidis* serotypes A, B, C, Y, and W-135 are available by using counterimmunoelectrophoresis, coagglutination, or latex agglutination. Cryptococcal antigen also can be directly detected in CSF. Polymerase chain reaction and nucleic acid amplification methods also are available to detect microorganisms in CSF.

Blood cultures often are requested along with CSF specimens to aid in the diagnosis of meningitis. Media that is inoculated for aerobic CSF cultures includes sheep blood, CNA, chocolate, MacConkey agars, and thioglycollate broth. Anaerobic or fungal plates are added when appropriate. The procedure for CSF analysis is found at the end of the chapter.

FIGURE 22-8 summarizes the identification of those organisms most frequently found in CSF.

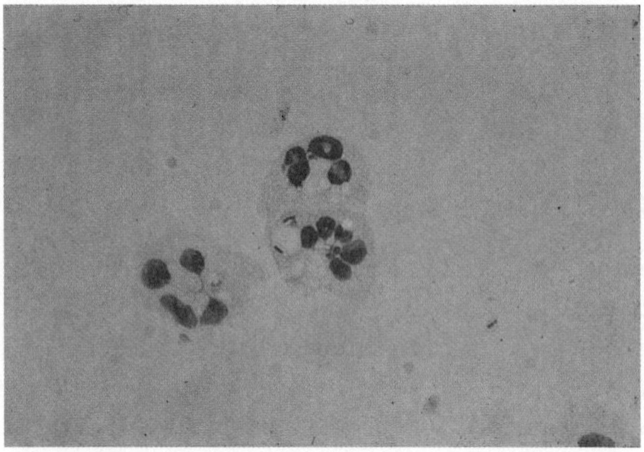

FIGURE 22-5 Gram stain of positive CSF specimen showing polymorphonuclear white blood cells with intracellular Gram negative bacilli.

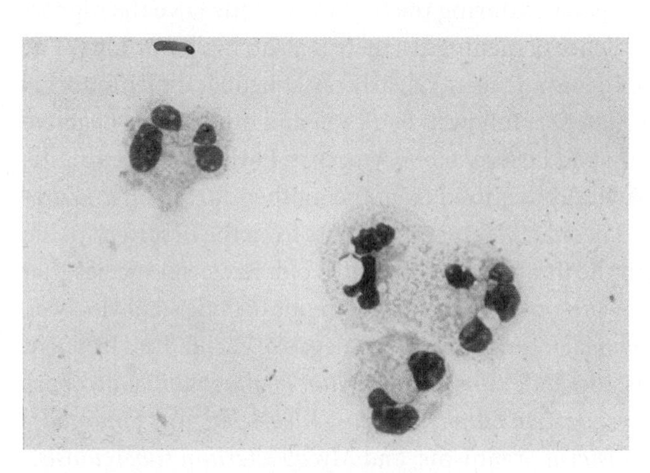

FIGURE 22-6 Wright's stain hematology smear of the specimen shown in Figure 22-5 showing vacuolated neutrophils and intracellular bacteria, indicative of bacterial meningitis.

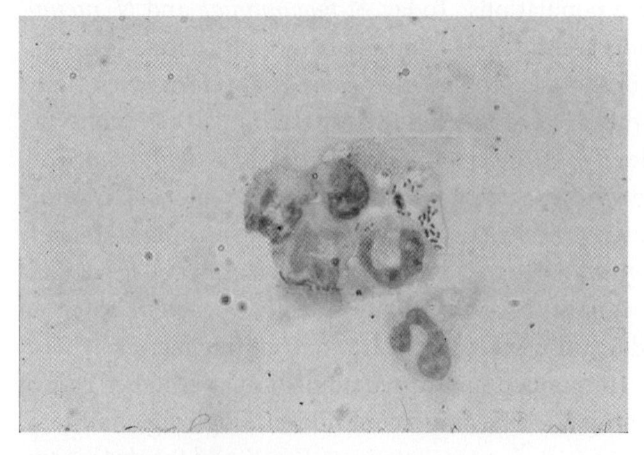

FIGURE 22-7 Gram-negative diplococci occurring intracellular to neutrophils in a CSF specimen.

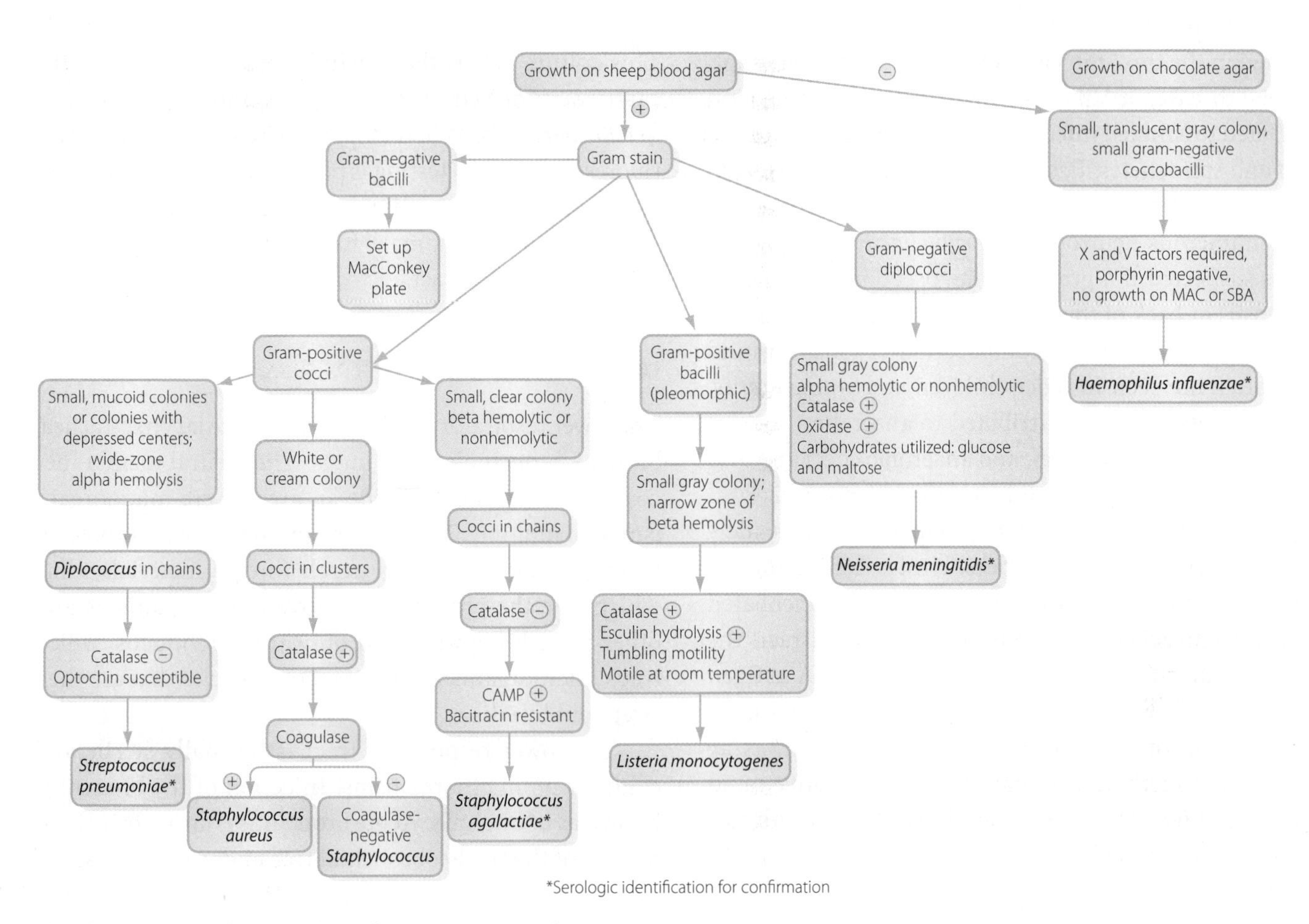

FIGURE 22-8 Identification scheme for common CSF pathogens.

Respiratory Tract Specimens and Infections

UPPER RESPIRATORY TRACT

The upper respiratory tract consists of the oral and nasal cavities, pharynx, and sinuses. Defense mechanisms of the upper respiratory tract include cilia and mucus, which can trap foreign particles and microorganisms and move them upward and out of the respiratory tract.

Because of the large number and species of normal bacterial flora, it often is difficult to determine the significance of the isolation of an organism from the upper respiratory tract. One should always report if normal flora is absent, present, or decreased and also provide a semiquantitation of any suspected pathogen, such as few, moderate, or heavy. The major normal flora of the upper respiratory tract includes the viridans streptococci, nonpathogenic *Neisseria*, coagulase-negative *Staphylococcus*, the *Enterococcus*, *Moraxella*, some *Haemophilus* species, *Lactobacillus*, a few *Candida albicans*, and nonpathogenic *Corynebacterium*. Also, small numbers of *S. pneumoniae* may be carried as normal flora in some individuals.

THROAT SPECIMENS

Throat cultures are plated on sheep blood agar, with a chocolate agar plate added for children less than 5 years of age to detect *Haemophilus*. Throat cultures are primarily requested to determine the presence of *Streptococcus pyogenes* (group A streptococci). Generally, two swabs are collected, with one used for rapid antigen testing and the other used for traditional culture. *Haemophilus influenzae*, a cause of epiglottitis and tracheobronchitis in nonimmunized individuals, also may be isolated from a throat culture. *C. albicans* in moderate to large numbers indicates thrush, a yeast infection found in newborns, infants, and immunosuppressed patients. Thrush appears as whitish patches on the tongue, the mucous membranes of the cheeks, and oropharynx. *Neisseria gonorrhoeae* may be detected in the throat in cases of oral gonorrhea. Fusospirochetal disease, or Vincent's angina, is an oral infection attributed to a mixed infection of the anaerobe *Fusobacterium* and spirochetes. Fusospirochetal disease is detected through a Gram stain, which shows the bacteria and many numerous neutrophils. *Corynebacterium diphtheriae* is suspected if a gray to white pseudomembrane on the tonsils or back of the pharynx is present. Peritonsillar abscesses may occur as a complication of tonsillitis and most often are seen in older children and young adults. These abscesses may be attributed to anaerobes, such as *Fusobacterium*, *Bacteroides*, and anaerobic cocci and also to *Streptococcus pyogenes* and viridans streptococci.

Direct antigen testing for the group A antigen is widely performed in physicians' offices, clinics, and laboratories. In direct antigen testing, throat swabs are incubated with either an acid or an enzyme reagent that extracts the group A antigen. Next, antibody against group A antigen is reacted with the extracted antigen, using either latex agglutination or enzyme-linked immunosorbent assay (ELISA) as a method of visualization. All negative rapid tests for group A streptococci must be confirmed with culture onto sheep blood agar. A variety of rapid GAS methods are available.

The throat culture procedure is described at the end of the chapter.

Other Upper Respiratory Tract Specimens

The sinuses are usually sterile, but colonization from the upper respiratory tract can occur. Sinus infection is generally diagnosed through clinical symptoms, with cultures being requested only in unique circumstances. Rhinoscleroma is a chronic, granulomatous infection of the sinus and sometimes the pharynx. This infection produces nasal obstruction as a result of large and extended growths and often is attributed to infection with *Klebsiella rhinoscleromatis*.

The anterior nares may be cultured to determine the carrier state of *Staphylococcus aureus*. Approximately 10% to 20% of the general population and up to 50% of those who work in the health care setting have been estimated to carry the organism asymptomatically, which serves as a route of nosocomial infection. These specimens generally are plated onto agar selective to isolate MRSA.

Nasopharyngeal cultures are collected by inserting a small, flexible wire swab through the nostril, across the bottom of the nasal passage, and into the nasopharynx. This culture also is the specimen of choice to detect the carrier state of *Neisseria meningitidis* and presence of *Bordetella pertussis*. When *B. pertussis* is suspected, direct fluorescent antigen testing is performed and Reagin-Lowe or Bordet-Gengou medium is inoculated. **FIGURE 22-9** is an identification summary for common pathogens of the upper respiratory tract.

LOWER RESPIRATORY TRACT

The lower respiratory tract consists of the larynx, trachea, bronchi, bronchioles, and lungs. The pleural membranes cover the lungs and provide an area where microorganisms can multiply. The lower respiratory tract is protected through coughing, which expels foreign materials; cilia, which line the bronchi and move microorganisms and other particles upward and outward; and mucus, which traps microorganisms and foreign particles that are then swept out by cilia.

The lower respiratory tract is normally sterile and contains no microorganisms. Infection of the bronchi is known as **bronchitis**. Acute bronchitis is an acute inflammation of the tracheobronchial tree and usually is caused by viruses; it often occurs following an upper respiratory infection, such as from the influenza virus or rhinovirus, the cause of the common cold. Symptoms include cough, fever, and the production of sputum. Chronic bronchitis is found in adults and characterized by excessive mucous production. Those at risk for chronic bronchitis include cigarette smokers, those who inhale toxic fumes or dust, and those who have frequent infections. Organisms associated with chronic bronchitis include *Streptococcus pneumoniae*, *Haemophilus influenzae* (nonencapsulated forms), and *Moraxella catarrhalis*.

Inflammation of the lower respiratory tract, including the lung, is known as **pneumonia**. Agents may be bacterial, viral, fungal, or parasitic.

Pneumonia may result from bacteria that colonize the upper respiratory tract and then enter the lung. Another route is from inhalation of large numbers of microorganisms that are in airborne droplets. Pneumonia may be categorized as either community-acquired pneumonia (CAP) or hospital-acquired or ventilator-associated pneumonia. CAP is acquired outside of the hospital or health care setting; hospital-associated pneumonia occurs within the hospital or health care setting or following treatment or therapy within a health care setting. Ventilator-associated

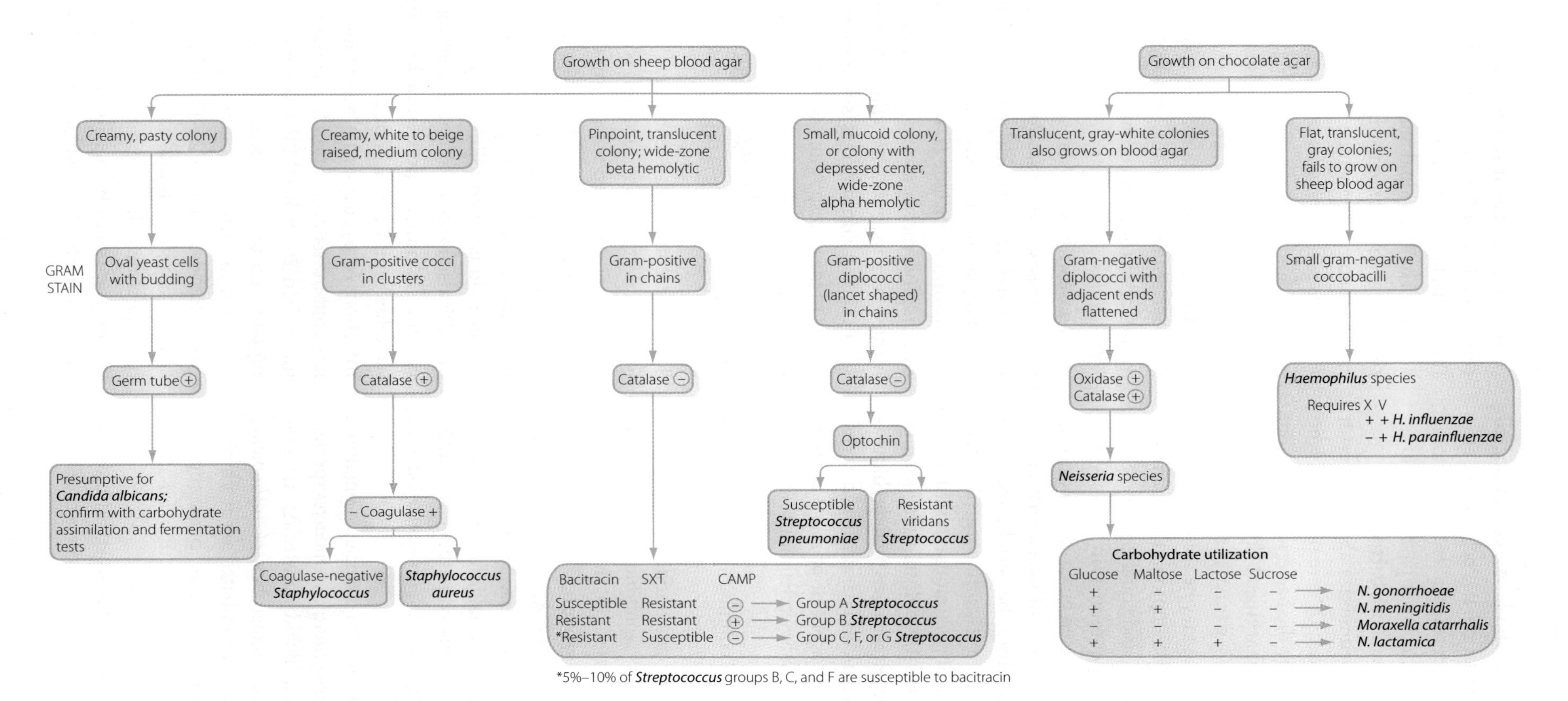

FIGURE 22-9 Identification scheme for upper respiratory tract pathogens.

pneumonia occurs in patients who have been intubated and undergo mechanical ventilation. It is believed that the infection occurs because the endotracheal or tracheostomy tube permits bacteria to enter the lower parts of the lung; these tubes also can be colonized with bacteria.

Health care–associated pneumonias also may result from contact with patients or health care providers who either are infected with or carry the bacteria. Aspiration, the inhalation of normal oropharyngeal flora or gastric contents into the lower respiratory tract, is another route for pneumonia. Finally, the lung may be seeded by bacteria that are present in the blood. Symptoms of pneumonia include fever, chills, chest pain, and cough.

Community-acquired pneumonia in infants and young children most often is caused by viruses, including respiratory syncytial virus (RSV), influenza virus, parainfluenza virus, and adenoviruses. Bacterial pneumonia in children may be attributed to *H. influenzae*, *S. pneumoniae*, or *S. aureus*. Causes of pneumonia in school-age children most commonly are *Mycoplasma pneumoniae* and *Chlamydia pneumoniae*; viral causes include rhinovirus, adenovirus, influenza virus, and parainfluenza virus. *Mycoplasma pneumoniae*, the agent of primary atypical pneumonia, most frequently causes pneumonia in young adults less than 30 years of age.

The most common cause of community-acquired bacterial pneumonia in adults is *Streptococcus pneumoniae*, which typically produces lobar pneumonia. Other organisms include *H. influenzae*, *C. pneumoniae*, *M. pneumoniae*, and respiratory viruses. In those older than 60 years, *S.aureus* and gram-negative bacilli also are associated with CAP. Viral causes of CAP in adults include influenza virus, parainfluenza virus, adenovirus, and cytomegalovirus. Secondary bacterial infections may follow viral pneumonia, and associated pathogens include *S. aureus*, β-hemolytic streptococci, *S. pneumoniae*, and *H. influenzae*.

Agents of hospital and ventilator-associated pneumonia include *Pseudomonas aeruginosa*; *Enterobacter* species; *Klebsiella* species; *S. aureus*, including MRSA; *Acinetobacter* species; *S. pneumoniae*; anaerobes; *H. influenzae*; and *Legionella*. Patients who are intubated are at a higher risk of nosocomial pneumonia; however, pneumonia is a common health care–associated infection for many patients.

Aspiration pneumonia may occur when an individual becomes unconscious as a result of seizures or alcohol or substance abuse or during surgery. It also happens in those who have difficulty swallowing, as might be seen in those with head trauma or neurological damage following a stroke. The individual may aspirate her or his oral secretions or gastric contents. Bacteria associated with aspiration pneumonia include the oral anaerobes, including *Prevotella* and *Porphyromonas* species; *Fusobacterium*; and anaerobic and microaerophilic streptococci. Other bacteria associated with aspiration pneumonia include *S. aureus*, the Enterobacteriaceae, and *Pseudomonas aeruginosa*.

Chronic lower respiratory tract pathogens include *Mycobacterium tuberculosis*, the agent of tuberculosis. Other agents of chronic infections are *Mycobacterium avium-intracellulare*, *M. kansasii*, *Actinomycetes*, and *Nocardia*.

Those with cystic fibrosis (CF) may have chronic respiratory disease from *Pseudomonas aeruginosa*, especially the mucoid strain, which produces large amounts of capsular polysaccharide. Other organisms found in those with CF pneumonia include *H. influenzae*, *Burkholderia cepacia*, *Staphylococcus aureus*, respiratory syncytial virus, influenza virus, and *Aspergillus*.

BOX 22-3 summarizes some of the more common agents of lower respiratory tract infections.

DIAGNOSIS OF LOWER RESPIRATORY TRACT INFECTIONS—SPUTUM SPECIMENS

The most common specimen collected for diagnosis of lower respiratory tract infections is sputum. Sputum often may be contaminated with normal oropharyngeal flora, and it is necessary to evaluate the quality of the sputum specimen. A Gram stain is performed on all sputum samples, and the number of squamous epithelial cells per low-power field is noted (SECs/LPF). The number of WBCs per LPF also is noted, although caution must be exercised because immunosuppressed or leukopenic patients may have low numbers of WBCs in the sputum, even with infection. As a general rule, acceptable specimens that are not contaminated contain fewer than 10 SECs/LFP and more than 25 WBCs/LPF. **FIGURE 22-10** shows an unacceptable sputum specimen with SECs and no WBCs; this specimen most likely is contaminated with oropharyngeal secretions. Figures 22-11 and 22-12 show acceptable sputum samples. **FIGURE 22-11** is a Gram stain of a sputum specimen showing a mixed flora of gram-positive bacilli, gram-negative bacilli, and yeast. The lack of WBCs may be attributed to neutropenia or a diminished immune

BOX 22-3 Lower Respiratory Tract Pathogens

Bacterial

Streptococcus pneumoniae: Most common cause in geriatric population; agent of community-acquired pneumonias; presence of capsule facilitates attachment and resistance to phagocytosis

Klebsiella pneumoniae: Agent is serious gram-negative pneumonia; produces "currant jelly" sputum; encapsulated; may be nosocomial

Other members of the Enterobacteriaceae associated with lower respiratory tract infections include *Serratia marcescens* and *Escherichia coli*.

Staphylococcus aureus: Agent in community-acquired and nosocomial pneumonias; may be acquired through the aspiration route

Pseudomonas aeruginosa: Agent in nosocomial pneumonias; acquired through aspiration and nonaspiration routes; mucoid strain associated with severe pneumonia in patients with cystic fibrosis

Haemophilus influenzae: Agent of infections in nonimmunized infants and children and immunosuppressed adults; presence of capsule facilitates infection

Mycobacterium tuberculosis: Agent of chronic lung infections and tuberculosis

Legionella pneumophila: Agent of Legionnaires' disease; acquired through inhalation of contaminated water aerosols; most often found in middle-aged males with an underlying medical problem

Mycoplasma

Mycoplasma pneumoniae: Agent of primary atypical pneumonia; most common cause of pneumonia in young adults

Viral

Myxoviruses (influenzae and parainfluenza viruses): Agents of bronchitis and pneumonia; occur in endemics or epidemics

Respiratory syncytial virus: Most often seen in children less than 5 years of age as cause of bronchitis and pneumonia

Fungal

Coccidioides immitis: Agent of coccidioidomycosis

Histoplasma capsulatum: Agent of histoplasmosis

Blastomyces dermatitidis: Agent of blastomycosis

Cryptococcus neoformans: Agent of cryptococcosis

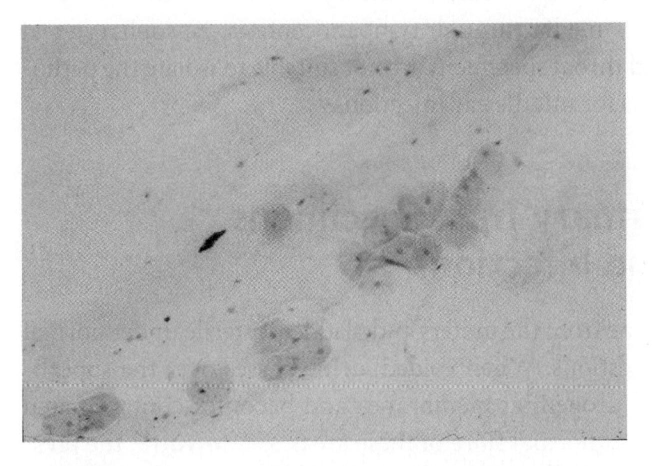

FIGURE 22-10 Unacceptable Gram stain of sputum showing squamous epithelial cells, indicating collection of saliva and not sputum.

response in the host. **FIGURE 22-12** is a Gram stain of a sputum sample showing the typical morphology of *Streptococcus pneumoniae*, gram-positive diplococci, and many segmented neutrophils.

Acid-fast stains are performed when *Mycobacterium* infection is suspected, and the Gomori-methenamine silver stain is performed when the fungus *Pneumocystis jiroveci* (formerly the parasite *Pneumocystis carinii*) pneumonia is suspected. Direct fluorescent antibody staining for *Legionella* and several viruses is performed when appropriate.

Sputum is ideally collected in the morning, when it is most concentrated. Gastric contents may be collected from children who cannot produce a sputum sample.

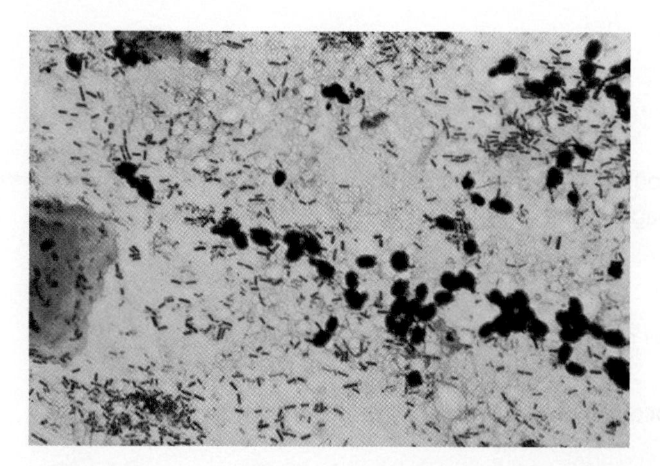

FIGURE 22-11 Gram stain of a sputum specimen showing a mixed flora of Gram-positive and Gram-negative bacilli and yeast.

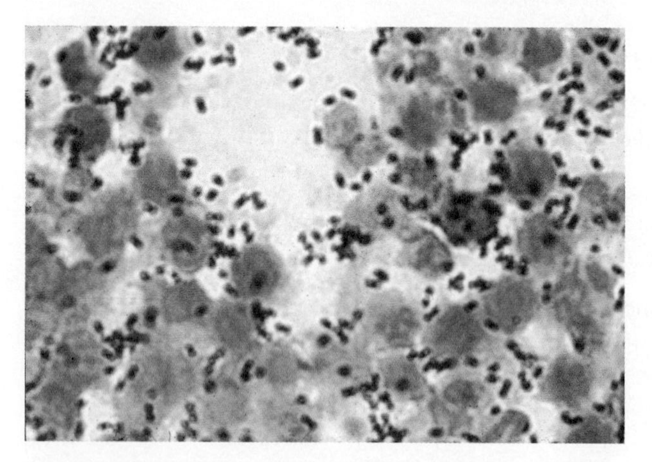

FIGURE 22-12 Gram stain of a sputum sample showing the typical morphology of *Streptococcus pneumoniae* and many segmented neutrophils.

The procedure for the sputum culture is described at the end of the chapter.

Other collection methods, which are more invasive but produce a less-contaminated specimen, include bronchoalveolar lavage, in which saline is injected through a bronchoscope into the bronchi and then aspirated and cultured. Bronchial brushings use a catheter telescoped into the bronchi. The area is then brushed and the specimen collected. Invasive procedures include transtracheal and thin-needle aspirations and open-lung biopsy. Transtracheal aspiration is a risky procedure that involves the insertion of a needle, connected to a catheter, into the trachea. Pleural fluid, collected through thoracentesis, also is suitable for the diagnosis of lower respiratory tract infection.

FIGURE 22-13 summarizes the identification of lower respiratory tract pathogens.

Eye and Ear Specimens and Infections

Eye infections may be caused by aerobic and anaerobic bacteria, fungi, viruses, and amoebas. These infections may be characterized by conjunctival discharge, redness, ocular pain, or the presence of pink eye. Examination of a swab or corneal scrapings may reveal the agent of the infection. If chlamydial infection is suspected, a direct antigen detection procedure is performed.

Bacterial agents of eye infection include *Haemophilus influenzae*, *Haemophilus aegyptius* (pink eye), *Moraxella*, *Neisseria gonorrhoeae*, and *Pseudomonas aeruginosa*. The free-living amoeba of the genus *Acanthamoeba* is a cause of **keratitis** in soft contact lens wearers. It can be observed in a direct mount of the specimen.

Tympanocentesis, the puncture of the tympanic membrane with a needle to aspirate middle ear fluid, is reserved for complicated cases of ear infection. Because the infecting organisms are predictable in childhood ear infections and the procedure for collection is complicated, most ear infections are treated by the physician without culture. *Streptococcus pneumoniae*, *H. influenzae*, and *Moraxella catarrhalis* account for most cases of acute otitis media in infants and children. Other bacteria less frequently associated with ear infections include *Streptococcus pyogenes*, *Staphylococcus aureus*, *P. aeruginosa*, *Klebsiella pneumoniae*, and *Escherichia coli*. In complicated cases it may be necessary to identify the agent of recurrent or chronic otitis media through tympanocentesis. Nasopharyngeal and throat specimens are not suitable to isolate the pathogens for middle ear infections.

Urinary Tract Specimens and Infections

Urine from the ureters and bladder is sterile under normal conditions. When voided, urine passes over the superficial urogenital membranes and becomes contaminated by the normal flora of these areas. **Bacteriuria**, the presence of bacteria in the urine, is not necessarily indicative

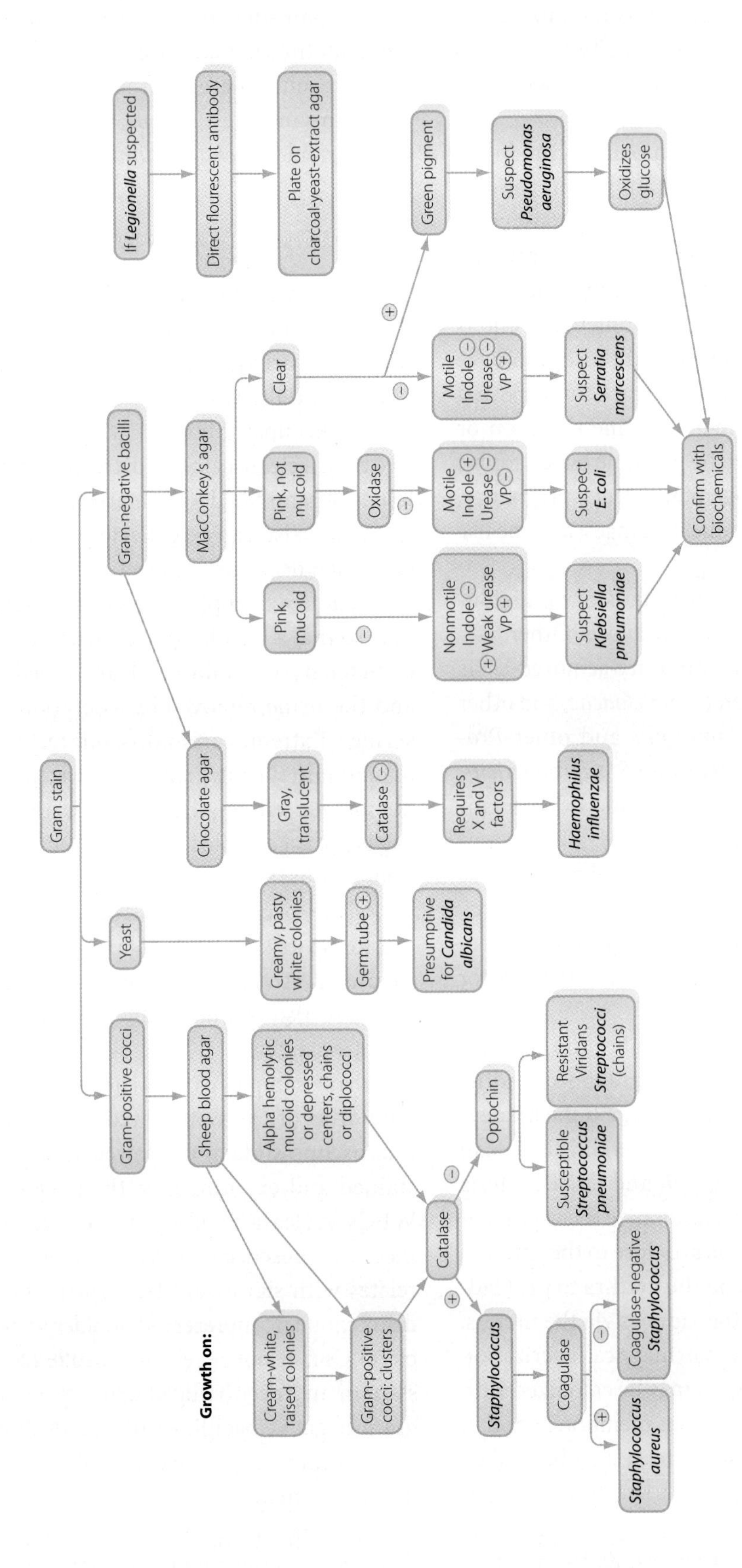

FIGURE 22-13 Identification scheme for common lower respiratory tract pathogens.

of a urinary tract infection (UTI) unless the number or colony count of the bacteria is significant. Types of UTIs include cystitis, urethritis, pyelonephritis, glomerulonephritis, and pyelitis.

Urinary tract infections are common bacterial infections in both the ambulatory population and in patients in the health care setting. In fact, UTIs are the most common type of health care–associated infection. In general, UTIs are more common in females than in males; they also are found more often in pregnant women. Infections are found in those who are diabetic and those who have anatomic abnormalities in the urinary tract. Predisposing factors associated with UTIs include urine retention or compromised urine flow caused by prostatic hypertrophy, tumors, kidney stones, or congenital defects; pregnancy, because of hormonal and anatomical changes; and the use of urinary catheters.

Community-acquired UTIs in ambulatory individuals most often are caused by *Escherichia coli*. Other bacteria frequently implicated in community-acquired UTIs include *Klebsiella* species, *Enterobacter cloacae*, and other *Enterobacter* species; *Proteus mirabilis* and other *Proteus* species; *Staphylococcus aureus* and *S. saprophyticus*; *Enterococcus*; *Pseudomonas aeruginosa* and other members of the Enterobacteriaceae.

Nosocomial UTIs are most often caused by *E. coli*, as well as by *Klebsiella* species, *Proteus* species, staphylococci, *Pseudomonas aeruginosa*, *Enterococci*, and *Candida* species. Urinary catheters significantly increase the risk for urinary tract infections.

UTIs can result from different routes and circumstance. The most common route is known as an ascending kidney infection, in which the bacteria reach the kidneys from the bladder through the ureters. Ascending UTIs can occur when coliforms, such as *E. coli* and other bacteria found in the gastrointestinal tract, colonize the vaginal or periurethral areas. These bacteria are close to the external urethral surfaces and may ascend the urethra to the bladder and may eventually reach the kidneys via the ureters. Many ascending UTIs result from urinary catheterization or cystoscopy. The hospital patient may be colonized with bacteria on his or her skin and mucous membranes and in the gastrointestinal tract. These bacteria may be pushed into the bladder by the catheter, or the bacteria may colonize the catheter.

A descending kidney infection results from hematogenous spread resulting from bacteremia. The microorganisms are deposited by the blood in the kidneys, multiply there, and are shed in the urine. Descending UTIs are much more rare than ascending UTIs; implicated organisms include *S. aureus*, *Candida albicans*, *Salmonella* species, and *Mycobacterium tuberculosis*.

URINE COLLECTION AND PROCESSING

The specimen of choice for bacterial culture of urine is the clean-catch midstream sample. Specimens collected through a urinary catheter for urine culture should be requested only when the patient cannot produce a midstream specimen. Straight catheterized urine is more invasive than a clean-catch midstream sample but is less likely to be contaminated. Catheterized urine is sterile.

Urine also can be collected from an indwelling catheter when necessary. Collection from an indwelling catheter requires clamping off the catheter tubing above the port so that a freshly voided sample can be collected. The catheter port should be cleaned well with 70% alcohol and the urine removed by aspiration with a needle and syringe. Extreme care and aseptic techniques must be used to maintain the integrity of the system so that bacteria are not introduced into the bladder. Urine from the collection bag is not acceptable for culture because bacteria can multiply within the urine in the bag.

Urine specimens should be preserved or refrigerated at 4°C for up to 24 hours if not processed and tested. Chemical preservatives include boric acid, glycerol, and formate; there are also commercially available collection and preservative systems.

Urine samples can be screened using the Gram stain. One drop of the well-mixed sample is pipetted onto a microscope slide and allowed to air-dry. The smear is stained and examined for the presence of bacteria and WBCs. At least 20 oil-immersion fields should be examined; the presence of at least one organism per field correlates with significant bacteriuria. Because WBCs may disintegrate in unpreserved or older urine, the quantitation of WBCs may not be reliable. **FIGURE 22-14** shows the Gram stain of an uncentrifuged urine specimen with moderate gram-negative bacilli. **FIGURE 22-15** shows a mixed infection of gram-negative bacilli and gram-positive cocci in a urine specimen.

Pyruria, the presence of WBCs in urine, can be detected by observing the urinary sediment microscopically. However, pyruria also may indicate other diseases,

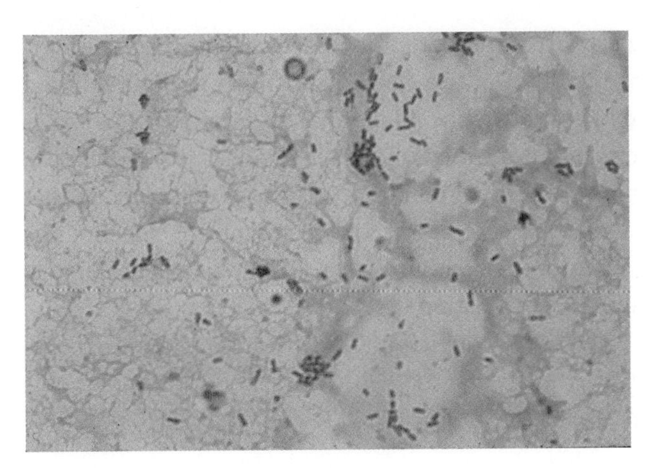

FIGURE 22-14 Gram stain of an uncentrifuged urine specimen with moderate gram-negative bacilli.

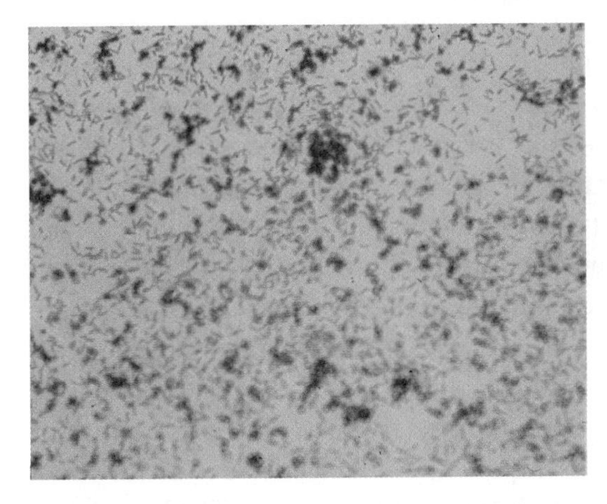

FIGURE 22-15 Gram stain of mixed infection of gram-negative bacilli and gram-positive cocci in a urine specimen.

such as vaginitis, and thus does not always indicate a UTI. Leukocyte esterase, an enzyme produced by WBCs and other inflammatory cells, can be detected using chemical strips for urinalysis. These strips also detect urinary nitrite, which is useful to identify those bacteria that can reduce nitrate to nitrite. Members of the Enterobacteriaceae, including *E. coli*, *Enterobacter* species, and *Proteus* species, give a positive nitrite reaction on the chemical strips. Urinalysis chemical strips can serve as an adjunct in screening urine specimens for infection.

COLONY COUNT

Urine specimens with significant bacteriuria noted through the screening must be cultured. A colony count is performed on all samples to be cultured to determine the

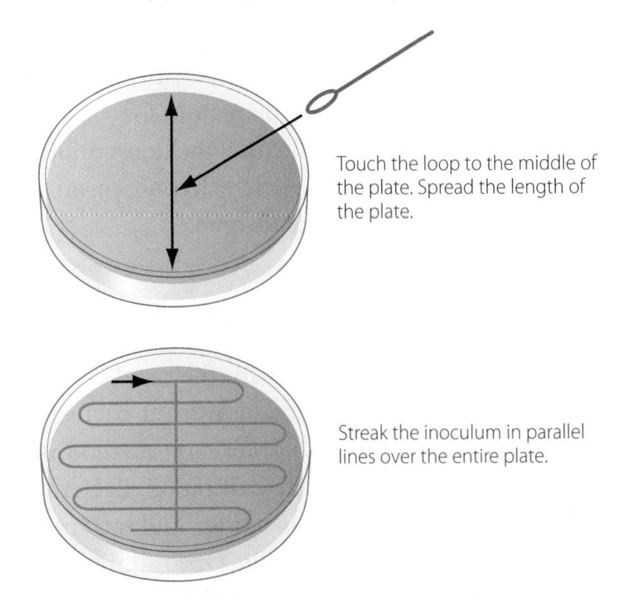

FIGURE 22-16 Colony count procedure and diagram.

number of colony-forming units per milliliter (CFU/ml). The colony count is usually performed on sheep blood agar in the technique shown in **FIGURE 22-16**. For clean-catch midstream specimens, the 1 μl calibrated loop is generally used; the number of colonies growing at 24 hours is multiplied by 1,000 to determine the CFU/ml. When culturing specimens that will likely contain a low number of bacteria, such as urine collected from a catheterization or suprapubic aspiration, a larger volume of urine should be cultured. For these specimens, it is better to use the 10 μl calibrated loop. The number of colonies growing at 24 hours is then multiplied by 100 to determine the CFU/ml. Before inoculation, the urine is mixed well and the calibrated loop inserted vertically into the cup or tube. Colony counts greater than 10^5 CFU/ml are considered to be positive for infection. However, this guideline may vary based on institutional policy, the organism isolated, the collection method, and host factors. For example, lower CFU/ml may be considered significant in suprapubic aspirates or straight catheterized specimens.

Most UTIs are caused by a single pathogen; yet, in some cases, two different organisms may be responsible for the infection. However, the isolation of three or more different species with a colony count in the range of 10^4 to

10^5 CFU/ml may indicate that the specimen is contaminated. In such cases a repeat specimen, which is collected and processed correctly, is requested. The isolation of a single species with a colony count of 10^4 CFU/ml also may be considered positive for a UTI. Explanations for a lower colony count in the presence of infection include a dilute urine sample, a partially treated UTI, dehydration, chronic pyelonephritis, or acute urethral syndrome.

AUTOMATED URINE SCREENING METHODS

Automated instruments are available for the rapid detection of bacteriuria, the presence of significant bacteria in the urine. The Bac-T-Screen (bioMérieux) method is based on the principle of colorimetric filtration. Bacteria and white blood cells are trapped on a filter, and safranin O stain is used to dye the trapped cells. One milliliter of urine is added to a filter in one well of the instrument. The instrument automatically adds acetic acid and dye. The acetic acid functions as both a diluent and a decolorizer, removing unbound dye. The filter card is removed and placed in the spectrophotometric reader. Results are compared against a negative control and are available in 1 to 2 minutes.

The Coral UTI Screen System (Coral Biotechnology) uses the principle of bioluminescence, the enzymatic reaction of adenosine triphosphate (ATP) with luciferin and luciferase. Bacterial ATP is measured after the removal of somatic ATP. Somatic releasing agent and 25 ml of urine are added to a test tube, which incubates at room temperature for 15 to 45 minutes. After the addition of reagents, the tube is read for bioluminescence, using a luminometer.

The IRIS 939 UDx System (International Remote Imaging System, Inc.) consists of a flow microscope and a view station (video camera) with a computer and monitor. Urine specimens are placed on the carousel, the specimens are mixed, and 3 ml of the urine is analyzed. The specimen is strained and moves to the flow microscope. A laminar flow system produces a wide planar stream for the focal plane of the microscope. The particles in the urine are differentiated in the flow by a high-resolution monitor. Asymmetric particles align with the narrowest cross section perpendicular to the flow of sheath fluid, which differentiates particles in the stream. The flow cell is aligned in the focal plane of the attached microscope. Light is provided by a strobe, and a video camera attached to the microscope is synchronized to the strobe. The captured photographic images are stored. The software identifies entire elements, which are digitized and then identified by the image analysis program. The specimen is first examined under a low-power (10×) objective, and if no particles are found, analysis is complete on that specimen. If there are particles present, the specimen is examined under a high-power (40×) objective to enable accurate identification.

FIGURE 22-17 depicts an identification scheme of common urinary tract pathogens. The procedure for urine culture is described at the end of the chapter.

Gastrointestinal Tract Specimens and Infections

The gastrointestinal (GI) tract consists of the esophagus, stomach, small and large intestines, and anus. The lining of the GI tract is known as the mucosa; mucosal surfaces differ along the various parts of the GI tract, which affects the types of infections. Normal flora in the small and large intestines also protects other bacteria from colonizing or establishing infection in the area. Although the upper small intestine harbors small numbers of normal flora, including *Streptococcus*, *Lactobacillus*, and yeast, the number of bacteria in the lower small intestine increases exponentially and includes members of the Enterobacteriaceae and *Bacteroides*. The large intestine contains immense numbers of normal flora bacteria, including the anaerobes *Bacteroides*, *Clostridium*, and *Peptostreptococcus* and the aerobes *Escherichia coli* and other members of the Enterobacteriaceae, such as *Proteus*, *Klebsiella*, and *Enterobacter*; enterococci; and streptococci. Interestingly, anaerobes outnumber aerobes by a factor a high as 1,000:1 in the large intestine. When the normal intestinal flora is reduced from antibiotic use or in other conditions, organisms can multiply in larger numbers. This can result in an overgrowth of other microorganisms, such as *Candida* species, staphylococci, *Pseudomonas* species, and members of the Enterobacteriaceae. In pseudomembranous colitis, *Clostridium difficile* multiplies and produces harmful toxins. This condition is found most frequently in hospital-acquired infections when the patient's normal flora has been suppressed by antibiotics.

Diarrheal diseases are important causes of infection and mortality throughout the world. Many of these

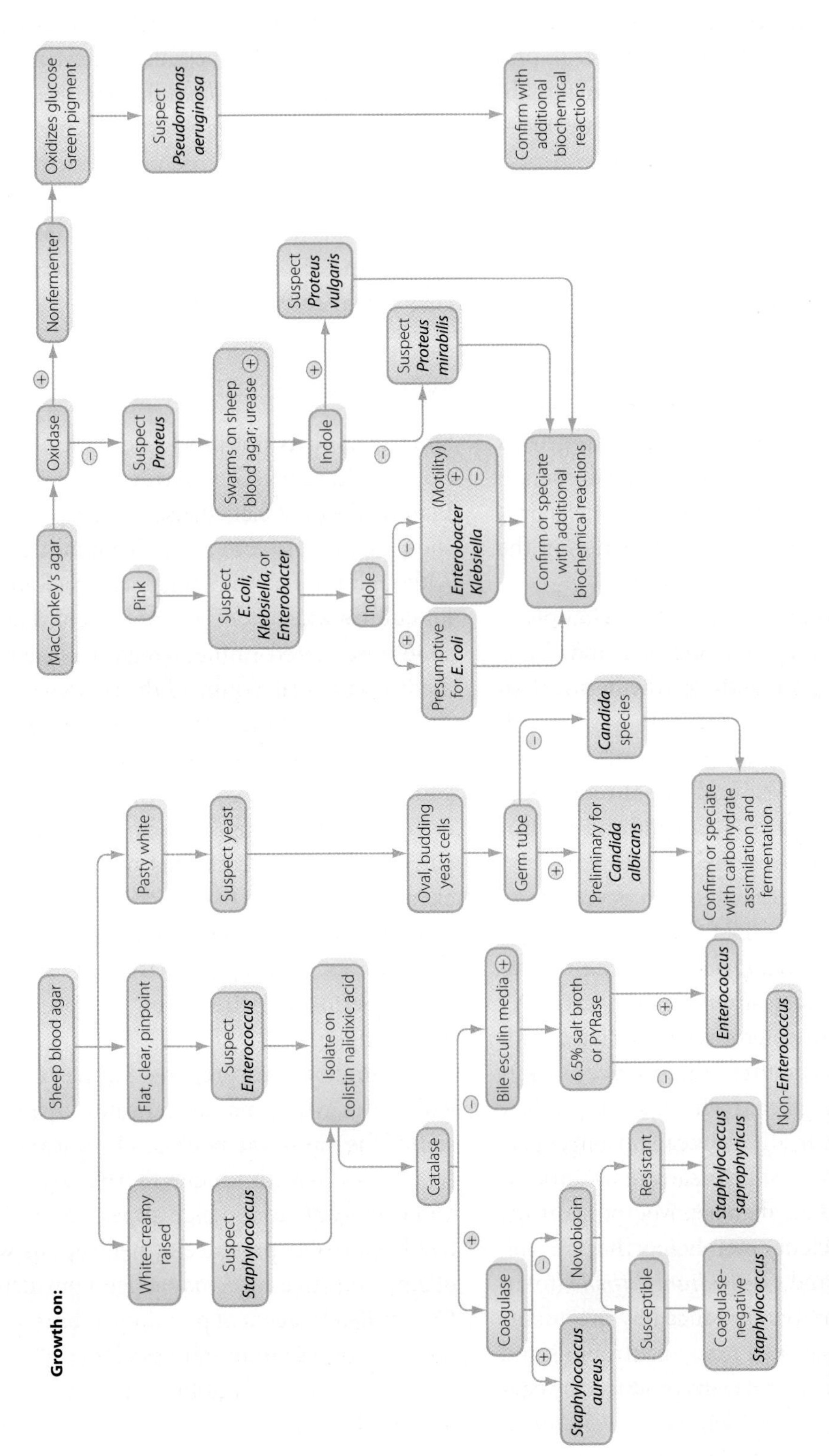

FIGURE 22-17 Identification scheme for common urinary tract pathogens.

diseases are found in developing countries in Africa and Asia. However, there is also significant diarrheal disease in the United States and other developed countries. Many enteric pathogens are acquired through the fecal–oral route and related to the individual's personal hygiene habits. These infections also are acquired through the ingestion of contaminated food and water and person-to-person and animal-to-person transmission. Host immune factors also play a role in the acquisition and severity of gastrointestinal infections.

Mechanisms that protect the GI tract from infection first include the acidic pH of the stomach. Also, peristalsis pushes organisms along the GI tract for removal in the feces. The mucous membranes that line the GI tract contain various protective cells. The Peyer's patches are groups of follicle cells in the small and large intestines that contain macrophages and T and B lymphocytes. These cells produce secretory IgA; phagocytic cells also function in the destruction of microorganisms.

Those microorganisms that can survive the low pH of the stomach, such as *Shigella*, verotoxic *E.coli*, and *C. difficile*, more often are associated with gastroenteritis than are those that are sensitive to the acidic pH.

Microorganisms associated with **gastroenteritis** may cause infections in several ways, including through production of toxins. Enterotoxins produce fluid and electrolyte loss by their action on the epithelial cells. Examples of microorganisms that produce enterotoxins are *Vibrio cholerae*, enterotoxigenic *E. coli* (ETEC), *Salmonella* species, *Staphylococcus aureus*, *Campylobacter jejuni*, *Clostridium perfringens*, and *Clostridium difficile* (toxin A). *Bacillus cereus* produces an enterotoxin associated with diarrhea, as well as an emetic toxin that induces vomiting. Cytotoxins attack the epithelial cells, resulting in their destruction. When this occurs, the cells can no longer perform secretion or absorption, which leads to an inflammatory condition, with tissue damage. Microorganisms that produce cytotoxins include enterohemorrhagic *E. coli* (EHEC), *Shigella* species, and *Clostridium difficile* (toxin B). The inflammatory condition produced by cytotoxins is associated with the presence of many neutrophils and red blood cells in the stool. Neurotoxins produced by bacteria include botulinum toxin of *Clostridium botulinum*; this preformed toxin is ingested and blocks the release of acetylcholine at the cholinergic nerve junctions, resulting in paralysis.

Other microorganisms initiate infection through attachment to or colonization of the gastrointestinal tract. Enteropathogenic *E. coli* attaches and adheres to the intestinal epithelium in the small intestine and colon. The parasite *Giardia lamblia* adheres to the small bowel epithelial cells through its ventral sucking disk. *Giardia* is an important cause of gastroenteritis and is acquired through contact with contaminated water. *Cryptosporidium* and *Isospora* species are parasites associated with diarrheal disease and also are able to adhere to intestinal epithelial cells and affect their function.

SPECIMEN COLLECTION AND PROCESSING

Stool specimens not processed within 2 hours of collection should be placed into transport media, such as Cary-Blair medium. When viruses are suspected, the specimen should be placed into a suitable viral transport medium. Although not recommended, rectal swabs are acceptable for culture when stools cannot be collected. Rectal swabs should be plated immediately or placed into transport media to prevent drying of the specimen.

Stools can be examined directly by emulsifying in broth, saline, or water for the presence of *Campylobacter*, which exhibits a typical darting motility. A suspension is made on a microscope slide and a coverslip applied. Viral pathogens, such as rotavirus and Norwalk agent, must be examined using electron microscopy. Because such methods are beyond the scope of many clinical microbiology laboratories, latex agglutination or ELISA for rotavirus can be performed directly on the specimen to detect the viral antigens.

Gram stains are prepared for the examination of fecal leukocytes, which may be indicators of infection and invasion of the intestinal mucosa. The smear can be examined for pathogens with unique morphologies, such as *Vibrio* and *Campylobacter*, which appear as curved gram-negative bacilli. The presence of neutrophils with aggregates of gram-positive cocci may suggest purulent enterocolitis. *C. difficile*, the agent of pseudomembranous colitis, can be observed in the Gram stain as a large, gram-positive bacillus. After prolonged antibiotic therapy, *C. difficile* appears in the stool, where the organism multiplies to large numbers. The organism produces a cytotoxin, which also can be detected in the stool. The predominance of yeast also can be detected through the Gram stain. **FIGURE 22-18**

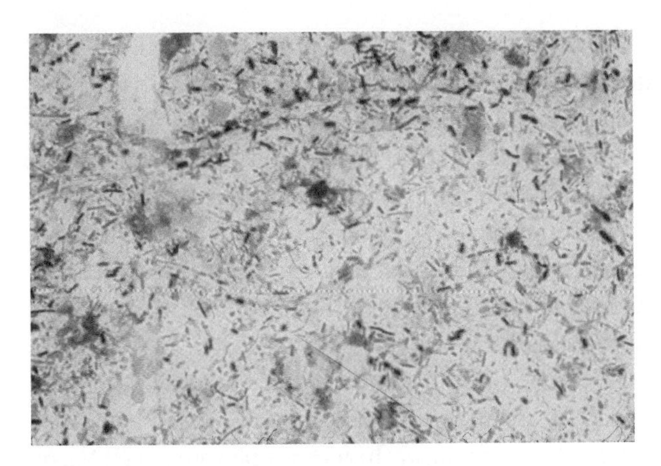

FIGURE 22-18 Gram stain of normal stool.

shows the Gram stain of a normal stool that shows the variety of bacteria that are normally present.

Most laboratories routinely screen stool samples for *Salmonella*, *Shigella*, and *Campylobacter.* Screening for verotoxic *E. coli* on sorbitol MacConkey agar is included by some laboratories but may be based on the incidence of the infection in other laboratories. On request or when epidemiological information suggests, screening also is done for *Yersinia enterocolitica*, *Vibrio cholerae*, *Vibrio parahaemolyticus*, and verotoxic *E. coli*. For example, in eastern and southeastern U.S. coastal areas, agar for the detection of *Vibrio*, which is an occupational hazard for fishermen and a contaminant of shellfish, might be recommended.

When evaluating the primary culture characteristics from a stool specimen, it is important to note the absence of normal flora coliforms. This may be a significant finding, especially if there are large amounts of other microorganisms, such as nonlactose fermenters, yeast, *Pseudomonas aeruginosa*, or *Staphylococcus aureus*.

Viruses associated with gastroenteritis include rotavirus and Norwalk virus. During epidemics, especially in infants, screening to detect rotavirus antigen is recommended.

The diagnosis of the type of lower intestinal tract infections is greatly facilitated by knowledge of the patient's medical history, of epidemiological considerations, and of any travel to foreign countries. Information about the individual's meals and whether a similar infection occurred in family members also is helpful in determining the source and type of infection. The method for the examination of stool cultures is described at the end of the chapter.

FIGURE 22-19 presents an identification scheme for common lower intestinal tract pathogens.

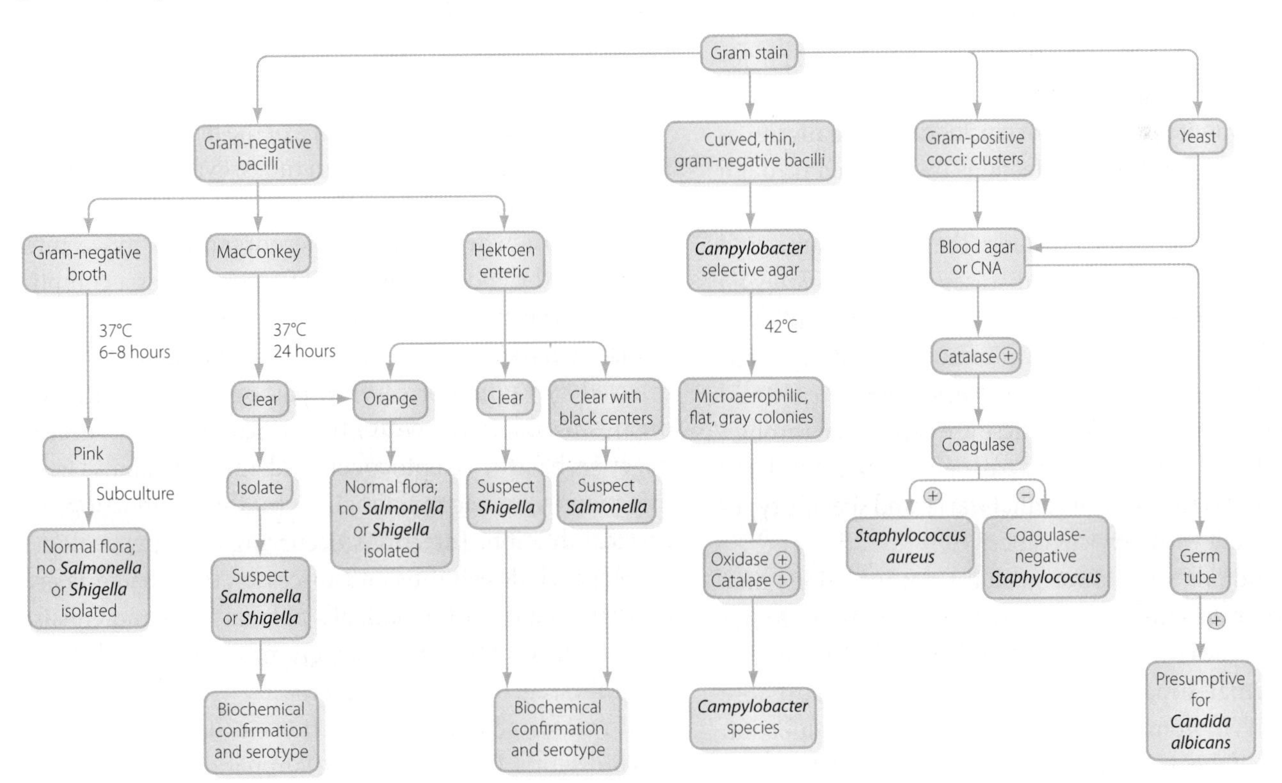

FIGURE 22-19 Identification scheme for common pathogens of the lower gastrointestinal tract.

Genital Tract Specimens and Infections

Genital tract specimens are cultured to determine the causative agents of urethritis, vaginitis, and cervicitis, as well as childbirth infections. Most often, genital tract specimens are collected to determine the presence of *Neisseria gonorrhoeae*, the agent of gonorrhea, and *Chlamydia trachomatis*, a common cause of cervicitis.

The mucosal surfaces of the female genital tract are normally colonized with several species of bacteria, which are usually considered to be normal flora and may even protect the host from the establishment of infection from pathogens. The normal flora of the female genital tract varies with age, hormonal levels, and pH. In adult females an acidic environment exists, and the normal flora includes Enterobacteriaceae, streptococci, staphylococci, *Peptococcus*, *Peptostreptococcus*, and anaerobic non-spore–forming bacilli, in addition to lactobacilli, which predominate. Yeasts, especially *Candida albicans*, often are isolated from the normal female genital tract. Group B streptococci also may be present as normal vaginal flora but may cause infections in the neonate during delivery. The normal flora in the penis includes small numbers of yeasts, corynebacteria, and coagulase-negative staphylococci. The normal flora of the urethra includes coagulase-negative staphylococci, corynebacteria, and some anaerobes.

Infections of the genital tract include the sexually transmitted diseases and other infections transmitted through other routes. In females, these infections are found in the lower genital tract, which includes the vulva, vagina, and cervix. Sexually transmitted diseases include *Chlamydia trachomatis*, *Neisseria gonorrhoeae*, *Treponema pallidum*, *Trichomonas vaginalis*, human immunodeficiency virus (HIV), *Mycoplasma hominis*, *Ureaplasma urealyticum*, and herpes simplex virus (HSV). These are contracted through sexual activity with an infected partner. Human papilloma virus (HPV) is the cause of genital warts, and specific types are associated with cervical cancer.

Individuals with lower genital tract infections may have few or no symptoms or may be symptomatic. Males with gonorrhea or chlamydia usually have a urethral discharge; females may or may not have symptoms. Those who are asymptomatic may serve as a source of infection for others; if these infections are not treated, they can result in pelvic inflammatory disease or infertility in the female.

Urethritis caused by *N. gonorrhoeae* is known as gonococcal urethritis. Nongonococcal urethritis may be caused by *C. trachomatis*, *Mycoplasma hominis*, *M. genitalium*, *Ureaplasma urealyticum*, and *Trichomonas vaginalis*. Males with urethritis have symptoms of urethral discharge and burning urination. Symptoms in females include a purulent vaginal discharge, burning urination, and lower abdominal pain, although some infections are asymptomatic.

Cervicitis (the inflammation of the cervix), usually a sexually transmitted disease, may be caused by *C. trachomatis*, *N. gonorrhoeae*, herpes simplex virus (HSV), or the parasite *Trichomonas vaginalis*. Cervicitis is characterized by a purulent discharge, which contains many polymorphonuclear neutrophils in cases of the endocervix. In females, *N. gonorrhoeae* most frequently is isolated from the endocervix. Often, individuals may be infected with both *N. gonorrhoeae* and *C. trachomatis*.

Vaginitis is the inflammation of the vaginal mucosa and includes vaginal candidiasis, trichomoniasis, and bacterial vaginosis. *Candida albicans* is the cause of most cases of vaginal candidiasis. Trichomoniasis is caused by the parasite *Trichomonas vaginalis*. Bacterial vaginosis is a polymicrobic condition associated with the overgrowth by *Gardnerella vaginalis* and the presence of various aerobes and anaerobes. There is also a decrease in the normal flora bacteria lactobacilli.

Organs involved in infections of the female upper genital tract are the uterus, fallopian tubes, ovaries, and sometimes the abdominal cavity. Pelvic inflammatory disease (PID) occurs when cervical microorganisms move into and infect the endometrium. PID may occur as a complication of infection caused by *N. gonorrhoeae* or *C. trachomatis* when the endometrium or fallopian tubes have been infected by vaginal or cervical pathogens. Other microorganisms associated with PID include anaerobes, gram-negative bacilli, streptococci, and mycoplasma. These infections may occur following childbirth, abortion, or cervical dilation. Infections occurring after gynecologic surgery include cellulitis and abscesses; these bacteria are generally a part of the patient's normal flora and consist of staphylococci; streptococci; gram-negative bacilli; and anaerobes, such as *Peptostreptococcus*.

In males, genital tract infections include epididymitis and prostatitis. Epididymitis, inflammation of the epididymis, is associated with fever, pain, and swelling. Prostatitis may result from invasion of sexually transmitted pathogens or those transmitted through the urinary tract. Most often implicated in these infections are members of the Enterobacteriaceae, *N. gonorrhoeae*, *C. trachomatis*, and *Pseudomonas aeruginosa*.

Infections of the external genitalia, characterized by the presence of lesions or chancres, include syphilis (*Treponema pallidum*), chancroid (*Haemophilus ducreyi*), and herpes genitalis (HSV type 2). Genital or venereal warts caused by papillomavirus are also an important sexually transmitted disease (STD).

SPECIMEN COLLECTION FOR UROGENITAL INFECTIONS

Specimens collected from females with suspected genital infections most frequently are from the uterine cervix and urethra. Urethral specimens are obtained by inserting a urogenital swab into the urethra and gently rotating and allowing it to remain for a few seconds to saturate the swab with exudate. Urogenital swabs that are cotton or rayon must contain charcoal to absorb fatty acids and other compounds that are toxic to gonococci. It is important that the specimen contain epithelial cells when testing for chlamydia.

To collect cervical specimens, cervical mucus is cleared with a swab, and then the sample is collected using a smaller swab with a Dacron or polyester tip. The endocervix is revealed and the specimen collected with the aid of a speculum. The swab is rotated to collect cervical cells and exudate and is positioned to avoid touching the vaginal canal. Endometrial specimens or aspirates from laparoscopy or culdoscopy are collected to diagnose PID.

For male patients the urethral exudate is usually collected. When there is insufficient material to collect, a narrow cotton, rayon, or Dacron swab on a plastic or aluminum shaft can be inserted into the urethra. The swab is left in place for a few seconds to saturate the fibers. For *Chlamydia* the swab is rotated in a circular motion to collect some epithelial cells because *C. trachomatis* is an intracellular pathogen.

Because *N. gonorrhoeae* is very susceptible to temperature fluctuations, such as cooling, and does not sustain drying or low levels of CO_2 very well, it is imperative to smear, plate, and transport the specimen quickly. Direct smears for gonorrhea should be made immediately after collection. If immediate inoculation is not possible, the specimen must be placed into transport media and sent to the laboratory. The use of charcoal in transport systems neutralizes toxic materials in the specimen or on the swab. Agar plate transport systems, such as the JEMBEC™ (Becton Dickinson), provide a medium selective for *Neisseria gonorrhoeae* as well as a disposable, plastic zippered bag with a CO_2 activator. The JEMBEC™ plate is inoculated by rolling the swab across the agar so that all parts of the swab contact the surface of the agar. Next, the inoculum is spread out in a "W" pattern. Upon receipt in the laboratory, the plate is cross-streaked and incubated at 35°C ± 2°C in 5% CO_2.

DIRECT EXAMINATION

The Gram stain for gonorrhea is prepared by rolling the swab over the microscope slide. The Gram stain from male patients has a high degree of sensitivity for the diagnosis of gonorrhea. The presence and estimation of the amount of gram-negative diplococci occurring intracellularly or extracellularly to an estimation of the amount of segmented neutrophils are noted. However, because of normal flora of the female genital tract, including coccobacilli such as *Acinetobacter* and *Moraxella* and the anaerobic gram-negative coccus *Veillonella*, the Gram stain is less reliable. **FIGURE 22-20** illustrates a Gram stain showing the presence of many gram-negative diplococci occurring intracellularly and extracellularly to segmented neutrophils.

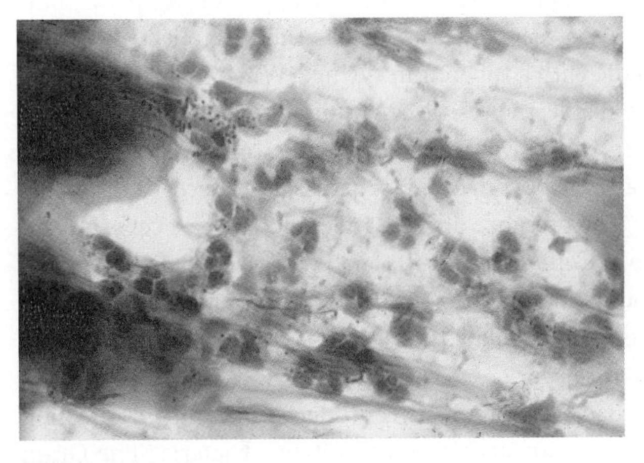

FIGURE 22-20 Gram stain showing the presence of many gram-negative diplococci occurring intracellularly and extracellularly to segmented neutrophils.

The Gram stain must always be confirmed by culture, antigen testing or molecular testing. Specimens are plated onto a medium selective for *N. gonorrhoeae* and onto chocolate agar. To inoculate these plates, use the same method as described for the JEMBEC™ plate. The plates are incubated at 35°C ± 2°C for 24 hours, examined for growth, and incubated for another 24 hours. *Neisseria* species are oxidase and catalase positive. Confirmation is made through carbohydrate utilization of only glucose using cystine trypticase agar (CTA) sugars or a commercially available method.

The antigen of *N. gonorrhoeae* may be detected directly in the specimen through ELISA. Culture is used to confirm the presence of the organism.

C. trachomatis is the agent of lymphogranuloma venereum (LGV), a rare cause of genital ulcers in North America but a common agent of nongonococcal urethritis, mucopurulent cervicitis, epididymitis, and PID.

Chlamydia specimens preferably are collected using Dacron swabs with plastic or aluminum shafts. Calcium alginate and wooden shafts should be avoided because they may inhibit the replication of the organism. Because chlamydiae are intracellular parasites that live in columnar and cuboidal epithelial cells, collection of epithelial cells greatly enhances the recovery of the organism. The swabs are immediately placed into sucrose-phosphate medium with 5% fetal calf serum or Hank's solution with fetal calf serum. Antimicrobials are added to inhibit other microorganisms. Direct ELISA and fluorescent methods to detect chlamydial antigen are commercially available.

Herpes simplex virus type 2 infections usually appear as vesicular lesions on the vulva, perineum, penis, buttocks, or cervix. The vesicular fluid is collected using a needle with a tuberculin syringe. When insufficient fluid is available, the vesicle can be unroofed and the base of the ulcer firmly swabbed to collect cells. Immediate transfer to viral transport medium is necessary to recover the virus.

The presence of yeast and budding yeast cells, indicative of *Candida vaginitis*, can be observed in direct vaginal mounts or in Gram-stained preparations. *Candida albicans* can be isolated on sheep blood agar or Sabouraud's dextrose agar.

Bacterial vaginosis is produced by a mixed infection involving anaerobic and facultative bacteria. The Gram stain reveals mixed flora, including a heavy amount of *G. vaginalis*, which is observed as pleomorphic, gram-positive to gram-variable, diphtheroid-like bacterium.

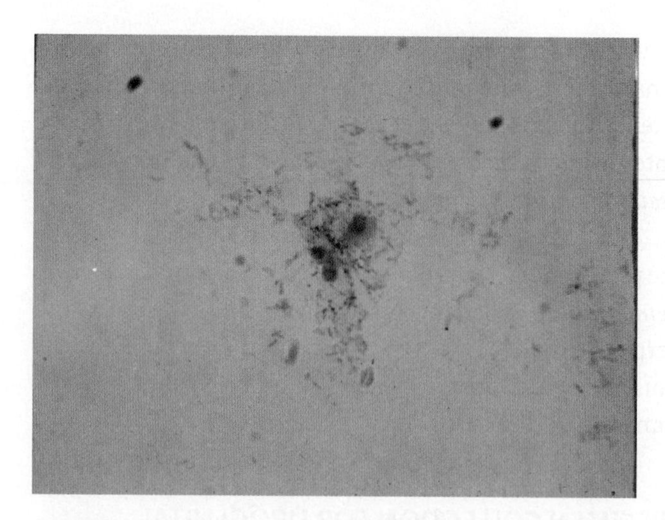

FIGURE 22-21 Gram stain showing clue cells.

Mobiluncus, curved gram-negative or positive bacilli with tapered ends, also may be present. Other organisms that may be present in bacterial vaginosis include *Peptostreptococcus*, *Porphyromonas*, and *Mycoplasma hominis*. The lack of lactobacilli and WBCs also is seen in cases of bacterial vaginosis. The presence of clue cells, which are squamous epithelial cells dotted with *Gardnerella* (**FIGURE 22-21**), also may be present in the Gram stain in cases of bacterial vaginosis. Culture is usually not indicated.

T. pallidum, the agent of syphilis, is detected through darkfield examination of the primary chancre. Nontreponemal serological tests, such as the rapid plasma reagin (RPR) and Venereal Disease Research Laboratories (VDRL), are used to detect reagin in the patient's serum during late primary and secondary syphilis. Because these tests are nonspecific, all positive results are confirmed by performance of a specific treponemal test, such as the fluorescent treponemal antibody (FTA).

H. ducreyi is the agent of soft chancre or chancroid, found most often in the tropics and Africa. Purulent exudate of the lesion is examined in a Gram stain smear for the presence of gram-negative bacilli arranged in parallel chains, known as the "school of fish" arrangement. Identification can be confirmed after culturing on chocolate agar with IsoVitaleX, gonococcal fetal calf serum, or rabbit–horse blood in 2% to 5% CO_2 at 35°C for up to 7 to 14 days. Important reactions include negative catalase, positive oxidase, X factor dependent, and porphyrin negative.

Human papillomavirus is the agent of genital warts, or condyloma acuminatum. *M. hominis* and *Ureaplasma urealyticum* also have been associated with nongonococcal urethritis and PID.

Skin and Wound Specimens and Infections

The skin has three layers: the epidermis, dermis, and subcutaneous tissue. The deepest layer is the subcutaneous tissue, which has fat cells, hair follicles and sweat glands. The middle layer is the dermis, which contains connective tissue, nerves, and blood vessels as well as oil glands and shorter hair follicles. The top layer of the skin is the epidermis and is made up of squamous epithelial cells. The supportive tissue below the subcutaneous tissue, known as fascia, consists of bands of fibrous tissue that cover the muscles and other connective tissue.

The skin constitutes the first protective barrier of the body against microorganisms. Fatty acids prevent drying of the hair and skin and are also antimicrobial. Lysozyme, present in perspiration, also serves as a defense mechanism. However, if the skin is damaged through trauma, wounds, surgery, or burns, then microorganisms in the environment can gain entrance into the body. Ducts of sweat and oil glands, as well as hair follicles, can serve as routes of infection for microorganisms to gain access to the deeper layers of the skin tissue.

Normal flora of the skin includes *Staphylococcus epidermidis* and other coagulase-negative staphylococci, *Micrococcus*, and some *Corynebacterium* species or diphtheroids. The anaerobe *Propionibacterium acnes* grows in hair follicles, aided by the presence of oil secreted from the sebaceous glands. This organism produces large amounts of propionic acid and maintains the pH of the skin between 3 and 5, creating an antimicrobial effect.

Clinical signs of wound infections include the accumulation of pus within the abscess or under the surface of the skin, redness, pain, and swelling. Nonsurgical wound infections often involve damage to the skin, as occurs with traumatic wounds, burns, abrasions, and bites.

Staphylococcus aureus is the most common cause of superficial skin infections, which also may reach the dermis and spread through the blood or lymphatics to other tissues. Folliculitis, an infection of the hair follicle, often is caused by infection from *S. aureus* or *Pseudomonas aeruginosa*.

Boils, furuncles, carbuncles, acne, and bedsores (decubitus ulcers) are frequently attributed to *S. aureus*. These infections can result in deep-seated infections, such as cellulitis, pneumonia, osteomyelitis, meningitis, and peritonitis.

The dermatophytic fungi also can infect the epidermis, causing ringworm (tinea) infection.

Infections of deeper parts of the epidermis and dermis include impetigo, erysipelas, erysipeloid, and cellulitis. **Impetigo**, a superficial and contagious pyoderma frequently found in children, first appears as a flaccid vesicle, which may rupture, and is most often caused by *S. pyogenes*. Secondary infections from *S. aureus* are common complications of impetigo. **Erysipelas**, also caused by infection from *S. pyogenes*, is an inflammatory disease characterized by painful, red, swollen eruptions of the skin. There is fever and lymphadenopathy; erysipelas most often occurs in infants and young children. **Erysipeloid**, caused by *Erysipelothrix rhusiopathiae*, is an uncommon skin infection characterized by a spreading red rash. The infection is occupational in those who work with animals; there is itching, fever, and other systemic effects.

Cellulitis, an infection of the dermis and subcutaneous tissue, is most often attributed to *S. aureus* and *S. pyogenes*. Less frequent causes include *Candida albicans* and *P. aeruginosa*. Anaerobes isolated as agents in cellulitis include *B. fragilis*, *Prevotella*, *Porphyromonas*, *Peptostreptococcus*, and *Clostridium*. Anaerobic infections often are accompanied by the presence of gas in the subcutaneous tissue, which is described as "gas gangrene." Cellulitis of the deeper tissues often involves mixed flora of aerobes and anaerobes, including *E. coli*, streptococci, *S. aureus*, *S. pyogenes*, and other Enterobacteriaceae.

Infections of the subcutaneous tissue include abscesses, ulcers, and boils. *Staphylococcus aureus* is the most common cause of subcutaneous abscesses. These infections often are polymicrobic and also may contain anaerobes or aerobes based on the site of infection.

Necrotizing fasciitis is a rare but extremely severe infection of the fascia, which covers muscle tissues and surrounding soft tissues. These infections spread rapidly, causing devastating destruction of muscle and other tissues. *Streptococcus pyogenes* most often is implicated in necrotizing fasciitis. *Staphylococcus aureus* and anaerobes such as *Bacteroides* species and *Clostridium* species are also causes of necrotizing fasciitis.

Deeper wound infections occur after there is a break in the skin from surgery, traumatic wounds, bites, and other diseases. Pathogens associated with deep wounds, surgical wounds, and abscesses often represent normal flora near the site of infection. For example, infection secondary to surgery or trauma of the bowel is often attributed to the normal flora of the lower gastrointestinal tract, including *Escherichia coli*, *Bacteroides fragilis*, anaerobic gram-negative bacilli, anaerobic gram-positive non-spore–forming bacilli, *Peptostreptococcus*, and *Clostridium*.

Postoperative wound infections are caused by nosocomial pathogens or from the patient's own normal flora. These may result following a medical procedure, which may cause a break in the skin or mucous membranes. Aerobic bacteria associated with postoperative wound infections include *S. aureus*, coagulase-negative staphylococci, enterococci, *E. coli*, *Proteus* species, *Pseudomonas aeruginosa*, *Enterobacter* species, *Klebsiella* species, and viridans streptococci. Anaerobic bacteria associated with postoperative wound infections include *Bacteroides* species, *Prevotella* and *Porphyromonas* species, *Fusobacterium* species, *Clostridium* species, *Peptostreptococcus* species, and non-spore–forming gram-positive bacilli.

Human bite infections reflect the normal flora of the oral cavity. Microorganisms that cause human bite infections are *Streptococcus anginosis*, α-hemolytic streptococci, *Staphylococcus aureus*, *Eikenella corrodens*, and *Streptococcus pyogenes*. Anaerobes associated with human bite infections include *Prevotella* species, *Fusobacterium* species, *Veillonella* species, and *Peptostreptococcus* species.

Bites from cats and dogs may result in infection from *Pasteurella* species, *Staphylococcus intermedius*, *S. aureus*, *Enterobacter cloacae*, anaerobic gram-positive cocci, *Fusobacterium* species, *Bacteroides* species, *Porphyromonas* species, and *Prevotella* species.

Patients with circulatory problems, such as diabetic persons and those with poor arterial circulation, peripheral vascular disease, and peripheral neuropathy, are especially susceptible to skin ulcers and cellulitis. Bacteria frequently attributed to such infections include *S. aureus*, *S. pyogenes*, *E. coli*, and other members of the Enterobacteriaceae and *P. aeruginosa*. Anaerobes also often are isolated from sites that are necrotic and poorly oxygenated; these organisms include *B. fragilis*, *Prevotella*, *Porphyromonas*, *Clostridium*, and *Peptostreptococcus*.

Decubitus ulcers, bedsores, and pressure sores often are infected with normal bowel flora. Common infectious agents include *E. coli* and other enteric bacilli, *B. fragilis*, *Clostridium*, *Enterococcus*, *P. aeruginosa*, and *S. aureus*.

Burn infections carry a high mortality and often result in secondary bacteremia. Hospitalized patients may be colonized with gram-negative bacilli, which often are resistant to several antibiotics. Microorganisms isolated from burn sites include *Streptococcus*, *S. epidermidis*, *P. aeruginosa*, *C. albicans*, and members of the Enterobacteriaceae. Antibiotic-resistant strains of these bacteria, such as methicillin-resistant *Staphylococcus aureus* (MRSA), are frequently observed as nosocomial burn pathogens.

SPECIMEN COLLECTION FOR WOUND AND SKIN INFECTIONS

Superficial wounds often contain many normal flora bacteria, which can obscure the isolation of the true pathogen. For this reason it is recommended that, whenever possible, the specimen be collected with a needle and syringe. Wound infections are frequently polymicrobic, with a mix of aerobic and anaerobic bacteria.

The Gram stain is very important in the initial identification of wound pathogens. For example, if a superficial wound reveals possible anaerobes, an anaerobic blood plate can be added to the initial isolation media. Wound and skin specimens are plated onto sheep blood agar, CNA, and MacConkey agar to isolate aerobes. When anaerobes are suspected, anaerobic blood agar, KV, and PEA are added. Sabouraud dextrose agar is added for dermatophytes. **TABLE 22-2** summarizes the identification of common anaerobic pathogens found in wounds and abscesses.

FIGURE 22-22 is a Gram stain of a wound showing gram-positive cocci that were identified as *S. aureus*. **FIGURE 22-23** is a Gram stain of an anaerobic gram-negative bacillus that was isolated from a peritoneal abscess and identified as *B. fragilis*.

Pleural, Peritoneal, Pericardial, and Synovial Fluids

Body fluids that are normally sterile are blood and cerebrospinal fluid, as discussed earlier, and pleural, peritoneal, pericardial, and synovial fluids. The accumulation of fluid in a cavity is known as an **effusion**. Effusions that have a low specific gravity and low levels of protein and cells are termed **transudates**. Effusions that have a high specific gravity, have high levels of protein, and contain many cells are known as **exudates**. Transudates usually

TABLE 22-2 Characteristics of Anaerobes Isolated from Wounds and Abscesses

Organism	Important characteristics
Bacteroides fragilis group	Gram-negative bacillus; grows on AB, PEA, and KV; enhanced growth in 20% bile; esculin hydrolysis positive; no pigment produced
Prevotella melaninogenica	Gram-negative bacillus; grows on AB, PEA, and KV; inhibited by 20% bile; lactose fermented; esculin hydrolysis negative; brick-red fluorescence under ultraviolet light; older colonies brown to black
Fusobacterium nucleatum	Gram-negative bacillus with tapered ends; opalescent colonial morphology when viewed microscopically; grows on AB and PEA; may or may not grow on KV; indole positive but basically biochemically inactive; lipase negative; glucose not fermented
Fusobacterium necrophorum	Gram-negative bacillus with tapered ends; grows on AB and PEA; may or may not grow on KV; indole positive; lipase positive; glucose fermented
Clostridium tetani	Gram-positive bacillus with round, terminal spores; rarely cultured from living wounds; diagnosis usually through clinical signs; unable to ferment most carbohydrates
Clostridium perfringens	Gram-positive bacillus; spores usually not observed; grows on AB and PEA; double-zone hemolysis on AB; lecithinase positive, ferments glucose, lactose, maltose, and fructose; reverse CAMP reaction positive
Clostridium ramosum	Gram-positive bacillus but usually stains gram negative; grows on AB and PEA; grows well on 20% bile; esculin hydrolysis positive; lecithinase negative; lipase negative; very fermentative

AB, anaerobic blood agar; PEA, phenylethyl alcohol agar; KV, kanamycin-vancomycin agar

occur as a result of hepatic or renal disease and hemodynamic changes that lead to the accumulation of fluid in the cavity. Exudates may result from infection by bacteria and other microorganisms, as well as from malignancy, trauma, toxic compounds, and other sources of inflammation in the cavity itself.

These fluids are collected through percutaneous needle aspiration after a thorough disinfection of the skin. In some cases, multiple tubes are filled for analysis. Normal body fluids are clear and slightly yellow in color. A turbid or cloudy fluid often indicates inflammation. On receipt of the fluid in the laboratory, the color, transparency, and volume are recorded. Because the yield of microorganisms from body fluids may be low, often a large volume of specimen is needed to isolate the pathogen. For fluids that are visually purulent, a Gram stain is performed directly from the specimen. When the fluid is clear or if the volume is greater than 1 ml, the fluid should be centrifuged at 2,500 rpm for 15 minutes. The sediment is resuspended in approximately 0.5 ml of supernatant,

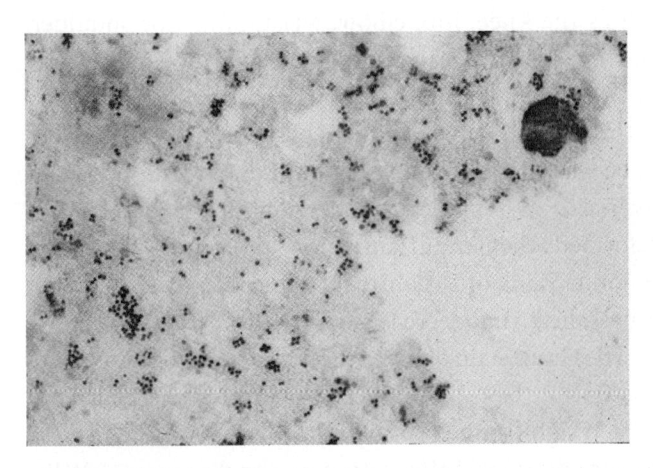

FIGURE 22-22 Gram stain of a wound showing gram-positive cocci that were identified as *S. aureus*.

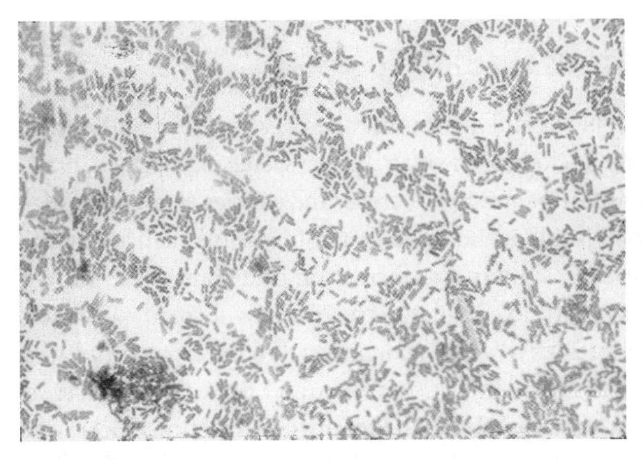

FIGURE 22-23 Gram stain of an anaerobic gram-negative bacillus that was isolated from a peritoneal abscess and identified as *B. fragilis*.

which is used to prepare the smear for the Gram stain and for culture.

Sterile fluids are routinely tested for protein and glucose values. In inflammatory states the protein is increased to more than 50% of the serum level, and the glucose level is decreased. Cell counts and differential WBC counts also are helpful in the diagnosis. Effusions with predominance of segmented neutrophils often reflect a bacterial infection, whereas those with a predominance of lymphocytes often indicate a viral infection.

PLEURAL FLUID

Pleural fluid lines the pleural space, which is between the lungs and chest cavity; normally, few cells are present. **Thoracentesis** is the collection of pleural fluid. Infections usually create an exudate. Pleural effusions may occur secondarily as a result of pneumonia; bacteria typically isolated as the pathogen include *Streptococcus pneumoniae*, *Staphylococcus aureus*, *Haemophilus influenzae*, *Pseudomonas aeruginosa*, various members of the Enterobacteriaceae, and several anaerobes. When associated with aspiration pneumonia, frequently there is a polymicrobic infection of aerobes and anaerobes.

Specimens are routinely plated on 5% sheep blood agar (SBA), MacConkey agar (MAC), anaerobic blood agar (AB), kanamycin-vancomycin blood agar (KV), and phenylethyl alcohol agar (PEA), as well as into thioglycollate broth. If yeast or a dimorphic fungus, such as *Coccidioides immitis*, is suspected, a KOH preparation and inoculation onto brain-heart infusion agar (BHI) also should be done. In cases of suspected tuberculosis, an acid-fast smear is performed, and Löwenstein-Jensen and Middlebrook media are inoculated.

PERITONEAL FLUID

Peritoneal fluid surrounds the organs of the abdominal cavity, including the liver, kidneys, spleen, stomach, bladder, intestinal tract, pancreas, and ovaries. The accumulation of fluid secondary to systemic disease, such as hepatic disease, results in the formation of a transudate known as ascitic fluid. Exudates are generally formed as a result of infectious disease, which may develop from surgery or trauma to the bowel or abdominal cavity, liver abscess, ruptured appendix, malignancy, obstruction, ulcerative colitis, or peritoneal or bowel abscess. The agents of **peritonitis** generally include *Escherichia coli*, *Bacteroides fragilis*, *S. aureus*, *Streptococcus*, *Enterococcus*, and other members of the Enterobacteriaceae. Because the normal bowel flora includes a high number of anaerobes, it is essential to collect and maintain the specimen free of oxygen. The collection of peritoneal fluid is known as a **paracentesis**. Peritoneal fluids are routinely plated on 5% SBA, chocolate agar, MAC, AB, KV, and PEA, as well as into thioglycollate broth.

PERICARDIAL FLUID

Pericardial fluid fills the pericardial space, which is contained in the pericardium, the protective sac of the heart. The fluid is normally clear with a volume of 10 ml to 20 ml. The volume of fluid may accumulate because of hemodynamic changes, such as those caused by congestive heart failure or by systemic edema from hepatic or renal failure. Inflammation resulting from infection also leads to a pericardial effusion. Viruses are the most common infecting organisms of the pericardium, including coxsackie viruses A and B, echovirus, and influenza viruses. Bacteria are less frequently associated with pericarditis and include *S. aureus*, *S. pneumoniae*, members of the Enterobacteriaceae, *Mycobacterium tuberculosis*, various anaerobes, and *Nocardia* species.

Pericardial fluid is plated on the primary media SBA, MAC, AB, KV, and PEA, as well as into thioglycollate broth.

SYNOVIAL FLUID

Synovial, or joint, fluid is secreted by the synovial cells, which line the joints, and functions to lubricate the joint space. Infections typically involve one of the large joints, such as the knee, hip, elbow, wrist, ankle, or shoulder. Infections usually reach the joints from the blood. However, secondary infections from noninfectious arthritis also may occur. Rapid diagnosis of septic arthritis is essential because destruction of the joint may occur quite rapidly. **Arthrocentesis**, the collection of synovial fluid, is performed when an inflammatory response is present in the joint. Signs of inflammation include swelling, pain, redness, heat, and decreased mobility.

The Gram stain of the specimen is examined for bacteria and white blood cells, such as neutrophils. A cell count and a Wright-stained differential white blood cell smear provide additional information for the diagnosis. A WBC count of fewer than 200 cells/μl is considered normal, and counts less than 2,000/μl are considered noninflammatory. WBC counts greater than 2,000/μl are categorized as inflammatory and generally associated with the infection septic arthritis. A predominance of segmented neutrophils suggests a bacterial infection.

The most common cause of septic arthritis is *S. aureus*, which accounts for more than half of all cases. Other gram-positive cocci, including *S. pneumoniae* and β-hemolytic streptococcus, as well as Enterobacteriaceae, *Neisseria gonorrhoeae*, and the anaerobes *Fusobacterium* and *Bacteroides*, also are associated with septic arthritis.

Infections of prosthetic joints occur rarely, but the agents vary from those associated with other joint infections. The most common pathogens are coagulase-negative *Staphylococcus* and anaerobic bacilli, such as *Propionibacterium*. As normal skin flora, these organisms may be introduced during surgery.

Synovial fluid is routinely inoculated onto chocolate agar, AB, KV, and PEA and into thioglycollate broth. SBA also may be added.

Laboratory Procedures

Procedure

Blood culture and collection of blood specimen

Materials

70% alcohol swab
Povidone iodine or 2% tincture of iodine
Gloves
Vacuum tube containing SPS or blood culture bottles (one aerobic and one anaerobic)
Appropriate needle, syringe, or vacuum tube holder to perform phlebotomy and a tourniquet

Procedure

1. Observe standard precautions at all times during the procedure. Do not change needles at any time during the procedure.
2. Inspect both arms of the patient to select an appropriate vein.
3. Cleanse the patient's skin over the venipuncture site by wiping with 70% alcohol in a circular motion from the site outward. Allow the alcohol to air-dry.
4. Using 2% tincture of iodine or povidone iodine, vigorously wipe the site in a circular motion from the site outward. Allow the iodine to air-dry on the skin for at least 1 minute.
5. Optional: Cleanse the area again, this time with 70% alcohol in the method described. Alternatively, this can be done after the needle has been removed on completion of the phlebotomy.
6. Disinfect the stopper of the collection bottle(s) or tube(s), using povidone iodine or tincture of iodine.
7. Apply the tourniquet and have the patient make a fist. If the site must be probed again, disinfect the tips of the glove's fingers, using the procedure described to prepare the site.
8. Insert the needle and collect the blood. Depending on the system being used, collect one SPS vacuum tube or aerobic and anaerobic culture bottles.
9. Release the tourniquet, remove the needle, and apply pressure to the site.
10. Gently invert the tube(s) or bottle(s) to ensure anticoagulation. Label completely with patient's name, date and time of collection, and specific site of collection (such as right forearm). Apply a bandage to the site.
11. Immediately transport blood culture(s) to microbiology laboratory.

Procedure

Specimen analysis

Materials

Gram stain reagents
Clean microscope slides
35°C to 37°C incubator
Chocolate agar
CO_2 incubator or candle jar

Procedure

1. Inoculate the blood culture medium if this was not done during the venipuncture.
2. Incubate the aerobic and anaerobic bottles at 35°C to 37°C. Vent one bottle of the set by carefully inserting a sterile cotton-plugged needle into the rubber septum of the bottle to release the vacuum if separate aerobic and anaerobic bottles were not used. The vented bottle is the aerobic bottle.
3. Visually examine each bottle daily, including the day of collection, for signs of growth. These include turbidity, production of gas, hemolysis of RBCs, or bacterial colonies forming on the RBC surface. Record

results under "Daily Observations"; list any indications of growth or indicate "no change."

4. Perform a Gram stain on all suspected positive cultures. Also, routinely perform a Gram stain on each bottle at 6 to 17 hours of incubation. Record results under "Gram stain."
5. The aerobic bottle should be blind subcultured daily. The first blind subculture should be performed 6 to 17 hours after collection. Plate a chocolate agar for each subculture and incubate at 35°C to 37°C in increased CO_2 or in the candle jar. Record results under "Subculture."
6. Re-incubate bottles after each daily subculture. Inspect the chocolate agar plates for any signs of growth.
7. It is not necessary to perform blind subcultures on the anaerobic bottle. Inspect each anaerobic bottle daily for signs of bacterial growth. Perform a Gram stain on any suspected positive and subculture any suspected positive to anaerobic blood agar. Incubate in an anaerobic jar and examine daily for 7 days.
8. Identify any organisms by performing the appropriate biochemical procedures.
9. Perform the appropriate antibiotic susceptibility panel using the Kirby-Bauer disk diffusion method.
10. Record all results on the worksheets provided.

Blood Culture Results

Specimen identification: ______

Date and time of collection: ______

Site of collection: ______

Collected by: ______

Media inoculated: ______

Aerobic: ______

Anaerobic: ______

Aerobic Results

Daily

Day	Date	Observations	Gram stain subculture
1			
2			
3			
4			
5			
6			
7			

Identification of Aerobe

Media	Colony type		Possible organisms	Additional testing
	Description and number	Gram stain		
Sheep blood				
Chocolate				
MacConkey				
Other				

Isolate	Tests performed	Observations	Interpretation

Identification: ______

Rationale: ______

______

Anaerobic Results

Record any sign of growth in the anaerobic bottle:

______

Date: ______

Observations: ______

List any media inoculated to identify the anaerobe. Describe your observations and interpret your results.

Media	Colony type		Possible organisms	Additional testing
	Description and number	Gram stain		
Anaerobic blood				
Thioglycollate				
KV				
PEA				

Isolate	Tests performed	Observations	Interpretation

Identification: ______

Rationale: ______

______

Antibiotic Susceptibility Testing

Isolate: ______________________________

Antibiotic concentration/code	Zone diameter	Interpretation (S, I, R)

Questions

1. Explain why the skin preparations for blood cultures differ from those for routine phlebotomy.

   ____

   ____

2. Compare the results obtained on the Gram stain with those obtained on the plated media. What conclusions can be made?

   ____

   ____

3. Are the organisms isolated considered to be contaminants or pathogens? Justify your response.

   ____

   ____

4. Why is it necessary to vent one bottle of the culture set when separate aerobic and anaerobic bottles are not used?

   ____

   ____

Procedure

Cerebrospinal fluid culture

Materials

5% sheep blood agar
Chocolate agar
Thioglycollate broth
MacConkey agar
Gram stain reagents
Centrifuge
Autoclaved slides or slides dipped in alcohol and then flamed
Sterile Pasteur pipette or vortex

Procedure

1. On receipt of the CSF, examine the specimen for volume, color, and transparency.
2. Centrifuge CSF tube 3 (if multiple tubes are collected). The specimen should be spun for 15 minutes at 1,500 to 2,000 g to concentrate the specimen if the volume is greater than 0.5 ml.
3. Decant the supernatant, leaving approximately 0.5 ml over the precipitate. The supernatant can be reserved for further testing.
4. Thoroughly mix the sediment either using a vortex or aspirating with a sterile Pasteur pipette.
5. Aspirate a large drop of the well-mixed CSF onto a sterile microscope slide. The slides are cleaned either by dipping into alcohol and flaming or by autoclaving. Do not flatten the drop or apply a coverslip. Allow the drop to air-dry. Then heat fix or fix with methanol.
6. Perform the Gram stain on the smear.
7. Examine the smear for the presence of bacteria, fungi, WBCs (neutrophils, lymphocytes), and RBCs. Record your observations.
8. Label all plates to be inoculated accurately and completely. Using the well-mixed or vortexed sediment, inoculate a sheep blood agar plate and a chocolate agar plate by pipetting several drops of the specimen onto the agar surfaces. Streak each plate for isolation. Incubate at 35°C ± 2°C under increased CO_2 for 72 hours. Examine plates daily for growth.
   a. Inoculate the thioglycollate broth with several drops of the sediment and incubate with a loosened cap for 5 days at 35°C ± 2°C.
   b. If gram-negative bacilli are seen in the Gram stain, also inoculate a MacConkey agar plate and incubate in atmospheric oxygen at 35°C ± 2°C.
   c. If the Gram stain suggests anaerobes, inoculate an anaerobic blood agar plate and incubate in either an anaerobic jar or bag.
9. Examine all plates and broth daily for growth. Perform a Gram stain on any growth.
10. Perform appropriate identification procedures on each colony type.
11. Perform the appropriate antibiotic susceptibility panel using the disk diffusion method on all pathogens.
12. Report any positive findings immediately to the physician.

CSF Culture Results

Specimen identification: ______________________

Number of tubes submitted: ______________________

Total volume of CSF: ______________________

Appearance:

Color: __________ Transparency: __________

Note any differences in appearance in tubes 1, 2, and 3:

____

Gram stain results: ______________________

____

Growth Characteristics

Media	Colony type		Possible organisms	Additional testing
	Description and number	Gram stain		
Sheep blood				
Chocolate				
MacConkey				
Thioglycollate				
Other:				
Other:				

Perform and interpret all necessary tests to identify any pathogens present.

Test	Observations	Interpretation	Possible organisms

Identify any microorganisms present in the specimen:

____

Provide a rationale for your identification:

____

Antibiotic Susceptibility Testing

Isolate: ______________________

Antibiotic concentration/code	Zone diameter	Interpretation (S, I, R)

Questions

1. Compare the results of the Gram stain with those obtained in culture: ______________________

   ____

2. What would you expect to see in a Wright-stained smear of CSF in which gram-positive cocci were observed in the Gram stain? ______________________

   Explain. ______________________

   ____

3. What is the purpose of the thioglycollate broth? ______

   ____

4. What is the normal appearance of CSF? ______________________

   ____

   How might CSF appear if there is a bacterial infection? ______________________

   ____

Procedure

Throat culture

Materials

5% sheep blood agar

Chocolate agar (if patient is less than 5 years old or if request for *Haemophilus*)

Loeffler agar slant and cystine-tellurite agar (if request for *Corynebacterium diphtheriae*)

Modified Thayer-Martin agar (if request for *Neisseria gonorrhoeae*)

Sterile tongue depressors

Sterile Dacron swabs

Sterile latex gloves

Procedure

1. Identify patient correctly.
2. Wearing sterile latex gloves, press patient's tongue with a sterile tongue depressor and have patient say "ah." This will expose the posterior pharynx.
3. Swab areas of inflammation or irritation over the posterior pharynx. Swab any red or swollen sites, as well as any exudate. Avoid touching the tongue, lips, and sides and roof of the mouth. Collect two swabs in this manner if direct antigen testing is to be performed.
4. Label swab(s) and transport to laboratory in a Culturette or in transport media if plates are not to be inoculated at this time.

5. For routine throat cultures, streak one sheep blood agar plate for isolation. Make three to five stabs into the growth so that subsurface hemolysis can be noted.
6. Streak any additional media for special requests for isolation.
7. Incubate blood agar at 35°C ± 2°C for 24 hours. Incubate all chocolate agar plates in increased CO_2. Some laboratories prefer to incubate the blood agar in increased CO_2 as well.
8. Examine plates for growth and hemolysis at 24 hours of incubation. Note the presence of any β-hemolytic streptococci. Also, determine whether normal flora is present. Describe each type of colony (size, color, hemolysis) present on the blood agar plate and estimate the number of each. Perform a Gram stain on each colony type.
9. Perform the bacitracin (and sulfamethoxazole-trimethoprim [SXT] if desired) susceptibility test on any colonies suggestive of group A streptococci.
10. Determine a possible genus and species for the other organisms present.
11. If the direct antigen test was performed, correlate these results with those observed on the culture plate.

Throat Culture Results

Specimen identification: ____________________

Date and time of collection: ____________________

Collected by: ____________________

Direct Antigen Testing

	Observations	Interpretation
Patient		
Positive control		

Sheep Blood Agar

	Present/absent	Description	Possible organisms
β-hemolytic streptococci			
Normal flora			

Characteristics of colonies on sheep blood agar	Gram stain	Normal flora or pathogen	Possible organisms

Colony type	Bacitracin		SXT	
	Diameter (mm)	Interpretation S or R	Diameter	Interpretation S or R

Questions

1. Identify any pathogens present in the throat culture.
____
2. Does the throat culture indicate normal flora or an infection? Explain. ____________________
____
____
3. Compare the results of the rapid antigen testing and throat culture. Explain any differences in the results.
____
____

Procedure

Sputum culture

Materials

5% sheep blood agar
Chocolate agar
MacConkey agar
Gram stain reagents

Procedure

1. Working in a biological safety cabinet, prepare a Gram stain smear from the specimen.
2. Examine the slide under the low-power (10×) objective for the presence of SECs and WBCs. Specimens containing less than 10 SECs/LPF or more than 25 WBCs/LPF are considered to be acceptable.
3. Switch to the oil-immersion objective and examine the smear to determine the morphology and Gram stain reaction of any bacteria present. Describe your observations.
4. Correctly and completely label all plates to be inoculated. Dip a swab in the sputum sample and roll over the surface of the blood, chocolate, and MacConkey agar plates. Streak each plate for isolation; stab the blood agar.
5. Incubate the blood and chocolate agar plates at 35°C under increased CO_2. Incubate the MacConkey agar plate in atmospheric oxygen at 35°C.

6. Examine the plates after 24 hours of incubation. Determine whether normal flora is present, absent, or decreased. Describe the various colony types, noting the color, size, and type of hemolysis.
   a. Perform a Gram stain on each colony type. Record your results.
   b. Note any mucoid colonies or those with depressed centers, which are α-hemolytic and may indicate *Streptococcus pneumoniae.*
7. Prepare a flow chart to identify all pathogenic isolates. Perform the required tests to identify any pathogen. The optochin susceptibility test should be performed on any colony suspected to be *S. pneumoniae.*
8. Perform the appropriate antibiotic panel on all pathogens using the Kirby-Bauer method.
9. Record all results.

Sputum Culture Results

Specimen identification: ______________________

Date and time of collection: ______________________

Collected by: ______________________

Gram Stain Screening

SEC/LPF	WBC/LPF	Interpretation

Gram Stain Observations (Oil-Immersion Objective)

Gram stain reaction and morphology	Possible organisms

Colonial Morphology

Media	Colony type		Possible organisms	Additional testing
	Description and number	Gram stain		
Sheep blood				
Chocolate				
MacConkey				

Perform the optochin susceptibility test on any organism suspected to be *S. pneumoniae.* Record your results.

Colony type	Optochin susceptibility	
	Diameter (mm)	Interpretation (S or R)

Perform the germ-tube test on any yeast if it is the predominant organism or present in large numbers. Record your results. Any yeast that is germ-tube positive can be presumptively identified as *Candida albicans.*

Colony type	Germ tube	
	Description	Interpretaton

Perform and interpret all necessary tests to identify any pathogens present.

Test	Observations	Interpretation	Possible organisms

List any normal flora or pathogens present in the specimen: ______________________

____

____

Antibiotic Susceptibility Testing

Isolate: ______________________

Antibiotic concentration/code	Zone diameter	Interpretation (S, I, R)

Questions

1. Does the isolation of S. *pneumoniae* from a sputum sample always indicate a pathologic state? Explain.

   ____

   ____

2. Why are sputum samples incubated under increased CO_2? ______________________

   ____

Procedure
Urine culture

Materials
Clean-catch midstream urine specimen(s)
MacConkey agar 5% sheep blood agar
Colistin-nalidixic acid (CNA) agar (optional)
1 μl or 10 μl calibrated, disposable inoculating loop
Gram stain reagents
Microscope slide

Procedure

Specimen Screening and Gram Stain

1. Mix the urine sample and deliver one drop of the well-mixed sample to a clean microscope slide.
2. Allow the specimen to air-dry.
3. Fix the slide with methanol or by heat fixation.
4. Perform the Gram stain on the smear.
5. Examine a minimum of 20 fields under the oil-immersion objective (1,000×). Note all bacteria, including number, morphology, and Gram stain reaction. Also note the number of WBCs seen. Significant bacteriuria is indicated by the presence of one or more bacteria per oil-immersion field.
6. Record the results of the Gram stain.

Colony Count and Culture

1. Label all plates completely and accurately. Dip the sterile, disposable, calibrated loop vertically into the well-mixed urine specimen.
2. Touch the loop to the center of the blood agar plate and spread in a vertical line across the plate.
3. Using the same loop (do not flame or enter urine sample again), draw the loop across the plate, crossing the initial streak several times. Lines should be parallel and should not overlap.
4. If desired, rotate the plate 90° and spread inoculum at right angles to the first set of parallel lines.
5. Streak the MacConkey (and CNA) plate(s) for isolation.
6. Incubate all plates at 35°C to 37°C for 24 hours.
7. Count the colonies present on the blood agar plate. Determine the CFU/ml of urine as follows:
   a. Multiply the number of colonies by 1,000 if the 1 μl loop was used.
   b. Multiply the number of colonies by 100 if the 10 μl loop was used.
   c. Convert the number to scientific notation; for example, if 150 colonies were counted and a 1 ml loop was used, the count would be 150,000, or 1.5×10^5, CFU/ml of urine.
   d. Colony counts greater than 10^5 CFU/ml are considered to be positive for UTIs. Those in the range of 10^4 to 10^5 CFU/ml may be contaminated or indicate a partially treated UTI. Dehydration, chronic pyelonephritis, and low urine specific gravity also may produce counts in this range in the presence of infection. Counts in the area of 10^3 CFU/ml are usually considered to be negative.
8. Examine the other plates for growth. Determine whether gram-positive or gram-negative bacteria are present. Give possible species for each colony type.
9. Perform all necessary tests to identify any pathogen(s) present.
10. Perform the appropriate antibiotic panel using the Kirby-Bauer method on all pathogens.
11. Record all results.

Urine Culture Results

Specimen identification: ____________________

Specimen type: ____________________

Date and time of collection: ____________________

Collected by: ____________________

Gram stain results: ____________________

Colonial Morphology

	Colony type			
Media	Description and number	Gram stain	Possible organisms	Additional testing
Sheep blood				
Colony count__________CFU/ml				
Chocolate				
MacConkey				
CNA				

Perform and interpret all necessary tests to identify any pathogens present.

Test	Observations	Interpretation	Possible organisms

Identification: ____________________

Rationale: ____________________

____

____

Antibiotic Susceptibility Testing

Isolate: ______________________

Antibiotic concentration/code	Zone diameter	Interpretation (S, I, R)

Questions

1. Correlate the results of the Gram stain with your observations on the primary isolation medium.

____

____

2. A urine specimen submitted to the laboratory by a patient who collected the sample at home produced 59 colonies when a 1 μl calibrated loop was used. On sheep blood agar, three distinct colony types were noted. What is your action? Explain.

____

____

Procedure

Stool culture

Materials

MacConkey agar (or eosin-methylene blue)

Hektoen enteric (HE) agar (or *Salmonella–Shigella* or xylose-lysine-desoxycholate)

Gram-negative (GN) broth (or selenite broth)

Campylobacter blood agar

5% sheep blood agar

Gram stain reagents

Optional media

Cefsulodin-irgasan-novobiocin (CIN) medium if *Yersinia enterocolitica* suspected

Sorbitol-MacConkey agar if verotoxic *Escherichia coli* suspected

Thiosulfate-citrate-bile salts-sucrose (TCBS) agar if *Vibrio* suspected

Cycloserine-cefotixin-fructose (CCF) egg yolk agar if *Clostridium difficile* suspected

Brilliant green (BG) or bismuth sulfite (BS) agar if *Salmonella typhi* suspected

Procedure

1. Insert a swab into the stool culture and prepare a smear. Allow it to air-dry and then fix using heat or methanol. Perform the Gram stain on the smear.
2. Examine the smear for the presence of WBCs, RBCs, and any abnormal bacterial forms, including curved gram-negative bacilli, which may indicate *Vibrio* or *Campylobacter*. A normal stool contains numerous gram-negative bacilli, some gram-positive cocci, and gram-positive bacilli. Record your observations.
3. Insert another swab into the specimen and roll it over the surfaces of the blood agar, MacConkey agar, HE agar, and *Campylobacter* blood agar plates. Streak each plate for isolation. Insert the swab into the GN broth and cap the tube. Streak any other optional plates for isolation if indicated.
4. Incubate all plates, except the *Campylobacter* blood agar, and the broth at 35°C to 37°C for 24 hours. The *Campylobacter* blood agar is incubated at 42°C in a microaerophilic environment, such as in a *Campylobacter* bag.
5. At 6 to 8 hours of incubation, subculture the GN broth to fresh MacConkey and HE plates.
6. At 24 hours of incubation, examine the plates for growth.
   a. Examine the MacConkey plate for the presence of normal flora, which appears as pink lactose fermenters. Scan the plate closely to detect any colorless, nonlactose fermenters that are likely pathogens.
   b. Note the inhibition of the normal flora on the HE plate. Examine the plate for any colorless colonies with or without a black pigment, which indicates a pathogen.
   c. Record all results.
7. Examine the blood agar plate for growth. Note the number of colonies that are not members of the Enterobacteriaceae. In particular, examine the plate for yeast and *Staphylococcus aureus*.
8. Examine the *Campylobacter* blood agar for flat, gray colonies typical of *Campylobacter*. Perform a Gram stain and the oxidase and catalase tests on any suspicious growth. *Campylobacter* appears as a thin, curved, gram-negative bacillus; it is oxidase and catalase positive.

9. Re-incubate any plates without growth for another 24 hours.
10. Examine the plates after 48 hours of incubation, as well as those subcultured from the GN broth. Record your results.
11. Prepare a flow chart for the identification of any pathogens that are isolated.
12. After consulting with your instructor, perform all tests that are necessary to identify the pathogen(s).
13. Perform the Kirby-Bauer antibiotic susceptibility test on all pathogens identified.

Stool Culture Results

Specimen identification: ____________________

Date and time of collection: ____________________

Collected by: ____________________

Gram stain results: ____________________

Colonial Morphology

Media	Description		Number	Possible organisms	Normal flora/ pathogen
	Lactose	H_2S			
MacConkey					
HE					
MacConkey (subculture from broth)					
HE (subculture from broth)					
Other:					

Compare your observations on the Gram stain with the growth on the agar plates. Perform a Gram stain on each distinct colony type. Record your results.

Media	Colony type		Possible organisms	Additional testing
	Description and number	Gram stain		
MacConkey				
HE				
Other:				

Perform and interpret all necessary tests to identify any pathogens present.

Test	Observations	Interpretation	Possible organisms

Identification: ____________________

Rationale: ____________________

____

Antibiotic Susceptibility Testing

Isolate: ____________________

Antibiotic concentration/code	Zone diameter	Interpretation (S, I, R)

Questions

1. Contrast the growth on the MacConkey plate with that on the HE plate.
   What differences do you note? ____________________
   ____
   Why do these occur? ____________________
   ____
2. Contrast the growth on the MacConkey plate streaked from the swab with that streaked from the subculture from the GN broth. Are there any differences?
   ____
   Explain why or why not: ____________________
   ____
   State the purpose of enrichment broth: ____________________
   ____

Case Studies and Review Questions

Case Study 1

A 65-year-old male is admitted to the hospital with high fever, shaking chills, nausea, and vomiting. His medical record indicates that he has a history of emphysema and has been a heavy cigarette smoker since he was a teenager.

A complete blood cell count, differential, and chemistry profile are ordered by the physician. The CBC reveals a WBC count of 15,000/μl, with 40% bands, 46% segmented neutrophils, 11% lymphocytes, and 3% monocytes.

Breathing was labored, and a chest X-ray film revealed consolidation of the upper part of the lung. Sputum and blood cultures were performed.

1. The Gram stain from the sputum specimen revealed numerous segmented neutrophils, many gram-negative bacilli, and few gram-positive cocci. An occasional squamous epithelial cell was seen. What can be said about the quality of this specimen?
   a. It is suitable for culture and does not seem to be contaminated.
   b. It is unsuitable for culture and definitely contaminated; it should be re-collected.
   c. Its quality cannot be determined until the specimen is plated and incubated and the growth examined.
   d. None of the above
2. Which of the following media indicate the most appropriate plating for the sputum specimen?
   a. 5% sheep blood agar, MacConkey agar, chocolate agar, anaerobic blood agar
   b. Chocolate agar, Bordet-Gengou, MacConkey agar, thioglycollate
   c. 5% sheep blood agar, MacConkey agar, chocolate agar, CNA
   d. 5% sheep blood agar, MacConkey agar, anaerobic blood agar, CNA
3. Examination of the plates at 24 hours of incubation reveals heavy growth of a mucoid lactose fermenter on the MacConkey plate. A few α-hemolytic colonies are observed on the CNA plate. Which statement most likely describes these observations?
   a. The colonies on MacConkey and CNA are both pathogens.
   b. The colonies on MacConkey and CNA are both normal flora.
   c. The colonies on MacConkey should be considered to be pathogenic and those on CNA normal flora.
   d. The colonies on CNA should be considered to be pathogenic and those on MacConkey normal flora.
4. Which of the following tests are most appropriate in the identification of the pathogen(s)?
   a. Catalase, coagulase, optochin
   b. Indole, motility, decarboxylase patterns
   c. Indole, urease, deaminase
   d. Oxidase, catalase, porphyrin
5. The blood cultures were positive. What do you think a Gram stain performed on a subculture of the blood culture would reveal?
   a. Gram-positive diplococci
   b. Gram-positive cocci in clusters
   c. Gram-negative diplococci
   d. Gram-negative bacilli

Case Study 2

A 26-year-old female patient reports to her obstetrician during her seventh month of pregnancy for a routine visit. Her only concern is that she has experienced painful, burning, and frequent urination for the past few days. The routinely voided urine sample yielded positive results for nitrate and leukocyte esterase.

6. What can be said about the quality of the specimen for culture?
   a. A pathogen is obviously present so there is no need to be concerned about normal flora or contaminants—it is a suitable specimen.
   b. A Gram stain should be performed to see whether normal flora contaminants are present to determine whether it is suitable.
   c. Normal flora contaminants are causing the positive nitrate and esterase reactions. Re-collect for a clean-catch midstream specimen.
   d. A clean-catch midstream specimen should be collected to determine the presence of a urinary tract infection.

Upon receipt of the specimen in the laboratory, a colony count is performed using a 1 μl calibrated inoculating loop on 5% sheep blood agar; a MacConkey agar plate also is inoculated. At 24 hours, heavy growth of a lactose fermenter is observed on the MacConkey plate. The colonies are counted on the blood agar plate, revealing 140 colonies, which are flat, grayish, and nonhemolytic.

7. Determine the colony count per milliliter of urine.
   a. 1.4×10^2/ml
   b. 1.4×10^3/ml
   c. 1.4×10^4/ml
   d. 1.4×10^5/ml
   e. 1.4×10^6/ml
8. A rapid indole test is performed on the lactose fermenter, with a positive result. This organism can be presumptively identified as:
   a. *Enterobacter cloacae*
   b. *Klebsiella pneumoniae*
   c. *Escherichia coli*
   d. *Proteus mirabilis*
   e. *Enterococcus*
9. Which of the following tests are *most* helpful in the final identification of this organism?
   a. VP, citrate, motility
   b. Urease, deaminase, motility
   c. Lysine decarboxylase, VP, urease
   d. Glucose fermentation, citrate, deaminase

Case Study 3

A 9-month-old infant boy is brought to the emergency room by his mother. She states that the child has been listless and hasn't been interested in eating or taking his bottle for the past 2 days. She says the baby has been sleeping long hours and that she has difficulty waking him from his nap. The baby has had a low-grade fever, which she was treating with acetaminophen. While taking the medical history, the physician notes that the baby has not received any immunizations.

A CBC and differential are performed, revealing a WBC of 14,500/μl with 90% neutrophils, including 35% bands. The infant's condition worsens, and a cerebrospinal fluid collection is performed. The Gram stain reveals few gram-negative coccobacilli and 3 to 4 segmented neutrophils/oil-immersion field. A tentative diagnosis of meningitis is made.

10. Which of the following should be considered as the possible pathogen?
    a. *Streptococcus pneumoniae* or *Neisseria meningitidis*
    b. *Haemophilus influenzae* or *Staphylococcus aureus*
    c. *E. coli* or *Neisseria meningitidis*
    d. *Haemophilus influenzae* or *Neisseria meningitidis*
11. The specimen was plated onto 5% sheep blood agar, chocolate agar, CNA, MacConkey agar, and anaerobic blood and into thioglycollate. After 48 hours of incubation, growth was observed only on the chocolate agar. Which of the following tests are most appropriate in the identification?
    a. Oxidase, X and V factors, porphyrin
    b. Oxidase, carbohydrate utilization tests
    c. Oxidase, indole, VP, motility
    d. Catalase, coagulase, optochin

Case Study 4

A 60-year-old male diabetic patient received a puncture wound on his finger with a screwdriver while repairing his car. He cleaned the wound with soap, water, and peroxide; he then applied a local antibiotic. Three days later, he noticed the area was red, hot, and swollen. He also developed a low-grade fever, and he decided to call his physician.

The physician noted the development of cellulitis; he cultured the site using a needle and syringe and debrided the site. He also prescribed an oral broad-spectrum antibiotic.

Upon receipt in the laboratory, the specimen was Gram stained and plated onto sheep blood agar and MacConkey agar, which were incubated at 35°C; anaerobic blood, PEA, KV, and thioglycollate samples were inoculated and incubated anaerobically.

The Gram stain revealed the presence of many gram-positive cocci in clusters, moderate gram-positive bacilli, and many segmented neutrophils.

12. The aerobic plates revealed a moderately heavy growth of a medium-sized, creamy white colony with narrow zone β-hemolysis on the blood agar plate. No growth was seen on the MacConkey agar. Which of the following is the most appropriate action to identify this organism?
    a. Perform Gram stain and catalase
    b. Plate on CNA to isolate anaerobic gram-positive cocci
    c. Re-collect the specimen because normal skin flora has been isolated
    d. Perform CAMP and bacitracin tests to speciate
13. To differentiate normal skin flora from the pathogenic *Staphylococcus*, which of the following tests is most appropriate?
    a. Novobiocin
    b. Coagulase
    c. Bile-esculin hydrolysis
    d. Bacitracin

14. Growth was evident on the anaerobic blood agar and PEA plates; no growth was observed on the KV. Growth was observed in the lower third of the thioglycollate tube, and a foul odor was very evident in this tube. Which group of anaerobes can be eliminated as the possible infecting organism?
    a. Gram-negative cocci
    b. Gram-positive cocci
    c. Gram-negative bacilli
    d. Gram-positive non-spore–forming bacilli
    e. Gram-positive spore-forming bacilli
15. Results of the isolated were as follows:
    Indole –
    Esculin hydrolysis +
    Catalase –
    Lecithinase +
    Starch hydrolysis –
    Milk digested –
    DNAse +
    Gelatinase +
    Glucose and lactose fermented
    This anaerobe is most likely:
    a. *Bacteroides fragilis*
    b. *Clostridium tetani*
    c. *Clostridium perfringens*
    d. *Peptostreptococcus anaerobius*
    e. *Fusobacterium nucleatum*
16. What observation of the anaerobic blood agar would have been an important clue to this bacterium's identification?
    a. Brown to black pigmentation
    b. Wide zone of β-hemolysis
    c. Pearly, opalescent growth
    d. Double zone of hemolysis

Case Study 5

A 34-year-old female is transported to the emergency room by ambulance after reporting that she was severely burned in a kitchen fire. Examination by the emergency room physician reveals second- and third-degree burns to her forearm and upper arm. The burns are cleansed and dressed, and the patient is immediately given intravenous antibiotics. She is admitted to the hospital. A specimen is obtained from the burn site for culture and susceptibility testing. After 3 days of hospitalization, an exudate is observed at the burn site. Although no pathogens were isolated from the specimen, the burn remains red and painful and does not seem to be improving. The attending physician questions the initial culture results, and another specimen from the site is sent to the laboratory. The Gram stain of the second specimen reveals many gram-negative bacilli.

17. How do you account for the discrepancy between the first and second specimens?
    a. Poor culture technique was used for the initial specimen.
    b. Second specimen is contaminated with normal skin flora.
    c. Patient developed an infection while in the hospital.
    d. All of the above are possible explanations.

    The second specimen revealed the presence of a nonlactose fermenter and a lactose fermenter on MacConkey agar. The CNA plate showed no growth, and no anaerobes were isolated.
18. The nonlactose fermenter produced a bluish-green pigment on MacConkey agar and may be presumptively identified as:
    a. *Serratia marcescens*
    b. *Pseudomonas fluorescens*
    c. *Pseudomonas aeruginosa*
    d. *Chryseobacterium meningosepticum*
19. Which of the following biochemical profiles most likely correlates with the correct identification of the nonlactose fermenter?

	Oxidase	Growth at 42°C	Glucose Oxidized	LDC	ADH	ODC
a.	+	–	+	–	+	–
b.	+	+	+	+	–	+
c.	+	–	+	–	–	+
d.	+	+	+	–	+	–
e.	–	+	+	–	+	–

20. The lactose fermenter was determined to be indole negative by the spot indole test. Which of the following organisms is *not* a possible choice for identification of this isolate?
    a. *Enterobacter cloacae*
    b. *Enterobacter aerogenes*
    c. *Klebsiella pneumoniae*
    d. *E. coli*
    e. Responses a, b, and c
21. The following biochemical profile was obtained for the lactose fermenter:
    VP + Citrate + Motile
    LDC – ADH + ODC +

Urease –
Fermented sucrose, mannitol, sorbitol, arabinose, raffinose
Failed to ferment dulcitol and adonitol
It can most likely be identified as:
a. *Klebsiella pneumoniae*
b. *Enterobacter aerogenes*
c. *Enterobacter cloacae*
d. *Pantoa (Enterobacter) agglomerans*
e. *Escherichia coli*

Case Study 6

A 68-year-old male is examined in the hospital emergency room with complaints of a fever and worsening shortness of breath. He had been diagnosed a few years earlier with chronic obstructive pulmonary disease. His vital signs showed a temperature of 100°F, pulse of 92 beats/minute, respiration of 22/minute, and a blood pressure of 124/78 mm Hg. Chest X-ray films revealed small infiltrates in both upper lobes and in many small cavities. A sputum specimen was collected for culture and acid-fast bacilli.

The Gram stain yielded more than 25 neutrophils/LPF, a rare squamous epithelial cell, moderate gram-positive cocci, a few gram-negative bacilli, and a few corynebacteria. The acid-fast stain revealed approximately 10 to 12 acid-fast bacilli on the entire slide. The patient was prescribed a therapy of isoniazid and ethambutol.

22. The sputum specimen:
    a. Appears to be contaminated
    b. Indicates the presence of one or more pathogenic organisms
    c. Reflects the normal oropharyngeal flora
    d. More than one response applies
23. Based on the patient's history and the findings in the smears, which of the following are the most appropriate media for primary plating?
    a. Sheep blood agar, MacConkey agar, chocolate agar, and Middlebrook
    b. Sheep blood agar, MacConkey agar, chocolate agar, thioglycollate
    c. CNA, MacConkey agar, anaerobic blood, selective Middlebrook
    d. CNA, MacConkey agar, chocolate agar, Sabouraud's dextrose agar
24. The routine culture showed a mixed flora of a moderate amount of viridans streptococci, a few *Haemophilus*, and a few corynebacteria. What is the next step toward working up this culture?
    a. Speciate *Streptococcus* and *Haemophilus*
    b. Speciate *Haemophilus* and corynebacteria
    c. Report findings that suggest normal mixed bacterial flora
    d. Report "no organisms isolated."
25. The acid-fast bacillus grew in 5 days when incubated in the dark at 35°C as tan to buff-colored colonies. The plate was exposed to direct light from a 100 watt light for 5 hours, then re-incubated. Within 48 hours, the colonies all developed an orange to yellow pigment. Which of the following is a possible species for this *Mycobacterium?*
    a. *M. kansasii*
    b. *M. marinum*
    c. *M. gordonae*
    d. *M. tuberculosis*
    e. More than one is correct.
26. This *Mycobacterium* is classified as a:
    a. Photochromogen
    b. Scotochromogen
    c. Nonphotochromogen
    d. Rapid grower
27. The *Mycobacterium* gave the following results:
    Heat-stable catalase +
    Nitrate reduction +
    Tween 80 hydrolysis +
    Niacin accumulation –
    It most likely can be identified as:
    a. *M. gordonae*
    b. *M. tuberculosis*
    c. *M. simiae*
    d. *M. marinum*
    e. *M. kansasii*

Case Study 7

A 55-year-old male patient recovering from surgery for a bowel obstruction had redness, swelling, pain, and tenderness at the surgical incision. The patient had been recovering well up to that time from the surgery, which was successfully performed 4 days earlier. A low-grade fever was noted, and both aerobic and anaerobic cultures were collected from the incision. Several hours later, the patient's condition worsened as the fever increased and shaking chills occurred. A stat complete blood cell count was performed, and blood cultures were collected. Results revealed the presence of moderate gram-positive cocci and gram-negative bacilli in the Gram stain from the cultures taken earlier in the day. The CBC revealed a WBC of 16,500/μl with 85% neutrophils (60% segmented and 25% banded). Subculture of the aerobic blood culture bottle at 8 hours of incubation revealed a moderate number of gram-positive cocci. The blood culture was subsequently subcultured to both blood and chocolate agar and incubated at 35°C. At 18 hours of incubation, heavy growth was noted of flat, gray, nonhemolytic colonies, which were determined to be catalase negative.

28. Which of the following tests are most needed to identify this isolate?
    a. CAMP, bacitracin, bile esculin, 6.5% salt broth
    b. Optochin, bile esculin, and PYRase
    c. Coagulase, bile esculin, and optochin
    d. CAMP, bile esculin, and PYRase
29. If the organism is bile-esculin positive, it can be classified as:
    a. Group D *Streptococcus*
    b. *Enterococcus*
    c. Group D *Streptococcus*—non-*Enterococcus*
    d. Viridans streptococci
30. The gram stain morphology of this isolate will most probably show gram positive:
    a. Cocci in clusters
    b. Cocci in chains
    c. Diplococci
    d. Coccobacilli
31. Turbidity and hemolysis were noted in the anaerobic blood culture vial at 18 hours of incubation. A Gram stain revealed many gram-negative bacilli. You would expect this anaerobe to grow on/in which of the following anaerobic media?
    a. Anaerobic blood only
    b. Anaerobic blood and thioglycollate
    c. Anaerobic blood, thioglycollate, and PEA
    d. Anaerobic blood, thioglycollate, PEA, and KV
32. Appropriate anaerobic media were inoculated and incubated. Lombard-Dowell medium was inoculated from colonies growing on the anaerobic sheep blood agar. At 48 hours, the following results were observed with anaerobic biochemical reactions.
    Indole –
    Enhanced growth and positive hydrolysis on 20% bile-esculin agar
    Catalase +
    Lecithinase –
    Lipase –
    Gelatin hydrolysis –
    Starch hydrolysis –
    Glucose and lactose fermented
    The anaerobic growth is most likely:
    a. *Fusobacterium nucleatum*
    b. *Clostridium perfringens*
    c. *Bacteroides fragilis*
    d. *Prevotella melaninogenica*
    e. *Porphyromonas asaccharolyticus*
33. The source of this pathogen is most likely:
    a. Nosocomial infection acquired from health care environment
    b. Nosocomial infection acquired from health care providers
    c. Endogenous infection from patient's normal flora
    d. Exogenous infection from unsterile wound dressings

Bibliography

Bowler, P. G., Duerden, B. I., & Armstrong, D. G. (2001). Wound microbiology and associated approaches to wound management. *Clinical Microbiology Reviews, 14,* 244–269.

Brouwer, M. C., Tunkel, A. R., & van de Beek, D. (2010). Epidemiology, diagnosis and antimicrobial treatment of acute bacterial meningitis. *Clinical Microbiology Reviews, 23,* 467–492.

Bryan, C. S. (1989). Clinical implications of positive blood cultures. *Clinical Microbiology Reviews, 2,* 329–353.

Carroll, K. C. (2002). Laboratory diagnosis of lower respiratory tract infections: Controversy and conundrums. *Clinical Microbiology Reviews, 40,* 3114–3120.

Cockerill, III, F. R., Wilson, J. W., Vetter, E. A., Goodman, K. M., Torgerson, C. A., Harmsen, W. S., . . . Wilson, W. R. (2004). Optimal testing parameters for blood cultures. *Clinical Infectious Diseases, 38,* 1724–1730.

Dreyer, A. W., Ismail, N. A., Nkosi, D., Lindeque, K., Matthew, M., van Zyl, D. G., & Hoosen, A. A. (2011). Comparison of the VersaTREK Blood Culture System against the Bactec 9240 System in patients with suspected bloodstream infections. *Annals of Clinical Microbiology and Antimicrobials, 10,* 1.

Forbes, B. A., Sahm, D. F., & Weissfeld, A. S. (2007). Genital tract infections. In *Bailey and Scott's diagnostic microbiology* (12th ed.). St. Louis, MO: Mosby Elsevier.

Gray, L. D., & Fedorko, D. P. (1992). Laboratory diagnosis of bacterial meningitis. *Clinical Microbiology Reviews, 5,* 130–145.

Hall, K. K., & Lyman, J. A. (2006). Updated review of blood culture contamination. *Clinical Microbiology Reviews, 19,* 788–802.

Hughes, C., & Roebuck, M. J. (2003). Evaluation of the IRIS 939 UDx flow microscope as a screening system for urinary tract infection. *Journal of Clinical Pathology, 56,* 844–849.

Kunin, C. M. (1994). Urinary tract infections in females. *Clinical Infectious Diseases, 18,* 1–12.

Mermel, L. A., & Maki, D. G. (1993). Detection of bacteremia in adults: Consequences of culturing an inadequate volume of blood. *Annals of Internal Medicine, 119,* 270–272.

Orenstein, R., & Wong, E. (1999). Urinary tract infections in adults. *American Family Physician, 59,* 1225–1234.

Semenuik, H., Noonan, J., Gill, H., & Church, D. (2002). Evaluation of the Coral UTI Screen system for rapid automated screening of significant bacteriuria in a regional centralized laboratory. *Diagnostic Microbiology and Infectious Disease, 1,* 7–10.

Warren, J. W. (1997). Catheter-associated urinary tract infections. *Infectious Disease Clinics of North America, 11,* 609–622.

Weinstein, M. P., Lee, A., Mirrett, S., & Barth Reller, L. (2007). Detection of bloodstream infections in adults: How many blood cultures are needed? *Journal of Clinical Microbiology, 45,* 3546–3548.

Winn, Jr., W., Allen, S., Janda, W., Konemen, E., Procop, G., Schreckenberger, P., & Woods, G. (Eds.). (2005). Introduction to microbiology: Part II: Guidelines for the collection, transport, processing, analysis and reporting of cultures from specific specimen sources. In *Koneman's color atlas and textbook of diagnostic microbiology* (6th ed.). Philadelphia, PA: Lippincott Williams & Wilkins.

Glossary

δ-aminolevulinic acid (δ-ALA) a precurser to prophryins and hemoglobin; it is used in the procedure that determines the ability of members of the genus *Haemophilus* to convert δ-ALA to porphyrins.

acid-fast bacilli (AFB) name given to bacteria in the genus *Mycobacterium* because of their ability to retain stain even after acid decolorization.

acquired immunity resistance resulting from prior exposure to the infectious agent; may be actively acquired from the actual infection or from vaccination or passively acquired, as from mother to fetus.

acquired immunodeficiency syndrome (AIDS) disease characterized by loss of immune compentency; opportunistic infections, such as *Pneumocystis carinii* infections, cryptococcosis, candidiasis; and unusual malignancies such as Kaposi's sarcoma and non-Hodgkin's lymphomas; caused by the retrovirus human immunodeficiency virus and transmitted by the exchange of body fluids, including semen or blood, or through the transfusion of contaminated blood or blood products.

acquired resistance ineffectiveness of an antimicrobial agent against a particular microorganism that results from prior exposure of the organism to the agent; may result from chromosomal mutations or effects of bacterial enzymes.

actinomycosis infection characterized by thick, lumpy abscesses or granulomas, which drain a thin granular pus through multiple sinuses, usually in the cervicofacial, thoracic, or abdominal areas in humans; attributed to infection by *Actinomyces israelii*.

acute-phase specimen serum specimen to determine specific antibody levels. Serum is collected early in the infection, when antibody levels are generally low.

additive effect two antimicrobial agents produce effects equal to the combined effect of the drugs when administered separately.

adsorption first step in the establishment of a viral infection, which involves the attachment of the virus to the host receptor site.

aerotolerance method to determine oxygen preference of a microorganism by determining its ability to grow on aerobic blood agar in the presence of oxygen and on anaerobic blood agar in the absence of oxygen.

affinity strength of the reaction between a single antigenic determinant and a single combining site on the antibody. It reflects cumulative effects of the forces of attraction and repulsion that occur between the antigen and antibody.

agglutination clumping or adhering of bacterial, viral, or fungal antigens to corresponding antibody evidenced by aggregation of the antigen and antibody. Antibody may be tagged for visualization of reaction with latex beads (latex agglutination) or red blood cells (hemagglutination).

alginate mucoid polysaccharide found in certain strains of *Pseudomonas aeruginosa* that may protect the organism from phagocytosis.

amastigote leishmanial or intracellular form of the hemoflagellates, which is small and oval, containing a kinetoplast and nucleus but lacking an undulating membrane and external flagellum; generally found in the host's reticuloendothelial tissue.

amplicon amplified target nucleic acid in molecular testing methods.

anaerogenic *E. coli* nongas-producing strains of *Escherichia coli*.

antagonistic effect effect of one antimicrobial agent opposes that of the second such that the resulting action is significantly less than the action of each agent alone.

anthrax infectious disease of farm animals, such as cattle, goats, pigs, and sheep, which is caused by the gram-positive bacillus *Bacillus anthracis* and may be transmitted to humans through direct contact or inhalation; also known as pulmonary anthrax or Woolsorter's disease.

antibacterial agents antimicrobial agents that prevent the growth of bacteria.

antibiogram unique pattern of susceptibility and resistance of a microorganism to a group of antibiotics; useful in epidemiology.

antibiotic a chemical derived from a microorganism that inhibits the growth of another microorganism; some are chemically modified.

antibiotic media agar that contains antibiotics as inhibitory agents that may suppress the normal flora or other bacteria and enhance the isolation of a particular organism or group of bacteria; for example, colistin-nalidixic acid inhibits gram-negative bacteria, and modified Thayer-Martin is selective for *N. gonorrhoeae.*

antibody protein that is induced by the introduction of antigen into the host and that reacts specifically with the antigen. The following immunoglobulins comprise the immune response: IgG, IgM, IgA, IgD, and IgE.

antibody titer amount of antibody present in a serum sample; the inverse of the highest dilution at which the antibody is detected.

antifungal agents antimicrobial agents that inhibit or prevent the growth of fungi.

antigen foreign compound capable of stimulating the production of antibodies.

antimicrobial agents agents that inhibit the growth or action of microbes.

antiviral antimicrobial agent that inhibits or prevents the growth of viruses.

arthrocentesis puncture of a joint, with the withdrawal of synovial fluid for diagnostic purposes, such as the diagnosis of infectious disease.

ascospore type of specialized spore involved in sexual reproduction of some fungi in which two to eight spores are contained in a sac-like ascus.

assimilation ability of microorganisms to utilize nutrients that are useful in the classification of yeasts and used to determine whether the yeast can grow in the presence of either an individual carbohydrate or a nitrate.

asymptomatic carrier an individual who harbors a microorganism without any harmful effects who may transmit the infection to others.

autonomous effect antibiotic interaction in which the combined effect of both drugs is equal to the result of the most effective drug used alone.

auxotype gonococcal strains that require specific nutrients for growth. For example, AHU auxotypes require arginine, hypoxanthine, and uracil for growth.

avidity indicator of the strength of binding of an antigen with many antigenic determinants and many antibody binding sites; sum total of all binding between antigen and antibody in a solution.

β-lactamases bacterial enzymes that destroy the β-lactam ring of penicillins and cephalosporins, leading to bacterial resistance; penicillinase.

bacitracin susceptibility selective inhibition of group A *Streptococcus* to 0.02–0.04 units of bacitracin; used in the identification of streptococci.

bacteremia the presence of bacteria in the blood.

bacterial vaginosis nonspecific vaginosis; mixed vaginal flora of anaerobes and aerobes with an absence of lactobacilli and white blood cells.

bacteriocidal agents antimicrobial agents that cause the death of bacteria.

bacteriostatic agents antimicrobial agents that inhibit the growth of bacteria without killing.

bacteriuria the presence of bacteria in the urine. The presence of more than 100,000 CFUs per milliliter of urine is generally diagnostic for a urinary tract infection.

Bartlett's classification scheme used to determine suitability of sputum specimens by a numerical comparison based on the amount of neutrophils and squamous epithelial cells observed in a Gram-stained smear prepared from the specimen.

basidiospore type of specialized spore involved in sexual reproduction of some fungi. The spores are contained in a club-shaped basidium.

bile esculin media used to select group D *Streptococcus* and *Enterococcus* based on their ability to grow in 40% bile and to hydrolyze esculin.

biohazard laboratory dangers that may be a source of infection to laboratory workers. Examples include exposure to microorganisms through the airborne route, ingestion, direct inoculation, mucous membrane contact, or arthropod vectors.

biological false-positives conditions that produce a false reaction for *T. pallidum* in nontreponemal screening tests for syphilis, including autoimmune diseases and infections that cross-react, producing a positive reaction in nontreponemal tests, such as the RPR (rapid plasma reagin), but a negative reaction in the treponemal tests.

biosafety level four levels of protocol to be followed when working with potentially pathogenic microorganisms. Protocol may include protective gloves, laboratory coats, biological safety cabinets, warning signs, and barrier controls.

blastomycosis infectious disease caused by the dimorphic fungus *Blastomyces dermatitidis*, which may infect the skin, lungs, kidneys, central nervous system, and bones and is most commonly found in North America, especially in the southeastern United States. The disease is characterized by cough, dyspnea, chills, and fever and is known also as Gilchrist's disease.

botulism often fatal form of food poisoning caused by the anaerobic spore-forming bacillus *Clostridium botulinum* and the ingestion of the powerful botulism toxin, which acts as a neurotoxin, causing eventual respiratory paralysis.

bound coagulase clumping factor; enzyme produced by *Staphylococcus aureus* that converts fibrinogen to fibrin and is useful in the identification of the organism.

bradyzoites slowly replicating trophozoites of the parasite *Toxoplasma gondii*. They are intracellular and encyst in the host's tissue.

brightfield microscopy type of microscopy in which the field is illuminated with a light source. The specimen appears dark against a light background. This type of microscopy is useful in examining stained smears.

broad-spectrum antibiotics type of antimicrobial agent that has a range of effectiveness against several types of bacteria, including both gram-positive and gram-negative microorganisms.

bronchitis acute or chronic inflammation of the tracheobronchial tree characterized by cough and fever and caused by any of several bacterial or viral pathogens.

Brown's classification scheme to identify *Streptococcus* that is based on the organisms type and pattern of hemolysis. Types of hemolysis include α-, β-, and α′-hemolytic and nonhemolytic.

CAMP reaction synergistic hemolysis observed between β-hemolytic *Staphylococcus aureus* and group B streptococci; named for Christie, Atkins, and Munch-Petersen.

capnophilic microorganisms that prefer an incubation environment with increased carbon dioxide (3%–10% CO_2).

capsid protein covering of the virus particle.

capsomer protein subunits that form the protein coat (capsid) of a virion or virus particle.

carbohydrate fermentation ability of microorganisms to utilize carbohydrates in the absence of oxygen; anaerobic breakdown of carbohydrates, such as glucose, into carbon compounds, such as pyruvic acid.

cell-mediated immunity type of acquired immunity associated with T lymphocytes that is involved in resistance to infectious diseases caused by viruses and some bacteria. Cell-mediated immunity is also involved in delayed hypersensitivity reactions, graft rejection, and certain autoimmune diseases.

cellulitis an infection of the skin or connective tissue characterized by local heat, redness, pain, and swelling.

cercaria stage of the trematode life cycle with a body and a tail that develops from germ cells in the sporocyst or rediae; this is the final stage that develops in the snail host.

cervicitis acute or chronic inflammation of the mucous membranes of the cervix characterized by redness, edema, and pain.

chancroid very contagious local venereal ulcer caused by *Haemophilus ducreyi*.

choleragen cholera enterotoxin that is associated with the loss of electrolytes and fluids.

chromoblastomycosis type of subcutaneous fungal infection caused by the dematiaceous fungi, which are dark, slow-growing fungi, such as *Fonsacaea* species, *Phialophora verrucosa*, *Cladosporium carrionii*, *Exophiala* species, and *Wangiella dermatitidis*. These fungi are found on vegetation and in the soil, and infection is generally transmitted through a puncture wound or skin trauma involving fungally contaminated vegetation.

clue cell adherence of small bacilli, usually *Gardnerella vaginalis*, to squamous vaginal epithelial cells; significant in the diagnosis of bacterial vaginosis.

coagulase-negative staphylococci (CoNS) those species of *Staphylococcus* that do not produce coagulase, including *S. epidermidis* and *S. saprophyticus*.

coccidioidomycosis infectious fungal disease caused by the inhalation of spores of the dimorphic fungus *Coccidioides immitis*, characterized by respiratory symptoms and later a low-grade fever, anorexia, weight loss, dyspnea, and pain in the joints and bones. The disease is found most commonly in the hot, dry climates of the southwestern United States and Central and South America and is known also as desert fever, San Joaquin fever, and valley fever.

cold agglutinins nonspecific immunoglobulin M (IgM) antibodies that may be produced in response to *Mycoplasma pneumoniae* infection that agglutinate human type O red blood cells at 4°C but not at 37°C; useful in the diagnosis of *Mycoplasma pneumoniae* infection when present in high titers or if a fourfold increase is noted between the acute and convalescent titers.

colonization presence and multiplication of a microorganism in or on a host without signs of infectious disease.

colony count colony-forming units per milliliter (CFU/ml) of urine determined by using a calibrated inoculating loop. Counts equal to or greater than 10^5/ml are diagnostic for urinary tract infections.

colorimetry quantitative analysis through comparison of the color development in an unknown sample with that of a known standard. Color absorbance is directly proportional to the concentration of the substance to be measured.

conidia asexual spores produced by some fungi either singly or multiply in long chains or clusters by specialized hyphae, known as conidiophores.

conidiogenesis conidia formation exhibited by some fungi.

convalescent-phase specimen serum sample collected to determine antibody level later in the infection when the antibody response is high; generally collected at least 2 weeks after the acute phase specimen.

coracidium free-living larval stage of the cestode *Diphyllobothrium latum*, which hatches in freshwater and is ingested by the first intermediate host—crustaceans or copepods of the genus *Diaptomus*.

counterimmunoelectrophoresis solid-phase system that uses electricity and the precipitin reaction to detect antigen or antibody. Antigen and antibody move in opposite directions in an electrical field and form precipitates in the area where their concentrations meet in optimal proportions.

cyst form immotile form of the protozoan parasites, which is protected by a cyst wall and may be transmitted to another host.

cytopathogenic effect (CPE) alteration, disruption, or damage to the cells of a cell monolayer, resulting from virus infection.

darkfield microscopy a form of microscopy in which the specimen appears light against a black background as a result of the field being illuminated by a peripheral light source. This technique is used to examine spirochetes, including *Treponema*, *Borrelia*, and *Leptospira*.

definitive host the host in which the sexual reproductive phase of a parasite occurs.

dematiaceous fungi a group of dark, slow-growing fungi, which are found on vegetation and associated with subcutaneous mycoses, including the development of chronic, warty, tumorlike lesions of the feet and lower legs. Examples include *Fonsacaea fedrosoi*, *F. compactum*, *Phialophora verrucosa*, *Cladosprorum carrionii*, *Exophilia* species, and *Wangiella dermatitidis*.

deuteromycetes division in botanical taxonomy that includes most medically important fungi; characterized by septate hyphae and asexual reproduction.

differential media class of primary isolation media that selects for a particular group of bacteria and also permits the classification of the organism based on distinct growth characteristics. An example is MacConkey agar, which selects for gram-negative bacteria by inhibition of gram-positive bacteria and also permits characterization of lactose-fermenting bacteria by a pink color.

digenetic sexual cycle of the trematodes, in which distinct patterns of reproduction occur in alternate generations.

dimorphic fungi those fungi that possess both a yeast phase, which grows at 35°C to 37°C, and a mold, or mycelial, phase, which grows at 25°C to 30°C.

diphtheroid pleomorphic morphology of some gram-positive bacilli, including *Corynebacterium*, characterized by club-shaped or branching forms that resemble Chinese characters.

diploid cell lines type of cell culture that must have at least 75% of the cells with the same karyotype as those from the normal cells from which the cell line was derived. Examples include MRC-5, HDF, and WE-38 cell lines.

direct immunofluorescence microscopic method to determine presence of an antigen by exhibition of fluorescence when the specimen is reacted with a fluorescein-labeled antibody.

disinfection the process of destroying pathogenic organisms or causing inhibition of their activity.

eclipse stage in the establishment of viral infection in which replication and expression of genetic material occur as the viral nucleic acid acts as a template for production of messenger RNA, which directs the synthesis of viral proteins.

ectoparasite parasite that lives on or in the external area of the host.

ectothrix infection fungal infection of the hair, involving the outside of the hair shaft.

effusion escape of fluid from the blood vessels or lymphatics, usually into a body cavity; may be associated with circulatory, hepatic, or renal disorders or from infection, malignancy, or other inflammatory states.

ELISA enzyme-linked immunosorbent assay; system to detect antigen or antibody; uses an enzyme that can react with a substrate to form a colored end product. The antigen (or antibody) is bound to an enzyme, such as horseradish peroxidase or alkaline phosphatase.

encephalitis inflammation of the brain, usually resulting from a viral infection.

endemic syphilis bejel; nonvenereal syphilis caused by the spirochete *Treponema pallidum* subspecies *endemicum*, which is transmitted through poor sanitation or poor personal hygiene.

endoparasite parasite that lives within the body of its host.

endothrix infection fungal infection of the hair, involving the inside of the hair shaft.

endotoxin lipopolysaccharide macromolecules that comprise the gram-negative bacterial cell wall; released only on cell lysis when the bacterium dies.

enrichment broth media used to enhance the growth of certain bacteria or groups of bacteria. Examples include gram-negative broth that destroys gram-positive bacteria and inhibits the early multiplication of coliforms and thioglycollate that permits the differentiation of bacteria based on oxygen requirements.

enterohemorrhagic *E. coli* (EHEC) verotoxic *E. coli*; serotypes of *E. coli* that produce verotoxin, which may result in mild diarrhea, nonbloody diarrhea, hemorrhagic colitis, or hemolytic uremic syndrome. The most frequently identified serotype is 0:157H:7, although more than 50 serotypes of verotoxic *E. coli* are known.

enteroinvasive *E. coli* (EIEC) diarrhea-producing serotypes of *E. coli* that invade the intestinal mucosal epithelial cells, resulting in a form of dysentery.

enteropathogenic *E. coli* (EPEC) serotypes of *E. coli* that attach to intestinal epithelial cells and are associated with acute diarrhea, especially in infants and children less than 2 years of age.

enterotoxigenic *E. coli* (ETEC) serotypes of *E. coli* associated with diarrhea and traveler's diarrhea, which result from the ingestion of the organism's heat-labile and heat-stable toxins.

enterotoxins cytotoxins that generally attack the cells of the mucous membranes of the small intestine, for example, enterotoxin A, produced by *Staphylococcus aureus.*

envelope outer membrane composed of a phospholipid bilayer, glycoproteins, and matrix proteins, which surround the nucleocapsid of some viruses.

envelope antigen antigenic determinant possessed by some members of the Enterobacteriaceae, which are capsular polysaccharides, surround the cell wall and are heat labile. Envelope, or K, antigens are possessed by *Salmonella, Klebsiella, E. coli,* and some *Citrobacter* species.

epimastigote crithidial, extracellular hemoflagellate form that is long and thin with an undulating membrane extending from the flagellum to the small kinetoplast, located near the larger nucleus; found in the arthropod host.

erysipelas an infectious skin disease or cellulitis with redness, vesicles, fever, pain, and lymphodema; caused most often by *Streptococcus pyogenes* and occurring most often on the face and legs.

erysipeloid an infection usually found on the hands and characterized by blue-red nodules or patches generally acquired by contact with animals, meat products, or fish contaminated with *Erysipelothrix rhusiopathiae.*

erythema chronicum migrans characteristic skin lesion of Lyme disease, a tick-borne borreliosis caused by *Borrelia burgdorferi.*

examthem subitum sixth disease, or roseola; viral disease of infants and children characterized by a rapid onset of fever and a fine macular rash caused by human herpesvirus type 6 (HHV-6).

exoerythrocytic schizogony preerythrocytic cycle of the malarial parasite *Plasmodium*, which occurs outside of the erythrocyte and is characterized by repeated nuclear division, followed by cytoplasmic division into daughter cells or merozoites.

exotoxin intracellular toxin generally released into the environment by living gram-positive bacteria.

exotoxin A exotoxin produced by virulent strains of *Pseudomonas aeruginosa*, which inhibits protein synthesis and is associated with tissue destruction.

exudates type of effusion resulting from an infection, malignancy, or other inflammatory state. Exudates generally contain many cells and have high specific gravities and protein levels.

facultative anaerobe having the ability to adapt to more than one oxygen level in the environment. Organisms are able to grow in the presence and absence of oxygen.

facultative parasites organisms that live on or in a host but may also survive independently.

fastidious bacteria that possess very complex or extensive nutritional requirements.

febrile agglutinin test bacterial agglutination test to determine presence of antibodies in serum; useful in the diagnosis of disease in which the agent is difficult to culture, such as with *Brucella* and *Francisella.*

fermentative ability of a microorganism to utilize a carbohydrate in the absence of oxygen.

fibrinolysin plasmin; proteolytic enzyme that lyses fibrin; includes staphylokinase produced by *Staphylococcus aureus* and streptokinase produced by *Streptococcus pyogenes.*

flagellar antigen antigenic determinant possessed by some motile members of the Enterobacteriaceae that are heat labile, composed of protein, and located in the flagellum.

fluorescent microscopy examination with a fluorescent microscope, which uses ultraviolet light to examine specimens that have been stained with a fluorescent dye.

fluorometry measurement of fluorescence emitted by compounds when exposed to ultraviolet radiation; useful in certain automated identification methods in microbiology.

free coagulase an extracellular enzyme produced by *Staphylococcus aureus* that converts fibrinogen into fibrin.

fungemia the presence of fungi in the blood.

fungi imperfecti the imperfect fungi; those fungi that do not exhibit a sexual phase and produce spores asexually from the mycelium.

gas-liquid chromatography method for separating and analyzing gaseous and chemical end products of metabolism through differences in their absorbency; used in the identification of anaerobes, which produce specific organic acids as end products of metabolism.

gastroenteritis inflammation of the stomach and intestines, resulting from various gastrointestinal disorders attributed to bacterial enterotoxins or invasion by viruses or bacteria.

general isolation media media such as trypticase soy agar or trypticase soy broth that supports the growth of most nonfastidious bacteria.

genetic probe method of identification in which sequences of deoxyribonucleic acid (DNA) or ribonucleic acid (RNA) form hybrids with the specific complementary strand of nucleic acid.

germ tube a hyphal-like extension of a yeast cell, showing no constriction at the point of origin; useful in the identification of *Candida albicans*.

glanders an infection caused by *Pseudomonas mallei*, which may be transmitted to humans from horses or other animals, such as sheep, goats, or dogs, and is associated with inflammation of the mucous membranes, ulcerating skin nodules, lymphadenopathy, pneumonia, or septicemia.

gonorrhea sexually transmittable disease that most often affects the genitourinary tract and less frequently the pharynx, conjunctiva, or rectum. Infection results from direct contact with the causative organism, *Neisseria gonorrhoeae*.

Gram stain commonly used differential staining method used to classify bacteria as gram-positive or gram-negative. Gram-positive bacteria retain the primary stain crystal violet and appear purple, whereas gram-negative bacteria lose the primary stain and retain the secondary stain of safranin O and appear pink.

gravid proglottids mature segments of a tapeworm that have fully developed reproductive structures and a uterus containing eggs.

***Haemophilus influenzae* serotype b** capsular serotype of *H. influenzae*, which is the most frequent cause of *H. influenzae* infections.

halophilic requiring increased chloride ions for growth.

Hansen's disease leprosy; chronic, communicable disease caused by *Mycobacterium leprae*, characterized by a thickening of the cutaneous nerves and round, saucer-shaped skin lesions or widespread plaques and nodules in the skin, eye, or bone.

hemagglutinin antigen viral surface antigen possessed by the influenza viruses and some parainfluenza viruses, which permits the virus to attach to glycoprotein on the surface of red blood cells and respiratory epithelial cells.

hematin or hemin degradation product of hemoglobin in red blood cells that is a nutrient requirement for several fastidious bacteria, such as *Haemophilus* and *Neisseria*.

hemolysins substances that lyse or dissolve red blood cells; produced by various bacteria, including certain staphylococci and streptococci.

hepatitis inflammation of the liver characterized by fever, nausea, vomiting, jaundice, and necrosis of liver cells caused by one of the following hepatitis viruses: hepatitis A, B, or C.

hermaphroditic containing both male and female reproductive organs. The mature proglottids of tapeworms are hermaphroditic.

heteroploid cell lines cell cultures whose cells contain more than 25% cells with an abnormal karyotype when compared with the normal cells of the primary culture. Heteroploid cell lines are derived from malignant tissue or other transformed cells. Examples include HeLA, Hep-2, and KB.

histoplasmosis fungal infection caused by inhalation of spores in soil contaminated with excreta from birds infected with the dimorphic fungus *Histoplasma capsulatum*. The disease is characterized by fever, malaise, cough, and lymphadenopathy, which may disseminate to ulcerations in the mouth and nose; enlargement of the spleen, liver, and lymph nodes; and severe lung infiltration. It most commonly is found in the Ohio and Mississippi Valleys.

humoral immunity type of defense mechanism against foreign antigen and tissue associated with the production of antibodies produced by the immunoglobulins. Humoral immunity includes antibody production against bacterial and viral antigens.

hyphae tubular filaments that are the microscopic units of the fungi and intertwine to form the mycelium.

immunoglobulin classes of humoral antibodies produced in response to foreign antigens. Five classes exist: IgA, IgD, IgE, IgG, and IgM. IgM is involved in the primary immune response, whereas IgG is found in the secondary immune response.

immunoserology diagnosis of infectious disease through analysis of antibody levels or titers in patient sera. Generally, acute and convalescent phase specimens are obtained and the titers compared.

immunosuppressive disease; irradiation; or use of chemical, pharmacologic, or physical agents that depresses the immune system, often resulting in an increased host susceptibility to infectious disease.

impetigo highly contagious skin infection generally attributed to *Streptococcus pyogenes*, which begins as an erythema and progresses to lesions, erosions, and crusts.

incidental host accidental host; infection of a host that is not considered to be the normal host such that the life cycle of the parasite may or may not be completed.

indirect immunofluorescence microscopic technique to detect the presence of antibody by permitting an antibody to react with its substrate and then adding a second fluorescein-labeled antibody that will bind to the first antibody in a positive reaction.

infection invasion of a host by multiplying microorganisms.

infectious disease structural or functional harm caused to a host by the effects of microorganisms that have multiplied and established disease.

inflammatory process protective response of the body to irritation or injury caused by a physical, chemical, or biologic agent; consists of complex cellular and histologic reactions in the local blood vessels and adjacent tissues. Cardinal signs of inflammation are *rubor* (redness), *calor* (heat), *tumor* (swelling), and *dolor* (pain).

innate immunity natural immunity; inborn resistance in an individual not immunized by previous infection or vaccination that is nonspecific and not stimulated by a particular antigen.

intermediate host the host in which the asexual reproductive or larval phase of the parasite occurs.

intrinsic resistance ability of a genus or species to remain unaffected by a particular antimicrobial agent; may delineate the antibiotic spectrum or be used as an identification tool, for example, resistance of *Staphylococcus saprophyticus* to novobiocin.

Kauffman-White classification method of classifying *Salmonella* species according to the presence of particular O, H, and Vi antigens. More than 2,200 serovars of *Salmonella* exist using this method.

Lancefield antigen grouping method to classify streptococci based on the type-specific cell wall carbohydrate, or C-substance.

late (slow) lactose fermenters those bacteria that possess β-galactosidase but not lactose permease, which results in the delayed or slow degradation of lactose. Late lactose fermenters are detected using the ONPG reaction.

latent viral infections viral infections that can become reactivated after months or years of dormancy; associated with the viral family Herpetoviridae. Viruses remain dormant in the white blood cells or peripheral nerves, and infection may reactivate in periods of physical stress or illness.

Legionnaires' disease severe type of legionellosis; an acute bacterial pneumonia and multisystemic disease caused by the gram-negative bacillus *Legionella pneumophilia*.

leptospirosis acute infectious disease caused by the spirochete *Leptospira interrogans*, which is transmitted in the urine of both wild and domestic animals. Humans may acquire the infection by direct contact with the animal's infected tissues or urine. The disease is characterized by fever, chills, jaundice, muscle aches, or hemorrhage into the skin.

leukocidan exotoxin produced by *Staphylococcus aureus*, which inhibits or lyses white blood cells.

listeriosis infectious disease caused by the gram-positive bacillus *Listeria monocytogenes* and may be transmitted to humans by contact with vegetation, food, or water infected with the organism. The disease is characterized by shock, endocarditis, hepatosplenomegaly, and meningitis or encephalitis.

Lyme disease acute, recurring inflammatory disease involving the joints; may progress, causing neurological effects caused by the spirochete *Borrelia burgdorferi*, generally acquired through the bite of an infected tick.

lymphogranuloma venereum (LGV) sexually transmitted disease caused by specific strains of *Chlamydia trachomatis* that is characterized by ulcerative genital lesions, swelling of the lymph nodes in the groin, headache, fever, and malaise.

macroconidia large, multicellular, club-, oval-, or spindle-shaped asexual fungal spores, which are usually septate.

macrogametes mature female sex cell that produces zygotes once fertilized by the male microgamete in the genus *Plasmodium* and the intestinal coccidia. Macrogametes develop from macrogametocytes.

melioidosis pneumonia-like disease caused by *Pseudomonas pseudomallei*, most commonly seen in Southeast Asia; also transported to the west by Asian immigrants and returning Vietnam war veterans. It is acquired through inhalation or direct contact through breaks in the skin.

meningitis infection or inflammation of the membranes covering the brain or spinal cord, usually purulent and involving the subarachnoid space.

meningococcemia the presence of the meningococci (*Neisseria meningitidis*) in the blood.

merogony schizogony; asexual life cycle of the sporozoan protozoa characterized by nuclear division, followed by cytoplasmic division. The dividing cell is known as the schizont and the daughter cells as merozoites.

merozoites trophozoites released from the host's red blood cells or hepatic cells on maturation during the asexual life cycle of *Plasmodium*.

mesophilic pertaining to a microorganism with an optimal growth temperature between 25°C and 40°C. Most human pathogens are mesophilic.

metacercaria infective stage of trematodes for humans, occurring when the cercaria loses its tail and encysts on water plants or a second intermediate host.

metachromatic granules Babes-Ernst bodies; irregularly staining granules believed to function as storage depots in *Corynebacterium* species. They appear as beads in the methylene blue stain.

microaerophilic microorganisms that grow only under reduced oxygen tension and are unable to grow either aerobically or anaerobically.

microconidia small, unicellular, round, elliptical, or pyriform asexual fungal spores.

microgametes mature male sex cells that fertilize the female macrogametes, producing zygotes in the malarial parasite *Plasmodium* and the coccidian protozoans. Microgametes develop from microgametocytes.

minimal bacteriocidal concentration (MBC) the lowest concentration of an antimicrobial agent that produces 99.9% killing or a reduction of 99.9% of the viable colony-forming units.

minimal inhibitory concentration (MIC) the lowest concentration of an antimicrobial agent that prevents visible growth; the lowest concentration of antimicrobial agent showing no visible growth in macrobroth or microbroth dilution procedure.

miracidium first-stage larvae of the trematodes, which are released from the egg and are ciliated and free swimming; are able to penetrate the snail tissue to continue its life cycle.

moderately obligate anaerobe those anaerobes that can grow at oxygen levels of 2% to 8%.

mold phase mycelial phase of a dimorphic fungus, which is usually observed on Sabouraud dextrose agar at 25°C to 30°C. The saprophytic phase is generally observed in nature.

monoclonal antibody antibody produced by the offspring of a single hybrid cell. Large amounts of antibodies of one molecule type are produced that react with a single epitope.

MRSA methicillin-resistant *Staphylococcus aureus.*

multidrug-resistant tuberculosis (MDR-TB) those strains of *Mycobacterium tuberculosis* that are resistent to two or more antimycobacterial agents used to treat tuberculosis infection.

multitest systems commercially available identification methods using several biochemical reactions and an identification index.

mumps acute viral disease characterized by swelling of the parotid glands and caused by a *Paramyxovirus.*

mycelium intertwining structure of fungi, composed of tubular filaments or hyphae.

mycetoma chronic granulomatous infection of the cutaneous and subcutaneous tissue and bone, characterized by tumorlike deformities of the subcutaneous tissue, with abscesses, draining sinuses, and granulomatous pus; caused by members of the aerobic *Actinomyces* or several septate fungi, such as *Aspergillus, Exophiala, Pseudoallescheria,* and *Curvularia.*

Mycobacteria other than tubercle bacilli (MOTT) method of classification proposed by Runyon for species of *Mycobacterium* other than tuberculosis, which groups these atypical mycobacterial species based on growth rate and pigment production.

mycoses fungal infections.

myonecrosis gas gangrene; irreversible damage to muscle tissue frequently caused by anaerobic bacteria, such as *Clostridium* species and characterized by pain, tenderness, the accumulation of gas within the muscle tissue, and blackish green colorization of the muscle tissue.

narrow-spectrum antibiotics antibiotics that are useful for treating a limited group of microorganisms, such as either gram-positive or gram-negative bacteria.

necrotizing fasciitis a rare but serious bacterial infection that rapidly spreads and usually is located in the fascial planes of the connective tissue, which results in rapid tissue necrosis. Commonly known as the flesh-eating bacteria, necrotizing fasciitis most commonly is caused by group A streptococci but also can be caused by other bacteria, such as *Klebsiella, Clostridium, E. coli, Staphylococcus aureus,* and *Aeromonas hydrophila.*

nephelometry quantitative method based on determining the amount of turbidity by measuring light scattering.

neuraminidase antigen antigen possessed by the influenza viruses and some parainfluenza viruses, which permits the virus to enter the host cell.

nicotinamide-adenine dinucleotide (NAD) coenzyme I; compound produced by certain bacteria, such as *Staphylococcus aureus,* and yeast, which is a nutrient requirement for certain fastidious bacteria, such as *Haemophilus.*

nonphotochromogens those mycobacteria that do not form a pigment even in the presence of a constant light source; Runyan Group III.

nonsaccharolytic asaccharolytic; inability of a microrganism to use carbohydrates even in the presence of oxygen

nonselective isolation media enriched media; primary isolation media that contain a nutrient supplement, for example, chocolate agar or sheep blood agar.

nontreponemal tests nonspecific screening tests, such as the RPR (rapid plasma reagin) and VDRL (Venereal Disease Research Laboratory), for syphilis, which detect reagin. Positive nontreponemal tests must be confirmed with a treponemal test.

normal flora microorganisms that are found in or on a particular body site and that usually do not cause infectious disease, for example, viridans streptococci in the oral cavity.

nosocomial of or pertaining to a health care setting. A nosocomial infection is one acquired in a hospital or other health care setting.

nucleic acid hybridization binding of a single-stranded nucleic acid probe with its DNA complement in an unknown sample.

nucleocapsid virus particle consisting of the viral nucleic acid (DNA or RNA) with its protein coat (capsid).

obligate aerobe microorganism that requires oxygen for growth and cannot grow in the absence of oxygen.

obligate anaerobe microorganism that cannot grow in the presence of oxygen, growing only in conditions with very little or no oxygen present.

obligate parasites parasites that require a host, depending on it for survival.

oocysts encysted form of the motile zygotes of *Plasmodium* species, which are formed when the microgamete fertilizes the macrogamete. The oocyst encysts in the stomach wall of the *Anopheles* mosquito.

oospore sexual reproductive spore in some fungi that involves the fusion of cells from two separate, nonidentical hyphae.

ophthalmia neonatorum gonococcal conjunctivitis of the newborn acquired from infected maternal secretions during delivery.

opportunistic normally nonpathogenic microorganisms that are capable of causing infection in an immunosuppressed host.

opportunistic mycoses fungal infections that are observed in immunocompromised individuals and include candidiasis, zygomycosis, and aspergillosis.

optochin test procedure to differentiate *Streptococcus pneumoniae* from other α-hemolytic streptococci. *Streptococcus pneumoniae* is inhibited by optochin (ethylhydrocupreine hydrochloride), whereas other α-hemolytic streptococci are resistant to optochin.

osteomyelitis infection of the bone or bone marrow usually caused by bacteria introduced by trauma, surgery, or extension of a nearby infection or from the blood; most commonly caused by *Staphylococcus aureus*.

oxidative ability of a microorganism to utilize a carbohydrate only in the presence of oxygen.

paracentesis removal of ascitic or peritoneal fluid from the abdominal cavity.

paracoccidioidomycosis chronic fungal infection caused by the dimorphic fungus *Paracoccidioides brasiliensis* and characterized by ulcers of the mouth and nose; enlarged, draining lymph nodes; cough; dyspnea; weight loss; and skin lesions. It occurs primarily in Mexico and South and Central America and is acquired through inhalation of fungal spores. It also is called South American blastomycosis.

parasitism relationship between two organisms in which the smaller lives on or in the larger, with a dependence on the larger host for survival.

partially acid fast ability of the genus *Nocardia* to retain carbolfuchsin during mild acid decolorization from the presence of unusual long-chain fatty acids in the cell wall. Other gram-positive branching bacilli cannot retain the stain.

pasteurellosis local wound infection caused by the gram-negative bacillus *Pasturella multicida,* which may be acquired through the bite or scratch of an infected animal, usually a cat.

pathogen any microorganism capable of causing infection.

peak specimen serum specimen collected to determine the level of a pharmaceutical agent, such as an antibiotic. Peak specimens, which represent the highest level of the agent in the blood, are generally collected one half hour after the dose is given intravenously or intramuscularly. Trough specimens represent the lowest level of the agent and are collected approximately one half hour before the next dose.

penetration stage in the establishment of a viral infection in which the viral genetic material enters the host cell either through fusion, phagocytosis, or injection.

penicilliosis an acute fungal infection of the lungs, bone marrow, and other organs in immunosuppressed individuals. It is caused by the dimorphic fungus *Penicillium marneffei* and is found primarily in Southeast Asia, China, India, and Hong Kong.

pertussis acute, highly contagious respiratory disease characterized by paroxysmal coughing that may end in a whooping inspiration; caused by the gram-negative bacillus *Bordetella pertussis.*

phaeohyphomycosis opportunistic fungal infections other than mycetoma and chromoblastomycosis, caused by the dematiaceous or darkly pigmented molds.

phagocytosis process of engulfing and destroying microorganisms by neutrophils, monocytes, and macrophages.

phase-contrast microscopy form of microscopy using a special condenser and objective with a phase-shifting ring, which permits viewing of small differences in the refractive index and differences in intensity. This type of microscopy is useful in viewing unstained specimens that appear transparent.

photochromogens those mycobacteria that are nonpigmented in the dark but produce a yellow pigment on constant exposure to light.

piedra fungal disease of the hair characterized by the presence of several small black or white nodules. White piedra is caused by *Trichosporon beigelii*, and black piedra is caused by *Piedraia hortae*.

pili short, hair-like projections on the bacterial cell that are involved in attachment, bacterial conjugation, and transfer of genetic material.

pinta ulcerative skin disease caused by the spirochete *Treponema carateum*, characterized by flat, red, nonulcerating skin lesions and spread through direct contact with infected lesions.

pityriasis versicolor tinea versicolor; a superficial fungal infection characterized by brownish or scaly areas on light skin and irregular patches of nonpigmented areas on dark skin; caused by the fungus *Malassesia furfur.*

plasmids extrachromosomal DNA that determines traits not necessary for the bacterium's survival but may aid its adaptation to adverse conditions. Certain plasmids enable the microorganism to resist particular antimicrobial agents.

plerocercoid second larval stage of the cestode *Diphyllobothrium latum*, which develops in the second intermediate host—the freshwater fish—and is the infective form for humans if ingested.

pneumolysin virulence factor produced by *Streptococcus pneumoniae*, associated with cytolysis.

pneumonia acute inflammation of the lungs attributed to infection by bacteria, commonly *Streptococcus pneumoniae*, viruses, or fungi, characterized by fever, chills, headache, cough, and chest pain.

polio poliomyelitis; acute inflammation of the gray matter of the spinal cord caused by the *Poliovirus* in the enterovirus family. Asymptomatic, mild, and paralytic forms of the disease occur.

polyclonal antibody heterogeneous antibodies that contain many different binding sites and capable of recognizing multiple epitopes on any single antigen.

polymerase chain reaction (PCR) procedure used to detect bacterial or viral nucleic acid in specimen using DNA polymerase to copy a DNA strand between two primer ends resulting in amplification of the original DNA strand.

polymicrobic infections containing more than one pathogenic organism, for example, an abscess that contains both an aerobe and an anaerobe.

PPNG penicillinase-producing *Neisseria gonorrhoeae*; those strains of *Neisseria gonorrhoeae* that are resistant to the effects of penicillin through the production of penicillinase or β-lactamase.

precipitin formation of an insoluable complex between an antibody and a specific soluable antigen.

primary atypical pneumonia acute, systemic disease involving the lungs; caused by *Mycoplasma pneumoniae* and characterized by fever and cough but relatively few physical symptoms.

primary cell cultures cell lines derived directly from parent tissue. Cells in primary culture must have the same karyotype and chromosome number as that of the original tissue. Examples include HEK, RK, and PMK.

procercoid the first larval stage that develops from the coracidium stage of *Diphyllobothrium latum*. It develops in the body of the first intermediate host, either crustaceans or copepods of the genus *Diaptomus*.

proglottids segments of tapeworms containing both male and female reproductive organs when mature.

promastigote leptomonal hemoflagellate form, which is long and thin and is found extracellularly in the midgut or pharynx of the arthropod host. This form resembles the epimastigote form except that the kinetoplast is located anteriorly and there is no undulating membrane.

psittacosis ornithosis; infectious disease of psittacine birds, including parrots and parakeets, caused by *Chlamydia psittaci*, which may be transmitted to humans and is characterized by headache, nausea, and fever preceded by chills; commonly known as "parrot fever."

pyocyanin a blue or blue-green water-soluble pigment, which may be extracted with chloroform and is produced by *Pseudomonas aeruginosa*.

pyogenic pus-forming; those bacteria associated with pus-forming infections.

pyogenic exotoxin extracellular toxin secreted by *Streptococcus pyogenes*, which may be associated with fever and the development of renal failure, respiratory distress, and necrosis.

pyoverdin a yellow pigment produced by some strains of *Pseudomonas aeruginosa*.

rabies an acute, usually fatal disease of the central nervous system transmitted from wild animals, such as skunks, bats, foxes, dogs, and raccoons infected with the *Lyssavirus* in the family Rhabdoviridae through an infected bite. The virus travels along nerves to the brain and other organs and incubates for days to months. Incubation is followed by fever; malaise; paresthesia; myalgia; and later severe encephalitis, delirium, muscle spasms, paralysis, and usually death.

rapid grower saprophytic mycobacteria that grow within 3 to 5 days; Runyan Group IV.

reactivation tuberculosis form of secondary tuberculosis that reoccurs as the result of the activation of a dormant endogenous infection. Reactivation may result from a diminished immune status, hormonal changes, poor nutrional status, or other debilitating states.

redia the elongated, saclike second or third larval stage of the trematode, which develops in the sporocyst and matures into many cercariae.

relapsing fever an acute infectious disease caused by the spirochete *Borrelia recurrentis* and spread through the bite of an infected tick that feeds on rodents and other animals.

resistant the ability of a microorganism to remain unaffected by an antimicrobial agent such that the organism is not inhibited by the agent.

retroviruses RNA-containing viruses characterized by possessing RNA-dependent DNA polymerases or reverse transcriptases, such as the human T cell lymphotrophic viruses (HTLV-1 and HTLV-2) and the human immunodeficiency virus (HIV-1 and HIV-2).

rostellum the anterior protruding portion of the scolex of a tapeworm, which may be armed with a row or several rows of hooklets.

rubella contagious viral infection occuring primarily in nonimmunized children and characterized by fever; upper respiratory infection; enlarged lymph nodes; arthralgia; and a fine, diffuse, red maculopapular rash; caused by the genus *Rubivirus* in the family Togaviridae and transmitted by infected respiratory droplets; also called German measles or 3-day measles because the symptoms generally last for 3 days.

rubeola measles; acute, contagious viral infection occuring primarily in nonimmunized children, involving the respiratory tract and characterized by a spreading maculopapular rash and caused by a *Paramyxovirus* and transmitted through infected respiratory droplets.

salt tolerant the ability of certain bacteria to withstand and grow well in high concentrations of sodium chloride. For example, *Enterococcus* can sustain 6.5% NaCl.

satellitism phenomenon of colonies of *Haemophilus* growing about β-hemolytic colonies of *Staphylococcus aureus* as a result of the latter's production of NAD and the presence of hematin.

schizogony merogony; form of asexual multiple fission seen in sporozoan protozoa in which the nucleus divides many times before the cytoplasm divides into as many parts as there are nuclei. The dividing cell is known as the schizont and the daughter cells as merozoites.

schizont sporozoan trophozoite that reproduces by schizogony to form daughter cells known as merozoites.

scolex the head, or anterior end, of a tapeworm, which enables the worm to attach by suckers and frequently by hooks on the rostellum to the intestinal wall.

scotochromogens those mycobacteria that are pigmented yellow to orange in the dark and on exposure to light intensify to an orange or orange-red color.

selective media primary isolation media that enhances the growth of a bacterium or group of bacteria while inhibiting the growth of another group or groups of bacteria. For example, Hektoen enteric agar is selective for *Salmonella* and *Shigella* while inhibiting the normal flora coliforms.

sensitivity the ability of a test system to detect small amounts of antigen or antibody. Systems with high degrees of sensitivity levels are better able to detect small quantities of the substance being analyzed.

septicemia systemic disease associated with the presence of pathogenic microorganisms and toxins in the blood; characterized by fever, chills, pain, prostration, and nausea.

serum bacteriocidal test Schlichter test; the lowest dilution of a patient's serum that kills a standard inoculum of an organism isolated from the patient.

shigellosis bacillary dysentery; acute, bacterial infection of the bowel, characterized by diarrhea, fever, and abdominal pain caused by bacteria in the genus *Shigella*.

smallpox highly contagious viral infection characterized by fever; prostration; and a vesicular, pustular rash caused by the smallpox or variola virus in the family Poxviridae. Smallpox was eradicated, and the world declared free of smallpox in 1979 by the World Health Organization.

somatic antigen antigenic determinant possessed by members of the Enterobacteriaceae that are present in the cell wall and associated with lipopolysaccharide. Somatic (body) antigens are heat stable and important in the serotyping of *E. coli*, *Shigella*, and *Salmonella*.

specificity the ability of a test system to distinguish between very similar antigens; a measure of the ability of an antibody to distinguish between epitopes.

sporangiospores asexual fungal spores contained in a sac or sporangium, which are produced terminally on sporangiophores or aseptate hyphae.

sporogony form of sexual reproduction whereby sporozoites form during the sexual stage of the life cycle of a sporozoan, primarily the malarial parasite, *Plasmodium*. The sex cells fuse in the body of the invertebrate host—the female *Anopheles* mosquito—where the encysted zygote divides and gives rise to sporozoites.

sporotrichosis chronic, subcutaneous fungal infection caused by *Sporothrix schenckii* and characterized by skin ulcers and subcutaneous nodules along the lymphatics. It is usually transmitted through a thorn prick or puncture wound from decaying vegetation, flowers, or soil.

sporozoites the form of the malarial parasite *Plasmodium* that develops in the sporocyst by mutiple fission of the zygote in the oocyst of the female *Anopheles* mosquito during the sexual reproductive phase of the parasite. After release from the oocyst, the sporozoites migrate to the mosquito's salivary glands, where they may be transmitted to humans.

standard precautions a set of safety regulations stating that blood, serum, or any body fluid or secretion containing blood should be handled as if it were capable of transmitting infectious disease.

sterilization method to destroy microorganisms in or on an object through heat, steam, chemicals, gas, or radiation.

streptokinase extracellular enzyme, produced by streptococci, that cleaves plasminogen into plasmin, resulting in the lysis of a fibrin clot.

streptolysin O hemolysin produced by streptococci. Streptolysin O is oxygen labile and antigenic.

streptolysin S hemolysin produced by streptococci. Streptolysin S is oxygen stable and nonantigenic.

strict obligate anaerobe an anaerobe that cannot grow in the presence of even 0.5% oxygen and is thus unable to grow on the surface of agar.

strobila chain of developing segments or proglottids of a tapeworm.

subcutaneous mycoses fungal infections of the subcutaneous tissue, which usually do not disseminate and include sporotrichosis, mycetoma, chromoblastomycosis, and phaeohyphomycosis.

superficial (cutaneous) mycoses fungal infections of the skin, hair, and nails, including dermatophytic infections, piedra, and tinea versicolor.

superinfection an infection that occurs as a result of the antimicrobial therapy for another infection. It results from a change in the normal flora that permits the multiplication of other microorganisms, for example, infection with *Candida albicans* resulting from penicillin treatment for streptococcal pharyngitis.

susceptible effectiveness of an antimicrobial agent against a particular microorganism indicated by inhibition of growth of the organism around the antibiotic disk.

SXT sulfamethoxazole-trimethoprim susceptibility test used to differentiate β-hemolytic streptococci. Lancefield groups A and B are resistant to SXT, whereas groups C, F, and G are susceptible.

synergistic antibiotic response in which the combined effect of two antibiotics is greater than the total of the individual effects.

systemic mycoses fungal infections of the lung and other organs, which generally disseminate and include histoplasmosis, coccidioidomycosis, histoplasmosis, and paracoccidioidomycosis.

tachyzoites the crescent-shaped, rapidly dividing, intracellular trophozoite form of *Toxoplasma gondii*.

tetanospasmin exotoxin produced by *Clostridium tetani*; the lethal neurotoxin that produces painful muscle spasms, resulting in lockjaw, laryngeal spasm, and tonic spasm of all muscles in the body.

tetanus acute, often fatal disease, of the central nervous system caused by infection from *Clostridium tetani*, which enters the body through a puncture wound, laceration, burn, or the umbical cord stump in a newborn. The disease is characterized by headache, fever, painful spasms of the muscles, and eventually tonic spasms of all muscules.

thallophytes those members of the plant family that possess true nuclei, lack stems and roots, do not possess chlorophyll, and absorb nutrients from the environment. The fungi are classified as thallophytes.

thoracentesis aspiration of pleural fluid for diagnostic purposes.

tinea ringworm; fungal skin, hair, and nail diseases caused by the dermatophytes and characterized by itching, scaling, and erythema of the skin; crumbling and destruction of the nails; and erythema, scaling, and crusting of the hair.

trachoma chronic, contagious infection of the conjunctiva caused by specific strains of *Chlamydia trachomatis* and characterized by inflammation, pain, photophobia, lacrimation, and, if untreated, blindness.

transposons "jumping gene"; genetic material that may move from one plasmid to another or from plasmid to chromosome.

transudates type of effusion that contains few cells; has a low specific gravity and protein level; and generally develops from renal, hepatic, or circulatory disorders.

treponemal tests specific tests for syphilis, such as the fluorescent treponemal antibody (FTA), which detect antigens to the spirochete *Treponema pallidum* and are used to confirm positive nontreponemal tests.

trophozoite form the motile stage of the protozoans that feeds and multiplies.

trough specimen serum specimen collected to determine the level of a pharmaceutical agent, such as an antibiotic. Trough specimens represent the lowest level of the agent and are collected approximately one half hour before the next dose.

trypanomastigote trypanosomal hemoflagellate form that is long and thin, with an undulating membrane and free flagellum; found extracellularly in the arthropod host.

tuberculosis chronic, granulomatous infection caused by the organism *Mycobacterium tuberculosis*, which is transmitted through inhalation of infected droplets; generally affects the lung, although other organs may be infected. Tuberculosis is characterized by pulmonary hemorrhage, dyspnea, purulent sputum, tubercles, and caseates in the lungs.

tularemia infectious disease of animals caused by the gram-negative bacillus *Francisella tularensis*, which may be transmitted by insect vectors or direct contact to humans causing lymph node enlargement, fever, skin ulcerations, or pneumonia.

tympanocentesis puncture of the tympanic membrane with a needle to aspirate middle ear fluid.

uncoating a stage in the establishment of a viral infection in which the virus loses its protein coat or capsid, exposing the viral nucleic acid, which will then be replicated and expressed in the eclipse stage.

undulant fever brucellosis; disease caused by gram-negative bacilli in the genus *Brucella*; primarily a disease of goats, pigs, and cattle and may be transmitted to humans through a break in the skin or by ingesting contaminated animal products.

urethritis inflammation or infection of the urethra characterized by dysuria.

varicella chickenpox; acute, highly contagious viral disease occuring primarily in children and caused by the varicella-zoster virus of the family Herpetoviridae; characterized by crops of pruritic vesicular skin eruptions and transmitted through either contaminated respiratory droplets or direct contact with the skin lesions.

vectors carriers, usually arthropods, that transmit a pathogenic microorganism, such as a parasite, from an infected to a noninfected host.

venereal syphilis sexually transmittable disease caused by the spirochete *Treponema pallidum* subspecies *pallidum*; usually transmitted through the sexual or congenital route. The disease usually consists of primary, secondary, latent, and tertiary stages.

viremia the presence of viruses in the blood.

viridans streptococci term applied to several species of streptococci that are α-hemolytic and make up the normal oropharyngeal flora.

virion elementary virus particle consisting of a central nucleic acid core of either DNA or RNA, which is surrounded by a protein coat, or capsid.

Weil-Felix reaction method of whole-cell agglutination that uses various *Proteus* surface antigens to detect cross-reacting antibodies to species of *Rickettsia*; useful in the speciation of *Rickettsia*.

yaws chronic, nonvenereal disease of the skin and bones caused by the spirochete *Treponema pallidum* subspecies *pertenue* and transmitted by direct contact with infected lesions.

yeast phase tissue or invasive phase of a dimorphic fungus, which is observed in vivo and grows on enriched media at 35°C to 37°C.

zoonoses diseases of animals that may be transmitted to humans from the primary animal host. Examples include pasturellosis, rabies, Lyme disease, and tularemia.

zygomycosis opportunistic fungal infection caused by the Zygomycetes (*Rhizopus*, *Absidia*, *Mucor*) and found in immunocompromised hosts; associated with infections of the nasal mucosa, sinuses, face, lung, liver, spleen, and brain.

zygospore sexual reproductive spore of some fungi, which involves the fusion of two identical cells arising from the same hypha.

Index

Note: Page numbers followed by *b*, *f*, or *t* indicate material in boxes, figures, or tables, respectively.

E

I

Q

R

S

U